SOFT TISSUE TUMORS

SOFT TISSUE TUMORS

Franz M. Enzinger, M.D.

Chairperson, Department of Soft Tissue Pathology,
Armed Forces Institute of Pathology,
Former Chief, World Health Organization,
International Center for the Histological Definition and
Classification of Soft Tissue Tumors,
Washington, DC

Sharon W. Weiss, M.D.

Professor of Pathology, Director of Anatomical Pathology,
The University of Michigan Medical Center and Hospitals,
Chairperson, World Health Organization,
Committee for the Histological Classification
of Soft Tissue Tumors,
Ann Arbor, Michigan

Third Edition

with 1750 illustrations, 30 in color

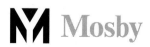

St. Louis Baltimore Berlin Boston Carlsbad Chicago London Madrid
Naples New York Philadelphia Sydney Tokyo Toronto

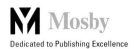

Executive Editor: Susan M. Gay
Senior Managing Editor: Lynne Gery
Project Manager: Linda McKinley
Design Coordinator: Elizabeth Fett
Manufacturing Supervisor: Kathy Grone

Third Edition

Printed in the United States of America

Mosby–Year Book, Inc.
11830 Westline Industrial Drive
St. Louis, Missouri 63146

Composition by Clarinda Company
Printing/binding by Maple-Vail Book Mfg. Group

Library of Congress Cataloging in Publication Data

Enzinger, Franz M.
Soft tissue tumors/Franz M. Enzinger, Sharon W. Weiss. --3rd ed.
p. cm.
Includes bibliographical references and index.
ISBN 0-8151-3132-1
1. Soft tissue tumors. I.Weiss, Sharon W. II. Title.
[DNLM: 1. Soft Tissue Neoplasms. WD 375 E61s 1994]
RC280.S66E56 1994
616.99'2--dc20
DNLM/DLC
for Library of Congress
94-32118
CIP

95 96 97 98 99 / 9 8 7 6 5 4 3 2 1

CONTRIBUTORS

Alfred E. Chang, M.D.

Professor of Surgery and Chief, Division of Surgical Oncology, University of Michigan Medical Center, Ann Arbor, Michigan

Jonathan A. Fletcher, M.D.

Associate Pathologist, Brigham and Women's Hospital; Assistant Professor Pathology and Pediatrics, Harvard Medical School, Boston, Massachusetts

John E. Madewell, M.D.

Professor and Chair, Department of Radiology, The Pennsylvania State University, Milton S. Hershey Medical Center, Hershey, Pennsylvania

Paul S. Meltzer, M.D., Ph.D.

Chief, Section of Molecular Genetics, Laboratory of Cancer Genetics, National Center for Human Genome Research, National Institutes of Health, Bethesda, Maryland

Richard P. Moser, Jr., M.D., F.A.C.R.

Professor of Radiology and Orthopedic Surgery; Chief, Division of Diagnostic Radiology, The Pennsylvania State University, Milton S. Hershey Medical Center, Hershey, Pennsylvania

Vernon K. Sondak, M.D.

Associate Professor of Surgery, University of Michigan Medical School; Director, Sarcoma Program, University of Michigan Cancer Center, Ann Arbor, Michigan

Richard J. Zarbo, M.D.

Head, Division of Surgical Pathology, Henry Ford Hospital, Detroit, Michigan; Professor of Pathology, Case Western Reserve University Medical School, Cleveland, Ohio

To our families

Inge, Bernie, Peter, and **Francine**

PREFACE TO THE THIRD EDITION

Since completion of the second edition of *Soft Tissue Tumors* in 1988, substantial advances have been achieved in the continuing exploration of soft tissue tumors, and many aspects of this complex subject have been amplified and clarified. In particular, rapid expansion of knowledge has been achieved in the immunopathological and cytogenetic diagnosis of these tumors, and many earlier diagnostic concepts had to be changed or modified. To accommodate these we have extensively revised and updated this edition of *Soft Tissue Tumors* and have added the following four new chapters: Molecular Biology of Soft Tissue Tumors (Chapter 4), Cytogenetic Analysis of Soft Tissue Tumors (Chapter 5), DNA Analysis of Soft Tissue Tumors (Chapter 6), and Approach to the Diagnosis of Soft Tissue Tumors (Chapter 7). Moreover, to cover new developments in the microscopic, immunohistological, and electron microscopic diagnosis of soft tissue tumors, it became necessary to expand or substantially modify many of the chapters, always keeping in mind the needs of the practicing pathologist. We also incorporated recent changes and modifications in soft tissue classification, including discussions and illustrations of several recently described entities, such as ossifying fibromyxoid tumor of soft parts, malignant extrarenal rhabdoid tumor, and malignant desmoplastic small cell tumor of childhood. The burgeoning literature also required us to update

the bibliography extensively and to increase the total number of listed references to over 5000. Also, the text was complemented and augmented by many new microscopic and radiographic illustrations, including some color plates, bringing the total number of illustrations to approximately 1800.

As with the first two editions, we are indebted to the many contributors who sent us many typical and not-so-typical soft tissue tumors for consultation. Without their contributions this book would not have been possible. We also owe special thanks to our colleagues at the Armed Forces Institute of Pathology and the Department of Pathology of the University of Michigan for their valuable support and help. We are also most grateful to Drs. Alfred E. Chang, Jonathan A. Fletcher, John E. Madewell, Paul S. Meltzer, Richard P. Moser, Vernon K. Sondak, and Richard Zarbo for devoting their efforts and valuable time to preparing or revising their chapters. As always we are indebted to our publisher for the editorial help received in the preparation and production of the third edition of this book. In particular we wish to express our thanks to Susan Gay and Lynne Gery for their patient cooperation and support.

Franz M. Enzinger
Sharon W. Weiss

CONTENTS

CHAPTER 1

GENERAL CONSIDERATIONS

Soft tissue can be defined as nonepithelial extraskeletal tissue of the body exclusive of the reticuloendothelial system, glia, and supporting tissue of various parenchymal organs. It is represented by the voluntary muscles, fat, and fibrous tissue, along with the vessels serving these tissues. By convention it also includes the peripheral nervous system because tumors arising from nerves present as soft tissue masses and pose similar problems in differential diagnosis and therapy. Embryologically, soft tissue is derived principally from mesoderm, with some contribution from neuroectoderm.

Soft tissue tumors are a highly heterogenous group of tumors that are classified on a histogenetic basis according to the adult tissue they resemble. Lipomas and liposarcomas, for example, are tumors that recapitulate to a varying degree normal fatty tissue, and hemangiomas and angiosarcomas contain cells resembling vascular endothelium. Within the various histogenetic categories, soft tissue tumors are usually divided into benign and malignant forms.

Benign tumors, which more closely resemble normal tissue, possess a limited capacity for autonomous growth. They exhibit little tendency to invade locally and are attended by a low rate of local recurrence following conservative therapy.

Malignant tumors or *sarcomas,* in contrast, are locally aggressive tumors that are capable of invasive or destructive growth, recurrence, and distant metastasis. Radical surgery is required to ensure total removal of these tumors. Unfortunately, the term *sarcoma* does not indicate the likelihood or rapidity of metastasis. Some sarcomas, such as dermatofibrosarcoma protuberans, rarely metastasize; others, such as malignant fibrous histiocytoma, do so with alacrity. For these reasons it is important to qualify the term *sarcoma* with a statement concerning the degree of differentiation or the histological grade. *Well differentiated* and *poorly differentiated* are qualitative and, hence, subjective terms used to indicate the relative maturity of the tumor with respect to the normal adult tissue. Histological grade is a means of quantitating the degree of differentiation by applying a set of histological criteria. Usually well-differentiated sarcomas are low-grade lesions, whereas poorly differentiated sarcomas are high-grade neoplasms. There are also borderline lesions in which it is difficult to determine the malignant potential, and there are benign neoplastic and nonneoplastic lesions that morphologically appear to be malignant but follow a benign clinical course *(pseudosarcomas).*

INCIDENCE

The incidence of soft tissue tumors, especially the relative frequency of benign to malignant ones, is nearly impossible to accurately determine.

Benign soft tissue tumors outnumber malignant tumors by a margin of about 100:1 in a hospital population, and their annual incidence is approximately 300 per 100,000 population.[60] The fact that many benign tumors, such as lipomas and hemangiomas, do not undergo biopsy makes the direct application of data from most hospital series invalid for the general population, however.

Malignant soft tissue tumors, on the other hand, ultimately come to medical attention. However, soft tissue sarcomas, compared with carcinomas and other neoplasms, are relatively rare tumors and constitute less than 1% of all cancers. Based on data from the National Cancer Institute's Surveillance, Epidemiology, and End Results Program, an estimated 5700 new soft tissue sarcomas developed in 1990 in the United States, and there were 3100 sarcoma-related deaths (Table 1-1). Another study, based on 240 soft tissue sarcomas of the extremities and limb girdles, indicates an annual incidence rate of 1.35 per 100,000 individuals in the Finnish population.[55] The incidence rate varies in different age-groups and also depends on the definition of soft tissue sarcomas and the types of neoplasms included among these tumors. For example, in one study of sarcomas of the locomotor system,[60] the overall annual incidence rate was 1.4 per 100,000, whereas the age-specific incidence rate for patients 80 years or older was 8 per 100,000. Moreover, in the National Cancer Survey,[20] retroperitoneal, mesenteric, and omental sarcomas are counted among the neoplasms of the digestive system, and pleural sarcomas (malignant me-

1

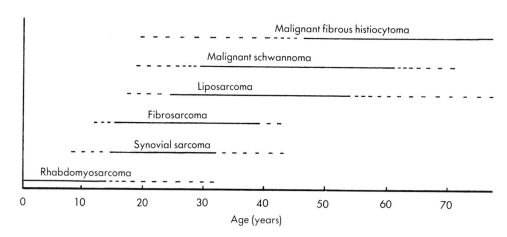

FIG. 1-1. Approximate relationship of age to incidence of various types of sarcomas. Continuous line indicates peak incidence of tumor. Dotted line indicates reduced incidence of tumor.

Table 1-1. Estimated new cases of cancer by site (United States, 1990)

Site	No. cases
Lung	157,000
Colon and rectum	155,000
Breast	150,900
Central nervous system	15,600
Soft tissue	5700
Bone	2100

Data from National Cancer Institute's Surveillance, Epidemiology, and End Results (SEER) Program.

sotheliomas) are included among the tumors of the respiratory tract.

There seems to be an upward trend in the incidence of soft tissue sarcomas, but it is not clear whether this represents a true increase or merely reflects better diagnostic capabilities and greater interest in this type of tumor. Judging from the available data, incidence and distribution of soft tissue sarcomas seem to be similar in different regions of the world.

Soft tissue sarcomas may occur anywhere in the body, but the majority arise from the large muscles of the extremities, the chest wall, the mediastinum, and the retroperitoneum. They occur at any age and, like carcinomas, are more common in older patients; about 15% affect persons younger than 15 years, and about 40% affect persons 55 years or older.

Soft tissue sarcomas occur more commonly in males, but both the sex and age incidences vary among different histological types (Fig. 1-1). For instance, embryonal rhabdomyosarcoma occurs almost exclusively in young individuals, whereas malignant fibrous histiocytoma is predominantly a tumor of old age and is rare in children younger

than 10 years. There is also no proven racial variation, even though the annual age-adjusted incidence rates have been reported to be higher for blacks than whites in the United States.[20]

PATHOGENESIS

As with other types of malignant neoplasms, the pathogenesis of most soft tissue tumors is still unknown. Recognized causes include various physical and chemical factors, exposure to ionizing radiation, and inherited or acquired immunological defects. Evaluation of the exact cause is often extremely difficult because of the long latent period between the time of exposure and development of sarcoma, as well as the possible effect of multiple environmental and hereditary factors during the induction period. Origin of sarcomas from benign soft tissue tumors is rare, except for malignant neural tumors (malignant schwannomas) arising in neurofibromas, which are nearly always in patients with the manifestations of neurofibromatosis.

Environmental factors

Trauma or *past injury* is frequently implicated in the development of sarcomas. However, many of these reports are anecdotal, and the integrity of the injured part was not clearly established before injury. Consequently, trauma often seems to be an event that merely calls attention to the underlying neoplasm. In occasional instances there is reasonable evidence to suggest a causal relationship. Rare examples of soft tissue sarcomas have been reported as arising in scar tissue following surgical procedures or thermal or acid burns, in fracture sites, and in the vicinity of plastic or metal implants, usually after a latent period of several years.[10,53]

Environmental carcinogens have been related to the development of sarcomas, but their role is largely unexplored, and only a few substances have been identified as playing a role in the induction of sarcomas in humans. However, it is well known that sarcomas of various types can be produced in laboratory animals following subcutaneous injection of polycyclic hydrocarbons. Tumor formation under these conditions depends on many factors, including the type of laboratory animals, site of inoculation, and length of time that the carcinogen is in contact with normal tissue. These tumors are rapidly growing, poorly differentiated sarcomas that are not easily compared with specific types of human sarcomas.

Asbestos, a hydrated silicate, is the most important known environmental carcinogen. Exposure to this substance, principally in the forms of crocidolite and chrysotile, occurs in asbestos miners, as well as in industrial workers who process, install, or repair electrical and thermal insulation, brake linings, cement tiles, and pipes. Inhaled as a microscopic particle, asbestos ultimately reaches the pulmonary parenchyma and pleural surface where, after many years, it may be associated with the development of pleural and peritoneal mesotheliomas or pulmonary carcinomas. Important risk factors are intensity and duration of asbestos exposure, as well as the type of asbestos and the submicroscopic fiber diameter.[61] The risk is greatest with crocidolite, the blue asbestos mined in South Africa; the risk is much less with chrysotile, the white asbestos chiefly found in Canada and Russia, which amounts to more than 95% of the asbestos used commercially[17-19] (see Chapter 30).

Dioxin exposure has also been implicated as a possible cause of sarcoma. In 1979 Swedish investigators reported an approximately sixfold increase in the incidence of soft tissue sarcomas in forestry and agricultural workers who had been exposed to dioxin-containing (2,3,7,8-tetrachlorodibenzo-p-dioxin, or TCDD) herbicides.[34] Subsequently, the possibility of an increased incidence of sarcomas was claimed for some of the 2 million soldiers stationed in Vietnam between 1965 and 1970 and exposed to Agent Orange, a defoliant that contained dioxin as a contaminant. Since 1980 several case control studies have been carried out, but so far none of these has found any significant association between Agent Orange exposure and development of sarcomas; all have been limited by the fact that follow-up periods in this group have been short and the level of exposure may be quite low.*

Analysis of workers exposed to dioxin in the industrial setting provides the advantage of higher levels of exposure and longer follow-up periods. In the study of Collins et al.,[15] which examined mortality rates among workers exposed to dioxin in an industrial accident, no sarcomas were noted in workers known to be exposed to dioxin alone. On the other hand, in an extremely large cohort study of 5172

workers at 12 plants, there was a slightly increased number of deaths due to cancer. Of greater interest was the fact that a statistically increased risk of mortality from soft tissue sarcomas was noted in the subset of workers with at least 1 year of exposure and a 20-year latent period. Although this study by no means establishes a relationship between dioxin exposure and soft tissue sarcoma, it suggests that dioxin may, in fact, be a human carcinogen, but at much higher levels than are observed in experimental animals.[30,69] Vinyl chloride exposure may be associated with hepatic angiosarcoma, but so far there is no evidence that it plays a role in the development of soft tissue sarcoma.[29]

Radiation has also been related to the development of sarcomas, but considering the frequency of radiotherapy, radiation-induced soft tissue sarcomas are definitely uncommon, and there is no doubt that the benefit of radiation in the treatment of malignant neoplasms outweighs the risk of developing sarcomas. About 0.1% of cancer patients treated with radiation who survive 5 years will develop a sarcoma of either bone or soft tissue. In order to qualify as a postradiation sarcoma, the criteria proposed by Cahan et al.,[11] and later modified by Arlen et al.,[4] must be met. These include documentation that the sarcoma developed within the radiated field, histological confirmation of the diagnosis, a period of latency of at least 3 years between the radiation and the tumor, and documentation that the region bearing the tumor was normal prior to the administration of the radiation. Nearly all postradiation sarcomas occur in adults, and women develop them more frequently, an observation which reflects the popular use of radiation in the treatment of breast and gynecological malignancies. In our experience, the most common disease for which patients receive radiation are lymphomas and breast, ovarian, and endometrial carcinomas. Although it was anticipated that the use of megavoltage radiation would reduce the incidence of postradiation sarcomas, this has not proved to be true. Both orthovoltage and megavoltage radiation may be associated with the subsequent development of sarcomas, and there do not appear to be differences in type of sarcoma or survival rates between the two groups, although the average dosages associated with orthovoltage radiation are lower and the latency periods longer. Interestingly, postradiation sarcomas do not display the wide range of appearances that are associated with sporadic nonradiation-induced tumors. The most common postradiation soft tissue sarcoma is malignant fibrous histiocytoma, which accounts for nearly 70% of cases, followed by osteosarcoma, fibrosarcoma, malignant peripheral nerve sheath tumor, chondrosarcoma, and angiosarcoma. Unfortunately, the majority of postradiation sarcomas are high-grade lesions and appear to be detected at a relatively higher stage compared with their sporadic counterparts. Thus, the survival rate associated with these lesions has been poor. In the experience of Robinson et al.,[56] based on review of all postradiation bone or soft

---

*References 5, 8, 31, 39, 69, 76.

tissue sarcomas culled from the literature, the 5-year survival rate was 5%. Laskin et al.[43] report a survival rate of 26% in a retrospective review of 53 radiation-associated soft tissue sarcomas accessioned at the AFIP. The interval between radiation and tumor development ranges from 2 to 25 years or more.[2,36,42] Extravasated thorotrast (thorium dioxide), while no longer used for diagnostic or therapeutic purposes, has induced soft tissue sarcomas at the site of injection.

Oncogenic viruses

The role of oncogenic viruses in the evolution of soft tissue sarcomas is still poorly understood. A significant number of patients with acquired immunodeficiency syndrome (AIDS) develop Kaposi's sarcoma. Although this has been interpreted by some as evidence that HTLV-III (HIV-I) may be oncogenic, the disparate incidence of Kaposi's sarcoma in the various AIDS risk groups raises the possibility that another agent, either alone or in concert with HIV-I, is responsible. A large body of circumstantial evidence implicating cytomegalovirus has been amassed, but no conclusive proof has been forthcoming (see Chapter 25).

Aside from their possible role in the development of Kaposi's sarcoma, there is no evidence that human transmissible viral agents constitute a major risk factor in the development of soft tissue sarcomas. However, with the use of the electron microscope, virus particles have been found repeatedly in a variety of soft tissue tumors.

Immunological factors

Immunodeficiency and therapeutic immunosuppression are also known to cause or influence the development of soft tissue sarcomas. Sarcomas of various types may be associated with therapeutic immunosuppression (long-term administration of cyclosporine and other immunosuppressive drugs) associated with organ transplantation, especially in renal and liver transplant recipients. Acquired regional immunodeficiency, or loss of regional immune surveillance, may also be the underlying mechanism in the development of the relatively rare angiosarcomas or lymphangiosarcomas that arise in the edematous extremity, either secondary to radical mastectomy (Stewart-Treves syndrome) or as a consequence of chronic lymphedema (see Chapter 25).

Genetic factors

A number of genetic diseases are associated with the development of soft tissue tumors, and the list will undoubtedly lengthen as we begin to understand the molecular underpinnings of mesenchymal neoplasia. Both neurofibromatosis 1 and neurofibromatosis 2, previously referred to as the peripheral and central forms of the disease, respectively, are classic examples of genetic disease associated with soft tissue tumors. Neurofibromatosis 1, which commences

early in life with the onset of café au lait spots, is later characterized by numerous neurofibromas. Inherited as an autosomal dominant trait the disease is primarily a neuroectodermal dysplasia, although nonneural tumors may occur as well. In 1% to 5% of cases, malignant peripheral nerve sheath tumors develop as a result of malignant degeneration of neurofibromas (see Chapter 32). The gene for neurofibromatosis 1 has been localized to the pericentromeric region of chromosome 17 and subsequently cloned. Its gene product, neurofibromin, ubiquitously distributed in normal tissues, appears to have tumor suppressor activity. Neurofibromatosis 2, while lumped with neurofibromatosis 1 in early clinical descriptions, is a clinically and genetically distinct disease. Characterized by bilateral acoustic neuromas, its gene has been localized to chromosome 22. The inherited or bilateral form of retinoblastoma has recently been associated with the development of sarcomas, usually osteosarcomas. In this disease, a germline mutation of the Rb1 locus occurs. When a "second hit" develops in the other allelic site within somatic cells (i.e., retinoblasts), tumors develop. For reasons that are still not clear, a late complication of the disease is the development of soft tissue sarcomas in regions that are well outside of any radiation field.

Polyposis coli, inherited as an autosomal dominant trait, may have as one of its stigmata retroperitoneal or mesenteric fibromatosis (Gardner's syndrome; see Chapter 10), but most of these tumors occur in surgically traumatized sites, suggesting an underlying combination of genetic and repair processes.[32,54] A number of other soft tissue tumors are known to occur in families, but the rarity of these reports indicates that collectively they do not account for a significant proportion of cases. These lesions, which are enumerated in Table 1-2, include various forms of fibromatoses, lipomas, xanthomas, leiomyomas, neurofibromas, neuroblastomas, and paragangliomas.[74] Rarely there are also patients with a familial cancer predisposition with increased risk of a second neoplasm[65] (see also Chapter 5).

CLASSIFICATION OF SOFT TISSUE TUMORS

Development of a useful and comprehensive histological classification of soft tissue tumors has been a relatively slow process. Earlier classifications have been largely descriptive and have been based more on the nuclear configuration than the type of tumor cells. Terms such as "round cell sarcoma," "spindle cell sarcoma," or "pleomorphic sarcoma" may be diagnostically convenient but should be discouraged because they are meaningless and convey little information as to the nature and potential behavior of a given tumor. Moreover, purely descriptive classifications do not clearly distinguish between tumors and tumorlike reactive processes.

More recent classifications have been based principally

Table 1-2. Soft tissue tumors occurring on an inherited basis or following a familial distribution

Tumor type	Comments
Fibrous tumors	
Palmar, plantar, and penile fibromatosis	Occasionally in several generations of one family and in twins
Deep fibromatosis (desmoid tumor)	Rare familial cases
Mesenteric fibromatosis	Frequently associated with familial polyposis coli and Gardner's syndrome
Fibromatosis colli	Occasionally in twins
Myofibromatosis	Rarely in siblings or increased familial incidence
Hyaline fibromatosis	Frequently in siblings
Fatty tumors	
Lipoma	About 5% familial
Multiple lipomas	Increased familial incidence
Angiolipoma	About 5% familial
Angiomyolipoma	Manifestations of tuberous sclerosis complex in about one third of patients
Fibrohistiocytic tumors	
Xanthoma tuberosum	Occurs in familial hyperlipidemia
Tendinous xanthoma	Occurs in familial hyperlipidemia and in cerebrotendinous xanthomatosis; autosomal recessive mode of inheritance
Muscular tumors	
Cutaneous leiomyoma	Occasional familial cases with pattern suggesting autosomal dominant mode of inheritance
Vascular tumors	
Glomus	Occasional familial cases following an autosomal dominant mode of inheritance
Osler-Weber-Rendu disease (hereditary hemorrhagic telangiectasia)	Autosomal dominant mode of inheritance
Blue rubber bleb nevus syndrome (cavernous hemangiomas of the skin and gastrointestinal tract)	Autosomal dominant mode of inheritance in some cases
Neural tumors	
Neurofibromatosis 1	Autosomal dominant mode of inheritance; NF1 gene localized to chromosome 17
Neurofibromatosis 2	Autosomal dominant mode of inheritance; NF2 gene localized to chromosome 22
Bilateral (inherited) retinoblastoma	Germline deletion of Rb1 locus on chromosome 13; associated with secondary sarcomas
Neuroblastoma	Rare familial cases
Paraganglioma	Occasional familial cases suggesting autosomal dominant mode of inheritance
Osseous tumors	
Fibrodysplasia ossificans progressiva	Occasionally increased familial incidence, including in homozygotic twins; autosomal dominant mode of inheritance
Miscellaneous tumors	
Tumoral calcinosis	Increased familial incidence; about 40% in siblings
Li-Fraumeni syndrome	Germline deletion of p53 locus resulting in familial rhabdomyosarcoma, early onset of breast carcinoma, and other neoplasms

on the line of differentiation of the tumor, that is, the type of tissue formed by the tumor rather than the type of tissue from which the tumor arose.

Over the past 2 or 3 decades there have been several attempts at reaching a useful and comprehensive classification of soft tissue tumors. These include the AFIP classifications published in the *Atlas of Tumor Pathology* in 1957,[64] 1967, and 1983,[44] and the World Health Organization classification published first in 1969[28] and revised in 1993.[78] The classification used herein is similar to the 1993 classification of the World Health Organization, a collective effort by pathologists in 10 countries.

Each of the histological categories is divided into a benign and malignant group, but this subdivision is not meant to imply that malignant soft tissue tumors tend to originate from their benign counterparts. In fact, malignant transformation of benign soft tissue tumors is an extremely rare event, with the exception of the occasional transformation of neurofibroma to malignant schwannoma. The various tumor types are named according to the histological type of the predominant cellular element, that is, the resemblance of the tumor to normal tissue or its embryonal counterpart. Rhabdomyosarcomas, for example, are tumors that show rhabdomyoblastic differentiation rather than tumors that arise from voluntary or striated muscle tissue. Most tumors retain the same pattern of differentiation in the primary and the recurrent lesions, but occasional ones change their pattern of differentiation or may even differentiate along several cellular lines. Specific subtypes are included in the classification whenever they are thought to be of value in diagnosing the tumor or in predicting its clinical behavior.

Malignant fibrous histiocytoma and liposarcoma are the most common soft tissue sarcomas of adults; together they account for 35% to 45% of all sarcomas. The incidence of the different types, however, varies in different series. For example, among 1116 soft tissue sarcomas reviewed by Hashimoto et al.,[35] malignant fibrous histiocytoma (25.1%) and liposarcoma (11.6%) were the most common, followed by rhabdomyosarcoma (9.7%), leiomyosarcoma (9.1%), synovial sarcoma (6.5%), malignant schwannoma (5.9%), and fibrosarcoma (5.2%). In the series by Markhede et al.,[48] the three most common sarcomas were malignant fibrous histiocytoma (28%), fibrosarcoma (14%), and liposarcoma (9%). Rhabdomyosarcoma, neuroblastoma, and extraskeletal Ewing's sarcoma are the most frequent soft tissue sarcomas of childhood. A histological classification of soft tissue tumors is presented in the box on pp. 7-9.

STAGING AND GRADING OF SOFT TISSUE SARCOMAS

The histological type of sarcoma does not always provide sufficient information for predicting the clinical course, and grading and staging of soft tissue sarcomas are essential for accurate prognosis, planning and evaluation of

therapy, and comparison and exchange of data. *Grading* determines the degree of malignancy and is based on an evaluation of several histological parameters. *Staging* provides shorthand information regarding the state or extent of the disease at a particular designated time, preferably at the time of the initial histological diagnosis. Grading and staging are complicated by numerous and often interrelated variables that are likely to affect clinical behavior. In fact, a grading or staging system that is comprehensive and gives full consideration to all factors that might affect the course of the disease and the results of therapy is too complex for practical purposes. On the other hand, a more limited and more practical system may suffer from the hazards of oversimplification and may result in data that are neither meaningful nor reliable and defeat the purpose for which the system was designed.

The accuracy of grading and staging obviously depends on the input of adequate and precise clinical and pathological data, and staging is best accomplished following biopsy and histological diagnosis of the primary tumor. Grading and staging of recurrent tumors are of much less significance because they are influenced by the preceding therapy. Moreover, the type of tumor, rather than its grade, provides information as to the likelihood of lymph node metastasis. For instance, lymph node metastasis is common in rhabdomyosarcoma and epithelioid sarcoma but is rare in liposarcoma and malignant schwannoma. As in all grading and staging systems, the data are recorded in a standard checklist or protocol.[58,66,67,72]

GRADING

Traditionally, as outlined by Broders et al.[9] in 1939, the grade of malignancy is determined by a combined assessment of several histological features: (1) degree of cellularity, (2) cellular pleomorphism or anaplasia, (3) mitotic activity (frequency and abnormality of mitotic figures), (4) degree of necrosis, and (5) expansive, or infiltrative and invasive growth. Additional factors include the amount of matrix formation and the presence or absence of hemorrhage, calcification, and inflammatory infiltrate. The amount of matrix formation, such as collagen or mucoid material, is usually inversely proportional to cellularity and degree of differentiation. Depth of the tumor is another important prognostic factor.

Because the various parameters are closely interrelated, almost any combination of them will provide useful information as to the grade of the tumor. The two most important parameters for grading soft tissue sarcomas, however, seem to be the number of mitotic figures and the extent of necrosis[1,25,46] (Table 1-3).

The number of grades varies in different staging systems: two, three, and four grades have been distinguished. Three-grade systems seem best suited for prediction of the different patterns of survival and likely response to therapy. Four-

Histological classification of soft tissue tumors

I. **Fibrous tumors**
   A. Benign tumors
      1. Nodular fasciitis (including intravascular and cranial types)
      2. Proliferative fasciitis and myositis
      3. Atypical decubital fibroplasia (ischemic fasciitis)
      4. Fibroma (dermal, tendon sheath, nuchal)
      5. Keloid
      6. Elastofibroma
      7. Calcifying aponeurotic fibroma
      8. Fibrous hamartoma of infancy
      9. Fibromatosis colli
      10. Infantile digital fibromatosis
      11. Myofibromatosis (solitary, multicentric)
      12. Hyalin fibromatosis
      13. Calcifying fibrous pseudotumor
   B. Fibromatoses
      1. Superficial fibromatoses
         a. Palmar and plantar fibromatosis
         b. Penile (Peyronie's) fibromatosis
         c. Knuckle pads
      2. Deep fibromatoses (desmoid tumor)
         a. Abdominal fibromatosis (abdominal desmoid)
         b. Extraabdominal fibromatosis (extraabdominal desmoid)
         c. Intraabdominal fibromatosis (intraabdominal desmoid)
         d. Mesenteric fibromatosis (including Gardner's syndrome)
         e. Infantile (desmoid-type) fibromatosis
   C. Malignant tumors
      1. Fibrosarcoma
         a. Adult fibrosarcoma
         b. Congenital or infantile fibrosarcoma
         c. Inflammatory fibrosarcoma (inflammatory myofibroblastic tumor)

II. **Fibrohistiocytic tumors**
   A. Benign tumors
      1. Fibrous histiocytoma
         a. Cutaneous fibrous histiocytoma (dermatofibroma)
         b. Deep fibrous histiocytoma
      2. Juvenile xanthogranuloma
      3. Reticulohistiocytoma
      4. Xanthoma
   B. Intermediate tumors
      1. Atypical fibroxanthoma
      2. Dermatofibrosarcoma protuberans (including pigmented form, Bednar tumor)
      3. Giant cell fibroblastoma
      4. Plexiform fibrohistiocytic tumor
      5. Angiomatoid fibrous histiocytoma

   C. Malignant tumors
      1. Malignant fibrous histiocytoma
         a. Storiform-pleomorphic fibrous histiocytoma
         b. Myxoid fibrous histiocytoma
         c. Giant cell fibrous histiocytoma (malignant giant cell tumor of soft parts)
         d. Xanthomatous (inflammatory type) fibrous histiocytoma

III. **Lipomatous tumors**
   A. Benign tumors
      1. Lipoma
         a. Cutaneous lipoma
         b. Deep lipoma
            (i) Intramuscular lipoma
            (ii) Tendon sheath lipoma
            (iii) Lumbosacral lipoma
            (iv) Intraneural and perineural fibrolipoma
         c. Multiple lipomas
      2. Angiolipoma
      3. Spindle cell or pleomorphic lipoma
      4. Myolipoma
      5. Angiomyolipoma
      6. Myelolipoma
      7. Chondroid lipoma
      8. Hibernoma
      9. Lipoblastoma or lipoblastomatosis
      10. Lipomatosis
         a. Diffuse lipomatosis
         b. Cervical symmetrical lipomatosis (Madelung's disease)
      11. Atypical lipoma
   B. Malignant tumors
      1. Liposarcoma
         a. Well-differentiated liposarcoma
            (i) Lipoma-like liposarcoma
            (ii) Sclerosing liposarcoma
            (iii) Inflammatory liposarcoma
         b. Myxoid liposarcoma
         c. Round cell (poorly differentiated myxoid) liposarcoma
         d. Pleomorphic liposarcoma
         e. Dedifferentiated liposarcoma

IV. **Smooth muscle tumors**
   A. Benign tumors
      1. Leiomyoma (cutaneous, deep and pleomorphic)
      2. Angiomyoma (vascular leiomyoma)
      3. Epithelioid leiomyoma
      4. Intravenous leiomyomatosis
      5. Leiomyomatosis peritonealis disseminata

Continued.

Histological classification of soft tissue tumors—cont'd

B. Malignant tumors
1. Leiomyosarcoma
2. Epithelioid leiomyosarcoma

V. **Skeletal muscle tumors**
A. Benign tumors
1. Adult rhabdomyoma
2. Genital rhabdomyoma
3. Fetal rhabdomyoma
4. Intermediate (cellular) rhabdomyoma
B. Malignant tumors
1. Rhabdomyosarcoma
a. Embryonal rhabdomyosarcoma
b. Botryoid rhabdomyosarcoma
c. Spindle cell rhabdomyosarcoma
d. Alveolar rhabdomyosarcoma
e. Pleomorphic rhabdomyosarcoma
2. Rhabdomyosarcoma with ganglionic differentiation (ectomesenchymoma)

VI. **Tumors of blood and lymph vessels**
A. Benign tumors
1. Papillary endothelial hyperplasia
2. Hemangioma
a. Capillary (including juvenile) hemangioma
b. Cavernous hemangioma
c. Venous hemangioma
d. Epithelioid hemangioma (angiolymphoid hyperplasia, histiocytoid hemangioma)
e. Granulation type hemangioma (pyogenic granuloma)
f. Tufted hemangioma
3. Deep hemangioma (intramuscular, synovial, perineural)
4. Lymphangioma
5. Lymphangiomyoma and lymphangiomyomatosis
6. Angiomatosis
7. Lymphangiomatosis
B. Intermediate tumors
1. Hemangioendothelioma
a. Epithelioid hemangioendothelioma
b. Endovascular papillary angioendothelioma (Dabska tumor)
c. Spindle cell hemangioendothelioma
C. Malignant tumors
1. Angiosarcoma and lymphangiosarcoma
2. Kaposi's sarcoma

VII. **Perivascular tumors**
A. Benign tumors
1. Glomus tumor

2. Glomangiomyoma
3. Hemangiopericytoma
B. Malignant tumors
1. Malignant glomus tumor
2. Malignant hemangiopericytoma

VIII. **Synovial tumors**
A. Benign tumors
1. Tenosynovial giant cell tumor
a. Localized tenosynovial giant cell tumor
b. Diffuse tenosynovial giant cell tumor (extraarticular pigmented villonodular synovitis, florid tenosynovitis)
B. Malignant tumors
1. Synovial sarcoma
a. Biphasic (fibrous *and* epithelial) synovial sarcoma
b. Monophasic (fibrous or epithelial) synovial sarcoma
2. Malignant giant cell tumor of tendon sheath

IX. **Mesothelial tumors**
A. Benign tumors
1. Solitary fibrous tumor of pleura and peritoneum (localized fibrous mesothelioma)
2. Multicystic mesothelioma
3. Adenomatoid tumor
4. Well-differentiated papillary mesothelioma
B. Malignant tumors
1. Malignant solitary fibrous tumor of pleura and peritoneum
2. Diffuse mesothelioma
a. Epithelial diffuse mesothelioma
b. Fibrous (spindled, sarcomatoid) diffuse mesothelioma
c. Biphasic diffuse mesothelioma

X. **Neural tumors**
A. Benign tumors
1. Traumatic neuroma
2. Morton's neuroma
3. Multiple mucosal neuromas
4. Neuromuscular hamartoma (benign Triton tumor)
5. Nerve sheath ganglion
6. Schwannoma (neurilemoma)
a. Cellular schwannoma
b. Plexiform schwannoma
c. Degenerated (ancient) schwannoma
d. Schwannomatosis
7. Neurothekeoma (nerve sheath myxoma)

Histological classification of soft tissue tumors—cont'd

8. Neurofibroma
   a. Diffuse neurofibroma
   b. Plexiform neurofibroma
   c. Pacinian neurofibroma
   d. Epithelioid neurofibroma
9. Granular cell tumor
10. Melanocytic schwannoma
11. Ectopic meningioma
12. Ectopic ependymoma
13. Ganglioneuroma
14. Pigmented neuroectodermal tumor of infancy (retinal anlage tumor, melanotic progonoma)

B. Malignant tumors
   1. Malignant peripheral nerve sheath tumor (MPNST) (malignant schwannoma, neurofibrosarcoma)
      a. Malignant Triton tumor (MPNST with rhabdomyosarcoma)
      b. Glandular MPNST (malignant glandular schwannoma)
      c. Epithelioid MPNST (malignant epithelioid schwannoma)
   2. Malignant granular cell tumor
   3. Clear cell sarcoma (malignant melanoma of soft parts)
   4. Malignant melanocytic schwannoma
   5. Gastrointestinal autonomous nerve tumor (plexosarcoma)
   6. Primitive neuroectodermal tumor
      a. Neuroblastoma
      b. Ganglioneuroblastoma
      c. Neuroepithelioma (peripheral neuroectodermal tumor)
      d. Extraskeletal Ewing's sarcoma

XI. Paraganglionic tumors
A. Benign tumors
   1. Paraganglioma
B. Malignant tumors
   1. Malignant paraganglioma

XII. Extraskeletal cartilaginous and osseous tumors
A. Benign tumors
   1. Panniculitis ossificans and myositis ossificans
   2. Fibroosseous pseudotumor of the digits
   3. Fibrodysplasia (myositis) ossificans progressiva
   4. Extraskeletal chondroma or osteochondroma
   5. Extraskeletal osteoma
B. Malignant tumors
   1. Extraskeletal chondrosarcoma
      a. Well-differentiated chondrosarcoma
      b. Myxoid chondrosarcoma
      c. Mesenchymal chondrosarcoma
   2. Extraskeletal osteosarcoma

XIII. Pluripotential mesenchymal tumors
A. Benign tumors
   1. Mesenchymoma
B. Malignant tumors
   1. Malignant mesenchymoma

XIV. Miscellaneous tumors
A. Benign tumors
   1. Congenital granular cell tumor
   2. Tumoral calcinosis
   3. Myxoma
      a. Cutaneous myxoma
      b. Intramuscular myxoma
      c. Juxtaarticular myxoma
   4. Angiomyxoma
   5. Amyloid tumor
   6. Parachordoma
   7. Ossifying and nonossifying fibromyxoid tumors
   8. Palisaded myofibroblastoma of lymph node
B. Malignant tumors
   1. Alveolar soft part sarcoma
   2. Epithelioid sarcoma
   3. Malignant extrarenal rhabdoid tumor
   4. Desmoplastic small cell tumor

XV. Unclassified tumors

---

grade systems usually show little difference between the two lowermost grades; two-grade systems, which distinguish only between low- and high-grade sarcomas, are more readily related to the two types of surgical therapy but make it difficult to accurately grade tumors of intermediate malignancy, such as well-differentiated fibrosarcomas.

The histological type and subtype may be used as a shortcut to establish the tumor grade.[16,24,52,57] Alveolar and embryonal rhabdomyosarcomas, neuroblastoma, extraskeletal Ewing's sarcoma, peripheral neuroepithelioma, and osteosarcoma, for example, are high-grade sarcomas. Well-differentiated and myxoid liposarcomas are low-grade tumors, whereas round cell and pleomorphic forms of liposarcoma are tumors of high-grade malignancy.

Table 1-3. Grading systems: histological parameters used in different grading systems

	Markhede[48]	Myhre Jensen[51]	Costa[16]	Coindre[14]
Cellularity	+	+	+	−
Differentiation	−	−	−	+
Pleomorphism	+	+	+	−
Mitotic rate	+	+	+	+
Necrosis	−	+	+	+

Ancillary procedures, such as special staining techniques, immunohistochemical studies, and electron microscopic studies, are useful in establishing the type of the tumor but are of little help in determining the grade of the tumor and its degree of malignancy.

LIMITATIONS AND PITFALLS OF GRADING

The significance and predictive value of the various histological parameters differ in various types of sarcomas. Mitotic activity, for example, is important in grading malignant schwannomas and leiomyosarcomas but is of much less significance in grading the various subtypes of malignant fibrous histiocytoma. Malignant granular cell tumor and alveolar soft part sarcoma behave more aggressively than is implied by their moderate degree of cellular pleomorphism and paucity of mitotic figures. Likewise, mitotic figures are rare in many diffuse and highly malignant mesotheliomas. Infantile fibrosarcoma, on the other hand, is a tumor of relatively low-grade malignancy despite its cellularity and prominent mitotic activity.

Occasional problems may also be caused by morphological variations in different portions of the same tumor. At times well-differentiated and poorly differentiated portions are encountered in leiomyosarcomas, malignant schwannomas, and liposarcomas (dedifferentiated liposarcomas). In these cases the grade should be determined on the basis of the least differentiated area, but the extent of the less–differentiated portion of the neoplasm must also be taken into consideration. For instance, a small focus of round cell liposarcoma in the center of myxoid liposarcoma does not necessarily indicate a poor prognosis but may change the grade from I to II. In a small percentage of cases, a higher degree of malignancy may be present in the recurrent or the metastatic growth. These changes may be spontaneous or may be the effect of treatment, particularly radiotherapy. On the other hand, there are also occasional rhabdomyosarcomas in which the recurrent lesion after therapy shows a higher degree of differentiation than the primary tumor.

Grading is not a substitute for a histological diagnosis and does not permit separating benign and malignant lesions; in fact, it may be misleading with tumors and tumorlike lesions of uncertain type and histogenesis. This applies not only to neoplasms but also to sarcoma-like lesions that display the conventional characteristics of malignancy but behave in a benign manner. Nodular and proliferative fasciitis and early stages of myositis ossificans are typical examples of these reactive, sarcoma-like lesions that are marked by a high degree of cellularity, markedly increased mitotic activity, and even, infrequently, areas of necrosis. Caution in this regard is particularly indicated because by no means have all of these benign mesenchymal lesions that occur in the guise of sarcomas yet been defined or recognized.

Grading, like diagnosing soft tissue sarcomas, requires representative, well-fixed, and well-stained histological material. Thick sections may be misleading as to the actual degree of cellularity and mitotic activity, and heavily stained sections may suggest less cellular differentiation than is actually present. Selection of the tissue sample and length of fixation may also influence artificially the degree of necrosis and the mitotic index. Necrosis may also be more prominent in ulcerated tumors or ones previously operated on.

GRADING SYSTEMS

Grading and staging systems should be based on soft tissue tumors of one specific type, since the predictive significance of the various grading and staging parameters varies in different types of sarcomas. However, in many systems assessment of the results and prognostic significance of grading and staging of soft tissue sarcomas is based on soft tissue tumors as a general group rather than on a specific tumor entity because of the relative rarity of these tumors and the difficulty of assembling a large number of sarcomas of any specific type. Therefore in many staging systems, the predictive value of the histological type is incorporated into the histological grade of the tumor.

Markhede et al.[48] published in 1982 a grading system that used four grades of malignancy based on cellularity, cellular pleomorphism, and mitotic activity. In their study, grade correlated well with survival rates. Patients with grade 1 and 2 tumors had similar clinical courses, and no patients died from these tumors. The 5- and 10-year survival rates with grade 3 tumors were 68% and 55%, respectively, and with grade 4 tumors 47% and 26%, respectively.

Myhre Jensen et al.[52] in 1983 graded 261 soft tissue sarcomas from the Aarhus Musculoskeletal Tumour Centre. They employed three grades, with 10-year survival rates of 97% for grade 1 tumors, 67% for grade 2 tumors, and 38%

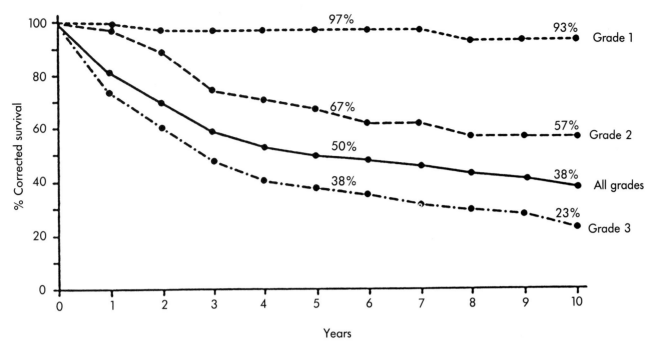

FIG. 1-2. Grading system of soft tissue sarcomas based on three grades of malignancy. (Myhre Jensen O et al: *Acta Pathol Microbiol Immunol Scand* 91A:145, 1983.)

for grade 3 tumors. The respective 10-year survival rates were 93%, 57%, and 23%. The authors concluded that mitotic activity was the main discriminating criterion but warned that delay in fixation, especially in the center of large tumors, may artificially reduce mitotic counts (Fig. 1-2).

Costa et al.[16] described a grading system based on a review of 163 sarcomas from the National Cancer Institute. They used a combination of histological diagnosis, cellularity, cellular pleomorphism, and mitotic rate as criteria for grading, but also included necrosis as an important determinant for predicting recurrence and survival rates. They employed a three-grade system and stressed that grade 2 and 3 tumors that exhibited moderate or marked necrosis had a significantly poorer prognosis; thus necrosis emerged as a major discriminating variable. The respective 5-year survival rates of patients with the three grades were 100%, 73%, and 46%.

Trojani et al.[72] and others[7,14] presented a grading system based on a study of 155 adult soft tissue sarcomas. On the basis of a multivariate analysis of the various histological features, they selected a combination of cellular differentiation, mitotic rate, and tumor necrosis for their grading system. The authors assigned a score of 0 to 3 to each of these parameters and added the scores together for a combined grade (Table 1-4). They concluded that the histological grade was the most important single factor in predicting survival rates; but they added that tumor depth (superficial versus deep) was another important prognostic parameter. The reproducibility of the system was tested among 15 pathologists, who reached agreement in 74% for tumor differentiation, 73% for mitotic rate, and 81% for tumor necrosis; the agreement as to histological type was only 61%.

Similar and more recent studies on the histological grading of soft tissue sarcomas were published by Tsujimoto et al. (236 cases),[73] Myhre Jensen et al. (278 cases),[51] and Hashimoto et al. (1116 cases).[35] Coindre et al.[13] applied their grading system to 123 spindle cell soft tissue sarcomas. Fig. 1-3 provides putative guidelines for grading soft tissue sarcomas; it gives the estimated range of malignancy for each type of sarcoma, which in turn serves as baseline for the determination of the histological grade by using standard cytological criteria such as cellularity, mitotic activity, and necrosis.

More recently, Ki-67 reactivity,[70,75] the argyrophilic stain for nucleolar organizer regions (AgNOR counts),[71,80] and mast cell counts[71] have been investigated as potential histological markers for the assessment of the proliferative activity of soft tissue sarcomas. The significance and utility of DNA flow cytometric analysis for grading and prognosis of soft tissue sarcomas is discussed in Chapter 6.

Table 1-4. Soft tissue sarcomas: definition of grading parameters

Parameter	Score
Degree of tumor differentiation	
Close resemblance to normal adult tissue (e.g., well-differentiated liposarcoma)	1
Tumor type clearly recognizable (e.g., alveolar soft part sarcoma)	2
Tumor type uncertain (e.g., undifferentiated sarcoma)	3
Tumor necrosis	
No tumor necrosis on any slide	0
Less than 50% tumor necrosis	1
More than 50% tumor necrosis	2
Mitotic count	
0-9 /per 10 HPF	1
10-19 /per 10 HPF	2
20+ / per 10 HPF	3
Histological grade	**Total score**
Grade 1	2, 3
Grade 2	4, 5
Grade 3	6, 7, 8

Modified from Coindre JM et al: *Cancer* 58:306, 1986.

STAGING SYSTEMS
American Joint Committee (AJC) staging system

The American Joint Committee on Cancer (AJC) system is based on the TNM staging system[6,57,58]; it uses the size and extension of the primary tumor (T), the involvement of lymph nodes (N), the presence of metastasis (M), and the type and grade of sarcoma (G). Three grades—low, moderate, and high—are distinguished, depending on the type of tumor, estimated degree of cellularity, and mitotic activity. The definitions of the four stages of malignancy are shown in the box below.

The survival curves for the four stages in Fig. 1-4 were obtained from a retrospective study of 702 sarcomas collected from 13 different institutions. The study included only tumors that were diagnosed during a 15-year period from 1954 to 1969, were histologically confirmed, had adequate follow-up information, and received primary treatment in the institution that contributed the specimen. Because the sample was too small to gain sufficient data on all well-defined soft tissue sarcomas, the staging system was limited to the eight most common types.[57,58]

AJC staging of soft tissue sarcomas: definitions of TNMG

T: Primary tumor
T1 Tumor less than 5 cm
T2 Tumor 5 cm or greater

N: Regional lymph nodes
N0 No histologically verified metastasis to regional lymph nodes
N1 Histologically verified regional lymph node metastasis

M: Distant metastasis
M0 No distant metastasis
M1 Distant metastasis

G: Histological grade of malignancy
G1 Low (well-differentiated)
G2 Moderate (moderately well-differentiated)
G3 High (poorly differentiated)
G4 Undifferentiated

From Beahrs OH et al: American Joint Committee on Cancer, 1992.

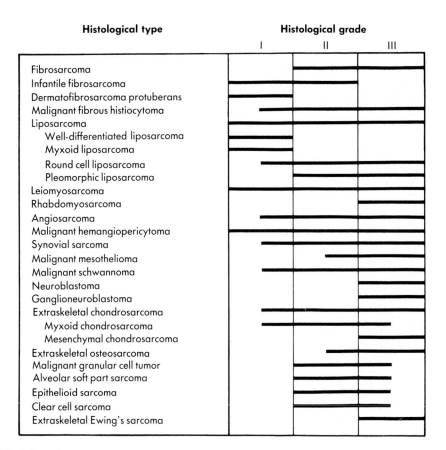

Histological type	Histological grade		
	I	II	III
Fibrosarcoma			
Infantile fibrosarcoma			
Dermatofibrosarcoma protuberans			
Malignant fibrous histiocytoma			
Liposarcoma			
Well-differentiated liposarcoma			
Myxoid liposarcoma			
Round cell liposarcoma			
Pleomorphic liposarcoma			
Leiomyosarcoma			
Rhabdomyosarcoma			
Angiosarcoma			
Malignant hemangiopericytoma			
Synovial sarcoma			
Malignant mesothelioma			
Malignant schwannoma			
Neuroblastoma			
Ganglioneuroblastoma			
Extraskeletal chondrosarcoma			
Myxoid chondrosarcoma			
Mesenchymal chondrosarcoma			
Extraskeletal osteosarcoma			
Malignant granular cell tumor			
Alveolar soft part sarcoma			
Epithelioid sarcoma			
Clear cell sarcoma			
Extraskeletal Ewing's sarcoma			

FIG. 1-3. Soft tissue sarcomas. Estimated range of degree of malignancy based on histological type and grade. Grade within the overall range depends on specific histological features such as cellularity, cellular pleomorphism, mitotic activity, amount of stroma, infiltrative or expansive growth, and necrosis.

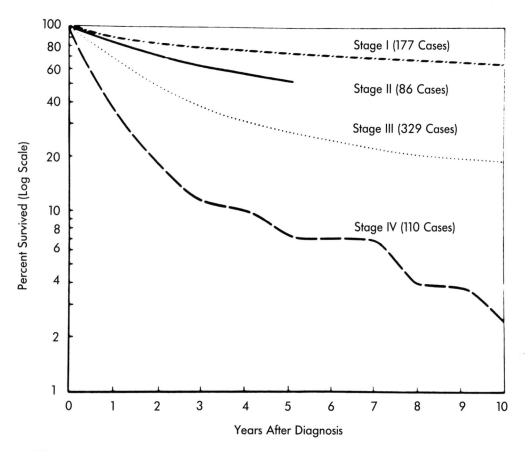

FIG. 1-4. American Joint Committee Staging System. Survival curves of 702 soft tissue sarcomas, stages I to IV.

AJC staging of soft tissue sarcomas: definitions of stages

Stage I

Stage Ia ($G_1T_1N_0M_0$): Grade 1 tumor less than 5 cm in diameter with no regional lymph node or distant metastasis

Stage Ib ($G_1T_2N_0M_0$): Grade 1 tumor 5 cm or greater in diameter with no regional lymph node or distant metastasis

Stage II

Stage IIa ($G_2T_1N_0M_0$): Grade 2 tumor less than 5 cm in diameter with no regional lymph node or distant metastasis

Stage IIb ($G_2T_2N_0M_0$): Grade 2 tumor 5 cm or greater in diameter with no regional lymph node or distant metastasis

Stage III

Stage IIIa ($G_{3,4}T_1N_0M_0$): Grade 3 tumor less than 5 cm in diameter with no regional lymph node or distant metastasis

Stage IIIb ($G_{3,4}T_2N_0M_0$): Grade 3 tumor 5 cm or greater in diameter with no regional lymph node or distant metastasis

Stage IV

Stage IVa ($G_{1-4}T_{1-2}N_1M_0$): Tumor of any grade or any size with regional lymph node metastasis but without distant metastasis

Stage IVb ($G_{1-4}T_{1-2}N_{0-1}M_1$): Tumor with distant metastasis

From Beahrs OH et al: American Joint Committee on Cancer, 1992.

A similar staging system has been used for pediatric soft tissue sarcomas, but in this system T_1 is being used for tumors limited to the organ or tissue of origin and T_2 for tumors that have invaded contiguous organs or tissues.[6]

Enneking system

The Enneking system, designed for sarcomas of both soft tissue and bone, distinguishes two anatomical settings: (1) T_1, intracompartmental tumors confined within the boundaries of well-defined anatomical structures such as a functional muscle group, joint, and subcutis; and (2) T_2, extracompartmental neoplasms that arise within or involve secondarily extrafascial spaces or planes that have no natural anatomical barriers to extension. There are two grades (G_1 and G_2) and three stages. Two grades are favored because they can be better related to the two types of surgical procedures (wide and radical excision) and because of the reported lack of any difference in the metastatic rate between intermediate- and high-grade tumors. The system distinguishes between stage I, low-grade sarcomas without metastasis; stage II, high-grade lesions without metastasis; and stage III lesions of either grade with metastasis. Each of these stages is subclassified according to the anatomical presentation of the lesion (T_1 or T_2); A signifies intracompartmental lesions and B signifies extracompartmental lesions. Clinical and radiological features are included in the assessment of the grade, and Enneking refers to the "surgical" rather than the "histological" grade of the tumor.[22,23]

Advantages and disadvantages of staging systems

Both of these staging systems serve as a valuable guide to therapy and provide useful prognostic information. The AJC system is applicable to soft tissue sarcomas at any site, whereas the Enneking system, with its emphasis on compartmentalization, is best suited for well-documented sarcomas arising in the extremities. It does not include the type, size, or depth of the tumor as separate parameters, and its two-tier grading system is probably too narrow for the wide biological range of soft tissue sarcomas. Because of the need for adequately defining compartmentalization, the system does not lend itself to retrospective staging. On the other hand, one drawback of the AJC system is its greater complexity (four stages with two subclassifications for each stage).

Another staging system, proposed by Hajdu in his textbook of soft tissue pathology,[33] uses a combined score of differentiation, cellularity, amount of stroma, vascularity, necrosis, and mitotic activity for determination of the histological grade (low, high) together with depth (superficial or deep) and size (small, big) of the tumor.

Obviously, staging of soft tissue sarcomas requires a multidisciplinary approach with close cooperation between clinician, oncologist, and pathologist. In view of the relative rarity of these tumors, staging and grading are ideally carried out in large medical centers with special interest and experience in the diagnosis and management of soft tissue sarcomas. Moreover, prospective rather than retrospective studies will be necessary to test the value of the various staging systems.

REFERENCES

1. Albus-Lutter CE, de Stefani E, van Unnik JAM: Clinicopathologic relations in soft tissue sarcomas. In *Management of soft tissue and bone sarcomas*, New York, 1986, Raven Press.

2. Amendola BE, Amendola MA, McClatchey KD, et al: Radiation associated sarcoma: a review of 23 patients with postradiation sarcoma over a 50 year period. *Am J Clin Oncol* 12:411, 1989.

3. Angervall L, Kindblom LG, Rydholm A, et al: The diagnosis and prognosis of soft tissue tumors. *Semin Diagn Pathol* 3:240, 1986.

4. Arlen M, Higinbotham NL, Huvos AG, et al: Radiation-induced sarcoma of bone. *Cancer* 28:1087, 1971.

5. Bailar JC: How dangerous is dioxin? *N Engl J Med* 324:260, 1991.

6. Beahrs OH, Henson DE, Hutter RVP, et al: *Manual for staging of cancer*. Third Edition. Philadelphia, ed 3, J.B. Lippincott Company 1992.

7. Boddaert A, Trojani M, Contesso G, et al: Soft tissue sarcomas of adults: study of pathological variables and definition of a histopathological grading system. In *Management of soft tissue and bone sarcomas*, New York, 1986, Raven Press.

8. Breslin P, Kang HK, Lee Y, et al: Proportionate mortality study of US Army and US Marine Corps veterans of the Vietnam war. *J Occup Med* 30:412, 1988.

9. Broders AC, Hargrave R, Meyerding HW: Pathological features of soft tissue fibrosarcoma with special reference to the grading of its malignancy. *Surg Gynecol Obstet* 69:267, 1939.

10. Burns WA, Kanhauwand S, Tillman L, et al: Fibrosarcoma occurring at the site of a plastic vascular graft. *Cancer* 29:66, 1972.

11. Cahan WG, Woodard HQ, Higinbotham NL, et al: Sarcoma arising in irradiated bone. *Cancer* 1:3, 1948.

12. Coindre JM: Pathology and grading of soft tissue sarcomas. *Cancer Treat Res* 67:1, 1993.

13. Coindre JM, Nguyen BB, Bonichon F, et al: Histopathologic grading in spindle cell soft tissue sarcomas. *Cancer* 61:2305, 1988.

14. Coindre JM, Trojani M, Contesso G, et al: Reproducibility of a histopathologic grading system for adult soft tissue sarcoma. *Cancer* 58:306, 1986.

15. Collins JJ, Strauss ME, Levinskas GJ, et al: The mortality experience of workers exposed to 2,3,7,8-tetrachlorodibenzo-p-dioxin in a tricholophenol process accident. *Epidemiology* 4:7, 1993.

16. Costa J, Wesley RA, Glatstein E, et al: The grading of soft tissue sarcomas: results of a clinicohistopathologic correlation in a series of 163 cases. *Cancer* 53:530, 1984.

17. Craighead JE: Current pathogenetic concepts of diffuse malignant mesothelioma. *Hum Pathol* 18:544, 1987.

18. Craighead JE, Abraham JL, Churg A, et al: The pathology of asbestos-associated diseases of the lung and pleural cavities: diagnostic criteria and proposed grading schema. *Arch Pathol Lab Med* 106:544, 1982.

19. Craighead JE, Mossman BT: The pathogenesis of asbestos associated diseases. *N Engl J Med* 306:1446, 1982.

20. Cutler SJ, Young IL: Third National Cancer Survey: incidence data. *NCI Monogr* 41:1, 1975.

21. Enjoji M, Hashimoto H: Diagnosis of soft tissue sarcomas. *Pathol Res Pract* 178:215, 1984.

22. Enneking WF: *Musculoskeletal tumor surgery*. New York, 1983, Churchill Livingstone.

23. Enneking WF, Spanier SS, Malawar MM: The effect of the anatomic setting on the results of surgical procedures for soft part sarcoma of the thigh. *Cancer* 47:1005, 1981.

24. Enzinger FM: Classification and prognostic factors of soft tissue sarcomas. In *Diagnostische und therapeutische Entwicklungen in der Hämatologie und Onkologie*, München, 1988, W. Zuckschwerdt Verlag.

25. Enzinger FM: Clinicopathological correlation in soft tissue sarcomas. In *Management of soft tissue and bone sarcomas*. New York, 1986, Raven Press.

26. Enzinger FM: Recent developments in the classification of soft tissue sarcomas. In *Management of primary soft tissue and bone tumors*. Chicago, 1977, Year Book Medical Publishers.

27. Enzinger FM: Recent trends in soft tissue pathology. In *Tumors of bone and soft tissue*. Chicago, 1965, Year Book Medical Publishers.

28. Enzinger FM, Lattes R, Torloni R: Histological typing of soft tissue tumours. International Histological Classification of Tumours. No. 3 Geneva, 1969, World Health Organization.

29. Evans DM, Williams WJ, Jung IT: Angiosarcoma and hepatocellular carcinoma in vinyl chloride workers. *Histopathology* 7:377, 1983.

30. Fingerhut MA, Halperin WE, Marlow DA: Cancer mortality in workers exposed to 2,3,7,8-tetrachlorodibenzo-p-dioxin. *N Engl J Med* 324:212, 1991.

31. Greenwald P, Kovasznay B, Collins DN, et al: Sarcomas of soft tissues after Vietnam service. *JNCI* 73:1107, 1984.

32. Haggit RC, Reid BJ: Hereditary gastrointestinal polyposis syndromes. *Am J Surg Pathol* 10:871, 1986.

33. Hajdu SI: *Pathology of soft tissue tumors*. Philadelphia, 1979, Lea & Febiger.

34. Hardell L, Sandstrom A: Case-control study: soft tissue sarcoma and exposure to phenoxyacetic acids or chlorophenols. *Br J Cancer* 39:711, 1979.

35. Hashimoto H, Daimaru Y, Takeshita S, et al: Prognostic significance of histologic parameters of soft tissue sarcomas. *Cancer* 70:2816, 1992.

36. Hatfield PM, Schulz M: Postirradiation sarcoma, including 5 cases after x-ray therapy of breast carcinoma. *Radiology* 96:593, 1970.

37. Heise HW, Myers MH, Russell WO, et al: Recurrence-free survival time for surgically treated soft tissue sarcoma patients: multivariate analysis of five prognostic factors. *Cancer* 57:172, 1986.

38. Hermanek P, Sobin LH: *UICC: Classification of malignant tumours*, ed 4, Berlin, New York 1987, Springer-Verlag.

39. Kang H, Enzinger FM, Breslin P, et al: Soft tissue sarcoma and military service in Vietnam: a case control study. *J Natl Cancer Inst* 79:693, 1987.

40. Kulander BG, Polissar L, Yang CY, et al: Grading of soft tissue sarcomas: necrosis as a determinant of survival. *Mod Pathol* 2:205, 1989.

41. Kuratsu S, Myoui A, Tomita Y, et al: Usefulness of argyrophilic nucleolar organizer staining for histologic grading of soft tissue sarcomas. *J Surg Oncol* 54:139, 1993.

42. Kuten A, Sapir D, Cohen Y, et al: Postirradiation soft tissue sarcoma occurring in breast cancer patients: report of seven cases and results of combination chemotherapy. *J Surg Oncol* 28:168, 1985.

43. Laskin WB, Silverman TA, Enzinger FM: Postradiation soft tissue sarcomas: an analysis of 53 cases. *Cancer* 62:2330, 1988.

44. Lattes R: Tumors of the soft tissue. In *Atlas of tumor pathology*. Second series. Fascicle 1/Revised. Armed Forces Institute of Pathology, 1983.

45. Malkin D, Li F, Strong L, et al: Germ line p53 mutations in a familial syndrome of breast cancer, sarcomas, and other neoplasms. *Science* 250:1233, 1990.

46. Mandard AM, Chasley JC, Mandard JC, et al: The pathologist's role in a multidisciplinary approach for soft part tissue sarcoma: a reappraisal (39 cases). *J Surg Oncol* 17:69, 1981.

47. Mandard AM, Petiot JF, Marnay J, et al: Prognostic factors in soft tissue sarcomas: a multivariate analysis of 109 cases. *Cancer* 63:1437, 1989.

48. Markhede G, Angervall L, Stener B: A multivariate analysis of the prognosis after surgical treatment of malignant soft tissue tumors. *Cancer* 49:1721, 1982.

49. Mazanet R, Antman KH: Sarcomas of soft tissue and bone. *Cancer* 68:463, 1991.

50. Meister P: Weichgewebssarkome: Klassifizierung und/oder Graduierung. *Zentralbl Allg Pathol* 134:355, 1988.

51. Myhre Jensen O, Høgh J, Østgaard SE, et al: Histopathological grading of soft tissue tumours: prognostic significance in a prospective study of 278 consecutive cases. *J Pathol* 163:19, 1991.

52. Myhre Jensen O, Kaae S, Madsen EH, et al: Histopathological grading in soft-tissue tumours: relation to survival in 261 surgically treated patients. *Acta Pathol Microbiol Immunol Scand* 91A:145, 1983.

53. Ott G: Fremdkörpersarkome. *Exp Med Pathol Klin* 32:1, 1970.

54. Pierce ER, Weisbord T, McKusick VA: Gardner's syndrome: formal genetic and statistical analysis of a large Canadian kindred. *Clin Genet* 1:65, 1970.

55. Rantakko V, Ekfors TO: Sarcomas of the soft tissues in the extremities and limb girdles: analysis of 240 cases diagnosed in Finland in 1960-1969. *Acta Chir Scand* 145:385, 1979.

56. Robinson E, Neugut AI, Wylie P: Clinical aspects of postirradiation sarcomas. *J Natl Cancer Inst* 80:233, 1988.

57. Russell WO, Cohen J, Cutler S, et al: Staging system for soft tissue sarcoma. In *American Joint Committee for Cancer Staging and End Results Reporting*. Task Force on Soft Tissue Sarcoma, Chicago, 1980, American College of Surgeons.

58. Russell WO, Cohen J, Enzinger FM, et al: A clinical and pathological staging system for soft tissue sarcomas. *Cancer* 40:1562, 1977.

59. Rydholm A: Management of patients with soft tissue tumors: strategy developed at a regional oncology center. *Acta Orthop Scand* (suppl) 203:13, 1983.

60. Rydholm A, Berg NO, Gullberg B, et al: Epidemiology of soft tissue sarcoma in the locomotor system: a retrospective population-based study of the interrelationships between clinical and morphological variables. *Acta Pathol Microbiol Immunol Scand* 92A:363, 1984.

61. Selikoff IJ, Churg J, Hammond EC: Asbestos exposure and neoplasia. *JAMA* 288:22, 1964.

62. Shiraki M, Enterline HT, Brooks JJ, et al: Pathologic analysis of advanced adult soft tissue sarcomas, bone sarcomas, and mesotheliomas: the Eastern Cooperative Oncology Group (ECOG) experience. *Cancer* 64:484, 1989.

63. Silverberg E, Boring CC, Squires TS: Cancer statistics, 1990. *CA Cancer J Clin* 40:9, 1990.

64. Stout AP: Tumors of soft tissue. AFIP *Atlas of tumor pathology*, Fascicle 1, First Series, Washington, DC, 1957, Armed Forces Institute of Pathology.

65. Strong LC, Williams WR, Lustbader E: Genetic etiology of second tumors in childhood soft tissue sarcoma survivors. *Proc Annu Meet Am Assoc Cancer Res* 27:204, 1986.

66. Suit HD, Russell WO: Soft part tumors. *Cancer* 39:830, 1977.

67. Suit HD, Russell WO, Martin RG: Management of patients with sarcoma of soft tissue in an extremity. *Cancer* 31:1247, 1973.

68. Suit HD, Russell WO, Martin RG: Sarcoma of soft tissue: clinical and histopathological parameter and response to treatment. *Cancer* 31:1247, 1973.

69. Suruda AJ, Ward EM, Fingerhut MA: Identification of soft tissue sarcoma deaths in cohorts exposed to dioxin and to chlorinated naphthalenes. *Epidemiology* 4:14, 1993.

70. Swanson SA, Brooks JJ: Proliferation markers Ki-67 and p 105 in soft tissue lesions: correlation with DNA flow cytometric characteristics. *Am J Pathol* 137:1491, 1990.

71. Tomita Y, Aozasa K, Myoui A, et al: Histologic grading in soft-tissue sarcomas: an analysis of 194 cases including AgNOR count and mast-cell count. *Int J Cancer* 54:194, 1993.

72. Trojani M, Contesso G, Coindre JM, et al: Soft tissue sarcomas of adults: study of pathological and prognostic variables and definition of a histological grading system. *Int J Cancer* 33:37, 1984.

73. Tsujimoto M, Aozasa K, Ueda T, et al: Multivariate analysis for histologic prognostic factors in soft tissue sarcomas. *Cancer* 62:994, 1988.

74. Tucker MA, Fraumeni JF: Soft tissue. In Schottenfeld D, Fraumeni JF Jr, editors: *Cancer epidemiology and prevention*. Philadelphia, 1982, WB Saunders.

75. Ueda T, Aozasa K, Tsujimoto M, et al: Prognostic significance of Ki-67 reactivity in soft tissue sarcomas. *Cancer* 63:1607, 1989.

76. USAF School of Aerospace Medicine: An epidemiologic investigation of health effects in Air Force personnel following exposure to herbicide: *Mortality update*. Brooks AFB, Texas, December 1984.

77. van Haelst-Pisani CM, Buckner JC, Reiman HM, et al: Does histologic grade in soft tissue sarcoma influence response rate to systemic chemotherapy. *Cancer* 68:2354, 1991.

78. Weiss SW, Sobin L: *WHO Classification of soft tissue tumors*, Berlin, Springer Verlag (in press).

79. Wiklund TA, Blomqvist CP, Raty J, et al: Postirradiation sarcoma: analysis of nationwide cancer registry material. *Cancer* 68:524, 1991.

80. Wrba F, Augustin I, Fertl H: Nucleolar organizer regions in soft tissue sarcomas. *Oncology* 48:166, 1991.

CHAPTER 2   ALFRED E. CHANG, VERNON K. SONDAK

CLINICAL EVALUATION AND TREATMENT OF SOFT TISSUE TUMORS

Soft tissue sarcomas are a heterogeneous group of malignant neoplasms that can arise from mesenchymal elements anywhere in the body. Despite the fact that soft tissues and bone comprise almost two thirds of the mass of the human body, sarcomas are uncommon tumors. Benign neoplasms of the soft tissues, in contrast, are commonplace and rarely consequential. These facts account for a number of observations about the clinical management of soft tissue sarcomas. Because of the relative rarity of sarcomas compared with benign soft tissue tumors, both patients and clinicians frequently fail to appreciate the significance of an enlarging soft tissue mass, and a tissue diagnosis is commonly obtained only after a significant delay. Few pathologists accumulate significant experience with these rare tumors, so once they are biopsied, pathological classification may be incomplete or inaccurate. Once the proper diagnosis is made, even clinicians experienced in cancer management may lack detailed knowledge of the behavior of specific soft tissue sarcomas and may be unable to provide appropriate therapy. The goal of this chapter is to review the clinical aspects of the evaluation and treatment of soft tissue tumors, in hopes of facilitating the prompt diagnosis and proper multimodality management of these challenging lesions. This chapter reflects current approaches to the treatment of adult soft tissue sarcomas. Treatment of childhood rhabdomyosarcomas is not reviewed; the management of these tumors differs significantly from those in adults (see Chapter 22).

Beginning with the initial biopsy, information provided by the pathologist assumes a critical role in the management algorithm of soft tissue sarcomas. Once the diagnosis of sarcoma has been established, the most important consideration in determining the treatment strategy is the histological grade of the tumor.[13] Sarcomas are usually assigned a grade from 1 to 3, with 1 being the lowest grade. Low-grade sarcomas rarely metastasize, although they can be locally aggressive. Higher-grade sarcomas (grade 2 or 3) pose a significant threat of metastasizing, and also

present problems of local control. Assigning a pathological grade to an individual tumor can be a difficult and subjective task, and the specific details of the criteria used to grade soft tissue sarcomas are discussed elsewhere. But the clinical importance of the tumor grade cannot be overstressed, and an ideal biopsy should allow for a confident grade assignment.

Next in importance to grade is the location of the primary tumor. The location of a soft tissue sarcoma influences the treatment options; for instance, retroperitoneal tumors require a very different approach than do lesions of an extremity. The sites of soft tissue sarcomas from four reported series are presented in Table 2-1. In virtually all series of adult soft tissue sarcomas, the extremities represent the predominant site of origin. Approximately 45% of soft tissue sarcomas occur in the lower extremity, 15% in the upper extremity, 10% in the head and neck region, 15% in the retroperitoneum, and nearly all the rest in the abdominal and chest wall. Visceral sarcomas, which arise from the connective tissue stroma found in all organs, account for a small minority of cases. Although their overall behavior may be similar to sarcomas found elsewhere, the treatment of a visceral sarcoma is highly dependent upon the organ within which it has arisen.

BIOPSY AND PREOPERATIVE EVALUATION

Both benign and malignant soft tissue tumors commonly present as a painless mass. There are no reliable findings on physical examination to distinguish whether a soft tissue mass is benign or malignant. Benign soft tissue tumors far outnumber their malignant counterparts. By virtue of these facts, prolonged delays before the institution of definitive treatment are common in patients with sarcoma. A survey of over 5800 sarcoma patients revealed that about half waited at least 4 months before seeing a physician, and 20% experienced delays of 6 months or more *after* seeking treatment before a correct diagnosis was made.[33] Often, sarcoma patients are diagnosed clinically as having a

Table 2-1. Anatomic sites of soft tissue sarcomas, based on recent large series

Author	Site					TOTAL
	Lower extremity	Upper extremity	Head and neck	Trunk	Retroperitoneum	
Abbas et al.[1]	81	42	24	66	38	251
Potter et al.[42]	152	59	12	48	36	307
Torosian et al.[63]	208	81	21	92	90	492
Lawrence et al.[33]	2110	594	406	872	568	4550
TOTAL	2551	776	463	1078	732	5600
(%)	(46%)	(14%)	(8%)	(19%)	(13%)	(100%)

"chronic hematoma" or "pulled muscle," and undergo prolonged observation or treatment for this. In fact, nonathletic adults rarely develop persistent soft tissue masses from either of these causes in the absence of a history of unusually strenuous activity. These diagnoses should only be entertained in the setting of clear-cut local trauma. When a soft tissue mass arises in a patient with no history of trauma or persists for more than 6 weeks after local trauma, biopsy is usually indicated.

Virtually all soft tissue masses over 5 cm in diameter, as well as any new, enlarging, or symptomatic lesions, should be biopsied. Only those small subcutaneous lesions which have persisted unchanged for many years should be considered for observation rather than biopsy. The best way to avoid undue diagnostic delay during the evaluation of a soft tissue mass is for the physician to always remain cognizant of the possibility of cancer.

Biopsy techniques

Properly performed, a timely biopsy is the critical first step in a multimodality treatment approach. Improperly done, it can complicate patient care and sometimes even eliminate treatment options. Several biopsy techniques are available to the clinician: fine-needle aspiration, core-needle biopsy, incisional biopsy, and excisional biopsy. The choice of biopsy is dictated by the size and location of the mass, as well as the experience of the pathologist. Excisional biopsy should be reserved for small (under 3 to 5 cm in greatest diameter) and superficial soft tissue masses where the chance of cancer is low and where complete excision would not jeopardize subsequent treatment in the event a sarcoma is found (Fig. 2-1).

Fine-needle aspiration is a cytological technique involving the use of a fine-gauge (usually 21 to 23 gauge) needle to aspirate individual tumor cells from a mass. Fine-needle aspiration cytology has a role to play in the diagnosis of some soft tissue lesions, but its use should be limited because even experienced cytopathologists will often be unable to discern the grade and histological type of a sarcoma from an aspirate. The advantage of fine-needle aspiration is that it is relatively atraumatic and hence can be used to

sample deep-seated tumors (i.e., retroperitoneal masses) under guidance with CT scan. Fine-needle aspiration minimizes the potential for tumor spillage within the peritoneal cavity that can accompany open surgical biopsy of a retroperitoneal sarcoma. Fine-needle aspiration guided by CT scan has proven to be very helpful in diagnosing intraabdominal and retroperitoneal tumors but is rarely needed for sarcomas of the extremities. Fine-needle aspiration biopsy is also acceptable to document local or distant recurrences in patients with a previously diagnosed sarcoma, where the cytological findings can be directly compared with the prior histological specimens.

A *core-needle biopsy* results in the retrieval of a thin sliver of tissue (approximately 1 by 10 mm). This procedure is most commonly performed with a Tru-Cut needle. Here again, the small sample size may make it difficult for a pathologist to accurately diagnose and grade the tumor, or the tissue obtained may not be representative of the entire tumor, leading to underestimation of the tumor grade. Tissue necessary for special staining or electron microscopic procedures may not be available with this technique. Previously expressed fears, however, that core-needle biopsy of extremity sarcomas would result in a significant number of hematomas—and thus dissemination of tumor cells beyond the confines of the primary site—appear to be groundless. Two recent series compared core-needle and open biopsies of soft tissue tumors, and documented that both the histological type and grade of a sarcoma could be correctly determined by core-needle biopsy in over 90% of cases.[3,4] These results have encouraged wider use of this technique, including core-needle biopsies guided by CT scan.

Excisional biopsy refers to removal of the entire grossly evident lesion, usually without any significant margin of normal tissue. Many sarcomas appear to be encapsulated at the time of open biopsy. In actuality, these tumors possess a "pseudocapsule" (Fig. 2-2), and removing the tumor in this apparent plane will leave gross or microscopic cancer behind in the majority of cases.[24] "Shellout," or excisional biopsy, should be reserved for lesions less than 3 to 5 cm in diameter, or for very superficial tumors. Excisional

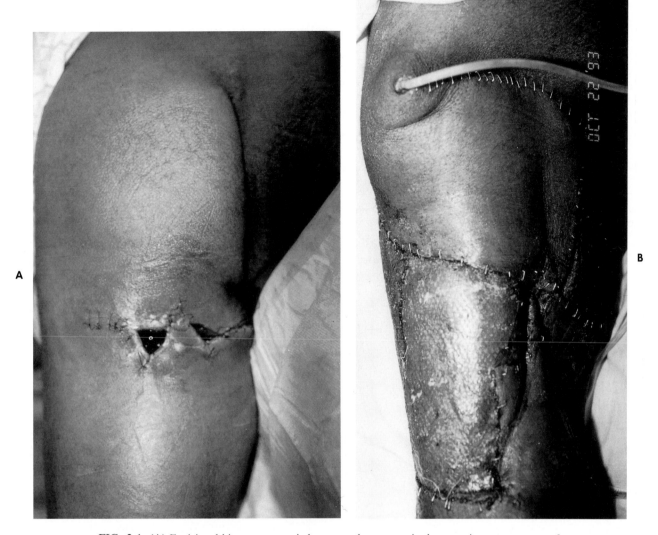

FIG. 2-1. (A) Excisional biopsy was carried out on a large mass in the posterior compartment of the upper thigh, using a transverse incision. The biopsy site subsequently became infected, leading to wound breakdown. The combination of the transverse orientation of the incision, the excisional biopsy with positive margins, and the postbiopsy wound complication all significantly compromised the ability to carry out a definitive resection. **(B)** Ultimately, wide excision of the biopsy site and surrounding normal tissue required reconstruction with a tensor fascia lata myocutaneous flap and split-thickness skin grafts for skin coverage.

biopsies of larger or deep sarcomas are undesirable since they can contaminate surrounding tissue planes, and this may compromise the subsequent definitive surgical procedure.

Incisional biopsy is the appropriate technique for diagnosing most soft tissue masses. This technique involves the removal of a generous wedge of tissue, which is minimally manipulated at the time of surgery. There are several important technical factors in the performance of an incisional biopsy. For extremity lesions, the incision should be oriented along the long axis of the extremity. For truncal or retroperitoneal lesions, the biopsy incision should be situated so that it can be readily excised along with the tumor if a diagnosis of sarcoma is made. The biopsy site should be directly over the tumor, at the point where the lesion is closest to the surface, and there should be no raising of flaps or disturbance of tissue planes superficial to the tumor (Fig. 2-3). Prior to wound closure, hemostasis should be achieved to prevent hematoma, which could disseminate tumor cells through normal tissue planes. Drains are not used routinely; in the uncommon case when a drain is required, it should exit either through or very near the biopsy incision. If cancer is diagnosed, the drain tract must be excised in continuity with the tumor mass.

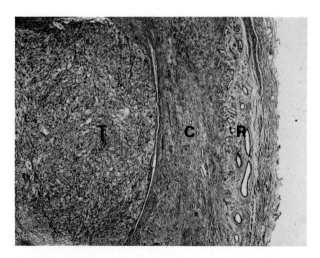

FIG. 2-2. High-grade sarcoma *(T)* surrounded by a pseudocapsule that is composed of a compression zone *(C)* and a reactive zone *(R)*. (×15.)

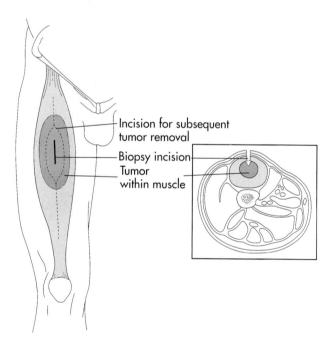

Incision for subsequent tumor removal
Biopsy incision
Tumor within muscle

FIG. 2-3. Technique for biopsy of an extremity soft tissue mass suspected of being a sarcoma. The mass should not be enucleated within the pseudocapsule; rather, incisional biopsy leaving the bulk of the lesion undisturbed should be carried out. (From Sondak VK: Sarcomas of bone and soft tissue. In Greenfield LJ, Mulholland MW, Oldham KT, et al, editors: *Surgery: scientific principles and practices,* Philadelphia, 1993, JB Lippincott. Used with permission.)

A *frozen section* at the time of biopsy can be useful to determine whether the specimen has adequate viable tissue for examination, as opposed to necrotic nonviable tumor or reactive zones of the pseudocapsule around the growing tumor. Because of the subtle criteria necessary to distinguish

Table 2-2. American Joint Commission on Cancer (AJCC) GTNM classification and stage grouping of soft tissue sarcomas

G: Tumor grade
- G_1 Well differentiated
- G_2 Moderately well differentiated
- G_3 Poorly differentiated

T: Primary tumor
- T_1 Tumor ≤ 5 cm in greatest diameter
- T_2 Tumor > 5 cm in greatest diameter

N: Regional lymph node involvement
- N_0 No known metastases to lymph nodes
- N_1 Verified metastases to lymph nodes

M: Distant metastasis
- M_0 No known distant metastasis
- M_1 Known distant metastasis

Stage grouping			
Stage IA	G_1	T_1	N_0	M_0
Stage IB	G_1	T_2	N_0	M_0
Stage IIA	G_2	T_1	N_0	M_0
Stage IIB	G_2	T_2	N_0	M_0
Stage IIIA	G_3	T_1	N_0	M_0
Stage IIIB	G_3	T_2	N_0	M_0
Stage IVA	Any G	Any T	N_1	M_0
Stage IVB	Any G	Any T	Any N	M_1

benign from malignant soft tissue tumors and the importance of proper grade assignment, treatment planning (including definitive resection) should almost always be delayed until a definitive report based on permanent sections is available.

Staging and preoperative evaluation

GTNM staging system. Because of the prognostic importance of histological grading, the staging of the primary tumor is based on both clinical and histological information. For soft tissue sarcomas, the familiar TNM classification is modified to a GTNM system (Table 2-2). Localized low-grade (G_1) tumors are classified as stage I, intermediate-grade tumors as stage II, and high-grade tumors as stage III. Any tumor with regional or distant metastatic disease, regardless of the grade of the primary tumor, is classified as stage IV. This staging system is clinically very useful, as it separates patients into groups with clearly differing prognoses (Fig. 2-4).

Following tumor grade in prognostic importance is tumor size. The larger the primary sarcoma, the greater the risk of metastasis and death. Size is also significant in determining whether local control can be achieved by surgery alone or with radiation.[12,43,48,60] When local control can be achieved, size also reflects the probability of developing distant metastases.[12,43,60] In the current American Joint Commission on Cancer (AJCC) system, tumors of 5 cm or

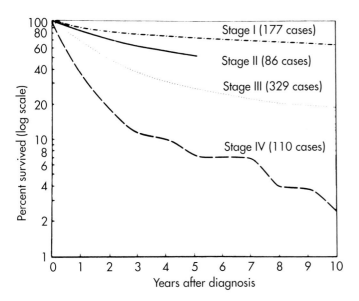

FIG. 2-4. Overall survival rates for soft tissue sarcoma patients based on AJCC stage at the time of presentation.

Table 2-3. Five-year disease-free survival rates by tumor size for patients with intermediate- and high-grade sarcomas treated with surgery and radiation (only patients in whom local control was achieved were included)

Tumor size (cm)	No. of patients	% disease-free at 5 years
<2.5	17	94
2.6-4.9	48	77
5.0-10.0	55	62
10.1-15.0	24	51
15.1-20.0	9	42
>20.0	6	17
TOTAL	159	65

From Suit HD, Mankin HJ, Wood WC, et al: Treatment of the patient with stage M_0 soft tissue sarcoma. *J Clin Oncol* 6:854, 1988.

less in greatest diameter are classified as T_1, while tumors exceeding 5 cm are classified as T_2. Each stage is subdivided into an A and B category, with T_1 tumors designated as subdivision A and T_2 tumors as subdivision B. Thus, an intermediate-grade sarcoma 7 cm in greatest diameter without evidence of regional or distant spread ($G_2T_2N_0M_0$) would be categorized as stage IIB. Although it is not specified in the GTNM system, tumors over 10 cm in diameter have an even worse prognosis than those over 5 cm. Table 2-3 documents the correlation between tumor size and 5-year disease-free survival rates in patients with intermediate- and high-grade sarcomas in whom local control was achieved with surgery and radiation. (Of note, in the same series from which Table 2-3 was taken, none of 38 grade 1 tumors successfully controlled locally developed distant metastases within 5 years.[60])

It is also recognized that superficially located tumors (i.e., those situated entirely above the deep or muscular fascia of the body) have a more favorable prognosis. Although the AJCC system does not address this factor, an alternative staging system used at the Memorial-Sloan Kettering does. In this system, size less than 5 cm, superficial location, and low histological grade are considered "favorable" factors, and the stage is assigned based on the number of unfavorable factors.[23] Hence, a small superficial low-grade tumor—which has no unfavorable factors—would be considered stage 0, while a large deep high-grade tumor would be classified as stage III. Although this system has some attractive aspects, it remains to be independently confirmed, and as yet has not been shown to be superior to the AJCC system. Problematical aspects include lack of recognition of an intermediate grade, as accepted by most pa-

thologists, and no indication that a small superficial high-grade sarcoma has a prognosis equivalent to that of either a small deep low-grade tumor or a large superficial low-grade tumor, even though all are lumped together in stage I. (Obviously, the same case can be made for tumors classified as stage II in this system.) Nonetheless, further investigation of this system is warranted, both to quantitate the contribution of tumor location relative to the muscular fascia as a prognostic factor, and to refine the relative contributions of individual prognostic factors to overall outcome.

Regional lymph node involvement is quite uncommon in soft tissue sarcomas, with less than 4% of cases having nodal metastases at presentation. When node involvement occurs, the prognosis is essentially the same as for distant metastatic disease and is therefore classified as stage IV (stage IVA if only nodal metastases are present; stage IVB if both regional and distant metastases are present). In a review of over 2500 patients in the world literature, the incidence of lymph node metastases from each of the major histological types of soft tissue sarcomas was analyzed.[64] Only 5% of patients with soft tissue sarcomas developed nodal metastases at any point in the course of their disease. The incidence of lymph node metastases was slightly higher in epithelioid sarcomas, rhabdomyosarcomas, and clear cell sarcomas, as compared with other histological types. Similar findings were noted in a review of a large prospective sarcoma database containing 1772 patients.[22] Forty-six patients (2.6%) developed lymph node metastases at some time during their lives. All but one of the 46 patients had a high-grade primary tumor, with epithelioid sarcomas, embryonal rhabdomyosarcomas, and angiosarcomas being the histological types most often associated with nodal involvement (13% to 17%). Because of the rarity of lymphatic involvement by sarcoma at the time of presentation, the differential diagnosis of spindle cell tumors presenting with lymph node metastases should always include carcinoma and melanoma.

Preoperative evaluation. Once a diagnosis of sarcoma is established, the extent of the primary tumor must be assessed and a search for the presence of metastatic disease conducted. Physical examination is important in determining the size of the tumor, any fixation to adjacent structures, the relationship of the tumor to the biopsy site, the functional status of the involved part, signs of lymph node involvement, and any confounding conditions that could compromise optimal surgical or radiation treatment. Distant metastatic disease is found in at least 10% of patients with soft tissue tumors at the time of presentation. A large-scale survey of 5800 patients with soft tissue sarcomas conducted by the American College of Surgeons found that 23% of patients had evidence of distant metastases at the time of presentation,[33] although the experience at large referral centers suggests a somewhat lower figure. By far the most frequent site of metastases is the lungs. In patients with sarcoma of an extremity who develop metastases, the lungs are involved over 75% of the time. About half of all sarcoma patients who die of metastatic disease have lung metastases as their only site of distant spread. Liver involvement is rare except in intraabdominal and retroperitoneal sarcomas, where it represents the second most common site of distant spread. Occasional patients develop bone or central nervous system metastases; these sites are uncommon in patients who do not already have lung metastases.[42]

For all patients with a newly diagnosed soft tissue sarcoma, a chest x-ray and chest CT scan are appropriate to search for pulmonary metastases. For intraabdominal or retroperitoneal tumors, a CT scan that includes the liver should be added. Other studies aimed at detecting metastases, such as radionuclide bone scans or CT scan or magnetic resonance imaging of the head, are not indicated in the absence of symptoms suggestive of metastatic involvement.

In addition to assessing the prognosis, the initial evaluation provides information about the extent of the primary tumor. Bone films may show cortical bone destruction or may reveal whether the mass is a primary bone tumor rather than a soft tissue tumor. Tumors adjacent to bone may result in a periosteal reaction, which can be detected by a bone scan.[18] In most cases, since soft tissue sarcomas rarely invade bone, neither plain radiographs of the bone nor bone scans prove helpful. CT scan and magnetic resonance imaging are the most important radiologic studies for assessing the extent and resectability of soft tissue sarcomas, regardless of the site of origin. These studies permit definition of the primary tumor in relation to bone, muscle, neurovascular structures, and adjacent organs—critical information when planning treatment. Both CT scan and magnetic resonance imaging can provide this information, and in most cases either study alone is sufficient. The choice between them is based primarily on availability, cost, and the experience of the radiologist; however, the advantages and disadvantages of each modality should be considered on a case-by-case basis.

CT scans are widely available, and both the primary site and the lungs (the major site of sarcoma metastasis) can be imaged at the same sitting. Most radiologists have more experience reading CT scans than magnetic resonance images. Tumor involvement of bone is generally more

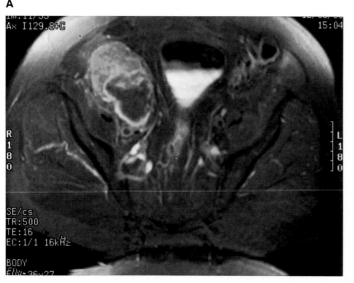

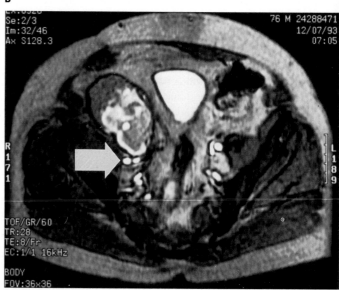

FIG. 2-5. **(A)** Standard magnetic resonance scan of a recurrent soft tissue sarcoma in the pelvic retroperitoneum. **(B)** To more precisely determine the relationship of the tumor to the iliac vessels *(arrow),* a magnetic resonance angiogram was performed.

clearly discernible on CT scan, while bone marrow invasion can be better defined by magnetic resonance imaging. Disadvantages of CT scanning include the use of ionizing radiation and the need for intravenous contrast administration.

Magnetic resonance imaging has several advantages in the evaluation of a primary sarcoma. The plane of imaging is not limited to the transverse (axial) plane of CT scanning. Coronal, sagittal, and even oblique planes may be imaged. Comparative studies have also suggested that magnetic resonance imaging may better define the relationship between tumor and muscle.[6,10] Because of the strong magnetic fields required for this type of imaging, it may not be feasible in patients with implanted metallic objects such as pacemakers, artificial joints, or some vena caval filters. While information obtained from CT scan and magnetic resonance imaging of the primary tumor may on occasion be complementary, for most patients either study alone will suffice.

Sarcomas have a characteristic arteriographic appearance, with prominent neovascularity and displacement of normal vessels. Angiography is rarely necessary for extremity lesions, although it may be more important for retroperitoneal tumors. Increasingly, information on the proximity of tumor to major vessels once provided by angiography is being obtained from specially sequenced magnetic resonance images (*magnetic resonance angiography*, Fig. 2-5).[31]

NATURAL HISTORY OF SOFT TISSUE SARCOMAS
Local recurrence

One of the major clinical problems in the treatment of soft tissue sarcomas is the propensity of the primary tumor to recur locally. Soft tissue sarcomas enlarge in a centrifugal fashion and compress normal tissue so as to give the appearance of encapsulation. This pseudocapsule, however, is actually composed of an inner compressed rim of normal tissue (compression zone) and an outer rim of edema and small newly formed vessels (reactive zone) (see Fig. 2-2). Fingers of tumor can extend into and through this pseudocapsule and give rise to satellite lesions. While the pseudocapsule provides surgeons with a tempting plane for dissection and invites a shellout procedure, such an excision leaves microscopic and often gross tumor in the wound.[24] Excision of any sarcoma within the pseudocapsule is inadequate therapy and will result in the development of local recurrences in up to 90% of patients.

The site of a soft tissue sarcoma can certainly influence the technical ease with which resectability can be accomplished, and hence affects the potential for local control. For instance, lesions of the head and neck regions, where abutment to vital structures is often the case, are less likely to be controlled compared with lesions in the extremities. In the extremity, the site of the tumor may also have prognostic implications. Local control is more difficult to achieve for proximal tumors compared with those more di-

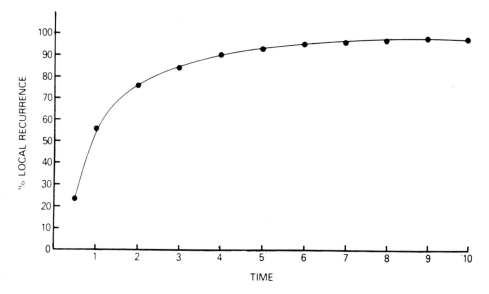

FIG. 2-6. Percentage of local recurrences versus time from definitive surgery for soft tissue sarcomas. (Adapted from Cantin J, McNeer GP, Chu FC, et al: The problem of local recurrence after treatment of soft tissue sarcoma. *Ann Surg* 168:47, 1968. Used with permission.)

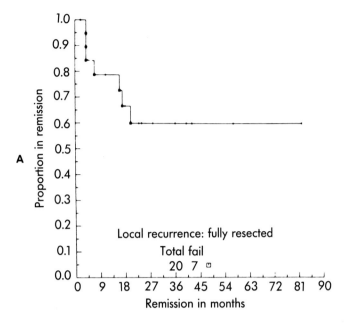

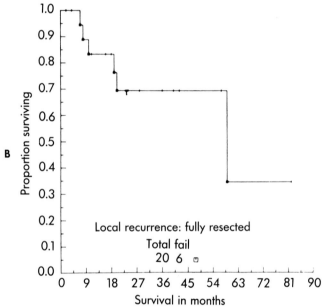

FIG. 2-7. Disease-free survival rates (**A**) and overall survival rates (**B**) in patients rendered free of disease after resection of isolated locally recurrent sarcoma. (From Potter DA, Glenn J, Kinsella T, et al: Patterns of recurrence in patients with high-grade soft-tissue sarcomas. *J Clin Oncol* 3:353, 1985. Used with permission.)

stally located, possibly because they achieve greater size before detection. Simon and Enneking[52] reported local recurrences following surgery alone in the buttock, groin, thigh, and areas below the knee to be 38%, 14%, 15%, and 0%, respectively. Potter et al.[43] reported that among 115 patients with thigh sarcomas, disease-free and overall survival rates were significantly worse for patients with tumor that had spread into the upper half of the thigh compared

with patients with tumor involvement limited to the distal thigh.

The time to local recurrence following surgery alone follows a predictable pattern. Approximately 80% of all lesions that are destined to recur locally will do so within 2 years (Fig. 2-6).[7] Simon and Enneking[52] reported that all of the local recurrences seen in 54 patients they treated surgically occurred within 30 months of resection. The impact of adjuvant therapy on local recurrences will be discussed subsequently.

Treatment of local recurrence. Isolated local recurrences of soft tissue sarcomas, regardless of site, should be considered for further resection. In one series of patients, 20 of 21 (96%) isolated local recurrences were surgically resectable.[42] A thorough evaluation for the presence of disseminated disease should be performed before resection of a local recurrence is contemplated. Fig. 2-7, *A*, shows the actuarial continuous disease-free survival rate for the 20 patients who underwent resection of isolated local recurrences: seven patients developed subsequent tumor recurrences. The median disease-free interval had not been reached. Fig. 2-7, *B*, shows the actuarial 3-year survival rate for these 20 patients, which was 69%. This encouraging rate of long-term survival after resection of isolated local recurrence has been documented by other investigators as well.[27]

Distant metastasis

Despite adequate local control of the primary tumor, many patients with high-grade and a few patients with low-grade soft tissue sarcomas will succumb to metastatic disease. Although most patients with soft tissue sarcomas present without obvious clinical metastases, many harbor occult micrometastases that eventually become clinically evident. These patients represent a population that could benefit from adjuvant systemic chemotherapy along with removal of the primary tumor (this topic is presented in more detail later).

As with local recurrence, the incidence and pattern of distant metastasis depends on the site of the primary sarcoma. Potter et al.[42] analyzed 307 patients who underwent complete resection of high-grade sarcomas followed with radiation therapy and chemotherapy. A total of 107 patients (35%) developed local recurrence or distant metastases and are listed in Table 2-4 according to site of the primary tumor. The predominant site of first recurrence was in the lung and occurred in 52% of patients who developed local or distant disease (75% of patients with primary tumors of an extremity). Patients with retroperitoneal sarcomas had a greater tendency for local recurrence and disseminated disease throughout the abdomen. Patients with head and neck and truncal sarcomas had a higher local recurrence rate than those with extremity sarcomas. Treatment options for patients with metastatic disease include surgical resection if

Table 2-4. Patterns of local recurrence and metastasis in patients with high-grade soft tissue sarcomas by site of primary tumor

Site of initial failure	Site of primary tumor					
	Extremity (%)	Breast (%)	Head and neck (%)	Trunk (%)	Retroperitoneum (%)	TOTAL (%)
Isolated local recurrence	7 (10)	0	2 (50)	7 (41)	5 (30)	21 (20)
Isolated lung metastases	43 (70)	3 (75)	2 (50)	5 (29)	3 (17)	56 (52)
Isolated other metastases	11 (15)	1 (25)	0	2 (12)	1 (6)	15 (14)
Multiple sites	4 (5)	0	0	3 (18)	8 (47)	15 (14)
TOTAL	65	4	4	17	17	107 (100)

From Potter DA, Glenn J, Kinsella T, et al: Patterns of recurrence in patients with high-grade soft-tissue sarcomas. *J Clin Oncol* 3:353, 1985.

the tumor is localized to one organ system or systemic cytotoxic chemotherapy if it is not. These treatment options are discussed in detail later in this chapter.

TREATMENT OF LOCALIZED TUMORS

Benign soft tissue tumors require only complete local excision for adequate treatment. By contrast, a variety of treatment approaches to localized primary and recurrent sarcomas have been reported, including surgery alone or in combination with radiation therapy or chemotherapy.

Treatment of extremity sarcomas

Surgical therapy. Surgery is the mainstay of any treatment approach for a clinically localized primary or recurrent soft tissue sarcoma. As has been described, however, removal of the gross tumor mass from within its pseudocapsule is associated with a prohibitively high likelihood of local recurrence. With the appreciation of the infiltrative nature of these tumors, radical procedures such as amputation came to be accepted as the standard for surgical therapy. Enneking has classified surgical procedures for sarcomas according to the margins that are achieved.[17] He describes four types of excisions:

1. *Intracapsular excisions* are performed inside the pseudocapsule and are often piecemeal in nature. An amputation that passes within the pseudocapsule is called an *intracapsular amputation*. The likelihood of local recurrence in this setting is virtually 100%.
2. *Marginal excisions* are en bloc excisions performed through the reactive zone (pseudocapsule) surrounding the tumor. Excisional biopsies and "shellout" procedures fall into this category. An amputation performed through this marginal zone is called a *marginal amputation*. Local recurrences are expected 60% to 80% of the time.
3. *Wide excisions* are en bloc excisions done through normal tissue beyond the reactive zone but within the muscular compartment of origin, leaving in place some portion of that compartment. The pseudocapsule is removed en bloc, and the tumor is never visualized during the procedure. Reported local recurrence

rates following wide excision without adjuvant therapy vary greatly depending on selection criteria and the adequacy of the margin as assessed histologically, but overall are approximately 30%. An amputation can be considered a *wide amputation* if it is performed through normal tissue proximal to the reactive zone but remains within the compartment of involvement.

4. *Radical excisions* are en bloc excisions of the tumor and the entire compartment of origin, leaving no remnant of the compartment intact. A radical amputation usually requires the disarticulation of the joint proximal to the involved compartment and results in the removal of the entire compartment at risk. Local recurrence rates are the lowest with these procedures and are discussed below.

The following types of surgical procedures are commonly employed when radical excision is chosen for the treatment of extremity soft tissue sarcomas:

Radical muscle compartment excisions. For those tumors that arise entirely within an anatomically defined muscular compartment, excision of the muscles comprising that compartment from origin to insertion is often successful in achieving local control. The thigh, which is the site of more than 50% of all extremity sarcomas, has three major compartments bounded by the fascia lata and its extensions. The anterior compartment includes primarily the quadriceps and sartorius muscles, which can be removed along with the femoral nerve. An anterior compartment excision results in knee weakness and instability, which can be improved with the use of the transplanted gracilis and short head of the biceps muscles. Even without such reconstruction, patients can ambulate after anterior compartment excision by using the hip flexors to throw the leg forward; gait is improved with the use of a locking knee brace. The medial thigh compartment consists of the gracilis, adductor minimus, adductor brevis, adductor longus, adductor magnus, and pectineus muscles. Medial compartment excision is generally well tolerated, with only limited functional deficit. Posterior compartment excision removes the hamstring muscles (semimembranosus and semitendinosus, and biceps femoris), as well as the posterior portion of the adductor magnus muscle. Ambulation is surprisingly well maintained after this surgery, with knee flexion brought about by the action of the gracilis and soleus muscles on the distal femur. Buttockectomy entails the removal of the entire gluteus maximus muscle, for tumors localized entirely within this muscle.

Radical amputations. Below-knee amputation is performed through the tibia and fibula and allows a stump to be used for fitting a prosthetic device. Rehabilitation from this procedure is usually very satisfactory. Below-knee amputation is the radical resection of choice for any soft tissue sarcoma of the foot. Above-knee amputation can be performed at any level distal to the lesser trochanter in order to allow enough stump for a prosthesis. This amputation does not constitute a radical excision for tumors occurring above the knee. Hip disarticulation entails the complete removal of the femur at the hip joint. Most muscles attached to the lower extremity are removed in their entirety. This procedure constitutes one option for radical excision for patients with lesions of the middle and lower thigh. Hemipelvectomy involves the removal of the entire lower extremity and hemipelvis, with disarticulation of the sacroiliac joint and pubic symphysis. This procedure is applicable for patients with proximal thigh and buttock tumors. The standard hemipelvectomy utilizes a posterior flap of skin and subcutaneous tissue overlying the buttock. For buttock and posterior thigh lesions, it is possible to construct an anterior myocutaneous flap based on the quadriceps muscles and superficial femoral artery to cover the surgical defect. Modified hemipelvectomy preserves the iliac wing, which allows improved patient rehabilitation. It is similar to the standard hemipelvectomy except the sacroiliac joint is preserved and the iliac bone is divided below the level of the sciatic notch. Because this involves transection of muscles in the buttock, it is not suitable for lesions in this area, but it does constitute a viable alternative to hip disarticulation for lesions of the mid-thigh. Internal hemipelvectomy is not generally employed for soft tissue tumors; it involves removal of the hemipelvis without amputation of the extremity, and can be useful in the management of bony tumors of the hemipelvis.

For tumors of the hand and wrist, below-elbow amputation is often used. Above-elbow amputation is used for tumors of the forearm. Shoulder disarticulation is reserved for distal arm and elbow lesions. Forequarter amputation (interscapulothoracic amputation) is applied to the treatment of lesions of the shoulder girdle, as well as the proximal arm. This procedure includes removal of the entire upper extremity along with the scapula and clavicle. Detailed descriptions of all these procedures are provided in atlases devoted to soft tissue tumor surgery.[29,34,59]

The means required to achieve a radical excision depend in part on the anatomical location of the tumor and its size. Many tumors of the extremities are not located within distinct anatomical compartments, and hence a radical excision cannot be achieved save by amputation. Similarly, large tumors that are localized to one compartment but also abut bone or major neurovascular structures cannot be radically excised without amputation. A radical excision, however, is *not* required for all sarcomas. With the use of adjuvant radiation therapy, local control rates with nonradical resections have improved to match those achievable with radical surgery. Currently, wide excision is the procedure of choice for low-grade sarcomas, or higher-grade tumors that will be treated with multimodality therapy. Marginal excision is frequently all that can be achieved in the treatment of retroperitoneal and head and neck sarcomas; intracapsular excision is not generally performed except for the occasional low-grade tumor for which any other type of excision would provide an unacceptable loss of function. Adjuvant radiation should almost always be considered when tumors must be treated with marginal or intracapsular excisions.

The experiences of Simon and Enneking[52] and Shiu et al.[50] using radical surgical procedures as single modality therapy are summarized in Table 2-5. Overall local control was obtained in approximately 80% of patients undergoing radical resection, regardless of whether or not amputation was performed. Unfortunately, even a "radical" excision is

Table 2-5. Local control and amputation rates in patients with soft tissue sarcomas of the extremity treated with radical surgery as the sole modality of therapy

	Simon and Enneking[52]	Shiu et al.[50]
Total number of patients	54	297
Radical compartment excision	25 (46%)	158 (53%)
Radical amputation	29 (54%)	139 (47%)
Percentage with local control		
Radical compartment excision	88%	72%
Radical amputation	79%	93%
Overall	83%	82%

Table 2-6. Local failure rates after radical excision with histologically negative versus positive margins

	Number of local failures per total number of patients	
Author	Negative margins	Positive margins
Simon and Enneking[52]	1/46	8/8
Markhede et al.[36]	5/76	16/19
TOTAL (%)	6/122 (5)	24/27 (89)

not always associated with an adequate margin when the resected specimen is examined histologically. When histological evaluation verified that adequate margins were obtained with the radical procedure, the local failure rate was 5% (Table 2-6). If, however, microscopic tumor was found at or within 1 mm of the surgical margin, the local failure rate rose to 89%. Inadequate margins were most commonly associated with large proximal thigh and groin tumors. With more distal extremity lesions there is rarely tumor remaining at or close to the surgical margin after appropriate radical excision, and the local control rate can be expected to approach 100% after radical amputation of these sarcomas.[39,42]

Although radical excisions that achieve a histologically negative margin are associated with high rates of local tumor control, the functional, psychological, and cosmetic costs can be high.[56] For this reason, radical surgery as single modality therapy has gradually been replaced by more conservative resection performed as part of multidisciplinary, multimodality treatment approaches. Nowhere is this trend more evident than in the treatment of extremity soft tissue sarcomas with multimodality limb-sparing therapy.

Limb-sparing procedures. Rosenberg et al. compared radical amputation to wide local excision plus postoperative radiation in a prospective, randomized trial. Patients who underwent limb-sparing surgery had a survival rate identical to those undergoing amputation, despite a slightly higher local recurrence rate (19% versus 6%, a difference that is not statistically significant).[47] This study demonstrated the merit of limb-sparing approaches to extremity sarcomas. Radical amputation is currently reserved for patients who are not suitable candidates for limb-sparing approaches, usually because of abutment of the tumor to bone or major neurovascular structures or very large tumor size.

Most current limb-salvaging protocols include wide excision as the definitive surgical procedure. Wide excision involves gross total removal of the tumor with a wide margin of normal tissue, but no attempt is made to resect an entire muscle compartment. Rather, a margin of 3 to 5 cm of normal tissue is obtained proximally and distally. This includes excision of some overlying skin to include all previous scars or areas of biopsy. Tumor should not be visualized during the surgical excision in order not to spill tumor cells into the surgical bed. On the lateral and deep margins, at least one grossly uninvolved fascial plane is resected en bloc with the tumor. For large or deep-seated tumors, resection of uninvolved periosteum or adventitia may represent the deep margin. If necessary, major vascular structures may be resected and reconstructed with graft material. On occasion, major nerves such as the sciatic nerve are sacrificed in order to preserve a functional albeit neurologically compromised extremity. Because of their less aggressive nature, when low-grade lesions are resected,

major vessels or nerves are not taken along with the tumor. Placement of titanium clips outlining the limits of the excision is essential as a guide to the radiation therapist in constructing the radiation treatment portal. Suction catheters are placed at the end of the dissection to allow evacuation of any blood and serous fluid from the operative bed and facilitate the adherence of skin flaps.

The use of multimodality therapy—particularly preoperative treatment—is associated with a high incidence of wound complications. These complications can be disastrous in an irradiated wound or if major vessels, nerves, or bone become exposed. To minimize the likelihood of wound breakdown, consideration should always be given to reconstruction of the surgical defect with free or pedicled myocutaneous flaps. Barwick et al.[5] have articulated the criteria for primary closure of a wide excision wound in patients undergoing multimodality therapy: the skin edges should be approximated without tensions, and the resection site must not have exposed bone, nerve, blood vessel, or tendon present. If the skin edges cannot be approximated without tension but the base of the resection is entirely muscle, then a split-thickness skin graft should be applied. Otherwise, a flap reconstruction is performed. Irradiated wounds in the trunk and retroperitoneum may present a formidable technical challenge to the reconstructive surgeon.[32]

Radiation therapy. For patients with small, superficial, or low-grade tumors, wide local excision alone is associated with a very low rate of local recurrence.[49] Most other patients undergoing surgical excision receive additional therapy to improve the chances for local control. In the majority of cases, this additional therapy includes radiation. Radiation has been shown to be effective as the sole therapy for extremity sarcomas in patients who refused or could not tolerate surgery. Of 26 patients treated with radiation alone (dose level of 65 Gy; 100 rad = 1 Gy), a local control rate of 61% was achieved at 4 years.[62] Although treatment with radiation alone was not as successful as treatment with radical surgery, success rates were high enough to suggest that radiation therapy should definitely be included in multimodality treatment approaches.

Postoperative radiation therapy. Postoperative radiation therapy after wide surgical excision provides excellent local control rates for primary extremity sarcomas up to 10 cm in size. The randomized trial of amputation versus wide local excision previously cited validated the concept of limb-sparing surgery combined with postoperative radiation. Generally, a dosage of 60 Gy or greater is required to ensure local control. At these dosages, the entire circumference of the extremity must not be irradiated, or massive lymphedema will result. In practice, a strip of skin and subcutaneous tissue away from the tumor is excluded from the treatment field to prevent this complication.

Postoperative radiation can also be delivered to the tumor

Table 2-7. Local control rates 5 years after wide excision with postoperative versus preoperative external beam radiation

Tumor size (cm)	Postoperative radiation		Preoperative radiation	
	No. of patients	% locally controlled	No. of patients	% locally controlled
<2.5	14	82	5	100
2.6-4.9	45	85	9	89
5.0-10.0	29	84	32	91
10.1-15.0	8	83	17	100
15.1-20.0	5	0	9	73
>20.0	1	0	6	100
TOTAL	102	80	78	92

Note: Allocation to therapy was by physician choice, not randomization.

From Suit HD, Mankin HJ, Wood WC, et al: Treatment of the patient with stage M_0 soft tissue sarcoma. *J Clin Oncol* 6:854, 1988.

Table 2-8. Local recurrence rates, disease-free survival rates, and functional result for extremity sarcoma patients after preoperative radiation followed by wide or marginal excision compared with stage-matched patients undergoing amputation or wide or marginal excision without radiation

Type of treatment	No. of patients	Local recurrence (%)	Disease-free survival (%)	Satisfactory function (%)
Amputation	16	2 (13)	11 (69)	2 (13)
Wide or marginal excision	19	7 (37)*	7 (37)	13 (68)
Preoperative radiation therapy plus excision	19	1 (5)	11 (58)	12 (63)

From Enneking WF, McAuliffe JA: Adjunctive preoperative radiation therapy in treatment of soft tissue sarcomas: a preliminary report. *Cancer Treat Symp* 3:37, 1985.

*$P < 0.05$ compared with preoperative radiation therapy plus excision; not significantly different from amputation group.

bed by means of implanted radioactive sources, a technique referred to as *brachytherapy*. This approach has the advantage of a much shorter time to initiation and completion of therapy (usually begun within a week of operation and completed in 4 or 5 days, as compared with 6 to 7 weeks of external beam radiation beginning a month or more postoperatively). On the other hand, brachytherapy is technically complex and requires the presence of an experienced radiation oncologist in the operating room. A randomized trial demonstrated a significant decrease in local recurrences for high-grade sarcomas after combined surgery and postoperative brachytherapy compared with surgery alone.[51] Patients with low-grade sarcomas did not benefit from adjuvant brachytherapy, although a recent retrospective review suggested that external beam radiation is effective in decreasing local recurrence in these tumors.[35] Otherwise, brachytherapy and external beam radiation appear to be equally effective when properly administered. The data from these studies provide strong support for the routine inclusion of radiation therapy (by some technique) in all patients with high-grade, and most patients with low-grade, extremity sarcomas undergoing limb-sparing surgery.

Preoperative radiation therapy. Preoperative radiation therapy followed by conservative surgery offers several theoretical advantages. The treatment volume is restricted to known or probable extension of tumor. This means that a smaller volume can be treated than is the case with postoperative radiation, since the latter must cover all tissues manipulated or handled during the surgical procedure. The resection may be of a lesser magnitude if regression of tumor is obtained with preoperative radiation. Seeding of the surgical bed with viable tumor cells may be reduced. Several centers have used this approach; local control rates for large tumors appear to be improved with preoperative treatment (Table 2-7), and in some cases tumors initially considered unresectable without amputation shrank sufficiently to permit limb-sparing resection.[60]

Enneking and McAuliffe[19] have reported their experience with preoperative radiation followed by wide or marginal resection of low- and high-grade extremity sarcomas. They compared their results with matched controls who had similarly staged tumors and underwent either a limb-sparing or amputation procedure without preoperative radiation (Table 2-8). Local recurrence rates were highest in the group undergoing limb-sparing surgery alone (37%) and were significantly higher than in the group undergoing preoperative radiation plus surgery (5%). In the same series, patients undergoing limb-sparing procedures had substantially better

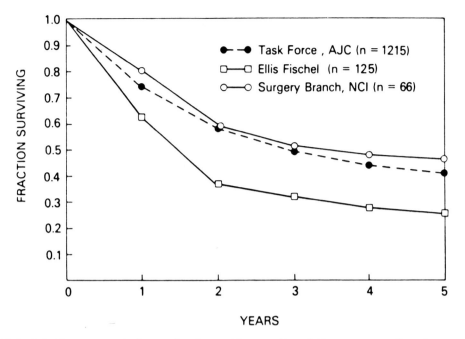

FIG. 2-8. Five-year survival rate of patients with extremity soft tissue sarcomas from three reported series. (From Rosenberg SA, Suit HD, Baker LH: Sarcomas of soft tissues. In DeVita VT, Hellman S, Rosenberg SA, editors: *Cancer: principles and practice of oncology,* ed 2, Philadelphia, 1985, JB Lippincott. Used with permission.)

postoperative function than those undergoing amputation. The use of preoperative treatment for large sarcomas of the extremities has increased the number of patients who can be considered for limb-sparing surgery.

Adjuvant chemotherapy. Although multimodality treatments achieve local control without amputation in a high percentage of patients with intermediate- and high-grade soft tissue sarcomas, metastatic disease ultimately develops in 50% of patients in most reported series (Fig. 2-8). This figure is even higher if stage IIIB tumors are considered. For this reason, the use of effective systemic adjuvant chemotherapy would be desirable following definitive treatment of local disease. To date, however, there is no conclusive evidence that administration of adjuvant chemotherapy to patients with extremity sarcomas can increase overall survival rates. Several prospective, randomized, controlled trials—as well as numerous retrospective studies—examining the role of adjuvant chemotherapy in sarcoma patients have been reported. A variety of factors limit the extent to which definitive conclusions can be drawn from these studies, including (1) the relatively small numbers of patients enrolled in each study, and hence the diminished significance of the statistical data; (2) the variety of eligibility criteria used, particularly in regard to tumor size, grade, and primary site; (3) the differing and often relatively ineffectual chemotherapeutic regimens employed; and (4) variations among study pathologists in the histopathological grading of the tumors.[65]

Retrospective reviews employing historical controls are difficult to interpret because of the selection factors used; this has been amply demonstrated in adjuvant studies of osteosarcoma patients.[61] Although some authors have cited a benefit from adjuvant therapy, many have not. On occasion, subsequent updates of patients from the same institution where initially favorable results were reported have shown a lack of overall effect. In any case, virtually all these retrospective series are sufficiently flawed that only prospective, randomized, controlled trials can be looked upon to provide information regarding the effectiveness of adjuvant chemotherapy. To date, all the randomized trials conducted in this area have used postoperative chemotherapy, administered after the performance of and successful recovery from amputation or wide excision (generally along with radiation).

Doxorubicin is the most commonly used cytotoxic drug for the management of metastatic sarcoma. Consequently, this agent has undergone extensive evaluation as single-agent adjuvant chemotherapy for resected soft tissue sarcomas. Randomized trials, however, demonstrate that adjuvant doxorubicin does not improve overall survival rates compared with surgery alone.[16] A randomized controlled trial of multiagent chemotherapy (doxorubicin, cyclophosphamide, and methotrexate) after surgery showed improved disease-free survival rates for patients with high-grade extremity sarcomas (but not those of the trunk or retroperitoneum).[46] Toxicity of this regimen proved substantial.

Symptomatic cardiac toxicity developed in 14% of patients, and many asymptomatic patients demonstrated decreased cardiac function on noninvasive testing. A subsequent study comparing this regimen with one having a lower dosage of doxorubicin (to limit cardiotoxicity) suggested that the less toxic program was as effective as the higher-dosage regimen.[9]

Despite the favorable findings from these two trials, other studies of adjuvant multidrug chemotherapy in soft tissue sarcomas have failed to demonstrate any improvement in overall survival rates. A recent metaanalysis of existing randomized trials pooled the available data to minimize the limitations imposed by sample size in any one study. These data suggest that adjuvant chemotherapy does lessen the likelihood of death and disease recurrence in patients with high-grade extremity sarcomas.[65] Whether the benefit is sufficient to justify the significant toxicity of adjuvant chemotherapy remains to be determined.

Increasingly, preoperative chemotherapy regimens are being employed in patients with extremity sarcomas.[15] This approach has become the treatment of choice for most patients with osteosarcomas of the extremity[38] but has yet to be established as superior to conventional therapy in soft tissue tumors. The use of preoperative chemotherapy has been termed *neoadjuvant chemotherapy;* this has been used alone or with preoperative radiation therapy. One of the main theoretical advantages of neoadjuvant chemotherapy is that the effectiveness of the drug regimen can be assessed by monitoring the clinical response and evaluating the degree of necrosis of the primary tumor at the time of resection.[8,41] As yet, however, there is no proof that patients whose primary tumor responds to the preoperative regimen are protected from developing metastases, or that patients whose tumor fails to respond should be switched to alternate therapy postoperatively. Given the numerous remaining questions regarding both preoperative and postoperative adjuvant chemotherapy, patients with high-grade extremity sarcomas should be enrolled in an established clinical trial whenever possible.

Treatment of nonextremity sarcomas

Unlike sarcomas of the extremities, lesions that arise in the head and neck, thoracic or abdominal wall, mediastinum, or retroperitoneum are rarely amenable to true "radical" resection. Furthermore, many of these tumors are situated in areas where nearby normal tissues impose limitations on the dosage of radiation that may be delivered to the tumor or tumor bed. Because of these factors, multimodality therapy approaches have in general been less successful for sarcomas in these sites than for sarcomas of the extremities. Local recurrences are more common, and—particularly for retroperitoneal tumors—often lead to the demise of the patient before disseminated metastases become evident. Given the current state of the art, improve-

ments in techniques for achieving local control of nonextremity tumors offers promise for greater increases in patient survival rates than is the case with primary tumors of the extremities.

General principles of evaluation and management of nonextremity sarcomas parallel those for extremity tumors. Long delays before diagnosis and initiation of therapy can only be avoided by maintaining a high index of suspicion and promptly performing a biopsy for any new, persistent, or enlarging soft tissue mass. Fine-needle and core-needle biopsies play a somewhat greater role, especially for relatively inaccessible sites such as the peritoneum. There is no situation in which definitive surgical therapy should be carried out without a precise diagnosis based on analysis of tissue, and frozen-section examination should rarely be relied upon to provide a definitive diagnosis. Particularly with tumors of the thoracic wall and those abutting or involving major bony structures (e.g., the vertebrae or the pelvic bones), the possibility that the tumor is actually a primary bone sarcoma or a metastasis from a carcinoma located elsewhere should always be kept in mind; this will avoid the pitfall of applying radical surgical resection to lesions best treated in another fashion. Characteristic features of soft tissue sarcomas at various sites other than the extremities are given below.

Sarcomas of the head and neck. Approximately 8% to 10% of all soft tissue sarcomas are located in the head and neck region (Table 2-1). In the soft tissues of the neck, it may at times be possible to obtain wide or radical margins by procedures similar to those employed for neck dissection, but sarcomas arising in the region of the mandible, maxilla, and base of the skull may prove extremely challenging (Fig. 2-9). Farr reported on 285 patients with soft tissue sarcomas of the head and neck with an absolute 5-year survival rate of 32%.[21] This was a diverse group of patients who received different forms of therapy over an extended period of time. A more recent review from the same institution focused on 176 adult patients treated between 1950 and 1985, and followed for a minimum of 2 years.[20] In this cohort, the 5-year survival rate was 55%, with 40% of patients alive at 10 years. Patients with high-grade tumors, however, had a 10-year survival rate of only 20%. Univariate analysis of prognostic factors identified tumor size of 5 cm or larger, positive margins, bone involvement, and high histological grade to be significantly associated with decreased survival rates. In the absence of multivariate analysis, it is impossible to know to what extent these adverse features are independent prognostic factors (e.g., large size, positive margins, and bone involvement were all far more common in high-grade than low-grade tumors in this series).

Sarcomas of the body wall. Sarcomas of the thoracic or abdominal wall constitute approximately 15% of all soft tissue sarcomas. These lesions can usually be adequately en-

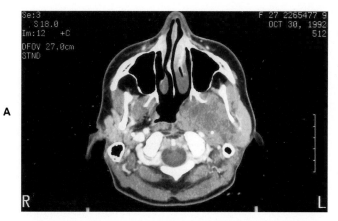

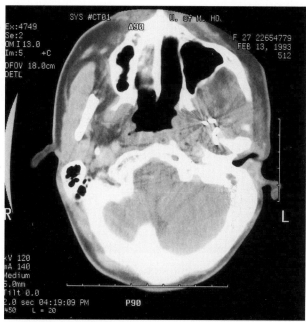

FIG. 2-9. (A) CT scan demonstrating a large high-grade fibrosarcoma involving the left mandible, infratemporal fossa, and masticator space. In order to facilitate resection, the patient was treated with preoperative external beam radiation along with the radiation sensitizer iododeoxyuridine. **(B)** Appearance after resection and reconstruction with bone grafts.

compassed by a wide full-thickness excision in order to achieve negative margins. Abdominal wall defects can be reconstructed in straightforward fashion with the use of a mesh prosthesis. Significant portions of the bony thorax can be resected without compromising respiratory function, even though nonrigid prosthetic materials are used. Very extensive defects of the thoracic cage will require a rigid reconstruction, generally employing a shaped prosthesis formed of methylmethacrylate cement between two pieces of polypropylene mesh.[40] Reconstruction of most chest wall and some large abdominal wall defects also requires coverage with myocutaneous flaps, which have better blood supply compared with standard skin flaps or split-thickness grafts and are associated with fewer wound complications even if postoperative radiotherapy is required.

Sarcomas of the retroperitoneum. Retroperitoneal sarcomas are perhaps the most difficult sarcomas to manage.[55,58] These tumors do not come to the attention of the patient until they are very large; retroperitoneal sarcomas under 5 cm are rarely seen.[57] Even massive tumors may present with only minimal symptoms (Fig. 2-10). Most retroperitoneal sarcomas are liposarcomas, leiomyosarcomas, or malignant fibrous histiocytomas[14,58] and may weigh several kilograms at the time of excision. Clinical evaluation of these tumors should include CT scan of the abdominal wall and chest; magnetic resonance imaging is helpful if the extent of vascular involvement requires definition, and may replace the need for arteriography and vena cavography.

The surgical approach to these tumors requires exploration through a transperitoneal approach, using either a midline or bilateral subcostal incision. Experience has shown

that retroperitoneal approaches via the flank, as are often used for nephrectomy, do not allow adequate visualization to perform safe resection.[57] The approach to resection of retroperitoneal sarcomas has been nicely outlined by Storm and Mahvi[58] and is shown in Fig. 2-11. The initial maneuver is to establish a plane of dissection of the tumor from major intraabdominal vascular structures. Subsequently, a retroperitoneal plane is established to allow complete tumor removal. When resecting a retroperitoneal sarcoma, it is nearly impossible to achieve the type of wide or radical margins that would be considered standard in the excision of an extremity tumor. Nonetheless, gross total resection of all visible tumor should be the goal of any surgical procedure, even if it involves resection of other intraabdominal structures. Incomplete resection or "debulking" of a retroperitoneal tumor is not associated with improved long-term survival rates compared with biopsy only with subsequent nonsurgical treatment.[37,58] Unfortunately, even with aggressive surgical approaches and a willingness to resect adjacent organs, only 50% to 60% of retroperitoneal sarcomas are amenable to complete excision.[14,28] With completely resected tumors, the major determinant of overall survival rates is the histological grade of the tumor (Fig. 2-12).[58] Unlike extremity sarcomas, where tumor-related deaths are rare in patients with low-grade tumors, only 42% of patients with completely resected low-grade retroperitoneal sarcomas were alive at 10 years. For patients with high-grade tumors, the prognosis is far worse: 24% were alive at 5 years and only 11% at 10 years despite complete tumor resection.

Local recurrence, with or without distant disease, is extremely common after surgical therapy of retroperitoneal

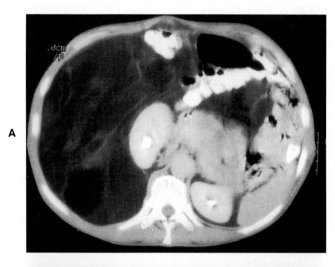

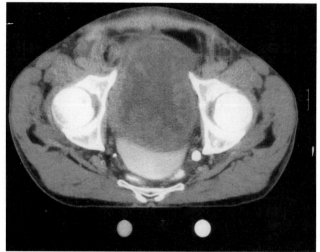

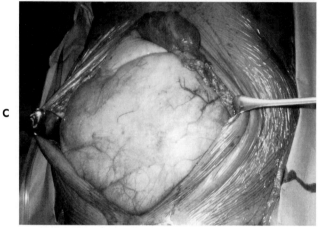

FIG. 2-10. (A-B) CT scans demonstrating massive retroperitoneal liposarcoma, which presented as an otherwise asymptomatic increase in abdominal girth. The tumor consisted predominantly of low-grade elements (A), but a 20-cm region of high-grade dedifferentiated liposarcoma was also present (B). (C) Appearance of the abdomen at laparotomy for tumor resection, showing the fatty tumor virtually filling the abdomen. Fifteen years previously, the patient had undergone a cholecystectomy and was told that he had "excessive fat" in the right retroperitoneum; no biopsy was obtained at that time.

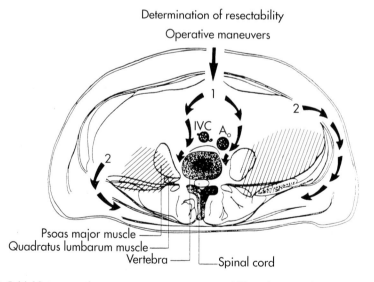

FIG. 2-11. Initial intraoperative maneuvers to assess resectability of retroperitoneal sarcomas (represented by cross-hatched regions). (1) A plane of dissection between the tumor and the major vascular structures is established. (2) A retroperitoneal plane is established to evaluate areas adjacent to the spinal foramina and allow resection of the tumor. (From Storm FK, Mahvi DM: Diagnosis and management of retroperitoneal soft-tissue sarcoma. *Ann Surg* 214:2, 1991. Used with permission.)

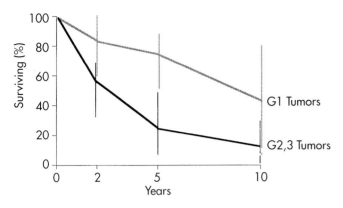

FIG. 2-12. Overall survival by tumor grade for completely resected retroperitoneal sarcomas, based on cumulative data from published series. In all, 49 low-grade (G1) and 80 high-grade (G2,3) sarcomas were included in this analysis. The range of valves reported in the individual series from which these data were derived is indicated by the vertical bars. (Modified from Storm FK, Mahvi DM: Diagnosis and management of retroperitoneal soft-tissue sarcoma. *Ann Surg* 214:2, 1991. Used with permission.)

sarcomas (Table 2-4). A randomized study was performed to investigate the effectiveness of intraoperative radiotherapy in decreasing local recurrence rates. Thirty-five patients were randomly chosen to receive either postoperative external beam radiotherapy (50 to 55 Gy) or intraoperative radiotherapy (20 Gy in a single dose delivered immediately after removal of the tumor) plus lower-dose postoperative external beam radiotherapy (35 to 40 Gy). All patients had large intermediate- or high-grade tumors, and were randomly chosen after exploration revealed no evidence of metastases and determined that the tumor was resectable. Overall survival rates were virtually identical between the two groups (median survival 52 months for external beam radiation only versus 45 months for intraoperative radiotherapy, an insignificant difference). After a median follow-up of 8 years, 26 of 35 patients had experienced disease recurrence, 16 of 20 patients in the external beam radiation group, all with local recurrence, and 10 of 15 patients in the intraoperative radiotherapy group. Only 6 of the 15 patients who received intraoperative radiotherapy had local recurrence, however, indicating that the intensive radiotherapy was able to sterilize residual tumor cells within the treatment field in some cases.[53] The logistic difficulties, expense, and toxicity of intraoperative radiotherapy are clearly not justified, given the minimal overall benefit. This trial clearly articulates the unsatisfactory results that are currently achieved with aggressive surgical resection and intraoperative or postoperative radiation in patients with retroperitoneal sarcomas.

Glenn et al. further explored the use of multimodality therapy with radiation and chemotherapy for retroperitoneal sarcomas.[26] Thirty-seven patients with completely resected high-grade retroperitoneal tumors went on to receive post-

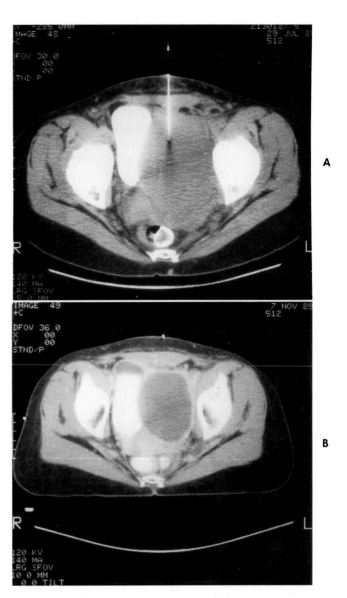

FIG. 2-13. (A) CT scan demonstrating a large high-grade pelvic malignant fibrous histiocytoma, considered unresectable because of involvement of the pelvic sidewall. (B) CT scan of the same patient after preoperative treatment with 62.5 Gy external beam radiation along with iododeoxyuridine. The tumor is significantly smaller, more homogenous, and has regressed away from the pelvic sidewall sufficiently to permit resection. The resected specimen was composed entirely of nonviable tumor tissue (100% necrosis after preoperative treatment). (From Sondak VK, Economou JS, Eilber FR: Soft tissue sarcomas of the extremity and retroperitoneum: advances in management. *Adv Surg* 24:333, 1991. Used with permission.)

operative adjuvant therapy. All 37 patients received postoperative radiotherapy (21 received chemotherapy, 16 did not). The actuarial 3-year survival rate was 43%, and it did not appear to be affected by chemotherapy. Both the radiation therapy and chemotherapy were poorly tolerated and associated with significant long-term toxicity in these patients, who were recovering from major operative procedures.

Recently, attention has turned to preoperative multimodality approaches for treatment of retroperitoneal sarcomas. Both cytotoxic chemotherapy[11] and radiation sensitizers[45,55] have been successfully administered along with external beam radiation prior to resection. Preoperative therapy is advantageous because it is administered when the patient is most able to withstand the rigors of therapy, and it also may cause the tumor to decrease in size, so that resection may be less extensive or a previously unresectable tumor may after all be resected (Fig. 2-13).

Adjuvant therapy for nonextremity sarcomas. Because nonextremity sarcomas rarely are amenable to resection with the wide or radical margins that are achievable in an extremity, radiation is employed after surgery in most cases. As with extremity tumors, there are clearly some cases in which postoperative radiation is not mandatory: low-grade tumors that are completely excised with histologically negative margins may be observed without adjuvant treatment, provided that any subsequent recurrence would again be amenable to excision. Most authorities advocate radiation therapy after resection of low-grade sarcomas with close or positive margins, and after resection of

any intermediate- or high-grade tumors. Some others, however, have reported good results with surgery alone for small and superficial high-grade tumors removed with wide margins.[30,49] Few randomized trials have been conducted to address this issue. For intermediate- and high-grade retroperitoneal sarcomas, a randomized trial of postoperative external beam radiation versus combined intraoperative and low-dosage postoperative external beam radiation showed no difference in overall survival rates, and local and regional failure was frequent in both groups.[53] A randomized trial of adjuvant radiation therapy delivered as brachytherapy included both extremity and body wall sarcomas but excluded retroperitoneal, mediastinal, and head and neck primary tumors. This trial demonstrated a significant reduction in local recurrence rates, but no difference in overall survival rates, for patients treated with brachytherapy.[51] The beneficial effect of brachytherapy was confined to the subset of patients with higher-grade tumors.

The efficacy of adjuvant chemotherapy for patients with nonextremity sarcomas has not been established to date. Results of a trial examining its efficacy in patients with soft tissue sarcomas of the head and neck, breast, and trunk wall, all of whom went on to receive postoperative radiotherapy, have been published.[25] Adjuvant chemotherapy

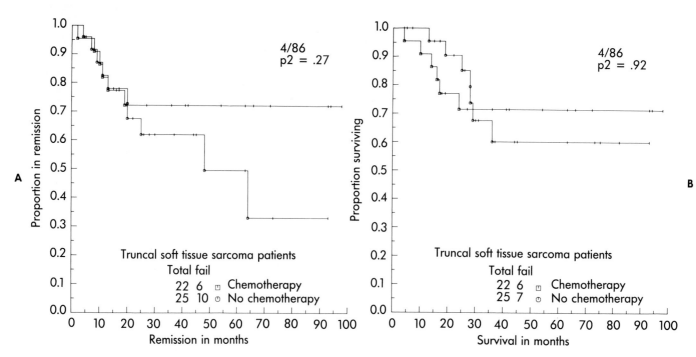

FIG. 2-14. Disease-free survival rates (**A**) and overall survival rates (**B**) in patients entered into a randomized trial of adjuvant chemotherapy versus observation after resection of high-grade truncal, breast, or head and neck sarcomas. After a median follow-up of 5 years, there are no significant differences between the two groups. (From Glenn J, Kinsella T, Glatstein E, et al: A randomized prospective trial of adjuvant chemotherapy in adults with soft tissue sarcomas of the head and neck, breast, and trunk. *Cancer* 55:1206, 1985. Used with permission.)

consisted of doxorubicin, cyclophosphamide, and methotrexate. The 3-year actuarial disease-free survival rate in the chemotherapy group was 72%, compared with 60% in the group without chemotherapy, and the 3-year overall survival rates were 71% and 60%, respectively (Fig. 2-14). The differences in these figures are statistically insignificant (P values of 0.27 and 0.92, respectively). Most other randomized trials of adjuvant chemotherapy have not distinguished patients with nonextremity sarcomas from those with extremity tumors. A review of all randomized trial data involving nonextremity tumors concluded that there was no evidence that adjuvant chemotherapy significantly improved overall survival rates.[16] Although single-institution nonrandomized trials have suggested benefit for adjuvant chemotherapy, its routine use in these patients cannot currently be supported, particularly in view of the substantial risk of significant long-term toxicity.

TREATMENT OF METASTATIC DISEASE
Surgical treatment

The sites of initial tumor recurrence in 307 patients after primary treatment of a soft tissue sarcoma were reviewed.[42] Primary therapy in these patients consisted of complete surgical resection, often in combination with postoperative chemotherapy and radiation therapy. A total of 107 patients (35%) had local recurrence or developed distant metastases at the sites identified in Table 2-4; the lung was the predominant site of disease in 52% of patients. Isolated local recurrences were the second most common, seen 20% of the time. As indicated earlier, the pattern of recurrence was dependent on the site of the primary sarcoma. Patients with sarcomas of the head and neck, retroperitoneum, and chest or abdominal wall had a higher local recurrence rate compared with those with tumors of the extremities. Approximately 80% of all local recurrences and disseminated metastases became evident within 5 years.

Removal of clinically normal lymph nodes generally has no role in the treatment of soft tissue sarcomas; dissection of tumor-containing lymph nodes, as proven on biopsy, should be performed if no other metastatic disease is evident. Radical lymphadenectomy for patients with nodal involvement in the absence of metastasis elsewhere was associated with a 34% 5-year survival rate, fully justifying an aggressive surgical approach in these patients.[22]

As is the case for patients with isolated local or regional recurrences, aggressive surgical treatment of pulmonary metastases should be attempted when technically feasible. Patients who are found to have pulmonary metastases by plain radiograph or CT scan of the chest should have a thorough evaluation for extrapulmonary tumor, particularly in the primary site, to determine whether operation is feasible. For sarcomas of the extremities and trunk, this can be accomplished by physical examination and CT scan or magnetic resonance imaging of the primary site, as well as a bone scan. For patients with retroperitoneal sarcomas, CT scan of the liver should be performed to exclude metastases there. Patients with extrapulmonary tumor are not considered candidates for curative resection of pulmonary metastases. The patient's pulmonary function should also be evaluated to ensure that the patient can tolerate a thoracotomy and will have adequate ventilatory reserve after resection. In one representative series, 40 of 56 patients (72%) with isolated pulmonary metastases were rendered disease-free with surgery, with an actuarial 3-year survival rate of 38%.[42] Several studies evaluating factors that might be significant in predicting outcome from pulmonary metastasectomy have been reported.[44] Univariate analyses have generally identified the number of metastatic nodules seen on preoperative CT scans (under 3 or 4 is considered most favorable), the disease-free interval prior to appearance of the lung nodules, and the tumor doubling time (more than 40 days is considered most favorable) as being correlated with length of postoperative survival. It should be noted that no single criterion appears sufficiently accurate to exclude any individual patient from resection; even patients with several unfavorable factors occasionally are long-term survivors. Overall 5-year survival rates range from 10% to 35% in most reported series. In osteosarcoma metastatic to the lung, adjuvant systemic chemotherapy after pulmonary resection appears to convey additional benefit[54]; whether this will prove relevant to soft tissue sarcomas remains to be determined.

Chemotherapeutic treatment

Systemic cytotoxic chemotherapy is generally not considered curative for patients with metastatic soft tissue sarcomas. Osteogenic sarcomas, Ewing's sarcomas, and childhood rhabdomyosarcomas all are associated with much higher response rates to chemotherapy. Nonetheless, for adult soft tissue sarcoma patients without a curative surgical option, chemotherapy represents the best currently available palliative treatment. Objective tumor regression and relief of symptoms can be achieved in a significant fraction of patients, with acceptable levels of toxicity. Cytotoxic drugs that are or have been commonly employed in the treatment of metastatic sarcomas include doxorubicin, cyclophosphamide, ifosfamide, methotrexate, vincristine, cisplatin, dactinomycin, and dacarbazine. Of these, doxorubicin and ifosfamide appear to have the highest degree of activity when administered as single agents. Most often, combination regimens are employed: the combination of doxorubicin and ifosfamide, with or without dacarbazine, appears to be particularly active (Fig. 2-15).

A multiinstitutional cooperative group study of 340 patients with metastatic soft tissue sarcoma compared response rates and survival times following treatment with doxorubicin and dacarbazine alone or combined with ifosfamide and mesna (a uroprotective agent used to minimize

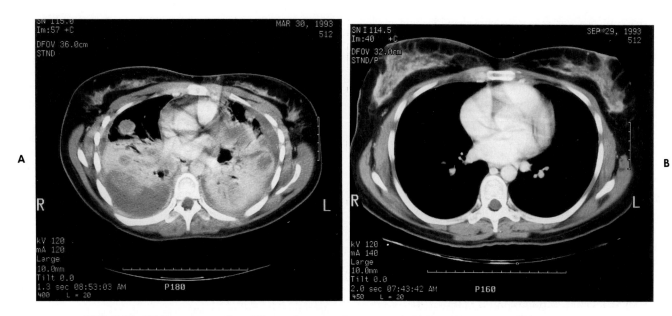

FIG. 2-15. (A) Pretreatment chest CT scan demonstrating metastatic high-grade sarcoma with associated malignant pleural effusion. **(B)** A CT scan obtained after 6 months of treatment with doxorubicin and ifosfamide shows complete resolution of the effusion, and virtually complete disappearance of the pulmonary parenchymal nodules. This response lasted 9 months and was associated with excellent palliation of the patient's symptoms of shortness of breath. (Courtesy Dean Brenner, M.D., Section of Hematology/Oncology, University of Michigan.)

the incidence of ifosfamide-induced hemorrhagic cystitis). The addition of ifosfamide increased the response rate significantly (32% versus 17% for doxorubicin plus dacarbazine). Toxicity was also greater, and overall survival rates did not differ significantly based on treatment.[2] The authors suggested ifosfamide be included in the initial therapy for patients receiving preoperative "induction" chemotherapy and for younger patients better able to tolerate the toxicity. For older patients, and those whose original tumor was of low or intermediate histological grade, they recommended the sequential use of doxorubicin and dacarbazine followed by ifosfamide upon progression.

Patients who achieve a partial response to chemotherapy but are left with one or several potentially resectable metastases should be considered for surgical excision. Conversion of a chemotherapy-induced partial response to a complete response can enhance the duration of response and is associated with a survival time equivalent to that obtained with complete response to chemotherapy alone. Similarly, the occasional patient with one or several metastatic lesions not amenable to resection can be treated effectively with localized radiation to consolidate the response to chemotherapy. To date, immunotherapeutic approaches, including monoclonal antibodies, cytokines, and adoptive cellular therapies, have demonstrated no efficacy in the management of metastatic sarcoma.

The clinical evaluation and treatment of patients with soft tissue sarcomas remains a challenge. Over the past 2 decades, aggressive treatment approaches by experienced multidisciplinary oncology teams have improved the outlook for these patients. The feasibility and appropriateness of limb-sparing therapies for patients with high-grade extremity sarcomas, many of whom would have been treated by amputation in the past, are now firmly established. The multidisciplinary team should include surgeons, radiation oncologists, medical oncologists, pathologists, radiologists, rehabilitation therapists, oncology nurses, and social workers. The contribution of the pathologist—and the need for a thorough and detailed enumeration of the histological features of the tumor relevant to therapy—cannot be overstressed. Because of the relatively low incidence of these tumors, patients with soft tissue sarcomas should generally be referred to medical centers with experience in sarcoma management. Nonetheless, it remains for every practicing physician to be aware of soft tissue sarcomas and their behavior, so that patients with soft tissue masses can be promptly and appropriately evaluated, a diagnosis made, and optimal therapy initiated.

REFERENCES

1. Abbas JS, Holyoke ED, Moore R, et al: The surgical treatment and outcome of soft-tissue sarcoma. *Arch Surg* 116:765, 1981.

2. Antman K, Crowley J, Balcerzak SP, et al: An intergroup phase III randomized study of doxorubicin and dacarbazine with or without ifosfamide and mesna in advanced soft tissue and bone sarcomas. *J Clin Oncol* 11:1276, 1993.

3. Ball AB, Fisher C, Pittam M, et al: Diagnosis of soft tissue tumours by Tru-cut biopsy. *Br J Surg* 77:756, 1990.

4. Barth RJ, Merino MJ, Solomon D, et al: A prospective study of the value of core needle biopsy and fine needle aspiration in the diagnosis of soft tissue masses. *Surgery* 112:536, 1992.

5. Barwick WJ, Goldberg JA, Scully SP, et al: Vascularized tissue transfer for closure of irradiated wounds after soft tissue sarcoma resection. *Ann Surg* 216:591, 1992.

6. Bland KI, McCoy DM, Kinard RE, et al: Application of magnetic resonance imaging and computed tomography as an adjunct to the surgical management of soft tissue sarcomas. *Ann Surg* 205:473, 1987.

7. Cantin J, McNeer GP, Chu FC, et al: The problem of local recurrence after treatment of soft tissue sarcoma. *Ann Surg* 168:47, 1968.

8. Casper ES, Gaynor JJ, Harrison LB, et al: Preoperative and postoperative adjuvant chemotherapy for adults with high grade soft tissue sarcoma. *Cancer* 73:1644, 1994.

9. Chang AE, Kinsella T, Glatstein E, et al: Adjuvant chemotherapy for patients with high-grade soft-tissue sarcomas of the extremity. *J Clin Oncol* 6:1491, 1988.

10. Chang AE, Matory YL, Dwyer AJ, et al: Magnetic resonance imaging versus computed tomography in the evaluation of soft tissue tumors of the extremities. *Ann Surg* 205:340, 1987.

11. Chawla SP, Rosen G, Eilber F, et al: Cisplatin and Adriamycin as neoadjuvant and adjuvant chemotherapy in the management of soft tissue sarcomas. In Salmon SE, editor: *Adjuvant therapy of cancer VI,* Philadelphia, 1990, WB Saunders.

12. Collin C, Friedrich C, Godbold J, et al: Prognostic factors for local recurrence and survival in patients with localized extremity soft-tissue sarcoma. *Semin Surg Oncol* 4:30, 1988.

13. Costa J, Wesley RA, Glatstein E, et al: The grading of soft tissue sarcomas. *Cancer* 53:530, 1984.

14. Dalton RR, Donohue JH, Mucha PJ Jr, et al: Management of retroperitoneal sarcomas. *Surgery* 106:725, 1989.

15. Eilber FR, Eckardt JJ, Rosen G, et al: Neoadjuvant chemotherapy and radiotherapy in the multidisciplinary management of soft tissue sarcomas of the extremity. *Surg Oncol Clin North Am* 2:611, 1993.

16. Elias AD, Antman KH: Adjuvant chemotherapy for soft-tissue sarcoma: a critical appraisal. *Semin Surg Oncol* 4:59, 1988.

17. Enneking WF: Staging of musculoskeletal neoplasms. In *Current concepts of diagnosis and treatment of bone and soft tissue tumors,* Heidelberg, 1984, Springer-Verlag.

18. Enneking WF, Chew FS, Springfield DS, et al: The role of radionuclide bone-scanning in determining the resectability of soft-tissue sarcomas. *J Bone Joint Surg* 63A:249, 1981.

19. Enneking WF, McAuliffe JA: Adjunctive preoperative radiation therapy in treatment of soft tissue sarcomas: a preliminary report. *Cancer Treat Symp* 3:37, 1985.

20. Farhood AI, Hajdu SI, Shiu MH, et al: Soft tissue sarcomas of the head and neck in adults. *Am J Surg* 160:365, 1990.

21. Farr HW: Soft part sarcomas of the head and neck. *Semin Oncol* 8:185, 1981.

22. Fong Y, Coit DG, Woodruff JM, et al: Lymph node metastasis from soft tissue sarcoma in adults: analysis of data from a prospective database of 1772 sarcoma patients. *Ann Surg* 217:72, 1993.

23. Geer RJ, Woodruff J, Casper ES, et al: Management of small soft-tissue sarcoma of the extremity in adults. *Arch Surg* 127:1285, 1992.

24. Giuliano AE, Eilber FR: The rationale for planned reoperation after unplanned total excision of soft-tissue sarcomas. *J Clin Oncol* 3:1344, 1985.

25. Glenn J, Kinsella T, Glatstein E, et al: A randomized prospective trial of adjuvant chemotherapy in adults with soft tissue sarcomas of the head and neck, breast, and trunk. *Cancer* 55:1206, 1985.

26. Glenn J, Sindelar WF, Kinsella T, et al: Results of multimodality therapy of resectable soft-tissue sarcomas of the retroperitoneum. *Surgery* 97:316, 1985.

27. Huth J, Eilber FR: Patterns of metastatic spread following resection of extremity soft-tissue sarcomas and strategies for treatment. *Semin Surg Oncol* 4:20, 1988.

28. Jaques DP, Coit DG, Hajdu SI, et al: Management of primary and recurrent soft-tissue sarcoma of the retroperitoneum. *Ann Surg* 212:51, 1990.

29. Karakousis CP: *Atlas of operations for soft tissue tumors,* New York, 1985, McGraw-Hill.

30. Karakousis CP, Emrich LJ, Rao U, et al: Selective combination of modalities in soft tissue sarcomas: limb salvage and survival. *Semin Surg Oncol* 4:78, 1988.

31. Kransdorf MJ, Jelinek JS, Moser RP: Imaging of soft tissue tumors. *Radiol Clin North Am* 31:359, 1993.

32. Ladin D, Rees R, Wilkins E, et al: The use of omental transposition in the treatment of recurrent sarcoma of the back. *Ann Plast Surg* 31:556, 1993.

33. Lawrence W Jr, Donegan WL, Natarajan N, et al: Adult soft tissue sarcomas: a pattern of care survey of the American College of Surgeons. *Ann Surg* 205:349, 1987.

34. Lawrence W, Neifeld JP, Terz JJ: *Manual of soft-tissue surgery,* New York, 1983, Springer-Verlag.

35. Marcus SG, Merino MJ, Glatstein E, et al: Long-term outcome in 87 patients with low-grade soft tissue sarcoma. *Arch Surg* 128:1336, 1993.

36. Markhede G, Angervall L, Stener B: A multivariate analysis of the prognosis after surgical treatment of malignant soft-tissue tumors. *Cancer* 49:1721, 1982.

37. McGrath PC, Neifeld JP, Lawrence W Jr, et al: Improved survival following complete excision of retroperitoneal sarcomas. *Ann Surg* 200:200, 1984.

38. Myers PA, Heller G, Healey J, et al: Chemotherapy for nonmetastatic osteogenic sarcoma: the Memorial Sloan-Kettering experience. *J Clin Oncol* 10:5, 1992.

39. Owens JC, Shiu MH, Smith R, et al: Soft tissue sarcomas of the hand and foot. *Cancer* 55:2010, 1985.

40. Perry RR, Venzon D, Roth JA, et al: Survival after surgical resection for high-grade chest wall sarcomas. *Ann Thorac Surg* 49:363, 1990.

41. Pezzi CM, Pollock RE, Evans HL, et al: Preoperative chemotherapy for soft-tissue sarcomas of the extremities. *Ann Surg* 211:476, 1990.

42. Potter DA, Glenn J, Kinsella T, et al: Patterns of recurrence in patients with high grade soft-tissue sarcomas. *J Clin Oncol* 3:353, 1985.

43. Potter DA, Kinsella T, Glatstein E, et al: High-grade soft tissue sarcomas of the extremities. *Cancer* 58:190, 1986.

44. Putnam JB Jr, Roth JA: Resection of sarcomatous pulmonary metastases. *Surg Oncol Clin North Am* 2:673, 1993.

45. Robertson JM, Sondak VK, Weiss SA, et al: Preoperative radiation therapy and iododeoxyuridine for large retroperitoneal sarcomas. *Int J Radiat Oncol Biol Phys* (in press).

46. Rosenberg SA, Tepper J, Glatstein E, et al: Prospective randomized evaluation of adjuvant chemotherapy in adults with soft tissue sarcomas of the extremities. *Cancer* 52:424, 1983.

47. Rosenberg SA, Tepper J, Glatstein E, et al: The treatment of soft-

tissue sarcomas of the extremities: prospective randomized evaluations of (1) limb-sparing surgery plus radiation therapy compared with amputation and (2) the role of adjuvant chemotherapy. *Ann Surg* 196:305, 1982.

48. Russell WO, Cohen J, Enzinger FM, et al: A clinical pathological staging system for soft tissue sarcomas. *Cancer* 40:1562, 1977.

49. Rydholm A, Gustafson P, Rööser B, et al: Limb-sparing surgery without radiotherapy based on the anatomic location of soft tissue sarcoma. *J Clin Oncol* 9:1757, 1991.

50. Shiu MH, Castro EB, Hajdu SI, et al: Surgical treatment of 297 soft tissue sarcomas of the lower extremity. *Ann Surg* 182:597, 1975.

51. Shiu MH, Hilaris BS, Harrison LB, et al: Brachytherapy and function-saving resection of soft tissue sarcoma arising in the limb. *Int J Radiat Oncol Biol Phys* 21:1485, 1991.

52. Simon MA, Enneking WF: The management of soft-tissue sarcomas of the extremities. *J Bone Joint Surg* 58A:317, 1976.

53. Sindelar WF, Kinsella TJ, Chen PW, et al: Intraoperative radiotherapy in retroperitoneal sarcomas: final results of a prospective, randomized, clinical trial. *Arch Surg* 128:402, 1993.

54. Skinner KA, Eilber FR, Holmes EC, et al: Surgical treatment and chemotherapy for pulmonary metastases from osteosarcoma. *Arch Surg* 127:1065, 1992.

55. Sondak VK, Economou JS, Eilber FR: Soft tissue sarcomas of the extremity and retroperitoneum: advances in management. *Adv Surg* 24:333, 1991.

56. Sondak VK, Leonard JA Jr, Robertson JM, et al: Limb-sparing surgery for extremity soft tissue sarcomas: functional and rehabilitation considerations. *Surg Oncol Clin North Am* 2:657, 1993.

57. Storm FK, Eilber FR, Mirra J, et al: Retroperitoneal sarcomas: a reappraisal of treatment. *J Surg Oncol* 17:1, 1981.

58. Storm FK, Mahvi DM: Diagnosis and management of retroperitoneal soft-tissue sarcoma. *Ann Surg* 214:2, 1991.

59. Sugarbaker PH, Nicholson TH: *Atlas of extremity sarcoma surgery*, Philadelphia, 1984, JB Lippincott.

60. Suit HD, Mankin HJ, Wood WC, et al: Treatment of the patient with stage M_0 soft tissue sarcoma. *J Clin Oncol* 6:854, 1988.

61. Taylor WF, Ivins JC, Pritchard DJ, et al: Trends and variability in survival among patients with osteosarcomas: a 7-year update. *Mayo Clin Proc* 60:91, 1985.

62. Tepper JE, Suit HD: Radiation therapy of soft tissue sarcomas. *Cancer* 55:2273, 1985.

63. Torosian MH, Friedrich C, Godbold J, et al: Soft tissue sarcomas: initial characteristics and prognostic factors in patients with and without metastatic disease. *Semin Surg Oncol* 4:13, 1988.

64. Weingrad DW, Rosenberg SA: Early lymphatic spread of osteogenic and soft-tissue sarcomas. *Surgery* 84:231, 1978.

65. Zalupski MM, Ryan JR, Hussein ME, et al: Systemic adjuvant chemotherapy for soft tissue sarcomas of the extremities. *Surg Oncol Clin North Am* 2:621, 1993.

CHAPTER 3

RICHARD P. MOSER, JR., JOHN E. MADEWELL

RADIOLOGIC EVALUATION OF SOFT TISSUE TUMORS

Soft tissue tumors are a large diverse group of pathological entities. Typically, the clinical findings associated with these tumors are disappointingly nonspecific. The patient frequently detects a soft tissue mass that may exhibit either slow or rapid growth, with coexistent pain as an inconstant finding. Examples include glomus tumors, leiomyomas, and lipomas. Infrequently, the clinical findings are highly suggestive of the specific nature of the tumor, as when an infant with a large arteriovenous malformation (Fig. 3-1) presents with congestive heart failure, or a patient with hyperpigmented cutaneous lesions presents with subcutaneous or deep-seated neurofibromas (Fig. 3-2) or, rarely, neurofibrosarcoma.

Predictably, the radiologic patterns manifested by soft tissue tumors are also diverse and frequently nonspecific. Exceptions are infrequent but include fatty tumors (Fig. 3-3)[*] and hemangiomatous neoplasms (Fig. 3-4).[†] Imaging studies for assessment of soft tissue tumors consist primarily of the triad of (1) conventional radiography, (2) magnetic resonance imaging, and (3) CT scanning. Less commonly, sonography or angiography are used. These imaging modalities play a major role in detecting, localizing, and determining the extent of the tumor. The two latter aspects are the primary functions of radiologic imaging of soft tissue tumors because they drastically affect the patient's surgical management.

Soft tissue tumors are usually round or oval in shape, although they are occasionally elliptical or even exhibit a dumbbell shape. They vary widely in size and may arise in the skin, subcutis, muscle, or other deep soft tissues. Superficial lesions of the skin are best assessed by clinical inspection and palpation. Masses arising in the subcutaneous and deeper soft tissues should be evaluated by radiologic studies, which can detect calcification, ossification, or radiolucency within the lesion and can determine the extent

of the mass, including involvement of adjacent bones, joints, neurovascular structures, or other soft tissues. The challenge to the radiologist is (1) to suggest an appropriate sequencing of radiologic studies that permits timely and accurate evaluation of the tumor while simultaneously minimizing expense and discomfort to the patient, and (2) to suggest an appropriate differential diagnosis. Unfortunately, radiologic features cannot reliably distinguish between benign and malignant soft tissue tumors.

SOFT TISSUE VERSUS BONY ORIGIN OF THE SOFT TISSUE MASS

Modern imaging modalities can usually easily determine whether the mass arises from the skeleton (marrow or cortex) or within the adjacent soft tissues (Fig. 3-5). The relationship between the soft tissue tumor and adjacent structures can be illustrated by several patterns (Fig. 3-6). First, the soft tissue mass may be completely separated from the adjacent bone by a noninvolved soft tissue plane. Furthermore, the margin of any soft tissue mass may be characterized as either sharp or ill defined (Fig. 3-7). Occasionally, the soft tissue mass barely touches or contacts the outer surface of the adjacent bone (Fig. 3-6), thereby creating an acute angle between the mass and the bone (Fig. 3-8). In the third situation, the mass directly affects the bone; this takes many forms, varying from extrinsic bony erosion to a periosteal reaction. Depending on the location of the soft tissue tumor, one or more bones can be affected. The area of extrinsic erosion of bone by the soft tissue mass may have sharp, well-defined margins which may be round or scalloped in contour (Fig. 3-9) and which may or may not exhibit sclerosis. Conversely, there may be an ill-defined interface between the soft tissue mass and the affected bone (Fig. 3-6), sometimes with ill-defined bony erosions (Fig. 3-10) or complete cortical destruction with associated extension of the tumor into the bone marrow (Fig. 3-11).

Soft tissue origin of the lesion should be suspected when multiple bones are eroded (Fig. 3-6). These bones are typ-

---

*References 3, 9, 18, 31, 50, 59, 62, 76, 81, 95, 98, 113, 138.
†References 16, 17, 23, 24, 35, 67, 73, 87, 92, 102, 106, 117, 124, 125.

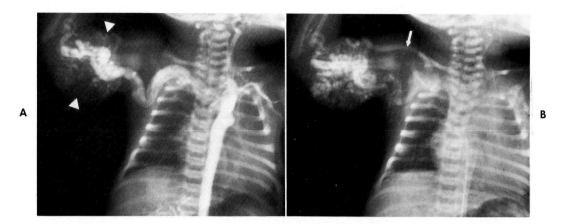

FIG. 3-1. An infant with an arteriovenous malformation presents with congestive heart failure. **A,** Aortogram demonstrates a massively hypertrophied feeding right subclavian artery. The subclavian artery is approximately equal in diameter to the descending thoracic aorta. The soft tissue mass *(arrowheads)* in the right arm is composed of tortuous vessels, seen to better advantage following contrast filling **(B)**; also note the large early draining vein *(arrow).*

ically adjacent to each other, with the tumor surrounding them or insinuated between them (Figs. 3-12 and 3-13). Predictably, this situation is encountered most frequently in the ribs, radius and ulna, carpals, metacarpals, tibia and fibula, tarsals, and metatarsals. An analogous situation exists when a soft tissue mass arises within or adjacent to a joint and secondarily erodes or invades the bony structures of the joint (Figs. 3-12 to 3-14).

The bone adjacent to a soft tissue mass may demonstrate periosteal new bone formation, with or without direct tumor invasion, characterized by indolent solid cortical thickening (Fig. 3-6) or more aggressive interrupted periosteal reaction (Figs. 3-6, 3-7, 3-14, and 3-15). Periosteal reactions are most commonly encountered in association with hypervascular soft tissue neoplasms. Both benign and malignant vascular soft tissue tumors may produce such periosteal reactions. The solid reaction is more typical of benign tumors, particularly hemangiomas. The interrupted reaction is more commonly noted in association with malignant soft tissue tumors.

These patterns (Fig. 3-6) are typical manifestations of soft tissue tumors restricted to soft tissue or secondarily affecting adjacent bone. In determining whether a lesion is primary in soft tissue or primary within bone, it can usually be assumed that the site of the most extensive abnormality represents the origin of the process. Comparison of plain radiographs with cross-sectional imaging studies such as CT scans, magnetic resonance images, and sonograms can usually localize the lesion primarily to soft tissue or bone, thereby resolving the dilemma of "inside out" (i.e., the situation in which the tumor arises in the bone and secondarily invades the adjacent soft tissues) or "outside in" (i.e., the situation in which the tumor arises in the soft tissues and secondarily invades the adjacent bone).

Bone tumors may be completely or partially contained within the affected bone. When radiologically detectable bone destruction occurs, the first indication of the presence of a bone tumor is endosteal cortical erosion. Eventually this can progress to complete cortical destruction with periosteal elevation and reaction and frank invasion of the adjacent soft tissues. The soft tissue mass associated with a primary skeletal neoplasm (inside out) has its epicenter within the affected bone, just the opposite of the situation that exists for a primary soft tissue tumor that subsequently affects the adjacent bone (outside in). In this latter situation (soft tissue tumor affecting bone), the epicenter of the soft tissue mass is outside of the bony structure (Fig. 3-16). Also, the outer cortical surface (rather than the inner endosteal surface) is eroded first by tumors of soft tissue origin. On extremely rare occasions, aggressive neoplasms such as Ewing's sarcoma, poorly differentiated chondrosarcoma, or leukemia may infiltrate through the microscopic haversian canals of cortical bone into the adjacent periosteal structures and present as a lesion of suspected soft tissue origin due to the absence of radiographically demonstrable cortical destruction. Because of the exquisite sensitivity of magnetic resonance scanning for detecting bone marrow involvement, however, the surgeon should rarely be mistaken as to the epicenter of the disease process.

RADIOLOGIC CRITERIA FOR BENIGN AND MALIGNANT SOFT TISSUE TUMORS

Imaging features that distinguish benign from malignant soft tissue tumors have been discussed extensively. There are numerous ways to radiologically characterize a soft tissue tumor such as size, shape, rate of growth, location, number of tumors, radiodensity, evidence of osseous involvement, and interface with adjacent soft tissues.[130,150]

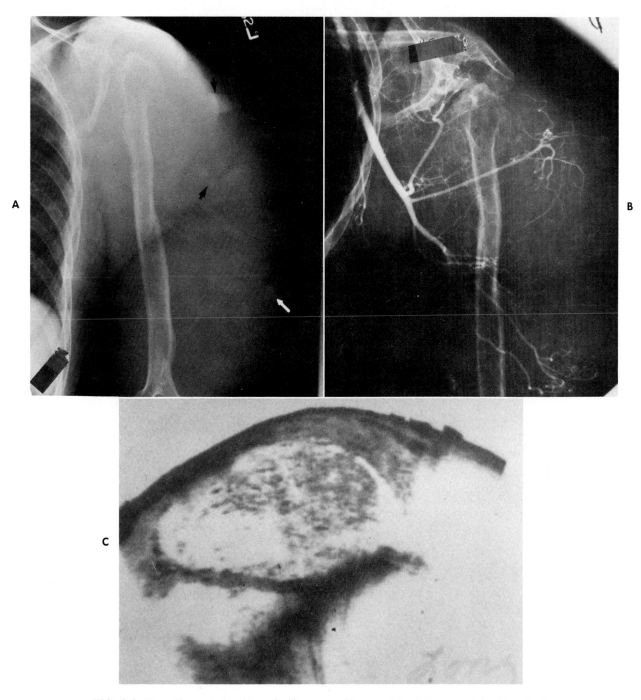

FIG. 3-2. Neurofibromatosis with a plexiform neurofibroma of the left arm and shoulder. **A,** On the radiograph, the large soft tissue neurofibroma causes secondary scalloping and cortical irregularity of the adjacent humerus. The shoulder joint is largely destroyed. Multiple smaller cutaneous neurofibromas are noted *(arrows).* **B,** Angiogram demonstrates displaced vessels and hypervascularity. **C,** Longitudinal sonogram demonstrates a sharply marginated, echogenic mass.

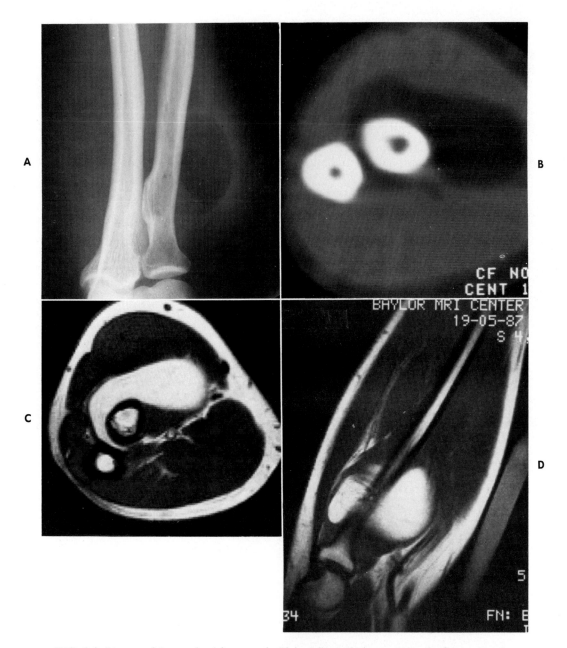

FIG. 3-3. Lipoma of the proximal forearm. **A,** Plain radiograph demonstrates the fatty nature (radiolucency) and sharp margins of the lipoma, adjacent to the proximal radius. **B,** The fatty nature of the tumor is readily apparent on CT scanning as a region of decreased attenuation (i.e., the attenuation of the lipoma is less than that of adjacent muscle) that partly envelops the radius. On the CT scan, the exact extent of the tumor is uncertain. **C,** Axial magnetic resonance scan at the same level as the CT scan (**B**) shows the excellent soft tissue contrast of magnetic resonance imaging and extension of the lipoma around the radius with insinuation between the radius and ulna. The bright or high-signal intensity of the lipoma on this T1-weighted image (TR-534ms TE-34ms) is typical of fatty tissue. **D,** Coronal T1-weighted magnetic resonance scan reveals to better advantage the three-dimensional nature of the lipoma, its sharp margins, and its significant encirclement of the radius. The radial cortex, which is black (due to absence of signal or signal void within the bony cortex) on the magnetic resonance scan, is intact and easily identified because of the contrasting high signal from the marrow fat within the bone.

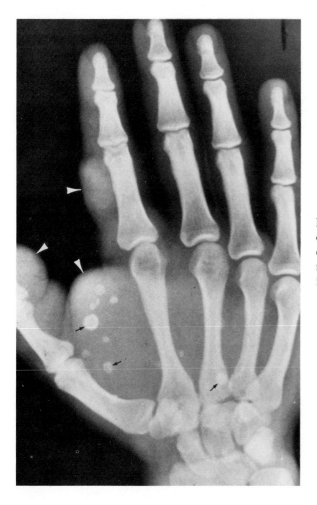

FIG. 3-4. Hemangioma with calcified phleboliths. The hemangioma causes extensive soft tissue swelling *(arrowheads)* with increased density involving the thumb, the index finger, and the thenar region. Multiple small calcified phleboliths are seen in a typical configuration of spherical rings *(small arrows).*

Unfortunately, none of these features is pathognomonic for benign or malignant tumors, but it is possible to characterize the "classic" benign soft tissue tumor and the "typical" malignant soft tissue tumor. This is helpful in preoperative staging and in alerting the treating physician, usually the surgeon, to the fact that the tumor has "predominantly" benign or malignant radiologic features. This will also affect the management of the neoplasm.

The margin or interface of the tumor with the uninvolved adjacent soft tissues may be either sharply demarcated or ill defined. Benign tumors are "usually" sharply circumscribed, whereas malignant tumors "usually" have an ill-defined interface. An important caveat must be added, however: both benign and malignant tumors may on occasion exhibit either sharp or ill-defined margins. Therefore, analysis of the margin of the soft tissue tumor is not absolute in determining the benign versus malignant status of the tumor. In fact, a sharp margin is not uncommon in malignant soft tissue tumors, and the inexperienced surgeon might inadvertently merely "shell out" the tumor when more extensive surgery is required. Understandably, merely "shelling out" the tumor is inadequate surgery for malig-

nant disease since this procedure leaves behind residual tumor, thereby increasing the likelihood of recurrence. Inflammatory and posttraumatic conditions within the soft tissues can also produce either sharp or ill-defined demarcation and, on occasion, can be confused with soft tissue tumors.

The tumor's size can vary significantly and is usually of minimal help in distinguishing benign from malignant soft tissue tumors. Ironically, some of the largest tumors recorded in the earlier literature were benign fatty tumors weighing as much or more than the patient.[3,28] The shape of the soft tissue tumor has no prognostic value in distinguishing benign from malignant tumors. The rate of growth of the tumor is an important feature to monitor (both clinically and radiologically) since benign tumors tend to either grow slowly or remain totally quiescent, whereas malignant tumors may grow rapidly (Fig. 3-15). Documentation of stable size for many years as opposed to progressive enlargement (either clinically or radiologically) can also be helpful. Stable size or very slow enlargement (Fig. 3-13, *C* and *D*) suggests a slowly growing, usually benign lesion, whereas rapid growth implies that the tumor is ma-

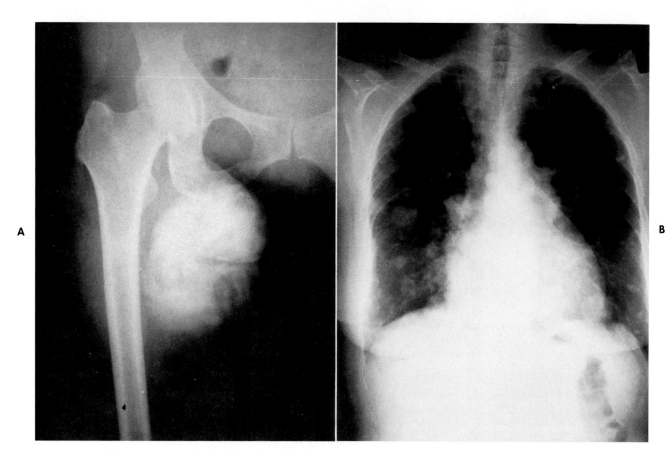

A   B

FIG. 3-5. Extraskeletal osteosarcoma of the thigh with several suspected skeletal metastases and extensive metastases to the chest. **A,** Frontal radiograph shows a large, densely calcified mass (diameter, 13 cm) in the medial soft tissues of the right thigh. **B,** Posteroanterior chest radiograph demonstrates diffuse bilateral pulmonary metastases of varying sizes. These metastases are disproportionately distributed adjacent to the heart. **C,** Methylene diphosphonate scintigram demonstrates marked radionuclide accumulation in the soft tissue lesion in the thigh and diffuse uptake in the chest. Based exclusively on the scintigram, it is impossible to localize precisely the sites of the lesions of the chest (e.g., pulmonary parenchymal, pericardial, or osseous). Also noted were three foci of increased radionuclide uptake in the proximal end of the right femur and right hemipelvis. Only two of these foci are apparent on this image. The third focus was near the right sacroiliac joint and was readily apparent on the posterior image. **D,** Axial CT scan with bone window demonstrates a large, sharply demarcated, densely but inhomogeneously calcified mass in the medial soft tissue of the right thigh. On all CT scan cuts, although the medial border of the mass is in close anatomical proximity to the adjacent femoral cortex, there was a distinct separation between the mineralized soft tissue mass and the femur. Overall, there was more extensive mineralization in the center of the soft tissue mass. **E,** Axial magnetic resonance scan (2500/30) demonstrates a large, sharply demarcated, inhomogeneous, soft tissue mass in the medial thigh. An interesting nodular pattern is noted within the lesion. **F,** Coronal magnetic resonance scan (600/30) also demonstrates inhomogeneous signal throughout the sharply demarcated soft tissue mass in the medial soft tissues of the right thigh. This case clearly demonstrates that malignant soft tissue masses can exhibit sharply demarcated margins on magnetic resonance scans.

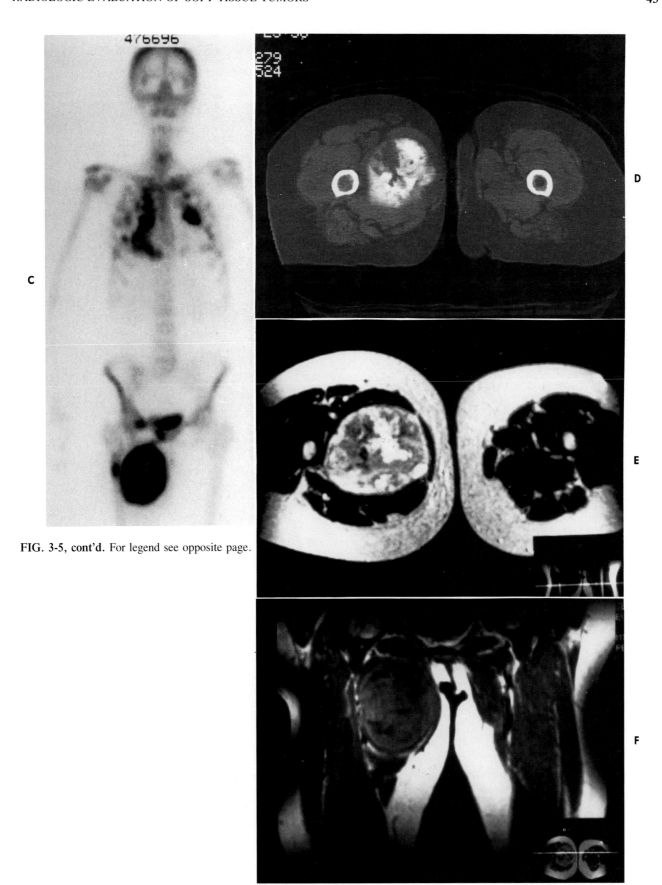

FIG. 3-5, cont'd. For legend see opposite page.

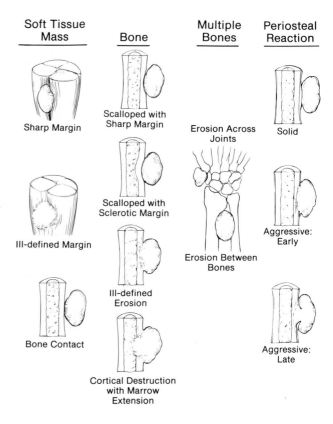

Soft Tissue Mass

Sharp Margin

Ill-defined Margin

Bone Contact

Bone

Scalloped with Sharp Margin

Scalloped with Sclerotic Margin

Ill-defined Erosion

Cortical Destruction with Marrow Extension

Multiple Bones

Erosion Across Joints

Erosion Between Bones

Periosteal Reaction

Solid

Aggressive: Early

Aggressive: Late

FIG. 3-6. Drawing illustrates the radiologic patterns of soft tissue tumors.

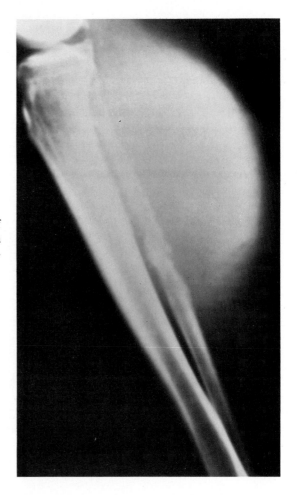

FIG. 3-7. Soft tissue leiomyosarcoma of the calf. The margins of the lesion are ill defined, especially distally. The leiomyosarcoma is invading the adjacent fibula, causing bony destruction and irregular periosteal reaction.

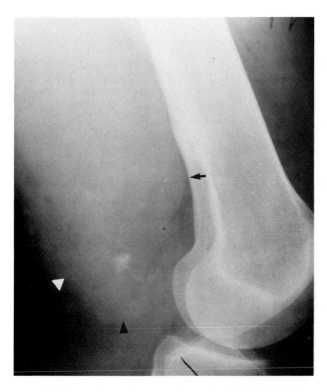

FIG. 3-8. Synovial sarcoma of the distal thigh in contact with the posterior femur. The contact point demonstrates an acute angle *(arrow)* between the tumor and the adjacent femur. Also of note, the mass has an ill-defined distal margin *(arrowheads),* and several small calcifications are noted within the tumor.

lignant (Fig. 3-15). Unfortunately, rapid growth is not completely specific for malignant tumors since benign tumors, with or without associated hemorrhage or infection within them, may occasionally demonstrate rapid enlargement.

The location of the soft tissue tumor can help in the proposed differential diagnosis. For instance, nodular synovitis (giant cell tumor of tendon sheath) and superficial fibromatoses predominate in the soft tissues of the hands and feet. Xanthomatosis usually affects the tendons about the elbows, hands, and heels. Synovial sarcomas frequently involve the soft tissues of the thigh and lower extremities near the knee but usually do not involve the joint. Also, non-neoplastic soft tissue masses (which could be confused with soft tissue tumors) occur in predictable locations. For example, popliteal cysts (Baker's cysts)[53,85,86,116] are characteristically located in the posterior aspect of the knee joint and exhibit a typical sonolucent pattern on sonography. However, there is such wide variation in the location of soft tissue tumors that location by itself is usually of little help in distinguishing benign from malignant tumors. The trite saying "it must be taken out to be spelled out" remains applicable.

Benign and malignant soft tissue tumors are most commonly solitary, but both can be multiple. Multiple benign lesions are more common and include fibromas, lipomas, hemangiomas, glomus tumors, xanthomas, myxomas, and neurofibromas. Multiple malignant lesions are less frequent and include soft tissue metastases, Kaposi's sarcoma, and angiosarcoma. The detection of multiple lesions is helpful in preoperative staging of the tumor since it is important for the surgeon, when planning the type of operation, to appreciate the extent of the disease. Unfortunately, by itself, multiplicity does not indicate whether the soft tissue lesion is benign or malignant.

The radiodensity of a soft tissue mass provides important clues to the preoperative diagnosis. The spectrum of radiodensity ranges from radiolucency to water (unit) density to radiopacity. Radiolucency is consistent with fat tissue (Figs. 3-17 and 3-18)[*] and sometimes myxomatous tissue. Rarely, air may be seen in the soft tissues, allowing the specific diagnosis of abscess (Fig. 3-19) (in the absence of a history of recent penetrating trauma). Water or unit density is nonspecific and typical of the vast majority of soft tissue tumors. Radiopacity can be due to calcification, chondrification, or ossification within the soft tissue tumor, depending on the specific radiologic pattern. These patterns of radiopacity, best demonstrated on plain radiographs, are important since they may allow a specific preoperative diagnosis. An example is the formation of phleboliths (Fig. 3-4), which is quite specific and may be detected in hemangiomas or occasionally in angiolipomas or hibernomas (Fig. 3-20). Mature chondroid matrix production[122] appears on plain radiographs as radiodense "rings" and curvilinear "arcs" (Fig. 3-21). This signifies that at least a portion of the soft tissue tumor is undergoing chondroid formation and

---

*References 3, 9, 31, 50, 59, 62, 95, 98.

Text continued on p. 54.

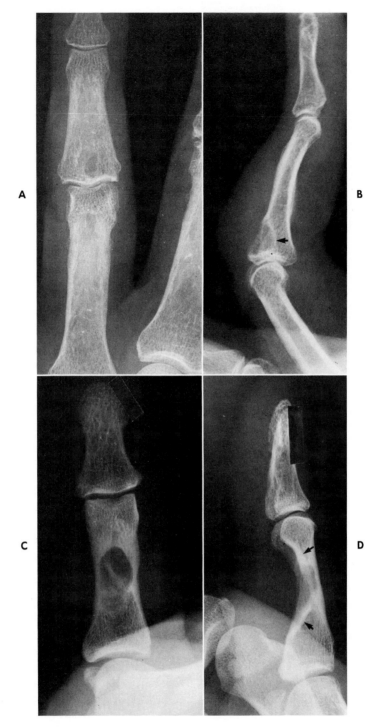

FIG. 3-9. Scalloped bony margins. **A** and **B**, Synovial chondromatosis of the finger exhibits a soft tissue mass adjacent to the middle phalanx, causing a scalloped, sclerotic margin *(arrow)*. The scalloping of the phalanx is due to the extrinsic erosion by the soft tissue mass and is seen best on the lateral view. **C** and **D**, A different patient presents with giant cell tumor of tendon sheath involving the thumb. The lesion could be easily mistaken for an intraosseous lesion on the frontal view **(C)**, but the extrinsic nature and scalloped sclerotic margins *(arrows)* are seen in excellent detail on the lateral view **(D)**.

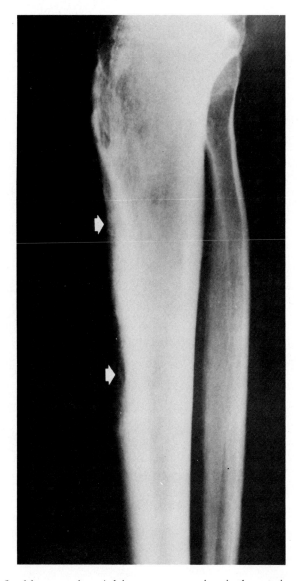

FIG. 3-10. Ill-defined bony erosion. A leiomyosarcoma arises in the anterior soft tissues of the lower leg. Bony destruction, with ill-defined margins *(arrows)*, is seen in the anterior tibial cortex.

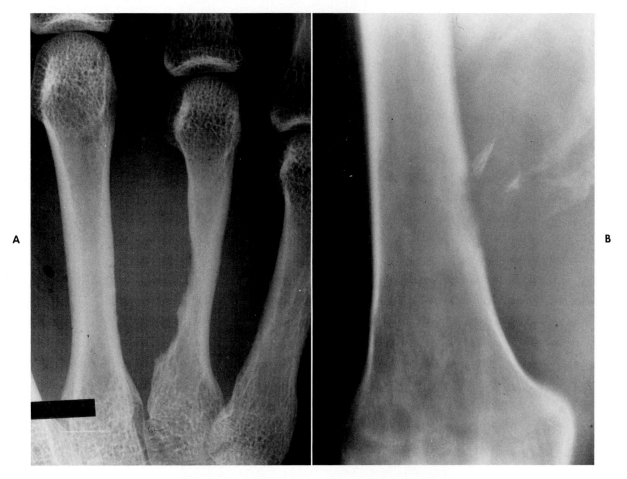

FIG. 3-11. Cortical destruction with marrow extension. **A** and **B,** Two different patients with synovial sarcoma show cortical destruction and marrow extension. The latter is indicated by destruction of endosteal cortex, although the marrow involvement can be imaged more convincingly on magnetic resonance scans. Both patients presented with a soft tissue mass. Coexistent calcification was noted in the synovial sarcoma of the thigh, where the tomogram (**B**) clearly demonstrates both the endosteal destruction and the areas of calcification.

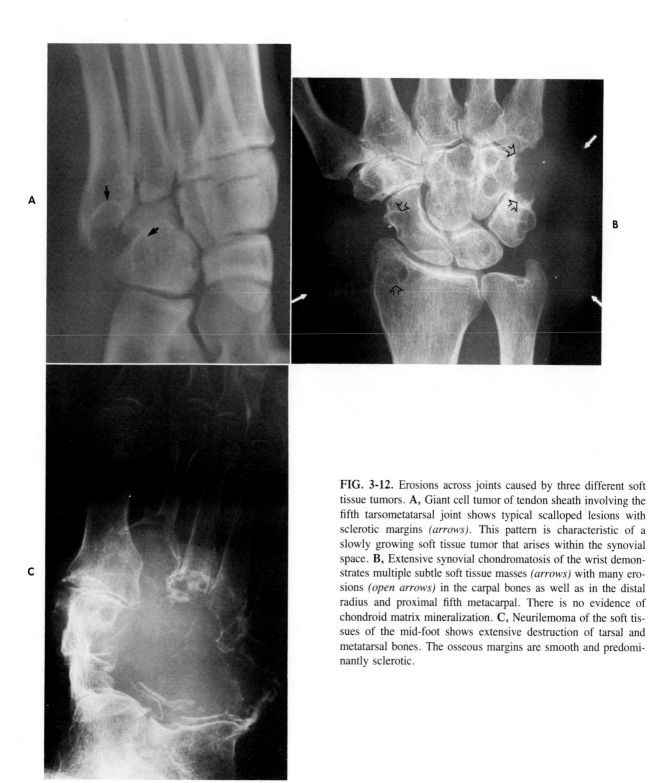

FIG. 3-12. Erosions across joints caused by three different soft tissue tumors. **A,** Giant cell tumor of tendon sheath involving the fifth tarsometatarsal joint shows typical scalloped lesions with sclerotic margins *(arrows)*. This pattern is characteristic of a slowly growing soft tissue tumor that arises within the synovial space. **B,** Extensive synovial chondromatosis of the wrist demonstrates multiple subtle soft tissue masses *(arrows)* with many erosions *(open arrows)* in the carpal bones as well as in the distal radius and proximal fifth metacarpal. There is no evidence of chondroid matrix mineralization. **C,** Neurilemoma of the soft tissues of the mid-foot shows extensive destruction of tarsal and metatarsal bones. The osseous margins are smooth and predominantly sclerotic.

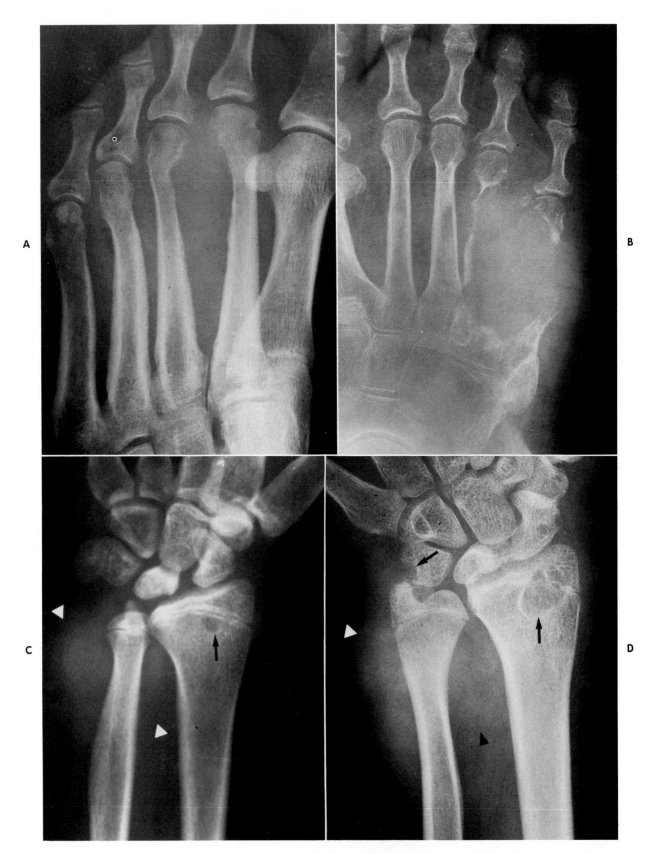

FIG. 3-13. Erosions between bones caused by three different soft tissue masses. **A,** Malignant schwannoma involving the soft tissues and bones of the foot. The soft tissue mass separates and erodes the second and third metatarsals with ill-defined cortical destruction of the affected bones. **B,** Chondrosarcoma of soft tissue shows aggressive and almost complete destruction of the fourth and fifth metatarsal bones by a large soft tissue mass. There are ill-defined bony erosions in the affected metatarsals. **C** and **D,** Pigmented villonodular synovitis of the wrist shows very slowly progressive bony destruction with smooth sclerotic margins *(arrows)* and enlargement of the soft tissue mass *(arrowheads)* between 1969 **(C)** and 1972 **(D).**

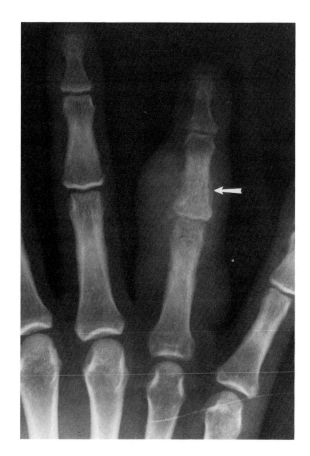

FIG. 3-14. Aggressive periosteal reaction due to chondrosarcoma of the synovium. Anterior view of the fourth finger shows a large soft tissue mass that extends from the base of the finger to the distal interphalangeal joint and contains several small subtle calcifications. The proximal interphalangeal joint is narrowed, and there is aggressive cortical destruction and periosteal reaction *(arrow)* involving both the middle and, to a lesser extent, the proximal phalanges.

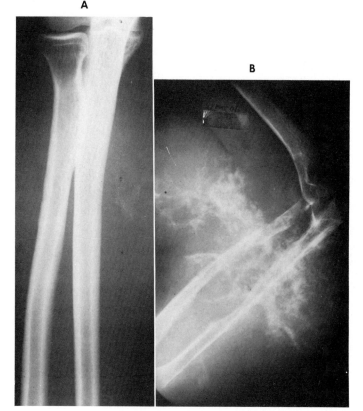

FIG. 3-15. Aggressive periosteal reaction and dramatic growth of a synovial sarcoma of the forearm. **A,** At clinical presentation, there is only extremely subtle calcification within the soft tissue mass on the radiograph of the proximal forearm. **B,** The follow-up radiograph approximately 1 year later reveals an extensive, rapidly growing tumor containing abundant calcification and evoking aggressive periosteal reaction in the radius and ulna. Both radial and ulnar cortices are destroyed, and there is marrow invasion. From an imaging perspective, the marrow invasion would be best demonstrated on magnetic resonance scans.

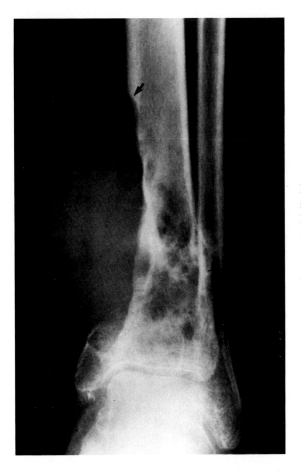

FIG. 3-16. Epicenter of lesion in soft tissue. A large soft tissue synovial sarcoma produces extrinsic erosion of the adjacent tibia. Note the oblique angle *(arrow)* at the proximal edge of bony erosion as the best, albeit subtle, clue that the epicenter of the mass is within the soft tissue. Even though there is extensive bone destruction, this pattern is still consistent with a tumor of soft tissue origin.

thus implies a cartilaginous tumor but, unfortunately, does not indicate whether it is benign or malignant. Osteoid matrix may form and mineralize in soft tissue tumors in a radiologic pattern of homogenous "cloudlike" densities or mature trabecular bone formation (Figs. 3-5 and 3-22). The latter pattern of mature trabecular bone is extremely reassuring because it suggests a very slowly maturing lesion that is typically benign such as ossifying lipoma, chondroma, hemangioma,[35] or, rarely, well-differentiated liposarcoma.

Calcification may occur in both benign and malignant soft tissue lesions.[151] Nodular (pseudosarcomatous) fasciitis[14,104] and myositis ossificans[45,54,75,115] are only two of the benign conditions that can demonstrate soft tissue calcification. Without a recognized structure (i.e., amorphous configuration), calcification is nonspecific (Fig. 3-14) and is merely another general feature of the tumor. However, amorphous calcifications are frequently present (up to 30% of patients) in synovial sarcomas (Figs. 3-8, 3-11, and 3-15),[*] and thus this entity should always be considered in the differential diagnosis of a soft tissue mass that contains amorphous calcification. Occasionally, peripheral maturation and calcification are seen as forming a well-developed shell, typical of healing myositis ossificans (Figs. 3-23 and 3-24).[45,115]

Tumoral calcinosis with homogeneous, extremely dense, lobulated calcific masses about the joint has a typical radiographic appearance (Fig. 3-25). This is a rare condition consisting of calcium salt deposition in extracapsular soft tissues about the joints,[*] most commonly the shoulders, hips, and elbows. Although usually idiopathic, tumoral calcinosis has been associated with metabolic disease (such as hyperparathyroidism), collagen vascular disease, and prior trauma. The deposits tend to enlarge gradually and may recur following surgery.

Bony involvement adjacent to a soft tissue tumor can be extremely informative. Smooth scalloping with an intact sclerotic bony margin separating the cortex from the adjacent soft tissue mass indicates slow growth (i.e., low biological activity) and is typically encountered in benign soft tissue tumors. However, this pattern can rarely be seen in slowly growing malignant neoplasms such as synovial sarcoma. Thus, when present, it implies a slowly developing

*References 6, 7, 19, 27, 56, 60, 66, 105, 111, 114.   *References 15, 30, 40, 48, 82, 109, 157.

Text continued on p.60.

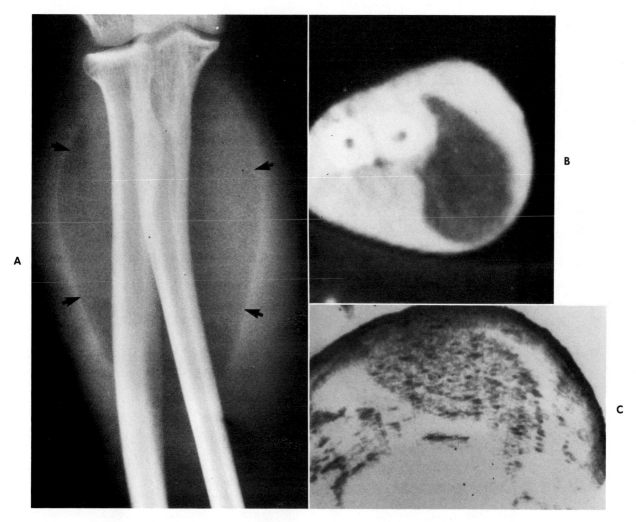

FIG. 3-17. Lipoma of the proximal forearm. **A,** Radiograph demonstrates the sharply marginated radiolucent mass *(arrows)* with uniform fatty density. **B,** The fatty nature, sharp margins, and typical homogenous fatty density of the lesion are confirmed on the CT scan. **C,** Sonography demonstrates the well-defined mass with uniform echogenicity throughout the lesion.

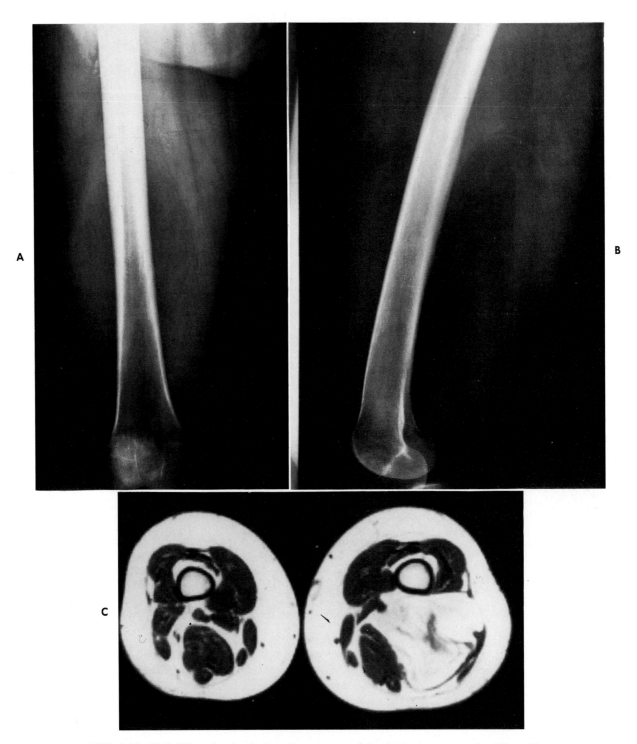

FIG. 3-18. Well-differentiated soft tissue liposarcoma of the thigh. Anteroposterior **(A)** and lateral **(B)** radiographs show an oval, fatty soft tissue mass in the posterior aspect of the distal thigh. The lesion is inhomogeneous, and its posterior and distal margins are indistinct, best appreciated on the lateral view **(B)**. Axial T1-weighted (600/15) **(C)** and T2-weighted (2500/90).

D

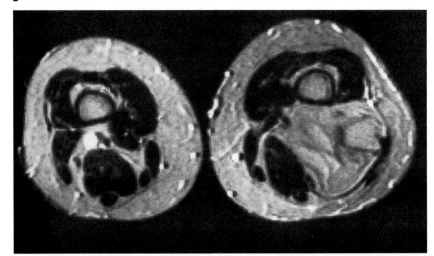

FIG. 3-18, cont'd. (D) Magnetic resonance scans define the borders of the liposarcoma to better advantage. Although the tumor is inhomogeneous, in most areas of the lesion the signal characteristics are identical to those in subcutaneous fat. Note how the liposarcoma abuts the adjacent posterior femoral cortex. (Courtesy Mark J. Kransdorf, MD.)

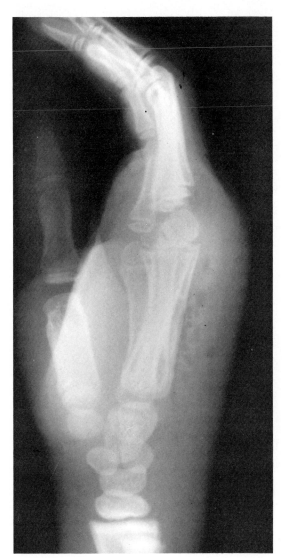

FIG. 3-19. Osteomyelitis of the hand with secondary soft tissue abscess. The lateral radiograph of the hand reveals soft tissue swelling with gas collection in the soft tissues surrounding the metacarpals of digits 2 through 5. (Courtesy Dr. Ruppert David.)

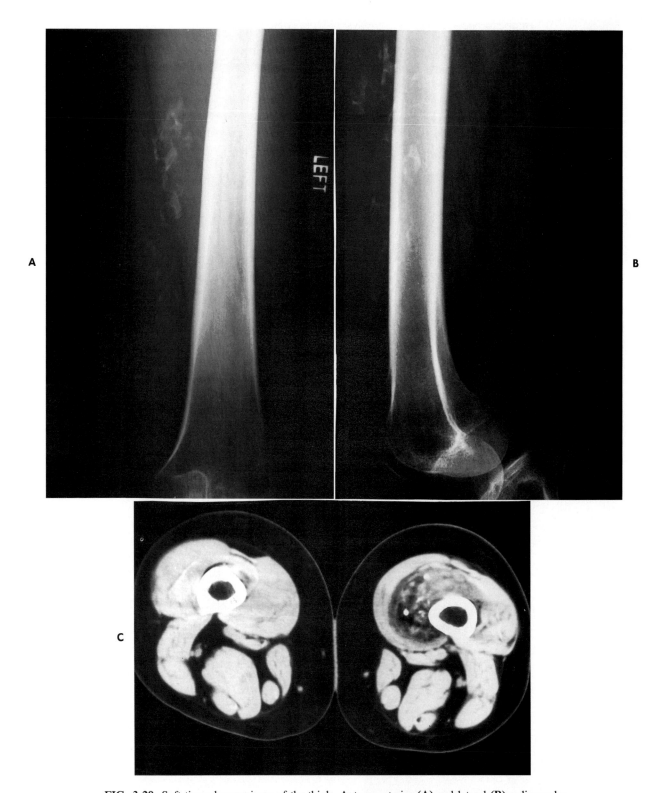

FIG. 3-20. Soft tissue hemangioma of the thigh. Anteroposterior (**A**) and lateral (**B**) radiographs show peculiar discrete "chicken-wire" calcifications in the anteromedial thigh. **C**, Axial CT scans with soft tissue and bone.

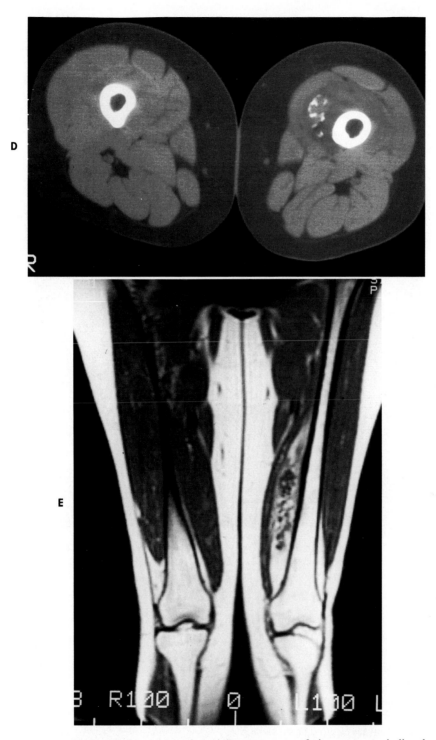

FIG. 3-20, cont'd. D, Windows show a large inhomogeneous soft tissue mass encircling the medial aspect of the femur. The margins of the mass are ill defined, particularly anteriorly. The configuration of some of the soft tissue calcifications is best appreciated on the bone windows. **E,** Coronal T1-weighted (350/10) magnetic resonance scan shows an interesting elliptical configuration to the inhomogeneous hemangioma. Note how the lesion abuts the medial femoral cortex.

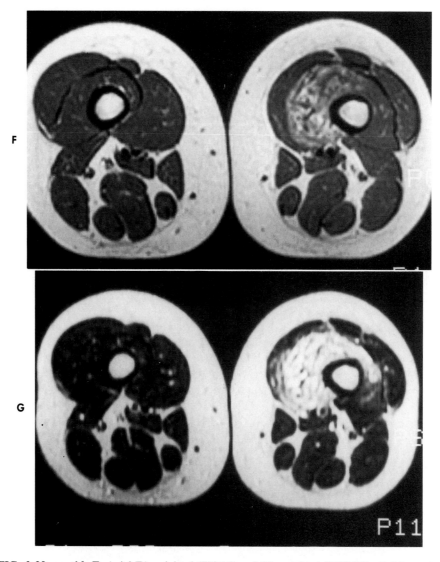

FIG. 3-20, cont'd. **F,** Axial T1-weighted (700/16) and T2-weighted (3000/85). **G,** Magnetic resonance scans also show the inhomogeneous nature of the soft tissue hemangioma and its relationship to the femoral cortex.

interface between the soft tissue mass and the adjacent bone and is usually seen in benign tumors. Irregular or ill-defined cortical destruction, whether limited to the cortex or associated with frank marrow invasion, is indicative of a rapidly growing lesion (i.e., high biological activity), suggesting a malignant soft tissue tumor. Other rapidly progressive disorders such as acute infection, arising either in bone or in soft tissue with secondary invasion of adjacent bone, may simulate this pattern; however, the clinical presentation differs markedly from that of a soft tissue tumor. Occasionally, bone adjacent to the soft tissue mass may not be eroded but may merely exhibit a periosteal reaction. If the periosteal reaction is a single-layered, multi-layered, or interrupted reaction (Fig. 3-15), then a malignant process should be the major consideration. If the periosteum is

thickened by a solid periosteal reaction and cortical hyperostosis, then the adjacent soft tissue process is usually benign. Frequently, this hyperostotic pattern occurs in association with vascular soft tissue tumors, especially hemangiomas.

IMAGING MODALITIES EMPLOYED TO EVALUATE SOFT TISSUE TUMORS

Multiple imaging modalities are useful in evaluating soft tissue masses.[*] These studies are invaluable in detecting the lesion, localizing its anatomical extent, and determining its

---

*References 5, 22, 31, 42, 55, 57, 58, 85, 86, 91, 92, 98, 118, 135, 146, 152, 154.

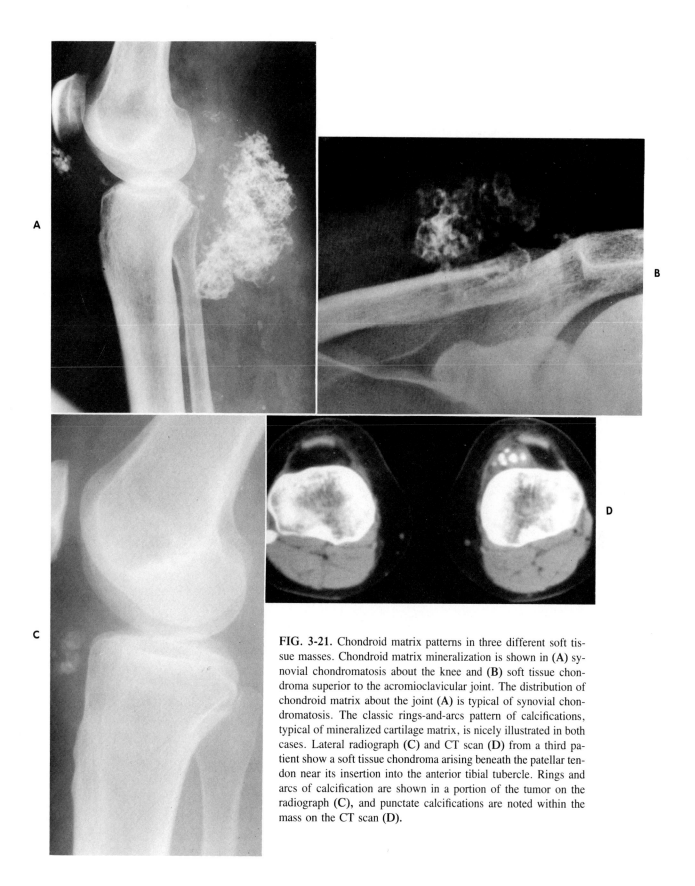

FIG. 3-21. Chondroid matrix patterns in three different soft tissue masses. Chondroid matrix mineralization is shown in (A) synovial chondromatosis about the knee and (B) soft tissue chondroma superior to the acromioclavicular joint. The distribution of chondroid matrix about the joint (A) is typical of synovial chondromatosis. The classic rings-and-arcs pattern of calcifications, typical of mineralized cartilage matrix, is nicely illustrated in both cases. Lateral radiograph (C) and CT scan (D) from a third patient show a soft tissue chondroma arising beneath the patellar tendon near its insertion into the anterior tibial tubercle. Rings and arcs of calcification are shown in a portion of the tumor on the radiograph (C), and punctate calcifications are noted within the mass on the CT scan (D).

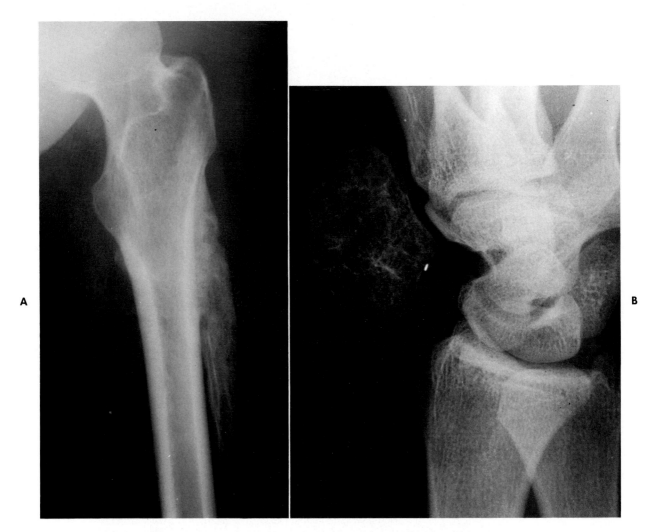

FIG. 3-22. Trabecular bone formation. **A,** Well-formed heterotopic bone formation with a trabecular pattern is seen along the muscle planes of the lateral thigh in this paraplegic patient. The proximal extent of the heterotopic bony mass is attached to the femur, and its margins are well defined. **B,** Chondroma of the soft tissue of the dorsum of the wrist also shows a well-developed trabecular pattern and a smooth peripheral shell. This is due to mature enchondral bone formation.

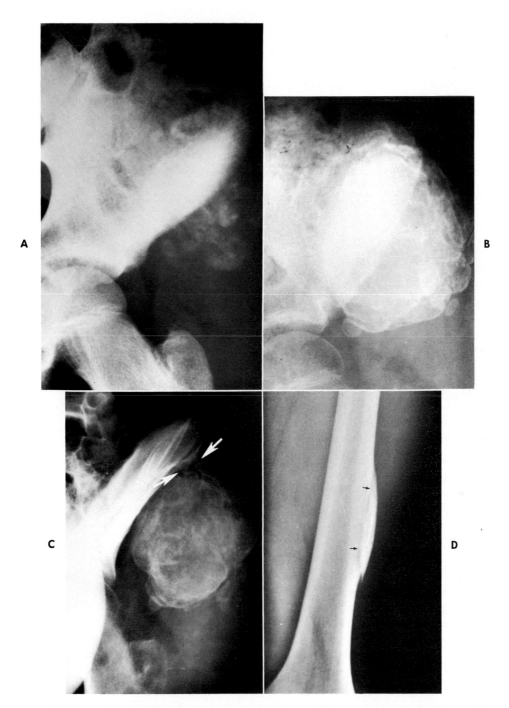

FIG. 3-23. Myositis ossificans in the healing stage in two different patients. Coned-down serial radiographs of myositis ossificans of the buttocks show progressive healing (over 8 weeks) with typical peripheral maturation and calcification. **A,** The initial film reveals a pattern of nonspecific amorphous calcification within the buttocks. **B,** A mature shell, along with small satellites, is seen on the follow-up film. **C,** The oblique film demonstrates attachment *(arrows)* to the superior ilium. **D,** In a different patient, a very mature dense myositis ossificans involving the deep soft tissue of the thigh has attached itself to the adjacent femoral cortex. The radiolucent line at its base *(arrows)* is a nonmineralized soft tissue band at the edge of the lesion.

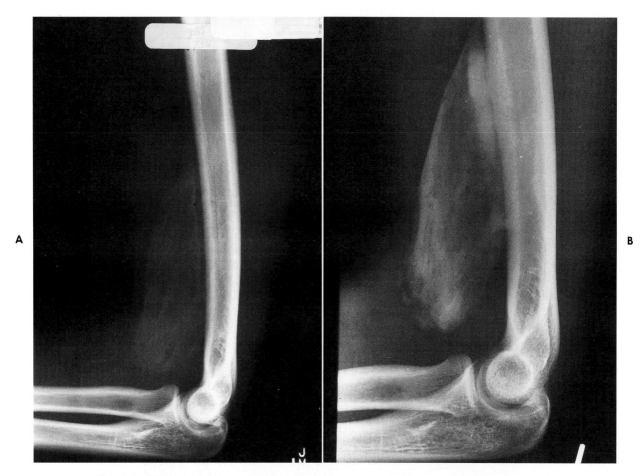

FIG. 3-24. Myositis ossificans of the arm. **A,** Lateral radiograph shows triangular calcification in the anterior soft tissues of the arm. **B,** Follow-up lateral radiograph 6 months later shows progressive "maturation" of the calcification within the soft tissue mass, and attachment of the lesion to the anterior humeral cortex.

effect on adjacent structures. Such findings are accurately predicted by radiologic imaging and are extremely helpful in staging the tumor and planning surgical or medical management.[36,37,128] A specific diagnosis, based exclusively on radiologic criteria, is usually not possible. However, as mentioned previously, radiologic findings indicating the presence of phleboliths (Fig. 3-4), fat (Figs. 3-3, 3-17, and 3-18), trabecular bone formation (Figs. 3-22, *A,* 3-23, and 3-24), or cartilage mineralization (Figs. 3-21, 3-22, *B,* and 3-27, *C*) are very important clues for identifying the lesion.

Conventional radiographic studies

The plain film radiograph obtained with low kilovoltage technique (below 50 kvp) enhances the difference in radiographic density between fat and muscle and accentuates soft tissue detail.[44,98,103,121] Routine (Fig. 3-26) or overpenetrated radiographs best demonstrate involvement of adjacent bone. Plain tomography is of particular value in assessing calcifications within soft tissue masses and in delineating

soft tissue abnormalities adjacent to complex bony structures (pelvis, spine, chest wall, and shoulder). Plain tomography augments, but does not replace, the plain radiograph.[98] The plain film is still superior to other techniques in predicting the presence and nature of bony involvement. Although the plain radiograph remains the best imaging modality for "naming" a bone tumor, magnetic resonance imaging is the best technique for making a preoperative diagnosis of a soft tissue mass because of its ability to discriminate fat from muscle and to clearly demarcate muscle groups, neurovascular structures, and other structures. When bone is involved by a slowly growing soft tissue mass, local pressure by the mass results in a scalloped pattern with a well-defined sclerotic margin (Figs. 3-2, 3-9, 3-12, and 3-13), which is most frequently seen in benign processes. Irregular cortical destruction is usually associated with fast-growing and frequently malignant lesions (Figs. 3-7, 3-10, 3-11, 3-13, *A* and *B,* and 3-14 to 3-16). Obliteration or displacement of normal fascial planes due to

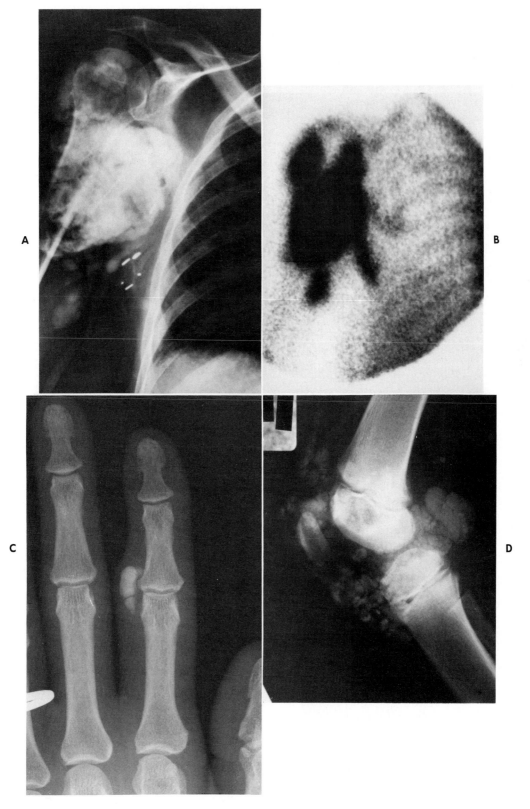

FIG. 3-25. Tumoral calcinosis in three different patients. Patient with renal osteodystrophy demonstrates tumoral calcinosis on the radiograph (**A**) with extensive homogenous calcification about the right shoulder. The bone scintigram (**B**) reveals increased radionuclide uptake. **C** and **D,** Two different patients with idiopathic tumoral calcinosis show the typical multiple lobules of homogeneous calcification about the joint. These are actually located outside of the joint capsule.

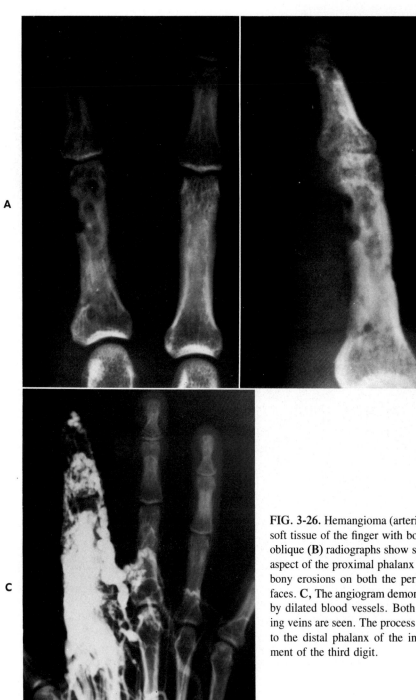

FIG. 3-26. Hemangioma (arteriovenous malformation type) of the soft tissue of the finger with bony involvement. Anterior (**A**) and oblique (**B**) radiographs show soft tissue swelling along the radial aspect of the proximal phalanx with extensive, tortuous scalloped bony erosions on both the periosteal and endosteal cortical surfaces. **C,** The angiogram demonstrates that the erosions are caused by dilated blood vessels. Both enlarged arteries and early draining veins are seen. The process extends from the palm of the hand to the distal phalanx of the index finger with minimal involvement of the third digit.

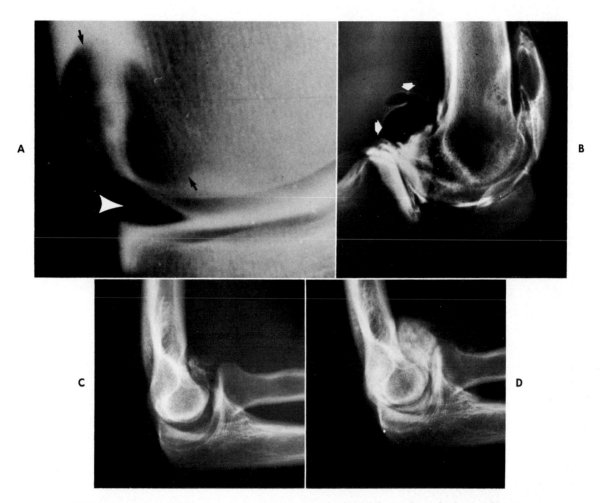

FIG. 3-27. Arthrographic studies of multiple cases. **A,** Coned-down view of a knee arthrogram shows the meniscus *(arrowhead)* and a large synovial mass *(arrows)* due to nodular synovitis. In another patient **(B),** a synovial cyst is seen posteriorly *(arrows)* on a lateral view from the arthrogram. In a third patient who complained of elbow pain, a plain film **(C)** shows the multiple ring-like calcifications suggesting a chondroid lesion anterior to the distal humerus. The elbow arthrogram **(D)** confirms the intraarticular location of the subtle chondroid filling defects (which are surrounded by dilute contrast medium that has been injected into the joint) and suggests the correct diagnosis of synovial chondromatosis.

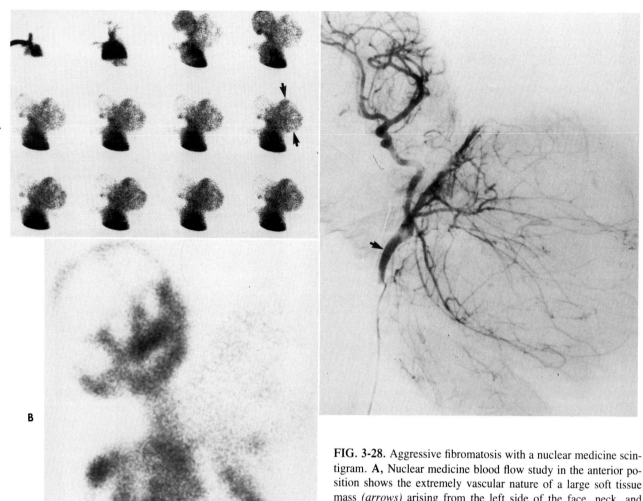

FIG. 3-28. Aggressive fibromatosis with a nuclear medicine scintigram. **A,** Nuclear medicine blood flow study in the anterior position shows the extremely vascular nature of a large soft tissue mass *(arrows)* arising from the left side of the face, neck, and upper chest. The static anterior bone scintigram **(B)** demonstrates subtle increased uptake in the mass. **C,** Angiogram reveals a dominant blood supply from the left carotid artery *(arrow)* on the selective injection, particularly from the external carotid artery.

soft tissue infiltration is common in both benign and malignant tumors. Occasionally, this interface may be lobulated and smooth, suggesting an encapsulated tumor. This is usually "pseudoencapsulation," however, since few soft tissue tumors possess a true capsule. Thus the margin about a soft tissue tumor, either benign or malignant, can be deceptive (Figs. 3-5 and 3-7), and inaccurate information may be disseminated if the presence of a smooth margin is automatically equated with a benign noninfiltrating tumor.

Arthrographic studies

Overall, arthrography plays a limited role in assessing soft tissue masses. Arthrography may be utilized to demonstrate synovial lesions (Fig. 3-27) and secondary involvement of the synovium by adjacent soft tissue or bony tumors. It is also helpful in showing synovial herniations or cysts that present as soft tissue masses.[53,85,86] When combined with CT scanning, arthrography can provide excellent visualization of the joint surface and its contact with adjacent structures.[86]

Scintigraphic studies

Radionuclide scanning with phosphate and other radiopharmaceutical agents demonstrates uptake in soft tissue tumors (Figs. 3-5, *C,* and 3-28).[*] However, detection is inconsistent, and if isotopic uptake occurs, the margins and local extent of the lesion are poorly defined and false-

---

*References 10, 30, 68, 99, 126, 127, 147.

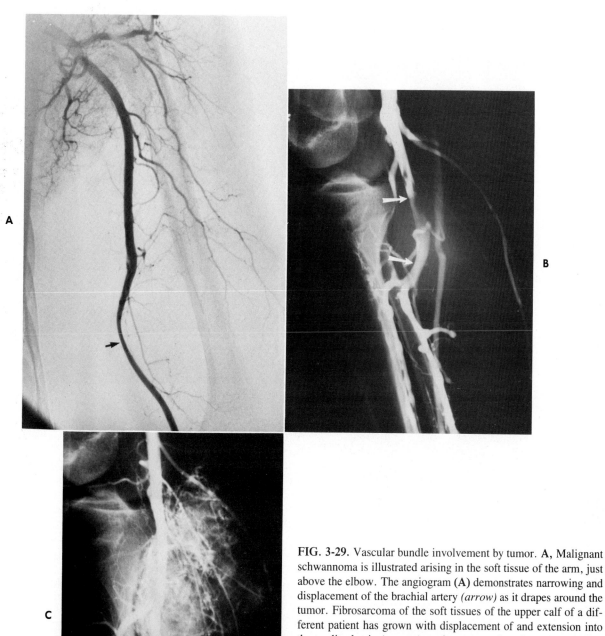

FIG. 3-29. Vascular bundle involvement by tumor. **A,** Malignant schwannoma is illustrated arising in the soft tissue of the arm, just above the elbow. The angiogram **(A)** demonstrates narrowing and displacement of the brachial artery *(arrow)* as it drapes around the tumor. Fibrosarcoma of the soft tissues of the upper calf of a different patient has grown with displacement of and extension into the popliteal vein *(arrows),* as demonstrated on the venogram **(B).** The angiogram **(C)** of this same patient reveals the hypervascular nature of the tumor, with tumor blush and multiple feeding arteries, mostly from the popliteal artery.

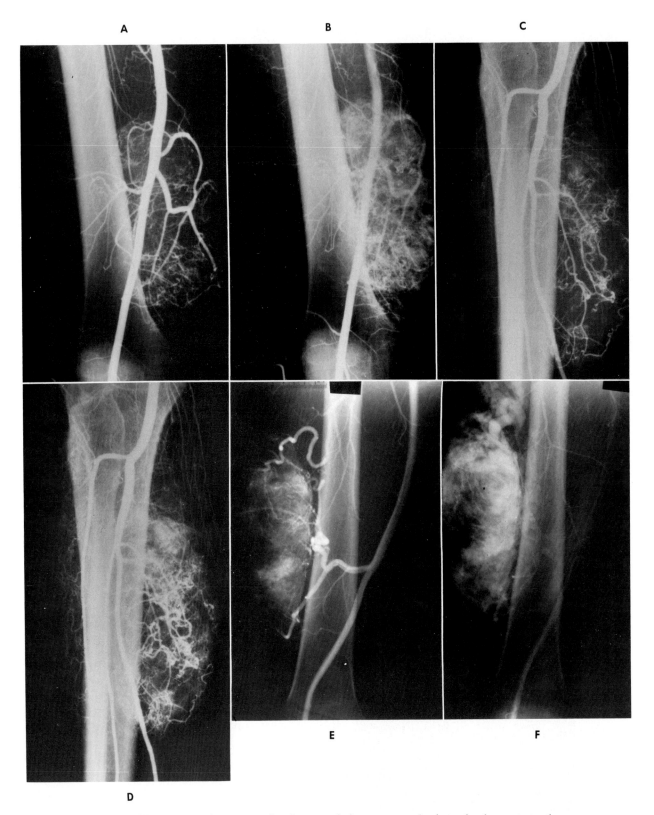

FIG. 3-30. Hypervascular pattern of malignant soft tissue tumors. Angiography demonstrates the hypervascularity, neovascularity, vascular displacement, and tumor blush most frequently seen in malignant tumors. Cases of malignant fibrous histiocytoma (**A** and **B**) of the thigh, leiomyosarcoma (**C** and **D**) of the calf, and synovial sarcoma (**E** and **F**) of the thigh are shown. The vascular pattern is similar in all three disease entities and is not unique for any specific diagnosis. A large draining vein is also seen near the superior aspect of the synovial sarcoma (**F**).

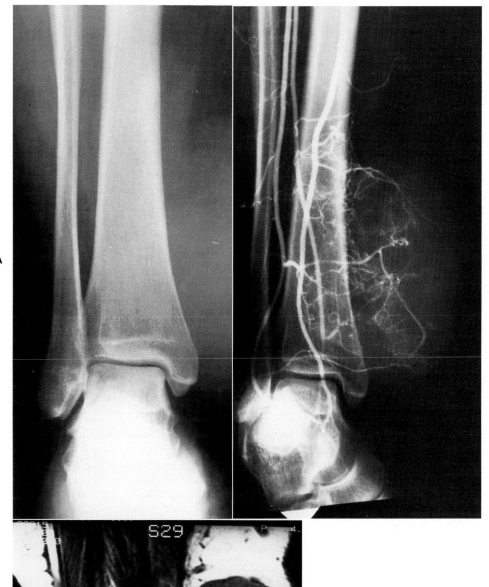

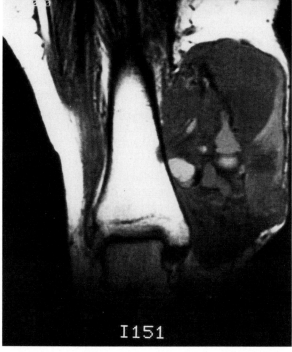

FIG. 3-31. Synovial sarcoma of the medial soft tissues above the ankle. **A,** Anteroposterior radiograph reveals a large nondescript soft tissue mass in the medial soft tissues just above the ankle. **B,** Angiogram shows hypervascularity and neovascularity within the lesion. **C,** Coronal T1-weighted (600/20) magnetic resonance scan shows a large heterogeneous soft tissue mass corresponding to the abnormalities noted on the radiograph and angiogram. The magnetic resonance scan also shows one small focus of tibial invasion that was not apparent on the radiograph. (Courtesy of Mark J. Kransdorf, MD.)

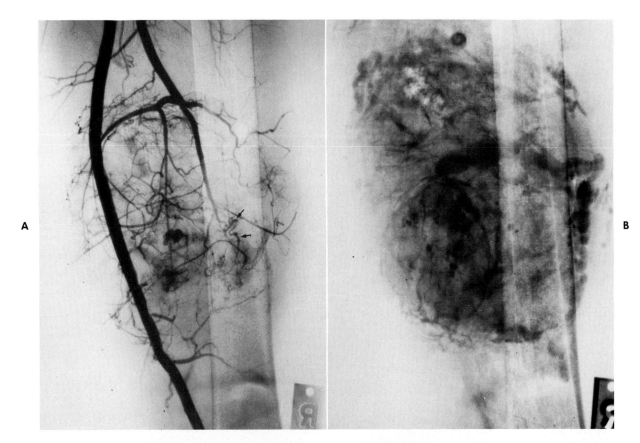

FIG. 3-32. Tumor neovascularity, puddling, and blush. Fibrosarcoma of the soft tissues of the thigh is illustrated on subtraction angiograms. The arterial phase angiogram **(A)** demonstrates a displaced femoral artery with extensive hypervascular blood supply to the tumor. Neovascularity *(arrows)* is extensive throughout the tumor and is recognized by the irregular tortuous course and changing caliber of the small arteries. The late angiogram **(B)** reveals both diffuse tumor blush and draining veins. Although strongly suggestive of a malignant tumor, these patterns are unfortunately still not specific.

negative scans do occur.[68,91,99] Although invasion of the adjacent bone is detectable by bone scanning, the bony involvement is usually already apparent on plain radiographs.[91] Dynamic scintigraphy clearly identifies vascular soft tissue lesions (Figs. 3-28, *A*, and 3-36, *A*). Positive scans can occur in many diverse diseases such as soft tissue neoplasm, infection, or in association with local or widespread soft tissue mineralization (Fig. 3-24, *B*). Scintigraphy is most helpful in identifying additional noncontiguous skeletal or soft tissue lesions that may not be either suspected clinically or detected on conventional radiographs. Such findings are significant for patient management, since they may alter the choice of therapeutic procedure.

Sonographic studies

Sonography provides an accurate method of detecting and determining the size (Figs. 3-2, *C,* and 3- 17, *C*) of the soft tissue mass in the extremities due to differential patterns of echoes detected in the mass in comparison to those noted in normal muscle and fascial planes.[*] This modality is less reliable than CT scanning or magnetic resonance imaging when the mass occurs in complex anatomical locations such as the pelvis, is located in deep soft tissues adjacent to bone, or occurs within the thorax surrounded by lung. When the soft tissue mass occurs in other locations, particularly in the abdomen or extremities, sonography precisely establishes anatomical relationships and tumor margins, but generally provides lesser detail than is available on CT scanning or magnetic resonance imaging. Most soft tissue tumors have an echogenicity distinct from the adjacent soft tissues, which provides an interface between the tumor and the surrounding soft tissues. An accu-

---

*References 5, 13, 43, 46, 50, 85, 91.

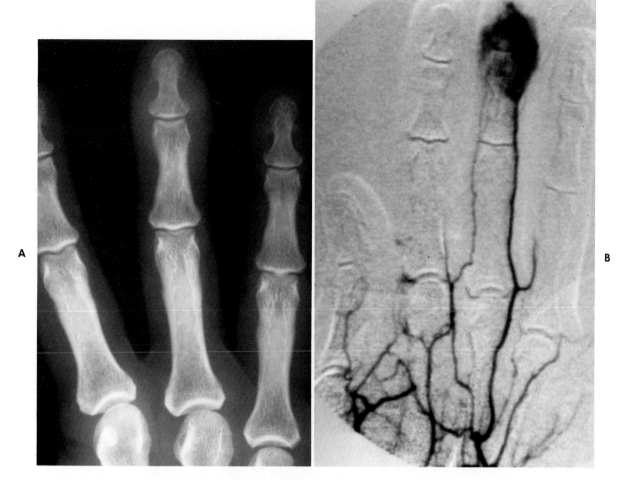

FIG. 3-33. Giant cell tumor of tendon sheath with diffuse tumor blush. **A,** Radiograph shows a soft tissue mass surrounding the distal interphalangeal joint of the middle finger. **B,** Digital subtraction angiogram demonstrates diffuse tumor blush in this benign lesion.

rate description of the size and configuration of the mass is obtained at sonography because the lesion can be visualized in both the transverse (axial) and longitudinal (sagittal) planes. Therefore, sonography is very useful in following either the size of the soft tissue mass on serial studies or the response of the lesion to treatment by nonsurgical means such as chemotherapy or radiation therapy. The echo pattern of solid masses is nonspecific, but a fluid-filled mass such as a synovial cyst (popliteal cyst) can be easily differentiated from a solid mass by sonography.[53,85]

Angiographic studies

Angiography is most helpful in evaluating the vascular supply of the soft tissue mass and the impact of the mass on adjacent vascular structures.* This modality can be es-

pecially useful when the lesion arises in the extremities, where fatty tissue is sparse.[58,89,91,98] The angiogram, performed with conventional cut film or digital subtraction technique (digital subtraction angiography), or both, provides information about the anatomical extent of the tumor, including its effect on adjacent structures, the arterial supply, and the venous drainage (Fig. 3-29). Since these features influence the choice of operative procedure, angiography is a valuable adjunct in patient management.[58,102] Much of this anatomical information can also be obtained via magnetic resonance angiography.[32,33] Since the patient with a soft tissue tumor is likely to undergo magnetic resonance scanning anyway, the referring physician should discuss with the radiologist the appropriateness of performing magnetic resonance angiography as a supplement to the routine magnetic resonance pulse sequences. Interventional angiographic procedures are sometimes necessary, occasionally to preoperatively embolize an extremely hypervas-

---

*References 17, 22, 42, 55, 61, 83, 84, 89, 91, 97, 98, 102, 135, 146, 152, 159.

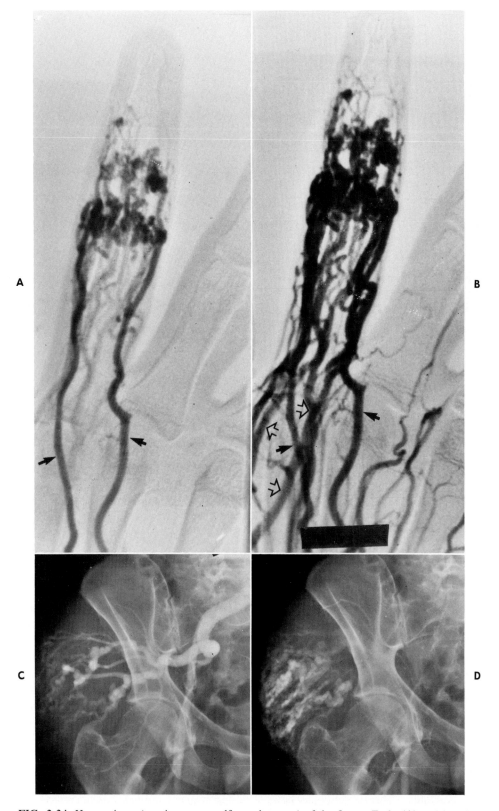

FIG. 3-34. Hemangioma (arteriovenous malformation type) of the finger. Early **(A)** and late **(B)** subtraction angiograms show dilated arteries *(arrows)* involving the soft tissue and adjacent bones. Shunting to the venous side is seen **(B)** with appearance of early draining veins *(open arrows)*. Hemangioma of the buttocks of a different patient. Early **(C)** and late **(B)** angiograms demonstrate enlarged tortuous vessels with an organized, parallel configuration. These findings are consistent with hemangioma.

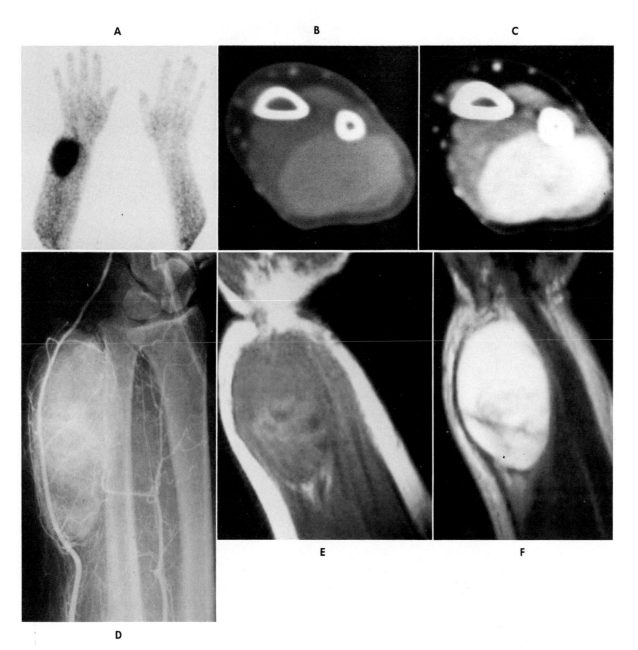

FIG. 3-35. Multiple imaging evaluation of a malignant fibrous histiocytoma. Malignant fibrous histiocytoma involving the soft tissues of the forearm demonstrated a sharply marginated soft tissue mass without bony erosion on the plain radiographs (not shown). The blood pool scan (A) shows focal increased tracer uptake in the tumor, consistent with its increased vascularity. The unenhanced CT scan (B) reveals muscle displacement by the mass, which is in contact with the ulna. The contrast-enhanced CT scan (C) shows the sharply marginated enhanced tumor. The late angiogram (D) demonstrates displaced vessels, neovascularity, and tumor blush. On the T1-weighted magnetic resonance study (E) the tumor is similar in signal intensity to the adjacent muscles, with little contrast resolution. However, on the T2-weighted scan (F), there is excellent contrast resolution, and the high signal of the tumor allows easy differentiation from the surrounding soft tissues.

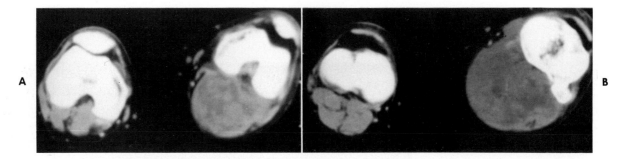

FIG. 3-36. CT scan of synovial sarcoma arising in the posterior soft tissues of the left knee. The transaxial CT scans are taken through the femoral condyles **(A)** and the upper calf **(B).** These CT scans show the extent of the tumor, which has a heterogeneous consistency, typically due to necrosis or hemorrhage. There is extension into the area of the popliteal artery, tibial nerve, and adjacent muscles.

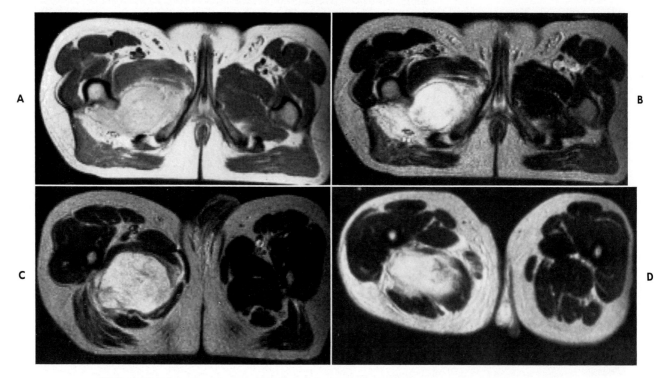

FIG. 3-37. Magnetic resonance imaging of a myxoid liposarcoma. The lesion involves the soft tissue of the upper medial thigh and extends into the right ischium. The T1-weighted, spin density mixed scan (TR-1600ms, TE-35ms) **(A)** also indicates involvement of the posterior aspect of the proximal femur. A T2-weighted scan **(B)** demonstrates increased contrast resolution and the high signal intensity of the tumor. Lower T2-weighted scans **(C** and **D)** show that although the femoral artery and vein are separate from the tumor, the mass is infiltrating adjacent muscle and soft tissue planes.

cular soft tissue mass or, rarely, to embolize a persistent arterial bleeder following surgical resection of the lesion.

Malignant soft tissue tumors display angiographic patterns that range from hypervascular (Figs. 3-30 and 3-31) to hypovascular. The angiographic features of neovascularity, puddling, and tumor blush are typical of malignant tu-

mors (Fig. 3-32). However, benign tumors may also occasionally demonstrate neovascularity (Fig. 3-33), and these less common associations should be kept in mind when patients afflicted with soft tissue tumors undergo angiography. Malignant soft tissue tumors are frequently heterogeneous and contain areas of hemorrhage and necrosis that tend to

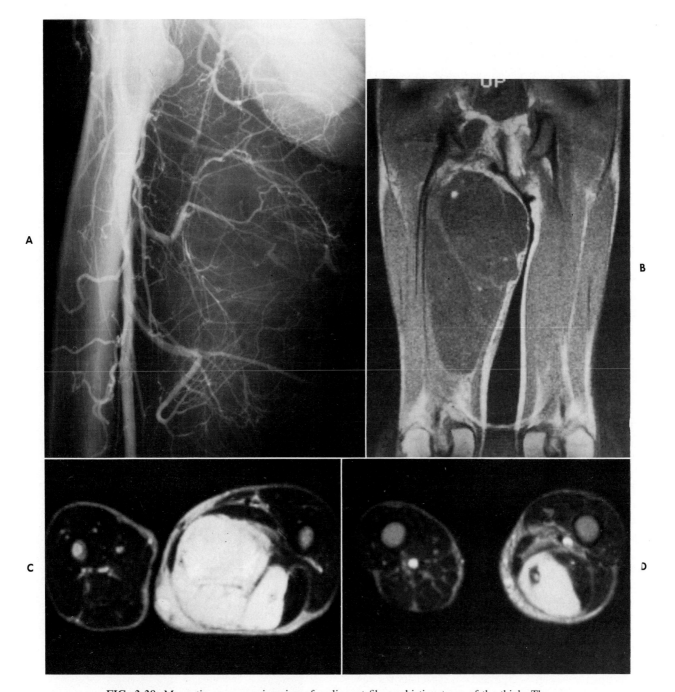

FIG. 3-38. Magnetic resonance imaging of malignant fibrous histiocytoma of the thigh. The angiogram (**A**) demonstrates the hypervascularity of the lesion. The coronal T1-weighted magnetic resonance scan (**B**) clearly demonstrates the extent of the tumor and its interface with adjacent structures. The two transaxial T2-weighted magnetic resonance scans (**C** and **D**) reveal the increased signal from the tumor as well as extensive edema and swelling of the subcutaneous tissue and fascial planes.

be less vascular on angiography, contrasting with areas of viable malignant tumor, which tend to have the greatest vascularity.[84,146] If the hemorrhagic or necrotic sites are inadvertently biopsied, confusing and erroneous conclusions may be drawn. Unsuspected satellite tumors about the pri-

mary mass may also be discovered by angiography.

Certain angiographic patterns are suggestive of specific histological diagnoses such as hemangiomas and vascular malformations (Fig. 3-34).[11,46,58] Hemangiopericytoma is another tumor that may exhibit a unique and striking hypervascular pattern.* A frequent angiographic feature of hemangiopericytoma is that early in the arterial phase the main arteries are displaced around the periphery of the tumor. Later, the feeding arteries spread in a meshwork pattern before actually penetrating the lesion. This peripheral vascular distribution noted at angiography correlates well with the plexiform meshwork of vessels covering the tumor that is seen on inspection of the gross specimen. This angiographic pattern is highly suggestive of hemangiopericytoma. However, in most soft tissue masses, a specific pathological diagnosis cannot be suggested by angiography. It is also difficult to differentiate benign from malignant soft tissue tumors by angiography.[58,91,98,152] Thus biopsy and resultant histological confirmation remain essential to establish the diagnosis.

CT scanning

Computed tomography (CT scanning) has proved extremely helpful in detecting soft tissue tumors and in monitoring the patient regarding both local recurrence and distant metastases (Figs. 3-35 and 3-36).[†] In this regard, if the patient is to undergo CT scanning or magnetic resonance imaging, it is imperative that a scan be obtained prior to biopsy or surgical intervention. If this principle is ignored, the value of the combined imaging studies is dramatically diminished since it becomes difficult, or even impossible, to distinguish how much of the soft tissue abnormality is due to the lesion itself and how much is due to hemorrhage or edema related to biopsy or surgery. CT scanning is most useful in defining the extent of the soft tissue mass (Figs. 3-35, B and C, and 3-36) and its relationship to adjacent structures, especially in complex anatomical sites such as the pelvis. This exquisite anatomical detail enables the surgeon to perform a more complete resection of the tumor or the radiotherapist to define a more precise radiation therapy field. Occasionally, CT scanning can help establish a diagnosis, especially with regard to the detection of adipose tissue (Figs. 3-3, B, and 3-17, B) in tumors whose fatty component may not be appreciated on plain radiographs. Contrast enhancement is valuable in assessing the vascularity of the soft tissue mass and in separating the mass from adjacent structures (Fig. 3-35, B and C), especially the vascular bundle. Soft tissue tumors can also be isodense with normal muscle on precontrast CT scans and become evident only following contrast infusion.[91] CT scanning is superior to magnetic resonance imaging in detecting and characterizing calcification within the soft tissue mass and detecting subtle cortical erosion and periosteal reaction in the bone adjacent to the soft tissue mass.[74,80] The ability of CT scanning to detect calcification within the soft tissue mass can prove invaluable in suggesting a specific diagnosis

(e.g., phleboliths suggest hemangiomas, calcified rings and arcs suggest a cartilaginous lesion, amorphous calcification within a large soft tissue mass might suggest a soft tissue osteosarcoma or synovial sarcoma, or peripheral calcification surrounding a soft tissue mass might suggest myositis ossificans, whereas calcification throughout the lesion might favor tumoral calcinosis).

Magnetic resonance imaging

Magnetic resonance imaging is a major technological innovation in medical imaging and has been the subject of

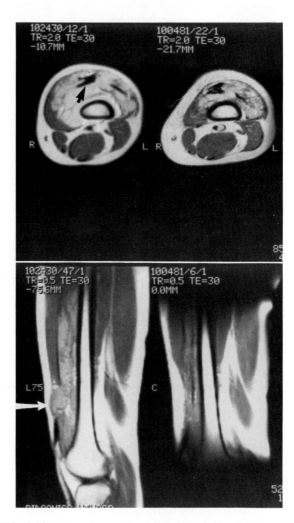

FIG. 3-39. Magnetic resonance imaging of a hemangioma. The scans on the left (top and bottom) were taken prior to surgery and the scans on the right (top and bottom) following surgery. The two top transaxial scans are spin density–weighted scans (TR-200ms, TE-30ms), and the two bottom sagittal scans are T1-weighted scans (TR-500ms, TE-30ms).[○○○] The preoperative scan (left, top and bottom) shows diffuse involvement about the femur with extension to the subcutaneous fat *(white arrow)*. There are linear branching signal voids representing large vessels *(black arrow)*. The postoperative scans (right, top and bottom) demonstrate a significant residual hemangioma. (Courtesy of Paul Weatherall and Jim Cohen, UTHSC at Dallas.)

---

*References 1, 61, 101, 112, 136, 159.
†References 1, 4, 5, 31, 34, 49, 50, 52, 59, 86, 91-94, 100, 118, 125, 129, 131, 134, 154-156, 158.

numerous publications.* Magnetic resonance imaging machines have proliferated rapidly since the mid 1980s despite their considerable expense. As might be anticipated, the images are severely degraded if the patient moves during the study, and since the patient must lie in a tunnel-shaped magnet, a small percentage of patients cannot be scanned due to claustrophobia. Low field strength, "open" magnets, best suited for scanning the extremities, have been introduced to eliminate problems related to claustrophobia. It is difficult to perform magnetic resonance scanning on critically ill patients who are receiving life support monitoring. Understandably, metal objects such as jewelry or a metallic life support apparatus must be removed before the patient approaches the magnet. Also, implanted metals such as cardiac pacemakers or surgical clips might preclude magnetic resonance scanning.

Both CT scanning and magnetic resonance scanning are

expensive and depend on sophisticated computers that rapidly analyze millions of extremely complex differential equations. There are significant differences between the two methods, however. CT scanning provides cross-sectional images primarily confined to the axial plane. Rarely, during imaging of the patient's face, coronal imaging can be accomplished directly with CT scanning. When other anatomical sites are scanned, however, computer-derived reconstructed images, usually of marginal quality, can be made in the coronal or sagittal plane. A major advantage of magnetic resonance imaging is its ability to directly image the region of anatomical interest in orthogonal planes (i.e., axial, coronal, and sagittal planes). This capability, as well as the excellent soft tissue contrast of the image, is invaluable in assessing the extent of a soft tissue mass.

Another major difference between CT scanning and magnetic resonance imaging is the underlying principles of physics responsible for the images. CT scanning, like x-ray, employs ionizing radiation that is attenuated by the physical characteristics of normal or diseased tissues. Magnetic resonance imaging is both different and more complicated.

---

*References 2, 8, 11, 12, 20, 21, 24-26, 29, 38, 39, 41, 51, 63-65, 69-72, 77-79, 88, 90, 96, 107, 108, 110, 119, 120, 123, 132, 133, 137, 139, 140-145, 148, 149, 153.

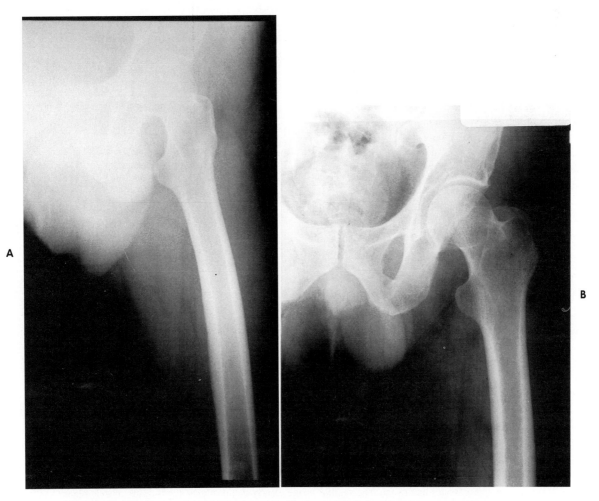

FIG. 3-40. Hibernoma of the thigh. **A** and **B,** Radiographs of the thigh demonstrate bizarre linear lucencies in the medial soft tissues of the left thigh.

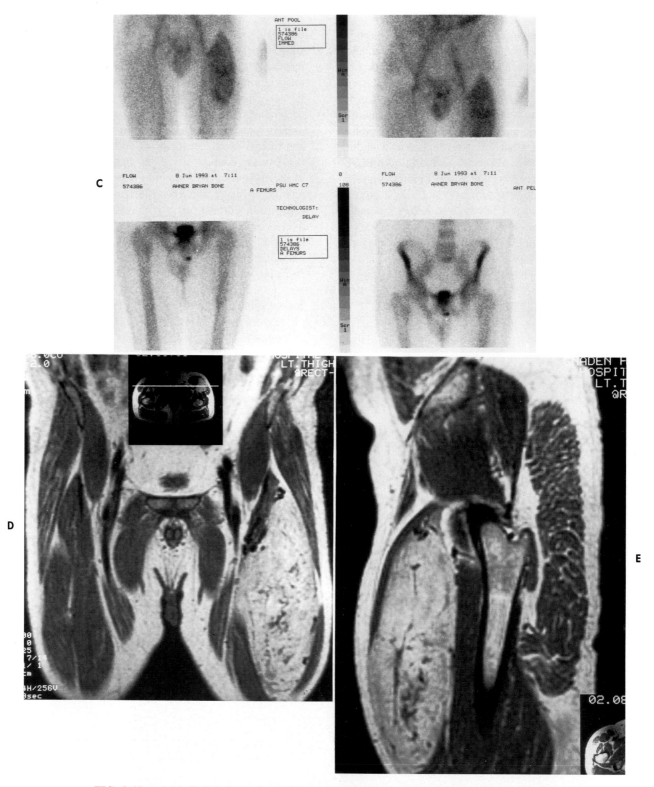

FIG. 3-40, cont'd. C, Scintigram demonstrates a large hypervascular soft tissue mass in the proximal thigh. The mass is readily apparent on the flow portion of the study but is very subtle on the delayed images. T1-weighted (600/25) coronal **(D)** and sagittal **(E)** scans demonstrate a large elliptical soft tissue mass in the proximal left thigh. The predominant signal in the inhomogeneous lesion approximates that of fat. The sagittal image clearly demonstrates a soft tissue muscle plane separating the mass from the underlining femoral cortex.

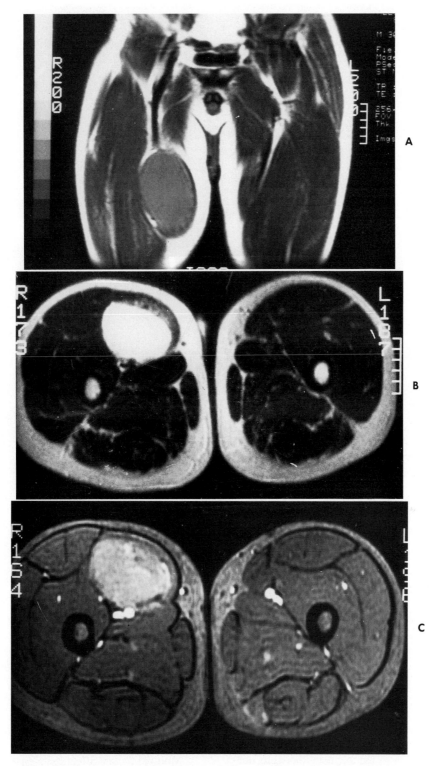

FIG. 3-41. Synovial sarcoma of the medial thigh. **A,** Coronal T1-weighted (600/20) magnetic resonance scan demonstrates a sharply marginated, oval soft tissue mass in the medial right thigh. At this pulse sequence, the signal of the mass is intermediate between that of subcutaneous fat and muscle. Axial T2-weighted scan (2000/80) **(B)** and GRE scan (33/13, with a 60-degree flip angle) **(C)** clearly demarcate the lesion, which is surrounded by a small amount of edema. There is evidence of muscle separating the mass from the femur. (Courtesy of Mark J. Kransdorf, MD.)

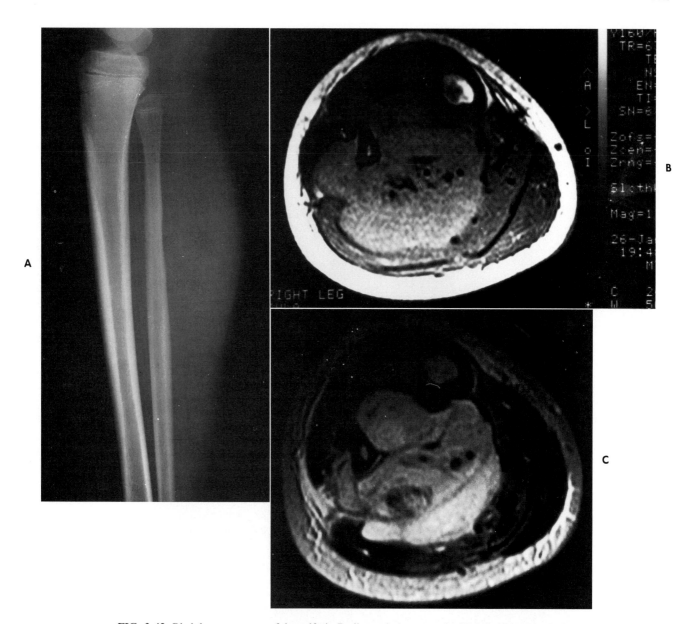

FIG. 3-42. Rhabdomyosarcoma of the calf. **A,** Radiograph demonstrates ill-defined increased density in the mid-portion of the calf without evidence of bony involvement. Axial T1-weighted (650/26) **(B)** and T2-weighted (2350/80) **(C)** magnetic resonance images demonstrate an ill-defined soft tissue mass in the calf. The lesion does not involve the tibia or fibula. The elliptical configuration of the lesion is appreciated to best advantage on the T2-weighted scan **(C).** (Courtesy of Mark J. Kransdorf, MD.)

It utilizes magnets weighing as much as several tons and having magnetic field strengths typically varying between 0.5 and 1.5 T. In addition to the magnets, there are transmitting and receiving antennas. The strong magnetic field causes the atomic nuclei (usually hydrogen nuclei) to line up and undergo precession, that is, the magnet causes the nucleus to wobble at a specific frequency rate. If the nuclei are exposed to pulses of radio waves, they absorb energy, and the excess energy in the nuclei is then released in the form of radio waves that serve as the magnetic resonance signal.

Multiple factors affect the signal: T1, the longitudinal or spin-lattice relaxation rate; T2, the spin-spin relaxation rate; TR, the pulse repetition time; and TE, the echo time. In general, short TR and TE times accentuate T1 differences between tissues and long TR and TE times accentuate T2 differences. The various parameters are selected by the radiologist, who then monitors the images. Since clinical

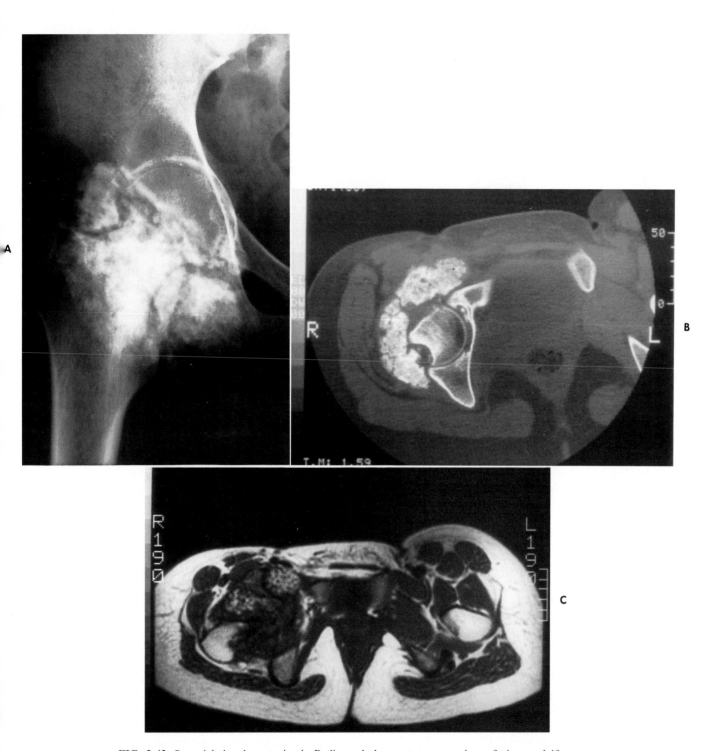

FIG. 3-43. Synovial chondromatosis. **A,** Radiograph demonstrates extensive soft tissue calcification overlying the right hip. **B,** Axial CT scan imaged at bone window demonstrates that the calcification is within the hip joint and causes some remodeling of the posterior aspect of the right femoral head. The appearance of the mineralization on both the radiograph and CT scan is strongly suggestive of a cartilaginous lesion. **C,** Axial T1-weighted (300/15) magnetic resonance scan demonstrates cartilaginous masses anterior to the right femoral neck. As is readily apparent, the CT scan (**B**) is much more suitable to characterize the calcification within the lesion. (Courtesy of Mark J. Kransdorf, MD.)

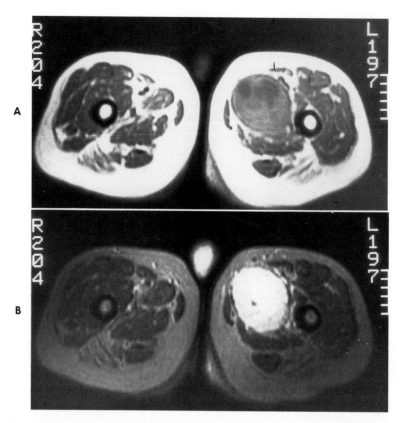

FIG. 3-44. Malignant fibrous histiocytoma of the thigh. Axial T1-weighted (800/20) **(A)** and T2-weighted (2000/80) **(B)** magnetic resonance scans demonstrate a large soft tissue mass in the medial aspect of the left thigh. On the T1-weighted scan **(A)**, the lesion is inhomogeneous. As is true of most soft tissue tumors, the lesion becomes much brighter on the T2-weighted scan **(B)**. The margins of the lesion are ill defined, particularly posterolaterally. The lesion closely approximates the cortex of the adjacent femur. (Courtesy of Mark J. Kransdorf, MD.)

magnetic resonance scanning was introduced in the United States in the early and mid 1980s, countless articles have been published in the literature addressing differing techniques and pulse sequences to be used in the procedure.

The majority of soft tissue tumors exhibit either a low signal intensity (i.e., they appear dark) or intermediate signal intensity on T1-weighted scans, and exhibit a high signal intensity (i.e., they are bright or white) on T2-weighted scans (Figs. 3-35 and 3-37 to 3-44). Therefore magnetic resonance imaging provides little diagnostic specificity for the majority of soft tissue tumors. However, there is a group of tumors that typically have a high signal on T1-weighted scans (Fig. 3-3, *C*), which includes hematomas, lipomas, liposarcomas, hemangiomas, and lesions complicated by hemorrhage into a preexisting tumor. These lesions vary in their histological picture, but all contain blood or fat. In contrast, flowing blood, unlike the stagnant blood in a hematoma, has a low signal intensity permitting assessment of vessel patency. Lesions that are predominantly fibrous exhibit low signal intensity on both T1- and T2-weighted images. Most soft tissue masses have a nonspecific appear-

ance on magnetic resonance imaging, but even so, this technique is the imaging modality of choice for determining (in three orthogonal planes) the extent of the lesion. If the plain radiograph obtained in the patient with a palpable soft tissue mass fails to demonstrate either bony involvement or calcification within the soft tissue lesion, then only magnetic resonance imaging (and not CT scanning) need be performed. Several investigators initially proposed that if magnetic resonance scanning showed a mass with a sharply defined margin, it was likely to be benign, but unfortunately, there are many exceptions to that "rule." Therefore, although the radiologist would prefer to encounter a sharply marginated soft tissue mass rather than one with ill-defined margins, the tumor can clearly exhibit well-defined margins on magnetic resonance scans and still be malignant. As a final caveat it must be said that in a cost-conscious era that has witnessed the proliferation of free-standing imaging centers, it is imperative that a final dictation of CT scanning or magnetic resonance scanning of musculoskeletal tumors must never be rendered until the radiologist correlates the cross-sectional imaging study with the plain radiograph.

CONCLUSION

In the surgical management of soft tissue tumors, several factors are important and influence the choice of operative procedure and its results. These factors include histological diagnosis, determination of anatomical extent of the tumor, and prevention of tumor spread into previously uninvolved compartments during the operative procedure.[34] Information pertaining to the latter two factors is best obtained by the multiple diagnostic imaging modalities outlined previously, that is, plain radiographs, magnetic resonance imaging, and CT scanning, and, to a lesser extent, sonography, angiography, and scintigraphy.

It is important to understand that even though all these modalities assist in obtaining significant morphological information about the soft tissue mass, the preoperative diagnosis usually remains unknown, and almost invariably biopsy is required to establish a specific diagnosis. If necessary, percutaneous biopsy can be successfully performed by the interventional radiologist under guidance with sonographic studies or CT scanning.

REFERENCES

1. Alpern MB, Thorsen MK, Kellman GM, et al: CT appearance of hemangiopericytoma. *J Comput Assist Tomogr* 10:264, 1986.
2. Balsara ZN, Stainken BF, Martinez AJ: MR image of localized giant cell tumor of the tendon sheath involving the knee. *J Comput Assist Tomog* 13:159, 1989.
3. Bartis JR: Massive lipoma of the foot: a case report. *J Am Podiatr Assoc* 64:874, 1974.
4. Berger PE, Kuhn JP: Computed tomography of tumors of the musculoskeletal system in children. *Radiology* 127:171, 1978.
5. Bernardino ME, Jing BS, Thomas JL, et al: The extremity soft tissue lesion: a comparative study of ultrasound, computed tomography, and xeroradiography. *Radiology* 139:53, 1981.
6. Bernreuter WK, Sartoris DJ, Resnick D: Magnetic resonance imaging of synovial sarcoma. *J Foot Surg* 29:94, 1990.
7. Berquist TH, Ehman RL, King BF, et al: Value of MR imaging in differentiating benign from malignant soft-tissue masses: study of 95 lesions. *AJR Am J Roentgenol* 155:1251, 1990.
8. Binkovitz LA, Berquist TH, McLeod RA: Masses of the hand and wrist: detection and characterization with MR imaging. *AJR Am J Roentgenol* 154:323, 1990.
9. Blacksin M, Barnes FJ, Lyons MM: MR diagnosis of macrodystrophia lipomatosa. *AJR Am J Roentgenol* 158:1295, 1992.
10. Blatt CJ, Hayt DB, Desai M, et al: Soft tissue sarcomas imaged with technetium-99m pyrophosphate. *N Y State J Med* 77:2118, 1977.
11. Bohndorf K, Reiser M, Lochner B, et al: Magnetic resonance imaging of primary tumours and tumour-like lesions of bone. *Skel Radiol* 15:511, 1986.
12. Bradley WG, Waluch V, Lai KS, et al: The appearance of rapidly flowing blood on magnetic resonance images. *AJR* 143:1167, 1984.
13. Braunstein EM, Silver TM, Martel W, et al: Ultrasonic diagnosis of extremity masses. *Skel Radiol* 6:157, 1981.
14. Broder MS, Leonidas JC, Mitty HA: Pseudosarcomatous fasciitis: an unusual cause of soft tissue calcification. *Radiology* 107:173, 1973.
15. Brown M, Thrall J, Cooper R, et al: Radiography and scintigraphy in tumoral calcinosis. *Radiology* 124:757, 1977.
16. Buetow PC, Kransdorf MJ, Moser RP, et al: Radiologic appearance of intramuscular hemangioma with emphasis on MR. *AJR Am J Roentgenol* 154:563, 1990.
17. Burrows PE, Mulliken JB, Fellows KE, et al: Childhood hemangiomas and vascular malformations: angiographic differentiation. *AJR* 141:483, 1983.
18. Bush CH, Spanier SS, Gillespy T: Imaging of atypical lipomas of the extremities: a report of three cases. *Skel Radiol* 17:472, 1988.
19. Cadman NL, Soule EH, Kelly PJ: Synovial sarcoma: an analysis of 134 tumors. *Cancer* 18:613, 1965.
20. Cerofolini E, Landi A, DeSantis G, et al: MR of benign peripheral nerve sheath tumors. *J Comput Assist Tomogr* 15:593, 1991.
21. Chang AE, Matory YL, Dwyer AJ, et al: Magnetic resonance imaging versus computed tomography in the evaluation of soft tissue tumors of the extremities. *Ann Surg* 205:240, 1987.
22. Cockshott WP, Evans KT: The place of soft tissue arteriography. *Br J Radiol* 37:367, 1964.
23. Cohen E, Kressel HY, Perosio T, et al: MR imaging of soft tissue hemangiomas: correlation with pathologic findings. *AJR Am J Roentgenol* 150:1079, 1988.
24. Cohen JM, Weinreb JC, Redman HC: Arteriovenous malformations of the extremities: MR imaging. *Radiology* 158:475, 1986.
25. Crim JR, Seegar LL, Yao L, et al: Diagnosis of soft tissue masses with MR imaging: can benign masses be differentiated from malignant ones? *Radiology* 185:581, 1992.
26. Dalinka MK, Zlatkin MB, Chao P, et al: Use of magnetic resonance imaging in the evaluation of bone and soft-tissue tumors. *Radiol Clin North Am* 28:461, 1990.
27. Davis B, Sundaram M, Kransdorf MJ: Synovial sarcoma: imaging findings in 34 patients. *AJR Am J Roentgenol* 161:827, 1993.
28. Delamater J: Mammoth tumor. *Cleveland Med Gaz* 1:31, 1859.
29. Demas BE, Heelan RT, Lane J, et al: Soft tissue sarcomas of the extremities: comparison of MR and CT in determining the extent of disease. *AJR Am J Roentgenol* 150:615, 1988.
30. Desai A, Eymontt M, Alavi A, et al: 99mTc-MDP uptake in nonosseous lesions. *Radiology* 135:181, 1980.
31. deSantos LA, Goldstein HM, Murray JA, et al: Computed tomography in the evaluation of musculoskeletal neoplasms. *Radiology* 128:89, 1978.
32. Dooms GC, Hricak H, Sotlitto RA, et al: Lipomatous tumors with fatty component: MR imaging potential and comparison of MR and CT results. *Radiology* 157:479, 1985.
33. Edelman RR: MR angiography: present and future. *AJR Am J Roentgenol* 161:1, 1993.
34. Edelman RR, Mattle HP, Atkinson DH, et al: MR angiography. *AJR Am J Roentgenol* 154:937, 1990.
35. Egund N, Ekelund L, Sako M, et al: CT of soft-tissue tumors. *AJR* 137:725, 1981.
36. Engelsted BL, Gilula LA, Kyriakos M: Ossified skeletal muscle hemangioma: radiologic and pathologic features. *Skel Radiol* 5:35, 1980.
37. Enneking WE: Staging of musculoskeletal neoplasms, from the Musculoskeletal Tumor Society. *Skel Radiol* 13:183, 1985.
38. Enneking WF, Spanier SS, Malawar MM: The effect of the anatomic setting on the results of surgical procedures for soft part sarcoma of the thigh. *Cancer* 47:1005, 1981.
39. Erlemann R, Reiser MF, Peters PE et al: Musculoskeletal neoplasms: static and dynamic Gd-DTPA-enhanced MR imaging. *Radiology* 171:767, 1989.
40. Erlemann R, Vassalio P, Bongartz G, et al: Musculoskeletal neoplasms: fast low-angle shot MR imaging with and without Gd-DTPA. *Radiology* 176:489, 1990.

41. Eugenidis N, Locher J: Tumoral calcinosis imaged by bone scanning: case report. *J Nucl Med* 18:34, 1977.

42. Feldman F, Singson RD, Staron RB: Magnetic resonance imaging of paraarticular and ectopic ganglia. *Skel Radiol* 18:353, 1989.

43. Finck EJ, Moore TM: Angiography for mass lesions of bone, joint, and soft tissue. *Orthop Clin North Am* 8:999, 1977.

44. Fornage BD, Rifkin MD: Ultrasound examination of the hand and foot. *Radiol Clin North Am* 26:109, 1988.

45. Frantzell A: Soft tissue radiography: technical aspects and clinical applications in the examination of limbs. *Acta Radiol* (suppl) 85:1, 1951.

46. Goldman AB: Myositis ossifcans circumscripta: a benign lesion with malignant differential diagnosis. *AJR* 126:32, 1976.

47. Grant EG, Gronvall S, Sarosi TE, et al: Sonographic findings in four cases of hemangiopericytoma. *Radiology* 142:447, 1982.

48. Greenfield GB, Arrington JA, Kudryk BT: MRI of soft tissue tumors. *Skel Radiol* 22:7, 1993.

49. Harkness J, Peters H: Tumoral calcinosis: a report of six cases. *J Bone Joint Surg* 49A:721, 1967.

50. Heelan RT, Watson RC, Smith J: Computed tomography of lower extremity tumors. *AJR* 132:933, 1979.

51. Heiken JP, Lee JKT, Smathers RL, et al: CT of benign soft-tissue masses of the extremities. *AJR* 142:575, 1984.

52. Hermann G, Abdelwahab IF, Miller TT, et al: Tumour and tumour-like conditions of the soft tissue: magnetic resonance imaging features differentiating benign from malignant masses. *Br J Radiol* 65:14, 1992.

53. Hermann G, Rose JS: Computed tomography in bone and soft tissue pathology of the extremities. *J Comput Assist Tomogr* 3:58, 1979.

54. Hermann G, Yeh HC, Lehr-James C, et al: Diagnosis of popliteal cysts: double-contrast arthrography and sonography. *AJR* 137:369, 1981.

55. Hernandez RJ, Keim DR, Chenevert TL, et al: Fat suppressed magnetic resonance imaging of myositis. *Radiology* 182:217, 1992.

56. Herzberg DL, Schreiber MH: Angiography in mass lesions of the extremities. *AJR* 111:541, 1971.

57. Horowitz AL, Resnick D, Watson RC: The roentgen features of synovial sarcomas. *Clin Radiol* 24:481, 1973.

58. Hudson TM, Hamlin DJ, Enneking WF, et al: Magnetic resonance imaging of bone and soft tissue tumors: early experience in 31 patients compared with computed tomography. *Skel Radiol* 13:134, 1985.

59. Hudson TM, Hass G, Enneking WF, et al: Angiography in the management of musculoskeletal tumors. *Surg Gynecol Obstet* 141:11, 1975.

60. Hunter JC, Johnston WH, Genant HK: Computed tomography evaluation of fatty tumors of the somatic soft tissues: clinical utility and radiologic-pathologic correlation. *Skel Radiol* 4:79, 1979.

61. Israels SJ, Chan HS, Daneman A, et al: Synovial sarcoma in childhood. *AJR* 142:803, 1984.

62. Jaffe N: Hemangiopericytoma: angiographic findings. *Br J Radiol* 33:614, 1960.

63. Jelinek JS, Kransdorf MJ, Shmookler BM, et al: Giant cell tumor of the tendon sheath: MR findings in nine cases. *AJR Am J Roentgenol* 162:919, 1994.

64. Jelinek JS, Kransdorf MJ, Shmookler BM, et al: Liposarcoma of the extremities: MR and CT findings of the histologic subtypes. *Radiology* 186:445, 1993.

65. Jelinek JS, Kransdorf MJ, Utz JA, et al: Imaging of pigmented villonodular synovitis with emphasis on magnetic resonance imaging. *AJR Am J Roentgenol* 152:337, 1989.

66. Jelinek JS, Kransdorf MJ, Utz JA, et al: Imaging of pigmented villonodular synovitis with emphasis on MR imaging. *AJR Am J Roentgenol* 152:337, 1989.

67. Jones BC, Sundaram M, Kransdorf MJ: Synovial sarcoma: MR imaging findings in 34 patients. *AJR Am J Roentgenol* 161:827, 1993.

68. Kaplan PA, Williams SM: Mucocutaneous and peripheral soft-tissue hemangiomas: MR imaging. *Radiology* 163:163, 1987.

69. Kaufman JH, Cedermark BJ, Parthasarathy KL, et al: The values of 67Ga scintigraphy in soft-tissue sarcoma and chondrosarcoma. *Radiology* 123:131, 1977.

70. Kilcoyne RF, Richardson ML, Porter BA, et al: Magnetic resonance imaging of soft tissue masses. *Clin Orthop Rel Res* 228:13, 1988.

71. Kransdorf MJ, Jelinek JS, Moser RP Jr, et al: Magnetic resonance appearance of fibromatosis: a report of 14 cases and review of the literature. *Skel Radiol* 19:495, 1990.

72. Kransdorf MJ, Jelinek JS, Moser RP, et al: MR appearance of fibromatosis: a report of 14 cases and review of the literature. *Skel Radiol* 19:495, 1990.

73. Kransdorf MJ, Jelinek JS, Moser RP Jr, et al: Soft tissue masses: diagnosis using MR imaging. *AJR Am J Roentgenol* 153:541, 1989.

74. Kransdorf MJ, McFarland DR, Moser RP, et al: Case report 649: arteriovenous malformation of the distal thigh with bone involvement. *Skel Radiol* 20:63, 1991.

75. Kransdorf MJ, Meis JM: Extraskeletal osseous and cartilaginous tumors of the extremities. *RadioGraphics* 13:853, 1993.

76. Kransdorf MJ, Meis JM, Jelinek JS: Dedifferentated liposarcoma of the extremities: imaging findings in four patients. *AJR Am J Roentgenol* 161:127, 1993.

77. Kransdorf MJ, Meis JM, Jelinek JS: Myositis ossifcans: MR appearance with radiologic-pathologic correlation. *AJR Am J Roentgenol* 157:1243, 1991.

78. Kransdorf MJ, Meis JM, Montgomery E: Elastofibroma: MR and CT appearance with radiologic-pathologic correlation. *AJR Am J Roentgenol* 159:575, 1992.

79. Kransdorf MJ, Moser RP, Jelinek J, et al: Intramuscular myxoma: MR features. *J Comput Assist Tomogr* 13:836, 1989.

80. Kransdorf MJ, Moser RP, Jelinek JS, et al: Soft tissue masses: diagnosis using MR imaging. *AJR Am J Roentgenol* 153:541, 1989.

81. Kransdorf MJ, Moser RP Jr, Madewell JE: Imaging techniques. In *Tumors of the hand and upper limb*. Bogumill GP, Fleegler EJ, McFarland GB, editors, New York, 1993, Churchill Livingstone.

82. Kransdorf MJ, Moser RP, Meis JM, et al: Fat containing soft tissue masses of the extremities. *RadioGraphics* 11:81, 1991.

83. Lafferty F, Reynolds E, Pearson O: Tumoral calcinosis: a metabolic disease of obscure etiology. *Am J Med* 38:105, 1965.

84. Lagergren C, Lindbom A: Angiography of peripheral tumors. *Radiology* 79:371, 1962.

85. Lagergren C, Lindblom A, Soderberg G: Vascularization of fibromatous and fibrosarcomatous tumors: histopathologic, microangiographic, and angiographic studies. *Acta Radiol* 53:1, 1960.

86. Lawson TL, Mittler S: Ultrasonic evaluation of extremity soft-tissue lesions with arthrographic correlation. *J Can Assoc Radiol* 29:58, 1978.

87. Lec KR, Cox GG, Neff JR, et al: Cystic masses of the knee: arthrographic and CT evaluation. *AJR* 148:329, 1987.

88. Levin DC, Gordon DH, McSweeney J: Arteriography of peripheral hemangiomas. *Radiology* 121:625, 1976.

89. Levin DC, Watson RC, Baltaxe HA: Arteriography in the diagnosis and management of acquired peripheral soft-tissue masses. *Radiology* 104:53, 1972.

90. Levin DN, Herrmann A, Spraggins T, et al: Improved visualization of musculoskeletal tumors using linear combinations of conventional MR images. In *Book of abstracts: Society of Magnetic Resonance in Medicine*, vol 5, Berkeley, California, 1986.

91. Levine E, Huntrakoon M, Wetzel LH: Malignant nerve-sheath neoplasms in neurofibromatosis: distinction from benign tumors by using imaging techniques. *AJR* 149:1059, 1987.

92. Levine E, Lee KR, Neff JR, et al: Comparison of computed tomog-

raphy and other imaging modalities in the evaluation of musculo-skeletal tumors. *Radiology* 131:431, 1979.

93. Levine E, Wetzel LH, Neff JR: MR imaging and CT of extrahe-patic cavernous hemangiogomas. *AJR* 147:1299, 1986.

94. Levinsohn EM, Bryan PJ: Computed tomography in unilateral ex-tremity swelling of unusual cause. *J Comput Assist Tomogr* 3:67, 1979.

95. Levitt RG, Sagel SS, Stanley RJ, et al: Computed tomography of the pelvis. *Semin Roentgenol* 13:193, 1978.

96. London J, Kim EE, Wallace S, et al: MR imaging of liposarcomas: correlation of MR features and histology. *J Compt Assist Tomogr* 18:832, 1989.

97. Mahajan H, Kim EE, Wallace S, et al: Magnetic resonance imaging of malignant fibrous histiocytoma. *Magn Reson Imaging* 7:283, 1989.

98. Margulis AR, Murphy TO: Arteriography in neoplasms of extremi-ties. *AJR* 80:330, 1958.

99. Martel W, Abell MR: Radiologic evaluation of soft tissue tumors. *Cancer* 32:352, 1973.

100. Matsui K, Yamada H, Chiba K, et al: Visualization of soft tissue malignancies by using 99mTc polyphosphate, pyrophosphate, and diphosphonate (99mTcP). *J Nucl Med* 14:632, 1973.

101. McLeod RA, Gisvold JJ, Stephens DH, et al: Computed tomogra-phy of soft tissues and breast. *Semin Roentgenol* 13:267, 1978.

102. McMaster MJ, Soule EH, Ivins JC: Hemangiopericytoma: a clini-copathologic study and long-term follow-up of 60 patients. *Cancer* 36: 2232, 1975.

103. McNeill TW, Chan GE, Capek V, et al: The value of angiography in the surgical management of deep hemangiomas. *Clin Orthop* 101:176, 1984.

104. Melson GL, Staple TW, Evens RG: Soft tissue radiographic tech-nique. *Semin Roentgenol* 8:19, 1973.

105. Meyer CA, Kransdorf MJ, Jelinek JS, et al: Case report 716: soft tissue metastasis in synovial sarcoma. *Skel Radiol* 21:128, 1992.

106. Meyer CA, Kransdorf MJ, Jelinek JS, et al: Radiologic appearance of nodular fasciitis with emphasis on MR and CT. *J Comput Assist Tomogr* 15:276, 1991.

107. Meyer JS, Hoffer FA, Barnes PD, et al: Biological classification of soft-tissue vascular anomalies: MR correlation. *AJR Am J Roent-genol* 157:559-564, 1991.

108. Mirowitz SA: Fast scanning and fat-suppression MR imaging of musculoskeletal disorders. *AJR Am J Roentgenol* 161:1147, 1993.

109. Mirowitz SA, Totty WG, Lee JK: Characterization of musculoskel-etal masses using dynamic GD-DTPA enhanced spin-echo MRI. *J Comput Assist Tomogr* 16:120, 1992.

110. Mitnick P, Goldfarb S, Slatopalsky E, et al: Calcium and phosphate metabolism in tumoral calcinosis. *Ann Intern Med* 92:482, 1980.

111. Moon KL, Genant HK, Helms CA, et al: Musculoskeletal applica-tions of nuclear magnetic resonance. *Radiology* 147:161, 1983.

112. Morton MJ, Berquist TH, McLeod RA, et al: MR imaging of syno-vial sarcoma. *AJR Am J Roentgenol* 156:337, 1991.

113. Mujahed Z, Vasilas A, Evans JA: Hemangiopericytoma: a report of four cases with a review of the literature. *AJR* 82:658, 1959.

114. Murphy WD, Hurst GC, Duerk JL, et al: Atypical appearance of lipomatous tumors on MR images: high signal intensity with fat-suppression STIR sequences. *J Magn Reson Imaging* 1:477, 1991.

115. Murray JA: Synovial sarcoma. *Orthop Clin North Am* 8:963, 1977.

116. Norman A, Dorfman HD: Juxtacortical circumscribed myositis os-sificans: evolution and radiographic features. *Radiology* 96:301, 1970.

117. Pathria MN, Zlatkin M, Sartoris DJ, et al: Ultrasonography of the popliteal fossa and lower extremities. *Radiol Clin North Am* 26:77, 1988.

118. Pearce WH, Rutherford RB, Whitehill TA, et al: Nuclear mag-netic resonance imaging: its diagnostic value in patients with congenital vascular malformations of the limbs. *J Vasc Surg* 8:64, 1988.

119. Petasnick JP, Turner DA, Charters JR, et al: Soft-tissue masses of the locomotor system: comparison of MR imaging with CT. *Radi-ology* 160:125, 1986.

120. Petterson H, Gillespy T, Hamlin DJ, et al: Primary musculoskeletal tumors: examination with MR imaging compared with conventional modalities. *Radiology* 164:237, 1987.

121. Petterson H, Hamlin DJ, Mancuso A, et al: Magnetic resonance im-aging of the musculoskeletal system. *Acta Radiol (Diagn) (Stockh)* 26:225, 1985.

122. Pirkey EL, Hurt J: Roentgen evaluation of the soft tissues in ortho-pedics. *AJR* 82:271, 1959.

123. Pope TL, Keats TE, de Lange EE, et al: Idiopathic synovial chon-dromatosis in two unusual sites: inferior radioulnar joint and ischial bursa. *Skel Radiol* 16:205, 1987.

124. Quinn SF, Erickson SJ, Dee PM, et al: MR imaging in fibroma-tosis: results in 26 patients with pathologic correlation. *AJR Am J Roentgenol* 156:539, 1991.

125. Rak KM, Yakes WF, Ray RL, et al: MR imaging of symptomatic peripheral vascular malformations. *AJR Am J Roentgenol* 159:107, 1992.

126. Rauch RF, Silverman PM, Korobkin M, et al: Computed tomogra-phy of benign angiomatous lesions of the extremities. *J Comput As-sist Tomogr* 8:1143, 1984.

127. Richman LS, Gumerman LW, Levine G, et al: Localization of Tc99m polyphosphate in soft tissue malignancies. *AJR* 124:577, 1975.

128. Rosenthal L: 99mTc-Methylene diphosphonate concentration in soft tissue malignant fibrous histiocytoma. *Clin Nucl Med* 3:58, 1978.

129. Russell WO, Cohen J, Cutler S, et al: Staging system for soft tissue sarcoma. American Joint Committee for Cancer Staging and End Re-sults Reporting: Task Force on Soft Tissue Sarcoma. Chicago, 1980, American College of Surgeons.

130. Savage RC, Mustafa EB: Giant cell tumors of tendon sheath (local-ized nodular tenosynovitis). *Ann Plastic Surg* 13:205, 1984.

131. Schumacher IM, Genant HK, Korobkin M, et al: Computed tomog-raphy: its use in space-occupying lesions of the musculoskeletal sys-tem. *J Bone Joint Surg* 60A:600, 1978.

132. Sherry CS, Harms SE: MR evaluation of giant cell tumors of ten-don sheath. *J Magn Reson Imaging* 7:195, 1989.

133. Shuman WP, Pattern RM, Baron RI, et al: Comparison of STIR and spin-echo MR imaging at 1.5T in 45 suspected extremity tumors: lesion conspicuity and extent. *Radiology* 179:247, 1991.

134. Soye I, Levine E, DeSmet AA, et al: Computed tomography in the preoperative evaluation of masses arising in or near the joints of the extremities. *Radiology* 143:727, 1982.

135. Stanley P, Miller JA: Angiography of extremity masses in children. *AJR* 130:1119, 1978.

136. Stout AP, Murray MR: Hemangiopericytoma: vascular tumor fea-turing Zimmerman's pericytes. *Ann Surg* 116:26, 1942.

137. Stull MA, Moser RP, Kransdorf MJ, et al: Magnetic resonance ap-pearance of peripheral nerve sheath tumors. *Skel Radiol* 20:9, 1991.

138. Sundaram M, Baran G, Merenda G, et al: Myxoid liposarcoma: mag-netic resonance imaging appearances with clinical and histologic cor-relation. *Skel Radiol* 19:359, 1990.

139. Sundaram M, McGuire MH, Fletcher J, et al: Magnetic resonance imaging of lesions of synovial origin. *Skel Radiol* 15:110, 1986.

140. Sundaram M, McGuire MH, Herbold DR, et al: High signal inten-sity soft tissue masses on T1 weighted pulsing sequences. *Skel Ra-diol* 16:30, 1987.

141. Sundaram M, McGuire MH, Herbold DR: Magnetic resonance im-aging of soft tissue masses: an evaluation of fifty-three histologically proven tumors. *Mag Res Imag* 6:237, 1988.

142. Sundaram M, McGuire MH, Schajowicz F: Soft tissue masses: his-

tologic basis for decreased signal (short T2) on T2-weighted MR images. *AJR* 148:1247, 1987.

143. Sundaram M, McLeod RA: MR imaging of tumor and tumorlike lesions of bone and soft tissue. *AJR Am J Roentgenol* 155:817, 1990.

144. Swensen SJ, Keller PL, Berquist TH, et al: Magnetic resonance imaging of hemorrhage. *AJR* 145:921, 1985.

145. Tehranzadeh J, Mnaymneh W, Ghavam C, et al: Comparison of CT and MR imaging in musculoskeletal neoplasms. *J Comput Assist Tomogr* 13:466, 1989.

146. Templeton AW, Stevens E, Jansen C: Arteriographic evaluation of soft tissue masses. *South Med J* 59:1255, 1966.

147. Thrall JH, Ghaed N, Geslien GE, et al: Pitfalls in Tc99m polyphosphate skeletal imaging. *AJR* 121:739, 1974.

148. Totterman S, Weis SL, Szumouski J, et al: MR fat suppression technique in the evaluation of normal structures of the knee. *J Comput Assist Tomogr* 13:473, 1989.

149. Totty WG, Murphy WA, Lee JKT: Soft-tissue tumors: MR imaging. *Radiology* 160:135, 1986.

150. Ushijma M, Hashimoto H, Tsuneyoshi M, et al: Giant cell tumor of the tendon sheath. *Cancer* 57:875, 1986.

151. Varma DG, Ayala AG, Guo SQ, et al: MRI of extraskeletal osteosarcoma. *J Comput Assist Tomogr* 17:414, 1993.

152. Viamonte M Jr, Roen S, Le Page J: Nonspecificity of abnormal vascularity in the angiographic diagnosis of malignant neoplasms. *Radiology* 106:59, 1973.

153. Weekes RG, Berquist TH, McLeod RA, et al: Magnetic resonance imaging of soft tissue tumors: comparison with computed tomography. *Mag Res Imag* 3:345, 1985.

154. Weekes RG, McLeod RA, Reiman HM, et al: CT of soft-tissue neoplasms. *AJR* 144:355, 1985.

155. Weinberger G, Levinsohn EM: Computed tomography in the evaluation of sarcomatous tumors of the thigh. *AJR* 130:115-118, 1978.

156. Wetzel LH, Levine E, Meuphy MD: A comparison of MR imaging and CT in the evaluation of musculoskeletal masses. *RadioGraphics* 7:851, 1987.

157. Wilbur J, Slatopalsky E: Hyperphosphatemia and tumoral calcinosis. *Ann Intern Med* 68:1044, 1980.

158. Wilson JS, Korobkin M, Genant HK, et al: Computed tomography of musculoskeletal disorders. *AJR* 131:55, 1978.

159. Yaghmai I: Angiographic manifestations of soft tissue and osseous hemangiopericytomas. *Radiology* 126:653, 1978.

PAUL S. MELTZER

CHAPTER 4

MOLECULAR BIOLOGY OF SOFT TISSUE TUMORS

The pathogenesis of cancer is one of the most complex problems in biology. Many aspects of the process by which a normal cell is transformed into a cancer cell remain elusive. However, modern cellular and molecular biology have had a profound impact on the understanding of carcinogenesis. This chapter will focus on the molecular biologic principles of soft tissue tumors, an aspect of tumor biology that has become central to the entire discipline. (For terms used in this chapter, see the glossary on p. 100.)

It has been suspected for decades that tumors arise by a multistep process involving sequential genetic alterations in normal progenitor cells. In this model, elaborated by Nowell, there is a selective advantage with each step, leading to clonal expansion and phenotypic transformation, until ultimately a fully malignant tumor develops.[90] It is now possible to assign specific genes to some of the steps involved in tumorigenesis, and techniques are available for elucidation of the remaining steps.[132] Even so, certain difficulties persist. For example, there is no single pathway by which all forms of cancer develop, but rather multiple genetic targets are altered in combination in a manner characteristic of each tumor category. The fact that multiple genetic alterations must occur before a cell becomes malignant explains the tendency of most cancers to occur in elderly people. Despite impressive technical advances, tumor biologists still are limited in their ability to study alterations in rare tumors or those that are difficult to cultivate in the laboratory, and there are still major gaps in the knowledge of the human genome. However, considering the current rate of progress, there is justifiable cause for optimism. It is reasonable to expect that the explosion of information in cancer genetics will lead to diagnostic refinements, reveal new prognostic markers, and ultimately identify novel therapeutic targets.

Many of the specific molecular events associated with human malignant tumors have been elucidated in hematopoietic neoplasms. Solid tumors have been less tractable, although in recent years, significant progress has been made

in the molecular analysis of these tumors as well. Despite their rarity compared with the intensively studied common solid tumors (such as colorectal carcinoma), important progress has been made in elucidating the molecular alterations present in soft tissue tumors. This has in part been due to the unanticipated relevance to soft tissue tumors of genes first recognized in other cancers. In other instances, highly tumor specific molecular genetic anomalies have been identified in individual soft tissue tumors.

TARGETS OF GENETIC ALTERATION IN HUMAN CANCERS
DNA recombinant technology

The development of recombinant DNA technology has tremendously facilitated analysis of the molecular events that occur during tumorigenesis. An understanding of the fundamental principles of molecular biology has become essential for readers of the current literature in oncology. The techniques used to characterize genes and gene expression in tumor cells all depend on the principle of base pair complementarity in the DNA double helix. DNA that has been rendered single stranded (denatured) readily returns to the double-stranded configuration, in which guanine is paired with cytosine and thymine with adenine (Fig. 4-1). Even though the human genome consists of over a billion base pairs, a segment of DNA corresponding to a specific gene will, under appropriate laboratory conditions, find the correct target sequence in single-stranded genomic DNA and form a double-stranded hybrid. If this segment of DNA is labelled so that it can be detected in the laboratory, it becomes a probe for the gene in question.

A DNA probe may be synthetic or may be a small segment of human DNA that has been propagated as a recombinant DNA clone in a microbial host. This cloned fragment can either be of genomic origin or prepared from messenger RNA (mRNA), in which case it is designated as complementary DNA (cDNA). Many human genes have been cloned and their DNA sequences determined. There is currently an international effort to identify the sequence of the entire human genome. Even now, while this process is incomplete, the intense interest in the genetic basis of cancer has made DNA sequences available for many genes related to cell growth and neoplasia.

Procedures based on the principle of DNA hybridization are exquisitely sensitive and can easily detect target molecules in the picogram range. Frequently these experiments are conducted using target nucleic acids (e.g., DNA or RNA extracted from tumor specimens) that have been immobilized to a solid support such as a nylon membrane. Detection of DNA that has been digested by a restriction endonuclease (an enzyme that cleaves DNA at a specific sequence) and size fractionated by gel electrophoresis and prior transfer to a solid support is referred to as Southern blot hybridization[120] (Fig. 4-2). The mRNA transcribed from a given gene can be similarly detected following electrophoresis and transfer to a membrane by means of the Northern blot procedure.

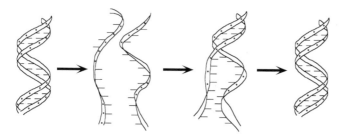

FIG. 4-1. The DNA double helix. Denaturing conditions dissociate the two strands, which can then reanneal to each other or to a complementary DNA probe.

Polymerase chain reaction. Recently, the polymerase chain reaction technique (PCR) has become extremely important in DNA analysis.[106] PCR uses specific synthetic oligonucleotides to amplify a section of a given gene in vitro. With automated equipment, it is possible to carry out this procedure in a few hours, starting with the DNA from a few cells (Fig. 4-3). This technique allows the analysis of genetic changes in DNA obtained by tumor biopsies, including paraffin-embedded material. PCR products can be analyzed for the presence of mutations by a variety of electrophoretic or hybridization techniques as well as DNA sequence analysis. With an additional step (reverse transcription), PCR can be carried out on RNA (RT-PCR). This is particularly useful in analysis of the abnormal mRNA that occurs in some tumors. Implementation of these and other related techniques has identified many of the genes that are critical for the growth of human cancers.

Genes contributing to tumorigenesis. Genes contributing to tumorigenesis fall into two broad categories: those that drive cells toward proliferation (oncogenes) and those that normally restrain cell proliferation (tumor suppressor genes).[61] The study of tumorigenic retroviruses in animal systems has led to the identification of numerous oncogenes.[12] Some retroviruses have acquired and subverted the function of host genes, which assist in growth and development when normally regulated but can cause neoplasia when aberrantly expressed or mutated. Other retroviruses inappropriately activate growth-promoting host genes on integration into the host genome. With a few important exceptions, the several dozen oncogenes identified in this fashion are not known to be targets of genetic alteration in human cancers. Their discovery has, however, contributed

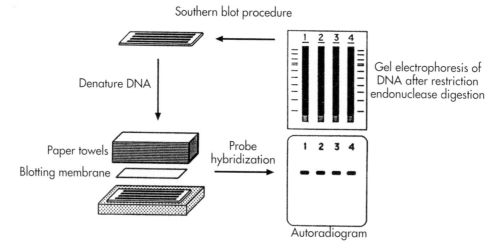

FIG. 4-2. The Southern blot procedure can be used to detect gross alterations in gene structure such as chromosome translocations and gene amplification. DNA fragments generated by restriction endonuclease cleavage are size fractionated by gel electrophoresis, transferred to a solid support, and detected by DNA hybridization.

tremendously to the elucidation of the complex regulatory networks that control the process of cell proliferation.

Mechanisms of oncogene activation in human cancers

Direct analysis of human tumors has led to the identification of a number of oncogenes of importance in human tumorigenesis. Two approaches have been particularly productive: DNA transfection and positional cloning.

DNA transfection. DNA transfection exploits the propensity of nontumorigenic immortalized cells (classically, NIH 3T3 cells) to take up exogenous tumor DNA and become transformed when they express a transferred oncogene.[95,126] Oncogenes identified by this process include the ras family of guanosine triphospate–binding proteins, which normally function in the transmission of mitogenic signals. Three members of this family, H-ras, K-ras, and N-ras, are now recognized in the human genome.[14] Remarkably, H-ras and K-ras had also been identified as retroviral oncogenes. DNA sequence analysis of the transforming ras genes has demonstrated that they have undergone point mutations. These mutations are not random but cluster in codons 12, 13, and 61, where they lead to amino acid substitutions that confer transforming activity by deregulating ras guanosine triphospatase activity. Analysis of ras mutations, which are now known to occur with varying frequency in a large variety of cancers, has provided decisive proof of the somatic mutation theory of cancer. These mutations are considered to be early steps in the development of colorectal and pancreatic carcinomas.

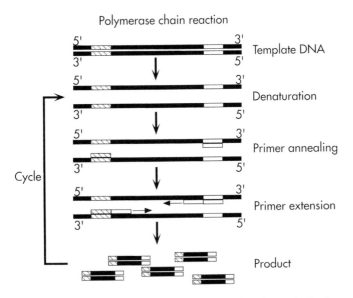

FIG. 4-3. The polymerase chain reaction (PCR) forms the basis of techniques used to analyze genes in minute specimens. PCR can generate microgram quantities of DNA starting from a few template molecules by successive cycles of denaturation, primer annealing, and primer extension.

Positional cloning. Although many human oncogenes fall outside the spectrum of sensitivity of the NIH 3T3 assay, alternative approaches have been productive. It would be a daunting task to search the billions of nucleotides in the human genome for oncogenic mutations. Fortunately, in many cases markers have been provided in the form of tumor-specific chromosome translocations. Although most of these have been described in hematopoietic neoplasms,[97] several have been described in solid tumors (see Chapter 5). The presence of a specific translocation facilitates the positional cloning of the gene at the breakpoint. Numerous translocation breakpoints have been analyzed in leukemias and lymphomas.[11] Two general categories of events have been described. One category of translocations leads to overexpression of an oncogene that has been translocated into a chromosomal region associated with immunoglobulin genes or T cell receptor genes. Because these gene clusters have been intensively studied, it is relatively straightforward to characterize translocations in these regions. Positive regulatory elements derived from lymphoid-specific genes presumably act on the translocated oncogene, leading to inappropriately high levels of oncogene expression. For example, in the t(8;14) translocation, which occurs in Burkitt's lymphoma, the myc oncogene is translocated into the immunoglobulin heavy chain locus.[23] The second category of translocations involves the juxtaposition of two genes, one from each translocation partner, resulting in the formation of a fusion gene product. This is an abnormal protein that is never seen in any normal cell and that is highly characteristic of the malignant disorder in which it is found. This is the underlying molecular event in the t(9;22) chromosome in chronic myelogenous leukemia, which fuses the bcr and abl genes.[27,44] All of the soft tissue tumor–specific translocations characterized to date result in the formation of fusion proteins (see discussion below).

Gene amplification. Gene amplification can be defined as the accumulation of additional copies of a gene out of proportion to a cell's modal chromosome number.[55] This phenomenon was originally studied in tissue culture cells that had acquired resistance to methotrexate through exposure to incrementally increased concentrations of the drug in the medium. Although a number of mechanisms may contribute to this phenomenon, resistance is frequently associated with accumulation of extra copies of the gene-encoding dihydrofolate reductase (dhfr), the target of methotrexate action. Increased transcription from the increased copies of the dhfr gene leads to increased production of the dhfr protein. Cytologically, the increased copies of the dhfr gene can be localized either extrachromosomally, as small paired chromatin bodies called double minutes (dmins), or intrachromosomally, as homogeneously staining regions (hsrs). Although originally described in the mtx/dhfr system, a similar phenomenon has been described with multiple additional selective agents. Gene amplification can be viewed as a mechanism by which cells can acquire increased expression of genes that confer a selective advantage. The propensity to undergo gene amplification is clearly enhanced in malignant cells. Although the mechanisms underlying this phenomenon are incompletely understood, gene amplification is a factor in the genetic instability of cancer cells that in some experimental systems can be related to specific abnormalities such as alterations in the p53 gene.[80] In view of these considerations, it is not surprising that amplification of several genes has been described in tumor specimens. However, in contrast to the in vitro systems described above, the targets of spontaneous amplification in tumor cells are oncogenes rather than drug resistance genes. In this situation, oncogene amplification can be viewed as a genetic alteration that contributes a proliferative advantage to a clone of tumor cells, which then comes to predominate in the tumor population. Amplification of a given gene can be readily determined in tumor specimens by the Southern blot procedure, PCR, or fluorescence in situ hybridization (FISH) analysis.

Oncogene amplification has been described in a wide variety of cancers, including soft tissue tumors.[3] Cytogenetic studies frequently show gene amplification through the identification of hsrs and dmins. Once amplified DNA has been identified in tumor cells, the next step is identification of the target gene encoded in the amplified sequences that drives the amplification process. When a well-known oncogene is mapped to the amplified region (e.g., N-myc in neuroblastoma), this may be straightforward, but not all genes are so easily found. Because the amount of DNA in dmins and hsrs may be extensive, several genes may be contained in the amplified region. Characterization of these genes and their patterns of amplification and expression in many tumors is necessary to define the actual target gene.

Tumor suppressor genes

If normal cells are induced to fuse with tumor cells, the hybrid cells frequently lose their ability to form tumors in experimental animals.[121] This effect depends on the introduction of specific normal chromosomes, suggesting that normal genes may suppress the ability of a cancer cell to form tumors. This is the operational definition of the term *tumor suppressor gene.* Tumor suppressor genes may be inactivated by somatic mutation, either by changes at the DNA sequencing level or by gross rearrangement. In the latter case, loss of an allele in tumor cells may be defined with polymorphic DNA markers. Such loss of heterozygosity studies are an important tool in mapping regions of chromosomal loss in tumors. Ideally this lengthy process concludes with identification of a gene that undergoes somatic mutation in tumors and suppresses tumorigenicity when reintroduced into tumor cells.

Rb tumor suppressor gene. Genetic analysis of tumors has identified several tumor suppressor genes. Two of these, p53 and Rb, are of particular relevance to soft tissue tumors. Rb, the hereditary retinoblastoma gene, is the prototypic tumor suppressor. Knudson's observations of the rate of onset of sporadic versus hereditary retinoblastoma led him to the "two-hit" hypothesis, which correctly predicted that two mutations were necessary for initiation of retinoblastoma.[62,63] In hereditary cases, one mutation has already occurred in the germline, accounting for early onset and high tumor probability (multifocality and bilaterality). In sporadic cases, the coincidence of two mutational events taking place in a single cell is much less frequent, resulting in unilateral disease of later onset. The Rb gene was identified by positional cloning relative to markers associated with hereditary retinoblastoma.[35,36,72] It is a nuclear phosphoprotein that appears to have a central role in cell cycle regulation.[45,79] It has binding affinity for other cell cycle proteins, and this affinity is modulated by cyclic phosphorylation during the cell cycle. It is not clear why germline mutations have such a strongly tissue-specific oncogenic effect resulting in early-onset retinoblastoma. Most likely, this is related to the existence of parallel regulatory pathways in most cell lines. It should be noted that in patients with hereditary retinoblastoma, the oncogenic propensity conferred by the Rb mutation is not strictly limited to retinoblastoma. These patients have a high risk of developing second cancers, particularly sarcomas.[31] Although some of these occur within prior orbital radiation fields, many originate outside of the field and must be related to the underlying genetic lesion. It is therefore not surprising, as discussed below, to find that sporadic cancers also acquire defects in the Rb gene.

p53 tumor suppressor gene. Among the most intensively studied tumor suppressor genes is the p53 gene, which was originally identified as a tumor antigen in SV40-infected cells.[74,133] Because of its increased expression in tumor cells, it was initially misclassified as an oncogene. Loss of heterozygosity analysis of colorectal cancer suggested the importance of a gene on chromosome 17p in the region where p53 had been previously mapped. When the DNA sequence of the remaining p53 allele was determined, inactivating mutations were identified.[6] It is now recognized that the normal p53 gene functions to restrain cell growth and that mutations in this gene can act to promote unregulated cell growth. Hundreds of examples of p53 mutations have been identified in a wide variety of human cancers.[47] The mutations are not distributed at random but cluster at certain highly conserved locations in the p53 gene. Mutations can exist in one p53 allele in tumors that also retain a normal allele. In these cases, biochemical evidence suggests that the mutant allele can act in a dominant negative fashion to inactivate the normal gene.[56] Some tumors have undergone complete inactivation of both genes, resulting in total loss of p53 function. Gene transfer experiments that restore a normal p53 gene to tumor cells carrying a defective p53 gene confirm that the p53 gene has tumor suppressor properties. Although the precise function of the p53 gene is as yet incompletely understood, current evidence suggests that the gene is a key regulator of the cell cycle through its function as a transcription factor regulating the expression of other genes. Recently WAF1, an important gene induced by p53, has been identified.[30] WAF1 exerts an inhibitory effect on the cyclin kinase/cyclin pathway and provides a direct biochemical connection between p53 and the cell cycle. Although somatic alterations of WAF1 have not been identified as yet in tumors, a similar negative regulator of the cyclin kinase/cyclin pathway, p16, has recently been identified and mapped to a region of chromosome 9 altered in melanoma.[113] This gene is also designated MTS1 (for multiple tumor suppressor) because it has been altered in a large number of cancers. Its role in soft tissue tumors is undefined at the present time.

Transgenic mouse technology. Transgenic mouse technology has become an important tool for studying gene function.[2] It is possible to both insert exogenous genes and delete normal genes from the mouse germline. Mice lacking a functional p53 gene are viable but highly prone to developing tumors.[29,41] In heterozygous mice (carrying only one functional p53 allele) osteosarcoma developed (32%), as did lymphoma (32%), hemangiosarcoma (10%), rhabdomyosarcoma (5%), undifferentiated sarcoma (3%), malignant schwannoma (3%), and a variety of less frequent tumors. In mice carrying homozygous defective p53 genes tumors developed more rapidly than those carrying heterozygous genes, with a preponderance of lymphoma (59%), hemangiosarcoma (18%), testicular tumors (7%), and undifferentiated sarcoma (5%). The mouse model can be compared with the phenotype observed in kindreds with the Li-Fraumeni cancer syndrome who carry germline mutations in the p53 gene.[83-85] These patients are predisposed to a characteristic constellation of tumors,[124] usually bone and soft tissue sarcomas, brain tumors, breast cancer, adrenal cortical carcinoma, and leukemia. As with all hereditary cancer syndromes, onset is early, with cancer risk near 50% by the age of 35 years. Fortunately, new germline mutations in p53 appear to be quite rare, and therefore account for only a minority of the sporadic tumors that fall within the Li-Fraumeni spectrum. It is reasonable to suspect germline p53 mutation in patients with a family history consistent with Li-Fraumeni syndrome or in individuals in whom two independent primary tumors with appropriate histologic characteristics develop.[75,84]

Defects in DNA mismatch repair

Recently, a new category of genetic alteration has been recognized in human cancers. Initial observations using PCR to amplify polymorphic dinucleotide repeat sequences in tumor specimens (a procedure used to identify loss of heterozygosity) unexpectedly revealed sequences of altered repeat length in tumor DNA that were not present in normal DNA.[1,50,128] These must have arisen from somatic mutation during DNA replication. This phenotype of somatic dinucleotide repeat instability has been associated with hereditary nonpolyposis colon cancer syndrome (HNPCC). Two genes have been identified, hMSH2 and hMLH1, which are mutated in HNPCC kindreds linked to chromosomes 2 and 3, respectively.[69,94] These genes are part of the DNA mismatch error repair system, and cells from HNPCC patients are highly defective in DNA repair.[96] This defect probably contributes to the evolution of cancer in these families through an increased rate of somatic mutation at other sites. The full scope of this phenomenon in the genetic basis of solid tumors is not yet established. The DNA replication error phenotype is not confined to HNPCC families or to the tumors associated with this syndrome (colorectal, endometrial, and ovarian carcinomas). It has also been found in apparently sporadic colorectal tumors as well as non-HNPCC tumors. It is not yet known if this phenomenon is important in soft tissue tumors.

GENETIC ALTERATIONS IN SOFT TISSUE TUMORS

As the genetic targets of tumorigenesis are uncovered, their role in the full spectrum of human tumors is gradually being defined. Because DNA is stable in banked frozen tissues, it is quite feasible to perform retrospective analyses. A few milligrams of tumor tissue provides enough DNA for several Southern blot procedures. PCR-based methods[106] require only a few cells for analysis and can be applied to paraffin-embedded material. Although PCR is capable of amplifying a given gene from minute specimens, PCR products typically span only a few hundred base pairs, and multiple reactions are necessary to fully characterize a given gene. Techniques for screening PCR products for mutation include differential oligonucleotide hybridization and gel electrophoresis techniques such as the single-stranded conformation polymorphism assay (SSCP) or denaturing gradient gel electrophoresis (DGGE).[42,48,82] The ultimate validation of SSCP or DGGE data as well as the precise characterization of mutations depends on DNA sequence analysis. All current techniques favor the analysis of smaller genes or those in which mutations tend to cluster (such as p53). Large genes (such as Rb) pose greater difficulties for screening. In general, unless the entire gene in question is sequenced, the data obtained by screening tests will tend to underestimate the true frequency of mutation.[43]

Tumor suppressor genes in soft tissue tumors

Although all of the currently recognized tumor suppressor genes were originally discovered in other cancers, several of these genes have considerable relevance to soft tissue tumors. Observations of p53 mutations in Li-Fraumeni syndrome, the occurrence of sarcomas in survivors of hereditary retinoblastoma, and the rare association of sarcomas with some familial cancer syndromes have motivated the study of these genes in soft tissue tumors.

p53 gene mutations. Because most inactivating mutations of p53 are concentrated in a relatively small region, the application of PCR-based techniques to p53 is particularly straightforward.[13] Additionally, immunohistochemical studies have frequently been used as surrogates for DNA analysis of p53.[11] Immunohistochemical procedures, which are less definitive than DNA sequencing, exploit the tendency of mutant forms of p53 to accumulate to much higher levels than are observed for the wild-type protein. Only relatively small series have been analyzed with either technique, limiting the precision with which the incidence of p53 mutation can be estimated in each diagnostic category. Nonetheless, there are sufficient data to establish a role for p53 mutation in the evolution of certain soft tissue tumors (Table 4-1). Both point mutation and gross defects of the p53 gene have been observed. In malignant fibrous histiocytoma, leiomyosarcoma, liposarcoma, and rhabdomyosar-

Table 4-1. Role of p53 mutation in evolution of some soft tissue tumors

Tumor	Abnormal genes per total tumors	Method
Angiosarcoma	2 of 4	PCR and sequencing[46]
Ewing's sarcoma	2 of 8	PCR and sequencing[64]
	1 of 19	PCR and sequencing[65]
	0 of 5	PCR and sequencing plus Southern[129]
Fibrosarcoma	1 of 2	PCR and sequencing plus Southern[129]
Leiomyosarcoma	2 of 6	PCR and sequencing[5]
	4 of 8	Immunohistochemical procedures[118]
	1 of 4	Immunohistochemical procedures[78]
Liposarcoma	1 of 4	Immunohistochemical procedures[118]
	1 of 4	PCR and sequencing plus Southern[129]
Malignant fibrous histiocytoma	4 of 11	Immunohistochemical procedures[134]
	4 of 14	Immunohistochemical procedures[118]
	3 of 12	PCR and sequencing[5]
	4 of 13	PCR and sequencing plus Southern[129]
Rhabdomyosarcoma	2 of 6	PCR and sequencing plus Southern[33]
Synovial sarcoma	0 of 5	PCR and sequencing plus Southern[129]

coma, p53 abnormalities are identifiable in 20% to 30% of cases.[5,33,78,118,129] In contrast, p53 mutations do not appear to be important in neuroblastoma.[25,49,64,131] There is a significant incidence of p53 mutation in osteosarcoma* and Ewing's sarcoma,[64,134] but there are insufficient data as to whether the extraosseous variants of these tumors have a similar pattern of mutation. In some instances, the precise pattern of p53 alteration may be relevant to mechanisms of damage by carcinogens. For example, in a study of angiosarcomas of the liver in patients exposed to vinyl chloride, two of four cases carried A to T missense transversions in p53.[46] Molecular epidemiological studies of this type may open new possibilities for cancer prevention.

Rb gene mutations. The retinoblastoma gene is significantly larger than p53 and is proportionately more difficult to study, so that only limited data are available. In sarcomas, total or partial gene deletions appear to be important mechanisms of Rb inactivation. This type of event is clearly important in osteosarcoma,[100] but less information is available for soft tissue sarcomas. In a study of the Rb gene at the gross structural level in DNA and RNA from a series of soft tissue sarcomas, Rb deletions were found in two of five malignant fibrous histiocytomas, two of four liposarcomas, one of one extraosseous osteosarcoma, and one of one mesenchymoma, and they were absent from the few cases studied of leiomyosarcoma, hemangiopericytoma, and extraosseous chondrosarcoma.[137] Expression of Rb was identifiable in normal muscle and adipose tissue but missing or aberrant in all tumors studied. Additional examples of deletion and rearrangement of Rb have been reported in single cases of spindle cell sarcoma, leiomyosarcoma, and fibrosarcoma.[123] Rearrangement was accompanied by loss of the normal allele. Of interest, spindle cell sarcoma also had rearrangement of the p53 gene. In contrast, genetic alteration or reduced expression of Rb was not found in 18 rhabdomyosarcoma specimens.[26] Given the spectrum of second cancers observed in survivors of bilateral retinoblastoma, it is likely that as improved procedures for scanning large genes become available, a significant role for Rb alteration will become apparent in some soft tissue tumors.

NF1 gene mutations. Neurofibromatosis type 1 (von Recklinghausen's disease) is now known to be due to defects in the NF1 gene on chromosome 17.[86] At the biochemical level, NF1 functions as a guanosine triphosphatase–associated protein (GAP) with a negative regulatory influence on the ras gene.[40] It therefore can be considered a candidate tumor suppressor gene. Interestingly, although the typical neurofibromas of NF1 patients are clonal in origin, they do not show loss of heterozygosity for chromosome 17 alleles.[101] In contrast, malignant tumors arising in NF1 patients have shown loss of chromosome 17 alleles consistent with the second "hit" predicted by Knudson's hypoth-

*References 5, 19, 108, 116, 129, 134.

esis.[38,76,81,138] In the best-studied example, a neurofibrosarcoma arising in an NF1 patient showed loss of heterozygosity in the NF1 region and a tumor-associated deletion in the NF1 gene in the remaining copy.[73] In addition, a few sporadic somatic mutations of NF1 have been identified in various cancers, including neuroblastoma (two cell lines), individual cases of anaplastic astrocytoma, myelodysplastic syndrome, and colorectal carcinoma.[52,76,127] Another study failed to find NF1 mutations by PCR-SSCP analysis of 50 neuroblastoma specimens.[49] It will be interesting to define the role of NF1 in sporadic tumors.

APC gene mutations. It is now recognized that both familial adenomatous polyposis and Gardner's syndrome are associated with mutations in the APC (adenomatosis polyposis coli) gene on chromosome 5q.[32,89] The APC gene has recently been implicated in cell adhesion by demonstration that it has affinity for the E-cadherin-binding protein β-catenin.[125] In the context of this volume, desmoid tumors are the principle soft tumor associated with Gardner's syndrome. Although there is limited information on alterations of the APC gene in sporadic desmoid tumors, deletions of 5q suggestive of loss of heterozygosity for the APC region have been described in sporadic desmoid tumors as well as those occurring in Gardner's syndrome.[15,112] APC mutation appears to be one of the earliest events in the progression of sporadic colorectal carcinoma found in some benign adenomas. In this regard it is particularly interesting to note the occurrence of germline mutations in the basement membrane collagen genes COL4A5 and COL4A6 in patients with Alport's syndrome with diffuse leiomyomatosis.[141] Alport's syndrome is an X-linked disorder characterized by renal failure, sensorineural deafness, and ocular lesions. Some families are also affected by diffuse leiomyomatosis of the esophagus, female genitalia, and trachea. Alport's syndrome without diffuse leiomyomatosis is characterized by defects in COL4A5, while Alport's syndrome with diffuse leiomyomatosis is characterized by defects in both genes. Although the mechanistic relationship between the basement membrane and smooth muscle proliferation is not fully defined, this observation is quite striking in view of the relationship of APC to desmoid tumors and highlights the relationship between the determinants of tissue structure and the regulation of cell proliferation.

Other tumor suppressor gene mutations. No significant data are available implicating any of the other known tumor suppressor genes in soft tissue tumors, and it is likely that many of the relevant genetic targets have yet to be identified. A number of approaches are being used to search for novel tumor suppressor genes in various cancers.[22,105,135] Polymorphic DNA markers can be used to compare normal and tumor tissues from the same individual, thereby detecting loss of chromosomal segments in a given tumor. A molecular cytogenetic technique, comparative genome hybridization, can be used to screen the entire genome of a tumor cell for chromosomal gains and losses.[54] Techniques based on gene expression, such as differential display, have been used to look for genes with reduced expression in tumor tissue relative to their normal progenitor.[77] Using these and other approaches, several chromosomal regions that may be relevant to soft tissue tumors are currently being characterized. Among the loci likely to contain a tumor suppressor gene is the 1p36 region, which is frequently deleted in neuroblastoma.[16] Although identification of genes that are inactivated in tumors remains a complex and challenging process, careful comparison of normal and tumor tissues can be expected to define additional specific targets of genetic loss in sarcomas.

Ras gene activation

Mutations of the ras gene are known to occur in soft tissue sarcomas, but studies to date are quite limited. In one recent study, H-ras mutations were found in codon 12 in two of six malignant fibrous histiocytomas and one of three embryonal rhabdomyosarcomas, and they were absent from one case each of alveolar rhabdomyosarocma, pleomorphic rhabdomyosarcoma, and leiomyosarcoma.[136] In angiosarcomas in workers exposed to vinyl chloride, K-ras mutations were identified in codon 13 in five of six tumors.[87] Given this information, it would be of some interest to thoroughly examine larger series for the full spectrum of ras mutations.

Tumor-specific translocations

Analysis of hematopoietic tumors was accelerated tremendously by the recognition of disease-specific chromosomal translocations such as t(9;22) in chronic myelogenous leukemia and t(8;14) in Burkitt's lymphoma. These examples illustrate the two basic themes developed by the analysis of many additional translocations. In one group of translocations, as exemplified by t(9;22), the rearranged chromosome leads to the generation of a chimeric fusion protein composed of sequences derived from two distinct genes, one of which is contributed by each of the partner chromosomes. This fusion product is never present in any normal cell, and its presence confers a proliferative advantage on the malignant cell. In the second category of translocation, as illustrated by t(8;14), an oncogene on one chromosome is juxtaposed with a positive regulatory element from another chromosome. The resultant oncogene overexpression is presumed to exert a growth-promoting effect. Several soft tissue tumor–specific translocations have now been characterized at the molecular level. Although it would be premature to make sweeping generalizations from these examples, to date all translocations cloned from soft tissue tumors resemble t(9;22) in that they lead to the creation of unique tumor-specific fusion proteins. The biochemical mechanisms by which these proteins contribute to tumor growth remain to be fully elucidated. However, their consistent presence in tumors of a given histological type and the nature of the genes involved provide a strong basis for concluding that these fusion proteins must be central to the pathogenesis of the tumors in which they occur. Four examples will be discussed below: t(12;16) in myxoid liposarcoma, t(11;22) in Ewing's sarcoma and peripheral neuroepithelioma, t(12;22) in clear cell sarcoma, and t(2;13) in alveolar rhabdomyosarcoma. The finding of these closely related translocations in clinically variable tumors raises important questions about the categorization of these disorders.

Myxoid liposarcoma. Myxoid liposarcoma is characterized by the presence of t(12;16). Through a candidate gene approach, a transcription factor designated CHOP was mapped to the breakpoint.[4] CHOP is a member of the C/EBP family of transcription factors, which is not expressed in proliferating cells but is induced by growth arrest or DNA damage and probably exerts an antiproliferative effect.[103] It contains a dimerization domain of the bZIP type through which it can interact with other proteins, its principle partner being the C/EBPβ transcription factor. Probes for CHOP recognize altered restriction fragments on Southern blot analysis of myxoid liposarcoma DNA (Fig. 4-4). The rearranged CHOP gene is joined to a previously unknown protein, which has been variably called TLS (translocated in liposarcoma) and FUS (Fig. 4-5).[24,98] Structural analysis of this protein reveals 55.6% identity with the EWS gene, target of the Ewing's sarcoma translocation (discussed below). The normal function of TLS/FUS is unknown. It is a nuclear protein, and its C-terminal portion, like that of EWS, contains an RNA-binding domain. The N-terminal domains of both genes contain multiple copies of the hexapeptide Ser/Gly-Tyr-Ser/Gly-Gln-Gln/Ser-Ser/Gln/Pro. In myxoid liposarcoma, a fusion transcript is expressed from t(12;16), in which the RNA-binding domain of TLS/FUS is replaced by CHOP sequences, including the bZIP dimerization domain. The few examples of fusion mRNA characterized to date predict the same peptide sequence at the TLS/CHOP junction. The mechanism by which the TLS/CHOP fusion protein promotes the proliferation of myxoid liposarcoma cells is not yet clear, but comparison with Ewing's sarcoma suggests that the operative mechanism will prove to be important in the growth of soft tissue tumors.

Ewing's sarcoma. A characteristic recurrent t(11;22) occurs in Ewing's sarcoma (both osseous and extraosseous) and peripheral neuroepithelioma. This is now the best-studied example of a solid tumor chromosome translocation. This rearrangement leads to the juxtaposition of a gene designated EWS on chromosome 22 with the FLI-1 gene on chromosome 11 (Fig. 4-6).[28] The normal function of EWS is unknown. However, it contains an RNA-binding domain in its C-terminal portion and a region with transcriptional activating properties in its N-terminal half. FLI-1 is

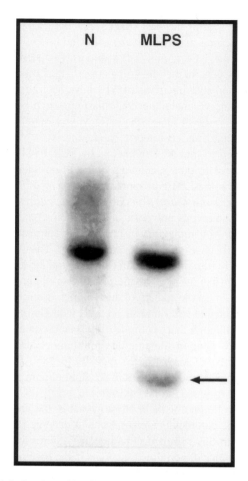

FIG. 4-4. Southern blot illustrating rearrangement of the CHOP gene in myxoid liposarcoma. Tumor DNA *(right lane)* contains an extra band derived from the t(12;16) translocation, which is not present in normal DNA *(left lane).*

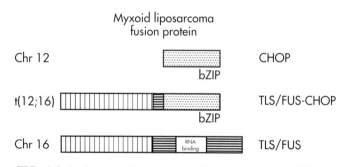

FIG. 4-5. In the myxoid liposarcoma fusion protein, the CHOP transcription factor provides sequences that replace the RNA-binding domain in TLS/FUS.

a member of the ETS family of transcription factors and is known to contain a DNA-binding domain.[99,140] The EWS-FLI fusion protein replaces the RNA-binding domain with sequences from FLI-1. In the initial cases studied, the entire DNA-binding domain and C-terminus of FLI-1 were

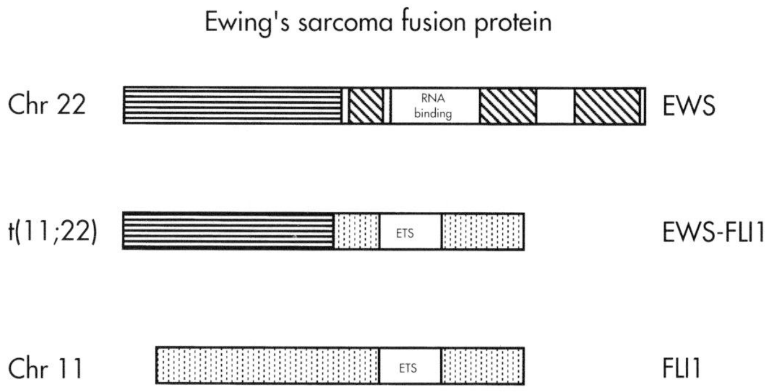

Ewing's sarcoma fusion protein

Chr 22 — EWS

t(11;22) — EWS-FLI1

Chr 11 — FLI1

FIG. 4-6. In the Ewing's sarcoma fusion protein, the ETS DNA-binding protein provides sequences that replace the EWS RNA-binding domain.

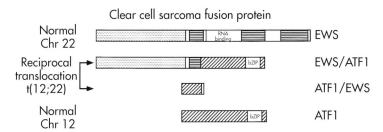

Clear cell sarcoma fusion protein

Normal Chr 22 — EWS

Reciprocal translocation t(12;22) — EWS/ATF1

ATF1/EWS

Normal Chr 12 — ATF1

FIG. 4-7. In the clear cell sarcoma fusion protein, DNA-binding sequences from ATF1 replace the EWS RNA-binding domain (EWS/ATF1). The shorter predicted mRNA from the reciprocal translocation (ATF1/EWS) is sometimes also expressed but probably is biologically inactive.

contributed to the fusion protein. This would suggest that an abnormal protein is formed that retains the effector portion of EWS, with its usual RNA-binding function replaced by the DNA-binding activity of FLI-1. Biochemical studies have demonstrated that the fusion protein is a potent transcriptional activator.[88] In a series of 89 Ewing's sarcomas and peripheral neuroepitheliomas, the breakpoints in the EWS and FLI-1 genes were identified in 80 and 66 cases, respectively. EWS always contributed at least its first seven exons, including the transcriptional activating domain, to the fusion protein, with the breaks tending to fall in a hinge region that joins this region to the RNA-binding domain.[143] The contribution of FLI-1 was considerably more variable. Of considerable interest, in 13 cases, EWS was joined not to FLI-1 but to a closely related gene, ERG, normally found on chromosome 21. Although occasional aberrations of chromosome 21 had been previously described, a balanced t(21;22) has not been described. The EWS-ERG fusion proteins have a similar structure and range of breakpoints within ERG to the EWS-FLI fusion proteins.

From a diagnostic perspective, the complexity of these rearrangements poses some problems. The ability to verify the presence of EWS rearrangements by molecular techniques means that it is possible to unambiguously place a

small round blue cell tumor in the group of disorders characterized by EWS rearrangements.[122] However, the variability of the breakpoints places significant demands on the laboratory performing the analysis. If Southern blot procedures are used, multiple probes that scan the EWS gene must be employed to be certain that a rearrangement will be detected. Determining the presence of a fusion protein by RT-PCR is more rapid, but the existence of multiple partners for EWS means that multiple primer pairs must be used to be assured of finding the fusion transcript.[67,119] In addition, samples must be processed in the operating room with appropriate techniques to allow preservation of RNA.

Clear cell sarcoma. Clear cell sarcoma (also referred to as malignant melanoma of soft parts) contains a t(12;22) translocation that, remarkably, also involves the EWS gene[142] (Fig. 4-7). As in Ewing's sarcoma, in clear cell sarcoma the RNA-binding domain of the EWS gene is replaced by sequences from the transcription factor ATF-1. With this example, the theme of replacement of an RNA-binding domain (in EWS or FUS/TLS) with sequences from a DNA-binding protein (ATF-1, CHOP, FLI-1, or ERG) becomes even more striking.

Alveolar rhabdomyosarcoma. Alveolar rhabdomyosarcoma cells exhibit a t(2;13) translocation. The genetic consequences of this rearrangement have been deter-

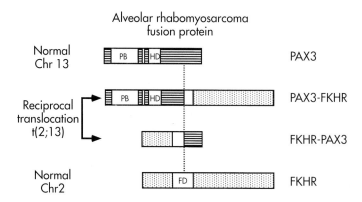

FIG. 4-8. In the alveolar rhabdomyosarcoma fusion protein, sequences from PAX3 are joined to sequences from FKHR, generating a chimeric transcription factor. Two chimeric proteins are potentially formed by the reciprocal translocation, but based on the pattern of expression, the PAX3-FKHR protein is the oncogenic product. *FD*, Forkhead domain; *HD*, homeodomain; *PB*, paired box.

mined[8,37,114] (Fig. 4-8). As in the case of myxoid liposarcoma, a candidate gene approach was successful in defining the translocation breakpoint, which involves the paired box transcription factor PAX3. Interestingly, mutations in PAX3 give rise to Waardenburg's syndrome (which is characterized by partial albinism and deafness). Sequence analysis of the chromosome 13 gene (which has been designated by different groups as FKHR or ALV) identifies it as a member of the forkhead (so named because of the phenotype caused by mutations in the *Drosophila* homolog) domain family of transcription factors. The predicted fusion transcript was found in each of eight alveolar rhabdomyosarcoma cell lines analyzed.[37] As in the translocation discussed above, the mechanism underlying the oncogenic impact of the PAX3-FKHR fusion product is unknown. While neither of these proteins has the RNA-binding domain found in EWS or TLS/FUS, the fusion protein is also a transcription factor. It is likely, therefore, that a common pathway in all of these examples will involve the impact of deregulated gene expression on cell proliferation.

Additional examples of tumor-specific recurrent translocations will soon be added to those discussed above. In one instance, the t(X;18) translocation found in synovial sarcoma, detailed molecular characterization is imminent. It can be anticipated with confidence that the genetic targets of multiple additional solid tumor translocations will be elucidated within the next several years.

Gene amplification in soft tissue tumors

Gene amplification is one of the more frequent molecular alterations in soft tissue tumors. The most intensively studied example is amplification of the N-myc oncogene in neuroblastoma. It might be expected that oncogene amplification would be associated with more aggressive clinical behavior. Initially recognized by virtue of its similarity to the c-myc oncogene, N-myc belongs to the helix-loop-helix family of transcription factors.[109] Amplified N-myc sequences in tumors are usually carried extrachromosomally as dmins that can integrate and form hsrs on culture.[110] A particularly striking feature of N-myc amplification is the high level of amplification, often several hundredfold, that can be reached in some neuroblastomas. Remarkably, the level of amplification tends to be consistent within a given patient, not changing on serial biopsies.[17] N-myc amplification is associated with high levels of N-myc protein expression, presumably leading to deregulated gene expression and a proliferative advantage to the tumor.[111] N-myc amplification is found in about half of patients with advanced disease with a poor prognosis.[111] Its prognostic significance is such that its status should be determined in every neuroblastoma.[16]

In contrast to neuroblastoma, where a single target gene was readily identified in the N-myc amplification unit, a more complex problem has been posed by the identification of amplified sequences from chromosome 12q in soft tissue tumors (Fig. 4-9). The histological categories affected include primarily malignant fibrous histiocytoma and well-differentiated liposarcoma. Osteosarcomas are also affected.[66] The region amplified varies in size from tumor to tumor but may be quite large, encompassing several genes, each of which may potentially have an effect on tumor growth. A number of interesting genes fall in the most consistently amplified region, including GLI, CHOP, SAS, CDK4, and MDM2. GLI was originally described in a dmin-bearing glioblastoma, and has been demonstrated to have transforming activity in an in vitro model.[58-60,102] However, GLI and CHOP[4] (the target of t(12;16) in myxoid liposarcoma) are only amplified in a subset of tumors with 12q amplification. This observation tends to exclude these two genes as targets. SAS (sarcoma amplified se-

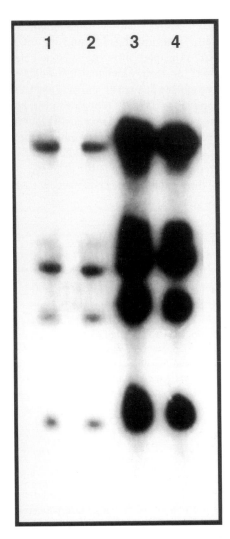

FIG. 4-9. Southern blot analysis illustrating amplification of MDM2 sequences in malignant fibrous histiocytoma. Note the increased intensity of hybridization in lanes 3 and 4 compared with lanes 1 (normal DNA) and 2 (malignant fibrous histiocytoma without amplification).

quence) is a member of the transmembrane 4 superfamily of membrane proteins (TM4SF).[51] Other TM4SF proteins include the melanoma antigen ME491 (CD63) and the lymphoma antigen TAPA-1. Although a role for these proteins in mitogenic signal transduction has been proposed, their function and therefore the effect of SAS overexpression remains unknown. A cyclin-dependent kinase gene, CDK4 is located in close proximity to SAS.[57] Because the equilibrium between cyclins, cyclin kinases, and their inhibitors (such as WAF-1) is central to cell cycle regulation, CDK4 overexpression may alter cell proliferation.

MDM2 (murine double minute 2), originally described in a murine dmin-bearing cell line, also falls within the chromosome 12q amplification unit.[91] MDM2 also has transforming activity in vitro, and its function has been studied in some detail since it has been recognized as a modulator of the tumor suppressor gene p53.[92] MDM2 protein interacts directly with p53 protein and exerts a negative effect on the transcriptional activation activity of p53. There is also evidence of transcriptional induction of MDM2 by normal p53, suggesting that there is a regulatory feedback loop involving these two proteins.[7] These observations have led to the hypothesis that MDM2 overexpression may be an alternative pathway to p53 inactivation. Supporting this concept, in a small series of MFH and liposarcoma specimens, p53 mutation and MDM2 amplification always occurred independently.[70] Antibodies are available for the MDM2 protein, and these have been applied in an immunohistochemical study of a series of 211 adult sarcomas also analyzed for p53 expression.[21] Of these cases, 37% overexpressed MDM2, while 26% expressed p53. These groups were not mutually exclusive, with approximately 10% of tumors expressing both antigens. Of some interest, not all tumors carrying apparent MDM2 amplification also exhibited high levels of immunochemically detectable MDM2 expression. In this cohort of patients, both p53 and MDM2 positivity were independent predictors of survival.

Remarkably, none of the chromosome 12 genes listed above is consistently amplified in all tumors carrying 12q amplification. In a study of 98 sarcomas, SAS and MDM2 were the most frequently amplified genes (10% and 9%, respectively).[34] These numbers are somewhat lower than those of other studies. For example, in another study using Southern blot analysis, seven of 22 malignant fibrous histiocytomas (32%) had amplification of SAS.[117] All retroperitoneal tumors showed amplification. Although CDK4 was not included in this study, its close linkage to SAS suggests that its frequency of amplification will be essentially the same as that for SAS. Studies using FISH, which are less affected by the presence of normal cells in the tumor specimen and which can detect low levels of amplification with high reliability, may be useful to refine these figures. Interestingly, tumors with amplification of one of these genes but without amplification of the other have been identified. This suggests that more than one gene may be the target of amplification in these tumors. Alternatively, the actual target gene, consistently amplified in every case, may remain to be identified. At this point, no single probe is adequate to characterize specimens for the presence of 12q amplification. A minimum of three probes, one for the MDM2 gene, one for the SAS-CDK4 region, and one for GLI, must be used.

Sporadic examples of amplification of myc family oncogenes have been described in a variety of soft tissue tumors, including malignant fibrous histiocytoma, chondrosarcoma, and rhabdomyosarcoma.* Aside from N-myc amplification

---

*References 9, 10, 18, 68, 93, 130.

in neuroblastoma, the clinical correlations with other gene amplification events in soft tissue tumors have not yet been drawn. However, as gene amplification has been among the strongest predictors of clinical outcome of all molecular alterations in those tumors, it is likely that this will be an important issue to clarify.

Clinical implications of molecular genetics

Rapid progress in the molecular characterization of human cancers leads to consideration of how this information might be applied in the diagnostic laboratory.[104] At the present time, it is clear that the major importance of molecular genetics is to investigators studying the fundamental biological principles of cancer. Nonetheless, DNA-based markers or their immunohistochemical surrogates clearly have valuable diagnostic and prognostic correlations in specific situations. Perhaps the most well-established example in a solid tumor is N-myc amplification in neuroblastoma. As usual in oncology, the importance of potential prognostic markers depends on the availability of effective therapeutic interventions for aggressive tumors. In this regard, the availability of bone marrow transplantation

---

Glossary of terms used in molecular biological study of soft tissue tumors

Codon: Fundamental unit of the genetic code, which specifies a single amino acid; composed of three "letters" selected from the four-letter "alphabet" that makes up a DNA sequence: G (guanine), A (adenine), T (thymine), and C (cytosine).

Denaturing gradient gel electrophoresis: Technique for screening PCR products for mutations by exploiting the subtle effects of sequence changes on the stability of double-stranded DNA.

Differential oligonucleotide hybridization: Technique for identifying mutations in PCR-amplified DNA, using small synthetic DNA probes (oligonucleotides) of known DNA sequence.

Loss of heterozygosity (LOH): Use of genetic markers to determine loss of chromosomal segments in tumor cells that may be associated with loss of a functional tumor suppressor gene during tumor progression.

Mismatch error repair: DNA normally contains two perfectly complementary strands in which G-C and A-T base pairs are matched at all positions. During DNA replication, errors may occur and later be corrected by a "proofreading" system, which scans the newly replicated DNA for mismatches in the normal pattern of basepairing.

Missense: Mutation that results in the substitution of an incorrect amino acid in a protein.

Nonsense: Mutation that results in the premature termination of a polypeptide.

Positional cloning: Isolation of a gene based on genetic information that determines its position on a given chromosome.

Positive regulatory element: DNA sequence in proximity to a given gene that provides recognition sites for the transcription factors controlling that gene's expression.

Single-stranded conformation polymorphism assay: Technique for screening PCR products for mutations by exploiting the abnormal migration of mutant DNA strands.

Transcription factor: Protein that binds to DNA at a specific site and promotes the expression of genes located in that region. Many distinct families of transcription factors have been identified, and aberrations of their function appear to be important events, both in solid tumors and leukemias. Transcription factors are multifunctional proteins that may be composed of several regions (domains), which interact with DNA or other components of the transcription apparatus. Among the several types of DNA-binding domains that have been identified is the ETS domain, named after the prototypical gene in this family. Structural alterations of genes of the ETS family have been identified in solid tumors. The bZIP (basic zipper) structural motif characterizes a family of transcription factors that function as dimers (either heterodimers or homodimers), with dimerization depending on the "zipper" sequence.

Transfection: Transfer of exogenous DNA into cells in tissue culture. Genes encoded in the transferred DNA may be expressed, altering the phenotype of the recipient cells.

Transgenic mouse: Animal in which a genetic alteration has been engineered by either the introduction of a foreign gene or the inactivation of an endogenous gene (knockout). This has proved to be an extremely powerful type of technology for the study of gene function.

Transition: Mutation in which one pyrimidine (T or C) or one purine (A or G) is substituted for the other.

Transversion: Mutation in which a purine (A or G) is substituted for a pyrimidine (T or C), or vice versa.

for neuroblastoma has provided impetus for identifying those patients with clinically low stage tumors who actually are at high risk because their tumors carry N-myc amplification. For many soft tissue tumors, their relative rarity and pathological complexity render meaningful clinical correlative studies more difficult. Additionally, several factors limit the clinical implementation of molecular genetics. At the present time, the technical expertise necessary for analysis of tumor DNA and RNA is usually available only at tertiary care centers. In the future, improved cost-effective molecular diagnostic techniques are likely to be widely disseminated. Much of the impetus for such technology development is related to the rapid progress in identifying human genes that may predispose to a wide variety of diseases, including, but not limited to, cancer.

Despite these considerations, several of the molecular alterations now recognized in soft tissue tumors are candidates for transfer into the clinical laboratory. Of particular importance are the fusion proteins derived from chromosome translocations. Because the anomalous mRNAs for these proteins are detected by RT-PCR, they are, in principle, detectable in tissue samples of minimal size. In addition, PCR-based technology does not suffer from the requirement of cytogenetic analysis for living cells and should facilitate the diagnosis of these translocations in a larger number of specimens than is presently possible. An additional application of PCR is the detection of minimal residual disease in the bone marrow transplantation setting. Pioneered in leukemias, this approach may prove valuable for some solid tumors such as Ewing's sarcoma. FISH is an alternative procedure that can detect specific translocations in small tissue specimens, which has proved valuable in leukemia and can easily be extended to solid tumors.[39,53,71,115,139] Another potential implication of tumor-specific fusion proteins is that, in theory, they may give rise to unique epitopes. These could be used to develop monoclonal antibodies that would allow the diagnosis of these translocations on tissue sections. Although many of these applications await further clinical correlative studies and technological development, the importance of molecular diagnostics will continue to increase. For example, most clinical correlative studies in soft tissue tumors have utilized only one or two molecular markers. However, a more complete genotypic analysis is clearly necessary to fully explore the relationship between clinical variables and tumor molecular genetics. It must be recognized that only parts of the puzzle posed by the molecular genetics of soft tissue tumors are in hand. As the remaining pieces of the puzzle are identified, the overall picture of molecular aberrations in cancer will inevitably become more apparent.

REFERENCES

1. Aaltonen LA, Peltomaki P, Leach FS, et al: Clues to the pathogenesis of familial colorectal cancer. *Science* 260:812, 1993.
2. Adams JM, Cory S: Transgenic models of tumor development. *Science* 254:1161, 1991.
3. Alitalo K, Schwab M: Oncogene amplification in tumor cells. *Adv Cancer Res* 47:235, 1986.
4. Aman P, Ron D, Mandahl N, et al: Rearrangement of the transcription factor gene CHOP in myxoid liposarcomas with t(12;16)(q13;p11). *Genes Chromosom Cancer* 5:278, 1992.
5. Andreassen A, Oyjord T, Hovig E, et al: p53 abnormalities in different subtypes of human sarcomas. *Cancer Res* 53:468, 1993.
6. Baker SJ, Fearon ER, Nigro JM, et al: Chromosome 17 deletions and p53 mutations in colorectal carcinomas. *Science* 244:217, 1989.
7. Barak Y, Juven T, Haffner R, et al: mdm2 expression is induced by wild type p53 activity. *Embo J* 12:461, 1993.
8. Barr FG, Galili N, Holick J, et al: Rearrangement of the PAX3 paired box gene in the paediatric solid tumour alveolar rhabdomyosarcoma. *Nat Genet* 3:113, 1993.
9. Barrios C, Castresana JS, Ruiz J, et al: Amplification of c-myc oncogene and absence of c-Ha-ras point mutation in human bone sarcoma. *J Orthop Res* 11:556, 1993.
10. Barrios C, Castresana JS, Ruiz J, et al: Amplification of the c-myc proto-oncogene in soft tissue sarcomas. *Oncology* 51:13, 1994.
11. Bennett WP, Hollstein MC, Hsu IC, et al: Mutational spectra and immunohistochemical analyses of p53 in human cancers. *Chest* 1992.
12. Bishop JM: Viral oncogenes. *Cell* 42:23, 1985.
13. Borresen AL, Hovig E, Smith SB, et al: Constant denaturant gel electrophoresis as a rapid screening technique for p53 mutations. *Proc Natl Acad Sci U S A* 88:8405, 1991.
14. Bos JL: The *ras* family and human carcinogenesis. *Mutat Res* 195:255, 1988.
15. Bridge JA, Sreekantaiah C, Mouron B, et al: Clonal chromosomal abnormalities in desmoid tumors: implications for histopathogenesis. *Cancer* 69:430, 1992.
16. Brodeur GM, Azar C, Brother M, et al: Neuroblastoma: effect of genetic factors on prognosis and treatment. *Cancer* 1992.
17. Brodeur GM, Hayes FA, Green AA, et al: Consistent N-myc copy number in simultaneous or consecutive neuroblastoma samples from sixty individual patients. *Cancer Res* 47:4248, 1987.
18. Castresana JS, Barrios C, Gomez L, et al: Amplification of the c-myc proto-oncogene in human chondrosarcoma. *Diagn Mol Pathol* 1:235, 1992.
19. Chandar N, Billig B, McMaster J, et al: Inactivation of p53 gene in human and murine osteosarcoma cells. *Br J Cancer* 65:208, 1992.
20. Cline MJ: The molecular basis of leukemia. *N Engl J Med* 330:328, 1994.
21. Cordon-Cardo CC, Latres E, Drobnjak M, et al: Molecular abnormalities of mdm2 and p53 genes in adult soft tissue sarcomas. *Cancer Res* 54:794, 1994.
22. Croce CM: Genetic approaches to the study of the molecular basis of human cancer. *Cancer Res* 1991.
23. Croce CM, Tsujimoto Y, Erikson J, et al: Chromosome translocations and B cell neoplasia. *Lab Invest* 51:258, 1984.
24. Crozat A, Aman P, Mandahl N, et al: Fusion of CHOP to a novel RNA-binding protein in human myxoid liposarcoma. *Nature* 363:640, 1993.
25. Davidoff AM, Pence JC, Shorter NA, et al: Expression of p53 in human neuroblastoma- and neuroepithelioma-derived cell lines. *Oncogene* 7:127, 1992.

26. De CA, T'Ang A, Triche TJ: Expression of the retinoblastoma susceptibility gene in childhood rhabdomyosarcomas. *J Natl Cancer Inst* 85:152, 1993.

27. de KA, van KA, Grosveld G, et al: A cellular oncogene is translocated to the Philadelphia chromosome in chronic myelocytic leukaemia. *Nature* 300:765, 1982.

28. Delattre O, Zucman J, Plougastel B, et al: Gene fusion with an ETS DNA-binding domain caused by chromosome translocation in human tumours. *Nature* 359:162, 1992.

29. Donehower LA, Harvey M, Slagle BL, et al: Mice deficient for p53 are developmentally normal but susceptible to spontaneous tumours. *Nature* 356:215, 1992.

30. el Deiry W, Tokino T, Velculescu VE, et al: WAF1, a potential mediator of p53 tumor suppression. *Cell* 75:817, 1993.

31. Eng C, Li FP, Abramson DH, et al: Mortality from second tumors among long-term survivors of retinoblastoma. *J Natl Cancer Inst* 85:1121, 1993.

32. Fearon ER, Vogelstein B: A genetic model for colorectal tumorigenesis. *Cell* 61:759, 1990.

33. Felix CA, Kappel CC, Mitsudomi T, et al: Frequency and diversity of p53 mutations in childhood rhabdomyosarcoma. *Cancer Res* 52:2243, 1992.

34. Forus A, Florenes VA, Maelandsmo GM, et al: Amplification and expression of genes in the q13-14 region of chromosome 12 in human sarcomas. *Cell Growth* 4:1065, 1993.

35. Friend SH, Bernards R, Rogelj S, et al: A human DNA segment with properties of the gene that predisposes to retinoblastoma and osteosarcoma. *Nature* 323:643, 1986.

36. Friend SH, Horowitz JM, Gerber MR, et al: Deletions of a DNA sequence in retinoblastomas and mesenchymal tumors: organization of the sequence and its encoded protein. *Proc Natl Acad Sci U S A* 84:9059, 1987.

37. Galili N, Davis RJ, Fredericks WJ, et al: Fusion of a fork head domain gene to PAX3 in the solid tumour alveolar rhabdomyosarcoma. *Nat Genet* 5:230, 1993.

38. Glover TW, Stein CK, Legius E, et al: Molecular and cytogenetic analysis of tumors in von Recklinghausen neurofibromatosis. *Genes Chromosom Cancer* 3:62, 1991.

39. Gray JW, Pinkel D: Molecular cytogenetics in human cancer diagnosis. *Cancer* 1992.

40. Gutmann DH, Wood DL, Collins FS: Identification of the neurofibromatosis type 1 gene product. *Proc Natl Acad Sci U S A* 88:9658, 1991.

41. Harvey M, McArthur MJ, Montgomery CJ, et al: Spontaneous and carcinogen-induced tumorigenesis in p53-deficient mice. *Nat Genet* 5:225, 1993.

42. Hayashi K: PCR-SSCP: a method for detection of mutations. *Genet Anal Tech Appl* 9:73, 1992.

43. Hayashi K, Yandell DW: How sensitive is PCR-SSCP? *Hum Mutat* 2:338, 1993.

44. Heisterkamp N, Stephenson JR, Groffen J, et al: Localization of the c-abl oncogene adjacent to a translocation break point in chronic myelocytic leukaemia. *Nature* 306:239, 1983.

45. Hollingsworth RJ, Hensey CE, Lee WH: Retinoblastoma protein and the cell cycle. *Curr Opin Genet Dev* 3:55, 1993.

46. Hollstein M, Marion MJ, Lehman T, et al: p53 mutations at A:T base pairs in angiosarcomas of vinyl chloride-exposed factory workers. *Carcinogenesis* 15:1, 1994.

47. Hollstein M, Sidransky D, Vogelstein B, et al: p53 mutations in human cancers. *Science* 253:49, 1991.

48. Hovig E, Smith SB, Brogger A, et al: Constant denaturant gel electrophoresis, a modification of denaturing gradient gel electrophoresis, in mutation detection. *Mutat Res* 262:63, 1991.

49. Imamura J, Bartram CR, Berthold F, et al: Mutation of the p53 gene in neuroblastoma and its relationship with N-myc amplification. *Cancer Res* 53:4053, 1993.

50. Ionov Y, Peinado MA, Malkhosyan S, et al: Ubiquitous somatic mutations in simple repeated sequences reveal a new mechanism for colonic carcinogenesis. *Nature* 363:558, 1993.

51. Jankowski SA, Mitchell DS, Smith SH, et al: SAS, a gene amplified in human sarcomas, encodes a new member of the transmembrane 4 superfamily of proteins. *Oncogene* 9:1205, 1994.

52. Johnson MR, Look AT, DeClue JE, et al: Inactivation of the NF1 gene in human melanoma and neuroblastoma cell lines without impaired regulation of GTP.Ras. *Proc Natl Acad Sci U S A* 90:5539, 1993.

53. Kallioniemi OP, Kallioniemi A, Kurisu W, et al: ERBB2 amplification in breast cancer analyzed by fluorescence in situ hybridization. *Proc Natl Acad Sci U S A* 89:5321, 1992.

54. Kallioniemi OP, Kallioniemi A, Sudar D, et al: Comparative genomic hybridization: a rapid new method for detecting and mapping DNA amplification in tumors. *Semin Cancer Biol* 4:41, 1993.

55. Kellems RE: *Gene amplification in mammalian cells: a comprehensive guide.* New York, 1993, Marcel Dekker.

56. Kern SE, Pietenpol JA, Thiagalingam S, et al: Oncogenic forms of p53 inhibit p53-regulated gene expression. *Science* 256:827, 1992.

57. Khatib ZA, Matsushime H, Valentine M, et al: Coamplification of the CDK4 gene with MDM2 and GLI in human sarcomas. *Cancer Res* 53:5535, 1993.

58. Kinzler KW, Bigner SH, Bigner DD, et al: Identification of an amplified, highly expressed gene in a human glioma. *Science* 236:70, 1987.

59. Kinzler KW, Ruppert JM, Bigner SH, et al: The GLI gene is a member of the Kruppel family of zinc finger proteins. *Nature* 332:371, 1988.

60. Kinzler KW, Vogelstein B: The GLI gene encodes a nuclear protein which binds specific sequences in the human genome. *Mol Cell Biol* 10:634, 1990.

61. Knudson AG: Antioncogenes and human cancer. *Proc Natl Acad Sci U S A* 90:10914, 1993.

62. Knudson AJ: Mutation and cancer: statistical study of retinoblastoma. *Proc Natl Acad Sci U S A* 68:820, 1971.

63. Knudson AJ, Hethcote HW, Brown BW: Mutation and childhood cancer: a probabilistic model for the incidence of retinoblastoma. *Proc Natl Acad Sci U S A* 72:5116, 1975.

64. Komuro H, Hayashi Y, Kawamura M, et al: Mutations of the p53 gene are involved in Ewing's sarcomas but not in neuroblastomas. *Cancer Res* 53:5284, 1993.

65. Kovar H, Auinger A, Jug G, et al: Narrow spectrum of infrequent p53 mutations and absence of MDM2 amplification in Ewing tumours. *Oncogene* 8:2683, 1993.

66. Ladanyi M, Cha C, Lewis R, et al: MDM2 gene amplification in metastatic osteosarcoma. *Cancer Res* 53:16, 1993.

67. Ladanyi M, Lewis R, Garin CP, et al: EWS rearrangement in Ewing's sarcoma and peripheral neuroectodermal tumor: molecular detection and correlation with cytogenetic analysis and MIC2 expression. *Diagn Mol Pathol* 2:141, 1993.

68. Ladanyi M, Park CK, Lewis R, et al: Sporadic amplification of the MYC gene in human osteosarcomas. *Diagn Mol Pathol* 2:163, 1993.

69. Leach FS, Nicolaides NC, Papadopoulos N, et al: Mutations of a MutS homolog in hereditary non-polyposis colorectal cancer. *Cell* 75:1215, 1993.

70. Leach FS, Tokino T, Meltzer P, et al: p53 Mutation and MDM2 amplification in human soft tissue sarcomas. *Cancer Res* 2231, 1993.

71. Lee W, Han K, Harris CP, et al: Use of FISH to detect chromosomal translocations and deletions: analysis of chromosome rearrangement in synovial sarcoma cells from paraffin-embedded specimens. *Am J Pathol* 143:15, 1993.

72. Lee WH, Bookstein R, Hong F, et al: Human retinoblastoma susceptibility gene: cloning, identification, and sequence. *Science* 235:1394, 1987.

73. Legius E, Marchuk DA, Collins FS, et al: Somatic deletion of the neurofibromatosis type 1 gene in a neurofibrosarcoma supports a tumour suppressor gene hypothesis. *Nat Genet* 3:122, 1993.

74. Levine AJ: The p53 tumor-suppressor gene. *N Engl J Med* 326:1350, 1992.

75. Li FP, Garber JE, Friend SH, et al: Recommendations on predictive testing for germ line p53 mutations among cancer-prone individuals. *J Natl Cancer Inst* 84:1156, 1992.

76. Li Y, Bollag G, Clark R, et al: Somatic mutations in the neurofibromatosis 1 gene in human tumors. *Cell* 69:275, 1992.

77. Liang P, Pardee AB: Differential display of eukaryotic messenger RNA by means of the polymerase chain reaction. *Science* 257:967, 1992.

78. Liu FS, Kohler MF, Marks JR, et al: Mutation and overexpression of the p53 tumor suppressor gene frequently occurs in uterine and ovarian sarcomas. *Obstet Gynecol* 83:118, 1994.

79. Livingston DM, Kaelin W, Chittenden T, et al: Structural and functional contributions to the G1 blocking action of the retinoblastoma protein (1992 Gordon Hamilton Fairley Memorial Lecture). *Br J Cancer* 68:264, 1993.

80. Livingstone LR, White A, Sprouse J, et al: Altered cell cycle arrest and gene amplification potential accompany loss of wild-type p53. *Cell* 70:923, 1992.

81. Lothe RA, Saeter G, Danielsen HE, et al: Genetic alterations in a malignant schwannoma from a patient with neurofibromatosis (NF1). *Pathol Res Pract* 189:465, 1993.

82. Makino R, Yazyu H, Kishimoto Y, et al: F-SSCP: fluorescence-based polymerase chain reaction-single-strand conformation polymorphism (PCR-SSCP) analysis. *Pcr Methods Appl* 2:10, 1992.

83. Malkin D, Friend SH: The role of tumour suppressor genes in familial cancer. *Semin Cancer Biol* 3:121, 1992.

84. Malkin D, Jolly KW, Barbier N, et al: Germline mutations of the p53 tumor-suppressor gene in children and young adults with second malignant neoplasms. *N Engl J Med* 326:1309, 1992.

85. Malkin D, Li FP, Strong LC, et al: Germ line p53 mutations in a familial syndrome of breast cancer, sarcomas, and other neoplasms. *Science* 250:1233, 1990.

86. Marchuk DA, Saulino AM, Tavakkol R, et al: cDNA cloning of the type 1 neurofibromatosis gene: complete sequence of the NF1 gene product. *Genomics* 11:931, 1991.

87. Marion MJ, Froment O, Trepo C: Activation of Ki-ras gene by point mutation in human liver angiosarcoma associated with vinyl chloride exposure. *Mol Carcinog* 4:450, 1991.

88. May WA, Lessnick SL, Braun BS, et al: The Ewing's sarcoma EWS/FLI-1 fusion gene encodes a more potent transcriptional activator and is a more powerful transforming gene than FLI-1. *Mol Cell Biol* 13:7393, 1993.

89. Nakamura Y, Nishisho I, Kinzler KW, et al: Mutations of the adenomatous polyposis coli gene in familial polyposis coli patients and sporadic colorectal tumors. *Princess Takamatsu Symp* 22:285, 1991.

90. Nowell PC: The clonal evolution of tumor cell populations. *Science* 194:23, 1976.

91. Oliner JD, Kinzler KW, Meltzer PS, et al: Amplification of a gene encoding a p53-associated protein in human sarcomas. *Nature* 358:80, 1992.

92. Oliner JD, Pietenpol JA, Thiagalingam S, et al: Oncoprotein MDM2 conceals the activation domain of tumour suppressor p53. *Nature* 362:857, 1993.

93. Ozaki T, Ikeda S, Kawai A, et al: Alterations of retinoblastoma susceptible gene accompanied by c-myc amplification in human bone and soft tissue tumors. *Cell Mol Biol (Noisy le grand)* 39:235, 1993.

94. Papadopoulos N, Nicolaides NC, Wei Y-F, et al: Mutation of a mutL homolog in hereditary colon cancer. *Science* 263:1625, 1994.

95. Parada LF, Tabin CJ, Shih C, et al: Human EJ bladder carcinoma oncogene is homologue of Harvey sarcoma virus ras gene. *Nature* 297:474, 1982.

96. Parsons R, Li GM, Longley MJ, et al: Hypermutability and mismatch repair deficiency in RER+ tumor cells. *Cell* 75:1227, 1993.

97. Pearson M, Rowley JD: The relation of oncogenesis and cytogenetics in leukemia and lymphoma. *Annu Rev Med* 36:471, 1985.

98. Rabbitts TH, Forster A, Larson R, et al: Fusion of the dominant negative transcription regulator CHOP with a novel gene FUS by translocation t(12;16) in malignant liposarcoma. *Nat Genet* 4:175, 1993.

99. Rao VN, Ohno T, Prasad DD, et al: Analysis of the DNA-binding and transcriptional activation functions of human Fli-1 protein. *Oncogene* 8:2167, 1993.

100. Reissmann PT, Simon MA, Lee W-H, et al: Studies of the retinoblastoma gene in human sarcomas. *Oncogene* 4:839, 1989.

101. Reynolds JE, Fletcher JA, Lytle CH, et al: Molecular characterization of a 17q11.2 translocation in a malignant schwannoma cell line. *Hum Genet* 90:450, 1992.

102. Roberts WM, Douglass EC, Peiper SC, et al: Amplification of the gli gene in childhood sarcomas. *Cancer Res* 49:5407, 1989.

103. Ron D, Habener JF: CHOP, a novel developmentally regulated nuclear protein that dimerizes with transcription factors C/EBP and LAP and functions as a dominant-negative inhibitor of gene transcription. *Genes Dev* 6:439, 1992.

104. Rowley JD, Aster JC, Sklar J: The impact of new DNA diagnostic technology on the management of cancer patients: survey of diagnostic techniques. *Arch Pathol Lab Med* 117:1104, 1993.

105. Sager R: Tumor suppressor genes in the cell cycle. *Curr Opin Cell Biol* 4:155, 1992.

106. Saiki RK, Gelfand DH, Stoffel S, et al: Primer-directed enzymatic amplification of DNA with a thermostable DNA polymerase. *Science* 239:487, 1988.

107. Scholz RB, Kabisch H, Weber B, et al: Studies of the RB1 gene and the p53 gene in human osteosarcomas. *Pediatr Hematol Oncol* 9:125, 1992.

108. Schreck RR: Tumor suppressor gene (Rb and p53) mutations in osteosarcoma. *Pediatr Hematol Oncol* 9:1992.

109. Schwab M, Alitalo K, Klempnauer KH, et al: Amplified DNA with limited homology to myc cellular oncogene is shared by human neuroblastoma cell lines and a neuroblastoma tumour. *Nature* 305:245, 1983.

110. Schwab M, Varmus HE, Bishop JM, et al: Chromosome localization in normal human cells and neuroblastomas of a gene related to c-myc. *Nature* 308:288, 1984.

111. Seeger RC, Wada R, Brodeur GM, et al: Expression of N-myc by neuroblastomas with one or multiple copies of the oncogene. *Prog Clin Biol Res* 271:41, 1988.

112. Sen GS, Van, der, et al: Somatic mutation of APC gene in desmoid tumour in familial adenomatous polyposis. *Lancet* 342:552, 1993.

113. Serrano M, Hannon GJ, Beach D: A new regulatory motif in cell-cycle control causing specific inhibition of cyclin D/CDK4. *Nature* 366:704, 1993.

114. Shapiro DN, Sublett JE, Li B, et al: Fusion of PAX3 to a member of the forkhead family of transcription factors in human alveolar rhabdomyosarcoma. *Cancer Res* 53:5108, 1993.

115. Shipley JM, Jones TA, Patel K, et al: Ordering of probes surrounding the Ewing's sarcoma breakpoint on chromosome 22 using fluorescent in situ hybridization to interphase nuclei. *Cytogenet Cell Genet* 64:233, 1993.

116. Smith SB, Gebhardt MC, Kloen P, et al: Screening for TP53 mutations in osteosarcomas using constant denaturant gel electrophoresis (CDGE). *Hum Mutat* 2:274, 1993.

117. Smith SH, Weiss SW, Jankowski SA, et al: SAS amplification in soft tissue sarcomas. *Cancer Res* 52:3746, 1992.

118. Soini Y, Vahakangas K, Nuorva K, et al: p53 immunohistochemistry in malignant fibrous histiocytomas and other mesenchymal tumours. *J Pathol* 168:29, 1992.

119. Sorensen PH, Liu XF, Delattre O, et al: Reverse transcriptase PCR amplification of EWS/FLI-1 fusion transcripts as a diagnostic test for peripheral primitive neuroectodermal tumors of childhood. *Diagn Mol Pathol* 2:147, 1993.

120. Southern E: Detection of specific sequences among DNA fragments separated by gel electrophoresis. *J Mol Biol* 98:503, 1975.

121. Stanbridge EJ: Functional evidence for human tumour suppressor genes: chromosome and molecular genetic studies. *Cancer Surv* 12:5, 1992.

122. Stephenson CF, Bridge JA, Sandberg AA: Cytogenetic and pathologic aspects of Ewing's sarcoma and neuroectodermal tumors. *Hum Pathol* 23:1270, 1992.

123. Stratton MR, Moss S, Warren W, et al: Mutation of the p53 gene in human soft tissue sarcomas: association with abnormalities of the RB1 gene. *Oncogene* 5:1297, 1990.

124. Strong LC, Williams WR, Tainsky MA: The Li-Fraumeni syndrome: from clinical epidemiology to molecular genetics. *Am J Epidemiol* 135:190, 1992.

125. Su LK, Vogelstein B, Kinzler KW: Association of the APC tumor suppressor protein with catenins. *Science* 262:1734, 1993.

126. Tabin CJ, Bradley SM, Bargmann CI, et al: Mechanism of activation of a human oncogene. *Nature* 300:143, 1982.

127. The I, Murthy AE, Hannigan GE, et al: Neurofibromatosis type 1 gene mutations in neuroblastoma. *Nat Genet* 3:62, 1993.

128. Thibodeau SN, Bren G, Schaid D: Microsatellite instability in cancer of the proximal colon. *Science* 260:816, 1993.

129. Toguchida J, Yamaguchi T, Ritchie B, et al: Mutation spectrum of the p53 gene in bone and soft tissue sarcomas. *Cancer Res* 52:6194, 1992.

130. Tsuda H, Shimosato Y, Upton MP, et al: Retrospective study on amplification of N-myc and c-myc genes in pediatric solid tumors and its association with prognosis and tumor differentiation. *Lab Invest* 59:321, 1988.

131. Vogan K, Bernstein M, Leclerc JM, et al: Absence of p53 gene mutations in primary neuroblastomas. *Cancer Res* 53:5269, 1993.

132. Vogelstein B, Kinzler KW: The multistep nature of cancer. *Trends Genet* 9:138, 1993.

133. Vogelstein B, Kinzler KW: p53 function and dysfunction. *Cell* 70:523, 1992.

134. Wadayama B, Toguchida J, Yamaguchi T, et al: p53 expression and its relationship to DNA alterations in bone and soft tissue sarcomas. *Br J Cancer* 68:1134, 1993.

135. Weinberg RA: Tumor suppressor genes. *Science* 254:1138, 1991.

136. Wilke W, Maillet M, Robinson R: H-ras-1 point mutations in soft tissue sarcomas. *Mod Pathol* 6:129, 1993.

137. Wunder JS, Czitrom AA, Kandel R, et al: Analysis of alterations in the retinoblastoma gene and tumor grade in bone and soft-tissue sarcomas. *J Natl Cancer Inst* 83:194, 1991.

138. Xu W, Mulligan LM, Ponder MA, et al: Loss of NF1 alleles in phaeochromocytomas from patients with type I neurofibromatosis. *Genes Chromosom Cancer* 4:337, 1992.

139. Zhang J, Meltzer P, Jenkins R, et al: Application of chromosome microdissection probes for elucidation of BCR-ABL fusion and variant Philadelphia chromosome translocations in chronic myelogenous leukemia. *Blood* 81:3365, 1993.

140. Zhang L, Lemarchandel V, Romeo PH, et al: The Fli-1 proto-oncogene, involved in erythroleukemia and Ewing's sarcoma, encodes a transcriptional activator with DNA-binding specificities distinct from other Ets family members. *Oncogene* 8:1621, 1993.

141. Zhou J, Mochizuki T, Smeets H, et al: Deletion of the paired alpha 5(IV) and alpha 6(IV) collagen genes in inherited smooth muscle tumors. *Science* 261:1167, 1993.

142. Zucman J, Delattre O, Desmaze C, et al: EWS and ATF-1 gene fusion induced by t(12;22) translocation in malignant melanoma of soft parts. *Nat Genet* 4:341, 1993.

143. Zucman J, Melot T, Desmaze C, et al: Combinatorial generation of variable fusion proteins in the Ewing family of tumours. *Embo J* 12:4481, 1993.

CHAPTER 5   JONATHAN A. FLETCHER

CYTOGENETIC ANALYSIS OF SOFT TISSUE TUMORS

Most malignant soft tissue tumors contain clonal chromosome aberrations, many of which are specific for particular tumor types.[35,98] Demonstration of characteristic chromosome abnormalities can be especially useful in diagnosis of undifferentiated small round cell or spindle cell soft tissue tumors.[35] The characteristic chromosome aberrations in these tumors appear to be critical in maintaining neoplastic transformation, and they are retained as a given tumor becomes progressively less differentiated. Hence, evaluation of specific chromosome abnormalities also can be useful in tumors that have lost diagnostic immunohistochemical or ultrastructural features. Unfortunately, cytogenetic analyses are labor intensive, and successful analyses depend on the ability of the cytogeneticist to culture the tumor cells in question.

GENERAL CONSIDERATIONS IN CYTOGENETIC ANALYSIS
Methodologic considerations

Normal human somatic cells contain two sex chromosomes and 22 pairs of autosomal chromosomes. Each chromosome has a shorter arm (designated p) and a longer arm (designated q), with a centromere separating the two arms. Before 1970 it was exceedingly difficult to assess cytogenetic aberrations because the various human chromosomes could only be distinguished based on the gross morphological features of overall chromosome size and centromere location. It was subsequently discovered that both fluorescent and nonfluorescent stains bind selectively and reproducibly to certain chromosome regions. This selective staining yields patterns of alternating light and dark bands in each chromosome arm, and knowledge of the characteristic normal banding patterns has facilitated studies of chromosomal alterations in neoplastic proliferations. Cytogenetic laboratories employ a number of staining techniques that highlight different chromosome regions, the most widely used being quinacrine staining for fluorescent studies[14] and Giemsa staining for nonfluorescent banding.[104] Soft tissue tu-

mors have been karyotyped extensively since the mid 1980s, and it is clear that virtually all malignant soft tissue tumors contain clonal chromosome aberrations[35,98] (Table 5-1). Although the presence of clonal chromosome aberrations was once assumed to be de facto evidence of cancer, it is now clear that such aberrations are found in many benign soft tissue tumors (Table 5-2). Cytogenetic aberrations are only one subset of all the genetic mutations found in malignant and benign soft tissue tumors. It is assumed that all neoplastic soft tissue tumors contain one or more clonal genetic mutations, which are responsible for deregulated cell growth. These mutations include cytogenetic aberrations (e.g., chromosome translocations or deletions of large chromosomal regions) and point mutations (e.g., deletions or substitutions of individual DNA nucleotides). Point mutations, by definition, cannot be detected at the cytogenetic level of resolution but can be evaluated by molecular biological studies.

The cytogenetic approach requires fresh, viable, tumor specimens, which should be processed rapidly and transported to the cytogenetics laboratory in sterile tissue culture media or in a physiological buffer such as Hank's Buffered Salt Solution. It is important that the cytogenetic sample be removed from the overall tumor specimen with sterile scalpel blades or scissors. Otherwise, bacterial or fungal contamination may lead to microbial overgrowth in the subsequent tissue cultures. Because viable tumor cells are essential in establishing the tissue cultures, it is also important that the specimen be selected carefully so as to contain a minimum of necrotic tissue. Finally, it is crucial to minimize nonneoplastic components, particularly fibroblasts, lest these cells overwhelm the tumor population after the cultures are established. The success of the cytogenetic analysis depends largely on the quality of the tumor specimen, whereas the amount of tumor is less important: thus, percutaneous needle biopsies of small round cell tumors can be karyotyped routinely.[35,54] At least 80% of all soft tissue tumors can be cultured successfully if the specimens are

Table 5-1. Characteristic cytogenetic aberrations in malignant soft tissue tumors

Histologic findings	Characteristic cytogenetic events	Frequency	Diagnostic utility?
Clear cell sarcoma	t(12;22)(q13;q12)	>75%	Yes
Dermatofibrosarcoma protuberans	Ring chromosome 17	>75%	Yes
Ewing's sarcoma	t(11;22)(q24;q12)	95%	Yes
Extraskeletal myxoid chondrosarcoma	t(9;22)(q31;q12)	50%	Yes
Fibrosarcoma, infantile	+8, +11, +17, +20	90%	Yes
Hemangiopericytoma	Translocation at 12q13	>25%	No
Intraabdominal desmoplastic small round cell tumor	t(11;22)(p13;q12)	>50%	Yes
Leiomyosarcoma	Deletion of 1p	75%	No
Liposarcoma			
Myxoid	t(12;16)(q13;p11)	75%	Yes
Pleomorphic	Complex*	90%	No
Well differentiated	Ring chromosome 12	80%	Yes
Malignant fibrous histiocytoma			
High-grade	Complex*	90%	No
Myxoid	Ring chromosomes	>50%	?
Malignant peripheral nerve sheath tumor	Complex*	90%	No
Mesothelioma	Deletions of 1p, 3p, and 22q	90%	Yes
Neuroblastoma			
Good prognosis	Hyperdiploid, no 1p deletion	90%	Yes
Poor prognosis	1p deletion,	90%	Yes
	double minute chromosomes	40%	Yes
Primitive neuroectodermal tumor	t(11;22)(q24;q12)	95%	Yes
Rhabdomyosarcoma			
Alveolar	t(2;13)(q35;q14)	80%	Yes
Embryonal	+2q, +8, +20	80%	?
Synovial sarcoma	t(X;18)(p11;q11)	95%	Yes

*Indicates the consistent finding of extremely complex karyotypes containing multiple numerical and structural chromosome aberrations.

Table 5-2. Consistent cytogenetic aberrations in benign soft tissue tumors

Histologic findings	Characteristic cytogenetic events	Frequency	Diagnostic utility?
Benign schwannoma	Monosomy 22	50%	Yes
Desmoid tumor	Trisomy 8	25%	No
	Deletion of 5q	10%	?
Hibernoma	Translocation at 11q13	?	?
Lipoblastoma	Rearrangement of 8q	>25%	Yes
Lipoma			
Solitary	Rearrangement of 12q14-15	75%	Yes
	Rearrangement of 6p	10%	?
	Deletion of 13q	10%	?
Multiple	None		
Neurofibroma	None		
Uterine leiomyoma	t(12;14)(q15;q24)	20%	Yes
	Deletion of 7q	15%	No
	Trisomy 12	10%	No

carefully selected so as to minimize necrotic and nonneoplastic components.

Chromosome banding is most successful during metaphase when the chromosomes are maximally contracted. To obtain metaphase cells, tumor specimens are first dis-

aggregated mechanically or enzymatically into single cells and small cell clusters.[63] Metaphase cells can often be extracted directly from disaggregated high-grade tumors if less than 1 hour has passed from time of biopsy.[35] Lower-grade tumors must be placed in tissue culture for several

Table 5-3. Cytogenetic abbreviations

Abbreviation	Meaning
cen	Centromere
del	Deletion
dmin	Double minute chromosome
hsr	Homogeneously staining region
ins	Insertion
inv	Inversion
mar	Marker chromosome (aberrant chromosome whose origin cannot be ascertained)
p	Chromosome short arm
q	Chromosome long arm
r	Ring chromosome
t	Translocation
tel	Telomere

days to improve the tumor cell mitotic index. It is imperative that the cytogeneticist be acquainted with the characteristic tissue culture morphologic characteristics of different tumor and nonneoplastic cell types. Daily inspection of the tissue cultures by inverted microscopy will reveal when the tumor population is growing rapidly, and a mitotic spindle inhibitor (e.g., Colcemid) can then be added to arrest growth of proliferating cells in metaphase. The time frame within which cytogenetic findings can be determined varies widely depending on the grade of the tumor. Metaphase preparations from high-grade tumors can often be obtained by direct harvesting or after 1 to 4 days in culture, and chromosome aberrations can be assessed the day after metaphase preparations are obtained. Low-grade tumors, by contrast, often must be cultured for up to 1 week before metaphase preparations can be obtained. Longer culture periods (e.g., 2 to 3 weeks) should be avoided assiduously because genetic artifacts often develop in long-term cultures. The most frequent artifact is loss of the neoplastic clone due to overgrowth by fibroblasts or other nonneoplastic cells; such overgrowth results in a spurious diploid karyotype.

Cytogenetic terminology

Karyotypes are described by means of an intricate shorthand system[49,77] (Table 5-3), which details both chromosome number and the location and mechanism of chromosome rearrangements. Numeric abnormalities are indicated by a plus or minus sign before a specific chromosome number (e.g., −22 . . . . .) indicating loss of one copy of chromosome 22. Chromosome rearrangements are indicated by abbreviations signifying the mechanism of the rearrangements. These rearrangement abbreviations are followed by one or more sets of parentheses that describe the actual chromosome bands affected by the rearrangements. An example of this shorthand is 47, XX, +8, t(12;16)(q13;p11), in which *47* indicates the total chromo-

some number, *XX* indicates a female cell, and *+8* indicates an extra copy, or trisomy, of chromosome 8. The *t* indicates a translocation, that is, a reciprocal exchange of material between two different chromosome arms, and the first set of parentheses indicates that chromosomes 12 and 16 are involved in the translocation. The second set of parentheses indicates that the translocation breakpoint on chromosome 12 is in the long arm *(q)* at band 13, whereas the translocation breakpoint on chromosome 16 is on the short arm *(p)* at band 11. The translocation (12;16) is a characteristic rearrangement in myxoid liposarcoma (Table 5-2), and trisomy 8 is a frequent secondary aberration in these tumors.[30,115,129] A useful guide to chromosome nomenclature International System for Human Cytogenetic Nomenclature, which was most recently updated in 1991.[49,77]

Molecular cytogenetics

Whereas conventional cytogenetic analyses are performed using various staining techniques that highlight chromosome bands, the newer discipline of molecular cytogenetics involves detection of specific DNA sequences by hybridization with complementary DNA probes.[62,90] These molecular cytogenetic assays are generally referred to as *FISH* (fluorescent in situ hybridization) when the hybridization reaction is detected by fluorescence microscopy, but the hybridizations can also be evaluated by brightfield microscopy using peroxidase or alkaline phosphatase detection strategies. Fluorescent detection is generally the most sensitive, whereas peroxidase or alkaline phosphatase reaction products are more stable and do not require fluorescent microscopy. FISH can be carried out using DNA probes that have been directly labeled with fluors such as fluorescein (FITC) and rhodamine. The sensitivity of FISH can often be enhanced by indirect detection, for example, hybridization with a biotinylated probe followed by incubation with avidin-FITC. The FITC signals in this indirect detection approach can then be amplified further by successive incubations with biotinylated antiavidin and avidin-FITC.

Fluorescent in situ hybridization to paraffin tissue sections is useful in demonstrating chromosome aberrations among particular cell populations,[29] but a drawback of this approach is that nuclei are often incomplete due to the necessary thinness (typically 4 to 6 μ) of the sections.[29,58] FISH can also be carried out against intact nuclei that have been disaggregated from thick (50 to 60 μ) paraffin sections[100,101] or frozen tumor specimens (Fig. 5-1). These hybridizations have been carried out successfully using tumor nuclei disaggregated from paraffin blocks that were more than 20 years old.[100] The DNA probes used in FISH can be directed against whole chromosomes or localized chromosome regions. "Cocktails" of probes that target an entire chromosome are referred to as chromosome "paints"; these are especially useful in confirming chromosome trans-

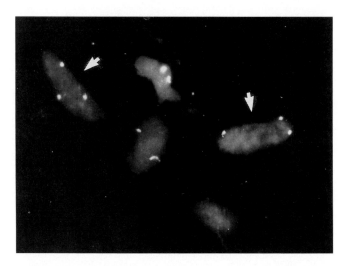

FIG. 5-1. Fluorescent in situ hybridization demonstration of trisomy 8 in nuclei disaggregated from a frozen desmoid specimen. In situ hybridization was carried out using a biotinylated chromosome 8 centromere probe, and probe detection was with avidin-FITC. Two nuclei (arrows) have triple hybridization signals.

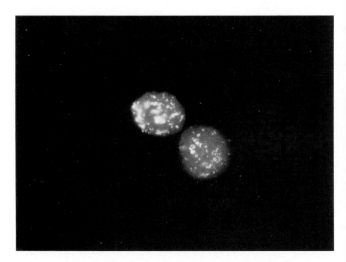

FIG. 5-2. Fluorescent in situ hybridization demonstration of N-myc amplification in neuroblastoma nuclei. In situ hybridization was carried out using a biotinylated N-myc probe, and probe detection was with avidin-FITC. Both nuclei have marked amplification of N-myc.

locations in metaphase preparations.[90,93] DNA probes that target specific chromosome regions are employed to demonstrate chromosome deviations in both metaphase and interphase cells. These localized probes are particularly useful for demonstration of chromosome translocations,[93,123] chromosome deletions,[72,119] and gene amplifications[107] in archival pathologic specimens (Fig. 5-2).

CYTOGENETIC ANALYSIS OF SPECIFIC TUMORS

Primitive neuroectodermal tumor and Ewing's sarcoma

More than 90% of extraskeletal Ewing's sarcomas and primitive neuroectodermal tumors contain an identical translocation of chromosomes 11 and 22 (Fig. 5-3).[13,126] The cytogenetic shorthand description of this translocation is t(11;22)(q12;q24), and the translocation results in fusion of the Fli-1 gene on chromosome 11 with the EWS gene on chromosome 22.[25,73,84] A minority of Ewing's sarcomas and primitive neuroectodermal tumors contain variant translocations of chromosome 22 in which the EWS gene is fused with genes on chromosomes other than chromosome 11.[110,112] The t(11;22) is often referred to as a "primary" genetic aberration because it is found in virtually all Ewing's sarcomas and primitive neuroectodermal tumors and is presumed to be the critical genetic aberration in both tumors. Other nonrandom cytogenetic abnormalities are seen in subsets of Ewing's sarcoma and primitive neuroectodermal tumor: these include trisomy 8 and translocation of chromosomes 1 and 16, which are found in approximately 50% and 20% of cases, respectively.[79] The clinical relevance of these secondary aberrations remains to be determined.

Several investigators have pointed out that the shared cytogenetic translocation in Ewing's sarcoma and primitive neuroectodermal tumors provides additional evidence of a close relationship between these tumors.[15,61,65,83] This argument has merit because specific chromosome translocations in cancers are generally observed only in closely related cell types. Such translocations are presumably nononcogenic in more distantly related cells. Thus, it is possible that Ewing's sarcoma and primitive neuroectodermal tumors result from transformation of closely related cells that differ only in their degree of neuroectodermal differentiation. It is also notable that an identical t(11;22)(q24;q12) translocation has been detected occasionally in other small round cell tumors, including several olfactory neuroblastomas (esthesioneuroblastomas),[130] one small cell osteosarcoma,[82] and one mesenchymal chondrosarcoma.[97] The t(11;22) translocation in olfactory neuroblastomas is perhaps not a surprising finding because these tumors often resemble primitive neuroectodermal tumor on clinical and histological evaluation.[75] Likewise, the description of chondroid differentiation in an experimental primitive neuroectodermal tumor model[46] suggests the possibility that mesenchymal chondrosarcomas with t(11;22)(q24;q12) translocation are simply Ewing's sarcomas with chondroid differentiation. Some small cell osteosarcomas and mesenchymal chondrosarcomas lack the t(11;22)(q24;q12) translocation, however, and these cases might be true osteosarcomas and chondrosarcomas.

The t(11;22)(q24;q12) translocation is detected readily by conventional cytogenetic methods because Ewing's sarcoma and primitive neuroectodermal tumor cells grow well in tissue culture. In fact, the translocation can generally be

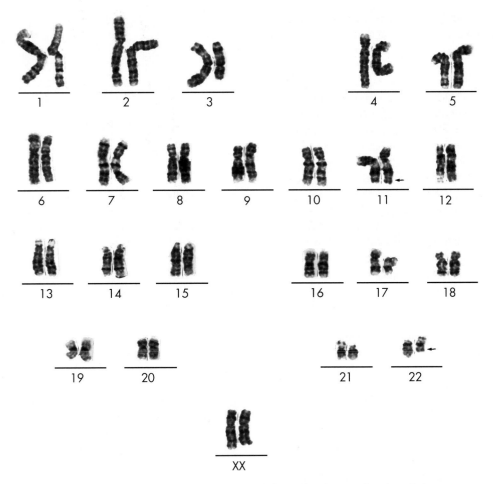

FIG. 5-3. Karyotype of a primitive neuroectodermal tumor showing translocation of chromosomes 11 and 22. Arrows indicate translocation breakpoints on the rearranged chromosomes. The chromosome 3 on the right is shorter than its partner because of a deletion; this was another clonal mutation in the tumor.

detected in needle biopsy specimens.[2,35,54] The translocation can also be detected by FISH, using probes to the EWS and Fli-1 regions,[26] as well as by reverse transcriptase PCR. One disadvantage of the FISH and molecular t(11;22) detection strategies is that neither method will detect the occasional "variant" translocations of chromosome 22.[110,112]

Clear cell sarcoma

Clear cell sarcomas of tendon and aponeuroses share many phenotypic features with cutaneous malignant melanomas and are also referred to as "melanomas of the soft parts." More than 75% of these tumors contain a translocation of chromosomes 12 and 22, t(12;22)(q13;q12) (Fig. 5-4).[33,89,117] The t(12;22) translocation fuses the ATF-1 gene on chromosome 12 with the EWS gene on chromosome 22.[133] Despite the histological similarities between clear cell sarcoma and cutaneous melanoma, these two tumors are quite different clinically. Clear cell sarcomas usually present as isolated masses located in deep soft tissues

without apparent origin from skin. Detection of the t(12;22) translocation might be a substantial aid in diagnosis of clear cell sarcoma because this translocation has not been observed in cutaneous melanoma or in any other tumor types.[76]

Intraabdominal desmoplastic small round cell tumor

Intraabdominal desmoplastic small round cell tumors contain undifferentiated malignant small round cell populations within a florid desmoplastic reaction. Although these tumors were only recently described as a distinct entity,[44] a novel translocation of chromosomes 11 and 22, t(11;22)(p13;q11-12), has already been reported in several cases.[6,92,99] The translocation breakpoint on chromosome 22 is in the same region as the breakpoint described above in Ewing's sarcoma and peripheral primitive neuroectodermal tumor. However, it is not yet known whether the EWS gene on chromosome 22 is rearranged in intraabdominal desmoplastic small round cell tumor. The chromosome 11 breakpoint in this tumor is on a different arm than the classic breakpoint in Ewing's sarcoma and primitive neuroectodermal tumor.

Rhabdomyosarcoma

Cytogenetic analyses have been useful in reaffirming the distinct nature of embryonal and alveolar forms of rhabdomyosarcomas. Most alveolar rhabdomyosarcomas contain a reciprocal translocation of chromosomes 2 and 13[28,108,124] (Table 5-1) that has not been described in other varieties of small round cell tumor. This translocation results in fusion of the PAX3 gene on chromosome 2 with the ALV gene on chromosome 13, and the resulting fusion gene can be detected readily by reverse transcriptase PCR.[4,106] PCR detection is an especially useful diagnostic approach for alveolar rhabdomyosarcomas, because the number of cases in which karyotyping can be successfully done appears to be less than 50%. However, a minority of alveolar rhabdomyosarcomas have "variant" translocations of chromosome 13 with chromosomes other than chromosome 2, and these cases will not be detected by the current PCR assay techniques.[27]

Embryonal rhabdomyosarcomas lack the translocation (2;13) of alveolar rhabdomyosarcoma but have several other nonrandom chromosome aberrations including extra copies of chromosomes 8 and 20 and of the chromosome 2 long arm.[108] These aberrations are typically accompanied by loss of genes from the short arm of chromosome 11. The chromosome 11 losses are readily demonstrated by molecular methods[103] but are usually not obvious on cytogenetical studies. The above-mentioned chromosome trisomies and 11 short arm losses are unusual in alveolar rhabdomyosarcoma and are highly suggestive of the embryonal subtype. However, similar aberrations are seen frequently in several other embryonal-type tumors, including hepatoblastoma and Wilms' tumors.[36,59,60] Malignant rhabdoid tumors lack the characteristic cytogenetic aberrations seen in either alveolar or embryonal rhabdomyosarcomas. As of yet, no diagnostically useful cytogenetic aberrations have been defined in soft tissue rhabdoid tumors.

Fibromatoses, fibrosarcomas, and related lesions

Trisomies of chromosomes 8, 11, 17, and 20 are characteristic aberrations in infantile fibrosarcomas.[1,20,101] It is interesting that one or more of this same group of trisomies is also found in the cellular variant of mesoblastic nephroma, which is an infantile renal tumor having substantial histological overlapping with infantile fibrosarcoma.[102] The cytogenetic parallels between infantile fibrosarcomas and mesoblastic nephromas are notable because both entities are associated with excellent prognosis after excisional biopsy despite being cellular undifferentiated tumors that are often mitotically active.[9,55,117,120,132] Several other fibrous tumors with a favorable prognosis share one

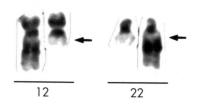

FIG. 5-4. Partial karyotype of a clear cell sarcoma showing translocation of chromosomes 12 and 22. Arrows indicate translocation breakpoints on the rearranged chromosomes.

or more of the above-mentioned trisomies, and these tumors will be discussed in the following paragraphs.

Dermatofibrosarcoma protuberans. The most striking cytogenetic abnormality in dermatofibrosarcoma protuberans is a ring chromosome of varying size that is often superimposed on an otherwise normal karyotype.[10,85,86,118] Ring chromosomes generally form when a given chromosome loses one or both of its telomeres. Telomeres ordinarily serve to stabilize the chromosome ends, and once they are lost the chromosome ends become "sticky" and tend to fuse with other chromosome ends. Fusion with the opposite chromosome arm results in the circular ring form. Portions of the ring chromosome in dermatofibrosarcoma protuberans appear to originate from chromosome 17,[86] but the tumorigenic role of this particular aberration remains to be determined. Additional cytogenetic abnormalities are seen in association with the ring chromosomes in some dermatofibrosarcoma protuberans tumors, the most frequent being trisomy for chromosome 8.[10,86] Although trisomy 8 and overrepresentation of chromosome 17 are seen in other fibrous tumors, the ring chromosome containing chromosome 17 appears to be a unique hallmark of dermatofibrosarcoma protuberans.

Desmoid tumors. Deep fibromatoses (desmoid tumors) often appear normal on cytogenetical studies, but trisomy for chromosome 8 has been reported in approximately 20% of these tumors[23,80] (Fig. 5-1). This trisomy is often found in a minority of the desmoid tumor cells (10% to 30%) and may be a secondary mutation rather than a primary tumorigenic event. Preliminary data suggest that desmoid tumors with trisomy 8 might be at increased risk of subsequent local recurrence.[80] A less common aberration in desmoid tumors is deletion of the chromosome 5 long arm, which is found in less than 10% of cases.[11] This deletion likely results in loss of the APC tumor suppressor gene: APC is the gene responsible for adenomatous polyposis coli, and a role for this gene in sporadic desmoid cases is supported by the high frequency of desmoid tumors in adenomatous polyposis kindreds with Gardner's syndrome.

Synovial sarcoma

Both biphasic and monophasic synovial sarcomas are characterized by a reciprocal translocation of chromosomes

X and 18, t(X;18)(p11;q11).[22,35,64,127] This translocation is found in more than 90% of synovial sarcomas, and the remainder have "variant" translocations of either chromosome X or chromosome 18 with a different partner.[64] The t(X;18) translocation is of particular diagnostic relevance because it is not found in potential histological mimics such as hemangiopericytoma, mesothelioma, leiomyosarcoma, or malignant peripheral nerve sheath tumor. Although the translocation (X;18) breakpoint has been cloned, the specific genes rearranged by the translocation have not been identified.[24]

Hemangiopericytoma

The most consistent cytogenetic abnormality in hemangiopericytoma is rearrangement of the chromosome 12 long arm, which is found in approximately 30% to 50% of cases[69,88,113] (Table 5-1). The chromosome 12 rearrangements are not diagnostic, however, because similar aberrations are found occasionally in other spindle cell sarcomas.[76]

Smooth muscle tumors

Leiomyosarcomas contain heterogeneous chromosome aberrations,[8,39,114] but the most consistent finding has been deletion of the chromosome 1 short arm (Table 5-1). These deletions are probably not useful diagnostically because similar deletions have been seen occasionally in malignant fibrous histiocytoma, rhabdomyosarcoma, and malignant peripheral nerve sheath tumors.[76] Most leiomyosarcomas contain very complex karyotypes with multiple clonal chromosome aberrations, and this complexity can be striking even in low-grade specimens[39] (Fig. 5-5). Most leiomyo-

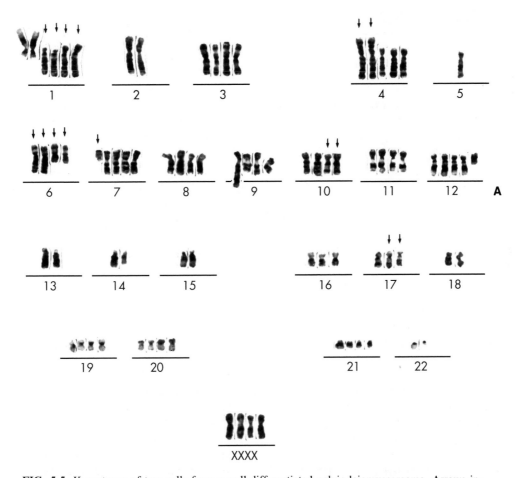

FIG. 5-5. Karyotypes of two cells from a well-differentiated pelvic leiomyosarcoma. Arrows indicate clonal chromosome rearrangements that were found in all cells analyzed from this tumor. "Mar" is an abbreviation for marker, which indicates an abnormal chromosome of uncertain origin. The karyotypes in **A** and **B** share numerous clonal abnormalities but differ in total chromosome number (80 versus 156 chromosomes). Chromosome rearrangements not designated by arrows (e.g., the bizarre chromosome 7 rearrangements at lower left in **B**) were not present consistently and reflect the genetic heterogeneity in this tumor. (From Fletcher JA, Morton CC, Pavelka K, et al: *Cancer Res* 50:4092, 1990.)

Continued.

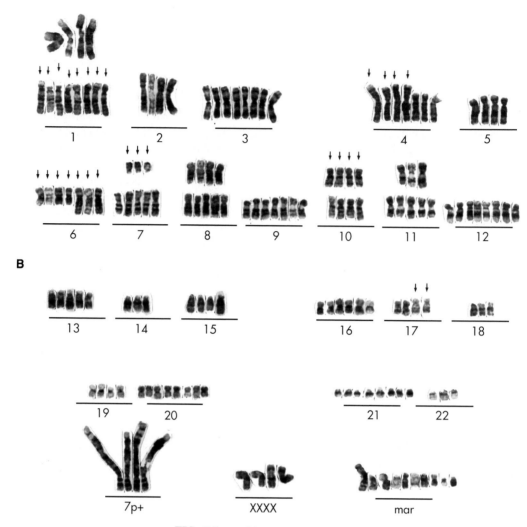

B

FIG. 5-5, cont'd. For legend see p. 111.

For legend see p. 111.

mas, by contrast, are either normal on cytogenetic studies or contain relatively simple cytogenetic aberrations.[71,81,92] Uterine leiomyomas, in particular, are known to have several recurrent chromosome aberrations. Translocation of chromosomes 12 and 14 and deletion of the chromosome 7 long arm (Table 5-2) are each found in 15% to 25% of cases, whereas trisomy 12 and rearrangements of the chromosome 6 short arm are each found in approximately 10% to 15% of cases.[71,81,92] These aberrations are not characteristic of leiomyosarcomas, and cytogenetic aberrations in leiomyomas do not appear to be associated with increased risk of cancer.

Adipose tumors

Characteristic cytogenetic profiles have been described for each of the common varieties of adipose tumor (Tables 5-1 and 5-2). The most diagnostically useful aberration is a translocation of chromosomes 12 and 16, t(12;16) (q13;p11), which is seen in the majority of myxoid liposarcomas.[30,115,129] The t(12;16) translocation results in fusion of the CHOP gene on chromosome 12 with the TLS gene on chromosome 16,[3,19] and this translocation can be detected either by cytogenetics or reverse transcriptase PCR. The t(12;16) translocation appears to be specific for myxoid liposarcoma and has not been found in other subtypes of liposarcoma or in other types of myxoid soft tissue tumors.[52,66,76,128] Well-differentiated liposarcomas (atypical lipomas) lack the t(12;16) translocation, but most cases contain large unidentifiable "giant marker" chromosomes[57,115] or ring chromosomes composed of chromosome 12 material,[21,57] or both (Fig. 5-6). The biological significance of these ring and "giant marker" chromosomes remains to be determined. Well-differentiated liposarcoma karyotypes are generally noncomplex, often containing ring

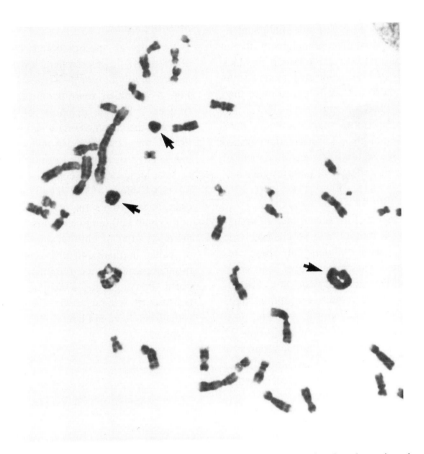

FIG. 5-6. Partial metaphase from a well-differentiated liposarcoma showing three ring chromosomes *(arrows)* of varying sizes.

or giant marker chromosomes, or both, as isolated aberrations. Pleomorphic liposarcomas, by contrast, have exceedingly complex karyotypes with multiple clonal chromosome aberrations.[35,57,115] These pleomorphic liposarcoma karyotypes are generally even more chaotic than the complex karyotypes seen in most high-grade leiomyosarcomas, malignant fibrous histiocytomas, and malignant peripheral nerve sheath tumors (see Table 5-1). The karyotypic complexity in pleomorphic liposarcomas has hampered attempts to define consistent chromosome aberrations that might be of diagnostic use.

Solitary typical lipomas contain rearrangements of the chromosome 12 long arm at a region distal to the characteristic translocation breakpoint of myxoid liposarcomas.[51,68,87] These rearrangements are generally translocations with a variety of partner chromosomes, and the most frequent translocation partner is the long arm of chromosome 3.[116] The chromosome 12 translocation breakpoint in typical lipomas is in the same region as a characteristic translocation breakpoint in uterine leiomyoma (Table 5-2). Thus, it is possible that a single gene on chromosome 12 contributes to cell proliferation both in leiomyomas and lipomas. Other nonrandom aberrations in lipomas include re-

arrangement of the chromosome 6 short arm and deletion of the chromosome 13 long arm, which are each seen in less than 10% of cases.[51] Given the high frequency of cytogenetic aberrations in solitary lipomas it is notable that multiple lipomas from the same patient invariably have normal karyotypes.[51] It is likely that most multiple lipomas arise by an oncogenetic mechanism which differs from that in solitary lipomas and which does not involve large-scale chromosomal rearrangement. Other nonrandom cytogenetic aberrations in benign adipose tumors include rearrangement of the chromosome 8 long arm in the pediatric tumor lipoblastoma[37] and rearrangement of the chromosome 11 long arm in hibernoma.[78]

Malignant fibrous histiocytoma

High-grade malignant fibrous histiocytomas have very complex karyotypes[35,66,67,96] containing numerous clonal chromosome abnormalities. Superimposed on the clonal aberrations are substantial nonclonal aberrations that are unique to individual metaphase cells. The cytogenetic complexity in these tumors suggests that specific factors are continually promoting chromosome disarray. This "genetic instability" might account for the morphological and immunohistochemical heterogeneity in high-grade malignant fibrous histiocytomas.[43,53,74] Most myxoid malignant fibrous histiocytomas, by contrast, are lower-grade tumors that lack the karyotypic complexity of high-grade malignant fibrous histiocytomas. Ring chromosomes are found in more than 50% of myxoid malignant fibrous histiocytomas.[66,85,96] No diagnostically useful chromosome rearrangements have been defined in high-grade malignant fibrous histiocytomas, but there are preliminary suggestions that rearrangement of chromosome 19 might be an indicator of poor prognosis.[96]

Peripheral nerve sheath tumors

Karyotypes have been reported for fewer than 20 malignant peripheral nerve sheath tumors, and no characteristic chromosome aberrations were evident in these tumors.[5,35,38,45] The reported karyotypes have been from high-grade tumors, and all have had very complex chromosome aberrations. Benign schwannnomas, by contrast, have noncomplex karyotypes, and monosomy 22 is found in at least 50% of cases.[5,7,18] The target of this chromosome 22 loss appears to be the neurofibromatosis 2 tumor suppressor gene.[95,125] Clonal cytogenetic aberrations are almost never found in neurofibromas, and it remains unclear whether most neurofibromas are true clonal neoplasms.[31,119]

Mesothelioma

Virtually all mesotheliomas contain clonal cytogenetic aberrations, the most characteristic being a group of deletions involving chromosomes 1, 3, and 22* (Table 5-1; Fig. 5-7). Other rearrangements found at slightly lower frequency include deletions of the chromosome 6 long arm and the chromosome 9 short arm.[34,121] The aforementioned chromosome deletions are found in mesotheliomas irrespective of primary location (pleural versus peritoneal) or histologic factors (epithelial versus sarcomatoid versus mixed).[34] None of the deletions is specific for mesothelioma; in fact, the same chromosome deletions are found in non–small cell lung carcinomas. Accordingly, cytogenetic demonstration of chromosome deletions is unlikely to be of value in distinguishing epithelial mesothelioma from bronchogenic adenocarcinoma. Cytogenetic analyses are useful in confirming a neoplastic proliferation, however, because the characteristic chromosome deletions of mesothelioma have not been found in reactive mesothelial hyperplasias.[47]

---

*References 32, 34, 35, 48, 91, 121, 122.

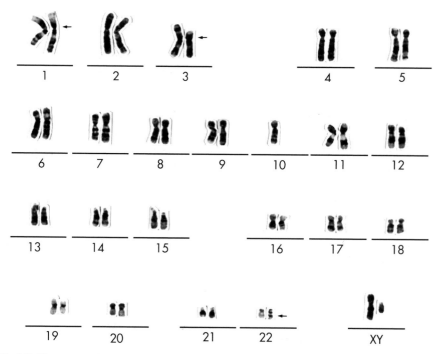

FIG. 5-7. Karyotype of a pleural mesothelioma in which arrows indicate rearrangements resulting in loss of material from the chromosome 1 short arm, chromosome 3 short arm, and chromosome 22 long arm.

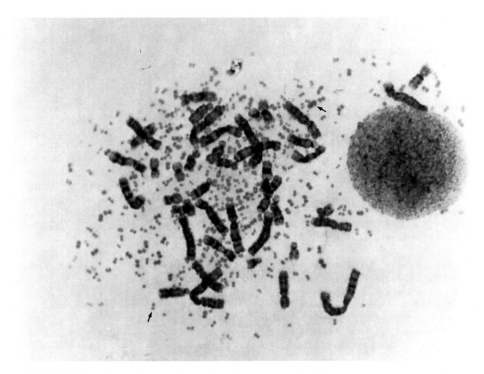

FIG. 5-8. Neuroblastoma metaphase cell with numerous double minute chromosomes of varying sizes *(arrows)*.

Neuroblastoma

Prognosis in many neuroblastomas can be established based on patient age and tumor stage. Advanced-stage neuroblastomas in children older than 2 years are rarely curable, whereas localized neuroblastomas, particularly in children younger than 2 years, are usually cured after resection and nonintensive chemotherapy. Advanced-stage neuroblastomas with a poor prognosis are invariably near-diploid or near-tetraploid with deletions of the chromosome 1 short arm, and approximately 40% of these cases have double minute chromosomes that contain amplified copies of the N-myc oncogene[12,16,56,105] (Figs. 5-2 and 5-8). Neuroblastomas with a favorable prognosis are generally near-triploid and lack chromosome 1 deletions or double minute chromosomes.[12,50,56] These genetic parameters can be useful in determining appropriate intensity of therapy for children whose prognoses cannot be established using clinical parameters.[12] Cytogenetic analyses of neuroblastoma have been difficult, however, because the tumor cells from neuroblastomas with the most favorable prognosis fail to divide in culture.[12] It is notable, therefore, that both N-myc amplification and chromosome 1 deletions can be demonstrated in interphase cells by in situ hybridization.[107,119]

Benign epithelial-mesenchymal tumors

Breast fibroadenomas, pulmonary chondroid hamartomas, and endometrial polyps are benign tumors composed of mesenchymal and epithelial cells. Some of these tumors have been considered historically as nonneoplastic hamartomas or hyperplasias, but recent cytogenetic studies have demonstrated clonal chromosome aberrations that indicate a neoplastic origin in some tumors from each of these categories.[13,40-42,70,111] Immunohistochemical analyses of the clonal aberrant metaphase cells from these tumors have shown that the clonal cells are mesenchymal.[40-42] These findings suggest that some breast fibroadenomas, pulmonary chondroid hamartomas, and endometrial polyps are true mesenchymal neoplasms, whereas the epithelial components in these clonal cases appear to be reactive hyperplasias.

REFERENCES

1. Adam LR, Davison EV, Malcolm AJ, et al: Cytogenetic analysis of a congenital fibrosarcoma. *Cancer Genet Cytogenet* 52:37, 1991.
2. Akerman M, Alvegard T, Eliasson J, et al: A case of Ewing's sarcoma diagnosed by fine needle aspiration. *Acta Orthop Scand* 59:589, 1988.
3. Aman P, Ron D, Mandahl N, et al: Rearrangement of the transcription factor gene CHOP in myxoid liposarcomas with t(12;16) (q13;p11). *Genes Chromosom Cancer* 5:278, 1992.
4. Barr FG, Galili N, Holick J, et al: Rearrangement of the PAX3 paired box gene in the paediatric solid tumor alveolar rhabdomyosarcoma. *Nature Genet* 3:113, 1993.

5. Bello MJ, de Campos JM, Kusak E, et al: Clonal chromosme aberrations in neurinomas. *Genes Chromosom Cancer* 6:206, 1993.

6. Biegel JA, Conrad K, Brooks JJ: Translocation (11;22)(p13;q12): primary change in intraabdominal desmoplastic small round cell tumor. *Genes Chromosom Cancer* 7:119, 1993.

7. Bijlsma EK, Brouwer-Mladin R, Bosch DA, et al: Molecular characterization of chromosome 22 deletions in schwannomas. *Genes Chromosom Cancer* 5:201, 1992.

8. Boghosian L, Dal Cin P, Turc-Carel C, et al: Three possible cytogenetic subgroups of leiomyosarcoma. *Cancer Genet Cytogenet* 43:39, 1989.

9. Bolande RP: Congenital mesoblastic nephroma of infancy. *Perspect Pediatr Pathol* 1:227, 1973.

10. Bridge JA, Neff JR, Sandberg AA: Cytogenetic analysis of dermatofibrosarcoma protuberans. *Cancer Genet Cytogenet* 49:199, 1990.

11. Bridge JA, Sreekantaiah C, Mouron B, et al: Clonal chromosome aberrations in desmoid tumors: implications for histogenesis. *Cancer* 69:430, 1992.

12. Brodeur GM, Azar C, Brother M, et al: Neuroblastoma: effect of genetic factors on prognosis and treatment. *Cancer* 70:1685, 1992.

13. Calabrese G, Di Virgilio C, Cianchetti et al: Chromosome abnormalities in breast fibroadenomas. *Genes Chromosom Cancer* 3:202, 1991.

14. Caspersson T, Zech L, Johansson C: Differential banding of alkylating fluorochromes in human chromosomes. *Exp Cell Res* 60:315, 1970.

15. Cavazzona A, Miser JS, Jefferson HTL, et al: Experimental evidence for a neural origin of Ewing's sarcoma. *Am J Pathol* 127:507, 1987.

16. Christianses H, Schlestag J, Christiansen NM, et al: Clinical impact of chromosome 1 aberrations in neuroblastoma: a metaphase and interphase cytogenetic study. *Genes Chromosom Cancer* 5:141, 1992.

17. Chung EB, Enzinger FM. Infantile fibrosarcoma. *Cancer* 38:729, 1976.

18. Couturier J, Delattre O, Kujas M, et al: Assessment of chromosome 22 anomalies in neurinomas by combined karyotype and RFLP analyses. *Cancer Genet Cytogenet* 45:55, 1990.

19. Crozat A, Aman P, Mandahl N, et al: Fusion of CHOP to a novel RNA-binding protein in human myxoid liposarcoma. *Nature* 363:640, 1993.

20. Dal Cin P, Brock P, Casteels-Van Daele M, et al: Cytogenetic characterization of congenital or infantile fibrosarcoma. *Eur J Pediatr* 150:579, 1991.

21. Dal Cin P, Kools P, Sciot R, et al: Cytogenetic and fluorescent in situ hybridization investigation of ring chromosomes characterizing a specific pathologic subgroup of adipose tissue tumors. *Cancer Genet Cytogenet* 68:85, 1993.

22. Dal Cin P, Rao U, Jani-Sait S, et al: Chromosomes in the diagnosis of soft tissue tumors. I. Synovial sarcoma. *Mod Pathol* 5:357, 1992.

23. Dal Cin P, Sclot R, Aly MS, et al: Some desmoid tumors are characterized by trisomy 8. *Genes Chromosom Cancer* 10:131, 1994.

24. Delattre O, Zucman J, Plougastel B, et al: Gene fusion with an ETS DNA-binding domain caused by chromosome translocation in human tumors. *Nature* 359:162, 1992.

25. de Leeuw B, Suijkerbujik RF, Balemans M, et al: Sublocalization of the synovial sarcoma–associated t(X;18) chromosomal breakpoint in Xp11.2 using cosmid cloning and in situ hybridization. *Oncogene* 8:1457, 1993.

26. Desmaze C, Zucman J, Delattre O, et al: Unicolor and bicolor in situ hybridization in the diagnosis of peripheral neuroepithelioma and related tumors. *Genes Chromosom Cancer* 5:30, 1992.

27. Douglass EC, Rowe ST, Valentine M, et al: Variant translocations of chromosome 13 in alveolar rhabdomyosarcoma. *Genes Chromosom Cancer* 3:480, 1991.

28. Douglass EC, Shapiro DN, Valentine M, et al: Alveolar rhabdomyosarcoma with the t(2;13): cytogenetic findings and clinicopathologic correlations. *Med Pediatr Oncol* 21:83, 1993.

29. Emmerich P, Jauch A, Hofmann M-C, et al: Interphase cytogenetics in paraffin-embedded sections from human testicular germ cell tumor xenografts and in corresponding cultured cells. *Lab Invest* 61:235, 1989.

30. Eneroth M, Mandahl N, Heim S, et al: Localization of the chromosomal breakpoints of the t(12;16) in liposarcoma to subbands 12q13.3 and 16p11.2. *Cancer Genet Cytogenet* 48:101, 1990.

31. Fialkow PJ, Sagebiel RW, Gartler SM, et al: Multiple cell origin of hereditary neurofibromas. *N Engl J Med* 284:298, 1971.

32. Flejter WL, Li FP, Antman KH, et al: Recurring loss involving chromosomes 1, 3, and 22 in malignant mesothelioma: possible sites of tumor suppressor genes. *Genes Chromosom Cancer* 1:148, 1989.

33. Fletcher JA: Translocation (12;22)(q13-14;q12) is a nonrandom aberration in soft tissue clear-cell sarcoma. *Genes Chromosom Cancer* 5:184, 1992.

34. Fletcher JA, Cibas E, Granados R, et al: Consistent chromosome aberrations and genetic stability in malignant mesotheliomas. *Lab Invest* 64:114A, 1991.

35. Fletcher JA, Kozakewich HP, Hoffer FA, et al: Diagnostic relevance of clonal chromosome aberrations in malignant soft-tissue tumors. *N Engl J Med* 324:436, 1991.

36. Fletcher JA, Kozakewich HP, Pavelka K, et al: Consistent cytogenetic aberrations in hepatoblastoma: a common pathway of genetic alterations in embryonal liver and skeletal muscle malignancies? *Genes Chromosom Cancer* 3:37, 1991.

37. Fletcher JA, Kozakewich HP, Schoenberg ML, et al: Cytogenetic findings in pediatric adipose tumors: consistent rearrangement of chromosome 8 in lipoblastoma. *Genes Chromosom Cancer* 6:24, 1993.

38. Fletcher JA, Lipinski KK, Corson JM, et al: Cytogenetics of peripheral nerve sheath tumors. *Cancer Genet Cytogenet* 41:224A, 1989.

39. Fletcher JA, Morton CC, Pavelka K, et al: Chromosome aberrations in uterine smooth muscle tumors: potential diagnostic relevance of cytogenetic instability. *Cancer Res* 50:4092, 1990.

40. Fletcher JA, Pinkus GS, Donovan K, et al: Clonal rearrangement of chromosome band 6p21 in the mesenchymal component of pulmonary chondroid hamartoma. *Cancer Res* 52:6224, 1992.

41. Fletcher JA, Pinkus JL, Lage JM, et al: Clonal 6p21 rearrangement is restricted to the mesenchymal component of an endometrial polyp. *Genes Chromosom Cancer* 5:260, 1992.

42. Fletcher JA, Pinkus GS, Weidner N, et al: Lineage-restricted clonality in biphasic solid tumors. *Am J Pathol* 138:1199, 1991.

43. Genberg M, Mark J, Hakelius L, et al: Origin and relationship between different cell types in malignant fibrous histiocytoma. *Am J Pathol* 135:1185, 1989.

44. Gerald WL, Miller HK, Battifora H, et al: Intra-abdominal desmoplastic small round-cell tumor: report of 19 cases of a distinctive type of high-grade polyphenotypic malignancy affecting young individuals. *Am J Surg Pathol* 15:499, 1991.

45. Glover TW, Stein CK, Legius E, et al: Molecular and cytogenetic analysis of tumors in von Recklinghausen neurofibromatosis. *Genes Chromosom Cancer* 3:62, 1991.

46. Goji J, Sano K, Nakamura H, et al: Chondrocytic differentiation of peripheral neuroectodermal tumor cell line in nude mouse xenograft. *Cancer Res* 52:4214, 1992.

47. Granados R, Cibas ES, Fletcher JA: Cytogenetic analysis of effusions for malignant mesothelioma: a diagnostic adjunct to cytology. *Acta Cytol* (in press).

48. Hagemeijer A, Versnel MA, Van Drunen EV, et al: Cytogenetic analysis of malignant mesothelioma. *Cancer Genet Cytogenet* 47:1, 1990.

49. Harnden DG, Klinger HP (editors): *ISCN 1985: an international system for human cytogenetic nomenclature.* Basel, 1985, S. Karger.

50. Hayashi Y, Inaba T, Hanada R, et al: Chromosome findings and prognosis in 15 patients with neuroblastoma found by VMA screening. *J Pediatr* 112:567, 1988.

51. Heim S, Mandahl N, Rydholm A, et al: Different karyotypic features characterize different clinicopathologic subgroups of benign lipogenic tumors. *Int J Cancer* 42:863, 1988.

52. Hinrichs SH, Jaramillo MA, Gumerlock PH: Myxoid chondrosarcoma with a translocation involving chromosomes 9 and 22. *Cancer Genet Cytogenet* 14:219, 1985.

53. Hirose T, Kudo E, Hasegawa T, et al: Expression of intermediate filaments in malignant fibrous histiocytoma. *Hum Pathol* 29:871, 1989.

54. Hoffer FA, Gianturco LE, Fletcher JA, et al: Percutaneous biopsy of peripheral primitive neuroectodermol tumors and Ewing's sarcomas for cytogenetic analysis. *Am J Radiol* 162:1141, 1994.

55. Howell CH, Othersen HB, Kiviat NE, et al: Therapy and outcome in 51 children with mesoblastic nephroma: a report of the National Wilms' Tumor Study. *J Pediatr Surg* 17:326, 1982.

56. Kaneko Y, Kanda N, Maseki N, et al: Different karyotypic patterns in early and advanced stage neuroblastomas. *Cancer Res* 47:311, 1987.

57. Karakousis CP, Dal Cin P, Turc-Carel C, et al: Chromosomal changes in soft-tissue tumors. *Arch Surg* 122:1257, 1987.

58. Kim SY, Lee JS, Ro JY, et al: Interphase cytogenetics in paraffin sections of lung tumors by nonisotopic in situ hybridization. *Am J Pathol* 142:307, 1993.

59. Koufos A, Grundy P, Morgan K, et al: Familial Wiedemann-Beckwith syndrome and a second Wilms' tumor locus both map to 11p15.5. *Am J Hum Genet* 44:711, 1989.

60. Koufos A, Hansen MF, Copeland NG, et al: Loss of heterozygosity in three embryonal tumors suggests a common pathogenetic mechanism. *Nature (London)* 316:330, 1985.

61. Ladanyi M, Heinemann FS, Huvos AG, et al: Neural differentiation in small round cell tumors of bone and soft tissue with the translocation t(11;22)(q14;q12): an immunohistochemical study of 11 cases. *Hum Pathol* 21:1245, 1990.

62. Lichter P, Chang Tang C, Call K, et al: High-resolution mapping of human chromosome 11 by in situ hybridization with cosmid clones. *Science* 247:64, 1990.

63. Limon J, Dal Cin P, Sandberg AA: Application of long-term collagenase disaggregation for the cytogenetic analysis of human solid tumors. *Cancer Genet Cytogenet* 23:305, 1986.

64. Limon J, Mrozek K, Mandahl N, et al: Cytogenetics of synovial sarcoma: presentation of ten new cases and review of the literature. *Genes Chromosom Cancer* 3:338, 1991.

65. Llombart-Bosch A, Carda C, Peydro-Olaya A, et al: Soft tissue Ewing's sarcoma: characterization in established cultures and xenografts with evidence of a neuroectodermic phenotype. *Cancer* 66:2589, 1990.

66. Mandahl N, Heim S, Arheden K, et al: Rings, dicentrics, and telomeric association in histiocytoma. *Cancer Genet Cytogenet* 30:23, 1988.

67. Mandahl N, Heim S, Willen H, et al: Characteristic karyotypic anomalies identify subtypes of malignant fibrous histiocytoma. *Genes Chromosom Cancer* 1:9, 1989.

68. Mandahl N, Hoglund M, Mertens F, et al: Cytogenetic aberrations in 188 benign and borderline adipose tissue tumors. *Genes Chromosom Cancer* 9:207, 1994.

69. Mandahl N, Orndal C, Heim S, et al: Aberrations of chromosome segment 12q13-15 characterize a subgroup of hemangiopericytomas. *Cancer* 71:3009-3013, 1993.

70. Johansson M, Dietrich C, Mandahl N, et al: Recominations of chromosome bands 6p21 and 14q24 characterise pulmonary hamartomas. *Br J Cancer* 67:1236, 1993.

71. Mark J, Havel G, Grepp C, et al: Chromosomal patterns in human benign uterine leiomyomas. *Cancer Genet Cytogenet* 44:1, 1990.

72. Matsumara K, Kallioniemi A, Kallioniemi O, et al: Deletion of chromosome 17p loci in breast cancer cells detected by fluorescence in situ hybridization. *Cancer Res* 52:3474, 1992.

73. May WA, Gishizky ML, Lessnick SL, et al: Ewing sarcoma 11;22 translocation produces a chimeric transcription factor that requires the DNA-binding domain encoded by FLI1 for transformation. *Proc Natl Acad Sci U S A* 90:5752, 1993.

74. Miettinen M, Soini Y: Malignant fibrous histiocytoma: heterogeneous patterns of intermediate filament proteins by immunohistochemistry. *Arch Pathol Lab Med* 113:1363, 1989.

75. Mills SE, Frierson HF: Olfactory neuroblastoma: a clinicopathologic study of 21 cases. *Am J Surg Pathol* 9:317, 1985.

76. Mitelman F: *Catalog of chromosome aberrations in cancer,* ed 4. New York, 1991, Wiley-Liss.

77. Mitelman F (editor): *ISCN (1991): Guidelines for cancer cytogenetics, supplement to an internation system for human cytogenetic nomenclature.* Basel, 1991, S. Karger.

78. Mrozek K, Karakousis CP, Bloomfield CD: Band 11q13 is nonrandomly rearranged in hibernomas. *Genes Chromosom Cancer* 9:145, 1994.

79. Mugneret F, Lizard S, Aurias A, et al: Chromosomes in Ewing's sarcoma. II. Nonrandom additional changes, trisomy 8 and der(16)t(1;16). *Cancer Genet Cytogenet* 32:239, 1988.

80. Naeem R, Fletcher JA: Trisomy 8 is a potential marker of high risk in desmoid tumors. *Am J Hum Genet* 51:A279, 1992.

81. Nilbert M, Heim S: Uterine leiomyoma cytogenetics. *Genes Chromosom Cancer* 2:3, 1990.

82. Noguera R, Navarro S, Triche TJ: Translocation (11;22) in small cell osteosarcoma. *Cancer Genet Cytogenet* 45:121, 1990.

83. Noguera R, Triche TJ, Navarro S, et al: Dynamic model of differentiation in Ewing's sarcoma cells: comparative analysis of morphologic, immunocytochemical, and oncogene expression parameters. *Lab Invest* 62:143, 1992.

84. Ohno T, Rao VN, Reddy ESP: EWS/Fli-1 chimeric protein is a transcriptional activator. *Cancer Res* 53:5859, 1993.

85. Orndal C, Mandahl N, Rydholm A, et al: Supernumerary ring chromosomes in five bone and soft tissue tumors of low or borderline malignancy. *Cancer Genet Cytogenet* 60:170, 1992.

86. Pedeutour F, Coindre J-M, Nicolo G, et al: Ring chromosomes in dermatofibrosarcoma protuberans contain chromosome 17 sequences: fluorescent in situ hybridization. *Cancer Genet Cytogenet* 67:149, 1993.

87. Pedeutour F, Suijkerbujik RF, Van Gaal J, et al: Chromosome 12 origin in rings and giant markers in well-differentiated liposarcoma. *Cancer Genet Cytogenet* 66:133, 1993.

88. Perez-Atayde AR, Kozakewich HP, McGill T, et al: Hemangiopericytoma of the tongue in a 10-year-old child: ultrastructural and cytogenetic observations. *Hum Pathol* 25:425, 1994.

89. Peulve P, Michot C, Vannier J-P, et al: Clear cell sarcoma with t(12;22)(q13-14;q12). *Genes Chromosom Cancer* 3:400, 1991.

90. Pinkel D, Landegent J, Collins C, et al: Fluorescence in situ hybridization with human chromosome-specific libraries: detection of trisomy 21 and translocations of chromosome 4. *Proc Natl Acad Sci U S A* 85:9138, 1988.

91. Popescu NC, Chahinian AP, DiPaolo JA: Nonrandom chromosome alterations in human malignant mesothelioma. *Cancer Res* 48:142, 1988.

92. Rein MS, Friedman AJ, Barbieri RL, et al: Cytogenetic abnormalities in uterine leiomyomata. *Obstet Gynecol* 77:923, 1991.

93. Ried T, Lengauer C, Cremer T, et al: Specific metaphase and interphase detection of the breakpoint region in 8q24 of Burkitt lymphoma cells by triple-color fluorescence in situ hybridization. *Genes Chromosom Cancer* 4:69, 1992.

94. Rodriguez E, Sreekantaiah C, Gerald W, et al: A recurring translocation, t(11;22)(p13;q11.2), characterizes intraabdominal desmoplastic small round-cell tumors. *Cancer Genet Cytogenet* 69:17, 1993.

95. Rouleau GA, Merel P, Lutchman M, et al: Alteration in a new gene encoding a putative membrane-organizing protein causes neurofibromatosis type 2. *Nature* 363:515, 1993.

96. Rydholm A, Mandahl N, Heim S, et al: Malignant fibrous histiocytomas with a 19p+ marker chromosome have increased relapse rate. *Genes Chromosom Cancer* 2:296, 1990.

97. Sainati L, Scapinello A, Montaldi A, et al: A mesenchymal chondrosarcoma of a child with the reciprocal translocation (11;22) (q24;q12). *Cancer Genet Cytogenet* 71:144, 1993.

98. Sandberg AA, Turc-Carel C, Gemmill RM: Chromosomes in solid tumors and beyond. *Cancer Res* 48:1049, 1988.

99. Sawyer JR, Tryka AF, Lewis JM: A novel reciprocal chromosome translocation t(11;22)(p13;q12) in an intraabdominal desmoplastic small round cell tumor. *Am J Surg Pathol* 16:411, 1992.

100. Schofield DE, Fletcher JA: Trisomy 12 in pediatric granulosa-stromal cell tumors: demonstration by a modified method of fluorescence in situ hybridization on paraffin-embedded material. *Am J Pathol* 141:1265, 1992.

101. Schofield DE, Fletcher JA, Grier HE, et al: Fibrosarcoma in infants and children: application of new techniques. *Am J Surg Pathol* 18:14, 1994.

102. Schofield DE, Yunis EJ, Fletcher JA: Chromosome aberrations in mesoblastic nephroma. *Am J Pathol* 143:714, 1993.

103. Scrable J, Witte D, Shimada H, et al: Molecular differential pathology of rhabdomyosarcoma. *Genes Chromosom Cancer* 1:23, 1989.

104. Seabright M: A rapid banding technique for human chromosomes. *Lancet* 2:971, 1971.

105. Seeger RC, Brodeur GM, Sather H, et al: Association of multiple copies of the N-myc oncogene with rapid progression of neuroblastomas. *N Engl J Med* 313:1111, 1985.

106. Shapiro DN, Sublett JE, Li B, et al: Fusion of PAX3 to a member of the forkhead family of transcription factors in human alveolar rhabdomyosarcoma. *Cancer Res* 53:5108, 1993.

107. Shapiro DN, Valentine MB, Rowe ST, et al: Detection of N-myc gene amplification by fluorescence in situ hybridization: diagnostic utility for neuroblastoma. *Am J Pathol* 142:1339-1346, 1993.

108. Sheng W-W, Soukup S, Ballard E, et al: Chromosomal analysis of sixteen rhabdomyosarcomas. *Cancer Res* 48:983, 1988.

109. Skuse GR, Kosciolek BA, Rowley PT: The neurofibroma in von Recklinghausen neurofibromatosis has a unicellular origin. *Am J Hum Genet* 49:600, 1991.

110. Sorensen PHB, Lessnick SL, Lopez-Terrada D, et al: A second Ewing's sarcoma translocation, t(21;22), fuses the EWS gene to another ETS-family transcription factor, ERG. *Nature Genet* 6:146, 1994.

111. Speleman F, Dal Cin P, Van Roy N, et al: Is t(6;20)(p21;q13) a characteristic chromosome change in endometrial polyps? *Genes Chromosom Cancer* 3:318, 1991.

112. Squire J, Zielenska M, Thorner P, et al: Variant translocations of chromosome 22 in Ewing's sarcoma. *Genes Chromosom Cancer* 8:190, 1993.

113. Sreekantaiah C, Bridge JA, Rao UNM, et al: Clonal chromosomal

114. Sreekantaiah C, Davis JR, Sandberg AA: Chromosomal abnormalities in leiomyosarcomas. *Am J Pathol* 142:293, 1993.

115. Sreekantaiah C, Karakousis CP, Leong SPL, et al: Cytogenetic findings in liposarcoma correlate with histopathologic subtypes. *Cancer* 69:2484, 1992.

116. Sreekantaiah C, Leong SPL, Karakousis CP, et al: Cytogenetic profile of 109 lipomas. *Cancer Res* 51:422, 1991.

117. Stenman G, Kindblom L-G, Angervall L: Reciprocal translocation t(12;22)(q13;q13) in clear-cell sarcoma of tendons and aponeuroses. *Genes Chromosom Cancer* 4:122, 1992.

118. Stephenson CF, Berger CS, Leong SPL, et al: Ring chromosome in a dermatofibrosarcoma protuberans. *Cancer Genet Cytogenet* 58:52, 1992.

119. Stock C, Abros IM, Mann G, et al: Detection of 1p36 deletions in paraffin sections of neuroblastoma tissues. *Genes Chromosom Cancer* 6:1, 1993.

120. Stout AP: Fibrosarcoma in infants and children. *Cancer* 15:1028, 1962.

121. Taguchi T, Jhanwar SC, Siegfried JM, et al: Recurrent deletions of specific chromosomal sites in 1p, 3p, 6q, and 9p in human malignant mesothelioma. *Cancer Res* 53:4349, 1993.

122. Tiainen M, Tammilehto L, Mattson K, et al: Nonrandom chromosomal abnormalities in malignant pleural mesothelioma. *Cancer Genet Cytogenet* 33:251, 1988.

123. Tkachuk DC, Westbrook CA, Andreeff M, et al: Detection of *bcr-abl* fusion in chronic myelogenous leukemia by in situ hybridization. *Science* 250:559, 1990.

124. Trent J, Casper J, Meltzer P, et al: Nonrandom chromosome alterations in rhabdomyosarcoma. *Cancer Genet Cytogenet* 16:189, 1985.

125. Trofatter J, MacCollin MM, Rutter JL, et al: A novel moesin-, ezrin-, radixin-like gene is a candidate for the neurofibromatosis 2 tumor suppressor. *Cell* 72:791, 1993.

126. Turc-Carel C, Aurias A, Mugneret F: Chromosomes in Ewing's sarcoma. I. An evaluation of 85 cases and remarkable consistency of t(11;22)(q24;q12). *Cancer Genet Cytogenet* 32:229, 1988.

127. Turc-Carel C, Dal Cin P, Limon J, et al: Involvement of chromosome X in primary cytogenetic change in human neoplasia: nonrandom translocation in synovial sarcoma. *Proc Natl Acad Sci U S A* 84:1981, 1987.

128. Turc-Carel C, Dal Cin P, Rao U, et al: Recurrent breakpoints at 9q31 and 22q12.2 in extraskeletal myxoid chondrosarcoma. *Cancer Genet Cytogenet* 30:145, 1988.

129. Turc-Carel C, Limon J, Dal Cin P, et al: Cytogenetic studies of adipose tissue tumors. II. Recurrent reciprocal translocation t(12;16)(q13;p11) in myxoid liposarcomas. *Cancer Genet Cytogenet* 23:291, 1986.

130. Whang-Peng J, Freter CE, Knutsen T, et al: Translocation t(11;22) in esthesioneuroblastoma. *Cancer Genet Cytogenet* 29:155, 1987.

131. Whang-Peng J, Triche TJ, Knutsen T, et al: Chromosome translocation in peripheral neuroepithelioma. *N Engl J Med* 311:584, 1984.

132. Wilson MB, Stanley W, Sens D, et al: Infantile fibrosarcoma: a misnomer? *Pediatr Pathol* 10:901, 1990.

133. Zucman J, Delattre O, Desmaze C, et al: EWS and ATF-1 gene fusion induced by t(12;22) translocation in malignant melanoma of soft parts. *Nature Genet* 4:341, 1993.

CHAPTER 6   RICHARD J. ZARBO

DNA ANALYSIS OF SOFT TISSUE TUMORS

The technology of automated cytometry has only recently been applied clinically to human medicine in the last decade with the advent of commercially available instruments and advanced computer software. The two different approaches to automated cytometry are those of *flow cytometry* and *digital image analysis*. The latter method has also gone by the names *microspectrophotometry* and *static cytophotometry*. Flow cytometry has become an accepted laboratory method of quantitating cell surface antigens (immunophenotyping) on hematolymphoid cells for diagnostic purposes. Quantitation of DNA content and cell cycle fractions remain an ongoing investigative application of both flow cytometry and image analysis with promising results in some solid human tumors. The potential applications of cytometric DNA measurements lie in the areas of diagnosis, prognosis, and therapeutic management of high-risk or unresponsive subsets of disease that would benefit from additional selected therapies. In this chapter, the present practical applications and technological state-of-the-art as applied to human soft tissue tumors will be reviewed.

After almost a decade of active clinical investigation, it is apparent that there is a misconception on the part of many, particularly the uninitiated, that this technology is presently capable of providing objective and reproducible data (both intralaboratory and interlaboratory) and that these data are of independent significance in the evaluation of human neoplasms. Suffice it to say that there are numerous quality control concerns that allow for the introduction of significant subjectivity to these automated cytometric techniques and detract from their clinical applicability. To be of clinical significance, DNA parameters should be analyzed in the context of other accepted clinical staging and histopathological features of prognostic import that are the present foundation of clinical decision making for patients with soft tissue sarcomas. To date, this multiparametric analysis has not been adequately performed for specific histological types of sarcomas controlled for similar anatomical site, tumor stage, histological grade, margin status, and therapeutic intervention to confirm a potential independent value for DNA analysis.

BASIC PRINCIPLES

Flow cytometry and image analysis make use of different technologies but use somewhat similar basic underlying principles of stoichiometric DNA staining reactions to quantitate relative DNA content distributions in human tumors. In flow cytometry, solid tissue or thick paraffin embedded tissue sections must be disaggregated into a single cell or nuclear suspension. The alternative is to use fine needle aspirates of in vivo tumors or ex vivo aspiration of excised tumors. Cell suspensions derived by any of these means are then "flowed" in a laminar stream past a focused laser beam for analysis. Light scatter resulting from intrinsic cell qualities and fluorescence emission from applied fluorochrome-labeled markers are detected from the examination of thousands of cells per minute by photodiode light detectors and photomultiplier tubes. Quantitation of DNA by flow cytometry makes use of dyes that either intercalate into double-stranded nucleic acids or interact with specific base pairs in a stoichiometric fashion. When stimulated by the incident laser light, the dye is excited to emit a fluorescent signal of a higher emission wavelength that is separated for detection from the incident light by mirrors and optical filters. The dye fluorescence intensity is proportional to the amount of nuclear DNA and related to DNA of normal cell standards for interpretation. Ordinarily, flow cytometry analysis that uses a single nuclear DNA fluorescence marker is "morphologically blind" to different cell types in the suspension. Use of additional markers bound to other fluorochromes, like fluorescein isothiocyanate, whose emission spectrum (green) can be separated from that of the wavelength of the DNA dye (red), allow for 2-color fluorescence multiparametric analysis, whereby different cell types within the cell suspension can be identified for separate analysis by phenotype-specific monoclonal antibodies.[51] Multiple correlated information parameters on

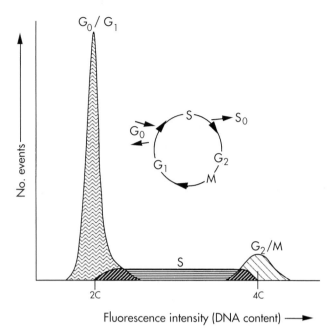

FIG. 6-1. Stylized DNA histogram and compartments of the cell cycle. Computerized mathematical models are employed to estimate S-phase and account for overlapping compartments.

each of thousands of cells, collected from light detectors and photomultiplier tubes, are stored in a computer for further data analysis using sophisticated software programs.

The DNA histograms from flow cytometry, usually composed of 10,000 to 20,000 cell events, are frequency distributions corresponding to light signals emitted by cell events. These histograms are relatively smooth and exhibit components that correspond to cells containing increasing amounts of DNA that relate to three separable phases of the cell cycle: (1) resting G_0 and cycling presynthetic G_1 phases, (2) synthetic (S) phase, and postsynthetic G_2 and mitotic (M) phases (Fig. 6-1). The DNA histogram is characterized by a dominant or modal peak (G_0/G_1) that in a normal human cell population corresponds to the amount of DNA seen in the 46 human chromosomes (equivalent designation 2C). The second smaller peak to the right, past the intervening plateau corresponding to S-phase, represents G_2- and M-phase cells that have twice the DNA content as the G_0/G_1 cells. These latter cells have a double copy or tetraploid chromosome complement and therefore are equivalent to the cytogenetic designation 4C.

It is by this logic of relative DNA staining related to fluorescence obtained with cells bearing a normal complement of chromosomes that flow and image cytometry measurements estimate "ploidy" values in neoplastic proliferations. Given the karyotypic quantitative and structural differences in the genome of tumors, the term *ploidy* is obviously a misnomer in these forms of cytometry and its usage should be restricted to cytogenetic analyses. However, the terms

diploid and *aneuploid* have become engrained in the cytometry literature. In cytometry, these ploidy terms should be prefaced as *DNA diploid* or *DNA aneuploid* to distinguish them from actual ploidy determinations by karyotypic analysis.

The S- and G_2/M-phases of the DNA histogram comprise the proliferative fraction of cells in the population sampled. Determination of tumor proliferation or S-phase fraction alone by software programs that model the DNA histogram is one distinct advantage of DNA analysis by flow cytometry. The large number of events sampled provide a statistically significant database for analysis. Smaller measurement coefficients of variation obtained with flow cytometry result in enhanced ability to resolve near-diploid genetic abnormalities compared with image analysis.

In image analysis, light microscope-based measurements are made on cells affixed to glass slides as cytological or cytocentrifuge preparations, touch imprints of fresh tumors, or nuclei from enzymatically disaggregated thick paraffin tissue sections of fixed tumors. Alternately, cells may be imaged in actual nondisaggregated thinner paraffin tissue sections that preserve histological architecture for morphological correlation. A video camera is used to "capture" an image (microscopic field), which is segmented into objects to be measured. In the case of DNA analysis, the objects are cell nuclei. Each object is stored in a computer as digitized "gray levels" or light intensity signals from pointlike picture elements or "pixels." Computer software is used to analyze the digitized images and display them on the video monitor. DNA content analysis by image densitometry makes use of the DNA-specific Feulgen staining reaction to stain DNA. The Feulgen reaction employs mild acid hydrolysis of DNA to detach free aldehyde groups that are then stained with Schiff's reagent. The transmitted light intensity is converted to an optical density value according to the Beer-Lambert law to develop a linear proportionality to the DNA concentration. Again, appropriate, normal DNA cell standards are measured to define the relative DNA content.

The DNA histograms from image analysis, based on several hundred cell events, are somewhat choppy in contour. The relatively few events in the S-phase portion of the histogram result in unreliable estimates of proliferation by image analysis. The chief advantage of image analysis is the ability to morphologically classify and identify rare cell events in conjunction with densitometric and/or morphometric analysis. The two types of DNA histograms obtained from examination of the same tumor by flow and image cytometry are illustrated in Fig. 6-2.

DNA ploidy and cytogenetic correlation

Measurements of DNA content by both flow and image cytometry can be correlated, with the use of appropriate normal DNA containing standards, to the relative DNA

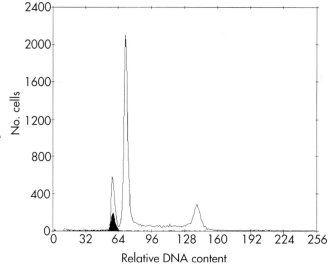

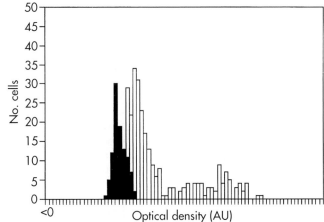

FIG. 6-2. Comparison of DNA histograms obtained by **(A)** flow cytometry of a disaggregated cell suspension, and **(B)** image analysis of touch imprints of the same malignant tumor. The flow cytometry histogram is composed of 20,000 cell events whereas the image analysis histogram is based on the analysis of 200 cells. The dark-shaded peaks within each histogram are from separate analyses, representing the superimposed reference DNA content of normal (diploid) G_0/G_1 cells within each tumor. The unshaded histograms represent DNA content of the tumor. The first unshaded peak in the flow cytometry histogram that overlaps the diploid control equates with G_0/G_1 cells, in this case nonneoplastic stroma, containing diploid DNA content. Tumor cells exhibiting a hyperdiploid DNA aneuploid stemline (DNA index = 1.2) compose the tallest unshaded peaks in each histogram (aneuploid G_0/G_1). The smallest unshaded peaks to the far right within each histogram are the G_2/M compartment of the DNA aneuploid cells.

content of a normal diploid complement of chromosomes. By convention, differences in DNA content from normal cells are expressed as the DNA index, calculated from the equation: Relative DNA fluorescence of tumor G_0/G_1 cells divided by the relative DNA fluorescence of DNA normal standard G_0/G_1 cells.[20] Thus a DNA index of 1 is equated with no change in DNA content detectable from normal cells, and a DNA index of 2 is equated with DNA content twice that of normal cells (tetraploidy). Increased DNA content less than twice normal would equate with hyperdiploidy. Loss of genetic material (hypodiploidy) would result in a DNA index of less than 1. Although good correlation of flow cytometry DNA index with estimates of quantitative chromosomal genomic changes from karyotypes has been demonstrated in soft tissue tumors,[26] discrepancies between the two techniques will exist. These differences will result for a number of reasons, including sampling differences of tumoral stemline heterogeneity, too few cells detected by flow cytometry, or lack of cell culture growth for cytogenetic detection. Therefore it is important to stress that flow cytometric DNA content (ploidy) cannot be equated to an actual determination of ploidy obtained from cytogenetically analyzed metaphases obtained from short-term cultures of tumor. In Mandahl et al.,[26] comparative study of bone and soft tissue tumors, peridiploid flow cytometric DNA indexes correlated with tumors bearing no karyotypic abnormality, karyotypic abnormalities without numerical chromosomal changes, and abnormalities with numerical chromosomal changes. On the other hand, of the flow cytometric DNA aneuploid tumors, almost 40% had normal karyotypes. This may reflect the inability to grow these tumors in culture for cytogenetic evaluation of metaphase chromosomes.

The resolving power of cytogenetics, with its morphological correlation, to detect small changes of genetic material is much greater than that of flow cytometry. It is estimated that by flow cytometry the best sensitivity that can be achieved is the detection of a minimum gain or loss of 5% of the human genome or the amount of DNA contained in approximately three average-sized chromosomes.[50] Because of the greater coefficients of variation obtained in image analysis measurements, the sensitivity of detection of near-diploid genetic abnormality with this technique should be even less. Therefore it should be understood that these cytometric DNA measurements are crude and relatively insensitive to all but large gains or losses of genetic material equivalent to greater than or equal to 3 to 4 chromosomes and are therefore unlikely to detect peridiploid abnormalities.[45] In general, flow cytometry DNA modal values are about 15% higher than those found on karyotype even when chromosome size is taken into account.[34,42] Given these caveats, I believe it is unwise to rely on DNA abnormalities detected by cytometric techniques for tumor diagnosis. A significant percentage of malignant tumors will be indistinguishable from normal ones and classified as DNA diploid because the near-diploid genetic abnormalities will not be detected.[48] In addition, chromosomal aberrations have been documented in a significant proportion of benign tumors including lipomas and leiomyomas.[8] Cytometric DNA abnormalities (aneuploidy) may be encountered not only in some types of benign soft tissue tumors but also in benign tumors of other organs (melanocytic nevi, colonic adenomas, endocrine adenomas). One can only conclude that flow cytometric DNA aneuploidy is neither a sensitive nor a specific marker of malignancy.

TECHNICAL AND QUALITY CONTROL ASPECTS OF DNA CYTOMETRY

There are numerous problematic areas in DNA flow cytometry that presently contribute considerable variation to the intralaboratory analysis and interlaboratory comparison of data. This is a significant limiting factor to the validation of DNA ploidy and proliferation measurements as indicators of prognosis and adjuncts in therapeutic decision making. This would include (1) the technical aspects of tumor sampling to ensure neoplastic cell representation from heterogeneous mixtures of normal cells and neoplastic tissue that may harbor multiple tumoral stemlines; (2) sample source (fixed or fresh tissue) and preparation; (3) tumor disaggregation into monodispersed cell suspensions; (4) cell fixation and DNA dye staining; (5) DNA histogram data analysis, mathematical modeling of overlapping cell cycle phases, and correction for background aggregates and debris; and (6) accepted criteria for classification of DNA histogram abnormalities.

For instance, optimization of tumor cell disaggregation from fresh soft tissue sarcomas, comparing mechanical and enzymatic disaggregation protocols with cell yields and rate of aneuploidy, has only recently been addressed by Zalupski et al.[47] The numerous quality control and technical considerations in flow cytometry are beyond the scope of this chapter but have been the subject of focused reviews by Bagwell,[4] Rabinovitch,[36] and Zarbo.[49]

Consensus guidelines for sampling, processing, instrument performance, and data and histogram analysis in human malignant neoplasms have recently been published by a DNA Cytometry Consensus Conference composed of 32 investigators from Europe and North America that was convened in October 1992 in Prouts Neck, Maine.[40] Useful information has been derived from retrospective studies like the majority of those using paraffin-embedded material, reviewed in this chapter. However, this Consensus Conference concluded that "Optimal analysis of deoxyribonucleic acid (DNA) ploidy and cell cycle phase fractions . . . will be obtained by prospective methods using fresh tissues and examination of whole cell preparations that allow for multiparametric analysis."[6] This is borne out in the DNA ploidy examination of soft tissue sarcomas by Zalupski et al.[47] who have documented a 14% error rate when nuclear preparations from formalin-fixed, paraffin-embedded specimens were compared with enzymatic disaggregation of fresh surgical specimens.[47]

Although cell cycle proliferation measurements in human

tumors are potentially more promising for the individual patient because of the continuous nature of this variable compared with the dichotomous variable of DNA ploidy (diploid versus aneuploid), at present, lack of standardization with numerous technical and methodological sources of variation severely limit clinical usefulness.[49] This makes published S-phase cut points defining prognostic subsets of

Table 6-1. DNA diploid soft tissue tumors

Benign entity	No. studied	Author/year
Fibroma	2	Kreicbergs et al. (1987)[21]
Fibromatosis	5	Kreicbergs et al. (1987)[21]; Kroese et al. (1990)[22]
Juvenile xanthogranuloma	1	Radio et al. (1988)[37]
Desmoid, classic	23	Matsuno et al. (1988)[27]
Desmoid, cellular	7	Matsuno et al. (1988)[27]
Dermatofibroma	9	Radio et al. (1988)[37]
Fibrous histiocytoma	2	Matsuno et al. (1988)[27]
Nodular fasciitis	1	Radio et al. (1988)[37]
Proliferative fasciitis	1	Akerman et al. (1987)[2]
Neuroma	1	Kroese et al. (1990)[22]
Neurofibroma	17	Kreicbergs et al. (1987)[21]; Kroese et al. (1990)[22]; Matsuno et al. (1988)[27]
Schwannoma	7	Kreicbergs et al. (1987)[21]; Kroese et al. (1990)[22]; Matsuno et al. (1988)[27]
Ganglioneuroma	1	Kroese et al. (1990)[22]
Leiomyoma	1	Kroese et al. (1990)[22]
Lipoma	19	Kreicbergs et al. (1987)[21]; Matsuno et al. (1988)[27]
Atypical lipoma	1	Akerman et al. (1987)[2]
Myxoma	1	Matsuno et al. (1988)[27]
Capillary hemangioma	37	Kroese et al. (1990)[22]; Matsuno et al. (1988)[27]; Eto et al. (1992)[15]; Fukunaga et al. (1993)[17]
Juvenile hemangioma	4	Eto et al. (1992)[15]
Epithelioid hemangioma	1	Fukunaga et al. (1993)[17]
Papillary endothelial hyperplasia	1	Fukunaga et al. (1993)[17]
Glomus tumor	6	Eto et al. (1992)[15]
Synovial cyst	2	Matsuno et al. (1988)[27]
Pigmented villonodular synovitis	6	Matsuno et al. (1988)[27]
Chondromatosis	2	Matsuno et al. (1988)[27]

disease inappropriate for extrapolation to results derived from laboratories using different techniques, procedures, and software models. To circumvent these problems and control for method variation, the Consensus Conference has recommended that each laboratory develop its own reference range of S-phase values for DNA diploid and DNA aneuploid tumors for a specific histological tumor type in order to evaluate numerical cut points of clinical significance.[40] Obviously, this present state-of-the-art is not functional for the optimal evaluation of patients with soft tissue sarcomas, which are rare neoplasms in the general population. Any one laboratory cannot possibly prospectively accumulate sufficient numbers of specific histological sarcoma types to generate a confident database of proliferation values to be stratified by ploidy subsets.

Although the technique of DNA measurement by image analysis has been performed for decades, it is currently less commonly applied in the clinical setting than flow cytometry. However, analogous quality control issues remain without consensus. These include tumor sampling, preparation, cell fixation and DNA staining, choice of appropriate controls, DNA histogram data analysis, and criteria for classification of DNA histogram abnormalities. Detailed aspects of quality control, methodological issues, and clinical applications of image analysis in tumor pathology have been the subject of reviews by Hall and Fu[19] and Mellin.[28]

Unfortunately, the present state-of-the-art in flow and image cytometry, lacking accepted methodology and quality control standards, makes cytometric evaluations of DNA ploidy and cell proliferation unreliable for individual patient care decisions. Nevertheless, there are a few selected and promising studies of human soft tissue neoplasms, mostly flow cytometry studies, that are worth considering.

Benign soft tissue tumors

Evaluation of DNA content in numerous histological types of benign soft tissue tumors has almost always resulted in a finding of DNA diploidy by flow cytometry (Table 6-1).[2,15,21,22,27] The only exception has been one case of juvenile angiofibroma, which was DNA aneuploid.[22] Again, with improved cytometry methods resulting in enhanced resolution, it would be unwise to equate the finding

of DNA aneuploidy with malignancy, given the fact that many benign tumors exhibit chromosomal aberrations.

Soft tissue sarcomas

Several general conclusions regarding DNA ploidy can be drawn from aggregate analysis of 354 soft tissue sarcomas from four flow cytometry studies.[3,5,21,22] These series are composed of heterogeneous histological types predominated by malignant fibrous histiocytoma (MFH) with significant numbers of fibrosarcomas, liposarcomas, leiomyosarcomas, and synovial sarcomas. A consistent finding is a correlation between increasing tumor grade and significantly higher frequencies of DNA aneuploidy in high-grade (III and IV) sarcomas (Table 6-2). Not unexpectedly, higher grade sarcomas also exhibit higher rates of tumor proliferation.[21,22] Studies of tumor proliferation by flow cytometry can be considered preliminary at best, given the paraffin material and more basic software analysis methods previously employed. At present, too few confident data have been generated to explore associations of tumor proliferation or S-phase fraction with clinical outcome.

Controlling for tumor grade (grades III and IV) and site (extremities and trunk), Alvegard et al.,[3] in a retrospective flow cytometry series of 148 soft tissue sarcomas of various histological types dominated by MFH (47%), have demonstrated with multivariate analysis that DNA aneuploidy determined by evaluation of paraffin blocks (one block per tumor) is an independent prognostic indicator of increased risk for the development of metastatic disease. In the Cox Proportional Hazards Model, DNA aneuploidy was the strongest prognostic factor (relative risk 3), followed by tumors of grade IV histology (relative risk 2.6), tumor size greater than 10 cm. (relative risk 2.2), intratumoral vascular invasion (relative risk 2.2), and male sex (relative risk 1.7). In this series, DNA aneuploidy correlated only with increased patient age but not with sex, tumor grade III versus grade IV, tumor size, degree of necrosis, or vascular invasion. Stratification of patients by risk factors was capable of prognosticating 5-year metastasis-free survivals of 79% for those with none or one risk factor, 65% with two risk factors, 43% with three risk factors, and 0% with four and five risk factors.

Table 6-2. Percentage of DNA aneuploid sarcomas (all types) by tumor grade

No. sarcomas	Grade I (%)	Grade II (%)	Grade III (%)	Grade IV (%)	Author/year
58	NE	8	72	89	Kreicbergs,[21] 1987
46	25	42	86	NGS	Kroese,[22] 1990
148	NE	NE	69	71	Alvegard,[3] 1990
102	33	26	71	80	Bauer,[5] 1991
TOTAL					
354	28	30	71	74	

NE, None examined; NGS, no grade scheme.

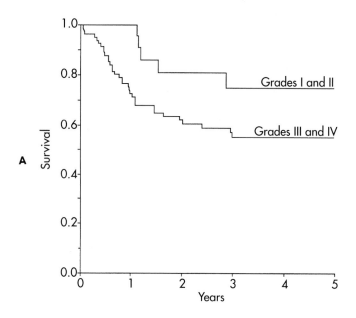

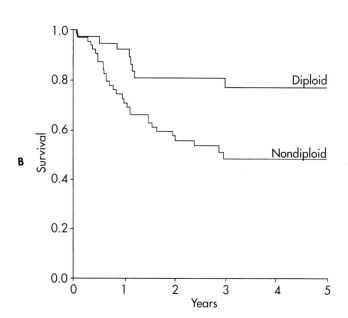

Additional evidence of the prognostic value of DNA flow cytometry is provided in a prospective series of 102 mixed soft tissue sarcoma histological types, again dominated by MFH (46%), performed on fresh tissues by Bauer et al.[5] They have demonstrated a significant difference ($P < 0.01$) in metastasis-free survival rates in surgically treated tumors between DNA diploidy (77%) and DNA nondiploidy, defined as aneuploid and tetraploid (48%), as well as a significant difference ($P < 0.05$) between grade I and II (74%) and grade III and IV (55%) tumors (Fig. 6-3). The frequency of DNA aneuploidy increased with higher tumor grade. This probably explains why tumor grade was not found to be an independent risk factor for metastasis in multivariate analysis. The three parameters of DNA aneuploidy, increased tumor size, and male sex were found by Cox regression analysis to be independent risk factors predictive of metastasis. Both nondiploid tumor status and tumor size of 5 to 10 cm had equivalent relative risk values of 4.5. These authors also found that the total risk of metastasis was strongly related ($P < 0.0001$) to the number of these latter two risk factors present such that 5-year survival was 90% for patients with neither of these two risk factors, 60% for patients with either risk factor present, and 30% for those possessing both risk factors of nondiploidy and tumor size greater than 10 cm (Fig. 6-4).

Applying image analysis to nuclei derived from enzy-

FIG. 6-3. Prospective flow cytometric DNA analysis of 102 heterogeneous types of soft tissue sarcomas. Life table curves of 5-year metastasis-free survival in relation to **A** (tumor grade) and **B** (ploidy). Analysis of difference in survival between patients with grade I and II and grade III and IV sarcomas ($P < 0.05$); and between patients with diploid and nondiploid (aneuploid and tetraploid) tumors ($P < 0.01$). Bivariate analysis showed that survival was related to both tumor grade and ploidy level, but only ploidy was identified as an independent risk factor for metastasis after Cox multivariate proportional regression analysis. (From Bauer CF, et al: DNA content prognostic in soft tissue sarcoma. 102 patients followed for 1-10 years. *Acta Orthop Scand* 62:187, 1991.)

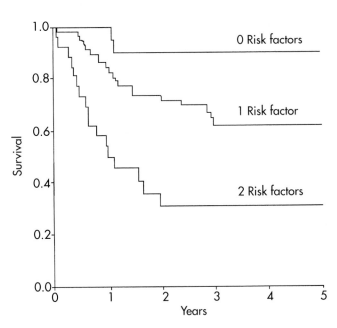

FIG. 6-4. Prospective flow cytometric DNA analysis of 102 heterogeneous types of soft tissue sarcomas. Life table curve of metastasis-free survival in relation to risk factors of none (90%), either nondiploidy or tumor size greater than 10 cm (60%) or both risk factors present (30%) ($P < 0.0001$). (From Bauer CF, et al: DNA content prognostic in soft tissue sarcoma. 102 patients followed for 1-10 years. *Acta Orthop Scand* 62:187, 1991.)

matic treatment of 50 μm paraffin sections, Pape et al.[31] have confirmed the association of DNA aneuploidy with histological grade and by univariate analysis of 64 patients have shown a modest difference in 5-year survival between DNA diploid (59%) and DNA aneuploid (43%) sarcomas of mixed histological types. Evaluation of ploidy patterns in 54 sarcoma specimens from multiple local recurrences of 18 patients revealed remarkable consistency when compared with the ploidy pattern of the primary tumors. However, this study was not controlled for multiple sampling to address innate tumoral stemline heterogeneity or affects of treatment modalities on ploidy of subsequent recurrences. Further prospective study of both of these issues would be fruitful.

It would appear from these studies of mixed soft tissue sarcoma histological types that determination of DNA aneuploidy in high-grade, soft tissue sarcomas may be a useful independent prognostic factor to be combined with other independent prognostic factors in identifying patients at increased risk for aggressive disease who may potentially benefit from additional therapies.

To date, flow cytometric DNA studies have focused on the most common as well as the rare and unusual histological types of soft tissue malignancies. There are insufficient data on some commonly occurring entities such as liposarcoma, fibrosarcoma, and malignant schwannoma to review in a clinically meaningful manner. The following sections address the best-studied sarcoma types.

Malignant fibrous histiocytoma

Malignant fibrous histiocytoma has been studied by cytometric techniques more often than the other soft tissue sarcomas. In general, there is a progressively higher frequency of DNA aneuploidy seen with increased tumor grade. Alvegard et al.[3] have demonstrated an 87% frequency of DNA aneuploidy in a large series of 70 grade III and grade IV MFH. This correlates with the summary data from four flow cytometry studies in the literature, accounting for 116 MFHs (all but 14 of which were high grade) in which the aggregate frequency of DNA aneuploidy was 86%.[2,3,21,22] Very few studies have been performed on low-grade MFH to cite a confident evaluation of DNA aneuploidy in these tumors.[2,3,21,22] However, using aggregate analysis, 6 out of 14 grade I and grade II MFHs have been DNA aneuploid by flow cytometry, accounting for a 43% frequency of DNA aneuploidy in these low-grade MFH.[1-3,21,22,46]

The large number of MFH studied by flow cytometry have not been segregated by histological subtype for correlation with DNA ploidy. Seven myxoid MFH, were briefly mentioned in an abstract by El-Naggar et al.,[13] 6 of which were DNA aneuploid.[13] No clinical correlation was attempted. Two flow cytometric studies of 13 angiomatoid MFH have been performed.[13,35] Retrospective flow cytometric evaluation of 6 cases by Pettinato et al.[35] and 7 tumors by El-Naggar et al.[13] revealed DNA diploidy in all primary and recurrent tumors examined. This purely diploid pattern is distinctly unlike the ploidy profiles of most MFH series summarized above. Too few cases of angiomatoid MFH have been examined by flow cytometry with appropriate clinical follow-up to draw any conclusion regarding the significance of DNA ploidy or proliferation in this low-grade sarcoma.

Although several large flow cytometry studies of heterogeneous sarcomas have evaluated numerous MFH, only one study has addressed clinical outcome in MFH alone. Preliminary evidence from the retrospective study by Radio et al.[37] of nine storiform-pleomorphic MFH suggests that DNA aneuploidy in MFH is associated with increased local recurrence and decreased survival in tumors of similar size, tumor grade, and clinical stage. Similar mean percentages of proliferating cells (%S + G_2/M phases) were observed in DNA aneuploid and diploid MFH. Therefore proliferation was not correlated with either DNA ploidy or survival in this small series. Further study of larger numbers of MFH using fresh tumors and the more sophisticated histogram-dependent software analysis models would do much to clarify the significance of these early findings in relation to the more conventional clinical and histological parameters of prognostic importance.

Flow cytometry studies of soft tissue sarcomas that analyze cell suspensions of dissociated sarcomas usually cannot discriminate between two morphologically distinct tumor cell populations, like the spindle cells and larger pleomorphic giant cells seen in MFH. Making use of digital image analysis, we have been able to document different hypertetraploid DNA contents of multinucleate pleomorphic tumor giant cells in a unique patient who developed two metachronous primary skeletal muscle MFHs arising 8 years apart,[29] lending ancillary support to the clinical and histological differences between these two metachronous MFH primaries.

Rhabdomyosarcoma

A prospective evaluation of pretherapeutic fresh tumor cell suspensions of unresectable rhabdomyosarcomas in children and adolescents by Shapiro et al.[41] has shown distinctive associations of DNA ploidy with histological subtype. Overall, one third of the 37 rhabdomyosarcomas studied displayed DNA diploid tumor stemlines. However, when categorized according to histological subtype, hyperdiploid DNA abnormalities (DI 1.1-1.8) were exclusively associated with embryonal rhabdomyosarcoma, whereas near-tetraploidy (DI 1.8-2.6) was commonly a feature of alveolar rhabdomyosarcoma. Corresponding chromosomal analyses revealed that DNA stemline indexes calculated by flow cytometry were highly correlated with modal chromosome numbers. Despite the DNA diploid flow cytometric findings in one third of the embryonal and one quarter of the alveolar rhabdomyosarcomas, all rhabdomyosarcomas displayed abnormal karyotypes undetectable by flow cytometry. S-phase fraction differences were also noted among the low proliferative DNA diploid (10.9%), high proliferative hyperdiploid (25.7%), and intermediate near-tetraploid (15.4%) tumors.

Unlike most adult malignant neoplasms, DNA aneuploidy with hyperdiploid stemlines conferred a significant survival advantage in pediatric rhabdomyosarcoma compared with the less favorable DNA diploid tumors (Fig. 6-5). This is attributed to lack of or only partial response to initial therapy in those patients with DNA diploid tumors compared with complete or partial responses to therapy by those patients with hyperdiploid tumors. The near-tetraploid group of patients had an intermediate prognosis between those of the favorable hyperdiploid and unfavorable diploid tumors. In these pediatric embryonal rhabdomyosarcomas, DNA ploidy remained a significant prognostic indicator after multivariate analysis and after adjustment for favorable sites (orbit and genitourinary tract) as well as tumor stage (stage 3 nonmetastatic versus stage 4 metastatic). Cox regression analysis revealed a 25.5 times greater relative risk of death for those with DNA diploid compared with those with aneuploid embryonal rhabdomyosarcomas. The relative risk of death in patients with DNA diploid alveolar rhabdomyosarcoma was 7.1 times greater than those with aneuploid tumors. Although the predictive power of DNA ploidy in alveolar rhabdomyosarcoma was of weaker

strength, the prognostic significance of DNA ploidy approached significance in both univariate and multivariate analyses.

Shapiro et al.[41] have suggested that the different patterns of DNA aneuploidy observed in these two histological subtypes of pediatric rhabdomyosarcoma may reflect different underlying genetic mechanisms leading to abnormal ploidy. It is possible that near-tetraploid stemlines arise by endoreduplication of the diploid DNA stemline, whereas hyperdiploid stemlines may arise by either selective chromosomal loss or chromosomal nondisjunction.

The direct association of higher S-phase fractions in patients with hyperdiploid rhabdomyosarcomas and a more favorable response to chemotherapy in this group compared with those with DNA diploid tumors is a clinical finding common to other pediatric malignancies such as acute lymphoblastic leukemia and pediatric neuroblastoma.[23-25] This probably relates to the fact that proliferating tumor cells are more susceptible to cytotoxic antineoplastic therapies compared with the more slowly growing DNA diploid tumors. This ability to prognosticate individual patients with pediatric rhabdomyosarcoma at high risk for treatment failure is an exciting potential clinical application for DNA flow cytometry that may identify patients who may benefit from additional therapies.

Synovial sarcoma

A retrospective flow cytometric evaluation of 46 primary synovial sarcomas by El-Naggar et al.[10] has shown a 33% overall rate of DNA aneuploidy. Using multiple sampling of 2 to 5 blocks per tumor, they have demonstrated a 15% rate of intratumoral DNA heterogeneity composed of separate zones of DNA diploid and aneuploid stemlines within the same neoplasm. DNA ploidy was highly correlated ($P <0.003$) with patient survival when subjected to univariate log-rank test (Fig. 6-6). In the multivariate Cox Proportional Hazards Model, DNA aneuploidy ranked second as an unfavorable independent prognostic factor with a relative risk ratio of 4.92, compared with tumor size greater than or equal to 5 cm with relative risk of 5.11, followed by age over 15 years that resulted in a relative risk of 4.92. In contrast to the significant survival advantage for patients with DNA diploid synovial sarcomas, there were no statistical differences in survival when differing S-phase fractions were considered. Furthermore, these authors have found no survival differences for patients segregated according to sex, tumor location, or histological subtypes of monophasic versus biphasic synovial sarcoma. Yet, mitotic counts were found to be a statistically significant but relatively weak predictor of patient outcome in multiparametric regression analysis. This would suggest a fruitful avenue for future evaluation of tumor proliferation antigens in synovial sarcoma as a potential prognostic marker to segregate tumors with different biological behaviors.

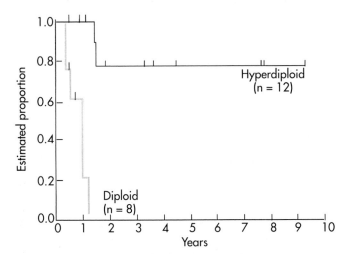

FIG. 6-5. Kaplan-Meier analysis of overall survival by ploidy classification at diagnosis for 20 patients with unresectable, nonmetastatic (group III) rhabdomyosarcoma. Patients with hyperdiploid tumors had significantly improved overall survival compared with those with diploid tumors ($P <0.0001$). Tick marks indicate patients remaining at risk. (From Shapiro DN, et al: Relationship of tumor-cell ploidy to histologic subtype and treatment outcome in children and adolescents with unresectable rhabdomyosarcoma. *J Clin Oncol* 9:159, 1991.)

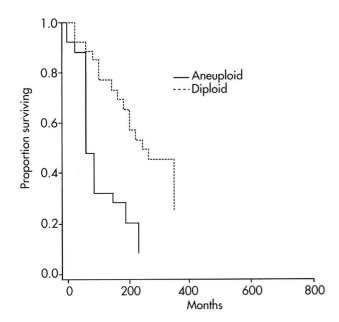

FIG. 6-6. Synovial sarcoma. Survival of patients with diploid neoplasms versus patients with aneuploid neoplasms. (From El-Naggar AK, et al: Synovial sarcoma: a DNA flow cytometric study. *Cancer* 65:2295, 1990.)

Clear cell sarcoma

Clear cell sarcoma (CCS), or malignant melanoma of soft parts, is a rare malignancy in which flow cytometric evaluation may also provide prognostic information. El-Naggar et al.[12] examined 11 CCS by flow cytometry, demonstrating an overall frequency of aneuploidy of 45%. DNA aneuploidy in CCS was associated with higher proliferative fractions, as is the case in other adult neoplasms. Interestingly, the mean survival of patients with DNA diploid CCS was approximately eight times that of those with aneuploid tumors (68.6 versus 8.2 months). To date, no other consistent prognostic parameters in CCS have been identified, and therefore the survival advantage conferred by DNA diploidy may be important in identifying those tumors with a different biological course that would benefit from additional therapies. The few neoplasms studied to date do not allow analysis of the significance of proliferative fraction as a predictor of clinical course or prognosis in CCS.

Epithelioid sarcoma

The largest study of epithelioid sarcoma has been performed by El-Naggar and Garcia,[11] employing retrospective evaluation of 20 primary epithelioid sarcomas. The overall rate of DNA aneuploidy was 40% (35% hyperdiploid and 5% tetraploid). Sampling of 2 to 5 blocks per tumor and analysis of tumor recurrences and/or metastases in 11 patients revealed no significant intratumoral or intertumoral DNA content heterogeneity between primary, recur-

rent, or metastatic lesions. The only significant predictors of favorable patient survival in this study were tumor size less than 5 cm and S-phase fraction percentage less than 5%. Neither patient age, sex, race, presence of metastasis, postsurgical therapy, nor DNA ploidy status were predictive of survival. No significant correlation was found between S-phase percentage and tumor size or histological tumor patterns composed of spindled versus epithelioid cell components. Given the quality control deficiencies of S-phase fraction determinations from paraffinized material, this one report paints a promising picture for this test in predicting patient outcome from a sarcoma whose biological behavior is typically indolent but unpredictable for the individual patient. Moreover, S-phase fraction determination may be helpful in identifying a subset of patients with otherwise favorable small tumors of less than 5 cm in diameter, which in this study behaved aggressively when characterized by a high S-phase fraction.

Superficial leiomyosarcoma

To date, no DNA studies limited to deep soft tissue, retroperitoneal, or vascular leiomyosarcomas have been performed. There are a handful of DNA studies of gastrointestinal and uterine leiomyosarcomas, which will not be reviewed here.[14a,33,43,44]

Superficial leiomyosarcomas have been the subject of one study of 14 tumors arising in the dermis and the subcutaneous tissues.[30] Although the tumors were separated for analysis into dermal and subcutaneous tumors, unfortunately, the authors failed to stratify the tumors by the often powerful predictors of tumor size, local extension, margin free excision, recurrence, and tumor necrosis. Also, there were too few cases to control for differences in therapy (e.g. simple excision versus amputation). Nevertheless, the authors report that all dermal leiomyosarcomas were DNA diploid, and none experienced metastatic spread. Of the 10 subcutaneous tumors, 4 also were diploid and devoid of metastases. In contrast, four of five DNA aneuploid subcutaneous leiomysarcomas had metastases to lung, and the fifth had a lymph node metastasis. Although DNA aneuploidy is a seemingly strong predictor of metastasis in superficial leiomyosarcoma in this small study, the metastatic disease was limited to the subcutaneous tumors, and DNA aneuploidy correlated with tumors of high grades (III and IV) and higher mitotic rate. Similar ranges of survival were also given for the DNA diploid and aneuploid subcutaneous leiomyosarcomas. The apparent correlation with progression to metastasis deserves to be restudied in a larger group of tumors with control for the other potential clinical and pathological parameters of prognostic significance cited above.

Kaposi's sarcoma

DNA analyses of Kaposi's sarcoma arising in the sporadic, acquired immunodeficiency syndrome (AIDS)-

Table 6-3. DNA content in Kaposi's sarcoma: summary of flow and image analyses

Kaposi's sarcoma clinical type	No. cases	No. aneuploid (%)	No. diploid/ peridiploid (%)	Author/year
Sporadic	125	8 (6)	117 (94)	Bisceglia et al. (1992)[7] Dictor et al. (1991)[9]
AIDS associated	33	0	33 (100)	Sanchez et al. (1988)[38] Dictor et al. (1991)[9]
African endemic	9	0	9 (100)	Fukunaga and Silverberg (1990)[18] Sanchez et al. (1988)[38] Eto et al. (1992)[15]

Table 6-4. DNA content in angiosarcomas: summary of flow cytometry studies

Angiosarcoma clinical type	No. cases	No. aneuploid (%)	No. diploid/ peridiploid (%)	Author/reference
Cutaneous	15	5 (33)	10 (67)	Dictor et al. (1991)[9]; Eto et al. (1992)[15]; Fukunaga et al. (1993)[17]
Stewart-Treves postmastectomy	8	6 (75)	2 (25)	Dictor et al. (1991)[9]; Eto et al. (1992)[15]; Fukunaga et al. (1993)[17]
Deep soft tissue and other sites	20	9 (45)	11 (55)	Dictor et al. (1991)[9]; Eto et al. (1992)[15]; Fukunaga et al. (1993)[17]

associated, and African endemic clinical settings have shown a relatively consistent DNA profile of DNA diploidy. The exception is a low frequency of DNA aneuploidy documented in cases of sporadic Kaposi's sarcoma (Table 6-3).[7,9,15,18,38] Although there is some evidence that the more advanced nodular phase and spindle predominant histological pattern of disease bear the highest proliferation rates, there are too few DNA aneuploid cases to associate this finding with advancing growth stages and histological patterns.[7] Although there may be some interlaboratory differences in methodology, similar median proliferative activity rates (%S + G_2/M) have been reported for sporadic and AIDS-associated cases using paraffin-embedded material.[7,18] Nevertheless, neither DNA analysis nor measurement of proliferative activity can address the basic question of the hyperplastic versus neoplastic biological nature of Kaposi's sarcoma.

Angiosarcoma

The overall frequency of DNA aneuploidy in angiosarcomas of all types distilled from three literature series is 47%, with some ploidy differences between the various clinical types (Table 6-4).[9,15,17] Although 75% of Stewart-Treves postmastectomy angiosarcomas are DNA aneuploid, there are too few reported cases to assess whether this apparent difference is significant. Fukunaga et al.[17] found no correlation of DNA ploidy status with location, histological pattern or staging parameters of tumor size, or the pres-

ence or absence of lung metastases. At present, cytometric DNA ploidy analysis is of no prognostic value in angiosarcomas, with nearly all patients dead of disease regardless of DNA ploidy status.

Hemangiopericytoma

In the Eto et al.[15] study of seven hemangiopericytomas, only one tumor was DNA aneuploid (14%). There was no prognostic significance for DNA ploidy and no correlation with histological features of prognostic significance such as degree of cellularity, tumor size, mitotic rate, or necrosis. Fukunaga et al.[17] also studied seven hemangiopericytomas. Two tumors considered to be histologically benign showed DNA diploidy, and the patients are alive without disease. Two of the other five histologically malignant tumors were DNA aneuploid; however, all patients with malignant hemangiopericytoma died of disease. Again, DNA ploidy did not correlate with clinical outcome in histologically malignant tumors. Finn et al.[16] found all 21 paraffin-embedded hemangiopericytomas (including seven angioblastic meningiomas) they examined to be DNA diploid, negating DNA ploidy as a useful discriminant. However, higher S-phase and proliferative (S + G_2/M) fractions determined with current histogram-dependent cell cycle and debris modeling software were observed in all tumors that showed aggressive biological behavior defined as exhibiting local recurrence, metastasis, or death from invasive disease.

Sinonasal hemangiopericytomas are a special histologi-

cal and biological low-grade variety of hemangiopericytoma. In their investigation of 14 tumors, El-Naggar et al.[14b] found all but one to be DNA diploid with low S-phase fractions. All patients were alive and free of disease, including the one patient with a DNA aneuploid neoplasm. The latter tumor differed in its display of nuclear pleomorphism and mitotic activity. However, the only recurrent tumor, 3½ years after surgery, was a DNA diploid neoplasm.

Spindle cell hemangioendothelioma

Fukunaga et al.[17] have reported two cases of spindle cell hemangioendothelioma, both of which were DNA diploid by flow cytometric evaluation of paraffin-embedded material. Both patients are alive and free of disease but there is insufficient follow-up and number of cases to correlate ploidy or proliferation in this low-grade vascular neoplasm with clinical outcome.

Malignant rhabdoid tumor

Schmidt et al.[39] have evaluated the ploidy status of 16 malignant rhabdoid tumors from the kidney (11), chest wall

(2), and head and neck (3) regions.[39] In this flow cytometry study of paraffin-embedded material, none of these tumors, including metastases, were DNA aneuploid. This is unexpected, given the marked nuclear cytological abnormalities seen in rhabdoid tumors. This homogeneity of ploidy precludes any role as a prognostic indicator in this aggressive neoplasm. Cell proliferation, although evaluated in six cases, was not correlated by the authors with outcome.

Alveolar soft part sarcoma

Image analysis of Feulgen-stained paraffin sections has been employed by Persson et al.[32] to evaluate the DNA content of 10 alveolar soft part sarcomas. Seven neoplasms of the usual histological type were all DNA diploid. However, abnormal DNA histograms, composed of diploid and aneuploid peaks, were noted in three tumors, all of which exhibited pleomorphic cytological features. Although definitive conclusions are compromised by the small size of the series, no correlation of DNA ploidy with clinical outcome was identified in this aggressive sarcoma.

REFERENCES

1. Agarwal V, Greenebaum E, Wersto R, et al: DNA ploidy of spindle cell soft-tissue tumors and its relationship to histology and clinical outcome. *Arch Pathol Lab Med* 115:558, 1991.
2. Akerman M, Killander D, Rydholm A: Aspiration of musculo-skeletal tumors for cytodiagnosis and DNA analysis. *Acta Orthop Scand* 58:523, 1987.
3. Alvegard TA, Berg NO, Baldetorp B, et al: Cellular DNA content and prognosis of high-grade soft tissue sarcoma: the Scandinavian Sarcoma Group Experience. *J Clin Pathol* 8:538, 1990.
4. Bagwell CB. Theoretical aspects of flow cytometry data analysis. In Bauer KD, Duque RE, Shankey TV eds., *Clinical flow cytometry: principles and application, Baltimore, 1993, Williams and Wilkins.*
5. Bauer HC, Kreicbergs A, Tribukait B: DNA content prognostic in soft tissue sarcoma: 102 patients followed for 1-10 years. *Acta Orthop Scand* 62:187, 1991.
6. Bauer KD, Bagwell CB, Giaretti W, et al: Consensus review of the clinical utility of DNA flow cytometry in colorectal cancer. *Cytometry* 14:486, 1993.
7. Bisceglia M, Bosman C, Quirke P: A histologic and flow cytometric study of Kaposi's sarcoma. *Cancer* 69:793, 1992.
8. Cooper CS, Stratton MR: Soft tissue tumours: the genetic basis of development. *Carcinogenesis* 12:155, 1991.
9. Dictor M, Ferno M, Baldetorp B: Flow cytometric DNA content in Kaposi's sarcoma by histologic stage comparison with angiosarcoma. *Anal Quant Cytol Histol* 13:201, 1991.
10. El-Naggar AK, Ayala AG, Abdul-Karim FW, et al: Synovial sarcoma: a DNA flow cytometric study. *Cancer* 65:2295, 1990.
11. El-Naggar AK, Garcia GM: Epithelioid sarcoma: flow cytometric study of DNA content and regional DNA heterogeneity. *Cancer* 69:1721, 1992.
12. El-Naggar AK, Ordonez NG, Sara A, et al: Clear cell sarcomas and metastatic soft tissue melanomas. *Cancer* 67:2173, 1991.
13. El-Naggar AK, Ro JY, Ayala AG, et al: Angiomatoid malignant fibrous histiocytoma: a DNA flow cytometric analysis of 7 cases. *Am J Clin Pathol* 90:502A, 1988.
14a. El-Naggar AK, Ro JY, McLemore D, et al: Gastrointestinal stromal tumors: DNA flow-cytometric study of 58 patients with at least five years of follow-up. *Mod Pathol* 2:511, 1989.
14b. El-Naggar AK, Batsakis JG, Garcia GM, et al: Sinonasal hemangiopericytomas: a clinicopathologic and DNA content study. *Arch Otolaryngol Head Neck Surg* 118:134, 1992.
15. Eto H, Toriyama K, Tsuda N, et al: Flow cytometric DNA analysis of vascular soft tissue tumors, including African endemic-type Kaposi's sarcoma. *Hum Pathol* 23:1055, 1992.
16. Finn WG, Goolsby CL, Rao MS: DNA flow cytometric analysis of hemangiopericytoma. *Am J Clin Pathol* 101:181, 1994.
17. Fukunaga M, Shimoda T, Nikaido T, et al: Soft tissue vascular tumors: a flow cytometric DNA analysis. *Cancer* 71:2233, 1993.
18. Fukunaga M, Silverberg SG: Kaposi's sarcoma in patients with acquired immune deficiency syndrome: a flow cytometric DNA analysis of 26 lesions in 21 patients. *Cancer* 66:758, 1990.
19. Hall TL, Fu YS: Biology of disease: applications of quantitative microscopy in tumor pathology. *Lab Invest* 53:5, 1985.
20. Hiddemann W, Schumann J, Andreeff M, et al: Convention on nomenclature for DNA cytometry: Committee on Nomenclature, Society for Analytical Cytology. *Cancer Genet Cytogenet* 13:181, 1984.
21. Kreicbergs A, Tribukait B, Willems J et al: DNA flow analysis of soft tissue tumors. *Cancer* 59:128, 1987.
22. Kroese MCS, Rutgers DH, Wils IS, et al: The relevance of the DNA index and proliferation rate in the grading of benign and malignant soft tissue tumors. *Cancer* 65:1782, 1990.
23. Look AT, Hayes FA, Nitschke R, et al: Cellular DNA content as a predictor of response to chemotherapy in infants with unresectable neuroblastoma. *N Engl J Med* 311:231, 1984.
24. Look AT, Melvin SL, Williams DL, et al: Aneuploidy and percentage S-phase cells determined by flow cytometry correlate with cell phenotype in childhood acute leukemia. *Blood* 60:959, 1982.
25. Look AT, Roberson PK, Williams DL, et al: Prognostic importance of blast cell DNA content in childhood acute lymphoblastic leukemia. *Blood* 65:1079, 1985.

26. Mandahl N, Baldetorp B, Ferno M, et al: Comparative cytogenetic and DNA flow cytometric analysis of 150 bone and soft-tissue tumors. *Int J Cancer* 53:358, 1993.

27. Matsuno T, Gebhardt MC, Schiller AL, et al: The use of flow cytometry as a diagnostic aid in the management of soft-tissue tumors. *J Bone Joint Surg* 70(A):751, 1988.

28. Mellin W: Cytophotometry in tumor pathology: a critical review of methods and applications, and some results of DNA analysis. *Pathol Res Pract* 185:37, 1990.

29. Nathanson SD, Zarbo RJ, Sarantou T: Metachronous second primary malignant fibrous histiocytoma in two skeletal muscles. *J Surg Oncol* 49:259, 1992.

30. Oliver GF, Reiman HM, Gonchoroff NJ, et al: Cutaneous and subcutaneous leiomyosarcoma: a clinicopathological review of 14 cases with reference to antidesmin staining and nuclear DNA patterns studied by flow cytometry. *Br J Dermatol* 124:252, 1991.

31. Pape H, Pottgen C, Ploem JS, et al: The prognostic value of DNA content measured by image cytometry in soft tissue sarcomas. *Ann Oncol* 3:S89, 1992.

32. Persson S, Willems JS, Kindblom LG, et al: Alveolar soft part sarcoma: an immunohistochemical, cytologic and electron-microscopic study and a quantitative DNA analysis. *Virch Arch A* 412:499, 1988.

33. Peters WS, Howard DR, Andersen WA et al: Deoxyribonucleic acid analysis by flow cytometry of uterine leiomyosarcomas and smooth muscle tumors of uncertian malignant potential. *Am J Obstet Gynecol* 166:1646, 1992.

34. Peterson S, Friedrich U: A comparison between flow cytometric ploidy investigation and chromosome analysis of 32 human colorectal tumors. *Cytometry* 7:307, 1986.

35. Pettinato G, Manivel JC, DeRosa G, et al: Angiomatoid malignant fibrous histiocytoma: cytologic, immunohistochemical, ultrastructural, and flow cytometric study of 20 cases. *Mod Pathol* 3:479, 1990.

36. Rabinovitch PS: Practical considerations for DNA content and cell cycle analysis. In Bauer KD, Duque RE, Shankey TV, eds., *Clinical flow cytometry: principles and application,* Baltimore, 1993, Williams and Wilkins.

37. Radio SJ, Wooldridge TN, Linder J: Flow cytometric DNA analysis of malignant fibrous histiocytoma and related fibrohistiocytic tumors. *Hum Pathol* 19:74, 1988.

38. Sanchez MA, Ames ED, Erhardt K et al: Analysis of DNA distribution in Kaposi's sarcoma in patients with and without the acquired immune deficiency syndrome. *Anal Quant Cytol Histol* 10:16, 1988.

39. Schmidt D, Leuschner I, Harms D, et al: Malignant rhabdoid tumor: a morphological and flow cytometric study. *Pathol Res Pract* 184:202, 1989.

40. Shankey TV, Rabinovitch PS, Bagwell B, et al: Guidelines for implementation of clinical DNA cytometry. *Cytometry* 14:472, 1993.

41. Shapiro DN, Parham DM, Douglass EC, et al: Relationship of tumor-cell ploidy to histologic subtype and treatment outcome in children and adolescents with unresectable rhabdomyosarcoma. *J Clin Oncol* 9:159, 1991.

42. Tribukait B, Granberg-Ohman I, Wijkstrom H: Flow cytometric DNA and cytogenetic studies in human tumors: a comparison and discussion of the differences in modal values obtained by the two methods. *Cytometry* 7:194, 1986.

43. Tsushima K, Rainwater LM, Goellner JR, et al: Leiomyosarcomas and benign smooth muscle tumors of the stomach: nuclear DNA patterns studied by flow cytometry. *Mayo Clin Proc* 62:275, 1987.

44. Tsushima K, Stanhope CR, Gaffey TA, et al: Uterine leiomyosarcomas and benign smooth muscle tumors: usefulness of nuclear DNA patterns studied by flow cytometry. *Mayo Clin Proc* 63:248, 1988.

45. Wang-Wuu S, Jacobs D, Soukup S: Comparison of chromosome analysis to DNA content by flow cytometry for pediatric tumors. *Pediatr Pathol* 10:671, 1990.

46. Xiang J, Spanier SS, Benson NA, et al: Flow cytometric analysis of DNA in bone and soft-tissue tumors using nuclear suspension. *Cancer* 59:1951, 1987.

47. Zalupski MM, Ryan JR, Ensley JF, et al: Development and optimization of tissue preparative methodology for DNA content analysis of soft tissue neoplasms. *Cytometry* 14:922, 1993.

48. Zarbo RJ: Flow cytometric DNA analysis of effusions: a new test seeking validation (editorial). *Am J Clin Pathol* 95:2, 1991.

49. Zarbo RJ: Quality control issues and technical considerations in flow cytometric DNA and cell cycle analysis of solid tumors. In Keren DF, Hanson H, Hurtubise P, eds., *Flow cytometry in clinical diagnosis*, Chicago, 1994, ASCP Press.

50. Zarbo RJ, Babu VR, Crissman JD: Sensitivity of flow cytometric DNA analysis of deparaffinized nuclei from urothelial carcinomas with near-diploid karyotypes. *Lab Invest* 60:109A, 1989.

51. Zarbo RJ, Visscher DW, Crissman JD: Two-color multiparametric method for flow cytometric DNA analysis of carcinomas using staining for cytokeratin and leukocyte-common antigen. *Anal Quant Cytol Histol* 11:391, 1989.

CHAPTER 7

APPROACH TO THE DIAGNOSIS OF
SOFT TISSUE TUMORS

CLINICAL INFORMATION

The diagnosis of a soft tissue lesion, as with other tumors, presupposes that the pathologist has a modicum of clinical information as well as adequate, well-processed tissue. At a minimum, the pathologist should be apprised of the age of the patient, location of the tumor, and its growth characteristics. In some cases, the results of radiographic studies, particularly CT scans may enhance his understanding of the clinical extent of the lesion (see Chapter 3).

Although age rarely, if ever, suggests a particular diagnosis, the real importance of this information is in knowing whether the patient is a child. In general, there is little overlap between soft tissue tumors occurring in children and those occurring in adults. Therefore, this critical piece of information essentially presents the pathologist with two different groups of tumors from which a differential diagnosis will be constructed. For example, pleomorphic forms of malignant fibrous histiocytoma are essentially unheard of in young children, and a pathologist would be better advised to consider other diagnoses for a pleomorphic tumor in a child. On the other hand, neuroblastoma and angiomatoid fibrous histiocytoma rarely occur after childhood, and such diagnoses should always be made cautiously in adults.

Location, too, provides ancillary help in differential diagnosis. Sarcomas, for the most part, develop as deeply located masses and infrequently present as superficial lesions. Exceptions occur, however, and include lesions such as dermatofibrosarcoma protuberans, epithelioid sarcoma, and angiosarcoma (see box on p.132). It is also useful to recall that when carcinomas or melanomas metastasize to soft tissue, it is usually as small superficial nodules rather than as large, deeply situated masses. In our experience, the most common carcinomas that present as soft tissue metastases are pulmonary and renal carcinomas, the former usually presenting as a subcutaneous mass on the chest wall and the latter presenting as a soft tissue mass in nearly any location.

Unfortunately, there is a great deal of overlap between the manner of presentation of benign and malignant soft tissue masses so that this information may be least helpful to the pathologist. Most soft tissue sarcomas of the extremities are detected by the patient as a slowly growing mass that has been present for about 6 months at the time of diagnosis. The duration of benign lesions may be quite similar, although such lesions are generally described as static or slowly growing. An exception to the foregoing observation is the rapid development of some cases of nodular fasciitis. These superficial, reactive lesions may develop rapidly over a period of 1 to 3 weeks, and we have even encountered some that evolved in a few days, a pattern of growth which is seldom, if ever, encountered in a sarcoma. Thus an astute general surgeon may sometimes suggest the diagnosis of a fasciitis in a rapidly evolving superficial lesion of the extremity.

Diagnostic material

Material for diagnosis can be obtained by needle or excisional or incisional biopsy, the choice being largely dependent on the size and location of the lesion (see Chapter 2). From a pathologist's perspective, the latter two specimens are preferable, since they yield a higher volume of tissue, but excisional biopsy of large, deep tumors is undesirable because it may interfere with further surgical procedures and may lead to complications such as a massive hematoma and disturbed wound healing. The biopsy procedure should always be planned in such a manner that the biopsy tract can be excised together with the tumor during the definitive surgical procedure. Needle biopsy may be quite adequate for documenting recurrent or metastatic disease in a patient with a known diagnosis of sarcoma but should used with caution when major surgical procedures depend on the diagnosis. In the past, frozen sections were performed commonly with the expectation that definitive surgery would be accomplished during the same intraoperative procedure; this trend is changing. Frozen sections are

---

Superficial soft tissue sarcomas

Dermatofibrosarcoma protuberans
Epithelioid sarcoma
Angiomatoid fibrous histiocytoma
Myxoid malignant fibrous histiocytoma
Angiosarcoma
Kaposi's sarcoma
Atypical fibroxanthoma

---

performed primarily to assure the surgeon that he or she has obtained representative and viable tissue that will be adequate for a permanent section diagnosis. This may be accomplished by freezing a portion of the biopsy material or sometimes, as in the case of a needle biopsy, performing a touch preparation. The presence of malignant cells in a nonnecrotic background on a touch preparation are reassuring that the specimen is adequate. However, a background of reactive or necrotic cells may suggest that a pseudocapsule has been biopsied or that the specimen is largely necrotic, requiring additional material depending on the clinical impression.

Since there is a growing tendency to perform limb sparing surgery for sarcomas of all types, the number of major amputation specimens received in the surgical pathology laboratory has markedly decreased compared to 1 or 2 decades ago. Most extremity sarcomas are excised with a wide local excision, sometimes combined with either preoperative or postoperative radiotherapy. As with many other types of surgical specimens, the margins should be marked with permanent ink and blotted dry prior to cutting. Once incised, the gross characteristics of the tumor should be noted. If malignancy is suspected, careful assessment of the tumor as to its surroundings is mandatory. This includes the location of the lesion (subcutis, muscle), size, relationship to vital structures (e.g., bone, neurovascular bundle), and the relative amount of necrosis present, if that can be judged grossly. Size is important in providing an accurate T descriptor for the surgeon if the lesion is a sarcoma. Lesions less than 5 cm are classified as T1, whereas those that are larger than 5 cm are classified as T2. Assessment of the degree of necrosis is important for untreated sarcomas because necrosis of greater than 15% has been associated with a worse clinical course in grade II and III sarcomas. The extent of necrosis in lesions treated with preoperative radiation or chemotherapy is also important since it aids the clinical staff in assessing the efficacy or preoperative radiation or chemotherapy, although it does not carry the same implication as necrosis occurring in an untreated lesion. Often, the gross appearance of the tumor may be deceptive. Sarcomas, for example, may appear to be well circum-

scribed, while some benign tumors may suggest an infiltrative or invasive growth pattern. Also, the term *encapsulation* is often misleading and may invite inadequate excision by shelling out or enucleation of the tumor.

There are no standard guidelines for sampling of soft tissue tumors, and to some extent, sampling is dictated by the specific case. In the case of a known benign lesion, a few representative sections suffice (or submitting the entire lesion if it is small). In the case of a sarcoma the questions to be answered will be different. For example, in a high-grade sarcoma, it may be less important to submit numerous sections than in a low-grade lesion in which the sampling is being driven by the need to document the presence of high-grade areas. We have generally taken one section for each centimeter of tumor diameter with no more than about 10 sections if the lesion appeared more or less uniform. Representative sections of the margins or sections designed to show impingement of vital structures are also submitted. We select blocks for margins judiciously, depending on the gross appearance of the lesion. Lesions that are several centimeters away from a margin seldom have positive margins microscopically, so extensive margin sampling in these situations is less critical than in excisions with grossly close margins. One exception, however, is the epithelioid sarcoma, a lesion that may be deceptive in its clinical extent grossly. Polaroid prints or Xerox impression of a specimen can be very useful in providing visual data as to the orientation of the specimen and sampling sites.

Most specimens are adequately handled as described above. However, in cases in which diagnostic difficulty is anticipated, it is useful to have glutaraldehyde-fixed tissue or frozen tissue in reserve in the event ancillary studies may be important. It should be emphasized that there are certain tumors in which ancillary studies are essential. Notably frozen tissue should be reserved for N-myc amplification studies in childhood neuroblastoma, and frozen tissue is highly recommended for use in national protocol studies for childhood rhabdomyosarcoma. Although we often perform cytogenetic studies in a wide variety of soft tissue lesions, these, for the most part, do not contribute directly to either diagnosis or therapy, an exception to this being the differential diagnosis of round cell sarcoma in which the question of an extraskeletal Ewing's sarcoma has been raised but in which the histological features do not permit an unequivocal diagnosis.

MICROSCOPIC EXAMINATION

The first and most important step in reaching a correct diagnosis is careful scrutiny of conventionally stained sections with the light microscope under low-power magnification. Useful microscopic features that can be identified at this point include the size and depth of the lesions, relationship to overlying skin and underlying fascia, and the nature of the borders (pushing, infiltrative).

Perhaps the most important question to ask at this juncture is whether the lesion under study is a reactive process or a neoplasm. Reactive lesions may occur in superficial or deep soft tissue but tend to be more frequent in the former location. There are a number of histological features that are suggestive of a reactive process. First, some reactive lesions display a distinct zonal quality. For example, in the case of fascial forms of nodular fasciitis, one encounters a cuff of proliferating fibroblasts that surround a central hypocellular zone of fibrinoid change. Myositis ossificans, too, displays a zonation that consists of centrifugal maturation of fibroblastic to osteoblastic mesenchyme. Cells comprising reactive lesions often have the appearance of tissue culture fibroblasts with large vesicular nuclei, prominent nucleoli, and striking cytoplasmic basophilia reflecting the presence of abundant rough endoplasmic reticulum. Although mitotic figures may be quite numerous, important negative observations include no atypical mitotic figures or nuclear atypia, as one would expect in a sarcoma (see the accompanying box).

Once satisfied that a reactive lesion can be excluded, the pathologist is justified in proceeding with an analysis of the neoplasm. With the microscope at low power, the pathologist is usually struck with the architectural pattern, appearance of the cells, and characteristics of the stroma. These characteristics can lend themselves to the development of a number of differential diagnostic categories such as those listed at right and in the boxes on p. 134.

1. Fasciculated, spindle cell tumors (e.g., fibromatosis, fibrosarcoma, synovial sarcoma, malignant peripheral nerve sheath tumor)
2. Myxoid lesions (e.g., myxoma, myxoid malignant fibrous histiocytoma, myxoid liposarcoma, myxoid chondrosarcoma)
3. Epithelioid tumors (e.g., alveolar soft part sarcoma, epithelioid sarcoma, epithelioid malignant schwannoma)
4. Small round cell tumor (neuroblastoma, extraskeletal Ewing's sarcoma, neuroepithelioma)
5. Pleomorphic tumors (malignant fibrous histiocytoma, pleomorphic rhabdomyosarcoma, pleomorphic liposarcoma, metastatic carcinoma)

Further study of the sections will provide important information about the growth pattern, degree of cellularity, and the amount and type of matrix formation. Growth patterns vary considerably and range from a fascicular, herringbone, or storiform (cartwheel, spiral nebula) patterns in fibroblastic, myofibroblastic, and fibrohistiocytic tumors to plexiform or endocrine patterns, palisading, and Homer-Wright and Flexner-Wintersteiner rosettes in various benign and malignant neural tumors. Biphasic cellular patterns, with epithelial and spindle cell areas are characteristic of synovial sarcoma and mesothelioma. Although not all growth patterns permit a definitive diagnosis, they are of great help in narrowing down the various differential diagnostic possibilities. Table 7-1 lists some of the most common architectural patterns in soft tissue pathology and relates them to the type of tumor in which they are most frequently found.

Other features that are clearly evident by scanning the

Reactive lesions simulating a sarcoma

Nodular fasciitis
Intravascular and cranial fasciitis
Proliferative fasciitis and myositis
Intravascular papillary endothelial hyperplasia
Myositis and panniculitis ossificans
Fibrodysplasia ossificans progressiva
Fibroosseous pseudotumor of the digits

Fasciculated spindle cell tumors

Fibromatosis (desmoid tumor)
Fibrosarcoma
Leiomyosarcoma
Spindle cell rhabdomyosarcoma
Synovial sarcoma
Malignant peripheral nerve sheath tumor

Myxoid soft tissue lesions

Myxoma, cutaneous, intramuscular*
Aggressive angiomyxoma
Myxoid neurofibroma
Neurothekeoma
Myxoid chondroma
Myxoid lipoma (including myxoid spindle cell lipoma)
Lipoblastoma
Ossifying fibromyxoid tumor of soft parts
Myxoid liposarcoma*
Myxoid chondrosarcoma*
Myxoid dermatofibrosarcoma protuberans
Myxoid malignant fibrous histiocytoma*
Botryoid embryonal rhabdomyosarcoma
Myxoid leiomyosarcoma

*Most commonly encountered myxoid tumors.

Epithelioid soft tissue tumors

Alveolar soft part sarcoma
Epithelioid sarcoma
Epithelioid angiosarcoma
Epithelioid hemangioendothelioma
Epithelioid leiomyosarcoma
Malignant epithelioid schwannoma
Malignant rhabdoid tumor
Malignant mesothelioma
Synovial sarcoma (biphasic and predominantly
    monophasic epithelial)

Round cell sarcomas

Alveolar rhabdomyosarcoma
Desmoplastic malignant small cell tumor of childhood
Embryonal rhabdomyosarcoma
Extraskeletal Ewing's sarcoma
Neuroblastoma
Peripheral neuropithelioma (PNET)
Round cell liposarcoma
Mesenchymal chondrosarcoma
Malignant hemangiopericytoma

Pleomorphic sarcomas

Malignant fibrous histiocytoma
Pleomorphic liposarcoma
Pleomorphic rhabdomyosarcoma
Pleomorphic peripheral nerve sheath tumor
Pleomorphic leiomyosarcoma

Table 7-1. Correlation of growth pattern and tumor type

Growth pattern	Tumor type
Alveolar	Alveolar soft part sarcoma alveolar rhabdomyosarcoma
Acinar	Synovial sarcoma, mesothelioma
Biphasic	Synovial sarcoma, mesothelioma
Cording	Epithelioid hemangioendothelioma myxoid chondrosarcoma, epithelioid malignant schwannoma, round cell liposarcoma (rare)
Fascicular	Fibromatosis (desmoid tumor) fibrosarcoma, malignant peripheral nerve sheath tumor, synovial sarcoma
Endocrinoid (Zell-ballen)	Paraganglioma, alveolar soft part sarcoma
Lobular, nodular nestlike	Lipoblastoma, liposarcoma epithelioid sarcoma, clear cell sarcoma fibrous hamartoma of infancy
Palisading	Schwannoma (neurilemoma), malignant peripheral nerve sheath tumor leiomyosarcoma, malignant Triton tumor (rare) synovial sarcoma (rare)
Plexiform	Neurofibroma, schwannoma (neurilemoma) plexiform fibrohistiocytic tumor
Plexiform capillary	Myxoid liposarcoma, myxoid malignant fibrous histiocytoma
Pericytoma	Hemangiopericytoma, synovial sarcoma mesenchymal chondrosarcoma, malignant peripheral nerve sheath tumor, myofibromatosis, juxtaglomerular tumor, solitary fibrous tumor of pleura and peritoneum, liposarcoma (rare)
Rosettes, pseudorosettes	Neuroblastoma, neuroepithelioma malignant peripheral nerve sheath tumor (rare)
Storiform (cartwheel)	Dermatofibrosarcoma protuberans fibrous histiocytoma, malignant fibrous histiocytoma neurofibroma
Tubulo-papillary	Mesothelioma

sections are the amount and type of extracellular matrix that is produced by the tumor cells, e.g., the presence and amounts of interstitial collagen and mucinous substances (glycosaminoglycans). Abundant myxoid material is produced by a variety of benign and malignant soft tissue tumors, ranging from myxoma and myxoid neurofibroma to myxoid liposarcoma and myxoid chondrosarcoma. It is usually an indication of a relatively slowly growing tumor, and it has been claimed that the degree of myxoid change in some malignant tumors is inversely related to the metastatic rate. Abundant collagen formation is also found more often in slowly growing tumors than in rapidly growing ones. However, this finding is not always significant and also may be a prominent feature of some highly malignant sarcomas such as synovial sarcoma and malignant fibrous histiocytoma and postirradiation sarcomas. Examination may also provide information as to the presence of calcification and metaplastic changes, especially metaplastic cartilage and bone formation. Table 7-2 summarizes these changes in a variety of soft tissue tumors.

Table 7-2. Calcification, chondroid and osseous metaplasia in soft tissue tumors.

	Calcification	Chondroid	Osteoid
Calcifying aponeurotic fibroma	+	+	−
Fibrodysplasia ossificans progressiva	+	+	+
Giant cell tumor	+	−	+
Hemangioma	+	−	+
Lipoma	+	+	+
Leiomyoma	+	−	−
Malignant fibrous histio-cytma	−	−	+
Melanocytic schwannoma	+	−	−
Mesencymal chondrosar-coma	−	+	+
Mesothelioma	−	+	−
Myofibromatosis	+	−	−
Myositis ossificans	−	+	+
Myxoid liposarcoma	−	+	−
Malignant mesenchy-moma	−	+	+
Malignant peripheral nerve sheath tumor	−	+	−
Myxoid chondrosarcoma	−	+	−
Ossifying fibromyxoid tumor	−	+	+
Osteosarcoma	+	+	+
Panniculitis ossificans	−	−	+
Synovial sarcoma	+	+	+
Tumoral calcinosis	+	−	−

+, Present (variable).
−, Usually absent.

Microscopic examination under higher magnification is required for obtaining information as to the degree and type of cellular differentiation, whether the tumor is well-, moderately, or poorly differentiated, and whether there are any specific cell types such as lipoblasts or rhabdomyoblasts. Lipoblasts, for example, are characterized by the presence of sharply defined intracellular droplets of lipid and one or more centrally or peripherally placed round or scalloped nuclei. Rounded and spindle-shaped rhabdomyoblasts can be usually identified in conventionally stained hematoxylin-eosin sections by their deeply eosinophilic cytoplasm with whorls of eosinophilic fibrillary material near the nucleus and cytoplasmic cross striations. Caution in the interpretation of these cells is indicated, however, because occasionally entrapped normal or atrophic fat or muscle tissue may closely resemble lipoblasts or rhabdomyoblasts respectively. Differentiated smooth muscle cells are characterized by their elongated shape, eosinophilic longitudinal fibrils, and long slender (cigar-shaped) nuclei, often with terminal juxtanuclear vacuoles. Other spindle cells are even more difficult to identify. Distinction of fibroblasts, myofibro-

---

Benign soft tissue tumors with nuclear atypia

Pleomorphic fibroma of the skin
Fibrous histiocytoma with bizarre cells
Pleomorphic lipoma
Pleomorphic leiomyoma
Ancient schwannoma (neurilemoma)

---

blasts, Schwann cells and the spindle cells of synovial sarcoma and mesothelioma is more often based on the location and growth pattern than on cytological characteristics; positive identification of these cells frequently requires immunohistochemical studies or electron microscopic analysis. Cellular inclusions are rare in soft tissue pathology; alveolar soft part sarcoma can be identified by the characteristic intracellular PAS-positive crystalline material, and digital fibromatosis can be identified by eosinophilic inclusions consisting of actinlike microfilaments.

High-power examination is also essential for mitotic counts, e.g., the number of mitotic figures per 10 HPF. Atypical mitotic figures are extremely rare in benign soft tissue tumors and almost always indicate malignancy. Mitotic counts are very useful in diagnosing benign and malignant nerve sheath tumors and tumors of smooth muscle tissue, but they are of little importance in the diagnosis of nodular fasciitis, localized and diffuse giant cell tumors, and malignant fibrous histiocytoma. Although nuclear atypia is more often associated with malignancy, it may occur as a degenerative feature in benign lesions (see the accompanying box).

SPECIAL STAINS

Although routine hematoxylin-eosin-stained sections from a well-sampled lesion are essential for diagnosis, ancillary methods such as special stains, immunohistochemical procedures, or ultrastructural studies are often indispensable for reaching a reliable diagnosis. Among the numerous special stains that are available to the pathologist, there are very few that need to be used on a routine basis and perhaps even fewer that substantially improve on the diagnosis suggested by routine methods. For example, special stains will distinguish a myxoid liposarcoma and myxoid chondrosarcoma on the basis of staining characteristics of the myxoid matrix, yet in most cases this distinction is easily made on routine preparations, and use of the special stain is an optional procedure. There are also situations in which the use of special stains may be quite misleading. Fat stains, for instance, must be interpreted with caution since intracellular fat is not only present in lipoblasts but also is demonstrable in a variety of non-lipomatous benign

Table 7-3. Intracellular glycogen in soft tissue sarcomas

Clear cell sarcoma	+
Epithelioid sarcoma	+
Extraskeletal Ewing's sarcoma	+
Fibrosarcoma	−
Leiomyosarcoma	+
Mesothelioma	+
Myxoid chondrosarcoma	+
Neuroblastoma	−
Neuroepithelioma	−
Rhabdomyosarcoma	+
Synovial sarcoma	−

+, Intracellular glycogen present in most cases.
−, Intracellular glycogen absent in most cases.

and malignant mesenchymal tumors and is a frequent complement of cellular degeneration regardless of tumor type.

The PAS-preparation with and without diastase digestion was formerly very useful in staining for glycogen in rhabdomyosarcomas, extraskeletal Ewing's sarcoma, mesothelioma and malignant melanoma, although currently there are more definitive immunohistochemical or ultrastructural methods for establishing these diagnoses. In contrast, intracellular glycogen tends to be absent or inconspicuous in neuroblastoma, peripheral neuroepithelioma and synovial sarcoma (Table 7-3). PAS preparations with diastase, however, are still the mainstay for identifying crystals in alveolar soft part sarcoma. Differentiation of mesothelioma from carcinoma is aided by the alcian blue preparation (with and without hyaluronidase predigestion) coupled with the PAS preparation, because the latter does not stain mesothelial mucin but does stain the neutral mucin present in many adenocarcinomas. The van Gieson and Masson's trichrome stains are used for separating collagen from smooth muscle tissue; the Grimelius stain is used for identifying neurosecretory (argyrophilic) granules in paraganglioma and related tumors.

IMMUNOHISTOCHEMISTRY

Although immunohistochemistry has improved the accuracy of diagnosis, one must be aware of the potential problems and limitations in the interpretation of these stains. Not only is it important to know the specificity of the antibody, but also it is important to be aware of the artifacts that may occur in these preparations, such as nonspecific staining of the edge of the tissue section (edge artifact) or necrotic zones, diffusion and/or uptake of some antigen into adjacent tissues or cells (e.g., myoglobin diffusion from necrotic muscle tissue into histiocytes), and cross-reactivity of some antibodies (a phenomenon more often encountered with monoclonal than polyclonal antibodies).

To use immunostains in the most effective and cost-efficient way, it is useful to have an algorithmic approach in mind when dealing with a given diagnostic problem. In

our laboratory, we encourage the use of panels of antibodies in a sequential fashion in order to systematically limit the differential diagnosis. For example, a panel of antibodies to differentiate a carcinoma, melanoma, sarcoma, and lymphoma from one another would be ordered before ordering a series of B- and T-cell markers. In our experience, immunohistochemistry is an important if not obligate part of the workup of certain basic problems that occur commonly in soft tissue pathology. These include evaluation of the following:

1. Round cell sarcomas
2. Pleomorphic tumors of the skin in which the diagnosis includes melanoma, carcinoma, and atypical fibroxanthoma
3. Undifferentiated malignant tumor in which the diagnoses include melanoma, carcinoma, sarcoma, and lymphoma.

Because of the complexity and importance of these methods they are discussed more fully in Chapter 8.

ELECTRON MICROSCOPY

Compared with the profound effect of immunohistochemistry on the diagnosis of soft tissue tumors, ultrastructural examination plays a lesser role in the assessment of soft tissue sarcomas. This can be explained in part by the sampling error inherent in this technique, the limited experience of many pathologists, and the relatively high cost of this procedure. Moreover, there are only a few ultrastructural markers that lead to a specific histological diagnosis, such as melanosomes in clear cell sarcoma and malignant melanoma and Weibel-Palade bodies in vascular tumors. In most instances the pathologist is called on to evaluate a constellation of less specific features and to decide, based on their frequency or prominence, the probability of a certain diagnosis, recognizing that a loss of differentiation by light microscopy is usually paralleled by a similar loss ultrastructurally.

Electron microscopy has shown itself to be most useful in the diagnosis of round cell sarcoma, such as the distinction of rhabdomyosarcoma from extraskeletal Ewing's sarcoma, neuroblastoma, and neuroepithelioma. The presence of thick (myosin) and thin (actin) microfilaments forms a hexagonal pattern in cross-section. Thick myosin microfilaments with linear arrays of ribosomes and/or intracellular Z-band material in an otherwise poorly differentiated sarcoma establishes the diagnosis of rhabdomyosarcoma, whereas multiple dendritic processes together with microtubules and small, dense-core granules within cytoplasmic processes are characteristic of neuroblastoma. Although extraskeletal Ewing's sarcoma has no specific ultrastructural features, the large rounded nuclei and paucity of organelles, coupled with cytoplasmic glycogen, suggests this diagnosis. In evaluating the ultrastructure of round cell sarcomas, it is important to guard against overzealous interpretation of electron micrographs, especially by inexperienced observers who have been known to diagnose nonspecific microfilaments as "myofilaments" and extracellular cross-banded collagen as intracellular "cross-striations."

Thus the success of electron microscopy in diagnosis obviously depends on the ability to limit the differential diagnoses by light microscopy and then to systematically search for relatively specific ultrastructural features that will favor one possibility over another. Electron microscopy, however, is of limited usefulness in distinguishing benign from malignant tumors and neoplastic from nonneoplastic lesions.

Alternative methodologies that are useful in the diagnosis of soft tissue tumors, and which provide even a greater degree of objectivity, are described and discussed in Chapter 5 (Cytogenetic analysis of soft tissue tumors) and Chapter 6 (DNA analysis of soft tissue tumors).

DIAGNOSTIC NOMENCLATURE AND FINAL REPORTING

Even with the complete sampling and ancillary studies, it may not be possible to accurately classify all sarcomas. In our consultation practice approximately 10% of all sarcomas do not lend themselves to a definitive classification. Nonetheless, it is often possible for the pathologist to provide the clinician with sufficient information so that therapy can proceed in an unencumbered fashion. For example, in the evaluation of moderately differentiated spindle cell sarcomas, one cannot always distinguish a malignant peripheral nerve sheath tumor from a fibrosarcoma. Yet this distinction is not clinically important if the pathologist is able to assure the clinician that the lesion is malignant and to provide a histological grade. Likewise, it is not worthwhile to labor exhaustively over classifying a pleomorphic sarcoma when the therapy will not differ. Thus in these am-

---

University of Michigan Hospital
Laboratory of Surgical Pathology
TEMPLATE REPORTING
OF SARCOMAS

Histologic type:
Grade: I, II, III
Size: Cm in greatest diameter
Location: Subcutis, muscle, body cavity
Margins: Positive, negative (if less than 1 cm, give measurement)
Necrosis: <15%, >15%
Ancillary studies: State if tissue was sent for cytogenetics, molecular diagnostics, flow cytometry, or tissue banking
TMN code:

---

biguous diagnostic situations, there is no substitute for a constructive dialogue among surgeon, pathologist, and oncologist to define the therapeutically relevant pathological information. When the pathologist cannot be certain of the exact diagnosis or even a precise grade, it is acceptable to use a generic diagnosis with a few modifying phrases. For example, low-grade myxoid sarcoma that does not seem to fall clearly into a specific diagnostic category could be labelled "low-grade myxoid sarcoma" with a comment that local recurrence rather than metastasis would be the expected behavior. Alternatively, the diagnosis "myxoid tumor with locally recurring potential" expresses the same information. To convey the pathological findings to the clinicians unambiguously, we have found it useful to standardize our reports. A sample template is given in the accompanying box.

REFERENCES

1. Albus-Lutter CE, de Stefani E, van Unnik JAM: Clinicopathologic relations in soft tissue sarcomas. In *Management of soft tissue and bone sarcomas.* New York, 1986, Raven Press.

2. Angervall L, Kindblom LG, Rydholm A, et al: The diagnosis and prognosis of soft tissue tumors. *Seminars in Diagn Pathol* 3:240, 1986.

3. Angervall L, Kindblom L-G: Principles for the pathologic diagnosis of soft tissue sarcomas. *Acta Oncologica* 28:suppl 2, 1989.

4. Enjoji M, Hashimoto H: Diagnosis of soft tissue sarcomas. *Pathol Res Pract* 178:215, 1984.

5. Enzinger FM: Recent trends in soft tissue pathology. In *Tumors of bone and soft tissue.* Chicago, 1965, Mosby.

6. Enzinger FM: Epithelioid sarcoma. A sarcoma simulating a granuloma or carcinoma. *Cancer* 26:1029, 1970.

7. Enzinger FM: Clinicopathological correlation in soft tissue sarcomas. In *Management of soft tissue and bone sarcomas.* New York, 1986, Raven Press.

8. Enzinger FM, Lattes R, Torloni R: Histological typing of soft tissue tumours. *International histological classification of tumours.* No. 3 Geneva, World Health Organization, 1969.

9. Enzinger FM, Shiraki M: Extraskeletal myxoid chondrosarcoma: an analysis of of 34 cases. *Human Pathol* 3:421, 1972.

10. Erlandson RA: *Diagnostic transmission electron microscopy of human tumors.* New York, 1981, Masson.

11. Erlandson RA: Cytoskeletal proteins including myofilaments in human tumors. *Ultrastr Pathol* 13:155, 1989.

12. Hajdu SI: *Pathology of soft tissue tumors,* Philadelphia, 1979, Lea & Febiger.

13. Laskin WB, Weiss SW, Bratthauer GL: Epithelioid variant of malignant peripheral nerve sheath tumor (malignant epithelioid schwannoma). *Am J Surg Pathol* 15:1136, 1991.

14. Lattes R: *Tumors of the soft tissue.* Atlas of Tumor Pathology. Second series. Fascicle 1/Revised. Armed Forces Institute of Pathology, Washington D.C., 1983.

15. Mackay B: Electron microscopy of soft tissue tumors, in *Management of primary bone and soft tissue tumors.* Chicago, 1977, Mosby.

16. Mackay B, Osborne BM: The contribution of electron microscopy to the diagnosis of tumors. *Pathol Annu* 8:359, 1978.

17. Mandard AM, Chasley J, Mandard JC: The pathologist's role in a

multidisciplinary approach for soft tissue sarcomas: a reappraisal. *J Surg Oncol* 1:69, 1981.

18. Markhede G, Angervall L, Stener B: A multivariate analysis of the prognosis after surgical treatment of malignant soft tissue tumors. *Cancer* 49:1721, 1982.

19. Rantakko V, Ekfors TO: Sarcomas of the soft tissues in the extremities and limb girdles: analysis of 240 cases diagnosed in Finland in 1960-1969. *Acta Chir Scand* 145:385, 1979.

20. Rydholm A: Management of patients with soft tissue tumors: strategy developed at a regional oncology center. *Acta Orthop Scand (suppl)* 203:13, 1983.

21. Shiraki M, Enterline HT, Brooks JJ, et al: Pathologic analysis of advanceed adult soft tissue sarcomas, bone sarcomas and mesotheliomas: The Eastern Cooperative Oncology Group (ECOG) Experience. *Cancer* 64:484, 1989.

22. Stout AP: *Tumors of soft tissue*. AFIP Atlas of Tumor Pathology, Fascicle 1, First Series, Armed Forces Institute of Pathology, Washington, D.C., 1957.

23. Suit HD, Russell WO, Martin RG: Sarcoma of soft tissue: clinical and histopathological parameter and response to treatment. *Cancer* 31:1247, 1973.

24. Taxy JB, Battifora H: The electron microscope in the study and diagnosis of soft tissue tumors. In Trump BF, Jones TT, eds: *Diagnostic electron microscopy*. New York, 1980, John Wiley & Sons.

25. Van Haelst UJGM: EM in the study of soft tissue tumors: diagnosis/differential diagnosis and histogenesis. In *Management of soft tissue and bone sarcomas*. New York, 1986, Raven Press.

26. Weiss SW, Enzinger FM: Malignant fibrous histiocytoma: an analysis of 200 cases. *Cancer* 41:2250, 1978.

27. Weiss SW, Enzinger FM: Epithelioid hemangioendothelioma: a vascular tumor often mistaken for a carcinoma. *Cancer* 50:970, 1982.

CHAPTER 8

IMMUNOHISTOCHEMISTRY OF SOFT TISSUE LESIONS

GENERAL CONSIDERATIONS

Immunohistochemical methods have become an accepted and necessary part of diagnostic pathologic studies. A variety of methods are available for the detection of antigens in tissue sections, and each has certain advantages and disadvantages. Immunofluorescent techniques, utilizing fluorescenated or rhodamine-coupled antibodies on frozen sections, have the advantage of superior antigen preservation but are less sensitive than immunoenzyme methods. Moreover, these methods are impractical for the general surgical pathology laboratory because frozen archival tissue is often not available, cytologic detail is less easily discerned, and the preparations are not permanent. For these reasons, immunoenzyme methods, specifically immunoperoxidase methods utilizing either peroxidase-antiperoxidase or avidin-biotin complex, have largely supplanted immunofluorescent methods for routine diagnoses. These methods have proven to be very sensitive and easy to interpret with standard light microscopy. The preparations are also permanent. Performed under optimal circumstances, the peroxidase-antiperoxidase and avidin-biotin complex methods yield comparable end results, although the latter method is more sensitive.[7]

Regardless of the method used, care must be taken to choose a fixative that will not destroy the antigen. Although formalin is an adequate fixative for most antigens, it is unacceptable, for instance, for detection of surface immunoglobulin and less than ideal for demonstration of intermediate filaments. For these reasons attention has been focused on means to enhance immunoreactivities in formalin-fixed, paraffin-embedded material. Pretreatment with proteolytic enzymes (e.g., trypsin, pepsin, chymotrypsin, protease type XIV, pronase) has been the most popular approach, although it is seldom required for alcohol-fixed tissue. Enzymatic predigestion probably increases antigenicity in a variety of ways. It may cause refolding of proteins to reveal hidden epitopes or remove macromolecules that aggregate near and prevent access to a given epitope.[9] The opti-

mal digestion time is empirically determined for each antigen and is influenced by the duration of previous fixation.[4] In our experience, it enhances immunoreactivities related to the intermediate filaments, factor VIII–associated antigen, cytoplasmic immunoglobulin, lysozyme, and alpha-1-antitrypsin, but is unnecessary and in fact contraindicated for demonstration of small peptide hormones, which are easily cleaved by proteases. An alternative antigen retrieval method is pretreatment of slides by lead or zinc salt solutions in a microwave oven.[16] Significant enhancement of a majority of antigens was noted, although others have reported that this technique offers no advantage over enzymatic digestion techniques.[11]

In general, antigens that have proven to be most useful in diagnosis of soft tissue tumors are those that are relatively restricted in their pattern of distribution (Table 8-1). Hence substances such as actin, myosin, and vimentin, which may be identified in a wide variety of mesenchymal and even epithelial lesions, are not very specific. In contrast, common leukocyte antigen, which is restricted to the surface of cells of leukocyte lineage, is exceedingly helpful in discriminating round cell sarcomas from lymphomas.[17] However, one must always be cognizant of the pattern and distribution of a given antigen both within normal and neoplastic tissue. For example, immunolocalization of common leukocyte antigen results in fine linear staining on the surface of a cell, S-100 protein in nuclear and/or cytoplasmic staining, and factor VIII–associated antigen in cytoplasmic staining only.

In selecting tissue for immunohistochemical sudies, it is also advisable to choose an area for staining that has normal tissues that can serve both as intrinsic positive and negative controls for the antigen. Nonetheless, it should always be borne in mind that intrinsic positive controls tend to have a higher density of antigen than neoplastic tissues and may sometimes be positive when the neoplastic cells are falsely negative due to inadequate method sensitivity. Utilization of high-quality antibodies is essential for diagnostic work.

Table 8-1. Distribution of common antigens in normal tissues and soft tissue neoplasms

Antigen	Normal tissue	Tumors
Actin (HHF-35)*	Skeletal, cardiac, and smooth muscle tissue Myofibroblasts Myoepithelial cells	Skeletal, cardiac, and smooth muscle tumors Variety of tumors and pseudotumors with myo-fibroblasts or myofibroblastic differentiation including, but not limited to nodular fasciitis, granulation tissue, scar tissue, fibromatosis, fibrosarcoma, malignant fibrous histiocytoma
CD-34	Hematopoietic stem cells Endothelium Dermal and periadnexal dendritic cells Endoneurial dendritic cells	Dermatofibrosarcoma protuberans Solitary fibrous tumor Gastrointestinal stromal tumorBenign nerve sheath tumor Epithelioid sarcoma
Cytokeratin	Epithelium, mesothelium	Epithelial tumors Mesothelioma Epithelioid sarcoma Synovial sarcoma Chordoma Rhabdoid tumor Rare to occasional sarcomas of diverse type including leiomyosarcoma, malignant fibrous histiocytoma, malignant peripheral nerve sheath tumor, rhabdomyosarcoma, desmo-plastic small cell tumor of childhood, epithe-lioid vascular tumors
Desmin	Skeletal, cardiac, and smooth muscle	Skeletal, cardiac, and smooth muscle tumors Aberrant expression in rare to occasional non-muscle tumors including angiomatoid fibrous histiocytoma, Ewing's sarcoma, liposarcoma, malignant fibrous histiocytoma
Epithelial membrane antigen	Epithelium, perineurium, meningothelial cells	Synovial sarcoma Epithelioid sarcoma Perineurioma Mesothelioma (variable) Neurofibroma (variable) Meningioma
Factor VIII–associated antigen (von Willebrand factor)	Vascular endothelium Lymphatic endothelium (variable)	Benign vascular tumors Lymphangioma (variable) Hemangioendothelioma Angiosarcoma (variable)
S-100 protein	Schwann cells, glial cells Skeletal muscle Chondrocytes Lipocytes Macrophage subsets Myoepithelial cells	Benign and malignant nerve sheath tumors Melanoma Chondromas, some chondrosarcomas Lipomas, some liposarcomas Histiocytosis X Sustentacular element in paragangliomas, neuroblastoma Rhabdomyoma, some rhabdomyosaroma
Vimentin	Most mesenchymal tissues	Most mesenchymal tumors Some carcinomas Melanoma

*Identifies alpha and gamma muscle actins.

Two types of antibodies are available: polyclonal and monoclonal (MoAb). A polyclonal antiserum consists of a heterogenous population of antibodies reacting with different epitopes of the antigen. The principal advantage of a polyclonal antiserum is that it reacts with the major immunodeterminants of a given antigen. However, the disadvantage is that it occasionally contains impurities. Affinity isolation, or passing the antiserum through a column containing pure antigen bound to insoluble substrate, removes these impurities. In contrast a MoAb is a homogenous population of antibodies reacting to a single epitope of an antigen. If chosen for its high-affinity binding to the antigen, it provides a theoretically unlimited, stable, pure antibody preparation of high quality. However, since it reacts with only one epitope, modification of that epitope may alter the binding and, hence, utility of the MoAb. A second problem is that it may cross-react with similar epitopes on an unrelated antigen and give rise to an unusual pattern of cross-reactivity. Hence performance testing should be carried out before using any new MoAb for diagnostic purposes.

The sausage technique, which combines a number of different tissues in one paraffin block, provides an expedient inexpensive means of testing a small amount of MoAb on a large number of tissues at one time (Fig. 8-1).[2]

INTERMEDIATE FILAMENTS

Intermediate filaments, so named because their size of 10 nm places them in an intermediate position between the thin (6 nm) microfilaments and thick (25 nm) microtubule filaments of the cell, are a major cytoskeletal system comprising five subgroups: the cytokeratins, vimentin, desmin, glial fibrillary acidic protein, and neurofilament protein.[22,23,25] Ultrastructurally similar, they appear as wavy unbranched filaments, which often occupy a perinuclear position in the cell. They share a variable degree of homology with one another as determined by biochemical and immunological means. In general, the expression of intermediate filaments by a cell is a reflection of the line of differentiation, although, as indicated below, other factors may influence the synthesis and modulation of these proteins.[20-22,26,28]

VIMENTIN

Vimentin (MW 57,000) is the intermediate filament traditionally associated with mesenchymal cells and mesenchymal tumors, although it is present in a wide variety of cells during early embryological development and is replaced by a type-specific intermediate filament in the course of differentiation.[22,116] It has been identified in fibroblasts, chondroblasts, smooth muscle cells, mesothelium, endothelium, and virtually all types of sarcomas. Its presumed absence from epithelium was formerly thought to be a reliable means of separating mesenchymal from epithelial tu-

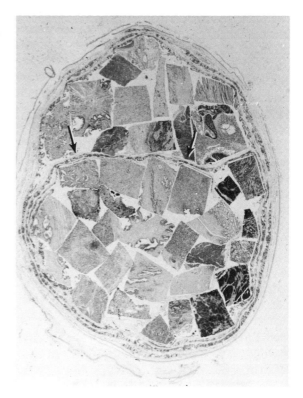

FIG. 8-1. Section generated from multitumor "sausage" block for testing antibodies on numerous tissues at one time. Block has been stained with MoAb to NSE. Intense staining is noted only in neuroendocrine carcinomas seen on right. Arrows indicate dividing septa. (Courtesy Dr. Hector Battifora.)

mors. However, several reports indicate that it can be identified in a variable percentage of normal epithelia and their neoplastic counterparts,[19,26,27] especially if alcohol-fixed material is used. Most adenocarcinomas of breast, lung, kidney, adrenal, and endometrium contain vimentin, whereas a smaller percentage of squamous carcinomas express the antigen.[19] Alterations in vimentin expression also occur within established cell lines under varying conditions.[21,28] For example, mesothelial cells reversibly lose keratin and increase vimentin production during periods of rapid growth in cell culture.[21] Expression of vimentin appears to be closely related not only to type and stage of differentiation but also to basic properties of cellular kinetics and contact. Although the diagnostic importance of vimentin has been diminished with respect to the other intermediate filaments, there are still a few instances where its strong expression may suggest a diagnosis. Strong expression of vimentin in the absence of keratin in an epithelioid tumor is very suggestive of melanoma, whereas coexpression of vimentin and keratin in a soft tissue tumor is very typical of epithelioid sarcoma. Since this intermediate filament is so ubiquitous, it also serves as an intrinsic positive control on which to evaluate the immunoreactivity of the intermediate filaments in the tissue section.[1]

EPITHELIAL ANTIGENS
Cytokeratin

Detection of cytokeratin is currently the most common method employed for documenting epithelial differentiation within a given lesion because these proteins are ubiquitously distributed within epithelia of various types and their neoplastic counterparts. One of the five classes of intermediate filaments, cytokeratin is collectively a group of 19 separate polypeptides, which range in molecular weight from 40 to 67 K. They can be further subdivided into acidic (type I) and basic (type II) subfamilies according to their charges, immunoreactivities, and amino acid sequences. The pattern or profile of keratins is determined by the type of epithelium and the degree of differentiation and follows certain rules recently elaborated by Cooper et al.[34] Keratins occur as pairs consisting of an acidic and basic form, the latter always exceeding the former in molecular weight. Stratified epithelium and simple epithelium have different patterns of pairs. Moreover, the various stratified epithelia differ from one another in having certain specific pairs indicative of their differentiation sequence (Fig. 8-2). Thus knowledge of the keratin profile of an epithelium gives some indication of its origin and, to a lesser extent, the tumors derived therefrom.

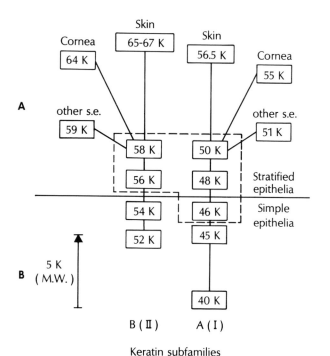

FIG. 8-2. Schematization of distribution of acidic (**A**) and basic (**B**) keratin subgroups within various tissues. (Modified from Cooper et al: *Lab Invest* 52:243, 1985.)

Antibodies to cytokeratin currently play an important role in diagnostic pathology. Monoclonal antibodies with limited specificities potentially allow for the subclassification of epithelial tumors, but, more importantly, monoclonal antibodies with broad reactivities often permit distinction of an epithelial from a nonepithelial tumor. Antibodies such as AE1, which react with the widely distributed low-molecular-weight keratins (40 to 56 K), have a very broad range of recognition.[3,34] With the use of this antibody, immunostaining is noted in most epithelial tumors, although variable results have been reported in renal and hepatocellular carcinoma.[3,57] Adequate results may be obtained with routinely fixed tissues, but full elucidation of the antigen usually requires enzymatic predigestion or, alternatively, fixation in alcohol.

The presence of cytokeratin does not absolutely indicate (as was formerly thought) epithelial origin. Mesothelium and mesotheliomas contain cytokeratin, and thus demonstration of this substance alone fails to discriminate mesotheliomas from adenocarcinomas. In fact, it appears that no antigen is an absolute discriminant in this difficult diagnostic problem. However, a panel of antibodies directed against a variety of antigens including keratin, carcinoembryonic antigen and TAG-72 (as defined by the monoclonal antibody B72.3) usually suggests one diagnosis over the other. Mesotheliomas usually express keratins of low and intermediate weight, usually lack carcinoembryonic antigen[30,44] and TAG-72,[59] and infrequently express epithelial membrane antigen except at the surface.[2,55] Adenocarcinomas usually contain only low-molecular-weight keratins, display surface or cytoplasmic epithelial membrane antigen, or both, and often express carcinoembryonic antigen.

However, the presence or absence of keratin as a sole antigen has proved helpful in our experience in distinguishing sarcomatoid mesotheliomas from true sarcomas; in separating unusual forms of mesothelioma, such as multicystic mesothelioma, from lesions that mimic them (e.g., lymphangioma) (Fig. 8-3); and in defining the fibroblastic nature of certain localized lesions of the pleura, formerly considered mesothelioma (i.e., fibrous mesothelioma).[37] It is also a valuable adjunct in the diagnosis of spindle cell tumors of the skin when the differential diagnosis includes atypical fibroxanthoma, spindle carcinoma, and malignant melanoma. Also, the punctate, paranuclear distribution of keratin within Merkel cell carcinomas may be a helpful feature in distinguishing this tumor from some round cell sarcomas and lymphomas (Fig. 8-4).

In addition to mesotheliomas, synovial sarcoma, epithelioid sarcoma, and extrarenal rhabdoid tumor consistently express cytokeratin.[32,35] In synovial sarcomas, cytokeratin can be localized to the glands and, to a lesser extent, the stroma, where its presence can serve as an independently reliable means of recognizing monophasic forms of the tumor (Fig. 8-5). In extrarenal rhabdoid tumors, cytokeratin is localized to the homogeneous eosinophilic zone adjacent to the nucleus (Fig. 8-6). In virtually all epithelioid sarcomas, cytokeratin is coexpressed with vimentin and provides an extremely helpful tool in distinguishing this tumor from granulomatous lesions with which it is occasionally con-

fused. It also appears that other sarcomas occasionally express cytokeratin. Keratin has been identified in leiomyosarcomas[39,45,47,56] and Ewing's sarcomas[38] by gel electrophoresis. The authors and others have also encountered cytokeratin expression sporadically in a variety of sarcomas, including malignant fibrous histiocytoma, liposarcoma, rhabdomyosarcoma, hemangiopericytoma, malignant peripheral nerve sheath tumor, epithelioid forms of hemangioendothelioma, and angiosarcoma.[10,41,42] The low frequency of this phenomenon, coupled with its reproducibility utilizing polyclonal and a variety of MoAbs, strongly suggests that it represents aberrant expression of the antigen rather than an unusual pattern of cross-reactivity with a minor epitope of another antigen. Nonetheless, observations such as the foregoing emphasize the need to evaluate all immunological staining results within the context of the other clinicopathological findings.

Problems in interpretation of cytokeratin preparations are twofold. Overlay of dandruff on slides can result in false-positive staining of the surrounding cells. This artifact is easily recognized by the localized nature of the staining (Fig. 8-7). A second more difficult problem in interpretation is infiltration of a tumor involving the pleural or peritoneal surface by reactive spindled mesothelial cells containing keratin (Fig. 8-8).[23] Care should always be taken to examine tumor distant from the mesothelial surface and to carefully observe the cytological characteristics of the immunoreactive cells.

Epithelial membrane antigen

Epithelial membrane antigen is the collective term given to a group of carbohydrate-rich, protein-poor, high-molecular-weight substances found on the surface of epithelial cells.[32,43] Antibodies to epithelial membrane antigen were prepared using delipidized human milk as the antigen, since it represents a rich source of milk-globule membranes. Early studies using polyclonal antisera with immunofluorescent techniques suggested that the antigens were restricted to mammary epithelium and its respective tumors,[32] but newer methods indicate that this antigen is widely distributed among epithelia and epithelial tumors of various types[43,53,56] and occasionally in other tissues.[36,53] In normal secretory epithelium, it can be localized to the apical or luminal surface of the cell and occasionally to intracytoplasmic lumina. However, in the neoplastic state it is present both on the surface of the cell and in the cytoplasm. According to one large series, the antigen can be demonstrated in virtually all epithelial tumors, but the intensity of immunoreactivity varies with the degree and type of differentiation as well as fixation.[53] Although initially thought to be quite specific for epithelial tumors, it, like keratin, has proved to have various notable exceptions. Epithelial membrane antigen or a substance like it can be identified on the surface of plasma cells, rare histiocytes, lymphomas (often

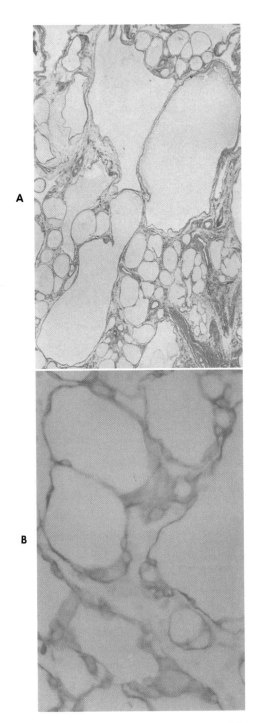

FIG. 8-3. Cystic mesothelioma (A) immunostained for cytokeratin (B). This stain provides easy separation from a cavernous lymphangioma. (A, × 25; B, antikeratin, PAP × 250.)

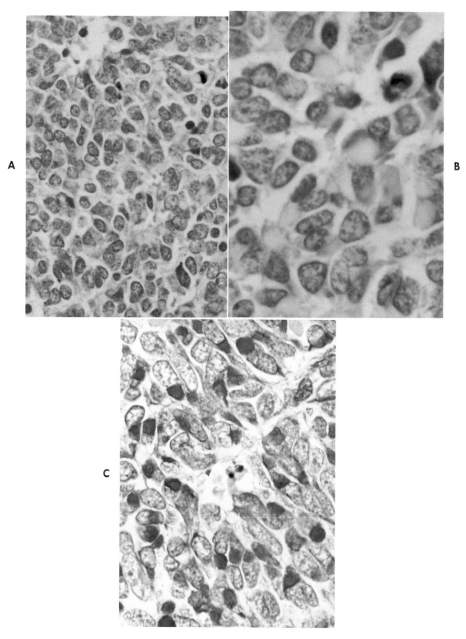

FIG. 8-4. Merkel cell carcinoma (A) showing characteristic perinuclear hyaline zone (B), which contains punctate keratin immunoreactivity (C). (A, × 100; B, × 400; C, antikeratin, PAP × 250.)

of the T cell type), and malignant histiocytoses.[36,53] Its presence in perineural cells (in the absence of S-100 protein) has become a means of recognizing nerve sheath tumors showing perineurial differentiation. The so-called perineurioma vaguely resembles a neurofibroma or fibrous histiocytoma but is characterized by nerve sheath cells that are positive for epithelial membrane antigen and negative for S-100 protein.[52] Since meningeal cells are closely related to perineurial cells it is not surprising that epithelial membrane antigen is commonly encountered in meningioma.[60] The antigen is also detected in some malignant nerve sheath tumors, synovial sarcomas (particularly in the luminal aspect of the glands), epithelioid sarcomas, and rarely in other types of sarcomas (e.g., leiomyosarcoma, malignant fibrous histiocytoma, rhabdomyosarcoma).[34] In our experience and that of others,[61] it has usually proved to be less sensitive than cytokeratin and, because of the foregoing exceptions, a less specific antigen.

Desmoplakin

Desmoplakins are highly conserved proteins present within the desmosomal plaques of epithelial cells. Utiliz-

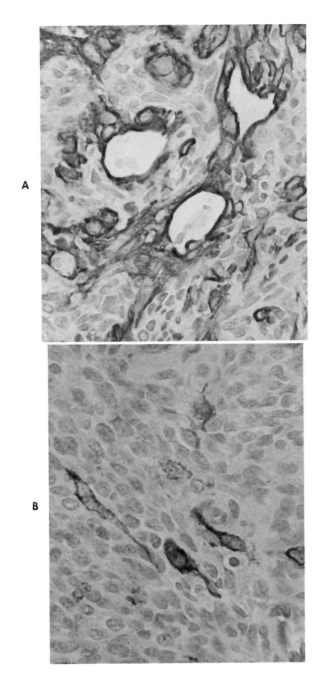

FIG. 8-5. Synovial sarcoma showing keratin immunoreactivity within glandular component (**A**) and, to a lesser extent within the spindled zones (**B**). (**A** and **B**, Antikeratin, PAP ×250.)

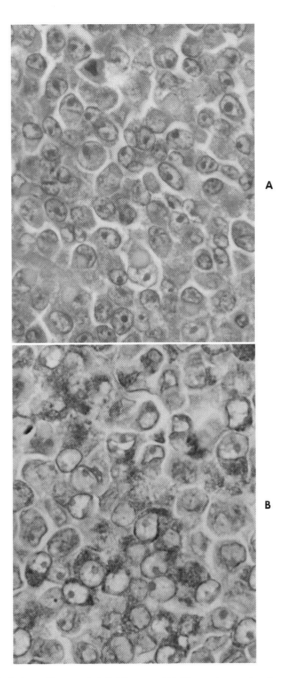

FIG. 8-6. Malignant rhabdoid tumor (**A**) illustrating perinuclear eosinophilic zone, which contains immunoreactive cytokeratin (**B**). (**A**, × 400; B, antikeratin, PAP × 400.)

ing antibodies directed against desmoplakin I and II, immunoreactivity can be localized to peripheral punctate regions in a wide variety of epithelial cells, meningeal cells, and mesothelium.[50] Desmoplakins can also be identified within the glandular component of synovial sarcomas but not in other sarcomas.[48] Thus desmoplakins represent an additional marker of epithelial differentiation independent of keratin.

MUSCLE ANTIGENS
Desmin

Desmin (MW 55,000), another in the family of intermediate filaments, serves as an integral part of the cytoskeleton of cardiac, skeletal, and smooth muscle fibers. In skeletal muscle it is localized to the Z zone between the myofibrils, where it presumably serves as a binding material for the contractile apparatus.[72] In smooth muscle it is associ-

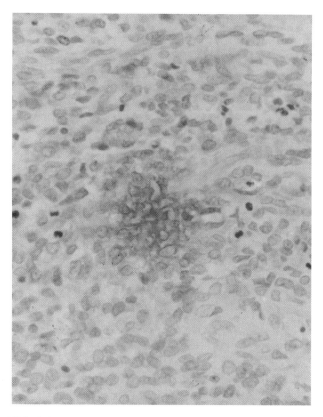

FIG. 8-7. Overlay of dandruff on slide creating intense focal immunostaining for cytokeratin. (Antikeratin, PAP × 250.)

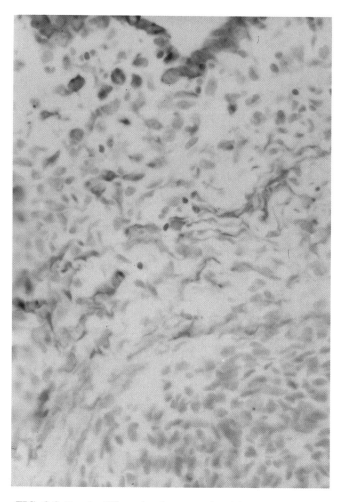

FIG. 8-8. Poorly differentiated sarcoma involving the abdominal mesothelial surface. Note the presence of cytokeratin-positive, spindled mesothelium adjacent to the tumor and rare cytokeratin-positive mesothelial cells within tumor. (Antikeratin, PAP × 100.)

ated with cytoplasmic dense bodies and subplasmalemmal dense plaques. Desmin can be readily identified immunohistochemically within skeletal, cardiac, and smooth muscle although its presence within vascular smooth muscle is variable. In addition, desmin is encountered in some subsets of myofibroblasts, reticulum cells of lymph node, endometrial stromal cells, fetal mesothelium, stromal cells of fetal kidney, and chorionic villi.

The prevalence of desmin immunoreactivity within a given tumor varies greatly depending on fixation. Immunoreactivity is best elicited when frozen tissues are utilized,[65,79] although adequate results can also be achieved with alcohol fixation or formalin fixation with enzymatic predigestion. Despite these variations, there is general agreement that antibodies to this antigen are useful, if not critical, in the differential diagnosis of round cell tumors, particularly rhabdomyosarcomas. Depending on the type of fixation, between 80% and 100% of rhabdomyosarcomas express this antigen, even in cells that appear relatively undifferentiated by light microscopy (Fig. 8-9). In one study desmin could be detected in over 90% of rhabdomyosarcomas when frozen tissue was used and in about 80% of cases with formalin-fixed tissue.[79]

Desmin has proven to be less useful in the diagnosis of smooth muscle tumors, however. Although it can be easily

detected in virtually all benign smooth muscle tumors, immunohistochemical studies are rarely needed to make the diagnosis of leiomyoma. Although it is potentially useful to identify leiomyosarcomas, the prevalence of this antigen in these tumors is far less than in rhabdomyosarcomas. Only about half of leiomyosarcomas express the antigen[62,63,80,74] and in some locations, such as the gastrointestinal tract, the incidence is even lower. (see Chapters 19 and 20).

Desmin immunoreactivity has also been documented in alveolar soft part sarcoma and intraabdominal desmoplastic small cell tumor. In the first instance the presence of desmin provides additional support for the growing presumption that these tumors represent a specific variant of skeletal muscle tumor. In the latter instance desmin is expressed along with a number of other marker substances in a tumor that bears little resemblance to other muscle tumors.

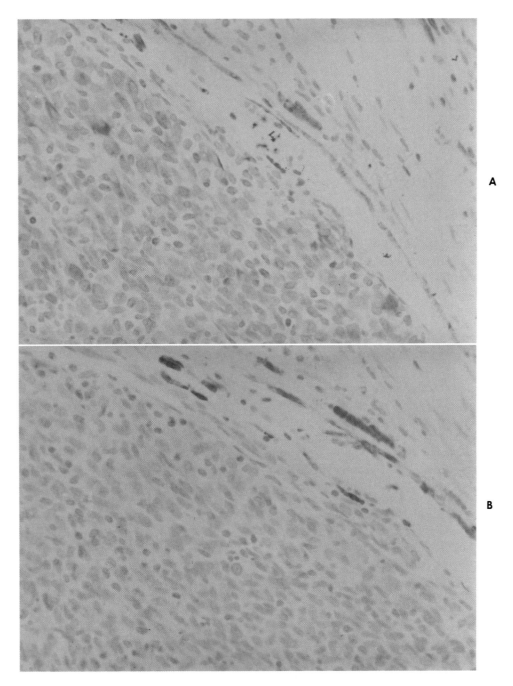

FIG. 8-9. Comparison of immunostaining for desmin (**A**) and myoglobin (**B**) on a serial section of rhabdomyosarcoma. Note that many of the tumor cells are desmin positive, but virtually no tumor cells are myoglobin positive. Adjacent normal muscle stains in both. (**A,** Antidesmin, PAP × 160; **B,** antimyoglobin, PAP × 160.)

With the increasing use of desmin antibodies there has been the growing realization that some myofibroblasts express this antigen. Thus, desmin immunoreactivity, identified focally within various spindle cell lesions not traditionally considered smooth muscle, has been interpreted as evidence of focal myofibroblastic differentiation. These include fibromatosis, malignant fibrous histiocytoma, and myofibroblastoma of the breast. Lastly, there is a growing list of sarcomas that have either no or at best a tenuous relationship to smooth muscle yet also contain desmin-positive cells. These cases are probably best interpreted as aberrant expression of the antigen. These include malignant peripheral nerve sheath tumor,[88] epithelioid sarcoma, peripheral neuroepithelioma,[79] liposarcoma, angiomatoid fibrous histiocytoma,[152] and rhabdoid tumor.

Myoglobin

Myoglobin is the oxygen-binding heme protein found in skeletal and cardiac cells. Before the advent of numerous monoclonal antibodies to desmin, antibodies for myoglobin were widely used for the diagnosis of benign and malignant skeletal muscle tumors (e.g., rhabdomyosarcoma).[65,67,72,75] Since myoglobin is not present within smooth muscle cells, it is a more specific antigen than desmin, but it has also proven to be less sensitive (Fig. 8-9). Less than half of rhabdomyosarcomas contain demonstrable myoglobin.[68,79] Although this protein appears early in muscle differentiation, it probably is not present in sufficient amounts to be readily detectable.[68] Errors in interpreting myoglobin immunostaining results can occur when myoglobin is released from damaged muscle cells and phagocytosed by adjacent neoplastic and nonneoplastic ones.[69]

Actin

Actins are a family of contractile proteins of similar molecular weight (42 kd) which are distributed ubiquitously in mammalian cells and which can be divided into alpha, beta, and gamma subtypes depending on electrophoretic mobility. There are three isoforms of alpha-actin (alpha-skeletal, alpha-cardiac, and alpha-smooth muscle), two forms of gamma-actin (gamma-smooth muscle and gamma-cytoplasmic), and one form of beta-actin (beta-cytoplasmic). Beta- and gamma-cytoplasmic actins are found in all cells, whereas the three alpha-actins and gamma-smooth muscle actin are expressed selectively as their respective names imply.

A variety of monoclonal antibodies are available that recognize epitopes of one or more actin isoforms. The most widely used actin antibody (HHF-35) reacts with alpha- and gamma-smooth muscle actins and will therefore decorate cardiac, skeletal, and smooth muscle cells from all sites.[87] In addition, it also recognizes pericytes, myoepithelial cells, and many subsets of myofibroblasts.[83] Consequently, this antibody can be used for immunostaining of myofibroblastic cells within granulation tissue, scar tissue, nodular fasciitis, and fibromatosis. Antibodies directed against alpha-smooth muscle actin have a more restricted spectrum of immunoreactivity in that they react with smooth muscle cells and some myofibroblasts but not cardiac and skeletal muscle.

Because most actin antibodies employed in general surgical pathologic studies also identify myofibroblasts, these reagents are not very useful for diagnosing smooth muscle tumors; this diagnosis is usually better made using a combination of conventional light microscopy and histochemical studies (Masson trichrome stain). However, antibodies directed against actin, like those directed against desmin, can play a role in the diagnosis of rhabdomyosarcoma. HHF-35, according to some authors, stains virtually all rhabdomyosarcomas. Thus in the context of round cell sarcoma, immunoreactivity for actin would be highly suggestive of rhabdomyosarcoma, especially since other round cell sarcomas such as neuroblastoma and Ewing's sarcoma are usually negative.[82]

Other muscle antigens

Antibodies to other muscle antigens have been used to identify myogenic tumors. These include antibodies to the muscle (M) subunit of creatine kinase (CK-M),[59] skeletal muscle myosin,[68,86] fetal heavy chain skeletal muscle myosin,[69] and titin.[66] The last is a large protein, comprising about 10% of the mass of sarcomeric muscle and localized to the junction of the AI bands. It appears later in myogenesis than desmin and is identified in more differentiated rhabdomyoblasts. With immunohistochemical methods titin can be localized to rhabdomyosarcomas, particularly the most differentiated ones. In the experience cited by Cavazzana et al., titin could be identified within 25%, 50%, and 100% of alveolar, embryonal, and spindled cell rhabdomyosarcomas respectively.[66]

VASCULAR ANTIGENS
Factor VIII–associated antigen (factor VIII–AG, von Willebrand factor)

Factor VIII is a complex of two components that have different biochemical, functional, and immunological properties.[94] Factor VIII-C, or antihemophilic factor, is synthesized by the liver and possesses procoagulant activity. Factor VIII–associated antigen, or von Willebrand factor, is a large multimeric protein that is synthesized by endothelial cells. Ultrastructurally the antigen has been localized to the Weibel-Palade body by means of immunoelectron microscopy. Although factor VIII–associated antigen can also be found in platelets and megakaryocytes, it has become a reasonably good marker of endothelial differentiation. However, full elucidation in tissue sections usually requires enzymatic predigestion. This antigen can be demonstrated, with some variability, in normal endothelium (Fig. 8-10, A) and endocardium and in most benign vascular tumors (e.g., hemangioma, pyogenic granuloma).[13,103,108] Although typically factor VIII–associated antigen is localized throughout the cytoplasm of the neoplastic cells, occasionally accentuation of factor VIII–associated antigen immunostaining is seen around vacuoles within neoplastic endothelium (Fig. 8-11, B). These vacuoles in actuality represent miniature lumina and are seen typically in certain low-grade vascular tumors (e.g., epithelioid hemangioendothelioma, spindle cell hemangioendothelioma). The presence of factor VIII–associated antigen in cardiac myxomas[97,102]

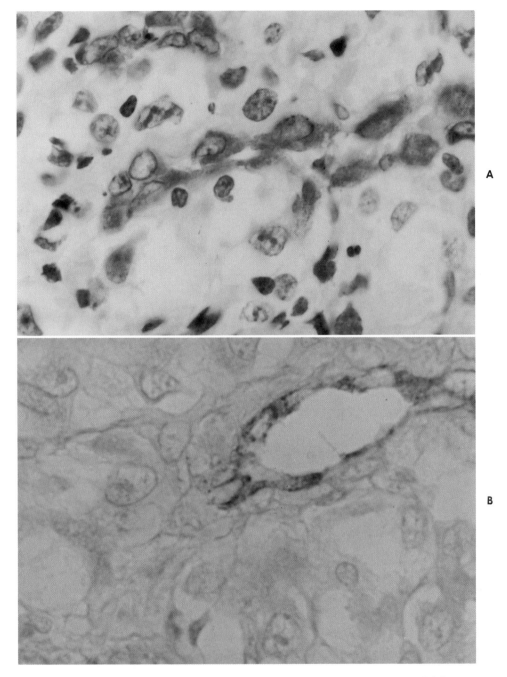

FIG. 8-10. **A,** Normal endothelium immunostained for factor VIII-AG. Note intense, slightly granular quality of cytoplasmic staining. **B,** Nonspecific uptake of factor VIII-AG by nonvascular tumor cells. Staining is homogeneous and of low intensity. Small vessel in upper right shows specific staining of endothelial cells. (**A, B,** Anti-factor VIII-AG, PAP × 250.)

and lymphangiomas is controversial, but differences may reflect differences in specificity of antiserum, enzymatic digestion, and interpretation. There is great variability of factor VIII-associated antigen within angiosarcomas, and the actual percentage of cells containing identifiable antigen is usually quite low (Fig. 8-12, *A*). In fact, some have suggested that the variability of factor VIII–associated antigen staining among angiosarcomas not only reflects the degree of differentiation but also histogenetic differences among angiosarcomas, some arising from lymphatic and others from capillary endothelium. In either event, the lack of this antigen in many angiosarcomas and the low percent-

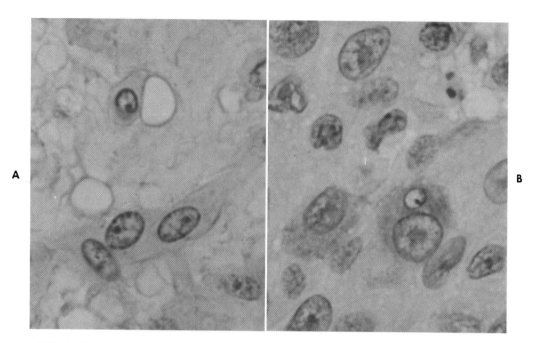

FIG. 8-11. Epithelioid hemangioendothelioma illustrating small intracytoplasmic vacuoles (lumina) **(A).** Cells express factor VIII, which is accentuated around cytoplasmic lumina **(B).** (**A,** × 400; **B,** Anti-factor VIII-Ag, PAP × 400.)

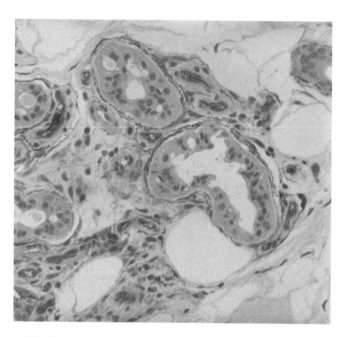

FIG. 8-12. CD-34 positive dendritic cells surrounding adnexal structures. (Anti-CD-34 × 160.)

age of positive cells make it evident that small biopsies of angiosarcomas could yield false-negative results on the basis of inadequate sampling.

Evaluation of other presumed vascular malignant tumors for factor VIII–associated antigen has provided new insights into differentiation. So-called proliferating angioen-

dotheliomatosis is currently regarded as a form of angiotropic lymphoma because of the absence of factor VIII–associated antigen and the presence of common leukocyte antigens. (see Chapter 25). Although Kaposi's sarcoma is regarded as a vascular lesion, it does not appear to express factor VIII–associated antigen,[101] despite earlier reports to the contrary.[104] Factor VIII–associated antigen can be localized to the supporting vessels within the tumor, however.

Faulty interpretation of stains for factor VIII–associated antigen represents a significant source of diagnostic error. Since factor VIII–associated antigen is a plasma protein, it may be endocytosed by nonendothelial cells, giving rise to potential false-positive interpretations. Nonspecific uptake can be suspected if many cells of a given tumor display diffuse homogenous staining in the nucleus or cytoplasm, or both (Fig. 8-11, *B*). Ideally immunostaining should be intense, finely granular, and confined to the cytoplasm (Fig. 8-11, *A*).

CD-34 (human progenitor cell antigen)

The CD-34 antigen is a protein with a molecular weight of 115- kD encoded by a gene on chromosome 1q that is expressed on the surface of hematopoietic progenitor cells of lymphoid and myeloid lineage in the bone marrow and in some acute leukemias. It has also been identified in vascular endothelial cells, particularly those engaged in active angiogenesis, dendritic cells that populate the mid and lower dermis and surround various adnexal structures (Fig. 8-12), and dendritic cells within the endoneurium (Fig. 8-13). Its localization to vascular endothelium resulted in

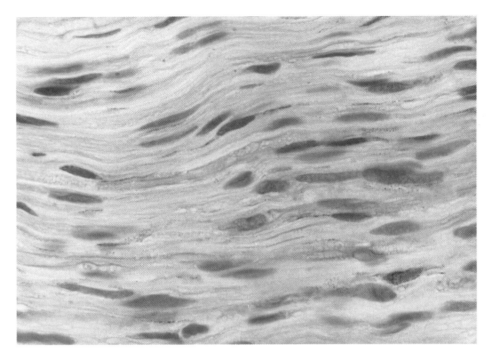

FIG. 8-13. CD-34 positive dendritic cells within endoneurium. (Anti-CD-34 × 400.)

early optimism that it would serve as a relatively specific marker of endothelial differentiation.[89,107,112] It can be detected in nearly all benign vascular tumors although it is not a sensitive antigen for identifying lymphatic endothelium and its respective tumors. About 80% to 90% of malignant vascular tumors including Kaposi's sarcoma also contain the antigen.[105] However, there are now a number of reports attesting to the fact that this antigen (or a closely related epitope) can be identified within a variety of nonvascular tumors.[141] These include dermatofibrosarcoma protuberans (Fig. 8-14), solitary fibrous tumors of pleura and peritoneum, benign nerve sheath tumors, epithelioid sarcoma, and epithelioid smooth muscle tumors of gastrointestinal and soft tissue origin. Since this potpourri of tumors seems to have little in common, the significance of this finding is not clear. Problems in differential diagnosis are not likely as a result of this immunostaining since these various tumors are seldom confused with one another by conventional microscopy. We have found this antigen quite useful when used with other vascular antigens to identify malignant vascular tumors. It also serves as a reasonably good discriminant between benign fibrous histiocytoma and dermatofibrosarcoma protuberans, although rarely benign fibrous histiocytomas contain tumor cells positive for CD-34 (Figs. 8-14 and 8-15).

CD-31 (platelet-endothelial cell adhesion molecule; PECAM-1)

CD-31 antigen is a transmembrane glycoprotein and member of the immunoglobulin superfamily that is present on the surface of endothelial cells as well as various hematopoietic cells, including megakaryocytes, platelets, and some plasma cells. It has only recently been used as a marker of endothelial differentiation[91,100] Virtually all benign vascular tumors express this antigen and in addition about 80% to 100% of angiosarcomas have identifiable immunoreactivity.[91] Unlike CD-34 it appears to have a very restricted distribution in nonvascular lesions, making it a more specific marker of vascular differentiation. However, a sporadic case of malignant mesothelioma, leiomyosarcoma, and occasional carcinoma possesses this antigen.[100] In the diagnosis of poorly differentiated tumors suspected of being angiosarcomas the prudent approach is to use a panel of antibodies, which collectively will identify virtually all angiosarcomas.

Blood group isoantigens (ABO)

The blood group isoantigens are a group of branching carbohydrate chains located on the surface of all cells but are traditionally associated with red blood cells, where their presence determines blood group compatibility. These antigens are derived from a common precursor substance, which is modified by the presence of certain allelic genes. In the presence of the H gene, the precursor substance is converted to the H antigen, which characterizes persons of blood group O. In the presence of the A gene or B gene, the H substance can be further altered to give rise to the A and B antigens, respectively. The immunocytochemical significance of these isoantigens lies in the fact that immunological or nonimmunological binding to these glycoproteins

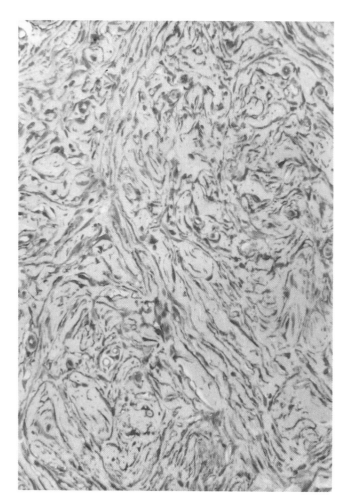

FIG. 8-14. Dermatofibrosarcoma protuberans showing diffuse immunoreactivity for CD-34. (Anti-CD-34 × 100.)

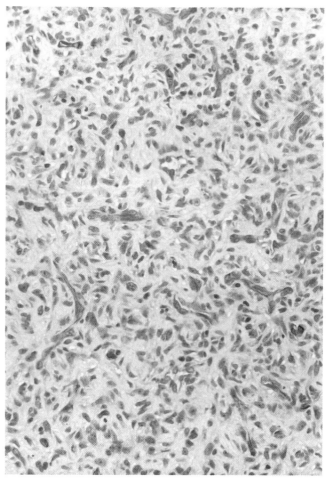

FIG. 8-15. Fibrous histiocytoma showing CD-34 positive capillary network. Tumor cells are negative in contrast to dermatofibrosarcoma protuberans. (Anti-CD-34 × 100.)

provides another means of identifying endothelial cells.

Ulex lectin, a plant protein derived from the seeds of the leguminous shrub *Ulex europaeus,* binds nonimmunologically to the H substance of the ABO system as well as other tissue glycoproteins independent of blood group type.[93] Several recent reports indicate that this lectin is more sensitive than factor VIII–associated antigen in recognizing normal endothelium and the cell of angiosarcomas.[93,98] However, *Ulex* binding is by no means specific for endothelium and it will also recognize antigens in various types of epithelium (e.g., lung, sweat glands, hair follicles)[106] and even in rare sarcomas.[113] Therefore, although its sensitivity is superior to that of factor VIII–associated antigen its diminished specificity renders it less effective as a diagnostic reagent. Monoclonal antibodies to the ABO isoantigens have recently been studied to evaluate their utility in diagnosis as compared with factor VIII–associated antigen.[111] Although results were equivalent to or better than those with factor VIII–associated antigen in benign or re-

active vascular lesions, their inability to recognize the majority of angiosarcomas offered little advantage over that of immunostaining for factor VIII–associated antigen. However, lymphatic endothelium was more readily identified with this method than with factor VIII–associated antigen.

Miscellaneous endothelial antigens

There are increasing numbers of monoclonal antibodies which identify either structural or synthetic components of the endothelial cells but which have been used only in a limited fashion for diagnostic work.[95,96,109] Antibodies directed against thrombomodulin, an antagonist of factor VIII, identify many benign and malignant vascular tumors but do not seem to offer any increased sensitivity compared with *Ulex* lectin.[114] The monoclonal antibody PAL-E[76] offers the advantage of selective immunoreactivity with certain types of endothelium and the potential to discriminate capillary from lymphatic endothelium (see Chapter 25).[109]

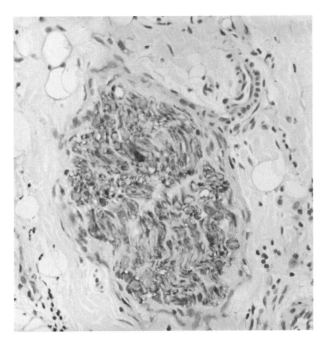

FIG. 8-16. Nerve illustrating S-100 protein immunoreactivity of schwann cells. Note that the perineurium does not stain. (Anti-S-100 protein × 250.)

NEURAL ANTIGENS
S-100 Protein

S-100 protein, so-named because of its 100% solubility in ammonium sulphate, is an acidic protein widely distributed in the central and peripheral nervous systems. Its function is unknown, but its partial sequence homology to calmodulin and its configurational alterations in response to potassium and calcium have led to the hypothesis that it plays a role in ionic regulation in the brain.

Although initially considered a brain-specific protein, S-100 protein has been demonstrated in a variety of nonneural cells as well.[139] Nonetheless, we have found it to be an empirically useful antigen as a marker of neuroectodermal tumors, given certain qualifications.[120,128,140] Using most commercially available antisera or monoclonal antibodies, S-100 protein is readily demonstrated in astrocytes, oligodendrocytes, Schwann cells (Fig. 8-16), folliculostellate cells of the adenohypophysis, satellite cells of the adrenal medulla, chondrocytes, adipocytes, myoepithelial cells, and various histiocytes, which include Langerhans' cells of the epidermis (Fig. 8-17) and interdigitating reticulum cells of the lymph nodes. It is not present in perineurial cells, however.

Perhaps its greatest use in the diagnosis of soft tissue lesions is in benign nerve sheath tumors and melanoma.[127,140] It is present in virtually all neurilemomas and neurofibromas, although the intensity and percentage of positive cells are far less in neurofibromas than in neurilemomas. This

observation parallels ultrastructural observations that neurilemomas are composed of a more uniform population of Schwann cells, whereas neurofibromas contain an admixture of perineurial cells and fibroblasts. S-100 protein immunostaining is invaluable in the diagnosis of cellular schwannoma (Fig. 8-18), a benign tumor often mistaken for fibrosarcoma or malignant peripheral nerve sheath tumor. Within cellular schwannomas S-100 protein is consistently diffuse and intense in contrast to the focal and sometimes weak staining in malignant Schwann cell tumors. S-100 protein can be identified within granular cell tumors[125,140] providing additional evidence of their neural origin. Unlike benign nerve sheath tumors, only about half of malignant nerve sheath tumors express the protein and in these cases the staining tends to be focal and spotty[140] (Fig. 8-19). Nonetheless, this protein is sometimes helpful in separating malignant peripheral nerve sheath tumors from other similar-appearing sarcomas (e.g., fibrosarcoma). Nearly all melanomas, regardless of the degree of pigmentation, express S-100 protein.[127,140] This has proven to be extremely helpful in the recognition of metastatic melanomas or melanomas having unusual growth patterns such as the neurotropic and desmoplastic forms. However, since some carcinomas (notably breast and lung) also may express S-100 protein, it is imperative that in the evaluation of any tumor in which the differential diagnosis includes both carcinoma and melanoma, immunostaining for both S-100 protein and cytokeratin should be done. Moreover, if coupled with staining for melanin or melanoma-associated antigen (HMB-45), the specificity of the method is improved. S-100 protein can also be identified within most of the traditional melanocytic tumors of soft tissue, including clear cell sarcoma of tendon and aponeurosis and melanocytic schwannoma, but interestingly it is lacking from the pigmented forms of dermatofibrosarcoma protuberans.[140]

S-100 protein is present within occasional nonneural tissues and tumors. It has been identified in normal adipocytes, lipomas, and occasional liposarcomas. However, the staining in liposarcomas is usually rather focal and weak. The antigen is identified within chondrocytes, chondromas, and a variable percentage of chondrosarcomas.[140] In our experience about 20% of synovial sarcomas may contain detectable amounts of the protein as well. The staining of normal skeletal muscle for this antigen is mirrored by the observation that immunoreactivity can also be detected in rhabdomyosarcomas, particularly in the most mature rhabdomyoblasts. Chordomas coexpress both cytokeratin and S-100 protein, a phenotype that allows for ready distinction from chondrosarcomas. Both normal Langerhans' cells and the cells of histiocytosis X strongly express the antigen, providing additional support of a common lineage. The presence of this antigen possibly may be of benefit in separating histiocytosis X from juvenile xanthogranuloma because the latter lacks the antigen.

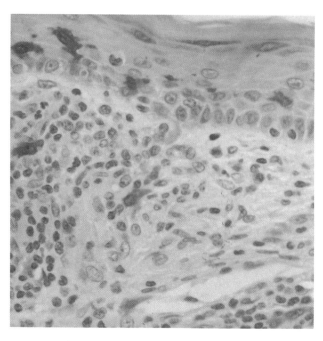

FIG. 8-17. Skin showing S-100 protein positive Langerhans' cells and macrophages in the dermis. The latter may infiltrate tumors and lead to the erroneous conclusion that the tumor expresses S-100 protein. (Anti-S-100 protein, × 250.)

Unlike many other antigens, valid staining for S-100 protein can be seen in the nucleus or cytoplasm, or both. The most significant source of error in interpreting S-100 staining results is mistaking the numerous macrophages which commonly infiltrate various tumors and which stain positively for S-100 protein as positively staining tumor cells. These cells must be carefully evaluated by the usual morphological criteria. They are typically small cells with a centrally placed rounded or folded nucleus and intensely staining multipolar or bipolar cytoplasmic processes (Fig. 8-15).

Neuron specific enolase

Enolase is an enzyme that converts 2-phosphoglycerate pyruvate to phosphoenolpyruvate in the glycolytic pathway. It exists as three distinct immunological subunits (alpha, beta, gamma), which can associate as three homodimers (alpha-alpha, beta-beta, and gamma-gamma) and at least one heterodimer (alpha-gamma). These isoenzymes differ in their distribution throughout the body. Beta-beta is found in skeletal muscle, alpha-alpha in glial cells of the brain, and gamma-gamma and gamma-alpha in neurons. Because the gamma subunit, referred to in the old literature as 14-3-2 protein, was present in such high concentrations in the brain relative to other tissues, it was termed neuron specific enolase, in contrast to the alpha subunit, known as nonneuronal enolase. The gamma subunit can be identified in neuronal and neuroendocrine cells, although the intensity of the immunoreactivity varies with the type of cell.

But many other cells also contain the gamma subunit, possibly in the form of the heterodimer.[106,125] It can also be identified within prostate tissue, loops of Henle, bronchial epithelium, plasma cells, and megakaryocytes.

Because of the wide distribution of this substance, it has limited use in the diagnosis of soft tissue tumors, particularly when polyclonal antibodies are used. With the use of monoclonal antibodies there appears to be better specificity[135,137] and less background staining but less sensitivity. Neuron specific enolase finds its greatest use in the identification of neuroblastic and neuroendocrine tumors. Thomas et al.,[137] utilizing a monoclonal antibody, noted staining of over half of neuroblastomas, paragangliomas, and various neuroendocrine tumors. About one third of malignant melanomas also produce the enzyme as well as 2% of nonneural tumors.

Neurofilament protein

Neurofilament protein, the intermediate filament characteristic of most, but probably not all, neuronal cells, is composed of three subunits: NF-H (200 kd), NF-M (160 kd), and NF-L (68 kd). Although most neuronal cells contain all three polypeptides, some appear to lack neurofilaments altogether or to contain only two of the three. Neurofilament protein has been identified within neuroblastoma, ganglioneuroma, and paraganglioma.[126,129] The amount and degree of staining appears to be roughly proportional to the amount of cytoplasm. Hence poorly differentiated neuroblastic cells are less apt to accept staining than ganglionic

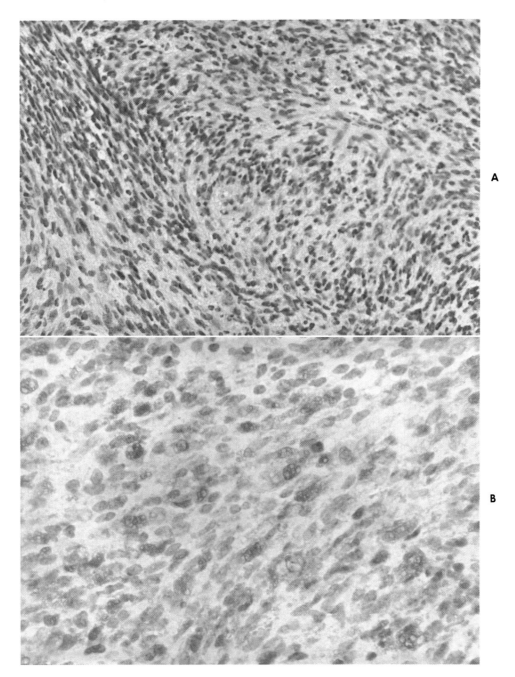

FIG. 8-18. Cellular schwannoma (**A**) showing vague palisading. Note that the majority of cells express S-100 protein. (**A,** × 160; **B,** Anti-S-100 protein × 250.)

cells.[126] Even so, great variability in the expression of neurofilament protein by neuroblastomas has been noted. This is probably due in part to differences in the type of antisera and fixation procedures. Mukai et al.[126] have shown that monospecific antibody to the 68-kd polypeptide is the most reliable antiserum for detection of neurofilament protein in neuroblastomas, and Osborn et al.[129] have shown rather conclusively that fixation and embedding substantially re-

duce antigenicity of neurofilament protein in neuroblastoma.

Glial fibrillary acidic protein

Glial fibrillary acidic protein is the intermediate filament characteristic of glial cells. Although it is a useful antigen in the diagnosis and distinction of glial versus nonglial tumors of the central nervous system, its use is restricted in

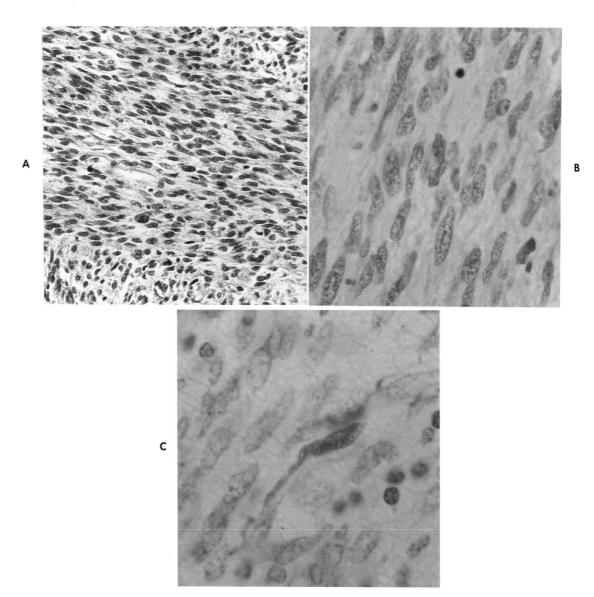

FIG. 8-19. Malignant peripheral nerve sheath tumor (**A**) composed of cells showing irregular or wavy nuclei (**B**). Note that in contrast to the cellular schwannoma, only an occasional cell is positive for S-100 protein (**C**). (**A**, × 60; **B**, × 400; **C**, Anti-S-100 protein, × 500.)

soft tissue. We use it primarily to distinguish glial hamartomas of soft tissue from nonglial lesions that may be confused with them, such as neurofibroma or extracranial meningioma, and to confirm the diagnosis of the rare cutaneous ependymoma. It should be pointed out that occasionally schwannomas will coexpress glial fibrillary acidic protein and S-100 protein,[121] and there has been a recent report of glial fibrillary acidic protein immunoreactivity in a melanotic schwannoma.[10]

Myelin basic protein

Myelin basic protein is a basic polypeptide that makes up about one third of the protein of the myelin sheath. It

can be identified in benign and malignant Schwann cell tumors and granular cell tumors.[13] It has been suggested that a practical use for this protein is the distinction of malignant schwannoma from malignant melanoma, since the latter does not produce this substance.[13] However, it is difficult to fully evaluate its use in view of the paucity of published reports.

Leu 7

Originally described as an antigenic marker for lymphocytes with natural killer activity, leu 7 (or a substance like it) can also be identified within benign and malignant nerve sheath tumors[132,142] as well as neuroendocrine tumors using the monoclonal antibody HNK-1. It is believed that this antibody detects an epitope that is associated with myelin proteins. This antigen is present in most schwannomas, and more than half of neurofibromas and malignant peripheral nerve sheath tumors. It does not act as a sole marker or have any advantage over S-100 protein in the diagnosis of malignant peripheral nerve sheath tumors but is best used in concert with it. Leu 7 immunoreactivity has been noted in a number of nonneural tumors including leiomyosarcomas, synovial sarcomas, and rhabdomyosarcomas.

Synaptophysin

Synaptophysin is a membrane protein found in the presynaptic vesicles of nerve cells. It can be identified within nerve cells of the peripheral and central nervous system as well as neuroendocrine cells. Consequently, it has proved to be a highly sensitive means of recognizing neuroendocrine tumors from a variety of sites.[117] Neuroblastic tumors (neuroblastoma, ganglioneuroblastoma, ganglioneuroma) and paragangliomas also contain this membrane protein.

Nerve growth factor receptor

Receptors to nerve growth factor can be identified in many benign and malignant nerve sheath tumors and neuroblastic tumors. Nerve growth factor receptor can be detected in nearly all granular cell tumors, neurofibromas, and schwannomas.[133] A somewhat lower percentage of malignant peripheral nerve sheath tumors, neuroblastomas, and paragangliomas express the receptor protein.[133] However, this protein may also be identifed in synovial sarcoma, hemangiopericytoma, smooth muscle tumors, and undifferentiated sarcoma.

HISTIOCYTIC ANTIGENS

The enzymes alpha-1-antitrypsin, alpha-1-antichymotrypsin, and muramidase (lysozyme) are the three most common substances utilized in the diagnosis of histiocytic and presumed histiocytic lesions. Alpha-1-antitrypsin is a glycoprotein (MW 57,000) synthesized chiefly by the liver and, to a lesser extent, by normal histiocytes and peripheral blood monocytes. It normally circulates with the alpha-1-globulin fraction of plasma, is increased during systemic infections, and possesses the ability to neutralize various proteolytic enzymes, including trypsin, chymotrypsin, elastase, and collagenase. It can also be detected in various body fluids, including mucus, saliva, and synovial fluid. The synthesis of alpha-1-antitrypsin is governed by a series of codominant alleles, M, S, and Z, where MM is the normal homozygous state and ZZ is the homozygous deficiency state associated with emphysema and cirrhosis in children. Alpha-1-antichymotrypsin is a proteolytic enzyme that neutralizes the effect of chymotrypsin. It can be localized to histiocytes, macrophages, and certain cells within the gastrointestinal tract. Muramidase

is a lysosomal enzyme present within various body secretions including tears, milk, and saliva.[148] It is also present within the serous cells of the bronchial and salivary glands, Paneth's cells, breast epithelium, and renal tubular cells. Like the other two enzymes, it is also present within histiocytes.

Several workers have endorsed the use of one or more of the above enzymes in the diagnosis of fibrohistiocytic tumors.[144,146,149] However, the actual percentage of fibrohistiocytic tumors that expresses one or more of these enzymes is highly variable. For example, du Boulay[144] found that all of 23 malignant fibrous histiocytomas contained Alph-1-antitrypsin, whereas Kindblom et al.[146] found that slightly over half of these tumors were positive. The presence of this enzyme in benign and intermediate fibrohistiocytic tumors is also variable with between one-quarter to three-quarters allegedly positive. Similar variability has been noted with Alpha-1-antichymotrypsin and muramidase is present in only a small percentage of malignant fibrous histiocytomas.[151,154]

In our opinion, these substances are not sufficiently specific to be used in the diagnosis of malignant fibrous histiocytoma, which remains principally a diagnosis based on hematoxylin-and eosin-stained material with judiciously chosen special stains to rule out other pleomorphic sarcomas or carcinomas. Both alpha-1-antitrypsin and alpha-1-antichymotrypsin can be identified in a variety of different sarcomas apart from malignant fibrous histiocytoma.[147,152] The observation that positive immunostaining often occurs in pleomorphic end-stage cells within malignant fibrous histiocytoma suggests that loss of structural integrity may allow passive influx of serum alpha-1-antitrypsin and alpha-1-antichymotrypsin, thereby accounting for positive immunoreactivity. This hypothesis is supported in our experience and that of others by the findings of alpha-1-antitrypsin positivity within pleomorphic cells in other types of sarcomas.[152] However, other investigators, who have been unable to demonstrate passive diffusion of other serum proteins into tumor cells, doubt this explanation.[147]

CD-68

CD-68 is a pan macrophage antigen, having a molecular mass of 110 kd, which may be a constituent of lysosomes. By means of the murine antibody KP1, derived following immunization with a lysosomal fraction of pulmonary macrophages,[150] the antigen can be localized within tissue macrophages in many body sites, in granulocytic precursors within bone marrow, and in neutrophil granulocytes weakly. Within neoplasms it is strongly expressed in some histiocytic, myeloid, and myelomonocytic malignant tumors and is also present as a minor dotlike immunoreactive substance in some lymphomas of B-cell lineage. However, we have noted this antigen occasionally within rare carcinomas and in granular cell tumors, which are characterized by a superabundance of large phagolysosomes.[153] Shortly after the commercial availability of this antibody it was quickly applied to a variety of fibrohistiocytic tumors to determine whether they exhibited histiocytic differentiation. It does not, for the most part, mark the tumor cells within malignant fibrous histiocytomas, although it does decorate multinucleated or osteoclast-like giant cells that may be encountered in malignant fibrous histiocytoma and plexiform fibrous histiocytoma. CD-68 is present within about half of angiomatoid fibrous histiocytomas, particularly those which display phagocytosis of hemosiderin.[153] Thus in the context of mesenchymal neoplasia the presence of this antigen may not necessarily imply true histiocytic differentiation so much as the acquisition of a phagocytic phenotype as reflected in the presence of lysosomes.

MISCELLANEOUS ANTIGENS
MIC2 gene product

The MIC2 gene, located on the short arm of the sex chromosome, encodes a surface protein (p30/32 ^{MIC2}), which was first described in T cell and null cell acute lymphoblastic leukemia using MoAb12E7. A more recent and popular monoclonal antibody (HBA-71),[157] identifying a different epitope of this protein, has shown that cells of Ewing's sarcoma and peripheral neuroectodermal tumors also express this protein in high amounts. Ambros et al.[155] detected the protein in 98% of Ewing's sarcomas and primitive neuroectodermal tumors as linear surface staining. Alveolar rhabdomyosarcomas, ependymomas, and islet cell tumors also express the protein, however. Provided one takes care in ruling out the diagnosis of rhabdomyosarcoma and leukemia by appropriate studies, this antigen has proven quite useful in the differential diagnosis of Ewing's sarcoma and peripheral neuroepithelioma.

Basement membrane antigens

Type IV collagen and laminin represent two of the principal components of basement membrane.[164] A variety of cells produce basement membrane, including epithelium, endothelium, Schwann cells, and smooth muscle cells. Not unexpectedly, laminin can be identified around cells within neurofibroma, neurilemoma, and leiomyoma.[165] It is more variable, however, in malignant schwannomas and leiomyosarcomas. Because of wide distribution of these substances in epithelial and mesenchymal lesions, there are relatively few situations in which localization of these antigens provides significant information. For example, the presence of type IV collagen and laminin would not necessarily discriminate carcinoma from many epithelioid sarcomas (e.g., epithelioid angiosarcoma, epithelioid malignant schwannoma).

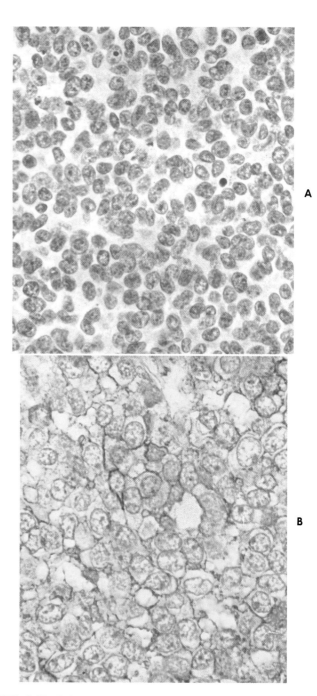

FIG. 8-20. Ewing's sarcoma (**A**) illustrating surface staining for the MIC-2 gene product p30/32. (**A**, × 250; **B**, anti-p30/32 ^{MIC2} × 400.)

Steroid receptor proteins

Although traditionally associated with hormonally sensitive tissues, steroid receptors can be identified in many types of tissues and tumors, including sarcomas. Their clinical significance in the latter tumors is not understood. The recent development of a specific monoclonal antibody to estrogen receptor protein allows the potential recognition and visualization of the protein within tissues. Our experience with this antibody indicates that low levels of the protein can be detected in soft tissue tumors of diverse types using an enzyme-linked immunosorbant assay.[167] Immunocytochemical localization of the protein has not been possible, probably because of the low levels of the protein. Nonetheless, the development of this antibody and the future development of monoclonal antibodies to the other steroid receptors offer the possibility of studying the issue further.

p53 gene product

The p53 gene is a tumor suppressor gene located on the short arm of chromosome 17 that encodes a nuclear phosphoprotein of 53 kD that binds DNA and negatively regulates cell division, preventing progression from G1 to S phase. Mutations of the p53 suppressor gene have been identified within a wide variety of tumors including carcinoma of the colon, esophagus, liver, breast, and lung. p53 mutations are also encountered in about 20% to 30% of soft tissue sarcomas of diverse type, notably leiomyosarcoma, malignant fibrous histiocytoma, liposarcoma, and synovial sarcoma.[156,158,160,166] There also appears to be a rough correlation between abnormalities of the p53 locus and increasing histological grade of soft tissue sarcomas.[159,160]

Missense mutations of the p53 locus increase the half-life of the protein product and allow it to be detected as nuclear immunoreactivity with appropriate antibodies. However, since there are a number of other types of mutations or mechanisms of p53 inactivation,[162] the incidence of missense mutations in sarcomas, as determined by immunohistochemical means, does not reflect the overall importance of this tumor suppressor locus in sarcomas. Moreover, there have been no studies that have determined whether p53 mutations in sarcomas are an independent prognostic indicator or whether they simply reflect other traditional parameters such as histological grade. The availability of antibodies directed against the gene product will undoubtedly give rise to a burgeoning literature in coming years attempting to define its role in tumor diagnosis and prognosis.

REFERENCES
General

1. Battifora H: Assessment of antigen damage in immunohistochemistry: the vimentin internal control. *Am J Clin Pathol* 96:669, 1991.
2. Battifora H: The multitumor (sausage) tissue block: novel method for immunohistochemical antibody testing. *Lab Invest* 55:244, 1986.
3. Battifora H: Recent progress in the immunohistochemistry of solid tumors. *Semin Diagn Pathol* 1:252, 1984.
4. Battifora H, Kopinski M: The influence of protease digestion and duration of fixation on immunostaining of keratins: a comparison of formalin and ethanol fixation. *J Histochem Cytochem* 34:1095, 1986.
5. DeLellis RA: *Diagnostic immunohistochemistry*. New York, 1981, Masson Publishing USA.
6. Erlandson RA: Diagnostic immunohistochemistry of human tumors: an interim evaluation. *Am J Surg Pathol* 8:615, 1984.
7. Hsu SM, Raine L, Fanger H: Use of avidin-biotin-peroxidase complex (ABC) in immunoperoxidase techniques: a comparison between ABC and unlabeled antibody (PAP) procedures. *J Histochem Cytochem* 29:577, 1981.
8. Kindblom LG: Histochemistry applied to pathologic diagnosis of soft tissue and bone tumors. In Spicer SS, editor: *Histochemistry in pathologic diagnosis*. New York, 1986, Marcel Dekker.
9. Larsson L-I: Tissue preparation methods for light microscopic immunohistochemistry. *Appl Immunohist* 1:2, 1993.
10. Miettinen M: Immunohistochemistry of soft-tissue tumors: possibilities and limitations in surgical pathology.
11. Momose H, Mehta P, Battifora H: Antigen retrieval by microwave irradiation in lead thiocyanate: comparison with protease digestion retrieval. *Appl Immunohist* 1:77, 1993.
12. Mukai K, Stollmeyer K, Rosai, J: Immunohistochemical localization of actin: applications in surgical pathology. *Am J Surg Pathol* 5:91, 1981.
13. Nadji M, Morales AR: *Immunoperoxidase techniques: a practical approach to tumor diagnosis*. Chicago, 1986, American Society of Clinical Pathologists Press.
14. Roholl PJM, De Jong ASH, Ramaekers FCS: Application of markers in the diagnosis of soft tissue tumours. *Histopathology* 9:1019, 1985.
15. Sheibani K, Tubbs RR: Enzyme immunohistochemistry: technical aspects. *Semin Diagn Pathol* 1:235, 1984.
16. Shi SR, Key ME, Kalra KL: Antigen retrieval in formalin-fixed paraffin-embedded tissues: an enhancement method for immunohistochemical staining based on microwave oven heating of tissue sections. *J Histochem Cytochem* 39:741, 1991.
17. Warnke RA, Gatter KC, Falini B, et al: Diagnosis of human lymphoma with monoclonal antileukocyte antibodies. *N Engl J Med* 309:1275, 1983.
18. Wick MR, Swanson PE, Manivel JC: Immunohistochemical analysis of soft tissue sarcomas: comparison with electron microscopy. *Appl Pathol* 6:169, 1988.

Intermediate filaments and vimentin

19. Azumi N, Battifora H: The distribution of vimentin and keratin in epithelial and nonepithelial neoplasms: a comprehensive immunohistochemical study on formalin and alcohol-fixed tumors. *Am J Clin Pathol* 88:286, 1987.
20. Ben-Ze'Ev A, Raz A: Relationship between the organization and synthesis of vimentin and the metastatic capability of B16 melanoma cells. *Cancer Res* 45:2632, 1985.
21. Connell ND, Rheinwald JG: Regulation of the cytoskeleton in mesothelial cells: reversible loss of keratin and increase in vimentin during rapid growth in culture. *Cell* 34:245, 1983.
22. Damjanov I: Antibodies to intermediate filaments and histogenesis. *Lab Invest* 47:215, 1982.
23. Denk H, Krepler R, Artliev U, et al: Proteins of intermediate filaments: an immunohistochemical and biochemical approach to the classification of soft tissue tumors. *Am J Pathol* 110:193, 1983.
24. Osborn M, Debusd E, Weber K: Monoclonal antibodies specific for vimentin. *Eur J Cell Biol* 34:137, 1984.
25. Osborn M, Weber K: Biology of disease: tumor diagnosis by inter-

mediate filament typing: a novel tool for surgical pathology. *Lab Invest* 48:372, 1983.

26. Ramaekers FCS, Haag D, Kant A, et al: Coexpression of keratin and vimentin-type intermediate filaments in human metastatic carcinoma cells. *Proc Natl Acad Sci USA* 80:2618, 1983.

27. Upton MP, Hirohashi S, Tome Y, et al: Expression of vimentin in surgically resected adenocarcinomas and large cell carcinomas of lung. *Am J Surg Pathol* 10:560, 1986.

28. Virtanen I, Lehto VP, Lehtonen E, et al: Expression of intermediate filaments in cultured cells. *J Cell Sci* 50:45, 1981.

Epithelial markers

29. Ariza A, Bilbao JM, Rosai J: Immunohistochemical detection of epithelial membrane antigen in normal perineurial cells and perinuerioma. *Am J Surg Pathol* 12:678, 1988.

30. Bolen JW, Hammar SP, McNutt MA: Reactive and neoplastic serosal tissue. *Am J Surg Pathol* 10:34, 1986.

31. Brown DC, Theaker JM, Banks PM, et al: Cytokeratin expression in smooth muscle and smooth muscle tumours. *Histopathology* 11:477, 1987.

32. Ceriani RL, Thomson K, Peterson JA, et al: Surface differentiation antigens of human mammary epithelial cells carried on the human milk fat globule. *Proc Natl Acad Sci USA* 74:582, 1977.

33. Chase DR, Enzinger FM, Weiss SW, et al: Keratin in epithelioid sarcoma: an immunohistochemical study. *Am J Surg Pathol* 8:435, 1984.

34. Cooper D, Schermer A, Sun TT: Classification of human epithelium and their neoplasms using monoclonal antibodies to keratins: strategies, applications, and limitations. *Lab Invest* 52:243, 1985.

35. Corson JM, Weiss LM, Banks-Schlegel SP, et al: Keratin proteins in synovial sarcoma. *Am J Surg Pathol* 7:107, 1983.

36. Delsol G, Stein H, Pulford KAF, et al: Human lymphoid cells express epithelial membrane antigen. *Lancet* 2:1124, 1984.

37. Erlandson RA: Proposed classification of pleural neoplasms. *Lab Invest* 54:19A, 1986.

38. Gould VE, Moll R, Berndt R, et al: Immunohistochemical analysis of Ewing's tumors. *Lab Invest* 56:28A, 1987.

39. Gown AM, Boyd HC, Chang Y, et al: Smooth muscle cells can express cytokeratins of "simple" epithelium: immunocytochemical and biochemical studies in vitro and in vivo. *Am J Pathol* 132:223, 1988.

40. Gown AM, Vogel AM: Monoclonal antibodies to human intermediate filament proteins. III. Analysis of tumors. *Am J Clin Pathol* 84:413, 1985.

41. Gray MH, Rosenberg AE, Dickersin GR, et al: Cytokeratin expression in epithelioid vascular neoplasms. *Hum Pathol* 21:212, 1990.

42. Gray MH, Rosenberg AE, Dickersin GR, et al: Glial fibrillary acidic protein and keratin expression by benign and malignant nerve sheath tumors. *Hum Pathol* 20:1089, 1989.

43. Heyderman E, Steele K, Ormerod MG: A new antigen on the epithelial membrane: its immunoperoxidase localization in normal and neoplastic tissue. *J Clin Pathol* 32:35, 1979.

44. Holden J, Churg A: Immunohistochemical staining for keratin and carcinoembryonic antigen in the diagnosis of malignant mesothelioma. *Am J Surg Pathol* 8:277, 1984.

45. Langloss JM, Kurman RJ, Bratthauer GL, et al: Expression of keratin by normal and neoplastic smooth muscle cells of the human uterus (in press).

46. Manivel JC, Wick MR, Swanson PE, et al: Epithelial membrane antigen in sarcomas. *Lab Invest* 56:46A, 1987.

47. Miettinen M: Immunoreactivity for cytokeratin and epithelial membrane antigen in leiomyosarcoma. *Arch Pathol Lab Med* 112:637, 1988.

48. Miettinen M: Keratin subtypes and desmosome plaque proteins in synovial sarcoma. *Lab Invest* 160:63A, 1989.

49. Miettinen M, Lehto VP, Badley RA, et al: Expression of intermediate filaments in soft tissue sarcomas. *Int J Cancer* 30:541, 1982.

50. Moll R, Cowin P, Kapprell H-P, et al: Desmosomal proteins: new markers for identification and classification of tumors. *Lab Invest* 54:4, 1986.

51. Norton AJ, Thomas JA, Isaacson PG: Cytokeratin-specific monoclonal antibodies are reactive with tumours of smooth muscle derivation: an immunocytochemical and biochemical study using antibodies to intermediate filament cytoskeletal proteins. *Histopathology* 11:487, 1987.

52. Perentes E, Nakagawa Y, Ross GW, et al: Expression of epithelial membrane antigen in perineurial cells and their derivatives: an immunohistochemical study with multiple markers. *Acta Neuropathol* 75:160, 1987.

53. Pinkus GS, Kurtin PJ: Epithelial membrane antigen: a diagnostic discriminant in surgical pathology. *Hum Pathol* 16:929, 1985.

54. Schlegel R, Banks-Schlegel S, McLeod JA, et al: Immunoperoxidase localization of keratin in human neoplasms. *Am J Pathol* 101:41, 1980.

55. Sheibani K, Battifora H, Burke JS: Antigenic phenotype of malignant mesothelioma. *Lab Invest* 54:57A, 1986.

56. Sloan JP, Ormerod MG: Distribution of epithelial membrane antigen in normal and neoplastic tissues and its value in diagnostic tumor pathology. *Cancer* 47:1786, 1981.

57. Spagnolo DV, Michie SA, Crabtree GS, et al: Monoclonal antikeratin (AE1) reactivity in routinely processed tissue from 166 human neoplasms. *Am J Clin Pathol* 84:697, 1985.

58. Swanson PE, Heffalumps, jaguars, and cheshire cats: a commentary on cytokeratins and soft tissue sarcomas. *Am J Clin Pathol* 95(suppl)PS2-7, 1991.

59. Szpak GA, Johnston WW, Roggli V, et al: The diagnostic distinction between malignant mesothelioma of the pleura and adenocarcinoma of the lung as defined by a monoclonal antibody (B72.3). *Am J Pathol* 122:252, 1986.

60. Theaker JM, Gillett MB, Fleming KA, et al: Epithelial membrane antigen expression by meningiomas and the perineurium of the peripheral nerve. *Arch Pathol Lab Med* 111:409, 1987.

61. Thomas P, Battifora H: Keratins versus epithelial membrane antigen: an immunohistochemical comparison of five monoclonal antibodies. *Hum Pathol* (in press).

Muscle antigens

62. Altmannsberger M, Osborne M, Treuner J, et al: Diagnosis of human childhood rhabdomyosarcoma by antibodies to desmin: the structural protein of muscle-specific intermediate filaments. *Virchows Arch (Cell Pathol)* 39:203, 1982.

63. Altmannsberger M, Weber K, Droste R, et al: Desmin is a specific marker for rhabdomyosarcomas of human and rat origin. *Am J Pathol* 118:85, 1985.

64. Bennett GS, Fellini SA, Toyama Y, et al: Redistribution of intermediate filament subunits during skeletal myogenesis and maturation in vitro. *J Cell Biol* 82:577, 1979.

65. Brooks JJ: Immunohistochemistry of soft tissue tumors: myoglobin as a tumor marker for rhabdomyosarcoma. *Cancer* 50:1757, 1982.

66. Cavazzana AO, Schmidt D, Ninfo V, et al: Spindle cell rhabdomyosarcoma: a prognostically favorable variant of rhabdomyosarcoma. *Am J Surg Pathol* 16:229, 1992.

67. Corson JM, Pinkus GS: Intracellular myoglobin: a specific marker for skeletal muscle differentiation in soft tissue sarcomas: an immunoperoxidase study. *Am J Pathol* 103:384, 1981.

68. DeJong ASH, van Unnik M, Albus, et al: Myosin and myoglobin as tumor markers in the diagnosis of rhabdomyosarcoma: a comparative study. *Am J Surg Pathol* 8:521, 1984.

69. Eusebi V, Bondi A, Rosai J: Immunohistochemical localization of myoglobin in nonmuscular cells. *Am J Surg Pathol* 8:51, 1984.

70. Eusebi V, Rilke F, Ceccarelli C, et al: Fetal heavy chain skeletal myosin: an oncofetal antigen expressed by rhabdomyosarcoma. *Am J Surg Pathol* 10:680, 1986.

71. Kahn HJ, Yeger H, Kassim O, et al: Immunohistochemical and electron microscopic assessment of childhood rhabdomyosarcoma: increased frequency of diagnosis over routine histologic methods. *Cancer* 51:1897, 1983.

72. Kindblom LG, Seidal T, Karlsson K: Immunohistochemical localization of myoglobin in human muscle tissue and embryonal and alveolar rhabdomyosarcoma. *Acta Pathol Microbiol Immunol Scand* 90:167A, 1982.

73. Manivel JC, Wick MR, Dehner LP, et al: Epithelioid sarcoma: an immunohistochemical study. *Am J Clin Pathol* 87:319, 1987.

74. Miettinen M, Lehto VP, Badley R, et al: Alveolar rhabdomyosarcoma: demonstration of the muscle type of intermediate filament protein, desmin as a diagnostic aid. *Am J Pathol* 108:426, 1982.

75. Mukai K, Rosai J, Hallaway BE: Localization of myoglobin in normal and neoplastic human skeletal muscle cells using an immunoperoxidase method. *Am J Surg Pathol* 3:373, 1979.

76. Mukai M, Iri H, Torikata C, et al: Immunoperoxidase demonstration of a new muscle protein (Z-protein) in myogenic tumors as a diagnostic aid. *Am J Pathol* 114:164, 1984.

77. Osborn M, Caselitz J, Weber K: Heterogeneity of intermediate filament expression in vascular smooth muscle: a gradient in desmin positive cells from the rat aortic arch to the level of the arteria iliaca communia. *Differentiation* 20:196, 1981.

78. Osborn M, Hill C, Altmannsberger M, et al: Monoclonal antibodies to titin in conjunction with antibodies to desmin separate rhabdomyosarcomas from other tumor types. *Lab Invest* 55:101, 1986.

79. Parham DM, Webber B, Holt H, et al: Immunohistochemical study of childhood rhabdomyosarcomas and related neoplasms: results of an Intergroup Rhabdomyosarcoma study project. *Cancer* 67:3072, 1991.

80. Rangdaeng S, Truong LD: Comparative immunohistochemical staining for desmin and muscle specific actin: a study of 576 cases. *Am J Clin Pathol* 96:32, 1991.

81. Roholl PJ, Elbers HRJ, Prinsen et al: Distribution of actin isoforms in sarcomas: an immunohistochemical study. *Hum Pathol* 21:1269, 1990.

82. Schmidt R, Cone R, Haas J, et al: Diagnosis of rhabdomyosarcomas using HHF35, an anti–muscle actin monoclonal antibody. *Lab Invest* 56:70A, 1987.

83. Skalli O, Schuerch W, Seemayer T, et al: Myofibroblasts from diverse pathologic settings are heterogeneous in their content of actin isoforms and intermediate filament proteins. *Lab Invest* 60:275, 1989.

84. Tokuyasu K, Dutton A, Singer S: Immunoelectron microscopic studies of desmin (skeletin) localization and intermediate filament organization in chicken skeletal muscle. *J Cell Biol* 96:1727, 1983.

85. Truong LD, Rangdaeng S, Cagle P, et al: The diagnostic utility of desmin: a study of 584 cases and review of the literature. *Am J Clin Pathol* 93:305, 1990.

86. Tsokos M, Howard R, Costa J: Immunohistochemical study of alveolar and embryonal rhabdomyosarcoma. *Lab Invest* 48:148, 1983.

87. Tsukada T, Tippens D, Mar H, et al: HHF 35, a muscle-actin-specific monoclonal antibody: I. Immunocytochemical and biochemical characterization. *Am J Pathol* 126:51, 1987.

88. Wick MR, Swanson PE, Scheithauer BW, et al: Malignant peripheral nerve sheath tumor: an immunohistochemical study of 62 cases. *Am J Clin Pathol* 87:425, 1987.

Vascular antigens

89. Aziza J, Mazerolles C, Selves J, et al: Comparison of the reactivities of monoclonal antibodies QBEND10 (CD34) and BNH9 in vascular tumors. *Appl Immunohistochem* 1:51, 1993.

90. Capo V, Ozzello L, Fenoglio CM, et al: Angiosarcomas arising in edematous extremities: immunostaining for factor VIII-related antigen and ultrastructural features. *Hum Pathol* 16:144, 1985.

91. De Young BR, Wick MR, Fitzgibbon JF, et al: CD 31: an immunospecific marker for endothelial differentiation in human neoplasms. *Appl Immunohistochem* 1:97, 1993.

92. Guarda LA, Ordonez NG, Smith L, et al: Immunoperoxidase localization of factor VIII in angiosarcoma. *Arch Pathol Lab Med* 106:515, 1982.

93. Holthoefer H, Virtanen I, Kariniemi AL, et al: *Ulex europaeus* I lectin as a marker for vascular endothelium in human tissues. *Lab Invest* 47:60, 1982.

94. Hoyer LW: The factor VIII complex: structure and function. *Blood* 58:1, 1981.

95. Jones RR, Spaull J, Spry C, et al: Histogenesis of Kaposi's sarcoma in patients with and without acquired immune deficiency syndrome (AIDS). *J Clin Pathol* 39:742, 1986.

96. Knowles DM, Tolidjiian B, Barboe C, et al: Monoclonal antihuman monocyte antibodies OKMI and OKMS possess distinctive tissue distribution including differential reactivity with vascular endothelium. *J Immunol* 132:2170, 1984.

97. McComb RD: Heterogenous expression of factor VIII/vWF by cardiac myxoma cells. *Am J Surg Pathol* 8:539, 1984.

98. Miettinen M, Holthofer H, Lehto VP, et al: Lectin as a marker for tumors derived from endothelial cells. *Am J Clin Pathol* 79:32, 1983.

99. Miettinen M, Lehto VP, Virtanen I: Postmastectomy angiosarcoma (Stewart-Treves) syndrome. *Am J Surg Pathol* 7:329, 1983.

100. Miettinen M, Lindenmayer AE, Chaubal A: Endothelial cell markers CD31, CD34, and BNH9 antibody to H- and Y-antigens: evaluation of their specificity and sensitivity in the diagnosis of vascular tumors and comparison with von Willebrand factor. *Mod Pathol* 7:82, 1994.

101. Millard PR, Yeryet AR: An immunohistochemical study of factor VIII–related antigen and Kaposi's sarcoma using polyclonal and monoclonal antibodies. *J Pathol* 146:31, 1985.

102. Morales AR, Fine G, Castro A, et al: Cardiac myxoma (endocardioma): an immunocytochemical assessment of histogenesis. *Hum Pathol* 12:896, 1981.

103. Mukai K, Rosai J, Burgdorf W: Localization of factor VIII related antigen in vascular endothelial cells using an immunoperoxidase method. *Am J Surg Pathol* 4:273, 1980.

104. Nadji M, Morales AR, Ziegel-Weissman J, et al: Kaposi's sarcoma: immunohistologic evidence for an endothelial origin. *Arch Pathol Lab Med* 105:274, 1987.

105. Nickoloff BJ: The human progenitor cell antigen (CD-34) is localized on endothelial cells, dermal dendritic cells, and perifollicular cells in formalin-fixed normal skin, and on proliferating endothelial cells and stromal spindle-shaped cells in Kaposi's sarcoma. *Arch Dermatol* 127:523, 1991.

106. Ordonez NG, Batsakis JG: Comparison of *Ulex europaeus* I lectin and factor VIII–related antigen in vascular lesions. *Arch Pathol Lab Med* 108:129, 1984.

107. Ramani P, Bradley NJ, Fletcher CDM: QBEND/10, a new monoclonal antibody to endothelium: assessment of its diagnostic utility in paraffin sections. *Histopathology* 17:237, 1990.

108. Schested M, Hou-Jensen K: Factor VIII–related antigen as an endothelial cell marker in benign and malignant diseases. *Virchows Arch (Pathol Anat)* 391:217, 1981.

109. Schlingemann RO, Dingjan GM, Emeis JJ, et al: Monoclonal antibody Pal-E specific for endothelium. *Lab Invest* 52:71, 1985.

110. Sirgi KE, Wick MR, Swanson PE: B72.3 and CD 34 immunoreactivity in malignant epithelioid soft tissue tumors: adjuncts in the recognition of endothelial neoplasms. *Am J Surg Pathol* 17:179, 1993.

111. Stephenson TJ, Mills PM: Monoclonal antibodies to blood group isoantigens: an alternative marker to factor VIII–related antigen for

benign and malignant vascular endothelial cells. *J Pathol* 147:139, 1985.

112. Traweek ST, Kandalaft PL, Mehta P, et al: The human hematopoietic progenitor cells antigen (CD-34) in vascular neoplasia. *Am J Clin Pathol* 96:25, 1991.

113. Wick MR, Manivel JC: Expression of *Ulex europaeus* I lectin binding and blood group isoantigens by epithelioid sarcomas: a diagnostic trap. *Lab Invest* 54:69A, 1986.

114. Yonezawa S, Maruyama I, Sakae K, et al: Thrombomodulin as a marker of vascular tumors: comparative study with factor VIII and *Ulex europaeus* I lectin. *Am J Clin Pathol* 88:405, 1987.

Neural and neuroectodermal antigens

115. Chesa PG, Melamed MR, Old LJ, et al: Expression of nerve growth factor receptor (NGF-R) and surface differentiation antigens in human sarcomas. *Lab* 58:33A, 1988.

116. Dahl D: The vimentin-GFA protein transition in rat neuroglia cytokeleton occurs at the time of myelination. *J Neurosci Res* 6:741, 1981.

117. Gould VE, Wiedenmann B, Lee I, et al: Synaptophysin expression in neuroendocrine neoplasms as determined by immunocytochemistry. *Am J Pathol* 126:243, 1987.

118. Gown AM, Thompson SJ, Bothwell M: Monoclonal antibody to nerve growth factor receptor: a new marker for nerve sheath tumors. *Lab Invest* 58:35A, 1988.

119. Haimoto H, Takahashi Y, Koshikawa T, et al: Immunohistochemical localization of gamma-enolase in normal human tissues other than nervous and neuroendocrine tissues. *Lab Invest* 52:257, 1985.

120. Kahn HJ, Marks A, Thom H, et al: Role of antibody to S-100 protein in diagnostic pathology. *Am J Clin Pathol* 79:341, 1983.

121. Kawahara E, Oda Y, Ooi A, et al: Expression of glial fibrillary acidic protein (GFAP) in peripheral nerve sheath tumors: a comparative study of immunoreactivity of GFAP, vimentin, S-100 protein, and neurofilament in 38 schwannomas and 18 neurofibromas. *Am J Surg Pathol* 12:115, 1988.

122. Michels S, Swanson PE, Robb JA, et al: Leu 7 in small cell neoplasms: an immunohistochemical study with ultrastructural correlations. *Cancer* 60:2958, 1987.

123. Miettinen M: Synaptophysin and neurofilament proteins as markers for neuroendocrine tumors. *Arch Pathol Lab Med* 111:813, 1987.

124. Moss TJ, Seeger RC, Kindler-Rohrborn, et al: Immunohistochemical detection and phenotyping of neuroblastoma cells in bone marrow using cytoplasm neuron specific enolase and cell surface antigens. *Adv Neuroblastoma Res*, Alan R. Liss. 1985.

125. Mukai M: Immunohistochemical localization of S-100 protein and peripheral nerve myelin proteins (P2 protein, PO protein) in granular cell tumors. *Am J Pathol* 112:139, 1983.

126. Mukai M, Torikata C, Iri H, et al: Expression of neurofilament triplet proteins in human neural tumors. *Am J Pathol* 122:28, 1986.

127. Nakajima T, Watanabe S, Sato Y, et al: Immunohistochemical demonstration of S-100 protein in malignant melanoma and pigmented nevus and its diagnostic application. *Cancer* 50:912, 1982.

128. Nakajima T, Watanabe S, Sato Y, et al: An immunoperoxidase study of S-100 protein distribution in normal and neoplastic tissues. *Am J Surg Pathol* 6:715, 1982.

129. Osborn M, Dirk T, Kaeser H, et al: Immunohistochemical localization of neurofilaments and neuron-specific enolase in 29 cases of neuroblastoma. *Am J Pathol* 122:433, 1986.

130. Pahlman S, Esscher T, Nilsson K: Expression of gamma-subunit of enolase, neuron specific enolase, in human nonneuroendocrine tumors and derived cell lines. *Lab Invest* 54:554, 1986.

131. Perentes E, Rubinstein LJ: Immunohistochemical recognition of human nerve sheath tumors by anti-leu7 (HNK-1) monoclonal antibody. *Acta Neuropathol* 68:319, 1985.

132. Perentes E, Rubinstein LJ: Recent applications of immunoperoxidase histochemistry in human neuro-oncology. *Arch Pathol Lab Med* 111:796, 1987.

133. Perosio PM, Brooks JJ: Expression of nerve growth factor receptor in paraffin-embedded soft tissue tumors. *Am J Pathol* 132:152, 1988.

134. Schmechel DE: Gamma-subunit of the glycolytic enzyme enolase: nonspecific or neuron specific? *Lab Invest* 52:239, 1985.

135. Seshi B, True L, Carter D, et al: Immunohistochemical characterization of a set of monclonal antibodies to human neuron-specific enolase. *Am J Pathol* 131:258, 1988.

136. Swanson PE, Manivel JC, Wick MR: Immunoreactivity for leu 7 in neurofibrosarcoma and other spindle cell sarcomas of soft tissue. *Am J Pathol* 126:546, 1987.

137. Thomas P, Battifora H, Manderino GL, et al: A monoclonal antibody against neuron-specific enolase: immunohistochemical comparison with a polyclonal antiserum. *Am J Clin Pathol* 88:146, 1987.

138. Tsokos M, Linnoila RI, Chandra RS, et al: Neuron-specific enolase in the diagnosis of neuroblastoma and other small round cell tumors in children. *Hum Pathol* 15:575, 1984.

139. Vanstapel MJ, Gatter KC, de Wolf-Peeters C, et al: New sites of human S-100 immunoreactivity detected with monoclonal antibodies. *Am J Clin Pathol* 85:160, 1986.

140. Weiss SW, Langloss JM, Enzinger FM: Value of S-100 protein in the diagnosis of soft tissue tumors with particular reference to benign and malignant Schwann cell tumors. *Lab Invest* 49:299, 1983.

141. Weiss SW, Nickoloff BJ: CD-34 is expressed by a distinctive cell population in peripheral nerve, nerve sheath tumors, and related lesions. *Am J Surg Pathol* 17:1039, 1993.

142. Wick MR, Swanson PE, Scheithauer BW, et al: Malignant peripheral nerve sheath tumor: an immunohistochemical study of 62 cases. *Am J Clin Pathol* 87:425, 1987.

Histiocytic antigens

143. Brecher ME, Franklin WA: Absence of mononuclear phagocyte antigens in malignant fibrous histiocytoma. *Am J Clin Pathol* 86:344, 1986.

144. du Boulay CEH: Demonstration of alpha-1-antitrypsin and alpha-1-antichymotrysin in fibrous histiocytomas using the immunoperoxidase technique. *Am J Surg Pathol* 6:559, 1982.

145. Isaacson P, Jones DB, Judd MA: Alpha-1-antitrypsin in human macrophages. *Lancet* 2:964, 1979.

146. Kindblom LG, Jacobsen GK, Jacobsen M: Immunohistochemical investigations of tumors of supposed fibroblastic-histiocytic origin. *Hum Pathol* 13:834, 1982.

147. Leader M, Patel J, Collins M, et al: Anti-alpha-1-antichymotrypsin staining of 194 sarcomas, 38 carcinomas, and 17 malignant melanoma: its lack of specificity as a tumour marker. *Am J Surg Pathol* 11:133, 1987.

148. Mason DY, Taylor CR: The distribution of muramidase (lysozyme) in human tissues. *J Clin Pathol* 28:124, 1978.

149. Meister P, Nathrath W: Immunohistochemical characterization of histiocytic tumors. *Diagn Histopathol* 4:79, 1981.

150. Pulford KAF, Rigney EM, Micklem KJ, et al: KP1: a new monoclonal antibody that detects a monocyte/macrophage associated antigen in routinely processed tissue sections. *J Clin Pathol* 42:414, 1989.

151. Roholl PJ, Kleyne, Elbers J, et al: Characterization of tumor cells in malignant fibrous histiocytomas and other soft tissue tumours in comparison with malignant histiocytes. I. Immunohistochemical study on paraffin sections. *J Pathol* 147:87, 1985.

152. Roholl PJM, Kleyne, Van Unnik JAM: Characterization of tumor cells in malignant fibrous histiocytomas and other soft tissue tumors, in comparison with malignant histiocytes. II. Immunoperoxidase study on cryostat sections. *Am J Pathol* 121:269, 1985.

153. Smith MEF, Costa MJ, Weiss SW: Evaluation of CD68 and other histiocytic antigens in angiomatoid malignant fibrous histiocytoma. *Am J Surg Pathol* 15:757, 1991.

154. Wood GS, Beckstead JH, Turner RR, et al: Malignant fibrous histiocytoma tumor cells resemble fibroblasts. *Am J Surg Pathol* 10:323, 1986.

Miscellaneous antigens

155. Ambros IM, Ambros PF, Strehl S, et al: MIC2 is a specific marker for Ewing's sarcoma and peripheral primitive neuroectodermal tumors: evidence for a common histogenesis of Ewing's sarcoma and peripheral primitive neuroectodermal tumors from MIC2 expression and specific chromosome aberration. *Cancer* 667:1886, 1991.

156. Andreassen S, Oyjord T, Hovig E, et al: p53 abnormalities in different subtypes of human sarcomas. *Cancer Res* 53:468, 1993.

157. Chaudhuri PK, Walker MJ, Beattie CW, et al: Distribution of steroid hormone receptors in human soft tissue sarcomas. *Surgery* 90:149, 1981.

158. Dei Tos AP, Doglioni C, Laurino L, et al: p53 protein expression in nonneoplastic and benign and malignant neoplasms of soft tissue. *Histopathology* 22:45, 1993.

159. Drobnjak M, Latres E, Pollack D, et al: Prognostic implications of p53 nuclear overexpression and high proliferation index of Ki67 in adult soft tissue sarcomas. *J Natl Cancer Inst* 86:549, 1994.

160. Goldblum JR, Frank TS, Poy ES, et al: p53 mutations and histologic progression in well-differentiated liposarcoma and dermatofibrosarcoma protuberans. Submitted to *Am J Surg Pathol*.

161. Hamilton G, Fellinger EJ, Schratter I, et al: Characterization of human endocrine tissue and tumor associated Ewing's sarcoma antigen. *Cancer Res* 48:6127, 1988.

162. Leach FS, Tokino T, Meltzer P, et al: p53 mutations and MDM2 amplification in human soft tissue sarcomas. *Cancer Res* 53:(10 suppl)2231, 1993.

163. Levy R, Dilley J, Fox RI, et al: A human thymus leukemia antigen defined by hybridoma monoclonal antibodies. *Proc Natl Acad Sci USA* 76:6552, 1979.

164. Martinez-Hernandez A, Amenta PS: The basement membrane in pathology. *Lab Invest* 48:656, 1983.

165. Miettinen M, Foidart JM, Ekblom P: Immunohistochemical demonstration of laminin, the major glycoprotein of basement membranes, as an aid in the diagnosis of soft tissue tumors. *Am J Clin Pathol* 79:306, 1983.

166. Soini Y, Vahakangas K, Nuorva K, et al: p53 immunohistochemistry in malignant fibrous histiocytoma and other mesenchymal tumors. *J Pathol* 168:29, 1992.

167. Weiss SW, Langloss JM, Shmookler BS, et al: Estrogen receptor protein in bone and soft tissue tumors. *Lab Invest* 54:689, 1986.

CHAPTER 9

BENIGN FIBROUS TISSUE TUMORS

FIBROUS CONNECTIVE TISSUE: STRUCTURE AND FUNCTION

Fibrous connective tissue consists principally of fibroblasts and an extracellular matrix containing both fibrillary structures (collagen, elastin) and nonfibrillary, gel-like extracellular matrix, or ground substance. Fibrous connective tissue may be characterized as loose or dense, depending upon the relative abundance of its fibrillary and nonfibrillary components. Dense fibrous connective tissue is mainly the tissue arranged in parallel bundles or sheets found in tendons, aponeuroses, and ligaments.

Fibroblasts vary in configuration. Most commonly they are spindle shaped, especially when stretched along bundles of collagen fibers, and have rather pale-staining, smoothly contoured, oval nuclei with small amounts of chromatin, one or two minute nucleoli, and, depending upon their state of activity, eosinophilic to weakly basophilic cytoplasm. The cytoplasmic borders are usually rather indistinct because the long, slender processes are difficult to discern with conventional stains and are visualized only with special stains such as iron hematoxylin or with the electron microscope. Fibroblasts, in loosely arranged, richly myxoid connective tissue, tend to assume a more stellate shape, with multiple slender cytoplasmic extensions that are discernible even in hematoxylin-eosin preparations. Fibroblasts are responsible for the intracellular assembly of various extracellular fibrillary and amorphous products such as procollagen, protoelastin, and glycosaminoglycans. The term *fibrocytes* is used for more quiescent cells that show the basic features of fibroblasts but have smaller nuclei and scantier amounts of cytoplasm. Functionally, they are less active than fibroblasts and are mainly engaged in the maintenance of the extracellular matrix.

Myofibroblasts are modified fibroblasts that show features common to both fibroblasts and smooth muscle cells. Their existence was first reported by Gabbiani et al. (1971)[4] in granulation tissue of healing wounds. Myofibroblasts also occur in a variety of reparative and proliferative fibrous lesions, such as nodular fasciitis and fibromatosis, and in numerous benign and malignant fibrous tumors, including fibrosarcoma and malignant fibrous histiocytoma. In view of the presence of myofibroblasts in most reactive and neoplastic fibrous lesions, the term *myofibroblastoma* is of little significance and should be used sparingly in describing and classifying fibrous tumors.

Fibroblasts and myofibroblasts produce procollagen and collagen (types I and III) and immunohistochemically stain for vimentin and actin, but actin is much more prominent in myofibroblasts. Desmin is expressed less commonly but has been reported in cells of plantar and extraabdominal fibromatosis (desmoid tumor).[5] The exact nature and function of myofibroblasts are still unknown. They probably play a role in cellular motility and in the contraction of fibrous tissue in healing wounds.[1,6-10]

Ultrastructurally, fibroblasts and myofibroblasts are marked by chromatin-poor, round or oval nuclei, and distinct profiles of well-developed rough endoplasmic reticulum, often with distended cisternae. Both tend to have a large Golgi complex that is associated with small vesicles filled with granular or flocculent material. There are also a few long, slender mitochondria, mainly in a perinuclear location, many free ribosomes, occasional fat droplets, and slender microfilaments. Golgi complex and dilated granular endoplasmic reticulum are much more prominent in those fibroblastic cells that are actively engaged in collagen formation. There are pinocytotic vesicles but no external lamina. Myofibroblasts, in addition, are characterized by indented nuclei and parallel arrays of microfilaments running along the axis of the cells, mostly beneath the cell membrane, dense bodies, and occasional intercellular junctions. They may also show basal lamina-like material and plasmalemmal attachment plaques.*

Collagen is the main product of fibroblasts and the main component of the extracellular matrix. It forms a heterogeneous group of closely related, noncontractile, fibrillary (banded) and nonfibrillary structures (glycoproteins) that vary in function and distribution. It has a high content of proline and hydroxyproline, is partly digested by pepsin and

---

*References 1, 2, 5, 6, 8, 10.

trypsin, and on boiling in water or acid solutions forms gelatin. Collagen fibers are acidophilic and birefringent, and stain a deep blue with Masson trichrome stain; occasionally, older fibers may also show some fuchsinophilia with this stain. Collagen is synthesized within the granular endoplasmic reticulum as procollagen from proline, lysine, and other amino acids. It is segregated in the Golgi complex, packed into secretory vesicles, and released at the cell surface where the collagen monomers are enzymatically cleaved and assembled to tropocollagen and collagen fibers. The precise lateral alignment and overlapping of the collagen molecules cause a distinct banding effect with a 64-nm periodicity that identifies collagen fibers under the electron microscope. Cross linking of the fibrils strengthens the fibers and makes them insoluble. Long-spacing collagen with 240-nm periodicity is occasionally encountered in normal and neoplastic tissues. Type IV collagen, the collagen of basal lamina, does not form banded fibers and does not undergo any further changes after secretion from the cell.

Several types of fibrillary or interstitial collagen are distinguished: *Type I collagen* is most ubiquitous, occurring not only in fibrous connective tissue but also in tendons, ligaments, bones, corneal tissue, and dentin. It is strongly birefringent and consists of two alpha-1 chains and one alpha-2 chain entwined in a helical configuration. *Type II collagen* is characteristic of cartilaginous tissue but is also found in the notochord, the nucleus pulposus, and the embryonic cornea. *Type III collagen* is usually associated with type I, and mainly occurs in the dermis, the blood vessels, and the intestinal tract. Among the nonfibrillary types, *type IV collagen* is the major component of the basal lamina. *Type V collagen* is primarily found in blood vessels and smooth muscle tissue. Other types of collagen *(types VII, VIII, and IX collagen)* are less common and less well defined. Reticular fibers form a delicate network of fibers that have the same cross banding as collagen (67 nm) but differ from collagen fibers by their small size (approximately 50 nm in diameter) and their argyrophilia. They are composed mainly of type III collagen.[2,7] "Amianthoid" fibers are fused, abnormally thick collagen fibers having a typical periodicity but measuring up to 1000 nm in diameter.

Elastic fibers are usually closely associated with collagen fibers and are important components of the dermis, large vessels, and internal organs such as the heart and the lung. They are slender branching, refractile, weakly birefringent fibers that form a characteristic wavy pattern. They stain with aldehyde-fuchsin, Weigert's resorcin-fuchsin, and Verhoeff's stains; ultrastructurally, they show no cross striations or banding. *Elastin,* the main component of elastic fibers, is synthesized and secreted as tropoelastin by fibroblasts and typically contains high amounts of glycine, alanine, valine, and desmosine, but little hydroxyproline. It is resistant to trypsin digestion but is hydrolyzed by elastase. In addition there is a microfibrillary component consisting of 10- to 12-nm fibrils that is found chiefly at the periphery of the elastic fibers. *Fibronectin* is a structural glycoprotein of high molecular weight that is synthesized by fibroblasts and a variety of other cells. It affects intercellular cohesion and cell shape and interacts as "molecular glue" between cells and the extracellular matrix.

Glycosaminoglycans (mucopolysaccharides) form the ground substance of connective tissue. They are intimately associated with fibroblasts and collagen fibers, play an important role in salt and water distribution, and serve as a link in various cellular interactions. They have a high molecular weight, are negatively charged, and are capable of binding large amounts of fluid. Glycosaminoglycans do not stain with hematoxylin-eosin preparations, but stain well with alcian blue, colloidal iron, and toluidine blue. Hyaluronic acid is depolymerized and decolorized by hyaluronidase. Antibodies specific for proteoglycans, which may be suitable for the differential diagnosis of myxoid tumors, have been developed.[3]

Glycosaminoglycans are synthesized within fibroblasts or chondroblasts, where they are polymerized and sulfated within the Golgi complex. Chemically, they are linear polysaccharide chains of hexosamines (glycosamino-) and various sugars (-glycans) that are (with the exception of hyaluronic acid) bound to proteins. The most important types are *hyaluronic acid,* a nonsulfate disaccharide chain composed of glucosamine and glucuronic acid; *chondroitin 4- and 6- sulfates,* combining galactosamine and glucuronic acid; *dermatan sulfate;* and *heparan sulfate.* Hyaluronic acid is abundant in fibrous connective tissue and is the major component of synovial fluid. Chondroitin sulfate predominates in hyaline and elastic cartilage, nucleus pulposus, and intervertebral disks; dermatan sulfate in dermis, tendons, and ligaments; and heparan sulfate in various structures rich in reticular fibers.[11,12]

BENIGN FIBROUS PROLIFERATIONS

Fibrous tumors and tumorlike lesions form a large and diverse group of distinct entities that differ greatly in their behavior. Some are perfectly benign lesions that remain localized and do not recur even after simple excision. Others are poorly circumscribed, grow in an infiltrative manner, and tend to recur, unless they are widely excised. Still others are frankly malignant tumors that recur and metastasize in a high percentage of cases. On these grounds and on the basis of age incidence, four separate categories of fibrous proliferations are distinguished: (1) *benign fibrous proliferations*, (2) *fibromatoses*, (3) *fibrosarcomas,* and (4) *fibrous proliferations of infancy and childhood.* The fourth category is included as a separate category because most fibrous lesions occurring during the first years of life have a characteristic structure and differ in their histological picture and behavior from those found in older children and adults.

The *benign fibroblastic proliferations* constitute a heterogenous group of relatively well defined entities that are for the most part reactive rather than neoplastic in origin. Some of these entities, such as nodular fasciitis, proliferative fasciitis, and proliferative myositis, grow rapidly and may reach their final size within 1 or 2 weeks. They are richly cellular and, not surprisingly, are often mistaken for sarcomas. Yet they rarely recur, never develop metastases, and are readily cured by local excision.

Other entities that have been included in this group differ by their slow, insidious growth and larger size. As a rule they are much less cellular and contain considerable amounts of collagen. Their incidence varies; fibroma of tendon sheath, for example, is a comparatively common tumor but is still poorly recognized. Elastofibroma and nasopharyngeal angiofibroma, on the other hand, are well-recognized, clearly defined entities, although they occur much less frequently than fibroma of tendon sheath. There are still other, less well defined fibroma-like lesions in the soft tissues, but these are rare and most likely constitute the richly collagenous end-stage of a reparative fibroblastic proliferation. Nonetheless, the term *fibroma* is often loosely applied to these lesions. One of these is a small, often-pedunculated fibrous growth of the corium that is found chiefly on the trunk and seldom reaches a size of more than 1 cm; traditionally it has been classified as *fibroma durum* or *molle*, depending on its relative content of collagen and fat. The term *fibroepithelial polyp* is usually applied to similar but pedunculated cutaneous nodules consisting of a mixture of dense fibrous tissue and fat covered by hyperplastic squamous epithelium. There are also fibromas with a prominent vascular component *(angiofibroma)*, focal smooth muscle differentiation *(myofibroma)*, and bone formation *(osteofibroma)*, as well as fibroma-like pseudotumors that arise from the testicular tunic and other sites. Kamino et al.[40] described a *pleomorphic fibroma*, a richly collagenous, polypoid growth marked by large pleomorphic and hyperchromatic nuclei occurring chiefly in the extremities of adults. Cutaneous fibroma-like lesions may be an occasional feature of Gardner's syndrome and the tuberous sclerosis complex *(periungual, subungual, and gingival angiofibromas)*.

There are also other collagen-producing tumors that may mimic a fibroma: fibrous histiocytoma, neurofibroma, and localized fibrous tumor of the pleura (fibrous mesothelioma) are the most common. The diagnosis of neurofibroma, in particular, is often used indiscriminately as a convenient label for any benign collagen-forming tumor arising in soft tissue.

Confusion in diagnosis is also frequently caused by reactive or reparative fibroblastic proliferations that are poorly defined and occur in association with chronic inflammation, wound healing, and organizing hemorrhage. Recognition of these lesions is usually possible if attention is paid to the cellular polymorphism and the zonal variations in the histological picture. In many examples of this kind, the presence of inflammatory elements, siderophages, and foci of hemorrhage helps to indicate the correct diagnosis.

NODULAR FASCIITIS

Nodular fasciitis, first reported by Konwaler et al.[42] in 1955, is a benign, quasineoplastic proliferation of fibroblasts that is often mistaken for a sarcoma because of its rapid growth, rich cellularity, and mitotic activity. It is one of the more common soft tissue lesions and exceeds in frequency any other tumor or tumorlike lesion of fibrous tissue. This is attested to by the more than 1000 cases that were reviewed at the Armed Forces Institute of Pathology (AFIP) in a 20-year period and the large number of cases reported in the literature.*

The exact cause of nodular fasciitis is still unknown, but there is little doubt that it is a self-limiting reactive process rather than a true neoplasm. Neither is it a true inflammatory process, and hence the term *nodular fasciitis* is somewhat of a misnomer. Other terms, such as *pseudosarcomatous fasciitis,*[19,22,36,54,68] *proliferative fasciitis,*[64] *infiltrative fasciitis,*[42] and *pseudosarcomatous fibromatosis*[61] have been synonymously used in the literature. Rare morphological variants of nodular fasciitis have been described as *parosteal, cranial,* and *intravascular fasciitis.*

Clinical findings

Most patients give a history of a rapidly growing mass or nodule that has been present for only 1 or 2 weeks. In

---

*References 13, 20, 23, 24, 26, 27, 39, 41, 46, 47, 60, 62.

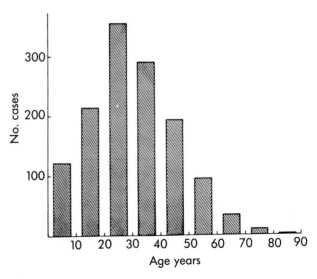

FIG. 9-1. Age distribution of nodular fasciitis (1317 cases).

Table 9-1. Anatomical distribution of nodular fasciitis (1319 cases)

Anatomical location	No. patients	Percent
Upper extremities	610	46
Head, neck	269	20
Trunk	235	18
Lower extremities	205	16
TOTAL	1319	100

about half of the cases there is associated soreness, tenderness, or slight pain. Numbness, paresthesia, or shooting pain is rare and develops only when the rapidly growing nodule exerts pressure on a peripheral nerve. Practically all lesions are solitary, and among the AFIP cases there are only three in which two or more nodules were found at the same site. We have never encountered nodular fasciitis at multiple sites as reported by Hutter et al.[38] in their series.

Nodular fasciitis is most common in adults between 20 and 40 years of age. It is less frequent in infants and children and rare in patients older than 60 years (Fig. 9-1). Males and females are about equally affected. Most of the lesions grow rapidly; in 45% of our cases the preoperative duration was less than 1 month, and in 30% less than 2 weeks. Only 7% of the patients had a lesion known to be present for more than 1 year.

Although nodular fasciitis may occur virtually anywhere on the body, there is a distinct predilection for certain sites; the most common locations are the upper extremities, especially the volar aspect of the forearm, followed by the trunk, particularly the chest wall and back. Nodular fasciitis in the head and neck is next in frequency, and is the most common site in infants and children.[67] Nodular fasciitis is less common in the lower extremities and infrequent in the hands and feet (Table 9-1). Rare examples have been reported in the oral region.[16,18,50,72]

Gross findings

Grossly, the lesion consists of a round to oval, nodular, nonencapsulated mass, which tends to be well circumscribed and usually measures less than 2 cm in greatest diameter. Larger examples occur but are uncommon, although we have encountered lesions measuring as much as 10 cm in greatest diameter. In these exceptional cases great caution must be exercised in making this diagnosis, since some fibrosarcomas closely resemble nodular fasciitis.[16]

The cut surface varies considerably and depends on the relative amounts of collagen and mucoid material within the lesion: it may be firm or soft and gelatinous. Generally, the more collagenous lesions are apt to be mistaken for fibromatosis or fibrosarcoma and the predominantly myxoid lesions for ganglion, myxoma, or schwannoma. In fact, as in most soft tissue tumors, the gross appearance is an un-

reliable criterion for diagnosis. Also, the appearance of nodular fasciitis on CT scan or MRI does not allow a specific diagnosis.[48]

Microscopic findings

Three different types of nodular fasciitis can be distinguished: the *subcutaneous type,* which forms a round or oval, relatively well circumscribed nodule in the subcutis (Fig. 9-2); the *intramuscular type,* which is larger and more ovoid in shape (Fig. 9-3); and the *fascial type,* which spreads along the superficial fascia and the interlobular septa of the subcutaneous fat, is less well circumscribed, and often assumes an irregular stellate appearance (Fig. 9-4). The relative incidence of the three types varies considerably, the subcutaneous type being about four times more common than either the intramuscular or fascial type.[32] The great majority of cases arise from the superficial fascia, but occasional lesions also originate in fibrous structures surrounding vessels or nerves. Depending upon the predominant cellular features, Price et al.[57] distinguished myxoid, cellular, and fibrous types.

All tumors consist predominantly of plump, immature-appearing fibroblasts bearing a close resemblance to the fibroblasts found in tissue culture or granulation tissue. In general, the fibroblasts vary little in size and shape and have oval, pale-staining nuclei with prominent nucleoli. Mitotic figures are fairly common, but atypical mitoses are virtually never seen (Figs. 9-5 to 9-7).

Characteristically, the fibroblasts are arranged in short irregular bundles and fascicles and are accompanied by a dense reticulin meshwork and only small amounts of mature birefringent collagen (Figs. 9-5 and 9-6). The intervening matrix is rich in mucopolysaccharides, which stain readily with alcian blue preparation and are depolymerized by hyaluronidase. The abundance of ground substance in most cases is responsible for the characteristic loosely textured, "feathery" pattern of nodular fasciitis; however, there are also cellular forms with only small amounts of interstitial myxoid material. Intermixed with the fibroblasts are scattered lymphoid cells and erythrocytes (Fig. 9-7, *A*), and, in the more central portion of the lesion, a small number of lipid macrophages and multinucleated giant cells (Fig. 9-7, *B*). Occasionally, there are associated areas of microhemorrhage, but siderophages are rare.

There are minor variations in the histological picture; sometimes the intramuscular form of nodular fasciitis contains residual muscle fibers and muscle giant cells; this feature, however, is much less pronounced in nodular fasciitis than in fibromatosis. Sometimes, in the fascial type of nodular fasciitis, the fibroblasts are arranged in a radial fashion around a central, poorly cellular, edematous area containing a mixture of mucoid material and fibrin. In this type the fibroblasts are closely associated with newly formed vessels of narrow caliber; they show considerable mitotic

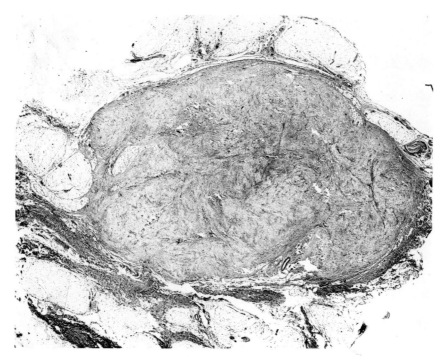

FIG. 9-2. Nodular fasciitis involving the subcutis. Note circumscription of the lesion and attachment to the superficial fascia. (×6.)

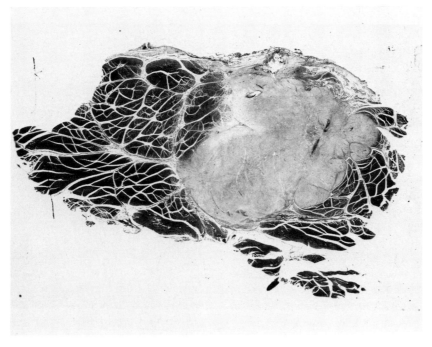

FIG. 9-3. Intramuscular nodular fasciitis. Like the subcutaneous type, the nodule is well circumscribed and seems to arise from the fascia. (×4.)

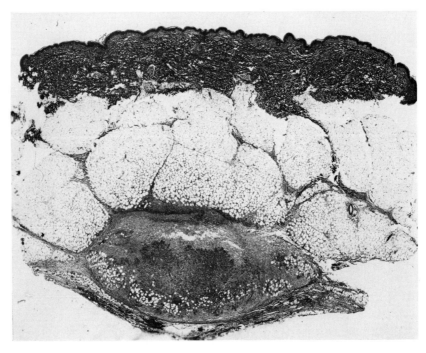

FIG. 9-4. Fascial type of nodular fasciitis. This lesion is usually less well circumscribed and tends to extend along the interlobular septa into the surrounding subcutis. (×5.)

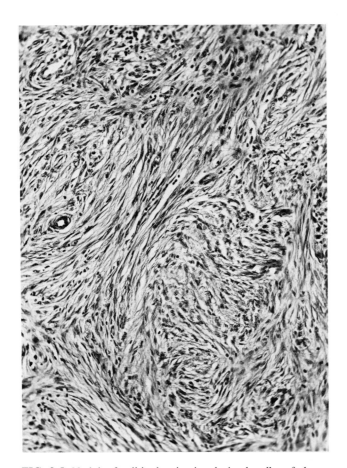

FIG. 9-5. Nodular fasciitis showing interlacing bundles of plump fibroblasts and a small number of scattered chronic inflammatory elements. (×210.)

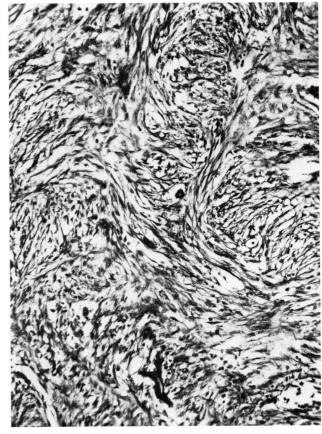

FIG. 9-6. Nodular fasciitis displaying a similar picture as in Fig. 9-5 but exhibiting a more loosely textured arrangement of the fibroblasts as a result of a more pronounced myxoid matrix. (×160.)

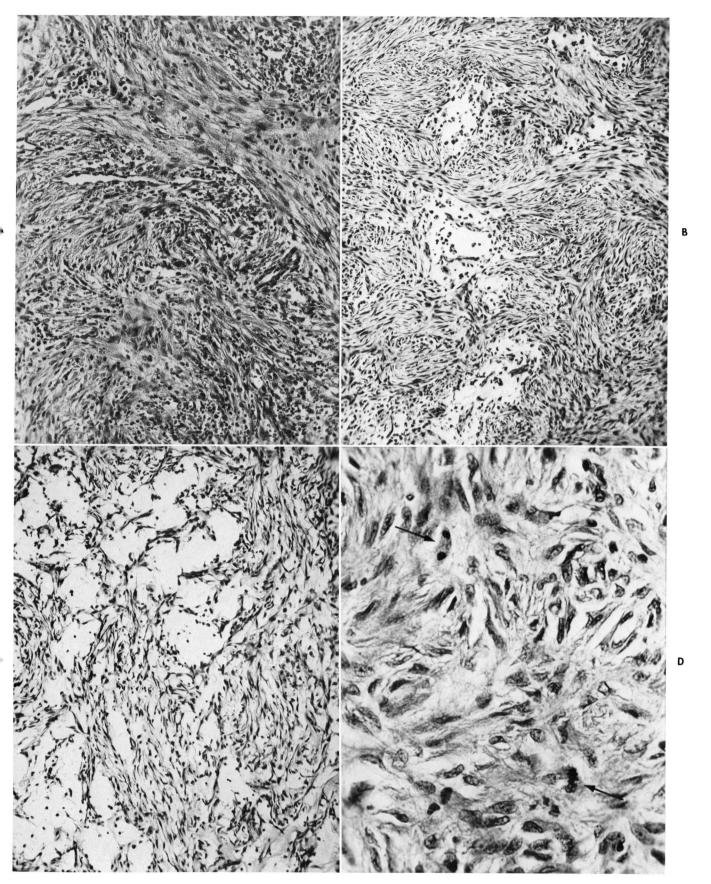

FIG. 9-7. Nodular fasciitis—variations in its histological picture. **A,** Microhemorrhages and inflammatory elements between bundles of fibroblasts. (×165.) **B,** Mucoid pools containing chronic inflammatory cells and occasional macrophages. (×90.) **C,** Richly mucoid form of nodular fasciitis. (×115.) **D,** Mitotic figures may be numerous *(arrows),* but atypical mitotic figures are virtually never seen. (×440.)

activity exceeding the average mitotic activity of the subcutaneous and intramuscular forms.

There is a close correlation between the microscopic picture and the preoperative duration of the lesions. Lesions of short duration tend to have a predominantly myxoid appearance, whereas those of longer duration are characterized by hyaline fibrosis (Fig. 9-8, *B*), tissue shrinkage, and formation of minute fluid-filled spaces, or microcysts, a sequence closely paralleling the cicatrization of granulation tissue. Sometimes, in cases of long duration, the microcysts fuse and form a large centrally located cystic space (*cystic nodular fasciitis*) (Fig. 9-8, *A*).[26,62]

Ossifying fasciitis

Nodular fasciitis-like fibroblastic proliferations with metaplastic bone have been described as *ossifying fasciitis*,[28] *fasciitis ossificans*,[43] and, when arising from the periosteum, as *parosteal fasciitis*.[37] Most of these lesions show features of both nodular fasciitis and myositis ossificans, but they are less well circumscribed than nodular fasciitis and lack the zonal maturation of myositis ossificans. Yet, occasionally, small foci of metaplastic bone may also be found in morphologically typical cases of nodular fasciitis. *Panniculitis ossificans* and *fibroosseous pseudotumor of the digits*[29] are closely related lesions that show a more irregular pattern and are akin to myositis ossificans (see Chapter 36).

Intravascular fasciitis

Intravascular fasciitis is a rare variant of nodular fasciitis characterized by involvement of small or medium-sized veins or arteries. The condition may present as a solitary nodule with focal intravascular extensions or as a predominantly intravascular growth that assumes a multinodular, plexiform, or serpentine configuration (Fig. 9-9). The intravascular growth closely resembles nodular fasciitis, but it has a less prominent mucoid matrix and often a greater number of multinucleate giant cells, a feature that may cause confusion with fibrous histiocytoma or a giant cell tumor of soft parts. More cellular examples may be mistaken for a fibrosarcoma or malignant fibrous histiocytoma. Intravascular fasciitis prevails in children, adolescents, and young adults. Despite the intravascular growth, there is no evidence of aggressive clinical behavior, recurrence, or metastasis.[54]

Cranial fasciitis

Cranial fasciitis is a rapidly growing, nodular fasciitis-like fibroblastic proliferation of varying size. It occurs chiefly, but not exclusively, in infants during the first year of life and involves the soft tissues of the scalp and the underlying skull. It usually erodes the outer table of the cranium but not infrequently also penetrates the inner table, and infiltrates the dura and sometimes even the leptomen-

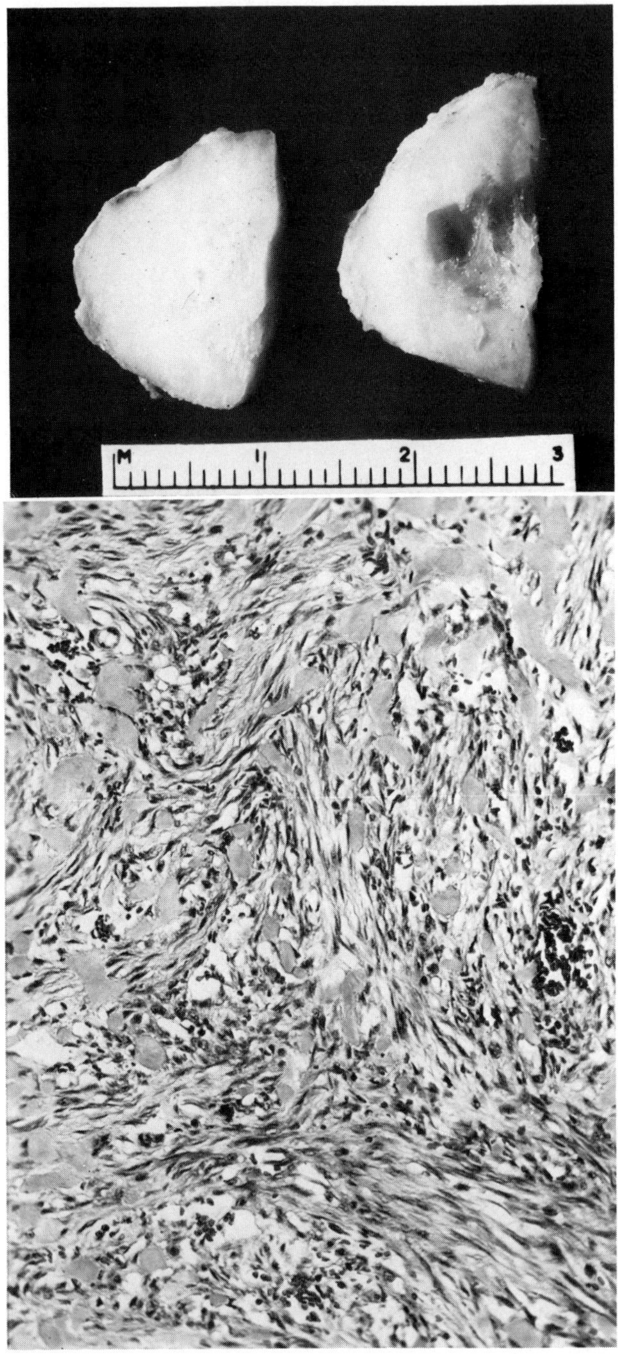

FIG. 9-8. A, Late form of nodular fasciitis with central cystlike space caused by cicatrization and tissue shrinking. B, Nodular fasciitis showing marked hyaline fibrosis, a feature that is usually encountered in lesions of long duration. (×165.)

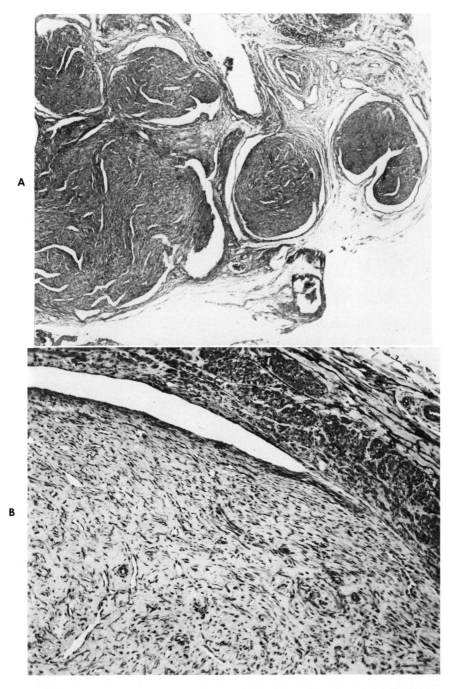

FIG. 9-9. Intravascular fasciitis. **A,** Low-power picture showing growth within several markedly dilated veins. Despite the intravascular growth, these lesions are benign. (×40.) **B,** Thick-walled vein with intravascular fibroblastic growth. (×100). (**A,** From Patchefsky AS, Enzinger FM: *Am J Surg Pathol* 5:29, 1981.)

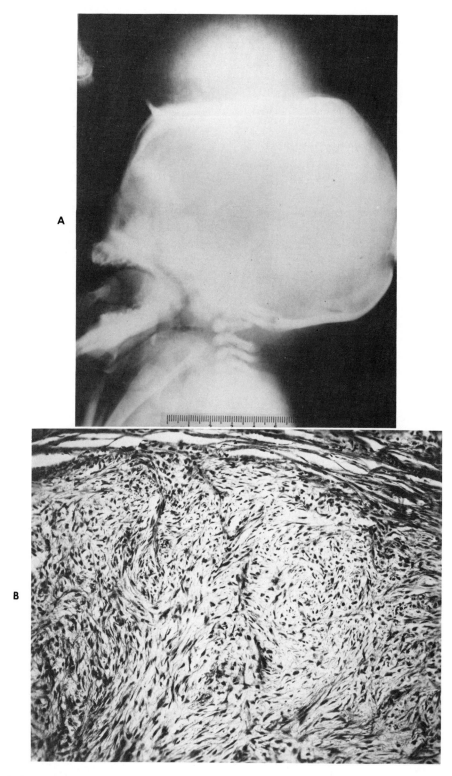

FIG. 9-10. Cranial fasciitis. **A,** Roentgenograph of large soft tissue mass attached to the inner table of the skull in an infant. **B,** Histological picture exhibiting proliferation of plump fibroblasts within a richly mucoid matrix. (×60.)

inges (Fig. 9-10). In addition to the proliferation of fibroblasts, there may be fragments of bone at the periphery and occasional multinucleate giant cells. The circumscription and the prominent myxoid matrix help to distinguish the lesion from infantile fibromatosis or myofibromatosis.*

Birth trauma may play a role in the development of the lesions; several of the affected children had been delivered by forceps. Cranial fasciitis is a benign and probably reactive process that seems to arise from the galea aponeurotica or the epicranial aponeurosis and infiltrates the incompletely formed cranial bone. One of the reported cases has been described as atypical fibrous histiocytoma.[17]

There is no relationship between cranial fasciitis and the "headbangers tumor," a fibrosing lesion of the forehead with pigmentation of the overlying skin.[64] Neither is there any association with an inherited fibrosing lesion of the scalp (cutis verticis gyrata) that occurs in adults and is associated with clubbing of the digits, enlargement of the distal extremities, and periosteal bone formation (pachydermoperiostosis).[56]

Immunohistochemical findings

Like other myofibroblastic processes, the cells of nodular fasciitis stain for vimentin, smooth muscle actin, and muscle-specific actin but not for desmin or S-100 protein. CD68 (KP1), a marker of lysosomes, is positive in macrophages and in some of the spindle cells.[51,52] According to Hasegawa et al.,[35] there are also occasional cases that are desmin positive.

Ultrastructural findings

Ultrastructurally, nodular pasciitis consists of elongated bipolar cells containing abundant intracytoplasmic, rough endoplasmic reticulum, often with cisternae filled with finely granular, electron-dense material. The nuclei have a smooth nuclear membrane and finely dispersed chromatin. In many of the cells there are also intracytoplasmic bundles of electron-dense microfilaments with focal condensation, as well as pinocytotic vesicles and occasional desmosomes. Collagen fibers and focal areas of basal lamina-like material surround many of the cells.[18,35,74]

All of these features are typical of myofibroblasts, a cell type that has been demonstrated in a variety of benign and malignant fibroblastic proliferations and that appears to play a role in cellular contraction and motility; it has been suggested that these cells are transitional stages between fibroblasts and smooth muscle cells, but we have never encountered evidence of smooth muscle differentiation in nodular fasciitis.

---

*References 14, 17, 30, 44, 53, 58.

Differential diagnosis

Hardly any other soft tissue lesion has caused as many problems and difficulties in diagnosis as nodular fasciitis. In several reports no less than half of the cases had been mistaken for a fibrosarcoma or some other malignant neoplasm, and evidently many cases of nodular fasciitis have been treated by unnecessary and overly radical surgery.

Although both nodular fasciitis and *myxoma* may display a prominent myxoid matrix, the latter is readily recognizable by its paucity of cells and its poor vascularization. *Fibrous histiocytoma* is less well circumscribed and is made up of spindle-shaped and rounded cells arranged in a whorled or storiform pattern, often in association with bundles of hyalinized collagen, chronic inflammatory cells, lipid macrophages, siderophages, and Touton-type giant cells. Yet it must be recognized that fibrous histiocytoma and nodular fasciitis are closely related lesions and that there are occasionally transitional forms between these two lesions.

Fibromatosis, a tumor that is usually less well circumscribed and larger and infiltrates muscle tissue, is characterized by slender spindle-shaped fibroblasts that are arranged in long sweeping fascicles and are separated by abundant collagen. Mitotic figures occur in both lesions, but they are much less frequent in musculoaponeurotic fibromatosis than in nodular fasciitis.[67]

Distinction from *fibrosarcoma* is primarily a matter of growth pattern and cellularity. The cells in fibrosarcoma are nearly always densely packed and are arranged in interweaving bundles, resulting in the characteristic "herringbone" pattern. Moreover, the individual cells are marked by a greater variation in size and shape, hyperchromatic nuclei, and a more pronounced mitotic rate, including atypical mitotic figures. The deep location, large size, and long duration of most fibrosarcomas will also help in differential diagnosis.

The myxoid type of *malignant fibrous histiocytoma,* a tumor that has also been classified as myxofibrosarcoma, occurs principally in patients older than 50 years and usually measures more than 3 cm when first excised. There are, however, sporadic examples that are of smaller size and affect younger patients. Microscopically, the main distinguishing features are the close association of myxoid and solid cellular areas and, especially, the striking cellular pleomorphism and the association with eosinophiles, plasma cells, and other inflammatory elements.

The term *fasciitis* has also been applied to several clinically and morphologically unrelated conditions. *Eosinophilic fasciitis,* a scleroderma-like process, presents with painful swelling and puckered induration of the arms and legs caused by inflammation and fibrosis of the fascia and subcutis, and tends to occur after unusual and strenuous physical exercise or after massive ingestion of

L-tryptophan.[45,73] The inflammatory infiltrate consists of a variable mixture of lymphocytes, plasma cells, and eosinophiles. In many of the cases there is also peripheral eosinophilia, hypergammaglobulinemia, and arthritis. Most patients with this lesion respond to treatment with corticosteroids.[15,33,34,49,63]

Necrotizing fasciitis is a rare, progressive, often fulminant inflammatory process with widespread inflammation and necrosis of fascia and subcutaneous tissues with undermining of the skin. It occurs mainly in debilitated persons with perineal infections or cutaneous ulcers or after operative procedures and is caused by a combination of multiple aerobic and anaerobic bacteria.[59,66] *Plantar fasciitis* refers to pain and tenderness in the region of the heel that radiates frequently over the entire plantar surface of the foot and principally affects obese persons.

Discussion

Although the cause of nodular fasciitis is unknown, it is likely that the fibroblastic proliferation is triggered by local injury or by a localized, nonspecific inflammatory process. If prior injury plays a role, however, it is difficult to explain why a history of trauma is given in no more than 10% to 15% of the cases and why the lesion is more common in the upper half of the body. On the other hand, there is little doubt that the basic features closely resemble those found in fat necrosis and granulation tissue.

The benign nature of nodular fasciitis is well documented. Nearly all examples of the lesion are effectively treated by local excision, and recurrence is rare (only 1% to 2% of all cases) and is usually seen soon after excision. Spontaneous regression has been observed, and once the diagnosis is made, no further treatment appears necessary. Despite its rapid growth, nodular fasciitis, as well as proliferative fasciitis and myositis, is diploid on DNA analysis.[31]

PROLIFERATIVE FASCIITIS

The term *proliferative fasciitis* is somewhat misleading because not all cases of proliferative fasciitis arise from the fascia and many are found in the subcutaneous fat without fascial attachment. Like its muscular counterpart *(proliferative myositis),* the microscopic appearance of the lesion is highly suggestive of a sarcoma, and many cases of this type have been misinterpreted in the past as embryonal rhabdomyosarcoma, ganglioneuroblastoma, or some other type of malignant neoplasm.[82]

Clinical findings

Proliferative fasciitis is a lesion of adult life, with a peak incidence between ages 40 and 70 years. Males and females are equally affected, and there is no preference for any particular race. About two thirds of the lesions occur in the extremities, especially in the forearm and the thigh, where they usually present as a firm palpable subcutaneous nodule that is movable and unattached to the overlying skin. Most lesions measure 1 to 5 cm in diameter, with a median of 2.5 cm. More often than not the lesion is tender but rarely causes pain. Like nodular fasciitis it grows rapidly and may reach its final size within 2 or 3 weeks. A history of trauma is given in about one third of cases.[76]

Pathological findings

The gross appearance of the lesion is never striking. In general, it is a poorly circumscribed, elongated or discoid mass of gray-white or red-tan tissue, which is embedded in the subcutaneous fat. Like the fascial type of nodular fasciitis, it extends along the fibrous septa separating the fat lobules (Figs. 9-11 and 9-12). Sometimes it encroaches on the superficial fascia, arises from it, or extends into the underlying muscle tissue, making it difficult to distinguish the lesion from proliferative myositis.

Microscopically, proliferative fasciitis may be the cause of considerable concern to the examining pathologist. Like nodular fasciitis it is composed of immature fibroblast-like spindle cells; in addition, there are numerous basophilic giant cells with one or two nuclei and occasional mitotic figures, superficially resembling ganglion cells. These cells are randomly oriented and are suspended in a matrix consisting of various proportions of mucoid material and collagen. The mucoid material appears to be more prominent in lesions of short duration. Intracytoplasmic inclusions having the staining characteristics of collagen are present in some of the giant cells. In older lesions the giant cells are often surrounded by mature hyalinized collagen, a feature that has been mistaken for neoplastic osteoid (Figs. 9-13 to 9-16). Ultrastructurally, the ganglion-like cells of both proliferative fasciitis and myositis appear to be modified fibroblasts with abundant rough endoplasmic reticulum, varying amounts of actinlike filaments, a distinct nuclear membrane, and a prominent nucleolus. Lipid inclusions are present in some of the cells (see Fig. 9-23).[77,87,88]

PROLIFERATIVE MYOSITIS

Proliferative myositis is a deep or intramuscular counterpart of proliferative fasciitis, a pseudosarcomatous process that was first described by Kern[81] in 1960. Like proliferative fasciitis it is a rapidly growing lesion that infiltrates muscle tissue in a diffuse manner and is characterized by bizarre giant cells bearing a close resemblance to ganglion cells.

Clinical findings

The symptoms are nonspecific, and the diagnosis always rests on the histological examination of tissue obtained by biopsy or excision. In the majority of cases the lesion is first noticed as a palpable, more or less discrete, solitary nodule or mass that measures 1 to 6 cm in diameter. It rarely

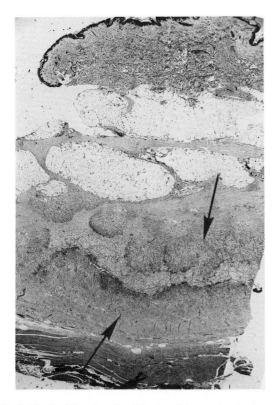

FIG. 9-11. Proliferative fasciitis involving subcutis *(arrows)*. Note central myxoid zone surrounded by a zone of greater cellularity and extension along the fibrous septa of the subcutaneous fat. (×8.)

causes tenderness or pain, even though it may double in size within a period of a few days. The duration between onset and excision is usually less than 3 weeks.[79,80,89]

The patients tend to be older than those with nodular fasciitis and are mostly in their forties or fifties. In fact, of the 33 cases of this condition that we reported in 1967, the median age was 50 years.[79] There seems to be no predilection for either sex or any particular race. The lesion mainly affects the flat muscles of the trunk and shoulder girdle, especially the pectoralis, latissimus dorsi, or serratus anterior muscle. Occasionally tumors are also found in the thigh.

Gross findings

As a rule, the process is poorly demarcated and appears as an area of pale gray scarlike induration involving muscle and overlying fascia (Fig. 9-17). In large, bulky muscles such as the quadriceps, these changes tend to be more superficially located; in smaller or flat muscles, they replace all or most of the musculature. Generally the extent of the lesion is greatest just beneath the muscle fascia. Nearly all of these lesions measure less than 6 cm in greatest diameter.

Microscopic findings

Two main features characterize this process: (1) a poorly demarcated fibroblastic proliferation involving the epimysium, perimysium, and endomysium; and (2) large, plump

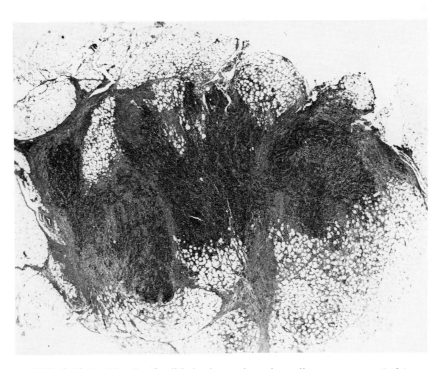

FIG. 9-12. Proliferative fasciitis having an irregular stellate appearance. (×9.)

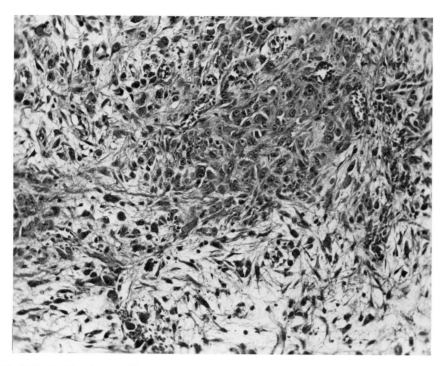

FIG. 9-13. Proliferative fasciitis composed of a mixture of fibroblasts and giant cells with abundant basophilic cytoplasm bearing some resemblance to ganglion cells. (×145.)

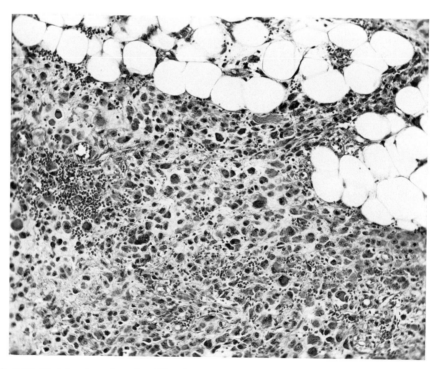

FIG. 9-14. Peripheral portion of proliferative fasciitis with beginning interstitial deposition of collagen. (×130.)

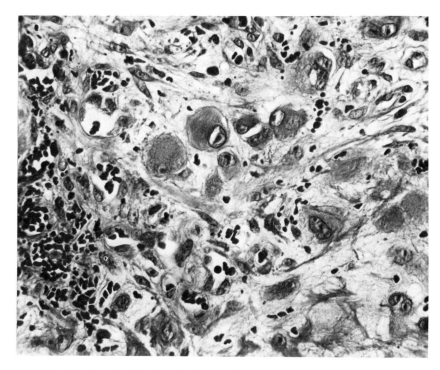

FIG. 9-15. Proliferative fasciitis showing large cells, associated focal hemorrhage, and a richly mucoid matrix. (×400.)

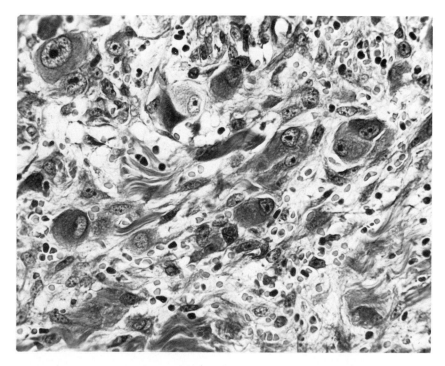

FIG. 9-16. Proliferative fasciitis. Characteristic mononuclear giant cells showing considerable variation in size and shape. The cells are associated with interstitial edema and extravasated erythrocytes. The lesion was initially diagnosed as rhabdomyosarcoma. There was no evidence of recurrence or metastasis after 13 years. (Masson trichrome stain; ×350.)

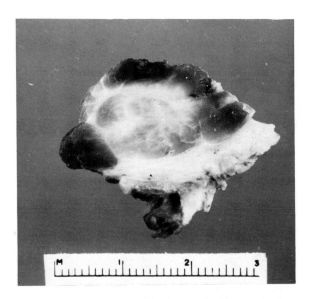

FIG. 9-17. Proliferative myositis characterized by poorly circumscribed scarlike fibrosing process involving both muscle and muscle fascia.

basophilic giant cells resembling ganglion cells or rhabdomyoblasts. The fibroblastic proliferation mainly affects the stromal tissue and, except for muscular atrophy, leaves the muscle tissue virtually uninvolved (Figs. 9-18 to 9-21). In particular, there is no sarcolemmal proliferation or attempted regeneration of muscle tissue. Complete replacement of muscle, as in nodular fasciitis or fibromatosis, is never seen. Under low power the alternating areas of proliferated fibroblasts and the remnants of the infiltrated muscle tissue create a vague checkerboard pattern (Fig. 9-19). Occasional cells are marked by eosinophilic inclusions characteristic of collagen (Fig. 9-22, *A*). Immunohistochemically, the cells stain positively for vimentin, actin, smooth muscle actin, factor XIIIa, fibronectin, and rarely for desmin and myosin. They do not stain for myoglobin. Ultrastructurally, they show the features of myofibroblasts.[75,78,85,90]

Focal ossification occurs but is always less conspicuous than in myositis ossificans (Fig. 9-22, *B*). Because of these features and the resemblance of proliferative myositis to nodular fasciitis and proliferative fasciitis, Dahl and Angervall[25] coined the term *pseudosarcomatous proliferative lesion of soft tissue without bone formation*.

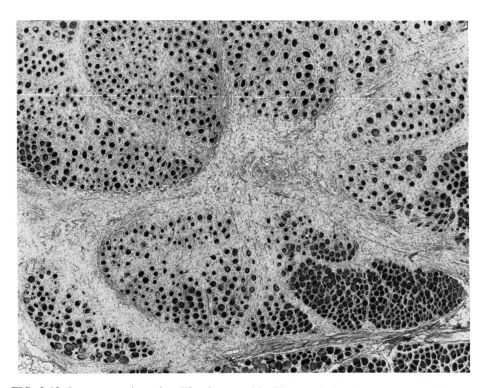

FIG. 9-18. Low-power view of proliferative myositis. The muscle bundles are separated by endomysial and epimysial proliferation of fibrous connective tissue in a checkerboard-like fashion. (×14.)

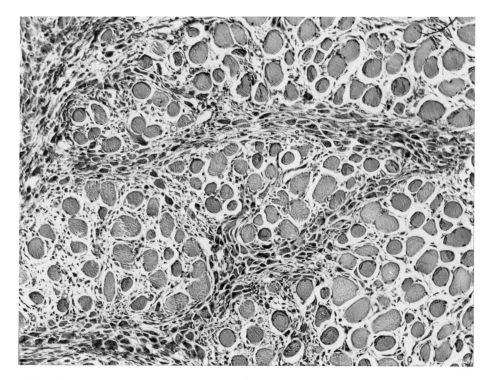

FIG. 9-19. Perimysial proliferation of basophilic giant cells in proliferative fasciitis simulating a sarcoma. The patient, a 60-year-old woman, was well and without recurrence 3 years after removal of lesion by simple excision. (×100.)

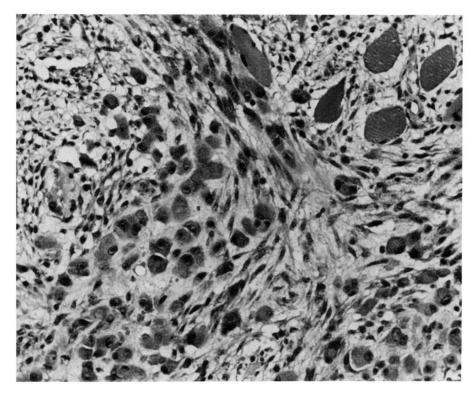

FIG. 9-20. Proliferative myositis. Giant cells—modified fibroblasts—have replaced muscle tissue. (×165.)

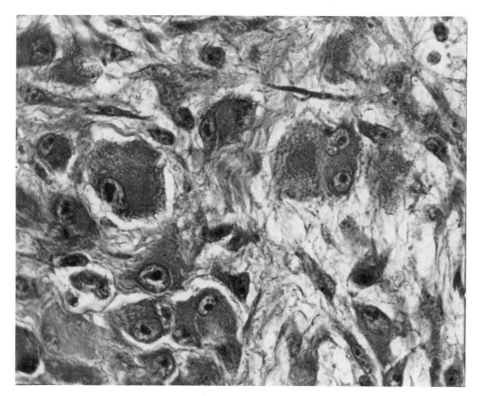

FIG. 9-21. Proliferation of large plump basophilic giant cells in proliferative myositis. (×480.)

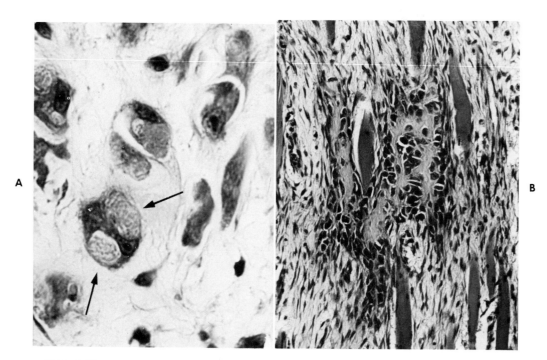

FIG. 9-22. **A,** Eosinophilic inclusions *(arrows)* having the staining characteristics of collagen within the giant cells. (×750.) **B,** Isolated focus of osteoid in proliferative myositis. (×150.)

Differential diagnosis

The large basophilic cells have been confused with ganglioneuroblasts and rhabdomyoblasts, but errors will be avoided if attention is paid to the clinical features and the small size of the lesion, the deep basophilia of the giant cells, and the absence of Nissl granules and immunoreactive desmin or myoglobin.

Discussion

Proliferative fasciitis and myositis, like nodular fasciitis, are self-limiting, benign, reactive processes that are adequately treated by local excision. The cause and mode of development remain unexplained, but it is likely that a lesion is preceded by some type of fascial or muscular injury directly or through local vascular impairment. The reported type of trauma varies: in some cases the lesion was preceded by a single episode of injury; in others trauma was mild and repeated in nature. Whatever the cause, there is little doubt that these are reactive processes rather than neoplasms. Despite their rapid growth and cellular pleomorphism, they are invariably cured by local excision. As expected, flow cytometric DNA analysis of nodular fasciitis, proliferative fasciitis, and myositis revealed a uniformly diploid pattern.[31]

PROLIFERATIVE FASCIITIS AND MYOSITIS IN CHILDHOOD

This process is closely related to the adult forms of proliferative fasciitis and myositis but occurs in infants and children and differs from the adult forms by its extreme cellularity and the presence of minute foci of acute inflammation and necrosis. According to the small number of cases reported,[83] the lesion is most common in the extremities and the head and neck region. It consists of large round or polygonal ganglion-like cells with prominent nucleoli that are arranged in a vague lobular architecture and, as in adult proliferative fasciitis, stain for vimentin and actin and are desmin negative (Fig. 9-23). Ultrastructurally, the large ganglion-like cells have the features of fibroblasts and myofibroblasts, with intracytoplasmic long-spacing collagen in one case. The process is that of a benign pseudosarcomatous lesion without any tendency toward progressive or metastatic growth. The circumscription of the lesion, the basophilia of the tumor cells, and the results of the immunostains help to exclude embryonal rhabdomyosarcoma and ganglioneuroblastoma.

ATYPICAL DECUBITAL FIBROPLASIA

Exuberant fibroblastic proliferation with large, plump fibroblasts, resembling proliferative fasciitis, is occasionally encountered in debilitated or immobilized, bedridden, or wheelchair-bound patients as the result of prolonged pressure and impaired circulation. These lesions are found chiefly over bony prominences, such as the region of the shoulder, sacrum, or greater trochanter, where they form a poorly circumscribed, painless soft tissue mass that is not infrequently mistaken for a neoplasm. They are slightly more common in women and have a peak incidence in the

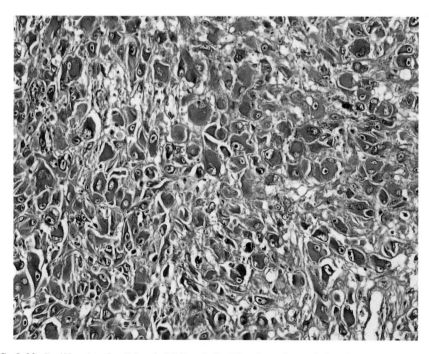

FIG. 9-23. Proliferative fasciitis of childhood. Proliferation of rounded and polygonal cells with abundant cytoplasm and prominent nucleoli. (×250.)

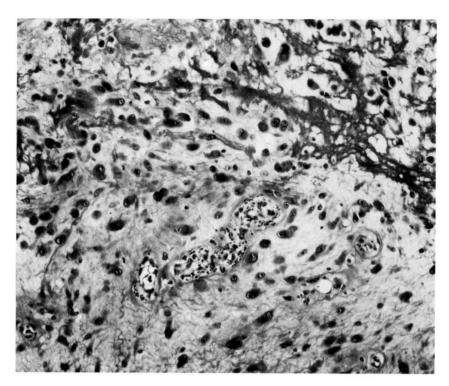

FIG. 9-24. Atypical decubital fibroplasia. Fibroblastic proliferation and fibrin deposition in the sacral region of a bedridden patient caused by prolonged pressure and impaired circulation. (×160.)

eighth and ninth decades of life.[84] Perosio and Weiss[86] described similar lesions as "ischemic fasciitis."

Microscopically, the lesions have a lobular or zonal pattern. In addition to the proliferation of plump fibroblasts with abundant basophilic cytoplasm, reminiscent of granulation tissue or proliferative fasciitis, there are a prominent myxoid stroma, deposits of fibrinous material, focal fibrinoid necrosis, a mild chronic inflammatory infiltrate, and areas of hemorrhage. Cystic changes and fibrosis may be prominent in older lesions. These changes involve chiefly the subcutis but may also affect the underlying muscle tissue (Fig. 9-24).

FIBROMA OF TENDON SHEATH

Whether fibroma of tendon sheath is a reactive fibrosing process or a neoplasm is not clear, but it is a distinct entity of characteristic location and histological appearance. It consists of a slow-growing, dense fibrous nodule that is firmly attached to tendon sheath and is found most frequently in the hands and feet. Its lobular configuration resembles that of a giant cell tumor of tendon sheath, but it is much less cellular and there are no xanthoma cells or giant cells.

The chief complaint is a small mass that has been present for some time and has increased only slowly in size. It is found most commonly in adults between the ages of 20 and

50 years and is more than twice as common in men as in women. Among the 138 cases in our series,[92] nearly all originated in the extremities, with the majority occurring in the fingers, hand, and wrist (the thumb being the most common single site). The mass rarely measures more than 2 cm in greatest diameter and is painless but may limit motion of the involved digit. A history of trauma is given in some cases.[91,95]

Gross findings

In general, the tumors are attached to tendon or tendon sheath, are well circumscribed, and are distinctly lobulated. They are firm and rubbery and on section have a uniform gray or pearly white, almost cartilaginous appearance. They range in size between 1 and 2 cm, but we have seen patients in whom lesions measured as large as 5 cm.

Microscopic findings

Under low-power examination most examples of this entity are well defined and are distinctly lobulated, a configuration similar to that of a giant cell tumor of tendon sheath. The individual lobules are often divided by narrow cleft-like spaces (Fig. 9-25). Under higher power the nodules are composed of scattered fibroblasts, narrow vessels, and large amounts of dense collagenous material, which is deeply eosinophilic and markedly hyalinized (Figs. 9-26 and 9-27).

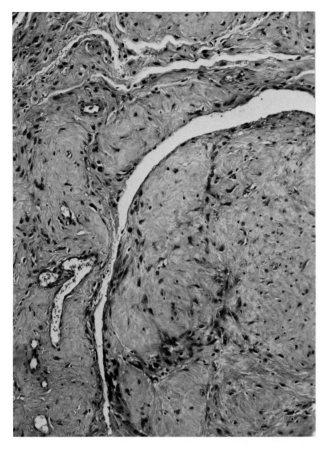

FIG. 9-25. Fibroma of tendon sheath showing lobular arrangement of dense fibrocollagenous tissue and an intervening cleftlike space. (×250.)

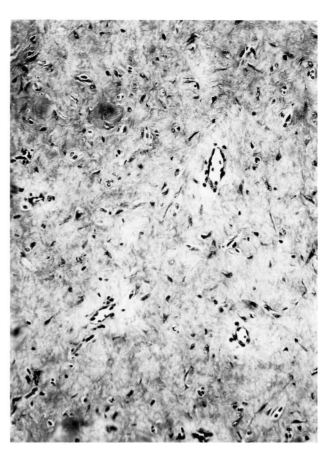

FIG. 9-26. Fibroma of tendon sheath composed of scattered spindle- to stellate-shaped fibroblasts within a sparsely cellular and richly collagenous stroma. (×160.)

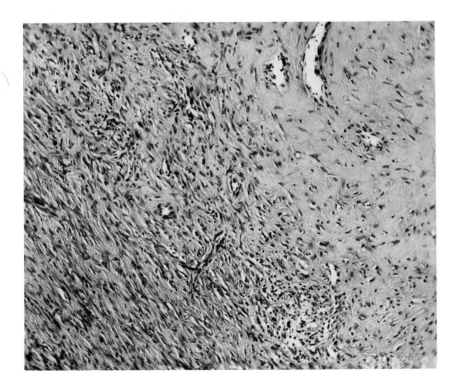

FIG. 9-27. Transition between cellular and collagenized portion of fibroma of tendon sheath. (×120.)

Foci of myxoid change with interspersed stellate-shaped fibroblasts may be a prominent feature. Occasionally, there is also a gradual transition between the poorly cellular hyalinized collagenous areas and more cellular areas; this probably represents an earlier stage in development (Fig. 9-27). Very rarely there is cellular pleomorphism[93] or focal osseous or chondroid metaplasia. The spindle cells are immunoreactive for vimentin and actin.

Confusion with other lesions is unlikely with the typical hyalinized and richly collagenous examples of the tumor. Confusion is possible, however, with more cellular forms, which may suggest nodular fasciitis, fibrous histiocytoma, and even fibrosarcoma. But even in these lesions, distinction will be readily apparent if attention is paid to the distinctly circumscribed or lobulated appearance, the attachment to tendon or tendon sheath, and the gradual transition between cellular and more hyalinized areas.

Electron microscopic findings

Ultrastructurally, the lesion consists of a mixture of myofibroblasts and fibroblasts. The myofibroblasts are more common in the cellular portions of the lesion and are characterized by actin-type intermediate filaments with focal condensation and multiple attachment sites. Typical fibroblasts prevail in the collagenized portions of the lesions.[91,96] Lundgren and Kindblom[94] also described an enclosing nuclear fibrous lamina that consists of a layer of moderately dense material within the nuclear envelope.

Discussion

Fibroma of tendon sheath is a perfectly benign process that recurs occasionally. Of 54 patients followed up in our series,[92] 24% of the fibromas recurred, but none caused any disturbance of movement or other complications, and all were treated effectively by local excision or reexcision of the growth.

The exact nature of this lesion is not clear. It is likely that there is an initial and rather transient cellular phase that resembles nodular fasciitis or fibrous histiocytoma and a collagenous phase that predominates and is typical and diagnostic of this entity. The exact cause of this biphasic development is not clear, but friction inherent in the location of the tumor or vascular impairment may account for the early onset of the sclerosing process.

NUCHAL FIBROMA

Nuchal fibroma is a rare and hitherto undescribed fibrous growth that occurs chiefly in the interscapular and paraspinal regions of patients between 25 and 60 years of age. It consists of broad bundles of collagen with only a few interspersed fibrocytes, is limited to the subcutis, and extends frequently with multiple short processes into the adjacent

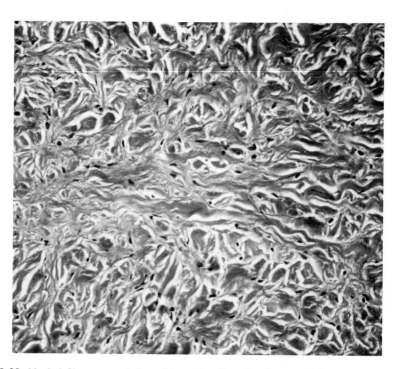

FIG. 9-28. Nuchal fibroma consisting of broad bundles of collagen and interspersed fibrocytes. The lesion was removed from the interscapular region of a 55-year-old man. (×160.)

subcutaneous fat, sometimes enclosing small foci of mature adipose tissue (Fig. 9-28). In rare instances, the collagen fibers display focal ossification.

Distinction from a *fibrolipoma* may be difficult, but the characteristic location in the paraspinal region, the absence of a fibrous capsule, and the small amounts of adipose tissue support the diagnosis of nuchal fibroma. More importantly, the subcutaneous location and the paucity of cells permit exclusion of *extraabdominal fibromatosis*. The lesion is benign but may recur if incompletely excised.

ELASTOFIBROMA

Elastofibroma is a peculiar tumorlike process that was first reported by Järvi and Saxén[113] in 1961. Typically, the lesion manifests as a slowly growing, solid, ill-defined mass of fibroelastic tissue occurring almost exclusively in elderly persons and arising chiefly from the connective tissue between the lower portion of the scapula and the chest wall. Because of its typical location, it was initially reported as *elastofibroma dorsi*, but because rare examples have also been found in other locations, the term *elastofibroma* is preferred.

Clinical findings

The lesion is easily overlooked because it causes few symptoms and usually manifests merely as a deep-seated mass that rarely causes tenderness, pain, or restriction of movement. On palpation it is firm and does not adhere to overlying skin. It is nearly always located in the lower subscapular area, deep to the rhomboid and latissimus dorsi muscles, where it is firmly attached to the chest wall, especially to the thoracic fascia, periosteum, and ligaments in the region of the seventh and eighth ribs. It is unilateral in the majority of cases.[101,106,122,130] Bilateral involvement is less common but is present in about 10% of all cases.[113,129] Elastofibroma has also been observed in the regions of the deltoid,[120] the greater trochanter,[99] the foot,[102] and, among our cases, the chest wall and the right breast. One tumor overlying the ischial tuberosity developed 3 months after fracture of the femur on the same side.[131] Kransdorf et al.[116] described the appearance of elastofibroma on CT scan and MRI.

Patients with elastofibroma are generally past the age of 55 years and more often are women than men. The majority are persons who have been involved for many years in heavy and repetitive manual labor. Elastofibroma has never been recorded in young adults, teenagers, or children. In general it is a very slow growing process, and there are several instances in which the lesion was known to be present for 5 or more years (Table 9-2).

Pathological findings

The excised mass is firm and spherical, with ill-defined margins; it averages 5 to 10 cm in greatest diameter. On section it has a gray-white, glistening surface with foci of cystic degeneration and interspersed fatty islands and streaks vaguely resembling a fibrolipoma (Fig. 9-29).

On microscopic examination the tumorlike mass consists of a mixture of intertwining swollen, eosinophilic collagen and elastic fibers in about equal proportions, associated with occasional fibroblasts, small amounts of interstitial mucoid material, and variously sized aggregates of mature fat cells. Typically the elastic fibers have a degenerated beaded appearance or are fragmented into small flowerlike, serrated discs or globules (chenille bodies) having a distinct linear arrangement (Figs. 9-30 to 9-32).

Elastin stains (Verhoeff's, Weigert's, Gomori's) reveal deeply staining, branched and unbranched fibers that have a central dense core and an irregular moth-eaten or serrated margin (Figs. 9-33 and 9-34). The elastin-like material is removed by prior treatment of the sections with pancreatic or bacterial elastase and pepsin, but collagenase or trypsin has no effect.[118] The altered fibers have a green fluorescence under ultraviolet light.

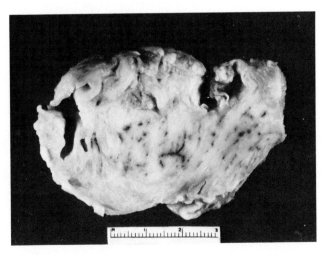

FIG. 9-29. Elastofibroma. The firm collagenous central portion blends with the surrounding fat.

Table 9-2. Age distribution of 49 cases of elastofibroma

Age (yr)*	No. cases	Percent
10-19	0	0
20-29	0	0
30-39	1	2
40-49	5	10
50-59	11	22
60-69	23	47
70-79	9	19
80-89	0	0
TOTAL	49	100

*Median age: 61 years. Two thirds were 59 years and older.

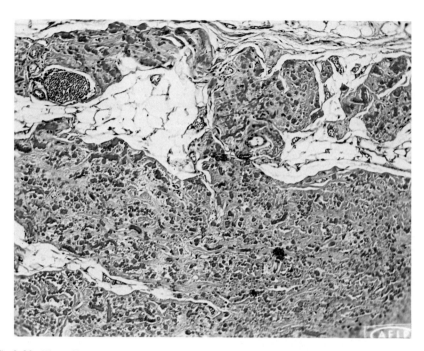

FIG. 9-30. Elastofibroma consisting of a mixture of collagen bundles, coarse elastic fibers, and residual fat. (×90.)

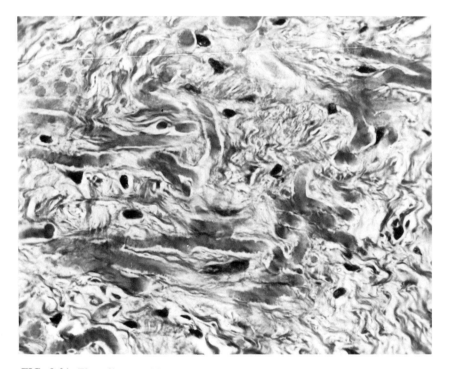

FIG. 9-31. Elastofibroma. Altered elastic fibers within a collagenous matrix. (×440.)

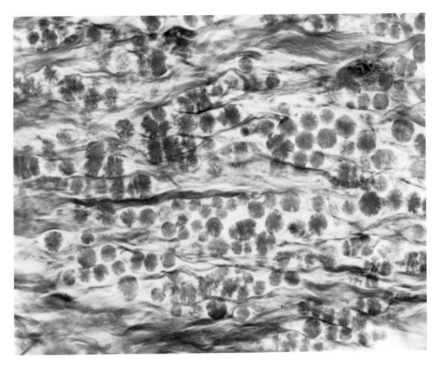

FIG. 9-32. Elastofibroma. Elastic fibers in cross-section showing characteristic serrated edge (petaloid globules). (×615.)

Ultrastructural findings

On examination with the electron microscope the fibers consist largely of granular or fibrillary aggregations of electron-dense material along a central core, surrounded by an amorphous matrix containing scattered microfibrils. The interspersed spindle cells show the characteristics of fibroblasts and myofibroblasts with a fibrous lamina within the nuclear envelope and a prominent and often dilated endoplasmic reticulum, pinocytotic vesicles, and fine cytoplasmic filaments without any periodicity. They also contain dense nonmembrane-bound granular bodies, ranging from 200 to 350 nm in diameter, presumably precursors of the extracellular elastin-like material.[98,108,115,132] Dixon and Lee[105] observed, in addition to the dense granular bodies, numerous coated vesicles measuring from 110 to 120 nm in thickness. Madri et al.[119] demonstrated collagen type II, in addition to collagen types I and III, in elastofibroma, Nakamura et al.[124] defined the biochemical characteristics of the elastin.

Discussion

Although it has been suggested that the entire process represents abnormal changes occurring in preexisting elastic fibers, it appears that elastofibroma is actually a degenerative pseudotumor and is the result of excessive forma-tion of collagen and especially abnormal elastic fibers secondary to repeated injury, more specifically injury caused by friction between the inferior edge of the scapula and the underlying chest wall. Opinions differ as to the exact nature of the fibers, but they seem to be formed by abnormal elastogenesis, as first suggested by Järvi et al.,[113,114] rather than by degeneration of preformed elastic fibers or collagen. Most believe that the basic cells are myofibroblasts, but it has also been suggested that the changes may be due to disturbance of elastic fibrillogenesis by periosteal derived cells.[117]

In keeping with the concept of a reactive process are the slow progression of the lesion, its occasional occurrence on both sides of the body, and its prevalence in patients who perform hard manual work. Because this particular response occurs in only a relatively small number of persons, it must be assumed that there is an underlying genetic disposition or inherent enzymatic defect. Although an increased familial incidence was not evident in the earlier reports of elastofibroma, Nagamine et al.[121,122] reported that about one third of the patients with this lesion in Okinawa gave such a history. Moreover, a systemic involvement is suggested by the finding of elastofibroma-like changes in the wall of a gastric ulcer in a Japanese woman with bilateral subscapular elastofibromas.[107]

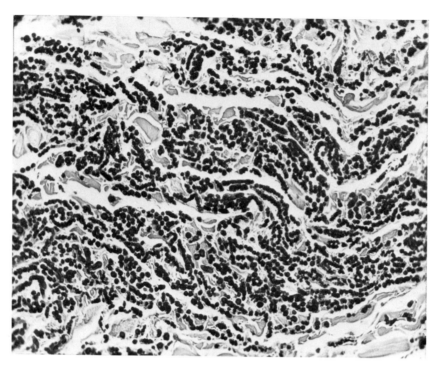

FIG. 9-33. Elastofibroma. Verhoeff elastin stain reveals globules of elastin in a linear arrangement. (×210.)

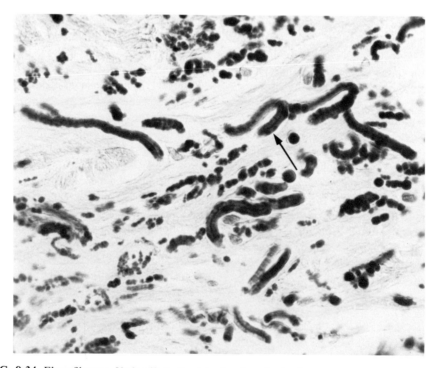

FIG. 9-34. Elastofibroma. Verhoeff elastin stain showing elastic fibers with a dense core *(arrow)*. (×210.)

Elastofibromalike changes have also been demonstrated in the thoracic fascia beneath the lower portion of the scapula in about 15% of routine autopsy cases,[112] in Morton's neuroma,[128] in a colonic polyp,[111] and in the submucosa of the rectum in a patient with multiple myeloma.[109] Benisch et al.[100] used the term *preelastofibroma* for a fibrous tumor that produced only weakly elastinophilic fibrillary material without progression to elastic tissue.

Confusion with other disorders of the elastic tissue are unlikely. *Pseudoxanthoma elasticum* is an autosomal recessive process presenting as multiple xanthoma-like yellow papules, chiefly in the neck, axilla, and inguinal region, which are composed of swollen, fragmented, sometimes calcified elastic fibers in the middermis. These alterations may be accompanied by similar changes in the cardiovascular system and angioid streaks in the retina. *Juvenile elastoma (nevus elasticus)* consists of white or yellow ill-defined plaques caused by accumulation of coarse, branching elastic fibers admixed with abnormal collagen.

Elastofibroma is a benign condition that has no tendency to recur and is best treated by surgical excision. Deutsch,[104] however, reported equally good results with radiotherapy.

NASOPHARYNGEAL ANGIOFIBROMA

Although it may be debated whether nasopharyngeal angiofibroma is a vascular or fibrous tumor, it is included here because of the predominance of the fibrous element and its resemblance to other fibrous tumors. It is, in fact, a unique process marked by a specific histological picture, exclusive occurrence in the nasopharynx, and specific age and sex incidence. Almost all cases occur in adolescent males, but the tumor may also have its onset during adult life. For this reason, the term *nasopharyngeal angiofibroma* may be more appropriate than juvenile nasopharyngeal angiofibroma.[133,162,168]

Clinical findings

The usual presenting complaints, as well as the two principal symptoms of the disease, are nasal obstruction affecting one or both sides and repeated epistaxis, which may be severe and life threatening and may require multiple blood transfusions and hospitalization.

In most cases physical examination reveals a protruding red or red-blue, rounded lobulated or polypoid mass that is firmly attached to the basilar process of the occipital bone or the body of the sphenoid. Frequently the mass extends into the anterior portion of the nasal cavity or laterally into the antrum. Less commonly it deflects the soft palate or involves the ethmoid and sphenoid sinuses. It may also erode the base of the skull or may extend from the antrum into the cheek and orbit, causing protrusion of the eye and visual disturbances, as well as swelling and bulging of the face (frog face). Inflammatory changes of neighboring structures, such as mastoiditis, sinusitis, and otitis media, are not uncommon.[147,152,158]

Most lesions occur in adolescent males between 10 and 17 years of age and usually have caused symptoms for 1 or 2 years when first seen. Rare microscopically verified cases have also been observed in slightly younger and older patients and in women.[150,154,157,160,165] The actual occurrence of the tumor in women, however, is still debated. It is conceivable that some of the reported cases in women were incorrectly diagnosed, especially since occasional richly vascular fibrotic polyps closely mimic the feature of nasopharyngeal angiofibroma.[149] In about half of the cases there is some evidence of delayed puberty and sexual underdevelopment.

In addition to transnasal biopsy, CT scan is essential for diagnosis. Also, angiography may be needed for adequate evaluation of large tumors. CT scan usually shows a well-circumscribed nasopharyngeal mass causing bowing of the posterior wall of the maxillary sinus and posterior displacement of the pterygoid plates. At a more advanced stage of the disease there is often extension into the adjacent sinuses, widening of the inferior and lateral portions of the superior orbital fissure, and sharply demarcated erosions of bone[139,141,151] (Fig. 9-35).

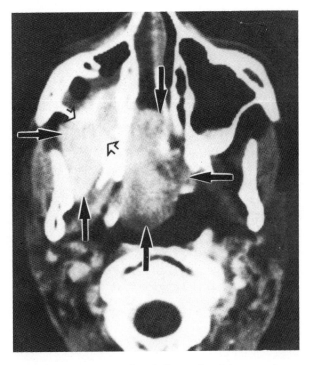

FIG. 9-35. Nasopharyngeal angiofibroma involving nasopharynx, nasal cavity, and right infratemporal fossa *(arrows)* and eroding through posterior wall of right maxillary antrum *(small arrows)*. (From Chandler JR, Goulding R, Moskowitz L, et al: *Ann Otol Rhinol Laryngol* 93:322, 1984.)

Gross findings

The resected tissue is firm and rubbery and has a smooth polypoid, gray to pink mucosal surface, which may be white in areas in which the mucosa has undergone squamous metaplasia or may be ulcerated. On section the tissue has a spongy appearance caused by the presence of numerous tiny gaping or cavernous vascular spaces surrounded by dense scarlike fibrous tissue.

Microscopic findings

Although there are minor variations in the microscopic picture of the growth, most of the lesions consist of dense fibrous tissue with interspersed slitlike or gaping vascular channels of different caliber. The vascular channels vary in number and configuration, are thin walled, and are lined by a single layer of endothelium with or without a narrow and often incomplete rim of smooth muscle tissue (Figs. 9-36 and 9-37). Characteristically, the vessels are devoid of an elastic membrane, a feature that may be responsible in part for the frequency and profusion of hemorrhage from areas of ulceration or when the lesion is incised at the time of surgical removal. Generally, the vascular component is more conspicuous at the periphery of the lesion and in tumors of short duration, especially those occurring in young persons.

The fibrous component varies in cellularity and collagen content and may show foci of hyalinization and myxoid degeneration. Sternberg,[162] in his classic review of this entity, noted the parallel arrangement of the collagen fibers that gives the fibrous tissue a fascialike appearance. Mast cells are common. There is often ulceration and squamous metaplasia of the overlying mucosal lining.

Electron microscopic findings

According to several ultrastructural studies,[142,149,166,168] the nuclei of the constituent fibroblasts are lobulated with marginal chromatin and frequent nucleoli and have at the periphery peculiar nuclear blebs and pockets. Typically there are also electron-dense intranuclear inclusions of granules of variable size surrounded by clear halos. The cytoplasm varies in appearance; in some cells there is a well-developed rough endoplasmic reticulum with a prominent Golgi complex; in others there are bundles of intracellular filaments with focal densities, pinocytotic vesicles, hemidesmosomes, and occasionally basal laminae, features characteristic of myofibroblasts. Stiller et al.[164] also reported occasional cells intermediate in appearance between fibroblasts and histiocytes. The vascular channels are lined by large endothelial cells of typical appearance, a distinct basal lamina, pericytes, and a small and variable number of smooth muscle cells.

Prognosis and treatment

In most cases the lesion grows aggressively, with extension into adjoining sinuses and destruction of bone. It re-

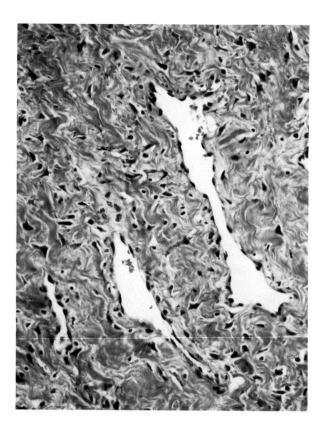

FIG. 9-37. Nasopharyngeal angiofibroma from the posterior nasopharynx of a 16-year-old boy. The lesion is composed of gaping, endothelial-lined vascular spaces surrounded by dense collagenous tissue. (×250.)

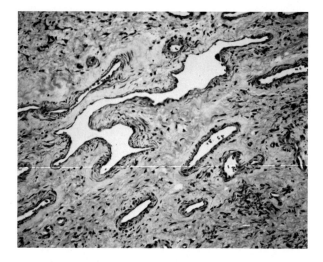

FIG. 9-36. Nasopharyngeal angiofibroma consisting of dense fibrocollagenous tissue with interspersed vascular channels of varying caliber. (×160.)

curs in about 36% to 60% of cases; the rate of recurrence depends on the completeness of the excision. Various surgical approaches have been used, but the transantral[134] and transpalatine[160,163,171] approaches seem to provide better surgical exposure than the transnasal approach. Radiotherapy is effective and even in moderate doses causes rapid relief of symptoms and regression of the tumor.[137,138,144] For instance, Cummings et al.[141] achieved permanent control in 80% of patients with external-beam megavoltage radiation. *Sarcomatous transformation*, however, has been observed in a small number of cases that received radiotherapy, generally after an interval of 10 or more years.[136,140,146,163] Development of squamous cell carcinoma and thyroid carcinoma has also been reported following radiotherapy of nasopharyngeal angiofibroma.[141,145] Androgen or testosterone therapy appears to be largely ineffective,[138,162] but Walike and Mackay[170] observed microscopic changes after treatment with stilbestrol.

KELOID

Keloid is a benign overgrowth of scar tissue occurring primarily in the corium of persons between 15 and 45 years of age. It may be solitary or multiple and has a predilection for dark-skinned individuals, especially blacks. Keloid (Greek, clawlike) was named for its multiple extensions, which bestow on the lesion an imaginary crablike appearance. There are, in addition to its common cicatricial forms, "spontaneous" or "idiopathic" forms of the condition, but these, too, are most likely the result of some minor infection or injury in areas with increased skin tension. *Hypertrophic scars*, lesions that remain confined to the original wound, should be distinguished from keloids because of their substantially lower recurrence rate.

Clinical findings

Keloids usually manifest as well-circumscribed round, oval, or linear elevations of the skin and often extend with multiple processes into the surrounding areas. They may be asymptomatic but more often are described by the patient as being itchy, tender, or painful. In their earlier phase keloids tend to be soft and erythematous; later they become increasingly indurated and turn white. They are found more commonly above than below the waist and have a predilection for the face, shoulders, forearms, and hands. About half of the "spontaneous" keloids occur as a transversal band in the presternal region, probably as the result of minor infection and increased skin tension in this region. In some patients keloids are limited to one portion of the body; thus keloids may develop after the piercing of ear lobes for earrings, but they may be absent in an appendectomy scar[181,186,187,190] (Figs. 9-38 to 9-40).

Keloids are induced by minor infections, especially acne and furuncles, smallpox and other vaccinations, tattooing, and cautery, as well as by laparotomies and various other surgical procedures. Sometimes even minor injuries, such as needle marks or mosquito bites, may produce small keloids of pinhead size. In some African countries keloidal scarification is produced deliberately in a special design, which is considered an adornment and beauty mark. The condition occurs mainly in the late teens and early adult life. It is found rarely in infants, small children, or the aged. Women are affected more commonly than men, a fact that may be related to the frequent occurrence of keloids in pierced ear lobes. There is a striking prevalence in dark-skinned persons, especially those of African and East Indian descent. In fact, keloids are about five to six times more common in blacks than in whites. Increased familial incidence has been repeatedly reported. Bloom,[177] for instance, described an Italian family in New York in which

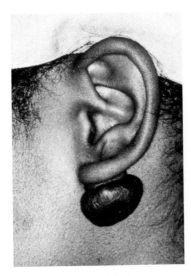

FIG. 9-38. Keloid in an 18-year-old black woman that occurred following piercing of earlobes for earrings.

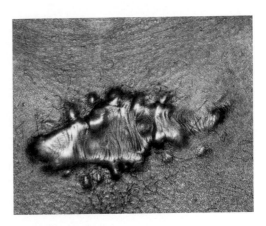

FIG. 9-39. "Spontaneous" keloid in the presternal region. These lesions may develop as the result of minor infection in an area of increased skin tension.

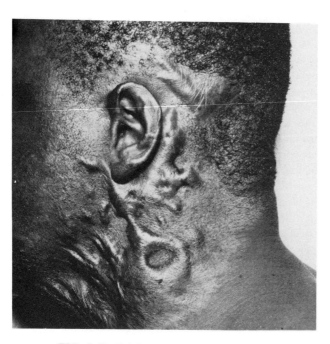

FIG. 9-40. Keloid following thermal injury.

14 members were affected over five generations. He found 31 familial cases of keloids in the literature.

As mentioned elsewhere, association of keloids with palmar, plantar, and penile fibromatosis has been observed. The possibility of an association between peptic ulcers and keloids has also been raised.[174]

Pathological findings

The disorder principally involves the corium and consists of thick, glassy, or hyalinized collagen fibers that are deeply acidophilic and haphazardly arranged. They are associated with comparatively small numbers of fibroblasts and a matrix rich in the mucinous material (Fig. 9-41). Early lesions tend to be more vascular, particularly at their periphery; late lesions are more prominently hyalinized, possess a less conspicuous vascular component, and consequently have a firm, white, scarlike gross appearance. Occasional keloids of long standing undergo calcification and osseous metaplasia. The epidermis overlying the lesion is either unaltered or shows mild acanthosis. Epidermal atrophy may be found in late stages of the disease. Ultrastructurally, keloids are composed of fibroblasts with prominent Golgi complexes and abundant rough endoplasmic reticulum.[192]

Hypertrophic scars share the microscopic picture of keloids in the early phase of the lesion, but in later stages, they flatten out and have a lesser amount of mucoid matrix and few or no glassy collagen fibers. The initial cellular

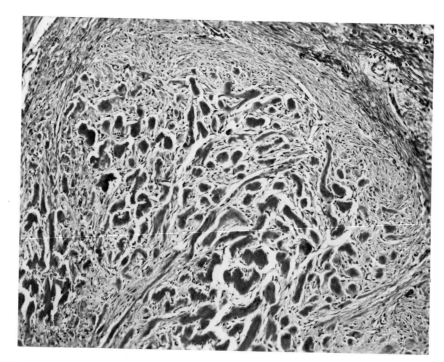

FIG. 9-41. Keloid displaying thick glassy eosinophilic fibers within fibroblastic tissue. (×100.)

phase is also marked by a greater proportion of myofibroblasts, which may play a role in the contraction and elevation of the scar tissue.[173,184] In contrast to keloid, the changes are strictly limited to the area of injury.[176,188] Kemble,[188] who examined keloids and hypertrophic scars with the scanning electron microscope, found a similar parallel arrangement of collagen fibers in both lesions.

Collagenoma, a "connective tissue nevus," is an intradermal fibrocollagenous nodule that microscopically resembles a hypertrophic scar or keloid, but there is no history of acne or dermal injury. The condition presents clinically as multiple discrete, asymptomatic, skin-colored nodules of small size that affect mainly the regions of the trunk and the proximal portion of the upper extremities. In general, they make their first appearance in the postpubertal period and are frequently found in two or more members of the same family. Their number is significantly increased during pregnancy.[183,197,199,200]

Circumscribed storiform collagenoma (sclerotic fibroma) and *fibrous papules of the face* are two other morphologically related lesions. The former presents as a solitary dermal nodule composed of glassy thickened collagen fibers arranged in a storiform pattern. It is identical to the fibrous nodules occurring in the multiple hamartoma syndrome or Cowden's disease.[191,194] The term *fibrous papules of the face* has been applied to a small dome-shaped fibrous nodule of the nose and face with an "onion skin" periadnexal or perivascular collagen pattern. This lesion has also been described as perifollicular fibroma and melanocytic angiofibroma.[182,193,196,198,203]

Scleroderma (morphea) is characterized by thickening and altered staining characteristics of existing collagen fibers but without new fiber formation and, consequently, without elevation of the skin.

Treatment

Keloids have been treated by various modes of therapy, ranging from application of pressure pads or topical injection of corticosteroids to surgery combined with interstitial irradiation or steroid therapy. Acne and postvaccination keloids have been noted to respond poorly to radiotherapy.[173,179,187,201] Obviously, as a general rule, elective cosmetic procedures should be avoided in patients having a tendency toward formation of keloids.

Discussion

Keloids remain stationary and do not regress or level off as ordinary scars do. Blackburn and Cosman,[176] who studied the histological picture of 116 keloids and 39 hypertrophic scars, reported recurrence in 64% of the former lesions and in only 10% of the latter.

Chemical analysis and comparison of the collagen in keloids and hypertrophic scars[172,178,180,185] revealed increased collagen, procollagen, and fibronectin synthesis and elevated proline hydroxylase in early keloids but only minor differences in their acid-soluble components and collagenolytic activity, indicating that the anabolic phase in keloids is disproportionately accelerated.

REFERENCES

Fibrous connective tissue: structure and function

1. Bhawan J: The myofibroblast. *Am J Dermatopathol* 3:73, 1981.
2. Bloom W, Fawcett DW: *A textbook of histology,* ed 10. Philadelphia, WB Saunders Co, 1986.
3. Caterson B, Baker JR, Christner JE, et al: Immunological methods for the detection and determination of connective tissue proteoglycans. *J Invest Dermatol* 79:45s, 1982.
4. Gabbiani G, Ryan GB, Majno G: Presence of modified fibroblasts in granulation tissue and their possible role in wound contraction. *Experientia* 27:549, 1971.
5. Hasegawa T, Hirose T, Kudo E, et al: Cytoskeletal characteristics of myofibroblasts in benign neoplastic and reactive fibroblastic lesions. *Virchows Arch (Pathol Anat)* 416:375, 1990.
6. Majno G: The story of the myofibroblasts. *Am J Surg Pathol* 3:535, 1979.
7. Rhodin JG: *Histology: A text and atlas.* New York, Oxford University Press, 1974.
8. Schürch W, Seemayer TA, Lagace R, et al: The intermediate filament cytoskeleton of myofibroblasts: an immunofluorescence and ultrastructural study. *Virchows Arch (Pathol Anat)* 403:323, 1984.
9. Seemayer TA, Lagace R, Schürch W, et al: The myofibroblast: biologic, pathologic, and theoretical considerations. *Pathol Ann* 15:443, 1980.
10. Seemayer TA, Schürch W, Lagace R: Myofibroblasts in human pathology. *Hum Pathol* 12:491, 1981.
11. Silbert JE: Structure and metabolism of proteoglycans and glycosaminoglycans. *J Invest Dermatol* 79:31 suppl 1, 1982.
12. Uitto J, Perejda A: *Diseases of connective tissue: the molecular pathology of the extracellular matrix.* New York, 1987, Marcel Deker.

Nodular fasciitis

13. Allen PW: Nodular fasciitis. *Pathology* 4:9, 1972.
14. Barohn RJ, Kasdon DL: Cranial fasciitis: nodular fasciitis of the head. *Surg Neurol* 13:283, 1980.
15. Bennet RM, Herron A, Keogh L: Eosinophilic fasciitis: case report and review of the literature. *Ann Rheum Dis* 36:354, 1977.
16. Bernstein KE, Lattes R: Nodular (pseudosarcomatous) fasciitis, a nonrecurrent lesion: clinicopathologic study of 134 cases. *Cancer* 49:1668, 1982.
17. Black SP, Adelstein E, Levine C: Atypical fibrous histiocytoma in the skull of an infant: case report. *J Neurosurg* 53:556, 1980.
18. Bodner L, Dayan D: Nodular fasciitis of the oral mucosa: light and electron microscopy study. *Head Neck* 13:434, 1991.
19. Bono JA: Nodular pseudosarcomatous fasciitis: two case reports and review of the literature. *Am Surg* 40:601, 1974.
20. Bückmann F: Tumorähnliche bindegewebige Proliferation in Subcutis und Muskulatur (noduläre Fasciitis). *Zbl Allg Path* 109:451, 1961.
21. Cramer SF, Kent L, Abramowsky C, et al: Eosinophilic fasciitis:

immunopathology, ultrastructure, literature review and consideration of its pathogenesis and relation to scleroderma. *Arch Pathol Lab Med* 106:85, 1982.

22. Culberson JD, Enterline HT: Pseudosarcomatous fasciitis. A distinctive clinical-pathologic entity: report of five cases. *Ann Surg* 151:235, 1960.

23. Dahl I, Akerman M: Nodular fasciitis: a correlative cytologic and histologic study of 113 cases. *Acta Cytol* 25:215, 1981.

24. Dahl I, Angervall L: Pseudosarcomatous lesions of the soft tissues reported as sarcoma during a 6-year period (1958-1963). *Acta Pathol Microbiol Scand* 85:917, 1977.

25. Dahl I, Angervall L: Pseudosarcomatous proliferative lesions of soft tissue with or without bone formations. *Acta Pathol Microbiol Scand* 85:577, 1977.

26. Dahl I, Angervall L, Magnusson S, et al: Classical and cystic nodular fasciitis. *Pathol Eur* 7:211, 1972.

27. Dahl I, Jarlstedt J: Nodular fasciitis in the head and neck: a clinicopathological study of 18 cases. *Acta Otolaryngol* 90:152, 1980.

28. Daroca PJ, Pulitzer DR, LeCicero J: Ossifying fasciitis. *Arch Lab Med* 106:682, 1982.

29. Dupree WB, Enzinger FM: Fibro-osseous pseudotumor of the digits. *Cancer* 58:2103, 1986.

30. Eckstein HB, Pincott JR: Cranio-spinal fasciitis in infancy. *Z Kinderchirurgie* 36:23, 1982.

31. El-Jabbour JN, Wilson GD, Bennett MH, et al: Flow cytometric study of nodular fasciitis, proliferative fasciitis, and proliferative myositis. *Hum Pathol* 22:1146, 1991.

32. Enzinger, FM: Recent trends in soft tissue pathology. In *Tumors of bone and soft tissue*, Chicago, 1965, Year Book Medical Publishers, pp 324 ff.

33. Fu TS, Soltani K, Sorensen LB, et al: Eosinophilic fasciitis. *JAMA* 240:451, 1978.

34. Gordon GV: Eosinophilic fasciitis: a case report and review of the literature. *Cutis* 28:271, 1981.

35. Hasegawa T, Hirose T, Kudo E, et al: Cytoskeletal characteristics of myofibroblasts in benign neoplastic and reactive fibroblastic lesions. *Virchows Arch (Pathol Anat)* 416:375, 1990.

36. Henny FA, Catone GA, Walker RB, et al: Pseudosarcomatous fasciitis: report of three cases. *J Oral Surg* 27:196, 1969.

37. Hutter RV, Foote FW, Francis KC, et al: Parosteal fasciitis. A self-limited benign process that simulates a malignant neoplasm. *Am J Surg* 104:800, 1962.

38. Hutter RV, Stewart FW, Foote FW Jr: Fasciitis: a report of 70 cases with follow-up proving the benignity of the lesion. *Cancer* 15:992, 1962.

39. Iwasaki H, Enjoji M: Nodular fasciitis: A clinicopathologic study of 84 cases. *Jpn J Cancer Clin* 18:793, 1972.

40. Kamino H, Lee JY, Berke A: Pleomorphic fibroma of the skin: a benign neoplasm with cytologic atypia: a clinicopathologic study of eight cases. *Am J Surg Pathol* 13:107, 1989.

41. Kleinstiver BJ, Rodriguez HA: Nodular fasciitis: a study of 45 cases and review of the literature. *J Bone Joint Surg* 50A:1204, 1968.

42. Konwaler BE, Keasbey L, Kaplan L: Subcutaneous pseudosarcomatous fibromatosis (fasciitis): report of 8 cases. *Am J Clin Pathol* 25:241, 1955.

43. Kwittken J, Branche M: Fasciitis ossificans. *Am J Clin Pathol* 51:251, 1969.

44. Lauer DH, Enzinger FM: Cranial fasciitis of childhood. *Cancer* 45:401, 1980.

45. Martin RW, Duffy J, Lie JT: Eosinophilic fasciitis associated with use of L-tryptophan: a case-control study and comparison of clinical and histopathologic features. *Mayo Clin Proc* 66:892, 1991.

46. Mehregan AH: Nodular fasciitis. *Arch Dermatol* 93:204, 1966.

47. Meister P, Bückmann FW, Konrad E: Nodular fasciitis (analysis of 100 cases and review of the literature). *Pathol Res Pract* 162:133, 1978.

48. Meyer CA, Kransdorf MJ, Jelinek JS, et al: MR and CT appearance of nodular fasciitis. *J Comput Assist Tomogr* 15:276, 1991.

49. Michet CJ Jr, Doyle JA, Ginsburg WW: Eosinophilic fasciitis: report of 15 cases. *Mayo Clin Proc* 56:27, 1981.

50. Miller R, Cheris L, Stratigos GT: Nodular fasciitis. *Oral Surg Oral Med Oral Pathol* 40:399, 1975.

51. Montgomery EA, Meis JM: Nodular fasciitis: its morphologic spectrum and immunohistochemical profile. *Am J Surg Pathol* 15:942, 1991.

52. Mozzicato P, Azumi N, Leslie K: Expression of alpha actin in non muscle sarcomas and sarcoma-like lesions. *Mod Pathol* 3:70A, 1990 (abstract).

53. Pasquier B, Keddari E, Pasquier D, et al: Fasciite cranienne de l'enfant: á propos d'un cas a révélation neonatale avec extension dure-mérienne. *Ann Pathol* 4:371, 1984.

54. Patchefsky AS, Enzinger FM: Intravascular fasciitis: a report of 17 cases. *Am J Surg Pathol* 5:29, 1981.

55. Phelan JT, Jurado J: Pseudosarcomatous fasciitis. *N Engl J Med* 266:645, 1962.

56. Polan S, Butterworth T: Cutis verticis gyrata: a review with report of seven new cases. *Am J Ment Defic* 57:613, 1953.

57. Price EB, Silliphant WM, Shuman R: Nodular fasciitis. *Am J Clin Pathol* 35:122, 1961.

58. Ringsted J, Ladefoged C, Bjerre P: Cranial fasciitis of childhood. *Acta Neuropathol* 66:337, 1985.

59. Rouse TM, Malangoni MA, Schulte WJ: Necrotizing fasciitis: a preventable disaster. *Surgery* 92:765, 1982.

60. Sengupta RP, So SC, Perry RH: Nodular fasciitis: an unusual cause of extradural spinal cord compression. *Br J Surg* 62:573. 1975.

61. Sherwin RP, Friedell GH: Pseudosarcomatous fibromatosis (infiltrative fasciitis). Report of two cases. *Boston Med Q* 10:49, 1959.

62. Shimizu S, Hashimoto H, Enjoji M: Nodular fasciitis: an analysis of 250 patients. *Pathology* 16:161, 1984.

63. Shulman LE: Diffuse fasciitis with hypergammaglobulinemia and eosinophilia. *J Rheumatol* 1(suppl.):46, 1974.

64. Sormann GW: The headbangers tumour. *Br J Plast Surg* 35:72, 1982.

65. Soule EH: Proliferative (nodular) fasciitis. *Arch Pathol* 73:437, 1962.

66. Stamencovic I, Lew DP: Early recognition of potentially fatal necrotizing fasciitis: the use of frozen-section biopsy. *N Engl J Med* 310:1689, 1984.

67. Stiller D, Katenkamp D: Die noduläre Fasziitis. *Zentralbl Chir* 98:885, 1973.

68. Stout AP: Pseudosarcomatous fasciitis in children. *Cancer* 14:1216, 1961.

69. Toker C: Pseudosarcomatous fasciitis: further observations indicating the aggressive capabilities of this lesion and justifying the inclusion of this entity within the category of the fibromatoses. *Ann Surg* 174:994, 1971.

70. Wallace RT, Wilson RS, Cain JR: Pseudosarcomatous fasciitis. *South Med J* 55:475, 1962.

71. Weiss SW: Proliferative fibroblastic lesions: from hyperplasia to neoplasia. *Am J Surg Pathol* 10 (suppl 1):14, 1986.

72. Werning JT: Nodular fasciitis of the oral region. *Oral Med Oral Pathol* 48:441, 1979.

73. Winkelmann RK, Connolly SM, Quimby SR, et al: Histopathologic features of the L-tryptophan-related eosinophilia-myalgia (fasciitis) syndrome. *Mayo Clin Proc* 66:457, 1991.

74. Wirman JA: Nodular fasciitis, a lesion of myofibroblasts: an ultrastructural study. *Cancer* 38:2378, 1976.

Proliferative fasciitis and proliferative myositis

75. Brooks JJ: Proliferative myositis. *Arch Pathol* 105:682, 1981.

76. Chung EB, Enzinger FM: Proliferative fasciitis. *Cancer* 36:1450, 1975.

77. Craver JL, McDivitt RW: Proliferative fasciitis: utrastructural study of two cases. *Arch Pathol Lab Med* 105:542, 1981.

78. El-Jabbour JN, Bennett MH, Burke MM, et al: Proliferative myositis: an immunohistochemical and ultrastructural study. *Am J Surg Pathol* 15:654, 1991.

79. Enzinger FM, Dulcey F: Proliferative myositis: report of 33 cases. *Cancer* 20:2213, 1967.

80. Gokel JM, Meister P, Huebner G: Proliferative myositis: a case report with fine structural analysis. *Virchows Arch (Pathol Anat)* 367:345, 1975.

81. Kern WH: Proliferative myositis: a pseudosarcomatous reaction to injury. *Arch Pathol* 69:209, 1960.

82. Kitano M, Iwasaki H, Enjoji M: Proliferative fasciitis: a variant of nodular fasciitis. *Acta Pathol Jpn* 27:485, 1977.

83. Meis JM, Enzinger FM: Proliferative fasciitis and myositis of childhood. *Am J Surg Pathol* 16:364, 1992.

84. Montgomery EA, Meis JM, Mitchell MS, et al: Atypical decubital fibroplasia: a distinctive fibroblastic pseudotumor occurring in debilitated patients. *Am J Surg Pathol* 16:708, 1992.

85. Pages A, Dossa J, Pages M: La myosite proliferante, un pseudo-sarcome musculaire: a propos d'un cas avec examen ultrastructural. *Ann Pathol* 3:161, 1983.

86. Perosio PM, Weiss SW: Ischemic fasciitis: a juxta-skeletal fibroblastic proliferation with a predilection for elderly patients. *Mod Pathol* 6:69, 1993.

87. Rose AG: An electron microscopic study of the giant cells in proliferative myositis. *Cancer* 33:1543, 1974.

88. Stiller D, Katenkamp D: The subcutaneous fascial analogue of myositis proliferans: electron microscopic examination of two cases and comparison with myositis ossificans localisata. *Virchows Arch (Pathol Anat)* 368:361, 1975.

89. Tennstedt A: Beitrag zur proliferativen Myositis, einer wahrscheinlichen Variante der pseudosarkomatösen Fasciitis. *Zentralbl Allg Pathol* 116:364, 1972.

90. Ushigome S, Takakuwa T, Takagi M, et al: Proliferative myositis and fasciitis. Report of five cases with an ultrastructural and immunohistochemical study. *Acta Pathol Jpn* 36:963, 1986.

Fibroma of tendon sheath

91. Azzopardi JG, Tanda F, Salm R: Tenosynovial fibroma. *Diagn Histopathol* 6:69, 1983.

92. Chung EB, Enzinger FM: Fibroma of tendon sheath. *Cancer* 44:1945, 1979.

93. Lamovec J, Bracko M, Voncina D: Pleomorphic fibroma of tendon sheath. *Am J Surg Pathol* 15:1202, 1991.

94. Lundgren LG, Kindblom LG: Fibroma of tendon sheath: a light and electron-microscopic study of six cases. *Acta Pathol Microbiol Immunol Scand* 92A:401, 1984.

95. Pulitzer DR, Martin PC, Reed RJ: Fibroma of tendon sheath: a clinicopathologic study of 32 cases. *Am J Surg Pathol* 13:472, 1989.

96. Smith PS, Pieterse AS, McClure J: Fibroma of tendon sheath. *J Clin Pathol* 35:842, 1982.

Elastofibroma

97. Akhtar M, Miller RM: Ultrastructure of elastofibroma. *Cancer* 40:728, 1977.

98. Banfield WG, Lee CK: Elastofibroma: an electron microscopic study. *J Natl Cancer Inst* 40:1067, 1968.

99. Barr JR: Elastofibroma. *Am J Clin Pathol* 45:679, 1966.

100. Benisch B, Peison B, Marquet E, et al: Pre-elastofibroma and elastofibroma (the continuum of elastic-producing fibrous tumors): a light and ultrastructural study. *Am J Clin Pathol* 80:88, 1983.

101. Brown RK, Clearkin KP, Nakachi K, et al: Elastofibroma dorsi. *N Engl J Med* 275:154, 1966.

102. Cross DL, Mills SE, Kulund DN: Elastofibroma arising in the foot. *South Med J* 77:1194, 1984.

103. Delvaux TC, Lester JP: Elastofibroma dorsi. *Am J Clin Pathol* 43:72, 1965.

104. Deutsch GP: Elastofibroma dorsalis treated by radiotherapy. *Br J Radiol* 47:621, 1974.

105. Dixon AY, Lee SH: An ultrastructural study of elastofibromas. *Hum Pathol* 11:257, 1980.

106. Enjoji M, Kikuchi J: Elastofibroma dorsi. *Acta Pathol Jpn* 18:239, 1968.

107. Enjoji M, Sumiyoshi K, Sueyoshi K: Elastofibromatous lesion of the stomach in a patient with elastofibroma dorsi. *Am J Surg Pathol* 9:233, 1985.

108. Fukuda Y, Miyake H, Masuda Y, et al: Histogenesis of unique elastinophilic fibers of elastofibroma: ultrastructural and immunohistochemical studies. *Hum Pathol* 18:424, 1987.

109. Goldblum JR, Beals T, Weiss SW: Elastofibromatous change of the rectum: a lesion mimicking amyloidosis. *Am J Surg Pathol* 16:793, 1992.

110. Gonzalez-Crussi F, Ramchand S, Molony R, et al: Elastofibroma dorsi. *Can Med Assoc J* 100:374, 1969.

111. Hayashi K, Ohtsuki Y, Sonobe H, et al: Pre-elastofibroma like colonic polyp: another cause of colonic polyp. *Acta Med Okayama* 45:49, 1991.

112. Järvi OH, Länsimies PH: Subclinical elastofibromas in the scapular region in an autopsy series. *Acta Pathol Microbiol Scand* 83:87, 1975.

113. Järvi OH, Saxén E: Elastofibroma dorsi. *Acta Pathol Microbiol Scand* 51:83, 1961.

114. Järvi OH, Saxén E, Hopsu-Havu VK, et al: Elastofibroma—a degenerative pseudotumor. *Cancer* 23:42, 1969.

115. Kindblom LG, Spicer SS: Elastofibroma: a correlated light and electron microscopic study. *Virchows Arch (Pathol Anat)* 396:127, 1982.

116. Kransdorf MJ, Meis JM, Montgomery E: Elastofibroma: MR and CT appearance with radiologic-pathologic correlation. *Am J Roentgenol* 159:575, 1992.

117. Kumaratilake JS, Krishnan R, Lomax-Smith J, et al: Elastofibroma: Disturbed elastic fibrillogenesis by periosteal-derived cells? An immunoelectron microscopic and in situ hybridization study. *Hum Pathol* 22:1017, 1991.

118. Mackenzie DH, Wilson JF, Cooke KB: Elastofibroma. *J Clin Pathol* 21:470, 1968.

119. Madri JA, Dise CA, Livolsi VA, et al: Elastofibroma dorsi: an immunochemical study of collagen content. *Hum Pathol* 12:186, 1981.

120. Mirra JM, Straub LR, Järvi OH: Elastofibroma of the deltoid: a case report. *Cancer* 33:234, 1974.

121. Nagamine N, Endo I, Genga K, et al: A clinicopathological study of elastofibroma. *Jpn J Cancer Clin* 24:1023, 1978.

122. Nagamine N, Miyagi Y, Endo J, et al: Elastofibroma: a clinicopathological study of 21 cases. *Jpn J Cancer Clin* 23:203, 1977.

123. Nagamine N, Nohara Y, Ito E: Elastofibroma in Okinawa: a clinicopathologic study of 170 cases. *Cancer* 50:1794, 1982.

124. Nakamura Y, Okamoto K, Tanimura A, et al: Elastase digestion and biochemical analysis of the elastin from an elastofibroma. *Cancer* 58:1070, 1986.

125. Peters JL, Fisher CS: Elastofibroma: case report and literature review. *J Thorac Cardiovasc Surg* 75:836, 1978.

126. Pierson RW, Jones HW: Elastofibroma. *Bull Mason Clin* 24:141, 1970.

127. Ramos CV, Gillespie W, Narconis RJ: Elastofibroma: a pseudotumor of myofibroblasts. *Arch Pathol Lab Med* 102:538, 1978.

128. Reed R, Bliss BO: Morton's neuroma. *Arch Pathol Lab Med* 95:123, 1973.

129. Stemmerman GN, Stout AP: Elastofibroma dorsi. *Am J Clin Pathol* 38:499, 1962.

130. Tighe JR, Clark AE, Turvey DJ: Elastofibroma dorsi. *J Clin Pathol* 21:463, 1968.

131. Waisman J, Smith DW: Fine structure of an elastofibroma. *Cancer* 22:671, 1968.

132. Winkelmann RK, Sams WM Jr: Elastofibroma: report of a case with special histochemical and electron microscopic studies. *Cancer* 23:406, 1969.

Nasopharyngeal angiofibroma

133. Acuna RT: Nasopharyngeal fibroma. *Acta Otolaryngol* 75:119, 1973.

134. Apostol JV, Frazell EL: Juvenile nasopharyngeal angiofibroma: a clinical study. *Cancer* 18:869, 1965.

135. Arnold JV, Huth F: Electron microscopic findings in four cases of nasopharyngeal fibroma. *Vichows Arch (Pathol Anat)* 379:285, 1978.

136. Batsakis JG, Klopp GT, Newman W: Fibrosarcoma arising in "juvenile" nasopharyngeal angiofibroma following extensive radiation treatment. *Am Surg* 21:786, 1955.

137. Bourne RG, Taylor RG: Treatment of a juvenile laryngeal angioma with a beta-ray therapy applicator. *Radiology* 103:423, 1972.

138. Briant TD, Fitzpatrick PJ, Book H: The radiological treatment of juvenile nasopharyngeal angiofibromas. *Ann Otol Rhinol Laryngol* 79:1108, 1970.

139. Chandler JR, Goulding R, Moskowitz L, et al: Nasopharyngeal angiofibromas: staging and management. *Ann Otol Rhinol Laryngol* 93:322, 1984.

140. Chen KTK, Bauer FW: Sarcomatous transformation of nasopharyngeal angiofibroma. *Cancer* 49:369, 1982.

141. Cummings BJ, Blend R, Keane T, et al: Primary radiation therapy for juvenile nasopharyngeal angiofibroma. *Laryngoscope* 94:1599, 1984.

142. Dorn A, Nowak R, Dietzel K, et al: Untersuchungen am juvenilen Nasenrachenfibrom. I. Mitteilung: Histochemie und Elektronenmikroskopie. *Acta Histochem* 39:162, 1971.

143. Figi FA, Davis RE: Management of nasopharyngeal fibroma. *Laryngoscope* 60:794, 1950.

144. Fitzpatrick PJ, Book H, Briant TD: The radiological treatment of juvenile nasopharyngeal angiofibromas. *Ann Otol Rhinol Laryngol* 79:108, 1970.

145. Fu YS, Perzin KH: Non-epithelial tumors of the nasal cavity, paranasal sinuses, and nasopharynx: a clinicopathologic study. I. General features and vascular tumors. *Cancer* 33:1275, 1974.

146. Gisselsson L, Lindgren M, Stenram WT: Sarcomatous transformation of juvenile nasopharyngeal angiofibroma. *Acta Pathol Microbiol Scand* 42:305, 1958.

147. Hazarika P, Nayak RG, Chandran M: Extra-nasopharyngeal extension of juvenile angiofibroma. *J Laryngol Otol* 99:813, 1985.

148. Heffner DK: Problems in pediatric otorhinolaryngic pathology. II. Vascular tumors and lesions of the sinonasal tract and nasopharynx. *Int J Pediatr Otorhinolaryngol* 5:125, 1983.

149. Hill DL: Morphology of nasopharyngeal angiofibroma: an electron microscope study. *J Submicrosc Cytol Pathol* 17:443, 1985.

150. Hiranandani LH, Melgiri RD, Juveker RV: Angiofibroma of the ethmoidal sinus in a female. *J Laryngol* 81:935, 1967.

151. Holman CB, Miller WE: Juvenile nasopharyngeal fibroma: roentgenologic characteristics. *Am J Roentgenol* 94:292, 1965.

152. Isherwood I, Dogra TS, Farrington WT: Extranasopharyngeal juvenile angiofibroma. *J Laryngol* 89:535, 1975.

153. Küttner K: Ultrahistochemische Untersuchungen an den Kerneinschlusskörpern des juvenilen Nasenrachenfibroms. *Z Laryngol Rhinol Otol* 52:748, 1973.

154. McGavran MH, Sessions DG, Dorfman RF, et al: Nasopharyngeal angiofibroma. *Arch Otolaryngol* 90:68, 1969.

155. Neel HB III, Whicker JH, Devine KD, et al: Juvenile angiofibroma: review of 120 cases. *Am J Surg* 126:547, 1973.

156. Nowak R, Dorn A, Reichel A: Elektronenmikroskopische Untersuchungen am juvenilen Nasen-Rachen-Fibrom. *Arch Otorhinolaryngol* 206:103, 1974.

157. Osborn DA, Sokolowski A: Juvenile nasopharyngeal angiofibroma in a female: report of a case. *Arch Otolaryngol* 82:629, 1965.

158. Perko M, Uehlinger E, Hjorting-Hansen E: Nasopharyngeal angiofibroma of the maxilla: report of a case. *J Oral Surg* 27:645, 1969.

159. Rodriguez H: A new surgical approach to nasopharyngeal angiofibroma. *Cancer* 19:458, 1966.

160. Rominger CJ, Santore FJ: Juvenile nasopharyngeal fibroma in female adult: report of a case. *Arch Otolaryngol* 88:85, 1968.

161. Seifert K: Elektronenmikroskopische Untersuchungen am juvenilen Nasenrachenfibrom. *Arch Klin Exp Ohren Nasen u Kehlkopfheilkd* 198:215, 1971.

162. Sternberg SS: Pathology of juvenile nasopharyngeal angiofibroma—a lesion of adolescent males. *Cancer* 7:15, 1954.

163. Spagnolo DV, Papadimitriou JM, Archer M: Postradiation malignant fibrous histiocytoma arising in juvenile nasopharyngeal angiofibroma and producing alpha-1-antitrypsin. *Histopathology* 8:339, 1984.

164. Stiller D, Katenkamp D, Küttner K: Cellular differentiations and structural characteristics in nasopharyngeal angiofibromas: an electron-microscopic study. *Virchows Arch (Pathol Anat)* 371:273, 1976.

165. Svoboda DJ, Kirchner F: Ultrastructure of nasopharyngeal angiofibromas. *Cancer* 39:1044, 1977.

166. Taxy JB: Juvenile nasopharyngeal angiofibroma. An ultrastructural study. *Cancer* 39:1044, 1977.

167. Thomsen KA: Surgical treatment of juvenile nasopharyngeal angiofibroma. *Arch Otolaryngol* 94:191, 1971.

168. Topilko A, Zakrzewski A, Pichard E, et al: Ultrastructural cytochemistry of intranuclear dense granules in nasopharyngeal angiofibroma. *Ultrastruct Pathol* 6:221, 1984.

169. Walike JW: Contrast nasopharyngography of angiofibromata. *Arch Otolaryngol* 86:676, 1967.

170. Walike JW, Mackay B: Nasopharyngeal angiofibroma. Light and electron microscopic changes after stilbesterol therapy. *Laryngoscope* 80:1109, 1970.

171. Ward PH, Thompson R, Calcaterra T, et al: Juvenile angiofibroma. A more rational therapeutic approach based upon clinical and experimental evidence. *Laryngoscope* 84:2181, 1974.

Keloid

172. Abergel RP, Pizurro D, Meeker CA, et al: Biochemical composition of the connective tissue in keloids and analysis of collagen metabolism in keloid fibroblastic cultures. *J Invest Dermatol* 84:384, 1985.

173. Arnold H Jr, Grauer F: Keloids, etiology and management by excision and intensive prophylactic radiation. *Arch Dermatol* 80:772, 1959.

174. Asboe-Hanson G: Hypertrophic scars and keloids. *Dermatologia* 120:178, 1960.

175. Baur PS, Larson DL, Stacey TR: The observation of myofibroblasts in hypertrophic scars. *Surg Gynecol Obstet* 141:22, 1975.

176. Blackburn WR, Cosman B: Histologic basis of keloid and hypertrophic scar differentiation. Clinicopathologic correlation. *Arch Pathol* 82:65, 1966.

177. Bloom D: Heredity of keloids: review of the literature and report of a family with multiple keloids in five generations. *N Y State J Med* 56:511, 1956.

178. Cohen IK, Keiser HP, Sjoerdsma A: Collagen synthesis in human keloid and hypertrophic scar. *Surg Forum* 22:488, 1971.

179. Cosman B, Crikelair GF, Gaulin MC, et al: The treatment of keloids. *Plast Reconstr Surg* 44:564, 1969.

180. Craig RD, Schofield JD, Jackson DS: Collagen biosynthesis in normal and hypertrophic scars and keloids as a function of the duration of the scar. *Br J Surg* 62:741, 1975.

181. Garb J, Stone JM: Keloids: review of the literature and a report of 80 cases. *Am J Surg* 58:315, 1942.

182. Graham JH, Sanders JB, Johnson WC, et al: Fibrous papule of the nose. *J Invest Dermatol* 45:194, 1965.

183. Hegedus SI, Schorr WF: Familial cutaneous collagenoma. *Cutis* 10:283, 1972.

184. Holmstrand K, Longacre JJ, DeStefano GA: The ultrastructure of collagen in skin, scar, and keloids. *Plast Reconstr Surg* 27:597, 1961.

185. Hoppes JE, Su CT, Im MJC: Enzyme activities in hypertrophic scars and keloids. *Plast Reconstr Surg* 47:132, 1971.

186. Hutchinson J: On keloids. *Arch Surg* 4:233, 1983.

187. Inalsingh CH: An experience in treating 501 patients with keloids. *Johns Hopkins Med J* 134:284, 1974.

188. Kemble JV: Scanning electronmicroscopy of hypertrophic and keloid scar. *Postgrad Med J* 52:219, 1976.

189. Ketchum LD, Cohen IK, Masters FW: Hypertrophic scars and keloids: a collective review. *Plast Reconstr Surg* 53:140, 1974.

190. King GD, Salzman FA: Keloid scars: analysis of 89 patients. *Surg Clin North Am* 50:595, 1970.

191. Maize J, Leidel G, Mullins S, et al: Circumscribed storiform collagenoma. *Am J Dermatopathol* 11:287, 1989 (abstract).

192. Matsuoka LY, Uitto J, Wortsman J, et al: Ultrastructural characteristics of keloid fibroblasts. *Am J Dermatopathol* 10:505, 1988.

193. Meigel WN, Ackerman AB: Fibrous papule of the face. *Am J Dermatopathol* 1:329, 1979.

194. Metcalf JS, Maize JC, LeBoit PE: Circumscribed storiform collagenoma (sclerosing fibroma). *Am J Dermatopathol* 13:122, 1991.

195. Pierard GE, Lapiere CM: Nevi of connective tissue: a reappraisal of their classification. *Am J Dermatopathol* 7:325, 1985.

196. Reed RJ, Hariston MA, Palomieque FE: The histologic identity of adenoma sebacceum and solitary melanocytic angiofibroma. *Dermatol Int* 5:3, 1966.

197. Rocha G, Winkelman RK: Connective tissue nevus. *Arch Dermatol* 85:722, 1962.

198. Rosen LB, Suster S: Fibrous papules: a light microscopic and immunohistochemical study. *Am J Dermatopathol* 10:109, 1988.

199. Smith AD, Weissman M: Connective tissue nevi. *Arch Dermatol* 102:390, 1970.

200. Uitto J, Santa Cruz D, Eisen A: Familial cutaneous collagenoma: clinical, histological, and genetic studies. In *Diseases of connective tissue: the molecular pathology of the extracellular matrix.* New York, 1987, Marcel Dekker.

201. Van Den Brenk HAS, Minty CCJ: Radiation of the management of keloids and hypertrophic scars. *Br J Surg* 47:595, 1960.

202. Wilson WW: Prophylaxis against postsurgical keloids: results in 500 patients. *South Med J* 58:751, 1965.

203. Zackheim MS, Pinkus H: Perifollicular fibromas. *Arch Dermatol* 82:913, 1960.

CHAPTER 10

FIBROMATOSES

Fibromatoses, as proposed by Stout,[129,130] are a broad group of benign fibrous tissue proliferations of similar microscopic appearance that are intermediate in their biological behavior between benign fibrous lesions and fibrosarcoma. Like fibrosarcoma they are characterized by infiltrative growth and a tendency toward recurrence, but unlike this tumor they never metastasize.

The various entities that constitute this group occur predominantly in adults and consist of highly differentiated fibrous tissue, which forms a firm, nonencapsulated, poorly circumscribed nodule or mass that may be solitary or multiple and has a predilection for certain anatomical sites. The term *fibromatosis* should not be applied to nonspecific reactive fibrous proliferations that are part of an inflammatory process or are secondary to injury or hemorrhage and have no tendency toward infiltrative growth or recurrence.

The fibromatoses can be divided into two major groups with several subdivisions (see accompanying box).

Classification of fibromatoses

I. Superficial (fascial) fibromatoses
  A. Palmar fibromatosis (Dupuytren's disease)
  B. Plantar fibromatosis (Ledderhose's disease)
  C. Penile fibromatosis (Peyronie's disease)
  D. Knuckle pads
II. Deep (musculoaponeurotic) fibromatoses
  A. Extraabdominal fibromatosis (extraabdominal desmoid)
  B. Abdominal fibromatosis (abdominal desmoid)
  C. Intraabdominal fibromatosis (intraabdominal desmoid)
    1. Pelvic fibromatosis
    2. Mesenteric fibromatosis
    3. Mesenteric fibromatosis in Gardner's syndrome

Superficial (fascial) fibromatoses are slow growing and of small size. These lesions arise from the fascia or aponeurosis and only rarely involve deeper structures. The clinical course usually can be divided into an early, rather cellular proliferative phase and a late, richly collagenous regressive or contractile phase. Allen[63] suggested the term *Dupuytren's fibromatoses* for this group of closely related lesions.

Deep (musculoaponeurotic) fibromatoses are rapidly growing tumors that often attain a large size. They tend to be more aggressive in their behavior than the superficial (fascial) fibromatoses, have a higher recurrence rate, and, as their name indicates, principally involve deeper structures, particularly the musculature of the trunk and the extremities. The descriptive term *desmoid tumor,* coined by Mueller in 1838 to emphasize the bandlike or tendonlike consistency of the lesions, is still widely used in the literature as a synonym for this type of fibromatosis. Another less common synonym is *nonmetastasizing fibrosarcoma.* The term *grade I fibrosarcoma* should be discouraged, since it is misleading as to the potential behavior of this tumor.

Although all fascial and musculoaponeurotic fibromatoses are capable of recurrence after excision, the recurrence rate of the individual entities varies substantially. It is governed less by the histological picture than by the location of the lesion, the age of the patient, and, of course, the mode of therapy. In fact, histological examination alone does not permit accurate prediction of the clinical course. Moreover, occasional examples of fibromatosis do regress spontaneously, but the incidence and likelihood of regression, like that of recurrence, is unpredictable in the individual case. As mentioned elsewhere, malignant transformation of fibromatosis has been reported but so far only in one case and years after massive radiotherapy.[127]

PALMAR FIBROMATOSIS

This condition, which is much better known as *Dupuytren's disease* or *Dupuytren's contracture,* is by far the most common type of fibromatosis. Its incidence in the general population ranges between 1% and 2%; it is rare in children and young adults but afflicts one out of five persons in the 65 years and older age group. It occurs less frequently in women than in men and, according to most reviewers, is rarely encountered in blacks and Orientals.

As one would expect, its relatively high incidence has generated a large number of reports and reviews in the literature. Some of these date back to the seventeenth century (Felix Plater, 1630),[29] but Dupuytren (1777-1835)[7] is generally credited with the first accurate description of the disease, which to this day bears his name. The term *palmar fibromatosis* is seldom used in the literature, although it characterizes more adequately the basic disease process: a nodular fibroblastic proliferation in the volar surface of the hand, closely resembling other forms of fibromatosis. In fact, the flexion contracture of the fingers, by which the disease is most widely known, is a late but important complication of the fibroblastic growth.

As in most forms of fibromatosis, the exact cause of the fibroblastic proliferation is still unknown. Age, sex, and a hereditary factor play definite roles in the pathogenesis, but there is little solid information as to whether the disease is triggered by injury or some other mechanisms. Its close relationship to plantar and penile fibromatosis and knuckle pads is well documented.

Clinical findings

In general, the onset of the disease is slow and insidious, and the initial manifestation consists merely of an isolated firm nodule in the palmar surface of the hand, which causes no symptoms except an occasional dull ache or a slight tingling sensation. At this stage of the disease most patients ignore the lesion and rarely are sufficiently concerned to seek therapy. In about half of the cases the nodule or nodules affect one hand, with a slight predominance of the right side. In approximately 40% to 60% of the cases, the lesion affects both hands, but the bilateral lesions rarely make their first appearance at the same time. Palmar fibromatosis is seldom seen in patients younger than 30 years, but its incidence increases rapidly with advancing age, and at age 65 years the lesion affects almost 20% of the general population. According to most reviewers, the condition is about three or four times more frequent in men than in women and is relatively rare in blacks and Asians.[22,24,33,41]

Several months or years after the appearance of the fibrous nodules, cordlike indurations or bands develop between nodules and adjacent fingers, often causing puckering and dimpling of the overlying skin (Fig. 10-1). As a rule, these changes are most prominent at the ulnar side of the palm and are accompanied by flexion contracture of increasing severity, which principally affects the fourth and fifth fingers of the hand. Other fingers may become involved; least often affected are the index finger and thumb. In rare instances, involvement of the extensor apparatus

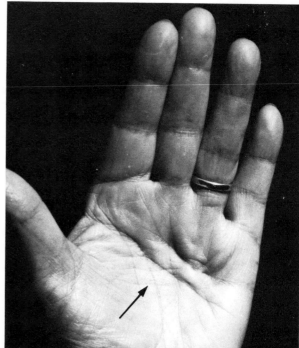

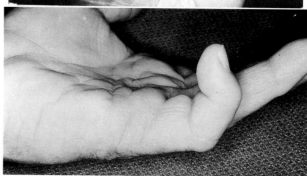

FIG. 10-1. A, Palmar fibromatosis with firm cordlike indurations and nodules causing puckering and dimpling *(arrow)* of the overlying skin. B, Flexion contracture of the fifth finger (Dupuytren's contracture).

causes hyperextension of one or more fingers. Eventually the flexion deformities or contractures of the fingers become so severe that normal function of the hand is greatly impaired, and patients find it increasingly difficult to handle tools or to shake hands. At this point therapy is usually sought. Without therapy, spontaneous improvement of the contractures is sometimes observed after a stationary period of 20 to 35 years. It is noteworthy that in some patients contractures never develop or are so slight that they cause little or no functional impairment.

There are also morphologically related but more diffuse fibrous lesions of the dorsum of the hands that have been variously described as *dorsal fibromatosis* or *peritendinous fibrosis of the dorsum of the hand (Secretan's disease).*[31]

Concurrence of palmar fibromatosis with other diseases

One of the most striking features of the disease is the coexistence with other forms of fibromatosis; in about 5% to 20% of cases, palmar fibromatosis is associated with plantar fibromatosis and in about 2% to 4% with penile fibromatosis (Peyronie's disease). Moreover, a higher incidence of knuckle pads has been observed.[23,36,68]

There is also an increased incidence in epileptic[1,2,21] and diabetic patients: according to Early's data,[8] the incidence of palmar fibromatosis is 5 times greater than normal in male epileptic patients and 11 times greater in female epileptic patients. Its incidence among diabetic patients is given as 10% by Weckesser.[39] The condition is also more common in patients suffering from chronic alcoholism and chronic liver disease[11,26,30,40] and patients having increased serum lipid levels.[34]

Gross findings

The excised tissue consists of a single small nodule or, when the tissue is obtained by fasciectomy, of an ill-defined conglomerate of several nodular masses intimately associated with portions of the thickened palmar aponeurosis and subcutaneous fat. The fibrous tissue is firm and scarlike on palpation and cuts with a gristly sensation, revealing a gray-yellow and gray-white surface; its color depends on the age of the lesion and its collagen content. The individual nodules are embedded in portions of the aponeurosis, which is readily recognized by its silvery glistening cut surface. The nodules rarely measure more than 1 cm in diameter. Occasionally they adhere to the overlying skin, and portions of the excised skin become part of the gross specimen.

Microscopic findings

The microscopic picture of the lesion varies little from case to case: in the earliest or proliferative phase of the disease it consists of one or more fibrous nodules that are strikingly cellular and are composed of plump, immature-appearing, spindle-shaped fibroblasts. The fibroblasts are of considerable uniformity and contain a variable number of mitotic figures; they are intimately associated with small to moderate amounts of collagen suspended in a matrix rich in glycosaminoglycans (mucopolysaccharides) (Figs. 10-2 and 10-3). The fibrous nodules originate within the palmar aponeurosis and extend into and replace the overlying subcutaneous fat. Because of their cellularity and mitotic activity, occasional examples of this lesion have been mistaken for fibrosarcoma (Fig. 10-4). Microhemorrhages, small deposits of hemosiderin, and scattered chronic inflammatory cells are present in some of the lesions.

Nodules that have been present for longer periods of

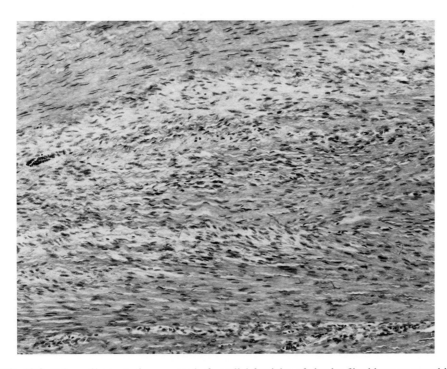

FIG. 10-2. Palmar fibromatosis composed of parallel fascicles of slender fibroblasts separated by variable amounts of collagen. (×100.)

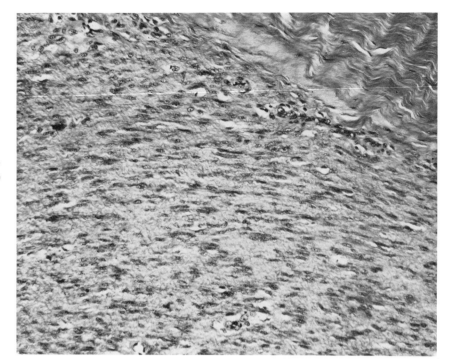

FIG. 10-3. Uniform fibroblastic proliferation in palmar fibromatosis. (×160.)

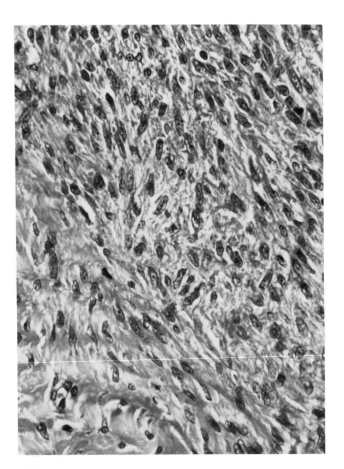

FIG. 10-4. Early, rather cellular form of palmar fibromatosis. Such lesions have been confused with fibrosarcoma, a tumor that is extremely rare in the palm of the hand. (×250.)

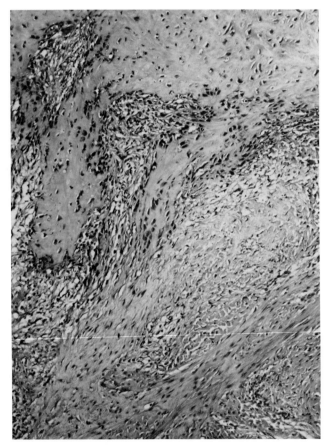

FIG. 10-5. Cartilaginous metaplasia in a late, rare form of palmar fibromatosis. (×100.)

time, ranging from 1 month to several years, are considerably less cellular and contain markedly increased amounts of dense birefringent collagen; in these cases the fibroblasts are more mature and are smaller and more slender in appearance. Similarly, the fascial or aponeurotic cords between nodules and fingers are composed of dense fibrocollagenous tissue that bears a close resemblance to tendons. Foci of osseous and cartilaginous metaplasia of the fibrous nodules are uncommon (Fig. 10-5).

Electron microscopic findings

Although ultrastructural studies of the disease were carried out prior to 1972,[5,15,27] Gabbiani and Majno[9] were the first to stress the presence of myofibroblasts; that is, a special type of fibroblast characterized by cytoplasmic extensions, well-developed rough endoplasmic reticulum, and bundles of 60- to 80-nm microfilaments with interspersed electron-dense patches (Fig. 10-6). Others also reported the presence of myofibroblasts together with typical fibroblasts, fibroblasts with lysosomes, and pericytes.[17] Kischer and Speer[18] noted at the periphery of the nodules occlusion of vascular lumina by multiple layers of basal lamina with proliferation of pericytes. They suggested that hypoxia, caused by the luminal occlusion, induces pericytes to differentiate into myofibroblasts. Like typical smooth muscle cells, the myofibroblasts have occasional basal lamina on the cellular surface and immunohistochemically react for nonmuscle myosin and fibronectin but not for smooth muscle my-

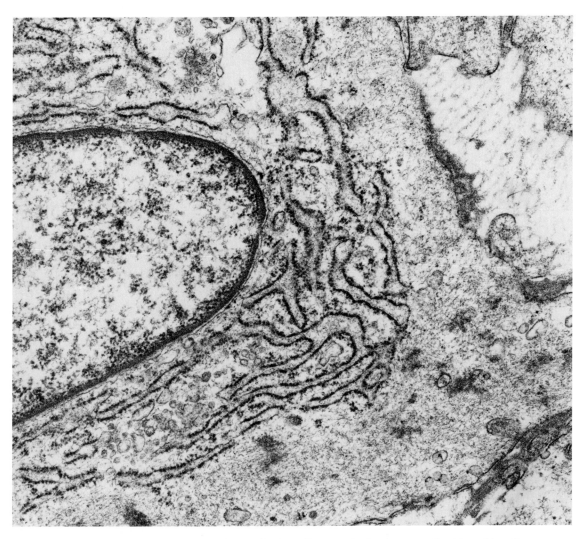

FIG. 10-6. Electron microscopic picture of palmar fibromatosis showing a myofibroblast with well-developed rough endoplasmic reticulum, interspersed and focally condensed microfilaments, and partial basal lamina. (×15,000.)

osin or laminin.[37] The myofibroblasts, under the influence of vasoactive prostaglandin, are thought to be responsible for the contraction of the lesion.[3,9] The overlying skin does not take part in the contraction and is only secondarily involved.[14,16,38]

Gokel et al.[10] distinguished three stages in the course of the disease: (1) a proliferative and predominantly fibroblastic stage, (2) an involutional myofibroblastic stage, and (3) a residual fibrocytic stage. Likewise, Hunter and Ogdon,[13] who studied the disease with the scanning electron microscope, demonstrated consecutive stages of maturation, with increasing deposition of collagen and parallel orientation of the collagen fibrils, ultimately resulting in tendonlike structures.

Differential diagnosis

Although *fibrosarcoma* of the hand is extremely rare, the cellularity and mitotic activity of the nodules in the initial stage of development may suggest malignancy. The cells of fibrosarcoma, however, tend to be arrayed in long fascicles, or a herringbone pattern, and show a greater degree of pleomorphism, with larger nuclei and a more pronounced mitotic rate, often associated with areas of necrosis. Most significantly, fibrosarcomas are nearly always deep seated, arise from muscle tissue, and affect the aponeurosis and subcutis only secondarily, while the cellular nodules in palmar fibromatosis arise within the aponeurosis and infiltrate the subcutis.

Treatment

Various forms of nonoperative therapy (cortisone, vitamin E) have been attempted in the past, but surgical extirpation remains the treatment of choice in patients with severe flexion contraction that impairs normal function of the hand. Fasciotomy, subcutaneous division of the fibrous bands, leads to immediate improvement of the contractures and can be carried out as an office procedure with little morbidity. Yet this procedure carries a high recurrence rate and may injure the digital arteries or nerves.

Fasciectomy or aponeurosectomy, complete extirpation of the palmar aponeurosis with wide exposure and skin graft when necessary, is the treatment of choice. It does not prevent recurrence in all cases, but there is a lower incidence of recurrence than in fasciotomy and much better long-term results. The advantages and disadvantages of the various therapeutic procedures have been reviewed in detail by Halliday et al.,[12] Krebs,[19] and others.[6,32,39]

Discussion

Several factors seem to play a role in the histogenesis of the disease, but their exact significance is still largely a matter of speculation. There is little doubt as to the existence of a hereditary disposition: the disease has been observed in identical twins[4] and in several generations of one fam-

ily[20,28]; it is often bilateral and, in a significant percentage of cases, is associated with plantar fibromatosis. Less often it develops together with penile fibromatosis[21,53] and knuckle pads[68]—fibrous thickening overlying the extensor surfaces of the metacarpophalangeal and proximal interphalangeal joints. Also, nonrandom cytogenetic abnormalities, similar to those in other forms of fibromatosis, have been observed.[35]

Trauma or microtrauma and reparative fibroblastic proliferation in a genetically predisposed person have been implicated as another causative factor.[42] In fact, as early as 1832 Dupuytren suggested repeated minor trauma as a major cause. Skoog[36] proposed that minor trauma causes partial rupture of the aponeurosis, followed by reparative fibroblastic proliferation, scarification, and contracture. Others, however, denied such a causative relationship, pointing out that the disease is equally common in clerical workers and manual laborers, affects not infrequently the left hand in right-handed persons, and occurs at a site—the ulnar portion of the palm—that is least exposed to traumatic injury.[25,41] Moreover, it develops predominantly in older persons, at a stage of life in which manual labor is normally greatly reduced.

It is still not clear, however, whether a genetic or acquired predisposition is responsible for the higher incidence of the disease in diabetic and epileptic patients as well as in alcoholics (and brewery workers), in persons suffering from alcoholic and nonalcoholic liver disease, and in patients with increased serum lipid levels.

PLANTAR FIBROMATOSIS

Like palmar fibromatosis, this process is characterized by a nodular fibrous proliferation arising within the plantar aponeurosis, but it is less frequent and, because of inherent differences in the anatomy of the hand and foot, is less likely to cause contractions of the digits. The lesion was described by Dupuytren and, later, in more detail by Ledderhose.[46] In fact, plantar fibromatosis is sometimes referred to as *Ledderhose's disease*. Its genetic linkage to palmar and penile fibromatosis is well established. There are few data as to its exact incidence. Yost et al.[41] found one case (0.23%) in a series of 430 consecutive patients.

Clinical findings

The lesion appears first as a single firm, subcutaneous thickening or nodule that adheres to the skin and is located in the middle and medial portion of the sole of the foot. It may be entirely asymptomatic, but not infrequently it causes mild pain after long standing or walking. For this reason, plantar fibromatosis is often biopsied or excised at an earlier and more cellular stage than palmar fibromatosis. Occasionally, when the superficial plantar nerve is involved, there is paresthesia of the distal portion of the sole of the foot and the undersurface of one or more toes. As a rule, the nodule grows slowly and in most cases is the only evidence of the disease. Contraction of the toes is rare, presumably because the distal extensions of the plantar aponeurosis to the toes are much less well developed than in the hand.

As in palmar fibromatosis the condition is about twice as common in men as in women, and it affects both feet in about 10% to 25% of cases.[47,48] Its age incidence differs slightly from that of palmar fibromatosis: as in palmar fibromatosis, there is a progressive increase in incidence with advancing age,[44] but there is a greater incidence in children and young persons. In Allen et al.'s[43] series, 35% were 30 years of age or younger, including two cases that were present at birth. Among 200 consecutive cases we saw in consultation at the AFIP, 111 (55%) occurred in patients under age 30 years, an unusually high incidence in younger patients, probably because earlier and hence more cellular lesions cause more problems in diagnosis and are more often submitted for consultation. Of the 111 cases, 22 were children 10 years of age or younger, the two youngest being a 4-year-old girl and a 2½-year-old boy.

Not infrequently, palmar and plantar fibromatoses affect the same patient, but the two lesions rarely occur at the same time; usually one precedes the other by an interval of 5 to 10 years. The reported incidence of plantar fibromatosis in patients with palmar fibromatosis ranges from 5% to 20%. Association with penile fibromatosis is much less common; Pickren et al.[48] found only one case among 104 cases of plantar fibromatosis. There are also reports of coexisting knuckle pads and keloids.

Pathological findings

Grossly and microscopically, the lesions are virtually indistinguishable from those found in palmar fibromatosis, although they are less often multinodular and only rarely contain the thick cords of fibrocollagenous tissue extending distally from the nodular growth (Fig. 10-7). Both palmar and plantar fibromatosis may be exceedingly cellular (Figs. 10-8 to 10-10), but in the majority of cases the cellular portions blend with fibrocollagenous tendonlike areas. Foci of inflammatory cells, sometimes in a perivascular arrangement, and deposits of hemosiderin are by no means rare, more so in the vicinity of the nodules than in the nodules themselves. Chondroid or osseous metaplasia is occasionally observed in lesions of long standing.

The differential diagnosis of plantar fibromatosis is essentially the same as that of palmar fibromatosis. As in the palm of the hand, fibrosarcoma in the planta pedis is infrequent.

Treatment

Many patients are unaware of the disease or consider it scar tissue, even without a history of injury. Most cases require no surgical therapy, unless the fibrous nodules cause discomfort or disability. Fasciectomy is the treatment of choice.[43,45]

Discussion

Trauma has frequently been considered an important factor in the pathogenesis of the disease. Obviously, the sole of the foot, more than most other sites, suffers a great variety of minor injuries over the years, and it is not surprising that a history of trauma is given in many cases. Yet the coexistence of the disease with other forms of fibromatosis, as well as its greater incidence in epileptic and diabetic patients, makes it very likely that a familial trait is the basic cause and that trauma plays only a secondary role. This concept is also supported by the absence of any occupational predilection and the fact that most examples of plantar fibromatosis arise in the medial portion of the plantar arch, an area least exposed to traumatic injury.

PENILE FIBROMATOSIS (PEYRONIE'S DISEASE)

Penile fibromatosis (Peyronie's disease), first described by Francois de la Peyronie in 1743,[56] is much less common than palmar or plantar fibromatosis. It occurs as an ill-defined fibrous thickening or mass in the shaft of the penis, alone or in conjunction with unilateral or bilateral palmar and plantar fibromatosis. Despite numerous studies of the disease, its exact cause and pathogenesis are still unknown. The condition is also referred to in the literature as *plastic induration of the penis*,[53,55,61] *fibrous cavernositis*,[52] and *fibrous sclerosis of the penis*.[58]

Clinical findings

The main complaint is a palpable induration or mass in the dorsal or lateral aspect of the shaft of the penis, causing the penis to curve toward the affected side. The mass

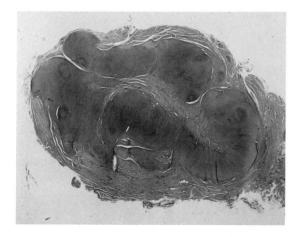

FIG. 10-7. Plantar fibromatosis showing characteristic nodular growth pattern. (×26.)

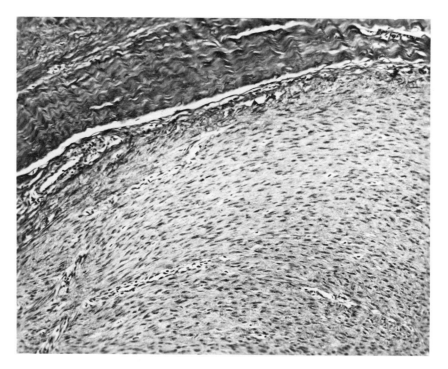

FIG. 10-8. Plantar fibromatosis firmly attached to the plantar aponeurosis. (×100.)

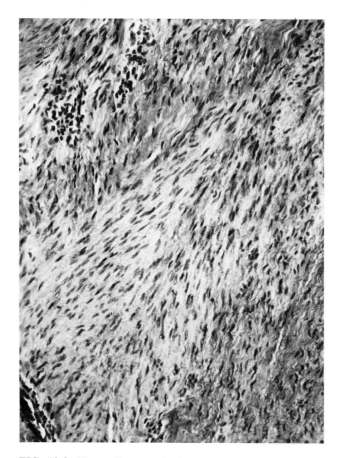

FIG. 10-9. Plantar fibromatosis showing considerable variations in the degree of cellularity and the amount of interstitial collagen. (×160.)

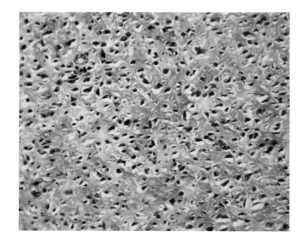

FIG. 10-10. Plantar fibromatosis. Round cell pattern caused by cross-section of spindle-shaped fibroblasts. (×160.)

is often associated with difficulties in passing urine and pain on erection and intercourse. The lesion, together with the abnormal curvature of the penis, develops slowly over many years, most commonly having its onset during the fifth decade of life. There are no reports of cases in children, but there are several in young adults between 20 and 30 years of age. Yet as in palmar and plantar fibromatosis, most patients are between 55 and 75 years of age. The clinical course varies: after many years of growth the lesion becomes stationary or, in about one third of untreated cases, resolves spontaneously.[60,62]

Penile fibromatosis is more common in patients with palmar and plantar fibromatosis than in the general population; its incidence varies from 2% to 4% in palmar fibromatosis and 1% to 2% in plantar fibromatosis. There is also an increased incidence in epileptic and diabetic patients and, according to Bivens et al.[51] in patients with carcinoids. Skoog[36] noted 7 cases of penile fibromatosis among 207 epileptic patients, and Lund[55] reported 3 cases among 361 epileptic patients. Corpus cavernosography may be helpful in outlining the extent of the disease.[50]

Gross findings

The fibrous mass chiefly involves fascial structures, corpus cavernosum, and rarely corpus spongiosum. It consists of dense pearly white to gray-brown tissue that is glistening on section and averages 2 cm in greatest diameter.

Microscopic findings

According to Smith,[58] who studied sections of 26 cases on file at the AFIP, the histological appearance varies considerably: in earlier lesions that have been present 3 months or less, there is a predominance of inflammatory infiltrate and relatively little fibrosis; whereas in older lesions, there is little inflammation and extensive fibrosis, with focal calcification or ossification in some cases. The fibrous proliferation involves mainly the connective tissue space beneath the tunica albuginea, as well as the wall and septa of the corpus cavernosum, and shows a less uniform pattern than that of other forms of fibromatosis (Fig. 10-11). In late stages of the disease there is extensive hyalinization of the fibrous tissue, with only a few chronic inflammatory cells surrounding occasional vascular spaces.

Treatment

Various modes of therapy have been recommended: chiefly, local excision, radiotherapy, cortisone, vitamin E, and ultrasound.[57,62] None of these seems to be effective in all cases, and surgical excision still appears to be the treatment of choice. Proper assessment of the various forms of therapy, however, is hampered by the relative rarity of the condition and the fact that some untreated cases resolve spontaneously.

Discussion

The exact cause of the disease is still not clear; an underlying inflammatory process has been suggested as a possible mechanism in its development, especially because of an occasional history of gonorrhea and prostatitis. Smith[59] found evidence of urethritis and fibrosis in 23 of 100 penises obtained at routine autopsies. He concluded that penile fibromatosis is preceded by an inflammatory phase and proposed the concept of "subclinical Peyronie's disease." He does not state, however, whether any of the 23 patients had an indwelling catheter before death.

Although it is conceivable that the fibrosing process is triggered by inflammation in a genetically predisposed person, it is unlikely that inflammation is the sole and principal cause of the disease, especially in view of the coexistence of the disease with other superficial forms of fibromatosis. As in other forms of superficial and deep fibromatoses, multiple chromosome abnormalities have been described in Peyronie's disease.[54]

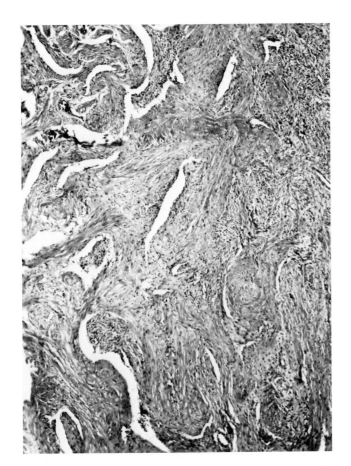

FIG. 10-11. Penile fibromatosis of the corpus cavernosum with narrowing of the vascular spaces by extensive fibrosis. (×60.)

KNUCKLE PADS

This entity is another lesion that is not infrequently encountered in conjunction with palmar or plantar fibromatosis.[23,65,71] The term was coined by Jones in 1923.[66] Knuckle pads consist of flat or dome-shaped noninflammatory fibrous thickening on the dorsal aspect of the proximal interphalangeal or metacarpophalangeal joints and the paratenon of the extensor tendons. It causes few symptoms other than occasional mild tenderness or pain and rarely requires surgical intervention. It may precede the onset of palmar or plantar fibromatosis and may spontaneously disappear after excision of these lesions[76] (Fig. 10-12); like palmar and plantar fibromatosis it chiefly affects patients in the fourth, fifth, and sixth decades of life and is more commonly observed in men than in women. It apparently does not occur in the toes. Microscopically, it resembles palmar fibromatosis, but there is no evidence of contraction.[64,67,69] Reichert et al.[70] described a rare variant of this condition, occurring mainly in adolescent males, as *pachydermodactyly*.

Knuckle pads should not be confused with padlike hyperkeratoses secondary to occupational trauma or self-manipulation and, of course, must be separated from Heberden's nodes of osteoarthritis.[69]

The reports as to its incidence in palmar fibromatosis vary considerably: in Weckesser's[39] series, 6% showed the lesion; in Skoog's[36] study, 44% had the lesion. An increased number of knuckle pads is found in conjunction with plantar fibromatosis[63] and in epileptic patients with and without palmar fibromatosis.[23]

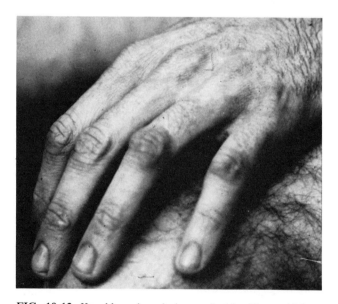

FIG. 10-12. Knuckle pads, a lesion marked by fibrous thickening over the extensor surfaces of the interphalangeal joints. It may be associated with both palmar and plantar fibromatosis.

EXTRAABDOMINAL FIBROMATOSIS (EXTRAABDOMINAL DESMOID)

Despite its relatively common occurrence, this tumor continues to present a difficult problem in recognition and management, especially because of the striking discrepancy between its deceptively harmless microscopic appearance and its potential to attain a large size, to recur, and to infiltrate neighboring tissues in the manner of a fibrosarcoma. It arises principally from the connective tissue of muscle and the overlying fascia or aponeurosis (*musculoaponeurotic fibromatosis*) and chiefly affects the muscles of the shoulder and pelvic girdles and the thigh of adolescents and young adults. The terms *extraabdominal desmoid, desmoid tumor,* and *well-differentiated nonmetastasizing fibrosarcoma* or *grade I fibrosarcoma* have also been used to describe this neoplasm. The term *aggressive fibromatosis* is often employed to emphasize its frequent aggressive behavior. Extraabdominal fibromatosis is one of the more common soft tissue lesions, and it is estimated that approximately 700 to 900 new cases (3 to 4 cases per million) occur in the United States annually.[80,119]

Clinical findings

Usually the presenting complaint is that of a deep-seated, firm, poorly circumscribed mass that has grown insidiously over several weeks and causes little or no pain. Tenderness or pain, however, may occur at a later stage of the disease and usually is associated with motion of the involved muscle or muscle group. Sometimes discomfort or pain is combined with numbness, hypesthesia, or motor weakness, especially when the aggressively growing tumor has infiltrated or encased a large nerve; rarely, numbness, tingling, or "stabbing" or "shooting" pain to the hand or foot is the first complaint, a clinical feature that has caused confusion with primary neoplasm of neural origin; at an advanced stage of the disease, the involved limb may become paralyzed.

Although the growth does occur in children younger than age 10 years, it is most common in patients between puberty and age 40 years, with a peak incidence between the ages of 25 and 35 years. It rarely affects infants or very old persons (Fig. 10-13). Women are slightly more commonly affected than men, but the literature data vary in this regard.[77,82,83,89,106] As in palmar fibromatosis, examples of increased familial incidence have been recorded, but this is rare and is seen in no more than perhaps 1% to 2% of all cases. There is no evidence, however, of any increased incidence in a particular race.[146]

Radiographic findings

The lesion presents as a soft tissue mass that interrupts the adjacent intermuscular and soft tissue planes. When the mass encroaches on bone it may cause pressure erosion or superficial defects of the adjacent cortex. The angiographic

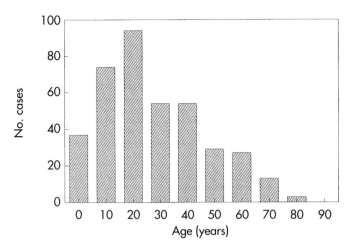

FIG. 10-13. Extraabdominal fibromatosis (extraabdominal desmoid). Age distribution of 383 cases.

Table 10-1. Anatomical distribution of 367 cases of extraabdominal (desmoid) fibromatosis

Anatomical site	No. patients	Percent
Head	7	1.9
Neck	28	7.6
Shoulder	81	22.1
Upper arm	21	5.7
Forearm	13	3.5
Hand	4	1.1
Chest wall; back	63	17.2
Mesentery	38	10.4
Buttock; hip	21	5.7
Thigh	46	12.5
Knee	27	7.4
Lower leg	17	4.6
Foot	1	0.3
TOTAL	367	100.0

picture, however, does not differ from that of other soft tissue tumors.[107] Occasionally there is a periosteal reaction consisting of "frondlike" spicules of bone that extend deep into the tumor.[72] Another peculiar and so far unconfirmed radiographic finding is the presence of multiple minor bone abnormalities at various sites in 80% of patients with fibromatoses.[91] These abnormalities include cortical thickening, exostoses, and translucent foci or compact islands of bone and alterations of the vertebral column (lumbarization of TH12 and sacralization of L5). These changes seem to occur in all age groups and are stated to be equally common in patients with abdominal and extraabdominal fibromatoses.

CT and MRI scans are helpful in diagnosis and in the assessment of margins prior to surgery; the similar density of surrounding muscle tissue, however, makes it sometimes difficult to determine the exact boundaries of the lesion and to distinguish it from other mesenchymal neoplasms.[102]

Anatomical location

Based on the anatomical distribution of 367 microscopically verified cases that we reviewed at the AFIP over a period of 20 years (Table 10-1), the principal location of the tumor is the musculature of the shoulder (22.1%), followed by that of the chest wall and back (17.2%), thigh (12.5%), mesentery (10.4%), and neck (7.6%). In the Rock et al.[121] review of 194 patients with fibromatosis, the shoulder, thigh, arms, back, and buttocks are the principal sites of involvement.

In the shoulder and neck region the growth presents most often in the deltoid, the scapular region, the supraclavicular fossa, or the posterior cervical triangle; it extends from these areas into the lower neck or the anterior or posterior portion of the axilla and the upper arm. Complete excision

in this location is often impossible without severing or injuring a portion of the brachial plexus, a major nerve, or a large vessel that has been infiltrated or entrapped by the tumor. In the subscapular region the tumor may extend into the adjacent chest wall and pleural space, sometimes simulating radiographically a primary pleural or pulmonary neoplasm.[77,81] Massive infiltration of the upper mediastinum from an extraabdominal fibromatosis of the neck has also been observed.[83]

Fibromatoses in the region of the pelvic girdle affect chiefly the gluteus muscle, those in the region of the thigh, the quadriceps muscle and muscles of the popliteal fossa. The hands or feet are rarely involved.[120] Fibromatoses of the head region, especially the mandible, maxilla, mastoid, tongue, and upper lip, are found foremost in children; they tend to be more cellular than those at other sites and may grow more aggressively, sometimes with encroachment of the trachea, massive destruction of the adjacent bone, or erosion of the base of the skull, sometimes with fatal outcome.[79,108,122,130,142] Fibromatosis of the breast[75,123,137] and thyroid[125] have also been described. Cases with bone involvement may be mistaken for desmoplastic fibroma of bone.[85,94]

Multicentric fibromatoses

Although there are no cases with metastasis in our material or in the literature, multicentric lesions do occur on rare occasions.[63,73,110,124,132] In most of these the second growth develops proximally to the primary lesion, but sometimes the tumor involves two or more distant and apparently independent sites. In general, however, multiple tumors occur in the same anatomical region. In the past we have seen several cases in which the foot or calf was the initial site of a fibromatosis, followed by a second tumor of similar microscopic appearance in the popliteal fossa, thigh, or inguinal region. There was also one case in which a tumor at the border of the right scapula developed following amputation of a similar tumor in the musculature of the forearm. In one of these patients, dissection of the amputated extremity revealed a dense fibrous cord along the neurovascular bundle, but the microscopic features of this tissue were quite different from those of the tumor, and multicentric growth rather than direct extension seems to be most likely. Association with extraabdominal fibromatosis at another site or abdominal fibromatoses has been observed but is rare.[110,160] We also reviewed one case in

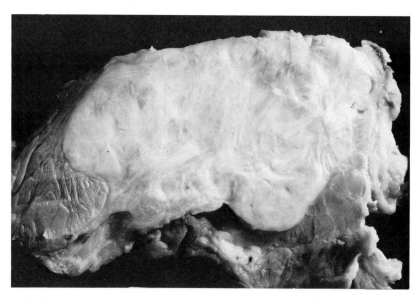

FIG. 10-14. Extraabdominal fibromatosis (desmoid tumor) involving the pectoralis muscle.

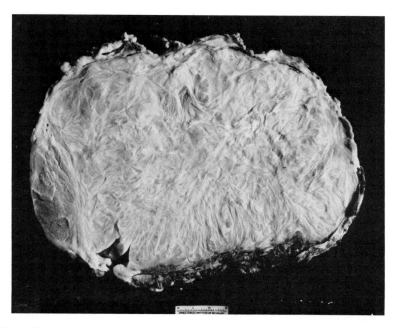

FIG. 10-15. Extraabdominal fibromatosis (extraabdominal desmoid) of the subscapular region in 16-year-old girl.

which multiple lesions of bone characteristic of fibrous dysplasia were present, in addition to a typical extraabdominal fibromatosis.

Gross findings

Nearly always the tumor is confined to the musculature and the overlying aponeurosis or fascia. Occasionally it extends along the fascial plane or infiltrates the overlying subcutaneous tissue, especially if it is a large tumor. Involvement of the periosteum is less common, but when it occurs, it may lead to bone erosion.

The average size of the tumor mass varies considerably, ranging between 5 and 10 cm in diameter. Examples measuring as large as 20 cm, however, are not particularly rare. In fact, we have encountered one case in which the entire lower leg was involved. In general, the tumor is firm, cuts with a gritty sensation, and on cross section reveals a glistening white, coarsely trabeculated surface resembling scar tissue (Figs. 10-14 and 10-15). Indeed, in recurrent tumors the operating surgeon may find it difficult to distinguish clearly between tumor and scar tissue.

Microscopic findings

Characteristically, the lesion is poorly circumscribed and infiltrates the surrounding tissue, usually striated musculature (Fig. 10-16). Invariably it consists of elongated slender spindle-shaped cells of uniform appearance surrounded and separated from one another by abundant collagen (Fig. 10-17). There are no cells with atypical or hyperchromatic nuclei, but nearly always there is some variation in cellularity when multiple sections are examined. The constituent nuclei are small, pale staining, and sharply defined and have one to three minute nucleoli (Fig. 10-17, *D*). Clearly defined cellular boundaries can be discerned only in those cases that have a more prominent mucoid matrix and relatively small amounts of collagen (Fig. 10-18).[83]

Cells and collagen fibers are usually arranged in sweeping bundles that are less well defined than those in fibrosarcoma. Glassy keloidlike collagen fibers or extensive hyalinization, which may obscure the basic pattern of the lesion, are occasional features that may cause difficulties in diagnosis (Fig. 10-19). Reticulin preparation and Masson trichrome stain clearly bring out the abundance of collagen between the individual tumor cells (Fig. 10-20). Immunohistochemically, the spindle cells stain with vimentin, α-smooth muscle actin, and muscle actin and, rarely, as in other myofibroblastic lesions, with polyclonal and monoclonal desmin.[92]

At the periphery of the growth, where the tumor has infiltrated muscle tissue, remnants of striated muscle fibers are frequently entrapped by the tumor tissue. As a result the muscle fibers undergo atrophy or form multinucleated giant cells that may be mistaken for evidence of malignancy (Fig. 10-21). Microhemorrhages and focal aggregates of

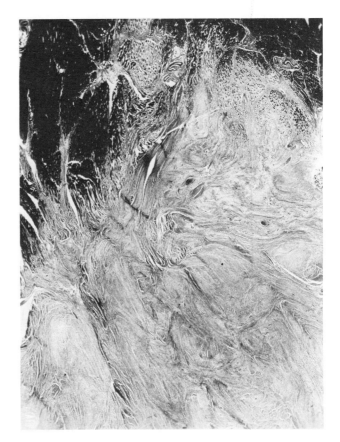

FIG. 10-16. Extraabdominal fibromatosis (extraabdominal desmoid) invading striated muscle tissue. (Masson-trichrome stain; ×6.)

lymphocytes are commonly seen. In rare instances there is calcification or chondroid or osseous metaplasia, but this is never a prominent feature of the tumor.[104]

Ultrastructural findings

As described by Taxy and Battifora[133] and others,[84,86,90,100,114] musculoaponeurotic fibromatosis consists of a uniform population of elongated fibroblast-like cells, often terminating in long and slender processes. The nuclei are rounded or oval and have an undulated outline and less frequently indentations, clefts, or deep infoldings. There is a prominent rough endoplasmic reticulum that is partly dilated and contains granular or fibrillary material within the dilated spaces. The cytoplasm possesses a small number of mitochondria, a prominent Golgi apparatus, free ribosomes, and occasional pinocytotic vesicles and microtubules (Fig. 10-22). Moreover, as in other fibrous proliferations, there are intracytoplasmic bundles of actin-type microfilaments measuring about 60 nm in diameter, often with areas of condensation (dense bodies); there are also occasional incom-

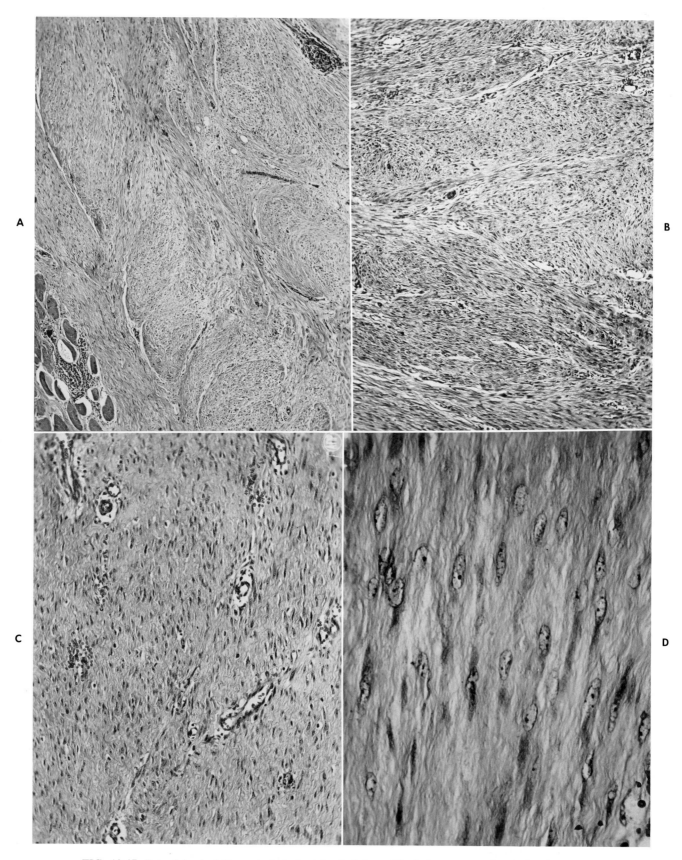

FIG. 10-17. Extraabdominal fibromatosis (extraabdominal desmoid). **A,** Low-power picture showing arrangement of tumor cells in ill-defined fascicles. (×35.) **B,** Interlacing bundles of fibroblasts separated by large amounts of collagen. (×100.) **C,** Another case showing the characteristic association of slender uniformly spindle-shaped nuclei and abundant collagen. (×145.) **D,** High-power picture showing vesicular nuclei with minute nucleoli, rather indistinct cytoplasm, and interstitial collagen. (×400.)

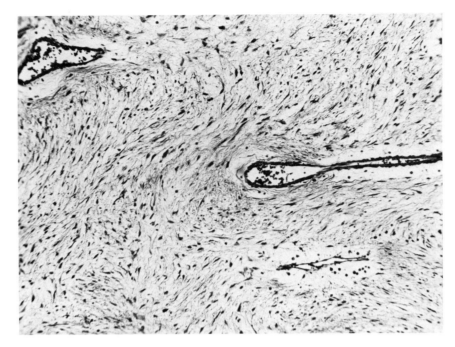

FIG. 10-18. Fibromatosis with relatively small amounts of collagen and a pronounced mucoid matrix. These features are most common in intraabdominal and mesenteric fibromatoses. (×90.)

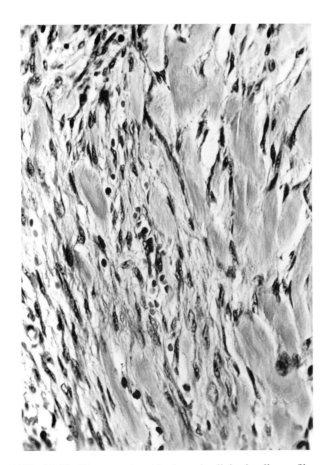

FIG. 10-19. Fibromatosis with glassy hyalinized collagen fibers reminiscent of keloid, a rare feature of this tumor. (×350.)

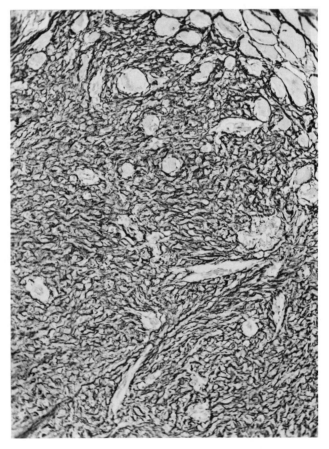

FIG. 10-20. Reticulin preparation of fibromatosis showing dense meshwork of collagen fibrils between individual tumor cells. (Reticulin preparation; ×100.)

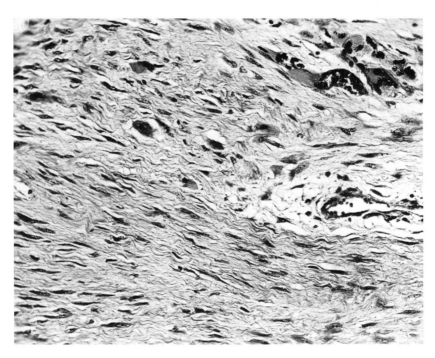

FIG. 10-21. Peripheral portion of a fibromatosis with entrapped muscle giant cells. (×210.)

plete or clumped basal lamina along the cell borders, all features characteristic of myofibroblasts. Considerable amounts of collagen and ground substance are always present in the intercellular spaces. Intracellular collagen formation has also been observed.[140] Typing of collagen seems to be of little value in the diagnosis of the disease.

Differential diagnosis

Two lesions must be primarily considered in differential diagnosis: (1) fibrosarcoma and (2) reactive fibrosis. Factors against *fibrosarcoma* are the uniform growth pattern, mature appearance of tumor cells, paucity of mitotic figures, and, paradoxically and only in tumors of small size, the more prominent infiltrative growth pattern of fibromatosis. Occasional mitotic figures do occur in musculoaponeurotic fibromatosis, but the finding of one or more mitotic figures per high-power field or the presence of atypical mitotic figures should be sufficient to arouse suspicion of malignancy. There is danger in using too small a biopsy specimen because occasional examples of fibrosarcoma contain hypocellular areas indistinguishable from fibromatosis.

Problems in diagnosis may also be caused by exuberant *fibroblastic proliferation* following injury such as trauma, minor muscle tear, or intramuscular injection. On a cellular level these lesions may closely resemble fibromatosis except for their more variable growth patterns and the pres-

ence of focal hemorrhage. In older lesions the only indication of hemorrhage may be deposition of hemosiderin in macrophages, which are usually situated along vascular structures. In cases of doubt, iron stains should be employed to verify the presence or absence of hemosiderin.

Desmoplastic fibroma of bone is indistinguishable from fibromatosis, especially when it presents as a soft tissue mass after breaking through the thinned or expanded cortex of the involved bone.[85,94] However, on closer scrutiny its predominant location in the metaphyseal or diaphyseal portions of long bone or in the jaw will reveal the correct diagnosis.

Confusion with *myxoma* or *nodular fasciitis* is possible, particularly if only a small amount of tissue (or needle biopsy) is available for examination. Fibromatosis always displays a greater degree of cellularity and more interstitial collagen than myxoma. It may focally exhibit a whorled or feathery cellular pattern, but this feature is never as prominent or as uniform as in nodular fasciitis.

Transformation of fibromatosis to fibrosarcoma is extremely rare, and we have never encountered such a case among several hundred examples of fibromatosis in the AFIP material. Soule and Scanlon,[127] however, described and illustrated such a case in which a typical fibromatosis of the inguinal region evolved into fibrosarcoma after a period of 10 years, and nine years following radiotherapy. Malignant transformation of fibromatosis may be errone-

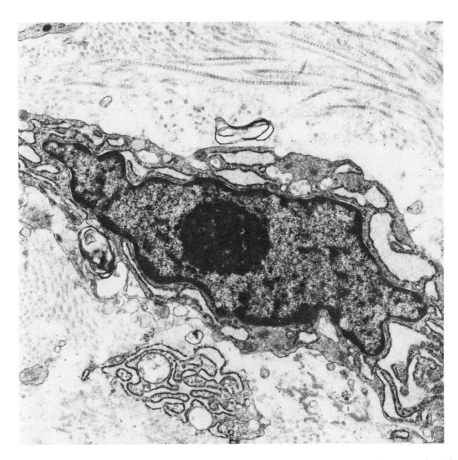

FIG. 10-22. Fibroblast from a typical extraabdominal fibromatosis. Note prominent rough endoplasmic reticulum and mature collagen fibrils in the extracellular space. (×11,400.) (From Taxy JB, Battifora H: The electron microscope in the study and diagnosis of soft tissue tumors. In Trump BF, Jones RT, eds.: *Diagnostic electron microscopy.* New York, 1980, John Wiley & Sons, Inc.)

ously suggested by occasional foci of increased cellularity and by exceptionally well-differentiated fibromatosis-like areas in some fibrosarcomas.

Clinical behavior

Despite its bland microscopic appearance, the tumor frequently behaves in an infiltrative, aggressive manner and, chiefly as the result of partial or marginal excision, recurs in a high percentage of cases. But there is no evidence that the tumor is capable of metastasis. In fact, in most studies the five-year survival rate is better than 90%.[77]

The recurrence rate in our cases and the literature averages 40% and ranges from as little as 29% to 65%,[77,82,83,107] but in one series as many as 90% of cases with marginal resection recurred.[121] Cases with two or more recurrences are not rare. Recurrence is more common in tumors located in the shoulder or pelvic girdle and neck and

in those affecting children and adolescents. Lopez et al.,[106] for instance, report a recurrence rate of 60% in adults and 88% in children. Recurrence usually becomes apparent during the first 2 or 3 years following the initial resection.

Spontaneous regression of the growth has been observed in sporadic cases. One of our patients, a 36-year-old man, refused further surgery after partial excision of a large tumor involving the supraclavicular fossa, the scalenus muscles, and the brachial plexus. There was no evidence of further growth, and the patient was well and without palpable tumor 9½ years later. A second patient, an elderly man suffering from a large recurrent tumor of the axilla and chest wall, declined further treatment because he was told that the lesion was a sarcoma and that "there was only a 30% chance of improvement." After 15 years there was continued pain and partial loss of mobility, but the tumor had substantially decreased in size and was no longer clearly palpable.[83] Likewise, Kofoed et al.[101] have seen 80% regression in a patient with untreated supraclavicular fibromatosis.

Treatment

Because the microscopic picture does not reliably reflect the growth potential of the tumor, therapy is predicated upon its extent and anatomical relationship. In view of the high and unpredictable recurrence rate and the fact that the incidence of recurrence is much greater in patients treated by local excision without adequate margins, it is mandatory to treat all tumors showing gross involvement of muscle by prompt radical excision, including excision of a wide margin of uninvolved structures around the grossly visible tumor.[80,93,111,118,146] Marginal resection is inadequate, except perhaps in those rare instances in which the tumor is very small, well circumscribed, and limited to the fascia or aponeurosis and occurs in older persons.

In view of the excellent prognosis in regard to patient survival, amputation or other mutilating procedures should be done only for palliative reasons if the tumor recurs repeatedly and does not respond to adjuvant radiation or endocrine therapy or if the extent of the tumor or threat of complications leaves no other choice.

Postoperative radiotherapy seems to be indicated in primary tumors that were incompletely excised, in recurrent tumors, and in tumors in which radical excision is impossible without major loss of function or significant morbidity. Radiotherapy without an attempt at resection may also achieve good results. Sherman et al.,[126] using megavoltage radiation therapy with a median dose of 50 Gy (5000 rad), and McCollough et al.[109] achieved local control rates of 75% and 83%, respectively. Others report similar beneficial results with primary or postoperative radiotherapy.[74,88,98,105,131] However, regression following radiotherapy is slow and may take as long as 2 or 3 years. Zelefsky et al.[145] treated 38 desmoids that were incompletely excised or had recurred with conservative resection and iridium-192 implantations with excellent long-term functional results. There is no reliable information as to the risk of malignant transformation following radiation therapy, but long-term follow-up in this regard is advisable.

The therapeutic usefulness of noninvasive antiestrogen therapy, especially tamoxifen and nonsteroidal antiinflammatory prostaglandin-inhibiting drugs (indomethacin, sulindac), is not fully established, but there are numerous reports that describe stabilization and regression not only of recurrent or unresectable tumors but also effective treatment of primary tumors.[99,103,134-136,141,174] In addition, complete or partial remissions were achieved with progesterone[103] and various chemotherapeutic agents.[138,178] Others, however, report little or no beneficial effect with these modes of therapy.[82]

Discussion

Genetic, endocrine, and physical factors seem to play an important role in development of the disease. Features suggesting an underlying genetic basis are the rare association of extraabdominal and abdominal fibromatosis in the same patient,[160] the occasional occurrence in siblings,[158] the finding of multiple minor osseous abnormalities in a high percentage of patients with fibromatosis,[90] and, most importantly, the common occurrence of mesenteric and other forms of fibromatosis in patients with hereditary familial colonic polyposis. Increased familial incidence in patients with extraabdominal fibromatosis is rare. However, Zayid and Dihmis[144] reported extraabdominal fibromatosis in three members (mother and her two children) of a Jordanian family; we encountered two other instances in which several members of one family were afflicted by the disease. So far there are only a few investigations as to the karyotype of patients with this tumor, but most suggest a common genetic basis for various types of fibromatoses. Bridge et al.[76] demonstrated absence of the Y chromosome and deletion of 5q in both extraabdominal and abdominal fibromatoses, including patients with Gardner's syndrome. Similar chromosomal abnormalities were described by others.[96,214,225]

In addition to genetic factors, endocrine factors probably play a role in the development of fibromatosis.[113] Unlike abdominal fibromatosis, which occurs mainly in young women during pregnancy and the postpartum period, we know of only two patients among our cases who developed the disease during gestation. Estrogen-related growth, however, is suggested by the reported inhibitory effect of an antiestrogen agent (tamoxifen) and the described cessation of growth and tumor regression after menopause.[80,110] Yet estrogen receptor levels do not seem to be a prognostically reliable yardstick of growth activity. Weiss et al.[139] studied three patients (two males and one female) for estrogen-receptor protein; two were within normal limits and one, a 22-year-old male, was marginally elevated. Häyry et al.[91] carried out a similar analysis in three patients with fibromatoses, but all had low levels that were within the range of normal.

Physical factors, such as trauma or radiation, may serve as a trigger mechanism. Among the many cases of fibromatosis that we have reviewed over the past 20 years, 13 occurred in a surgical scar (cicatricial fibromatosis) and four in a previously irradiated area (postirradiation fibromatosis). Additional examples developed in the region of a healed fracture, a burn scar (one after 34 years and another after 43 years), and a gunshot wound. Others were seen in areas injured previously in an automobile or motorcycle accident (six cases), football injury (three cases), and one or more injections (five cases). Some of these may be coincidental findings, but Lopez et al.[106] also elicited a history of trauma at the tumor site in 28% of cases. Similar examples of cicatricial and postirradiation fibromatoses are reported in the literature, including many cases in which an intraabdominal or abdominal fibromatosis developed in the region of an ileocolectomy for familial polyposis.[87,116,117]

ABDOMINAL FIBROMATOSIS (ABDOMINAL DESMOID)

Although this tumor is indistinguishable in its gross and microscopic appearances and its infiltrative growth from extraabdominal fibromatosis, it deserves separate consideration because of its characteristic location and its tendency to occur in women of childbearing age during or following pregnancy. Generally, the tumor arises from musculoaponeurotic structures of the abdominal wall, especially the rectus and internal oblique muscles and their fascial coverings. Identical tumors originating from the pelvic wall have been described as pelvic fibromatosis or intraabdominal desmoid.

Clinical findings

Abdominal fibromatosis manifests as a deeply located solitary mass that grows slowly but progressively. Usually it is firm on palpation and nontender and becomes much more prominent on muscle contraction. Unlike most intraabdominal tumors it does not move with respiration. The majority arise in the lower portion of the abdominal wall, especially the rectus muscle. Less commonly it takes origin from the internal or external oblique muscle and from the transversalis muscle or its fascia. Extension to the inner surface of the iliac crest and into the abdominal cavity takes place occasionally. In these cases the abdominal viscera may become adherent to the tumor. Sonography is helpful in the preoperative diagnosis of these cases.[164]

Typically, abdominal fibromatosis occurs in young, gravid, or parous women during gestation or, more frequently, during the first year following childbirth. Hence 7 out of 10 patients with the disease are women between 20 and 30 years of age.[167] In Pfeiffer's[169] large series, 87% of cases occurred in young women and 94% in women who had one or more children. There are also sporadic cases in adult males[153] and in children of both sexes, especially boys. In fact, of the five cases of abdominal fibromatosis in young children in the AFIP files, four were boys and only one a girl, 3 months of age. Similarly Booher and Pack[149] reported two cases in boys and one in a girl. Additional examples in infants and children are reported in the literature.[147,150,170]

In our material and in most studies, abdominal fibromatoses are less common than extraabdominal fibromatoses,[82] but in a study carried out in Finland,[119] abdominal fibromatoses (49%) outnumbered extraabdominal (43%) and mesenteric fibromatoses (8%). Most lesions are solitary, but

patients having both abdominal and extraabdominal fibromatoses have been described.[110,159]

Pathological findings

The gross and microscopic appearances are identical to those described under extraabdominal fibromatosis, except perhaps that the average tumor is smaller in size and behaves less destructively. In fact, most tumors measure 3 to 10 cm, and when arising in the rectus muscle or its fascia, they usually remain at the site of origin; that is, they do not cross the midline of the abdomen.

Under the microscope they show the characteristic features of fibromatosis: they are poorly cellular and poorly vascularized, infiltrate muscle tissue, and engulf muscle fibers. Despite their poor vascularity, degeneration or necrosis is hardly ever encountered.

Clinical behavior and therapy

In addition to its locally invasive growth, the tumor has the potential of recurrence. Its recurrence rate (15% to 30%), however, is slightly lower than that of extraabdominal fibromatosis (35% to 65%). Usually recurrence becomes evident within the first two years after excision or in connection with subsequent gestations or deliveries. Multiple recurrences are not particularly rare. Because recurrence is more common after limited or incomplete surgical removal, wide local excision with ample margins is the therapy of choice. As in extraabdominal fibromatosis, supplementary radiation may achieve control of recurrent or inoperable tumors. There is little information about the efficacy of endocrine (antiestrogen) or chemotherapy, but Hutchinson et al.[158] reported eradication of a nonresectable fibromatosis in the lower abdomen of a 15-year-old boy following treatment with dactinomycin, vincristine, and cyclophosphamide.

Discussion

The exact cause of abdominal fibromatosis is still uncertain. While endocrine factors are clearly implicated by the frequent occurrence of the tumor during or after pregnancy, there is no evidence of endocrine imbalance and there are occasional cases in which the tumor developed in nulliparous women and in children of both sexes and adult males. On the other hand, there are also reports of abdominal fibromatosis after prolonged and intensive estrogen therapy for prostatic cancer[163] and of extraabdominal fibromatosis occurring during pregnancy.[110] Trauma may serve as a contributing cause, especially since occasional examples of abdominal fibromatosis have arisen in the scars of appendectomies,[152] laparotomies,[148,154] and other abdominal operations (cicatricial fibromatosis). But since the majority of patients with abdominal fibromatosis have no history of gross injury, minor and undetected trauma such as a minute muscle tear may conceivably serve as a contributing etiological factor that triggers the fibrous growth in a hormonally or genetically predisposed patient.

INTRAABDOMINAL FIBROMATOSIS (INTRAABDOMINAL DESMOID)

As already indicated, this is a group of closely related lesions rather than a single entity that pose similar problems in histological diagnosis but can be distinguished by the clinical setting and location. It includes pelvic fibromatosis, mesenteric fibromatosis, and fibromatosis in Gardner's syndrome.

Pelvic fibromatosis

Although pelvic fibromatosis is essentially a variant of abdominal fibromatosis, it differs from the latter by its location in the iliac fossa and lower portion of the pelvis, where it manifests as a slow-growing palpable mass that is asymptomatic or causes slight pain. Clinically it is often mistaken for an ovarian tumor or a mesenteric cyst. Larger examples, which may be as large as 15 cm in greatest diameter, may encroach on the urinary bladder, vagina, or rectum, may cause hydronephrosis, and may even compress the iliac vessels.[91,155]

As in fibromatosis of the abdominal wall, the tumor arises from the aponeurosis or muscle tissue and occurs chiefly in young women between 20 and 35 years of age, but in the majority of cases it is unrelated to gestation or childbirth. Grossly and microscopically, the tumor is indistinguishable from other forms of fibromatosis, abdominal or extraabdominal (Fig. 10-23) and requires similar modes of therapy.

Mesenteric fibromatosis

Mesenteric fibromatosis occurs in mesentery of the small bowel or the retroperitoneum, or in both sites as separate tumors. Less commonly it originates from the ileocolic mesentery, gastrocolic ligament, and omentum. Diagnosis may be difficult in some cases because a reactive fibrosis following injury or hemorrhage may show a closely related histological picture. In fact, examples of idiopathic retroperitoneal or periureteric fibrosis (sclerosing retroperitonitis or periureteritis) have been repeatedly confused with mesenteric fibromatosis.[165,171]

As in pelvic fibromatosis, the lesion presents as an asymptomatic or slightly painful mass, which is usually palpable in the lower abdomen. Data as to age and sex incidence vary: In the AFIP series of 130 cases, 71 occurred in males and 59 in females, and patients ranged in age from 14 to 75 years.[151] Cases reported by Yannopoulos and Stout[178] affected males and females with equal frequency, and those reviewed by Kim et al.[160] occurred only in women. Like many other neoplasms in the retroperitoneum and abdomen, most mesenteric fibromatoses are of large size, with the majority measuring 10 cm or more in greatest diameter. Many grow rapidly and cause complications by compression of the small or large intestines or the ureter, sometimes complicated by intestinal perforation.[166,174]

Data as to the recurrence rate differ greatly. There seems to be no close correlation between the histological picture and behavior, but Burke et al.[151] report a slower growth rate in men than in women and a striking difference in recurrence rates between patients with (90%) and without (11%) familial polyposis. Treatment is similar to that described under extraabdominal fibromatosis, but excision is

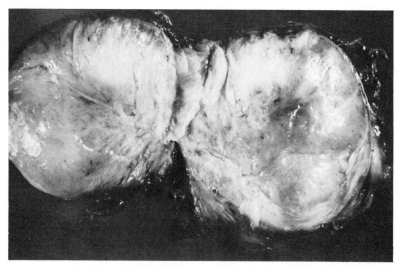

FIG. 10-23. Gross picture of pelvic fibromatosis. These lesions are indistinguishable from abdominal fibromatosis, except perhaps for their slightly more mucoid appearance.

often difficult because of the irregular growth pattern and intestinal attachment of the tumor. Jones[197] and others achieved regression or stabilization of several tumors with tamoxifen.

As in pelvic fibromatosis, the most likely cause appears to be tissue injury in a patient having a genetic disposition toward excessive fibrous growth. Frequently, abdominal surgery of various kinds precedes development of the tumor. In a few of these cases, a second and morphogically similar lesion develops in the scar of the abdominal incision.[147,172] Less commonly, mesenteric fibromatosis develops spontaneously without prior surgical intervention or soft tissue injury.[215] Some of the latter cases are incidental findings during abdominal exploration for some other cause. In fact, in one of our cases, mesenteric fibromatosis was found to be associated with Crohn's disease. There are also examples in which the lesion occurred during or after pregnancy.[151]

Mesenteric fibromatosis in Gardner's syndrome

While by no means all cases of mesenteric and retroperitoneal fibromatosis are examples of this disease, the association of fibromatosis with numerous colorectal adenomatous polyps, osteomata, cutaneous cysts, and other extracolonic manfestations is characteristic of Gardner's syndrome. Although patients with this syndrome were described prior to 1950,[208] Gardner was the first to recognize and correlate the genetic aspects of the disease, which he reported in a series of publications based on a detailed study of a family group in Utah.[187,189,209,214]

Gardner's syndrome is inherited as an autosomal dominant trait that occurs in approximately half of the children of afflicted parents. It is more common in women than men and is usually diagnosed in adults between 25 and 35 years of age. The incidence of fibromatosis in patients with familial polyposis ranges from 3.5% to 13%, with a slightly higher incidence in females than males.[180,197,206] Most tumors arise in the mesentery and retroperitoneum, but the abdominal wall may also be the primary site. Additionally, 40% to 50% of patients have cutaneous cysts, and 35% to 50% osteomata. The actual incidence of osteomata may be even higher, since a skeletal survey was done in only a few cases[196,220] (Fig. 10-24). Another common feature of the disease is pigmented ocular fundus lesions, which may be observed as early as 3 months of age.[216] Less common are richly collagenous fibromalike lesions, dental abnormalities, including impacted or supernumerary teeth, lipomata, leiomyomata, and carcinomas.[185,195,205-207,215] Maher et al.[206] reported the association of fibromatosis and nonpolyposis colon carcinoma in multiple members of one family over four generations.

As a rule, the onset of osteomata and cutaneous cysts occurs during childhood or the teens and precedes the onset of polyposis and fibromatosis by 10 to 15 years. Osteomata may occur anywhere in the skeleton but are usually found in the skull and facial bones, especially the maxilla, mandible, sphenoid, and frontal bone (Fig. 10-24, D). In long bones cortical thickening is more common than osteomata.[182,191,210,222]

Early cases tend to be asymptomatic or manifest with mild diarrhea and passage of small amounts of mucus or blood. At age 20 to 25 years, roentgenographic examination reveals in about half of cases numerous, discrete filling defects in the colon characteristic of multiple polyposis (Fig. 10-24, A-C). The ileum, duodenum, and stomach may also be affected. Transition from polyposis to adenocarcinoma, often at multiple sites, usually takes place at age 35 to 40 years, 10 or 15 years after the onset of polyposis. This is approximately 25 years earlier than the onset of colon carcinoma in the general population.

Mesenteric or retroperitoneal fibromatosis in Gardner's syndrome ordinarily has its onset 1 or 2 years following excision of the diseased portion of the intestinal tract; sometimes it is accompanied by a similar tumor in the abdominal wall arising in the scar of the preceding laparotomy. Not all cases of fibromatosis, however, develop as the result of surgical trauma, and a small number have been noted prior to surgical intervention.[194,196,204,211] A propensity toward fibrous adhesions has also been described[180] (Fig. 10-25).

Clinically the fibromatosis may be asymptomatic or may cause pain or intestinal obstruction as a result of impingement of the fibrous mass on the small or large bowel. Slow growth, as well as rapid growth, has been noted. Gold and Mucha,[190] for example, reported a mesenteric fibromatosis in a 40-year-old man, which grew in a period of 1 year from a 4-cm mass (observed but not removed at laparotomy) to an asymptomatic mass measuring 27 cm in greatest diameter (Fig. 10-25).

On histological examination the fibromatosis is virtually indistinguishable from those at other sites, but as in any fibromatosis occurring or extending into the abdominal cavity, the spindle-shaped cells or fibroblasts tend to be more loosely arranged and have a more prominent myxoid matrix (Fig. 10-26). At times a vague and focal storiform pattern is present, a feature that should not be confused with the much more pronounced storiform pattern found in benign and malignant fibrous histiocytomas.

The intestinal adenomatous polyps are indistinguishable from those in other forms of polyposis and are found throughout the intestinal tract, with the colon and the rectum being the two major sites of the disease. The polyps may be numerous; in some cases as many as one thousand polyps were counted (Fig. 10-24).[201]

Infrequently polyposis and other manifestations of Gardner's syndrome are associated with carcinomas (thyroid carcinoma[181] and basal cell carcinoma[203]), various soft tissue and bone sarcomas (fibrosarcoma,[187,191] osteosarcoma,[186]

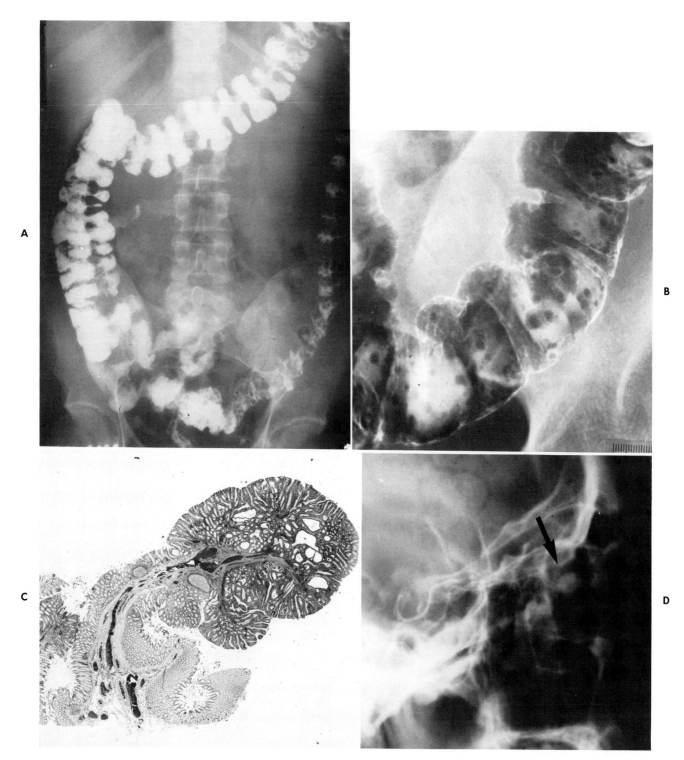

FIG. 10-24. Gardner's syndrome. **A, B,** and **C,** Familial polyposis of the colon. **D,** Osteoma of the frontal sinus *(arrow).*

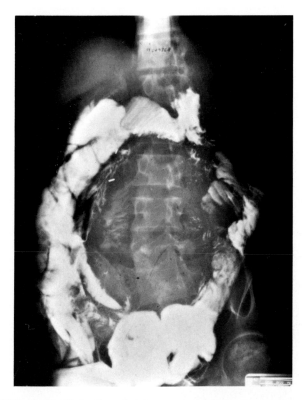

FIG. 10-25. Plain film of abdomen of a patient with mesenteric fibromatosis in Gardner's syndrome following total colectomy: loops of small bowel are displaced by mesenteric fibromatosis.

liposarcoma,[186] and chondrosarcoma[192]), and brain tumors (Turcot syndrome).[183,202]

Early detection of the disease permits proper surgical therapy before malignant transformation of the polyps takes place. Because the lesion usually does not manifest before the patient reaches reproductive age, genetic counseling and lifelong surveillance are an important part of therapy in patients with a positive family history.[184]

As in mesenteric fibromatosis without polyposis, complete excision of the tumor may be difficult, especially if the patient had a previous colectomy, and such a procedure may necessitate removal of a sizable segment of the intestines together with the fibrous growth. Yet in rapidly growing examples of this tumor, excision must be attempted in order to prevent complications caused by the presence of a massive, expanding, often recurring intraabdominal growth. Recurrence is common, and most reviewers report a recurrence rate in excess of 80%.[151,197] Fatal complications are also more frequent than in nonpolyposis fibromatoses.[193]

Endocrine therapy (tamoxifen and prednisolone), as well as noncytotoxic drug therapy (indomethacin and sulindac) and chemotherapy, was used with varying success in re-

current and inoperable tumors.[198,199,204,217-219] Spontaneous regression is rare but has been observed.

The exact nature of Gardner's syndrome is still not clear. It is a genetically determined autosomal dominant disease associated with defective genes, probably karyotypic abnormalities of the Y chromosome and 5q, similar to the findings in other forms of fibromatosis.[212,223] Constitutional markers may help in identifying individuals predisposed to the disease. Kopelovich and Gardner[200] analyzed the effect of tumor promoters (TPA) on the proliferation of cultured skin fibroblasts obtained from individuals with hereditary adenomatosis of the colon and rectum. Fibroblasts from gene carriers were less sensitive to the toxic effect of TPA than those from normal individuals.

IDIOPATHIC RETROPERITONEAL FIBROSIS (ORMOND'S DISEASE)

This is a rare fibromatosislike reactive process that may be confused with mesenteric fibromatosis. It was first described by Ormond in 1948.[232] It is characterized by a diffuse or localized fibroblastic proliferation and a chronic lymphocytic, plasmacytic infiltrate in the retroperitoneum causing compression or obstruction of the ureters, the aorta, or other vascular structures. Idiopathic retroperitoneal fibrosis is rare in children and is found mostly in adults, with a male predominance. The disease usually presents with a history of pain in the lower abdomen, the flank, or the lower back, sometimes associated with malaise, weight loss, fever, and hypertension. The proliferated fibrous tissue often encases and constricts one or both ureters, causing dilatation of the upper part of the ureter and hydronephrosis (fibrosing periureteritis). Less commonly it involves the adventitial tissues of the aorta (periaortitis), the vena cava, or the mesenteric or iliac vessels, occasionally resulting in collateral abdominal circulation. The fibrosing process may be diffuse or localized, sometimes presenting as a solid mass suggesting an enlarged lymph node or neoplasm.

Microscopic examination of the lesions reveals a fibrous proliferation, broad anastomosing bands of hyalinized collagen, and a plasmacytic and lymphocytic infiltrate of variable density, with occasional germinal centers. Simultaneous association of this process with fibrosing mediastinitis,[228,235] Riedel's thyroiditis,[234] sclerosing cholangitis,[224] and pseudotumor of the orbit[228] was reported and was referred to as "multifocal fibrosclerosis"[225] or "systemic idiopathic fibrosis."[230,231,233] Umemoto et al.[219] described the development of retroperitoneal fibrosis after prednisolone-induced regression of an abdominal and mesenteric fibromatosis in a patient with hereditary familial polyposis.

As the name idiopathic fibrosis indicates, the etiology is still not clear, but in about one third of cases various drugs have been associated with the disease, including methysergide and adrenergic-blocking agents.[237] This process was

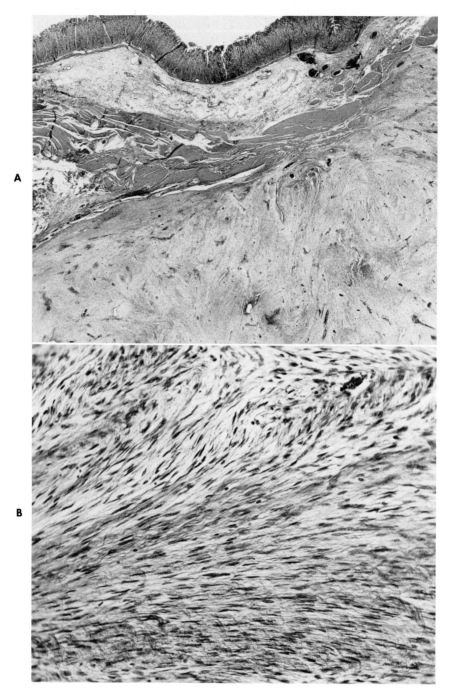

FIG. 10-26. Mesenteric fibromatosis in Gardner's syndrome. **A,** Low-power picture showing uniform fibrocollagenous growth attached to the muscular coat of the large bowel. (×8). **B,** Orderly arrangement of uniform fibroblasts associated with moderate amounts of collagen and mucoid material. (×145.)

also observed following therapeutic radiation and in association with various malignant neoplasms involving the retroperitoneal space. Although CT scan, MRI,[229] or ultrasonography is most useful in reaching a diagnosis, exploration and biopsy may become necessary for reaching an

unequivocal diagnosis. The treatment of choice is prolonged corticosteroid therapy, combined with ureterolysis and temporary nephrostomy in cases of renal outflow occlusion. In a few instances spontaneous regression has been observed.[227,228,236,237]

REFERENCES
Palmar fibromatosis

1. Arafa M, Noble J, Royle SG, et al: Dupuytren's and epilepsy revisited. *J Hand Surg [Br] 17:221, 1992.*
2. Arieff AJ, Bell J: Epilepsy and Dupuytren's contracture. *Neurology* 6:115, 1956.
3. Badalamente MA, Hurst LC, Sampson SP: Prostaglandins influence myofibroblast contractility in Dupuytren's disease. *J Hand Surg [Am]* 13:867, 1988.
4. Couch H: Identical Dupuytren's contracture in identical twins. *Can Med Assoc J* 39:255, 1938.
5. Dahmen G: Feingewebliche und submikroskopische Befunde beim Morbus Dupuytren. *Z Orthop Ihre Grenzgeb* 104:247, 1968.
6. Davis E: On surgery of Dupuytren's contracture. *Plast Reconstr Surg* 36:277, 1965.
7. Dupuytren G: De la retraction des doigts par suite d'une affection de l'aponeurose palmaire: description de la maladie, operation chirurgical qui convient dans de cas. *J Univ Med Chir Prat Paris* 5:348, 1831. Translated *Lancet* 2:222, 1834.
8. Early PE: Population studies in Dupuytren's contracture. *J Bone Joint Surg* 44B:602, 1962.
9. Gabbiani G, Majno G: Dupuytren's contracture: fibroblast contraction. *Am J Pathol* 66:131, 1972.
10. Gokel JM, Huebner G, Meister P, et al: Zur formalen Pathogenese des Morbus Dupuytren. *Verh Dtsch Ges Pathol* 60:474, 1976.
11. Graubard DJ: Dupuytren's contracture: etiologic study. *J Int Coll Surg* 21:15, 1954.
12. Halliday DR, Lipscomb PR, Seldon TH: Fasciectomy and controlled hypotension in treatment of Dupuytren's contracture. *Am J Surg* 111:282, 1966.
13. Hunter JAA, Ogdon C: Dupuytren's contracture: scanning electron microscope observations. *Br J Plast Surg* 28:19, 1975.
14. Iwasaki H, Müller H, Stutte HJ, et al: Palmar fibromatosis (Dupuytren's contracture): ultrastructural and enzyme histochemical studies of 43 cases. *Virchows Arch (Pathol Anat)* 405:41, 1984.
15. Jahnke A: Elektronenmikroskopische Untersuchungen über die Dupuytrensche Kontraktur. *Zbl Chir* 85:2295, 1960.
16. James WD, Odom RB: The role of the myofibroblast in Dupuytren's contracture. *Arch Dermatol* 116:807, 1980.
17. Katenkamp D, Stiller D: Die Dupuytrensche Palmarfibromatose—eine überschiessende Reaktion des Gefässmesenchyms? Ultrastrukturelle Untersuchungen. *Zentralbl Allg Pathol* 120:91, 1976.
18. Kischer CW, Speer DP: Microvascular changes in Dupuytren's contracture. *J Hand Surg* 9A:58, 1984.
19. Krebs H: Erfahrungen bei 350 operativ behandelten Dupuytrenschen Kontracturen. *Arch Chir* 338:67, 1975.
20. Ling RSM: The genetic factor of Dupuytren's disease. *J Bone Joint Surg* 45B:708, 1963.
21. Lund M: Dupuytren's contracture and epilepsy: clinical connection between Dupuytren's contracture, fibroma plantae, periarthrosis humeri, helodermia, induratio penis plastica and epilepsy with attempt at pathogenetic evaluation. *Acta Psychiatr Neurol* 16:465, 1941.
22. Mikkelsen OA: Dupuytren's disease: initial symptoms, age of onset and spontaneous course. *Hand* 9:11, 1977.
23. Mikkelsen OA: Knuckle pads in Dupuytren's disease. *Hand* 9:301, 1977.
24. Millesi H: Die Stellung der Dupuytrenschen Kontraktur in der Pathologie. *Handchirurgie* 1:15, 1970.
25. Moorehead JJ: Trauma and Dupuytren's contracture. *Am J Surg* 85:352, 1953.
26. Noble J, Arafa M, Royle SG, et al: The association between alcohol, hepatic pathology and Dupuytren's disease. *J Hand Surg* 17:71, 1992.
27. Patel JC: Constatation du microscope electronique dans la maladie de Dupuytren. *Presse Med* 69:793, 1961.
28. Pierce ER: Dupuytren's contracture in three successive generations. *Birth Defects* 10:206, 1974.
29. Plater F: Observationum Felici Plateri libri tres. Liber I. Basel, Johannis Ludovici Koenig & Johannis Brandmylleri, 1630.
30. Pojer J, Radivojevic M, Williams TF: Dupuytren's disease: its association with abnormal liver function in alcoholism and epilepsy. *Arch Intern Med* 129:561, 1972.
31. Redfern AB, Curtis RM, Wilgis EF: Experience with peritendinous fibrosis of the dorsum of the hand. *J Hand Surg* 7:380, 1982.
32. Rodrigo JJ, Neibauer JJ, Brown RL, et al: Treatment of Dupuytren's contracture. Long-term results after fasciotomy and fascial excision. *J Bone Joint Surg* 58A:380, 1976.
33. Rutishauser E, Lagier R: A propos de la Maladie de Dupuytren. *Schweiz Ztschr Allg Pathol* 18:1262, 1955.
34. Sanderson PL, Morris MA, Stanley JK, et al: Lipids and Dupuytren's disease. *J Bone Joint Surg* 74(B):923, 1992.
35. Sergovich FR, Botz JS, McFarlane RM: Nonrandom cytogenetic abnormalities in Dupuytren's disease (letter). *N Engl J Med* 308:162, 1983.
36. Skoog T: Dupuytren's contraction with special reference to aetiology and improved surgical treatment: its occurrence in epileptics: Note on knuckle-pads. *Acta Chir Scand* 96(suppl 139):1, 1948.
37. Tomasek JJ, Schultz RJ, Episalla CW, et al: The cytoskeleton and extracellular matrix of the Dupuytren's disease "myofibroblast": an immunofluorescence study of a nonmuscle cell type. *J Hand Surg [Am]* 11:365, 1986.
38. VandeBerg JS, Rudolph R, Gelberman R, et al: Ultrastructural relationship of skin to nodule and cord in Dupuytren's contracture. *Plast Reconstr Surg* 69:835, 1982.
39. Weckesser EC: Results of wide excision of palmar fascia for Dupuytren's contracture: special reference to factors which adversely affect prognosis. *Ann Surg* 160:1007, 1964.
40. Wolfe J, Summerskill JH, Davidson S: Thickening and contraction of the palmar fascia (Dupuytren's contracture) associated with alcoholism and hepatic cirrhosis. *N Engl J Med* 255:559, 1956.
41. Yost J, Winters T, Fett HC: Dupuytren's contracture. A statistical study. *Am J Surg* 90:568, 1955.
42. Zachariae L: Dupuytren's contracture: the etiological role of trauma. *Scand J Plast Reconstr Surg* 5:116, 1971.

Plantar fibromatosis

43. Allen RA, Woolner LB, Ghormley RK: Soft tissue tumors of the sole: with special reference to plantar fibromatosis. *J Bone Joint Surg* 37A:14, 1955.
44. Aviles E, Arlen M, Miller T: Plantar fibromatosis. *Surgery* 69:117, 1971.

45. Curtin JW: Fibromatosis of the plantar fascia: surgical technique and design of skin incision. *J Bone Joint Surg* 47A(8):1605, 1965.
46. Ledderhose G: Zur Pathologie der Aponeurose des Fusses und der Hand. *Arch Klin Chir* 55:694, 1897.
47. Pedersen HE, Day AJ: Dupuytren's disease of the foot. *JAMA* 154:33, 1954.
48. Pickren JW, Smith AG, Stevenson TW Jr, et al: Fibromatosis of the plantar fascia. *Cancer* 4:846, 1951.
49. Yost J, Winters TH, Fett HC Sr: Dupuytren's contracture. *Am J Surg* 90:568, 1955.

Penile fibromatosis (Peyronie's disease)

50. Billig R, Baker R, Immergut M, et al: Peyronie's disease. *Urology* 6:409, 1975.
51. Bivens CH, Marecek RL, Feldman JM: Peyronie's disease: a presenting complaint of the carcinoid syndrome. *N Engl J Med* 289:844, 1973.
52. Burford CE, Gleen JE, Burford EH: Fibrous cavernositis. *J Urol* 56:118, 1946.
53. Gossrau G, Sell W: The coexistence of plastic induration of the penis, Dupuytren contracture, and knuckle pads. *Derm Wschr* 151:1039, 1965.
54. Guerneri S, Stioui S, Mantovani F, et al: Multiple clonal chromosome abnormalities in Peyronie's disease. *Cancer Genet Cytogenet* 52:181, 1991.
55. Lund M: Dupuytren's contracture and epilepsy: clinical connection between Dupuytren's contracture, fibroma plantae, periarthrosis humeri, helodermia, induratio penis plastica and epilepsy with attempt at pathogenetic evaluation. *Acta Psychiatr Neurol* 16:465, 1971.
56. Peyronie de la F: Sur quelques obstacles qui s'opposent a l'ejaculation naturella de la semence. Section III, Chapter 19(4). *Memoires de l'acad. de Chir*, p. 425, 1743.
57. Seardino PL, Scott WW: The use of tocopherols in the treatment of Peyronie's disease. *Ann N Y Acad Sci* 52:390, 1949.
58. Smith BH: Peyronie's disease. *Am J Clin Pathol* 45(6):670, 1966.
59. Smith BH: Subclinical Peyronie's disease. *Am J Clin Pathol* 52(4):385, 1969.
60. Soiland A: Peyronie's disease or plastic induration of the penis. *Radiology* 42:183, 1944.
61. Wesson MB: Peyronie's disease (plastic induration), cause and treatment. *J Urol* 49:350, 1943.
62. Williams JL, Thomas GG: The natural history of Peyronie's disease. *J Urol* 103:75, 1970.

Knuckle pads

63. Allen PW: The fibromatoses: a clinicopathologic classification based on 140 cases, part I. *Am J Surg Pathol* 1:255, 1977.
64. Allison JR Jr, Allison JR Sr: Knuckle pads. *Arch Dermatol* 93:311, 1966.
65. Hueston JT: Some observations on "knuckle pads." *J Hand Surg* 9B:75, 1984.
66. Jones HW: Two cases of "knuckle pads." *Br Med J* 1:759, 1923.
67. Lagier R, Meinecke R: Pathology of "knuckle pads." *Virchows Arch (Pathol Anat)* 365:185, 1975.
68. Mikkelsen OH: Knuckle pads in Dupuytren's disease. *Hand* 9:301, 1977.
69. Morginson WJ: Discrete keratodermas over the knuckle and finger articulations. *Arch Dermatol* 71:349, 1955.
70. Reichert CM, Costa J, Barsky SH, et al: Pachydermodactyly. *Clin Orthop* 194:252, 1985.
71. Strobel H: Neuere Untersuchungen über die Fingerknöchelpölster. *Archiv Dermatologie u Syphilis* 187:91, 1949.

Extraabdominal fibromatosis

72. Abramowitz D, Zornoza J, Ayala AG, et al: Soft tissue desmoid tumors: radiographic bone changes. *Radiology* 146:11, 1983.
73. Barber HM, Galasko CSB, Woods CG: Multicentric extraabdominal desmoid tumours: Report of 2 cases. *J Bone Joint Surg* 55B:858, 1973.
74. Bataini JP, Belloir C, Mazabraud A, et al: Desmoid tumors in adults: the role of radiotherapy in their management. *Am J Surg* 155:754, 1988.
75. Bogomoletz WV, Boulenger E, Simatos A: Infiltrating fibromatosis of the breast. *J Clin Pathol* 30:533, 1985.
76. Bridge JA, Sreekantaiah C, Mouron B, et al: Clonal chromosomal abnormalities in desmoid tumors: Implications for histogenesis. *Cancer* 69:430, 1992.
77. Brodsky JT, Gordon MS, Hajdu SI, et al: Desmoid tumors of the chest wall: a locally recurrent problem. *J Thorac Cardiovasc Surg* 104:900, 1992.
78. Brooks MD, Ebbs SR, Colletta AA, et al: Desmoid tumours treated with triphenylethylenes. *Eur J Cancer* 28A:1014, 1992.
79. Conley J, Healey WV, Stout AP: Fibromatosis of the head and neck. *Am J Surg* 112:609, 1966.
80. Dahn I, Jonsson N, Lundh G: Desmoid tumours: a series of 33 cases. *Acta Chir Scand* 126:305, 1963.
81. Dashiell TG: Desmoid tumors of the chest wall. *Chest* 74:157, 1978.
82. Easter DW, Halasz NA: Recent trends in the management of desmoid tumors. Summary of 19 cases and review of the literature. *Ann Surg* 210:765, 1989.
83. Enzinger FM, Shiraki M: Musculo-aponeurotic fibromatosis of the shoulder girdle (extra-abdominal desmoid): analysis of 30 cases followed up for 10 or more years. *Cancer* 21:1131, 1967.
84. Feiner H, Kaye GI: Ultrastructural evidence of myofibroblasts in circumscribed fibromatosis. *Arch Pathol* 100:265, 1976.
85. Fisker AV, Philipsen HP: Desmoplastic fibroma of the jaw bones. *Int J Oral Surg* 5:285, 1976.
86. Goellner JR, Soule EH: Desmoid tumors: an ultrastructural study of eight cases. *Hum Pathol* 11:43, 1980.
87. Gonatas K: Extra-abdominal desmoid tumors. Report of six cases. *Arch Pathol* 71(2):214, 1961.
88. Greenberg HM, Goebel R, Weichselbaum RR, et al: Radiation therapy in the treatment of aggressive fibromatosis. *Int J Radiat Oncol Biol Phys* 7:305, 1981.
89. Harjola PT: Desmoid tumor compressing vital pelvic structures: a case report. *Ann Chir Gynaecol* 66:89, 1977.
90. Hasegawa T, Hirose T, Kudo E, et al: Cytoskeletal characteristics of myofibroblasts in benign neoplastic and reactive fibroblastic lesions. *Virchows Arch (Pathol Anat)* 416:375, 1990.
91. Häyry P, Reitamo JJ, Tötterman S, et al: The desmoid tumor. II. Analysis of factors possibly contributing to the etiology and growth behavior. *Am J Clin Pathol* 77:674, 1982.
92. Häyry P, Reitamo JJ, Vihko R, et al: The desmoid tumor. III. A biochemical and genetic analysis. *Am J Clin Pathol* 77:681, 1982.
93. Hunt RTN, Morgan HC, Ackerman LV: Principles in the management of extraabdominal desmoids. *Cancer* 13(4):825, 1960.
94. Inwards CY, Unni KK, Beabout JW, et al: Desmoplastic fibroma of bone. *Cancer* 68:1978, 1991.
95. Jewett ST, Mead JH: Extra-abdominal desmoid arising from a capsule around silicone breast implant. *Plast Reconstr Surg* 63:577, 1979.
96. Karlsson I, Mandahl N, Heim S, et al: Complex chromosome rearrangements in an extraabdominal desmoid tumor. *Cancer Genet Cytogenet* 34:241, 1988.
97. Khorsand J, Karkousis CP: Desmoid tumors and their management. *Am J Surg* 149:215, 1985.
98. Kiel KD, Suit HD: Radiation therapy in the treatment of aggressive fibromatosis (desmoid tumor). *Cancer* 54:2051, 1984.

99. Kinzbrunner B, Ritter S, Domingo J, et al: Remission of rapidly growing desmoid tumor after tamoxifen therapy. *Cancer* 52:2201, 1983.

100. Kiryu H, Tsuneyoshi M, Enjoji M: Myofibroblasts in fibromatoses: an electron microscopic study. *Acta Pathol Jpn* 35:533, 1985.

101. Kofoed H, Kamby C, Agnostaki L: Aggressive fibromatosis. *Surg Gynecol Obstet* 160:124, 1985.

102. Kransdorf MJ, Jelinek JS, Moser RP Jr, et al: Magnetic resonance appearance of fibromatosis. A report of 14 cases and review of the literature. *Skeletal Radiol* 19:495, 1990.

103. Lanari A: Effect of progesterone on desmoid tumors (aggressive fibromatosis). *N Engl J Med* 309:1523, 1983.

104. Lee YS, Sen BK: Dystrophic and psammomatous calcifications in a desmoid tumor: a light microscopic and ultrastructural study. *Cancer* 55:84, 1985.

105. Leibel SA, Wara WM, Hill DR, et al: Desmoid tumors: local control and patterns of relapse following radiation therapy. *Int J Radiat Oncol Biol Phys* 9:1167, 1983.

106. Lopez R, Kemalyan N, Moseley HS, et al: Problems in diagnosis and management of desmoid tumors. *Am J Surg* 159:450, 1990.

107. Markhede G, Lundgren L, Bjurstam N, et al: Extra-abdominal desmoid tumors. *Acta Orthop Scand* 57:1, 1986.

108. Masson JK, Soule EH: Desmoid tumors of the head and neck. *Am J Surg* 112(4):615, 1966.

109. McCollough WM, Parsons JT, van der Griend R, et al: Radiation therapy for aggressive fibromatosis: the experience at the University of Florida. *J Bone Joint Surg* 73(A):717, 1991.

110. McDougall A, McGarrity G: Extra-abdominal desmoid tumors. *J Bone Joint Surg* 61B:373, 1979.

111. McKinnon JG, Neifeld JP, Kay S, et al: Management of desmoid tumors. *Surg Gynecol Obstet* 169:104, 1989.

112. Miller LF, Durrani KM: Desmoid tumor in a child: report of case. *J Int Coll Surg* 36:561, 1961.

113. Musgrove JE, McDonald JR: Extraabdominal desmoid tumors: their differential diagnosis and treatment. *Arch Pathol* 45:513, 1948.

114. Navas-Palacios JJ: The fibromatoses: An ultrastructural study of 31 cases. *Pathol Res Pract* 176:158, 1983.

115. Nichols RW: Desmoid tumors. A report of 31 cases. *Arch Surg* 7:227, 1923.

116. Penick RM: Desmoid tumors developing in operative scars. *Int Surg Digest* 23:323, 1937.

117. Pettit VD, Chamness JT, Ackerman LV: Fibromatosis and fibrosarcoma following irradiation therapy. *Cancer* 7:149, 1954.

118. Posner MC, Shiu MH, Newsome JL, et al: The desmoid tumor: not a benign disease. *Arch Surg* 124:191, 1989.

119. Reitamo JJ, Häyry P, Nykyri E, et al: The desmoid tumor. I. Incidence, sex, age and anatomical distribution in the Finnish population. *Am J Clin Pathol* 77:665, 1982.

120. Ritter MA, Marshall JL, Straub LR: Extra-abdominal desmoid of the hand: a case report. *J Bone Joint Surg* 51A:1641, 1969.

121. Rock MG, Pritchard DJ, Reiman HM, et al: Extraabdominal desmoid tumors. *J Bone Joint Surg* 66A:1369, 1984.

122. Rodu B, Weathers DR, Campbell WG: Aggressive fibromatosis involving the paramandibular tissues. *Oral Surg Oral Med Oral Pathol* 52:395, 1981.

123. Rosen PP, Ernsberger D: Mammary fibromatosis: a benign spindle cell tumor with significant risk for local recurrence. *Cancer* 63:1363, 1983.

124. Sanders R, Bennet M, Walton JN: A multifocal extraabdominal desmoid tumor. *Br J Plast Surg* 36:337, 1983.

125. Schwarzlmüller B, Hofstädter F: Fibromatose der Schilddrüsenregion. Eine elektronenmikroskopische und enzymhistochemische Studie. *Virchows Arch (Pathol Anat)* 377:145, 1978.

126. Sherman NE, Romsdahl M, Evans H, et al: Desmoid tumors: a 20-year radiotherapy experience. *Int J Radiat Oncol Biol Phys* 19:37, 1990.

127. Soule EH, Scanlon PW: Fibrosarcoma arising in an extraabdominal desmoid tumor: report of a case. *Mayo Clin Proc* 37:443, 1962.

128. Stiller D, Katenkamp D: Cellular features in desmoid fibromatosis and well-differentiated fibrosarcomas, an electron microscopic study. *Virchows Arch (Pathol Anat)* 369:155, 1975.

129. Stout AP: The fibromatoses. *Clin Orthop* 19:11, 1961.

130. Stout AP: Fibrosarcoma, well-differentiated (aggressive fibromatosis). *Cancer* 7:953, 1954.

131. Suit H: Radiation dose and response of desmoid tumors. *Int J Radiat Oncol Biol Phys* 19:225, 1990.

132. Sundaram M, Duffrin H, McGuire MH, et al: Synchronous multicentric desmoid tumors (aggressive fibromatosis) of the extremities. *Skeletal Radiol* 17:16, 1988.

133. Taxy JB, Battifora H: The electron microscope in the study and diagnosis of soft tissue tumors. In *diagnostic electron microscopy*. New York, 1980, John Wiley & Sons.

134. Thomas S, Datta-Gupta S, Kapur BM: Treatment of recurrent desmoid tumour with tamoxifen. *Aust N Z J Surg* 60:919, 1990.

135. Waddell WR, Gerner RE, Reich MP: Non-steroidal anti-inflammatory drugs and tamoxifen for desmoid tumors and carcinomas of the stomach. *J Surg Oncol* 22:197, 1983.

136. Waddell WR, Kirsch WM: Testolactone, sulindac, warfarin, and vitamin K1 for unresectable desmoid tumors. *Am J Surg* 161:416, 1991.

137. Wargotz ES, Norris HJ, Austin RM, et al: Fibromatosis of the breast. A clinical study of 28 cases. *Am J Surg Pathol* 11:38, 1987.

138. Weiss AJ, Lackman RD: Low dose chemotherapy of desmoid tumors. *Cancer* 64:1192, 1989.

139. Weiss SW, Langloss JM, Shmookler BM, et al: Estrogen receptor protein in bone and soft tissue tumors. *Lab Invest* 54:689, 1986.

140. Welsh RA: Intracytoplasmic collagen formation in desmoid fibromatosis. *Am J Pathol* 49:515, 1966.

141. Wilcken N, Tattersall MH: Endocrine therapy for desmoid tumors. *Cancer* 68:1384, 1991.

142. Wilkins SA, Waldron CA, Mathews WH: Aggressive fibromatosis of the head and neck. *Am J Surg* 130:412, 1975.

143. Young ID, Fortt RW: Familial fibromatosis. *Clin Genet* 20:211, 1981.

144. Zayid I, Dihmis C: Familial multicentric fibromatosis: desmoids: a report of three cases in a Jordanian family. *Cancer* 24(4):786, 1969.

145. Zelefsky MJ, Harrison LB, Shiu MH, et al: Combined surgical resection and iridium 192 implantation for locally advanced and recurrent desmoid tumors. *Cancer* 67:380, 1991.

146. Ziarek S, Sawaryn T, Guzy R, et al: Zur Behandlung von Desmoidgeschwülsten. *Zentralbl Chir* 106:1046, 1983.

Abdominal, intraabdominal, and mesenteric fibromatoses

147. Bach C: Desmoid tumors of the abdominal wall in children. *Ann Pediatr* 11:239, 1964.

148. Berardi RS, Canlas M: Desmoid tumor and laparotomy scars. *Int Surg* 58:253, 1973.

149. Booher RJ, Pack GT: Desmoma of the abdominal wall in children. *Cancer* 4:1052, 1951.

150. Brockman DD: Congenital desmoid of the abdominal wall. *J Pediatr* 31:217, 1947.

151. Burke AP, Sobin LH, Shekitka KM, et al: Intraabdominal fibromatosis: a pathologic analysis of 130 tumors with comparison of clinical subgroups. *Am J Surg Pathol* 14:335, 1990.

152. Cahn A: Ein Fall von Fibrom der Bauchdecken in einer Appendektomienarbe. *Zentralbl Chir* 49:110, 1922.

153. Caldwell EH: Desmoid tumor: musculoaponeurotic fibrosis of the abdominal wall. *Surgery* 79(1):104, 1976.

154. Danforth WC: Occurrence of new growths in abdominal wall after laparotomy. *Surg Gynecol Obstet* 29:175, 1919.

155. Dong-Heup K, Goldsmith HS, Quan SH: Intraabdominal desmoid tumor. *Cancer* 27:1041, 1971.

156. Falletta JM, Steuber CP: Abdominal fibromatosis and thrombocytosis. *J Pediatr* 87:145, 1975.

157. Gaches C, Burke J: Desmoid tumor (fibroma of the abdominal wall) occurring in siblings. *Br J Surg* 58:495, 1971.

158. Hutchinson JR, Norris DG, Schnaufer L: Chemotherapy: a successful application in abdominal fibromatosis (letter to the editor). *Pediatrics* 63:157, 1979.

159. Keely J, DeRosario J, Schairer A: Desmoid tumors of the abdominal and thoracic walls in a child. *AMA Arch Surg* 80:144, 1960.

160. Kim DH, Goldsmith HS, Quan SH, et al: Intra-abdominal desmoid tumor. *Cancer* 27:1041, 1971.

161. Kirchmer JT Jr, Woma FJ Jr: Desmoid tumors of the abdominal wall. *South Med J* 70(9):1136, 1977.

162. Koppikar MG, Vaze AM, Patel MS, et al: Mesenteric fibromatosis. *J Postgrad Med* 26:196, 1980.

163. Little JS Jr, Foster RS: Intraabdominal desmoid tumor: an unusual case of recurrent tumor in a testis cancer patient. *J Urol* 147:1619, 1992.

164. Mantello MD, Haller JO, Marquis JR: Sonography of abdominal desmoid tumors in adolescents. *J Ultrasound Med* 8:467, 1989.

165. Morgan AD, Loughridge LW, Calne RY: Combined retroperitoneal and mediastinal fibromatosis. *Lancet* 1:67,1966.

166. Newmark H III, Ching G, Halls J: An abdominal mass caused by mesenteric fibromatosis. *Am J Gastroenterol* 77:885, 1982.

167. Pack GT, Ehrlich HE: Neoplasms of the anterior abdominal wall with special consideration of desmoid tumors. Experience with 391 cases and collective review of the literature. *Surgery* 45:77, 1959.

168. Panos TH, Poth EJ: Desmoid tumors of the abdominal wall: use of prednisone to prevent recurrence in a child. *Surgery* 45:77, 1959.

169. Pfeiffer C: Die Desmoide der Bauchdecken und ihre Prognose. *Beitr Klin Chir* 44:334, 1904.

170. Salmon M: Desmoid tumor of the abdominal wall in a young boy. *Ann Chir Infant* 5:107, 1964.

171. Sampliner JE, Paruleker S, Jain B, et al: Intraabdominal mesenteric desmoid tumors. *Am Surg* 48:316, 1982.

172. Schweitzer RJ, Robbins GF: A desmoid tumor of multicentric origin. *AMA Arch Surg* 80(3):488, 1960.

173. Sportiello DJ, Hoogerland DL: A recurrent pelvic desmoid tumor successfully treated with tamoxifen. *Cancer* 67:1443, 1991.

174. Stout AP, Hendry J, Purdie FJ: Primary solid tumors of the omentum. *Cancer* 16:231, 1963.

175. Strode JE: Desmoid tumors particularly as related to surgical removal. *Ann Surg* 139:335, 1954.

176. Svanvik J, Knutsson F, Jansson R, et al: Desmoid tumor in the abdominal wall after treatment with high dose estradiol for prostatic cancer. *Acta Chir Scand* 148:301, 1982.

177. Waddell WR: Treatment of intra-abdominal and abdominal wall desmoid tumor with drugs that affect the metabolism of cyclic 3,5-adenosine monophosphate. *Ann Surg* 781:299, 1975.

178. Yannopoulos K, Stout AP: Primary solid tumors of the mesentery. *Cancer* 16:914, 1963.

Gardner's syndrome

179. Berk T, Cohen Z, McLeod RS, et al: Management of mesenteric desmoid tumours in familial adenomatous polyposis. *Can J Surg* 35:393, 1992.

180. Bochetto JF, Raycroft JF, DeInnocentes LW: Multiple polyposis, exostosis and soft tissue tumors. *Surg Gynecol Obstet* 117:489, 1963.

181. Camiel MR, Mule JE, Alexander LL, et al: Association of thyroid carcinoma with Gardner's syndrome in siblings. *N Engl J Med* 278:1056, 1968.

182. Chang CH, Platt ED, Thomas KE, et al: Bone abnormalities in Gardner's syndrome. *Am J Roentgenol* 103:645, 1968.

183. Clarke TJ: Intraabdominal fibromatosis in polyposis coli syndrome (letter to editor). *Am J Surg Pathol* 15:413, 1991.

184. Coli RD, Moore JP, Lamarche PH, et al: Gardner's syndrome: a revisit to a previously described family. *Am J Dig Dis* 15:551, 1970.

185. Duncan BR, Dohner VA, Priest JH: The Gardner syndrome: need for early diagnosis. *J Pediatr* 72:497, 1968.

186. Fraumeni JF Jr, Vogel CL, Easton JM: Sarcomas and multiple polyposis in a kindred. A genetic variety of hereditary polyposis? *Arch Intern Med* 121:57, 1968.

187. Gardner EJ: Follow up study of a family group exhibiting dominant inheritance for a syndrome including intestinal polyps, osteomas, fibromas and epidermal cysts. *Am J Hum Genet* 14:376, 1962.

188. Gardner EJ, Richards RC: Multiple cutaneous and subcutaneous lesions occurring simultaneously with hereditary polyposis and osteomatosis. *Am J Hum Genet* 5:139, 1953.

189. Gardner EJ, Stephens FE: Cancer of the lower digestive tract in one family group. *Am J Hum Genet* 2:41, 1950.

190. Gold RS, Mucha SJ: Unique case of mesenteric fibrosis in multiple polyposis. *Am J Surg* 130:366, 1975.

191. Gorlin RJ, Chaudhry AP: Multiple osteomatosis, fibromas, lipomas and fibrosarcomas of the skin and mesentery, epidermoid inclusion cysts of the skin, leiomyomas and multiple intestinal polyposis: a heritable disorder of connective tissue. *N Engl J Med* 263:1151, 1960.

192. Greer JA Jr, Devine KD, Dahlin DC: Gardner's syndrome and chondrosarcoma of the hyoid bone. *Arch Otolaryngol (Chicago)* 103(7):425, 1977.

193. Haggitt RC, Reid BJ: Hereditary gastrointestinal polyposis syndromes. *Am J Surg Pathol* 10:871, 1986.

194. Halata MS, Miller J, Stone RK: Gardner syndrome: early presentation with a desmoid tumor: Discovery of multiple colonic polyps. *Clin Pediatr* 28:538, 1989.

195. Jalota R, Middleton RG, McDivitt RW: Epidermoid cyst of the testis in Gardner's syndrome. *Cancer* 34:464, 1974.

196. Jarvinen HJ: Desmoid disease as a part of familial adenomatous polyposis coli. *Acta Chir Scand* 153:379, 1987.

197. Jones IT, Jagelman DG, Fazio VW, et al: Desmoid tumors in familial polyposis. *Ann Surg* 204:94, 1986.

198. Kitamura A, Kanagawa T, Yamada S, et al: Effective chemotherapy for abdominal desmoid tumor in a patient with Gardner's syndrome: report of a case. *Dis Colon Rectum* 34:822, 1991.

199. Klein WA, Miller HH, Anderson M, et al: The use of indomethacin, sulindac, and tamoxifen for the treatment of desmoid tumors associated with familial polyposis. *Cancer* 60:2863, 1987.

200. Kopelovich L, Gardner EJ: The use of tumor promoter for the detection of individuals with the Gardner syndrome. *Cancer* 51:716, 1983.

201. Laberge MY, Saur WG, Mayo CW: Soft tissue tumors associated with multiple polyposis. *Proc Mayo Clin* 32:749, 1958.

202. Lewis JH, Ginsberg AL, Toomey KE: Turcot's syndrome: evidence of autosomal dominant inheritance. *Cancer* 51:524, 1983.

203. Lewis RJ, Mitchell JC: Basal cell carcinoma in Gardner's syndrome. *Acta Derm Venereol (Stockh)* 51:67, 1971.

204. Lotfi AM, Dozois RR, Gordon H, et al: Mesenteric fibromatosis complicating familial adenomatous polyposis: predisposing factors and results of treatment. *Int J Colorectal Dis* 4:30, 1989.

205. MacDonald JM, Davis WC, Crago HR, et al: Gardner's syndrome and periampullary malignancy. *Am J Surg* 113:425, 1967.

206. Maher ER, Morson B, Beach R, et al: Phenotypic variation in hereditary nonpolyposis colon cancer syndrome: association with infiltrative fibromatosis (desmoid tumor). *Cancer* 69:2049, 1992.

207. Martel AJ, Bonanno CA: Multiple polyposis of the gastrointestinal tract with osteoma and soft tissue tumors. *Am J Dig Dis* 13:588, 1968.

208. Miller RH, Sweet RH: Multiple polyposis of colon, a familial disease. *Ann Surg* 105:511, 1937.

209. Naylor EW, Gardner EJ, Richards RC: Desmoid tumors and mesenteric fibromatosis in Gardner's syndrome. *Arch Surg* 114:1181, 1979.

210. Neal CJ Jr: Multiple osteomas of the mandible associated with polyposis of the colon (Gardner's syndrome). *Oral Surg Oral Med Oral Pathol* 28:628, 1969.

211. Neale HW, Pickrell KL, Quinn GW: Extra-abdominal manifestations of Gardner's syndrome. *Plast Reconstr Surg* 56:92, 1975.

212. Okamoto M, Sato C, Kohno Y, et al: Molecular nature of chromosome 5Q loss in colorectal tumors and desmoids from patients with familial adenomatous polyposis. *Hum Genet* 85:595, 1990.

213. Pierce ER, Weisbord T, McKusick VA: Gardner's syndrome: formal genetics and statistical analysis of a large Canadian kindred. *Clin Genet* 1:65, 1970.

214. Richards RC, Rogers SW, Gardner EJ: Spontaneous mesenteric fibromatosis in Gardner's syndrome. *Cancer* 47:597, 1981.

215. Staley CJ: Gardner's syndrome: simultaneous occurrence of polyposis coli, osteomatosis and soft tissue tumors. *Arch Surg* 82:420, 1961.

216. Traboulsi EI, Krush AJ, Gardner EJ, et al: Prevalence and importance of pigmented ocular fundus lesions in Gardner's syndrome. *N Engl J Med* 316:661, 1987.

217. Tsukada K, Church JM, Jagelman DG, et al: Noncytotoxic drug therapy for intraabdominal desmoid tumor in patients with familial adenomatous polyposis. *Dis Colon Rectum* 35:29, 1992.

218. Tsukada K, Church JM, Jagelman DG, et al: Systemic cytotoxic chemotherapy and radiation therapy for desmoid in familial adenomatous polyposis. *Dis Colon Rectum* 34:1090, 1991.

219. Umemoto S, Makuuchi H, Amemiya T, et al: Intra-abdominal desmoid tumors in familial polyposis coli: a case report of tumor regression by prednisolone therapy. *Dis Colon Rectum* 34:89, 1991.

220. Weary PE, Linthicum A, Cawley EP, et al: Gardner's syndrome: a family group study and review. *Arch Dermatol* 90:20, 1964.

221. Weiner RS, Cooper P: Multiple polyposis of the colon, osteomatosis, and soft tissue tumors. Report of familial syndrome. *N Engl J Med* 253:795, 1955.

222. Witkop CJ Jr: Gardner's syndrome and other osteognathodermal disorders with defects in parathyroid functions. *J Oral Surg* 26:639, 1968.

223. Yoshida MA, Ikeuchi T, Iwama T, et al: Chromosome changes in desmoid tumors developed in patients with familial adenomatous polyposis. *Jpn J Cancer Res* 82:916, 1991.

Idiopathic retroperitoneal fibrosis (Ormond's disease)

224. Bartholomew LG, Cain JC, Woolner LB, et al: Sclerosing cholangitis: its possible association with Riedel's struma and fibrous retroperitonitis: A report of two cases. *N Engl J Med* 269:8, 1963.

225. Comings DE, Skubi KB, Van Eyes J, et al: Familial multifocal fibrosclerosis: findings suggesting that retroperitoneal fibrosis, mediastinal fibrosis, sclerosing cholangitis, Riedel's thyroiditis, and pseudotumor of the orbit may be different manifestations of a single disease. *Ann Intern Med* 66:884, 1967.

226. DuPont HL, Varco RL, Winchell CP: Chronic fibrous mediastinitis simulating pulmonic stenosis, associated with inflammatory pseudotumor of the orbit. *Am J Med* 44:447, 1968.

227. Hache L, Utz DC, Woolner LB: Idiopathic fibrous retroperitonitis. *Surg Gynecol Obstet* 115:737, 1962.

228. Hawk WA, Hazard JB: Sclerosing retroperitonitis and sclerosing mediastinitis. *Am J Clin Pathol* 32:321, 1959.

229. Hricak H, Higgins CB, Williams RD: Nuclear magnetic resonance imaging in retroperitoneal fibrosis. *Am J Radiol* 141:35, 1983.

230. Kerr WS Jr, Suby HI, Vickery A, et al: Idiopathic retroperitoneal fibrosis. Clinical experiences with 15 cases, 1956-1967. *J Urol* 99:575, 1968.

231. Mitchinson MJ: The pathology of idiopathic retroperitoneal fibrosis. *J Clin Pathol* 23:901, 1961.

232. Ormond JK: Bilateral ureteral obstruction due to envelopment and compression by an inflammatory retroperitoneal process. *J Urol* 59:1072, 1948.

233. Osborne BM, Butler JJ, Bloustein P, et al: Idiopathic retroperitoneal fibrosis (sclerosing retroperitonitis). *Hum Pathol* 18:735, 1987.

234. Rao CR, Ferguson GC, Kyle VN: Retroperitoneal fibrosis associated with Riedel's struma. *Can Med Assoc J* 108:1019, 1973.

235. Salmon HW: Combined mediastinal and retroperitoneal fibrosis. *Thorax* 23:158, 1968.

236. Tiptaft RC, Costello AJ, Paris AM, et al: The long-term follow-up of idiopathic retroperitoneal fibrosis. *Br J Urol* 54:620, 1982.

237. Utz DC, Rooke ED, Spittel JA Jr, et al: Retroperitoneal fibrosis in patients taking methysergide. *JAMA* 194:983, 1965.

CHAPTER 11

FIBROUS TUMORS OF INFANCY AND CHILDHOOD

Fibrous tumors of infancy and childhood can be divided into two large groups. The first group consists of lesions corresponding in clinical setting, microscopic picture, and behavior to similar lesions occurring in adults. Typical examples of such lesions are nodular fasciitis, palmar or plantar fibromatosis, and abdominal or extraabdominal fibromatosis. The second group consists of fibrous lesions that are peculiar to infancy and childhood and generally have no clinical or morphological counterpart in adult life. The latter are less common, and because of their unusual microscopic features, they pose a special problem in diagnosis. In fact, in this group of tumors the microscopic picture often fails to reflect accurately the biological behavior, and features such as cellularity and rapid growth may be mistaken for evidence of malignancy and sometimes may lead to unnecessary and excessive therapy. Accurate interpretation and diagnosis of these lesions are therefore of utmost importance for predicting clinical behavior and for selecting proper forms of therapy (Table 11-1).

FIBROUS HAMARTOMA OF INFANCY

Fibrous hamartoma of infancy is a distinctive fibrous growth first described by Reye[22] in 1956 as *subdermal fibromatous tumors of infancy*. After reviewing all cases of fibrous tumors of infancy on file at the AFIP, we reported 30 additional cases of this entity[12] and suggested the term *fibrous hamartoma of infancy* to emphasize its organoid microscopic appearance and its frequent occurrence at birth and in the immediate postnatal period. This term also affords clear distinction from Michelson's *nodular subepidermal fibrosis,* a benign tumor of adult life and a synonym for *cutaneous fibrous histiocytoma.*

Clinical findings

As a rule, the lesion develops during the first two years of life (median age, 10 months) as a small rapidly growing, soft to firm mass in the lower dermis or subcutis. Rare examples may also be encountered in older infants and children. Usually the mass is freely movable, but occasionally

Table 11-1. Clinicopathological characteristics of fibrous tumors of infancy and childhood

Histological diagnosis	Age (years)	Location	Solitary	Multiple	Recurrence	Regression
Fibrous hamartoma	B-2	Axillary and inguinal region	+	−	Rare	−
Myofibromatosis	B-A	Soft tissue, bone, viscera	+	+	Rare	+
Fibromatosis colli	B-2	Sternocleidomastoid muscle	+	Bilateral	Rare	+
Digital fibromatosis	B-2	Fingers and toes	+	+	Common	+
Infantile fibromatosis	B-4	Musculature	+	−	Common	−
Calcifying aponeurotic fibroma	2-A	Hands and feet	+	−	Common	+
Hyalin fibromatosis	2-A	Dermis and subcutis	(+)	+	−	−

A, Adult life; *B,* birth.

it is fixed to the fascia or muscle. Involvement of muscle, however, is rare, and when it occurs, it affects only its most superficial portion. There is nothing in the clinical history indicating that the lesions cause tenderness or pain. Like other fibrous tumors occurring in children, it is more than twice as common in boys as in girls. In about 15% to 20% of cases it is present at birth.[12,21]

The principal location is the region of the anterior or posterior axillary fold, followed in frequency by the upper arm, thigh, inguinal and pubic region, shoulder, back, and forearm. Lesions in the scrotum have also been described.[15,17] Apparently fibrous hamartoma never occurs in the hands or feet, a feature that helps to distinguish the tumor from digital fibromatosis and calcifying aponeurotic fibroma. Virtually all cases are solitary; multiple forms are exceedingly rare; there is only one such case on file at the AFIP—a fibrous hamartoma that manifested with multiple nodules in the groin. There is no evidence of increased familial incidence or of associated malformations or other neoplasms.

Gross findings

The excised lesion tends to be poorly circumscribed and consists of an intimate mixture of firm gray-white tissue and fat. The fatty component may be inconspicuous or may occupy a large part of the tumor. The latter forms may be confused with fibrolipoma, but they are never as well circumscribed or lobulated (Fig. 11-1). On average the mass measures 3 to 5 cm in greatest diameter, but we have seen large examples measuring 15 cm or more.

Microscopic findings

Invariably there are three different tissue components forming a vague, irregular, "organoid" pattern: (1) well-defined intersecting trabeculae of fibrous tissue of varying size and shape and composed of well-oriented spindle-shaped cells separated by varying amounts of collagen; (2) loosely textured areas consisting chiefly of immature small, rounded or stellate cells within a mucoid matrix that stains well with the alcian blue preparation and is removed by prior treatment of the section with hyaluronidase; and (3) interspersed mature fat, which may be present only at the periphery or may be the major component of the tumor (Figs. 11-2 to 11-4). Despite the lack of clear boundaries between the fat within the tumor and that in the surrounding subcutis, there is little doubt that the fat is an integral part of the lesion. In fact, in many cases its total amount exceeds many times the amount of fat normally present in the surrounding panniculus.[12]

Some tumors show an additional tissue component, a peculiar fibrosing process that has a superficial resemblance to a neurofibroma. It consists of thick collagen fibers and scattered fibroblasts and chiefly replaces the fat and the

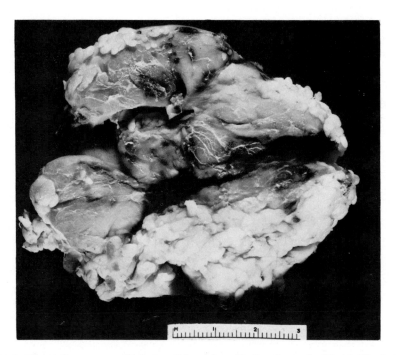

FIG. 11-1. Fibrous hamartoma of infancy of the right axilla in a 9-month-old girl. The lesion had been present for 4 months. The lesion is for the most part poorly circumscribed and blends with the surrounding subcutaneous fat.

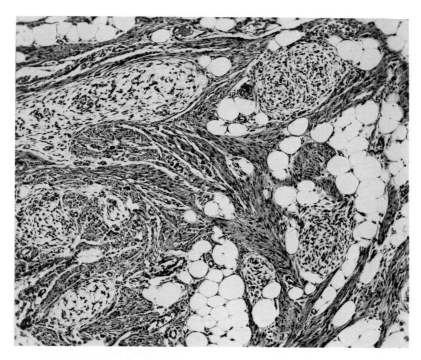

FIG. 11-2. Fibrous hamartoma of infancy in right upper arm of a 1½-year-old boy shows characteristic organoid pattern composed of interlacing fibrous trabeculae, islands of loosely arranged spindle-shaped cells, and mature adipose tissue. (×60.)

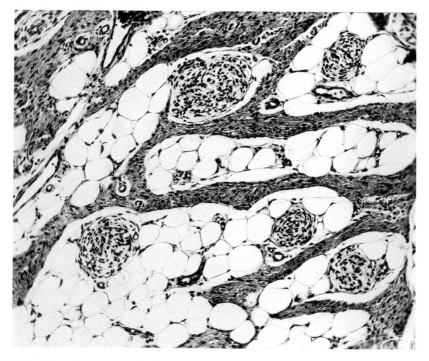

FIG. 11-3. Fibrous hamartoma of infancy showing distinct fibrous trabeculae and loosely textured nests of immature spindle cells. (×130.)

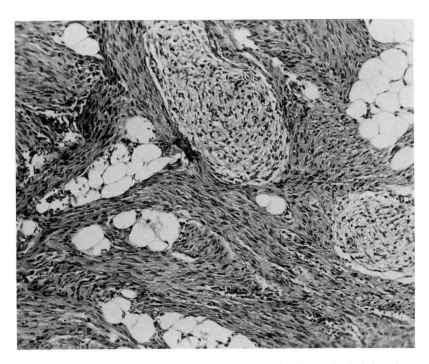

FIG. 11-4. Fibrous hamartoma of infancy in left upper arm of a 17-month-old infant shows typical association of well-defined fibrous and fatty elements. (×145.)

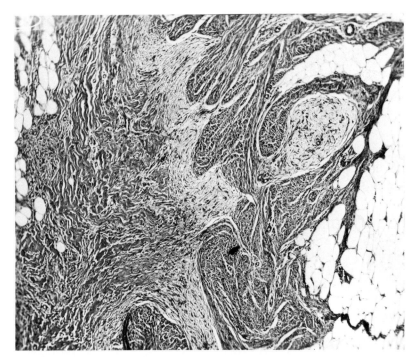

FIG. 11-5. Fibrous hamartoma of infancy. The central portion of the lesion is replaced by dense fibrosis, but there are remnants of the characteristic organoid features at the periphery. (×70.)

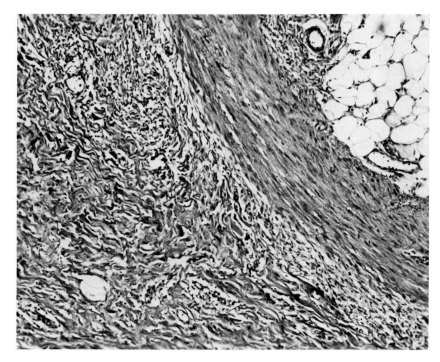

FIG. 11-6. Neurofibromalike fibrosis of fibrous hamartoma of infancy, a common feature of this lesion. Note diagnostic fibrous trabeculae. (Hematoxylin-eosin stain; ×100.)

loosely textured mesenchymal areas; sometimes it may be the principal component of the tumor (Fig. 11-5). In most of the latter cases, however, the presence of typical fibrous trabeculae at the periphery of the lesion and the clinical setting will provide the correct diagnosis (Fig. 11-6). Immunohistochemically, vimentin positivity is present in both the trabecular and loosely cellular areas, but actin and desmin reactivity is present only in the trabecular component.[13,15,19,24]

Ultrastructural findings

The lesion consists of a mixture of fibroblasts and myofibroblasts,[20] with abundant collagen fibrils in the fascicular fibrous areas and fibroblasts or primitive mesenchymal cells with stellate cytoplasmic processes, collagen fibrils, and fibrillar and granular material in the myxoid areas. Some of the vessels are surrounded by concentric layers of mesenchymal cells. Elastic fibers are absent.[14,15,20] Because of the myofibroblastic component, Aberer et al.[11] suggested the term *infantile subcutaneous myofibroblastoma.*

Differential diagnosis

Among the various proliferations of infancy, few are likely to be confused with this lesion. *Infantile fibromatosis* may encroach on the subcutis in a similar trabecular

manner, but this tumor arises primarily in muscle rather than in the subcutis and lacks the "organoid" pattern of fibrous hamartoma. Awareness of the characteristic "organoid" pattern also will facilitate distinction from *infantile fibrosarcoma* and *embryonal rhabdomyosarcoma.*[23] *Calcifying aponeurotic fibroma* may grow in the same trabecular manner, especially in its earliest phase, in which there is still little or no calcification. In these cases, however, the older age of the children and the location of the tumor in the palm of the hand will permit an unequivocal diagnosis. There are occasional fibrous tumors in adults that resemble fibrous hamartoma, but most of these have an additional smooth muscle component and most likely are examples of benign mesenchymoma.

Discussion

It is important to recognize and distinguish fibrous hamartoma of infancy from other forms of fibromatosis because it is a benign neoplasm that, despite its focal cellularity, is nearly always cured by local excision. There are recurrent cases, but these are rare and never cause clinical complications.

Its true nature and cause remain obscure. Reye[22] suggested that it may be a reparative process, but among the more than 120 cases at the AFIP, we have never encountered one that showed evidence of an early reactive or inflammatory phase. Indeed, it appears more likely that it is a dysontogenetic or hamartomatous process; in other words, it is an organoid growth of tissue indigenous to the area but different in quantity, arrangement, and cellular differentiation.

INFANTILE DIGITAL FIBROMATOSIS

As the name implies, *infantile digital fibromatosis* (or *infantile digital fibroma*) is a distinctive fibrous tumor of infancy characterized by its occurrence in the fingers and toes. It is further marked by its tendency to recur locally and the presence of characteristic inclusion bodies within the cytoplasm of the proliferated fibroblasts. Although the presence of intracellular inclusion bodies was first recognized by Reye[62] in 1965, typical examples of this tumor were reported earlier in the literature[40,50,60,63,65] under various terms, including *digital neurofibrosarcoma*.[48] We also briefly described a series of seven cases in 1963 as *infantile dermal fibromatosis*.[38]

Clinical findings

The fibrous nodules, which develop exclusively in the digits of the hands and feet, are hemispherical or dome-shaped, with a broad base and a smooth glistening surface that is skin colored or pale red. They usually are small and rarely exceed 2 cm in greatest diameter. Nearly always they are noted during the first year of life and in about one third of cases are already present at birth. Sporadic examples in older children, adolescents, and adults have also been reported.[27,30,59] Unlike most other forms of fibromatosis the condition seems to be slightly more common in girls than in boys, but there is no evidence of any hereditary trait.

The nodules are more often found in the fingers than the toes, and in most instances are located on the sides or dorsum of the distal or middle phalangeal joints, especially of the third, fourth, and fifth digits. In all cases thumbs and great toes are spared. The lesions may be single or multiple and often affect more than one digit of the same hand or foot (Fig. 11-7). Occasionally they involve both the fingers and toes of the same patient. They are very rare outside the hands and feet, but such a case with typical eosinophilic perinuclear inclusions was reported in the upper arm of a 2½-year-old child.[61]

There is no evidence that the nodules cause discomfort or pain, and many have been present for several weeks or months prior to excision. Associated functional impairment or joint deformities were noted in several instances, even in cases in which the nodules regressed spontaneously.

Pathological findings

The excised lesions are small firm masses that are covered on one side by intact skin and have a solid white cut surface. They show little variation in their microscopic appearance and, like the desmoid form of infantile fibroma-

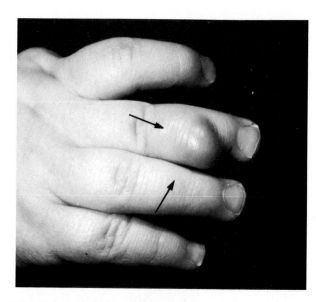

FIG. 11-7. Infantile digital fibromatosis of the middle finger of the right hand of a 7½-month-old boy.

tosis, consist of a uniform proliferation of fibroblasts surrounded by a dense collagenous stroma (Figs. 11-8 and 11-9). They are poorly circumscribed and extend from the epidermis down into the subcutis or deeper portions of the dermis surrounding dermal appendages. Changes in the overlying epidermis are usually minimal and consist only of slight hyperkeratosis or acanthosis.

Unquestionably the most striking feature of the tumor is the presence of small round inclusions within the cytoplasm of the proliferated fibroblasts. The relative number of the inclusions varies from case to case; in some they are numerous and easily detected; in others they are scarce and difficult to find with the hematoxylin-eosin preparation. Most are situated close to the nucleus, from which they are often separated by a narrow clear zone (Fig. 11-9). They are eosinophilic and resemble erythrocytes except for their more variable size (3 to 15 μ), their intracytoplasmic location, and lack of refringency. The inclusions stain a deep red with Masson trichrome stain and purple with PTAH, bright red with Lendrum's phloxine tartrazine stain, and black with iron-hematoxylin preparations; they do not accept the PAS, alcian blue, and colloidal iron stains. Moreover, they are negative for the Feulgen method, and, according to most reviewers, do not stain with methyl green-pyronine.[25,26,46,52,66] They also contain abundant sulfhydryl groups.[49]

Electron microscopic findings

Among the various investigators there is agreement that the constituent tumor cells are metabolically active fibro-

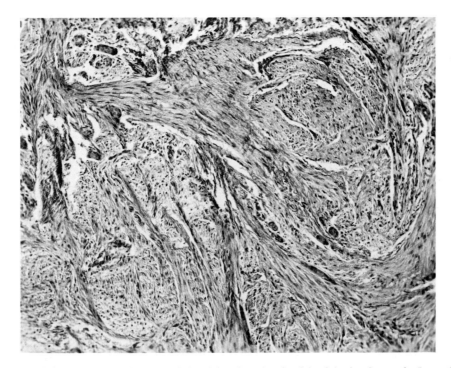

FIG. 11-8. Infantile digital fibromatosis involving the subcutis of the right ring finger of a 5-month-old child. (×60.)

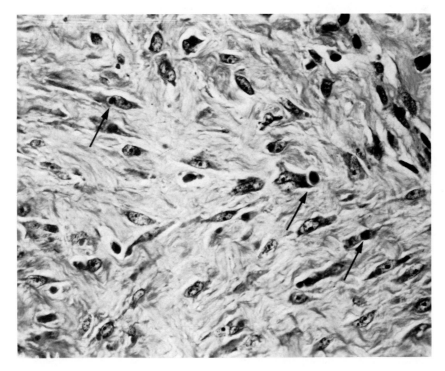

FIG. 11-9. Infantile digital fibromatosis. Fibroblasts with characteristic intracytoplasmic inclusions *(arrows).* (×400.)

blasts and myofibroblasts displaying a rich network of endoplasmic reticulum and a prominent Golgi zone. The myofibroblasts contain narrow intracellular bundles of 5 to 7-nm microfilaments with interspersed dense bodies and occasional patches of basal lamina. These straplike bundles of filaments are continuous with the juxtanuclear inclusion bodies, which also consist of fibrillary and granular material that has no limiting membrane and seems to originate in the endoplasmic reticulum (Fig. 11-10).* Identical intracellular inclusions were also observed in cultured spindle cells obtained from patients with digital fibromatosis.[45,66]

The results of immunohistochemical studies differ slightly: some investigators noted actin positivity in both cytoplasm and inclusions and suggested that the inclusions

---

*References 28, 31, 33, 34, 39, 42, 54.

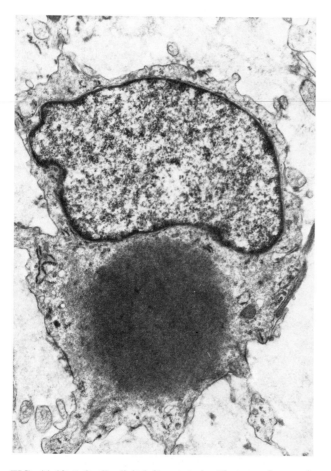

FIG. 11-10. Infantile digital fibromatosis. Electron microscopic picture showing inclusion within fibroblast. (From Taxy JB, Battifora H: The electron microscope in the study and diagnosis of soft tissue tumors. In Trump BF, Jones RT, editors: *Diagnostic electron microscopy,* New York, 1980, John Wiley & Sons, Inc.)

represent abnormal contractions of actinlike filaments.[37,39,41,44] Others found vimentin, actin, and myosin only in the cytoplasm but not in the inclusions, possibly because of degeneration of the actinlike filaments.[56,66,67]

Prognosis and therapy

Although 60% of cases recur locally, the ultimate prognosis is excellent. Recurrence takes place at the same site within a few weeks or months after the initial excision, or a second tumor develops in an adjacent finger or toe.[32] After the initial growth period, however, many of the lesions regress spontaneously.[43] For instance, in the case reported by McKenzie et al.[52] two of the three nodules were left untreated, and both regressed within a period of 3 years. Deviation deformities and contractures develop in some cases regardless of whether or not the lesions were removed surgically.[29,30,47] Because there is no evidence of aggressive behavior or malignant transformation, only surgical excision is needed, and, when necessary, correction of contractures and functional changes.

Discussion

The exact nature of the inclusions is not clear, but it is no longer thought that they are of viral origin. Attempts at viral isolation were unsuccessful, and both the immunohistochemical and ultrastructural findings strongly suggest that the intracellular inclusions are related to the intracellular bundles of microfilaments and represent densely packed masses of actin microfilaments.[44,58] Trauma may stimulate the development of the lesion: there are records of typical examples arising in scar tissue,[51,53] but there are also reports of similar inclusions in other tumors, including palisaded myofibroblastoma (see Chapter 18), a fibrous tumor of the tongue,[36] a dermal fibrous lesion occurring in the toxic oil epidemic syndrome,[57] and an endocervical polyp.[35]

MYOFIBROMA AND MYOFIBROMATOSIS

Myofibromatosis was first described by Stout[65] in 1954 as *congenital generalized fibromatosis.* Both of his patients were male infants who died soon after birth and had multiple fibrous nodules in soft tissues and internal organs. One of these cases was previously reported by Williams and Schrum[109] as a metastatic congenital fibrosarcoma.

Since Stout's original report, numerous additional examples of this entity were described in the medical literature. Most of them were infants with multiple fibrous nodules, and there were only a few patients with solitary lesions.[71,83,92-94,102,108] Yet, according to our experience,[79] solitary lesions seem to be several times as common as multiple ones, even taking into account that some lesions in the skeleton and internal organs are likely to be missed without a thorough roentgenographical examination. In fact, solitary tumors were found in 45 of the 61 patients in our series, and in 33 of the 34 patients reported by Smith et al.[103]

Most cases in the earlier literature were described as congenital generalized fibromatosis,[65] generalized hamartomatosis,[98] multiple congenital mesenchymal hamartomas,[71] and multiple vascular leiomyomas.[95] We prefer, however, the terms *myofibroma* and *myofibromatosis,* for the solitary and multiple lesions, respectively, not only because these lesions occur in infants and children but also in adults, and have a prominent myofibroblastic component, but also because of their behavior, which distinguishes them from other, more aggressive types of fibromatosis.

Clinical findings

Myofibroma manifests as a single swelling or mass in the dermis and subcutis and measures from a few millimeters to several centimeters in diameter. Solitary nodules are found most commonly in the general region of the head and neck, including the oral cavity,[104] the craniofacial bones,[85,87,89] and the shoulder girdle. They are less common in the extremities and rare in the viscera.[78,108] There are few symptoms, except for occasional pain caused by compression of nerves. The condition is almost twice as common in males as in females, and occurs not only in infants and children but also in adults.[79,80,110] In fact, Smith et al.[103] reported 28 cases with solitary lesions in patients older than 14 years.

Patients with multiple lesions *(myofibromatosis)* are less common than those with solitary ones; in our series of 61 cases only 16 had multiple lesions.[79] The individual nodules in these cases show essentially the same appearance as the solitary nodules, but occur not only in dermis and subcutis but also in muscle, the internal organs, and the skeleton. In most cases the visceral lesions are already present at birth. We are aware of only one report of multiple lesions in an adult.[103]

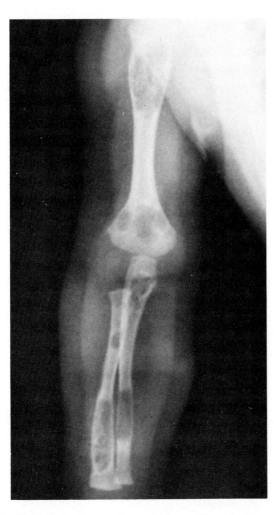

FIG. 11-11. Infantile myofibromatosis, multicentric type, with extensive bone involvement of the right arm. (From Brill, PW et al: *Pediatr Radiol* 12:771, 1982.)

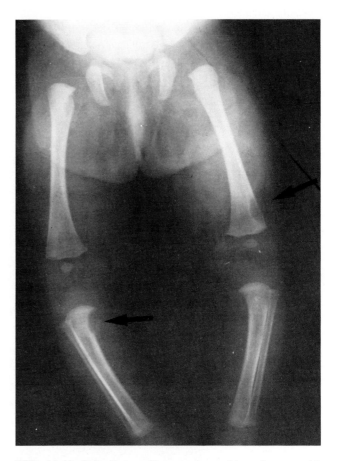

FIG. 11-12. Infantile myofibromatosis, multicentric type with multiple bone involvement *(arrows).* These osseous lesions tend to regress spontaneously and usually are no longer demonstrable after a few years.

The nodules may be numerous, especially when occurring in the subcutis, lung, or skeleton, and there are several examples in which more than 50 separate nodules were counted. For example, Schaffzin et al.[101] reported a newborn girl who had at birth 59 subcutaneous nodules. Heiple et al.[86] also described an infant who had more than 100 lesions in the skeleton that involved both flat and long bones. In the latter case the nodules were recognized only after the infant suffered a fracture in a minor fall and had a roentgenographic examination of the injured leg.

Apart from the soft tissues and the skeleton, the most common sites of the nodules are the lung, heart, gastrointestinal tract, and pancreas.[106] Internal lesions often cause symptoms such as severe respiratory distress, vomiting, or diarrhea, which often fail to respond to therapy and prove fatal within a few days or weeks after birth. Others cause few symptoms, making it likely that some internal lesions remain unrecognized. In rare instances the nervous system may be involved: we have seen two cases with multiple nodules of the brain, and Altemani et al.[68] reported a lesion of the spinal canal causing compression and flaccid paralysis of the lower limb. Orbital lesions may also encroach upon the adjacent dura or brain.[87] The nodules of myofibromatosis grow principally during the immediate perinatal period. Growth, however, is not restricted to this period, and continued enlargement or formation of new le-

sions may be observed during infancy or even later in life.[75,96,101] Daimaru et al.[80] reported examples of adult myofibroma that had been present for 10 or more years.

Roentgenographically, the bone lesions are circumscribed lytic areas with marginal sclerosis and without penetration of the cortex in most cases. Occasionally, however, a soft tissue lesion may extend into the underlying bone. Extraosseous lesions may show weak radiodensity as a result of focal calcifications (Figs. 11-11 and 11-12).[69,76,89] MRI of myofibromatosis was discussed by Moore et al.[97]

Pathological findings

As a rule, the nodules in the dermis and subcutis are better delineated than those in muscle, bone, or viscera. They are firm and scarlike in consistency and have a white-gray or pink surface; they vary greatly in size, averaging from 0.5 to 1.5 cm in greatest diameter. Plaschkes[99] described one case in which there were numerous minute skin lesions that "resembled the scars of healed chickenpox." Large lesions may become ulcerated.[90]

Microscopically, *myofibroma* and *myofibromatosis* display similar features, often showing a biphasic, nodular, or multinodular pattern, characterized by light-staining nodules separated by or associated with pericytoma-like richly vascular or spindle cell areas. The light-staining nodules consist mainly of plump spindle-shaped cells that often have

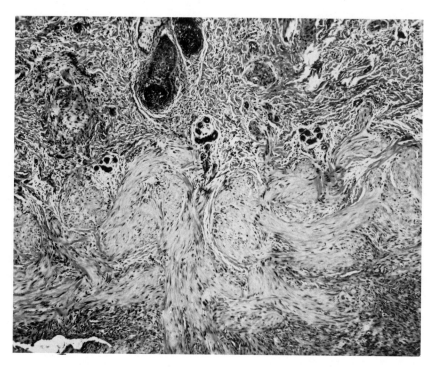

FIG. 11-13. Infantile myofibromatosis (solitary type) consisting of broad bundles of fibrous connective tissue in dermis and subcutis. (×60.)

a pronounced eosinophilic cytoplasm and are arranged in nodules or short bundles. The distinct margination of the tumor and the eosinophilia of the spindle-shaped cells are often reminiscent of leiomyoma (Figs. 11-13 to 11-17). With special stains these cells show features of both myoblastic and fibroblastic lesions; they contain fuchsinophilic and PTAH-positive intracellular longitudinal fibrils and are surrounded by considerable amounts of collagen (Fig. 11-15). Immunohistochemically, they are immunoreactive for vimentin and actin but do not stain for desmin or S-100 protein.[75,80,103]

The associated or intervening richly vascular areas are less well differentiated and consist either of round or polygonal cells with slightly pleomorphic hyperchromatic nuclei or small spindle cells; the cells are arranged in solid sheets or, more commonly, display a distinct pericytoma pattern, often with necrosis and calcification. In fact, in some tumors necrosis is so extensive that only a narrow rim of viable tissue is left at the periphery, resulting in a cyst-like lesion (Figs. 11-14 and 11-15). Because of these cellular and richly vascular areas and the extensive necrosis, some tumors have been mistaken for sarcoma. An erroneous diagnosis of sarcoma was also rendered in some childhood cases because of the presence of intravascular growth, a feature that was present in about one fifth of our cases and does not seem to have any prognostic significance (Figs. 11-18 to 11-20).

Ultrastructural findings

There is general agreement that the predominant cells are fibroblasts and myofibroblasts, with prominent endoplasmic reticulum, intracytoplasmic microfilaments, dense bodies, focal basal lamina, and occasional intercellular attachment sites (Fig. 11-21).* Fletcher et al.[84] however, reached the conclusion that the immunohistochemical and ultrastructural findings support a smooth muscle tumor.

---

*References 73, 74, 82, 90, 98, 104.

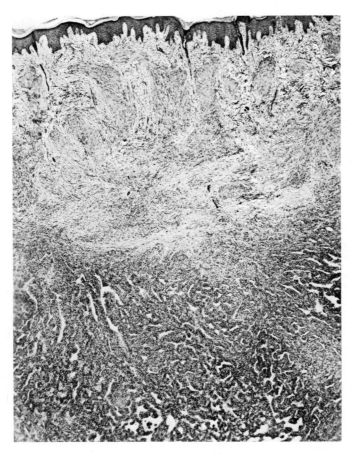

FIG. 11-14. Infantile myofibromatosis (solitary type). Note broad bundles of fibrous connective tissue surrounding a hemangiopericytomalike area in the center of the lesion. (×25.)

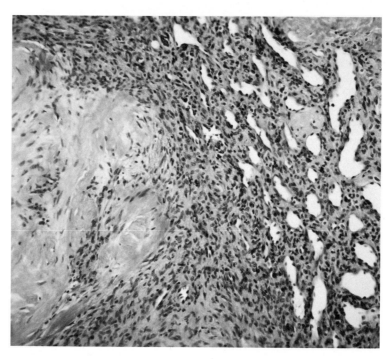

FIG. 11-15. Infantile myofibromatosis showing bundles of myofibroblasts associated with hemangiopericytomalike pattern. (×100.)

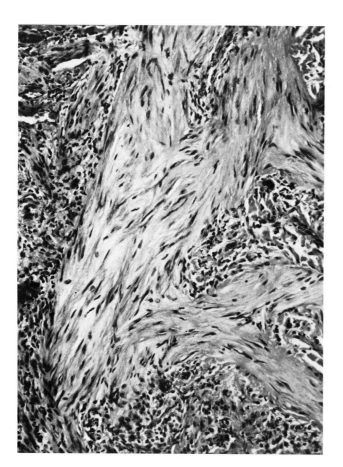

FIG. 11-16. Infantile myofibromatosis (solitary type). Bundles of well-oriented myofibroblasts superficially resembling smooth muscle tissue. (×160.)

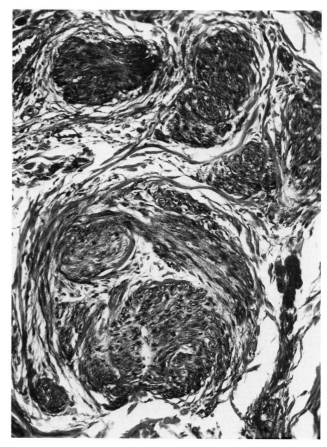

FIG. 11-17. Infantile myofibromatosis. Fuchsinophilic bundles of myofibroblasts in cross-section. (Masson-trichrome stain; ×160.)

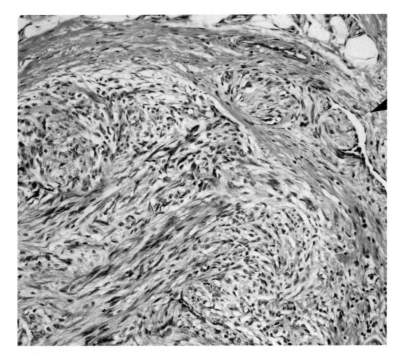

FIG. 11-18. Cellular portion of solitary form of myofibromatosis with focal intravascular growth *(arrow).* (×160.)

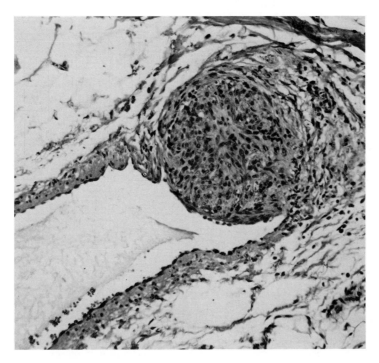

FIG. 11-19. Intravascular growth in solitary type of infantile myofibromatosis. Despite this feature these lesions are uniformly benign and are cured by simple local excision. (×160.)

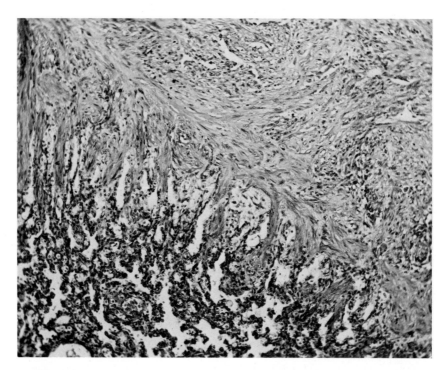

FIG. 11-20. Infantile myofibromatosis (multicentric type) involving lung. (×135.)

Differential diagnosis

Myofibroma may be confused with a variety of benign and malignant neoplasms. In general, the bundles or nodules of plump, eosinophilic myofibroblasts, often associated with a more centrally located vascular or small spindle cell component, will help to rule out *nodular fasciitis, fibrous histiocytoma, neurofibroma, hemangiopericytoma,* or *glomus tumor.* In particular, nodular fasciitis arises from the fascia and has a more prominent myxoid matrix and a chronic inflammatory cell infiltrate, and neurofibroma is positive for S-100 protein. Although mitotic figures are frequently increased and there may be intravascular growth, the alternating nodular and spindle cell pattern militates against *hemangiopericytoma, fibrosarcoma,* or some other malignant neoplasm. The scarcity of hemorrhage and necrosis in the adult forms of myofibroma may also help in differential diagnosis.[80,103]

Myofibromatosis, when it manifests with multiple nodules at birth or the first few weeks of life, is unlikely to be confused with other multicentric disease processes. As a rule, *neurofibromatosis* affects older children, and in addition to multiple tumors, there is evidence of multiple café au lait spots, and in about one half of cases a history of familial involvement. Likewise, *juvenile hyalin fibromatosis,* a much less common disease than myofibromatosis, makes its first appearance two or more years after birth, affects the dermis or subcutis exclusively, and is usually accompanied by joint deformities. Solitary forms of the disease may be mistaken for *infantile fibromatosis.* In the latter process, however, the tumors tend to be less well circumscribed, arise in muscle, and show a more uniform spindle cell pattern.

Discussion

The clinical course seems to be largely determined by the extent of the disease: solitary and multiple lesions confined to the soft tissues and bone carry an excellent prognosis; they tend to regress spontaneously and rarely need more than a diagnostic biopsy.* The prognosis is much less favorable in newborns and infants with multiple visceral lesions, and many of them die with signs of respiratory distress or diarrhea soon after birth. There are exceptions, however. Teng et al.[107] described a 4-month-old boy with a large mass in the kidney and multiple lesions in bone. The boy was well 18 months after excision of the renal tumor, and on x-ray examination the bone lesions had regressed and were no longer demonstrable. Likewise, Dimmick and Wood[82] reported a congenital myofibromatosis that involved numerous sites and caused respiratory distress and quadriplegia. They noted regression of the lesion, neurological improvements, and disappearance of most of the lesions within 9 months. Yet, occasionally, new lesions

_____

*References 71, 73, 79, 101, 102, 108

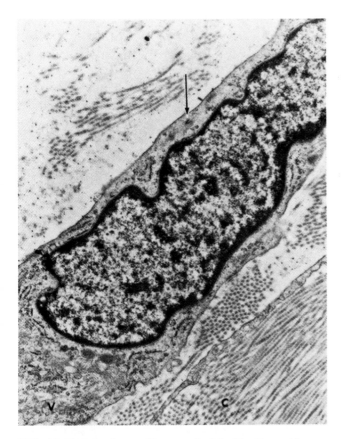

FIG. 11-21. Infantile myofibromatosis. Myofibroblast with condensed filamentous material *(arrow)*. (From Benjamin SP, Mercer RD, Hawk W: *Cancer* 40:2343, 1977.)

may develop years after regression of the primary tumor.[75] There is no evidence of a true metastasis. The metastasizing "myofibromatous tumor" described by Dictor et al.[81] seems to be more akin to malignant hemangiopericytoma than myofibroma.

Myofibroma and myofibromatosis are clearly the expressions of a benign, self-limiting, localized or generalized process, probably of hamartomatous origin, which consists to a large degree of cells having the characteristics of myofibroblasts and sometimes of pericytes. Although smooth muscle origin was suggested,[84,95] there is no evidence in our material or the reported cases that the tumor nodules ever evolve into leiomyomas.

The exact cause of this condition is not clear. The occasional occurrence of the disease in siblings and several members of one family supports a genetic disorder that has its onset during the last trimester of pregnancy and is inherited in an autosomal recessive or dominant mode.[70,75,88,90] Association with other lesions is exceedingly rare; Spraker et al.[105] observed the condition in a 6-week-old infant who suffered from porencephaly, hemiatrophy, telangiectasia, cutis marmorata, and glaucoma.

JUVENILE HYALIN FIBROMATOSIS

Juvenile hyalin fibromatosis is another rare hereditary disease that bears a superficial resemblance to myofibromatosis but differs by the cutaneous distribution of the tumor nodules and the histological picture, which is characterized by paucity of cells, a fibrillary matrix, and complete absence of mature collagen fibers. It is by no means a newly defined disease process: as early as 1873 Murray[121] described this condition in three siblings as *molluscum fibrosum in children,* an early synonym of neurofibromatosis. In 1903, 30 years later, Whitfield and Robinson[128] published a follow-up report of the same family. Since that time only about 30 cases of the disease have been recorded,[111-131] but it is likely that additional examples are hidden in the literature, especially among cases reported as neurofibromatosis. Yet the fact that there are only ten unpublished cases of juvenile hyalin fibromatosis on file at the AFIP testifies to the rarity of the disease.

Clinical findings

In contrast to the generalized form of fibromatosis the condition rarely occurs before the second month of life and is usually first noticed in children between 2 and 5 years of age. Typically it consists of multiple cutaneous papules, nodules, or tumor masses that vary in size from 1 millimeter to about 5 cm, are slowly growing and painless, and are found mainly in the regions of the head, back, and extremities, with a predilection for the nose, ears, scalp, back, and knees (Fig. 11-22). One of the two patients of Woyke et al.,[130] who was followed up for 19 years, had over 100 tumors removed surgically in 30 operations.

In some of the cases there is, in addition to the multiple cutaneous tumors, thickening of the gums, flexion contractures of large joints, poorly developed musculature, and muscle weakness. In fact, flexion contractures and gingival hyperplasia may be the first manifestation of the disease.[122] Moreover, the lesions may be associated with recurrent infections and retardation of growth and intellect. Roentgenographs may show, in addition to the soft tissue lesions, punched-out osteolytic lesions in bones, especially osteolysis of the distal phalanges of the fingers and toes, cortical defects, and delayed ossification.[111,123,126]

Pathological findings

The tumors are poorly circumscribed and consist of cords of spindle-shaped cells embedded in a homogeneous eosinophilic matrix (Figs. 11-23 to 11-25). They are found in the dermis, subcutis, and gingiva. Other sites, such as the joints, may also be involved.[126] One patient of Kitano et al.[119] died of fulminant hepatitis. Autopsy revealed an "amorphous substance" in the tongue, esophagus, intes-

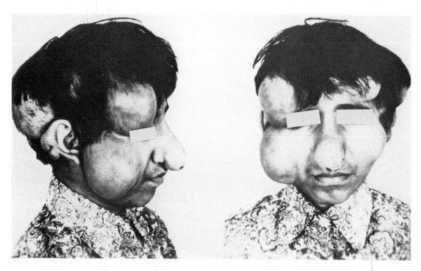

FIG. 11-22. Juvenile hyaline fibromatosis. Multiple masses involving scalp and face. (Courtesy Prof. Dr. Eduardo Carceres, Director, Instituto Nacional de Enfermades Neoplasicas, Lima, Peru.)

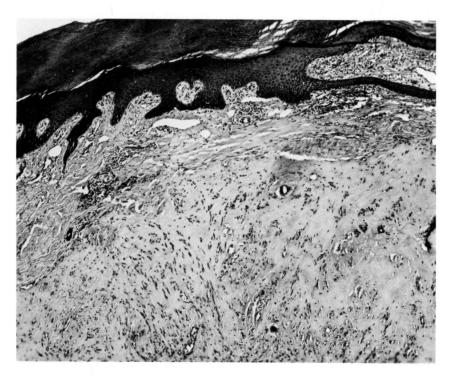

FIG. 11-23. Juvenile hyaline fibromatosis. Dermal nodule shows characteristic association of fibroblasts and large amounts of inspissated hyalinized material. (×55.)

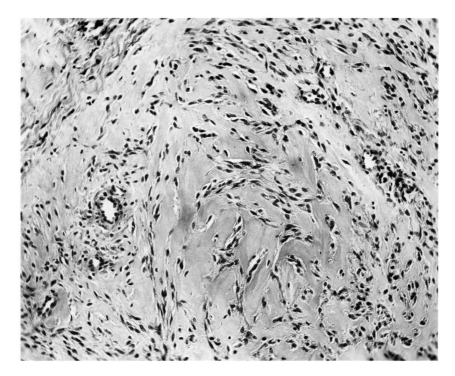

FIG. 11-24. Juvenile hyaline fibromatosis; cords of fibroblasts associated with large amounts of hyalinized collagen-like material. (×130.)

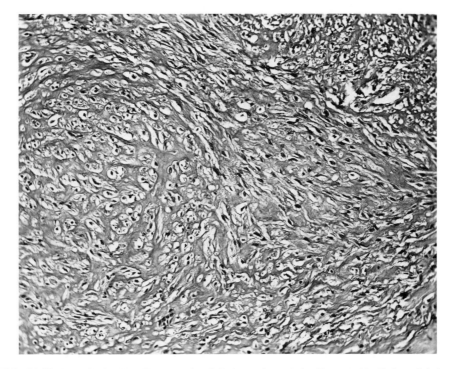

FIG. 11-25. Juvenile hyaline fibromatosis. Cellular variant of the disease with distinct shrinkage spaces around fibroblasts. (×130.)

tines, thymus, spleen, and lymph nodes. In general, the smaller and younger lesions tend to be more cellular, while the larger and older lesions contain more ground substance. The matrix is positive on staining with PAS and alcian blue but does not stain with toluidine blue or congo red. Reticulin preparations fail to demonstrate well-formed collagen fibers. Likewise, elastic tissue is absent. Occasional nodules are calcified.[120,126]

Electron microscopic examination reveals scattered fibroblastlike cells containing a prominent Golgi apparatus and aggregates of microfilaments or fibril-filled balls of varying size. Large amounts of similar microfibrillary material are present within the interstices, with occasional alignment of the fibrils to mature normal and long-spacing collagen fibers.[118,125-127,131]

Differential diagnosis

Multicentric infantile myofibromatosis is composed of multiple nodules that are present at birth or occur during the first year of life, are better circumscribed, and are found not only in the subcutis but also in muscle, bone, and viscera. Microscopically, they consist of broad, interlacing bundles of plump myofibroblasts, often with pericytomalike areas in the center of the lesion. The gums or joints are never involved. *Neurofibromatosis* tends to make its first appearance in slightly older children and is associated with café au lait spots; the tumors are composed of hyperchromatic serpentine nuclei and a fibrillary eosinophilic matrix, and are positive for S-100 protein. *Gingival fibromatosis*, a lesion that has a similar hereditary pattern, is limited to the gums of the upper and lower jaws and consists of dense, scarlike connective tissue rich in collagen. *Cylindromas*, or turban tumors, are confined to the head.

Winchester's syndrome, a rare autosomal hereditary disease, is characterized by densely cellular, poorly demarcated fibrous proliferations in the dermis, subcutis, and joints without deposition of a hyalin matrix, periarticular thickening and limitation of motion in the limbs and the spine, and corneal opacities. Severe radiographic changes of joints and bones are part of the disorder.[129] *Lipoid proteinosis (hyalinosis cutis et mucosae)* is another rare disorder, characterized by multiple cutaneous or mucosal plaques, papules, or nodules associated with dysphonia and hoarseness. These lesions lack the spindle cell proliferation of hyalin fibromatosis and consist of amorphous eosinophilic, PAS- and ORO-positive infiltrates located in the upper dermis and tending to surround sweat glands and small vessels.

Discussion

Although most lesions in hyalin fibromatosis are formed during childhood, new lesions may continue to appear into adult life. Over the years they show little change in size, shape, or microscopic appearance and persist unless they are excised for cosmetic or functional reasons. Woyke et al.,[130] who followed one patient for 19 years, reported successful surgical removal of over 100 tumors with good cosmetic results. Surgical removal of the finger lesions, however, may be difficult, since the tumors adhere to tendons. Joint function, however, has been slightly improved with cortisone and ACTH therapy. There is no response to radiotherapy.[123,124,130]

The condition is inherited as an autosomal recessive trait. It usually affects more than one sibling of the same family, and there is no predilection for either sex. We are not aware that it has ever been observed in more than one generation, but consanguinity of the parents of the afflicted children is on record in several cases.[112] Judging from electron microscopic examinations of the tumors, the basic defect appears to be a localized metabolic disturbance in the formation of collagen, presumably caused by incomplete alignment of precollagen or protocollagen, possibly due to increased or faulty synthesis of glycosaminoglycans by fibroblasts. Iwata et al.[117] demonstrated increased chondroitin synthesis by skin fibroblasts cultured from the lesion.

GINGIVAL FIBROMATOSIS

Gingival fibromatosis has been described under various synonyms, including *idiopathic or hereditary gingival fibromatosis*,[133,134,145] *hereditary gingival hyperplasia*,[136] *congenital idiopathic gingival fibromatosis*,[139,145] *generalized hypertrophy of the gums*,[138] and *gingival elephantiasis*.[144] It is a clinically distinct but rare disease that chiefly affects young persons of both sexes and has a tendency toward recurrent local growth. Idiopathic cases are slightly more common than familial ones. For instance, in a review of the literature by Takagi et al.[143] in 1991, 97 of 267 patients had a positive familial history.

Clinical findings

The principal complaint is a slow-growing, ill-defined enlargement or swelling of the gingivae, causing little pain but considerable difficulties in speaking and eating. In some cases the swelling is minimal and is limited to a small portion of the gum (*localized type*), but in most cases it is extensive and bilateral and involves the gingival tissues of both the upper and lower jaws and the hard palate (*generalized type*). The growth elevates the gingival mucosa in a nodular, ridgelike, or papillary manner and often covers the crowns of the teeth. Roentgenographs, however, show the teeth in their normal alveolar relationships. The condition occurs at any age, most often at the time of the eruption of the deciduous or permanent teeth. In fact, it was postulated that the erupting teeth trigger the fibrous growth.

Hypertrichosis is found in about 10% of patients with this condition. There may also be concomitant mental retardation, stunted growth, epilepsy, and cherubism (*Ramon's syndrome*).[138,141,143] Gingival fibromas or fibromatosis is also a feature of the *Zimmermann–Laband syndrome* (hepatomegaly with soft tissue and bone abnormalities) and *Cowden's disease* (multiple hamartoma syndrome).[133,140,143]

Pathological findings

Grossly, the growth consists of dense scarlike tissue that cuts with difficulty and has a gray-white glistening surface. On microscopic examination the specimens vary little in appearance and consist of poorly cellular and richly collagenous fibrous connective tissue beneath a normal or acanthotic squamous epithelium. If inflammatory changes are present, they are inconspicuous. Under the electron microscope the lesion is composed mainly of fusiform fibroblastlike cells and scattered myofibroblastlike cells with dilated endoplasmic reticulum; the cells are surrounded by abundant collagen and an interspersed finely granular substance.[143]

Differential diagnosis

There is a striking resemblance between gingival fibromatosis and hypertrophy of the gums following prolonged therapy with diphenylhydantoin sodium (Dilantin or phenytoin sodium).[132,135] Lesions of similar appearance may also be found during pregnancy and as the result of chronic gingivitis. In most of these cases a detailed clinical and family history will permit arriving at the correct diagnosis. Hyalin fibromatosis, a hereditary lesion that may also involve the gingiva in a similar manner, can be distinguished by its association with multiple cutaneous tumors and the characteristic microscopic appearance, especially the prominent PAS-positive hyalin matrix.

Discussion

Opinions as to the best mode of therapy vary. When the growth is massive and generalized, excision and reexcision of the overgrown gingiva may become necessary. Smaller lesions, however, may be effectively treated by simple extraction of the teeth, since this seems to remove the principal stimulus for further growth.

Gingival fibromatosis is inherited as an autosomal dominant or autosomal recessive disease that may affect several members of one family and may be traced over many generations.[136,142,144]

Sporadic cases without a family history are on record, however. Chromosomal analysis in two patients failed to show any specific changes.[143]

FIBROMATOSIS COLLI

Fibromatosis colli has long been recognized as a peculiar fibrous growth of the sternocleidomastoid muscle that usually appears during the first weeks of life and is often associated with muscular torticollis, or wryneck. It bears a close resemblance to other forms of infantile fibromatosis but is sufficiently different in its microscopic appearance and behavior to warrant its separation as a distinct entity. According to Coventry et al.[154] it occurs in 0.4% of newborns. Acquired torticollis, secondary to traumatic injury or muscle spasm, is an entirely different process that occurs in older persons and should not be confused with muscular torticollis complicating fibromatosis colli.

Clinical findings

Characteristically, the lesion manifests between the second and fourth weeks of life as a firm mass lying within or replacing the lower portion of the sternocleidomastoid muscle, especially its sternal or clavicular portion. It is movable only in a horizontal plane and never affects the overlying skin. Simultaneous involvement of both sternocleidomastoid and trapezius muscle does occur but is very rare.[159] It may develop in older children, but it is rarely noted at birth or before the second week of life. According to most authors, it more often affects the right than the left side, is rarely bilateral, and is more common in boys than in girls.[146,153,157,163]

Initially the mass grows rapidly, but after a few weeks or months the growth slows and becomes stationary. Later it begins to regress, and after a period of 1 or 2 years it may no longer be palpable. During the initial growth period, torticollis (rotation and tilting of the head to the affected side) occurs in only about one fourth to one third of cases and usually is mild and transient. Torticollis, however, often becomes much more pronounced at a later stage of development, generally having its onset at age 3 or 4 years. It appears that at this age the affected sternocleidomastoid muscle is incapable of keeping pace with the growth and elongation of the sternocleidomastoid muscle on the opposite side, causing functional imbalance and torticollis. Muscular torticollis, however, may also occur in children without a history of a mass in the sternocleidomastoid muscle, as, for example, in 11 of the 36 cases reported by Middleton.[161] Persistent, uncorrected torticollis may lead to asymmetry of the face and head (plagiocephaly) and facial asymmetry, which is usually marked by a prominent ipsilateral frontal eminence and slight bulge of the occipital bone.[149,150]

It is of interest that in about 40% to 50% of cases there is a history of complicated delivery. Coventry et al.,[154] for instance, state that 14 of 35 infants with fibromatosis colli had either a breech or forceps delivery. Similarly, in MacDonald's series,[160] 58% of the patients had complications at birth, including a 34% rate of breech deliveries. Associated congenital ipsilateral dislocation of the hip and pyloric stenosis also have been reported. Binder et al.[147] found hip dysplasia in 10.5% of cases.

There are rare instances of increased familial incidence. In MacDonald's series[160] of 51 cases, there were only two patients in which a second-degree relative was known to

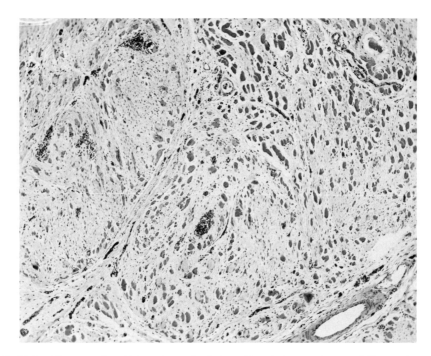

FIG. 11-26. Fibromatosis colli in a 2-month-old boy. Note intimate mixture of fibrous tissue and entrapped and partly atrophic muscle fibers. (×50.)

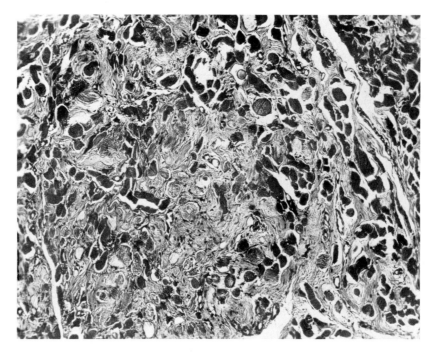

FIG. 11-27. Fibromatosis colli. Separation of atrophic muscle fibers by dense fibrous tissue. (Masson-trichrome stain; ×100.)

have torticollis. Campbell and Pedra,[151] as well as others, observed the condition in one of identical twins.

Pathological findings

When the growth is excised at an early stage, the operative specimen consists of a small mass of firm tissue averaging 1 to 2 cm in diameter. Its cut surface is gray-white and glistening and blends imperceptibly with surrounding skeletal muscle. Microscopic examination of the lesion discloses partial replacement of the sternocleidomastoid muscle by a diffuse fibroblastic process of varying cellularity. There is little cellular pleomorphism or mitotic activity. Scattered throughout the lesion are residual muscle fibers that have undergone atrophy or degeneration with swelling, loss of cross striations, and proliferation of sarcolemmal nuclei (Figs. 11-26 and 11-27). This intimate mixture of proliferated fibroblasts and residual muscle fibers is fully diagnostic of the lesion and should not be confused with the infiltrative growth of a malignant neoplasm. Lesions of long standing may show a lesser degree of cellularity and a greater amount of stromal collagen, but in general there is no reliable correlation between the histological picture and the age of the patient. Hemosiderin deposits are present in some cases but are never a prominent feature of the growth. Unlike fibrosing myositis there is no inflammatory infiltrate. More importantly, unlike fibrodysplasia ossificans progressiva there are no associated malformations of the hands or feet. According to some authors,[156,167] a reliable diagnosis can also be reached by fine-needle aspiration biopsy.

Prognosis and treatment

Following a stationary period of several months, the growth subsides in about two thirds of cases. It never recurs and at no time behaves aggressively. Recommendations as to the best type of therapy differ: while early excision of the lesion may prevent facial deformities, it seems best to use prolonged physical therapy and to reserve surgical correction (division of the lower attachment of the muscle) for the relatively small number of cases in which the lesion does not resolve spontaneously during the first year of life. Resection of the muscle may become necessary in older children with muscular torticollis.[148,152,158,159,162-164]

Discussion

The cause of the growth has been the subject of considerable debate in the literature. In view of the unusually high incidence of breech presentations and other complications at birth, birth injury may play an important role in the pathogenesis.[165] Yet there is little evidence that the growth represents merely an organizing form of hematoma or the late result of muscle tear; not only does the microscopic appearance of the lesion differ from that of proven cases of organizing hematoma, but there is also very little demonstrable hemosiderin. Vascular impairment or insufficiency as the result of prolonged venous stasis or ischemia or stretching of the muscle during labor appears a more likely cause that may be analogous to that of Volkmann's ischemic contracture. But it is also conceivable that the growth is a preexisting condition and is the cause rather than the effect of the abnormally high rate of complicated deliveries. Certainly, contributing genetic factors are suggested by the occasional examples of increased familial incidence[166] and the association of the growth with certain malformations.

INFANTILE (DESMOID-TYPE) FIBROMATOSIS

This tumor, which represents the childhood counterpart of musculoaponeurotic fibromatosis (abdominal or extraabdominal desmoid), usually arises as a solitary mass in skeletal muscle or in the adjacent fascia, aponeurosis, or periosteum. It chiefly affects children from birth to 8 years of age and is slightly more common in boys than girls. There are considerable variations in its morphological appearance, ranging from primitive mesenchymal forms to lesions that closely resemble adult desmoids, except perhaps for a less uniform pattern and a greater degree of cellularity.

Stout[189] was the first to identify and describe this childhood form of fibromatosis as a distinct entity, but since his report only a small number of cases have been added to the literature, many without detailed information as to their histological picture and behavior. Our data, therefore, are based mainly on a review of 136 cases from the files of the AFIP.

Clinical findings

In the majority of cases treatment is sought because of the presence of a firm solitary mass that is poorly circumscribed and deep seated and usually has grown rapidly during the preceding weeks or months. Nearly always the mass is noted during the first 8 years of life and is most commonly encountered in the first and second year after birth. Typical cases in older children do occur, however. Fleischmajer et al.,[178] for example, described such a tumor in a 15-year-old girl. In most cases the mass originates in skeletal muscle, especially in the muscles of the head and neck, the shoulder and upper arm, and the thigh (Table 11-2).

Table 11-2. Anatomical distribution of infantile (desmoid-type) fibromatosis (AFIP, 136 patients)

Anatomical location	No. patients	Percent
Head and neck	46	34
Upper extremities	44	32
Lower extremities	22	16
Trunk	24	18
TOTAL	136	100

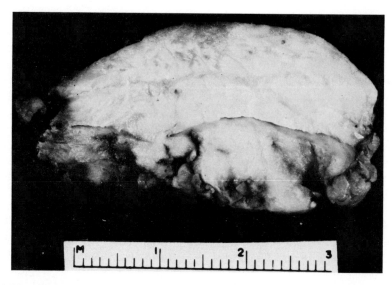

FIG. 11-28. Infantile fibromatosis. Replacement of muscle tissue by fibrous tissue and mature fat bearing a superficial resemblance to a lipomatous tumor. The lesion was excised from the right arm of a 2-year-old girl.

In the head and neck region the preferred sites are the tongue, the mandible, the maxilla, and the mastoid process.[170,180,183,187,190-192] As the lesion progresses, it may infiltrate adjacent muscles and may grow around vessels and nerves. This may result in tenderness, pain, or functional disturbances. Involvement of the joint capsule may lead to contracture and restriction of movement.

Roentgenographic examination merely shows a soft tissue mass that is sometimes associated with bowing or deformation of bone, especially in cases that had their onset during the first 2 or 3 years of life and were present for several months or years.[172] Lesions occurring in the regions of the mandible, maxilla, or mastoid frequently involve bone. In fact, in some of these cases it is difficult to determine whether the lesion arose in the soft tissues, periosteum, or bone.[171,177,182,184,193] Eady et al.[173] described a patient in whom congenital bowing of the ulna and dislocation of the radial head preceded the onset of fibromatosis.

Pathological findings

Grossly, the tumor consists of firm, ill-defined, scarlike masses of gray-white tissue measuring 1 to 10 cm or more in greatest diameter. The tumor is never encapsulated and usually is excised together with portions of the involved muscle and subcutaneous fat (Fig. 11-28). Occasionally the lesion may reach a large size and may occupy a large portion of the head and neck or a limb.

Microscopically, infantile fibromatosis has a wide morphological range reflecting progressive stages in the differentiation of fibroblasts. The least mature, most common

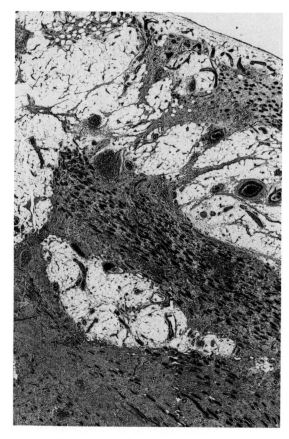

FIG. 11-29. Photomicrograph of infantile fibromatosis shown in Fig. 11-28. (×35.)

type of lesion, often described as the *diffuse, or mesenchymal, type* of infantile fibromatosis, is found chiefly in infants during the first few months of life; it is characterized by small haphazardly arranged round or oval cells within a myxoid background. The cells are intermediate in appearance between primitive mesenchymal cells and fibroblasts, and are often intimately associated with residual muscle fibers and lipocytes. The interspersed lipocytes are probably the result of ex vacuo fatty proliferation secondary to muscular atrophy of the infiltrated and immobilized muscle tissue (Figs. 11-29 to 11-32).

The diffuse type often blends with another and more cellular type *(fibroblastic type)*, which is chiefly composed of plump spindle-shaped fibroblasts arranged in distinct bundles and fascicles (Figs. 11-33 and 11-34). It also is found within muscle tissue, where it arises in the endomysium or epimysium or, in some cases, from the overlying fascia or aponeurosis. It may be very cellular and difficult to distinguish from infantile fibrosarcoma *(aggressive type)*.

There are also less cellular and more collagenous examples of this tumor *(desmoid type)* that are virtually indistinguishable from the adult forms of fibromatosis or desmoid tumor. They usually occur in children older than 5 years of age, and their behavior is similar to that of the adult form of fibromatosis. Cellular pleomorphism or giant cells are not a feature of the tumor. Secondary ossification is seen occasionally.[179]

Judging from the small number of ultrastructural studies, the tumor is made of a mixture of fibroblasts and myofibroblasts, with prominent and often dilated endoplasmic reticulum and bundles of peripherally placed microfilaments in some cells.[186,184]

Differential diagnosis

The diffuse, or mesenchymal, type of this tumor frequently causes problems in diagnosis. It may be confused with a myxoid or lipomatous tumor because of the large amounts of glycosaminoglycans (mucopolysaccharides) in its stroma and the partial replacement of the diffusely infiltrated muscle by lipocytes, which may be quite immature if the tumor occurs during the first year of life. *Myxoid liposarcoma,* however, is a rarity in children younger than 5 years of age, and usually is marked by lipoblasts and a plexiform capillary pattern. *Botryoid rhabdomyosarcoma* has a similar age incidence, but is uncommon in the musculature and nearly always occurs in the wall of mucosa-lined cavities such as the urinary bladder or vagina. *Lipoblastomatosis,* the infantile counterpart of lipoma, can be distinguished by its distinctly lobular pattern and the uniform appearance of the constituent lipoblasts. There may also be

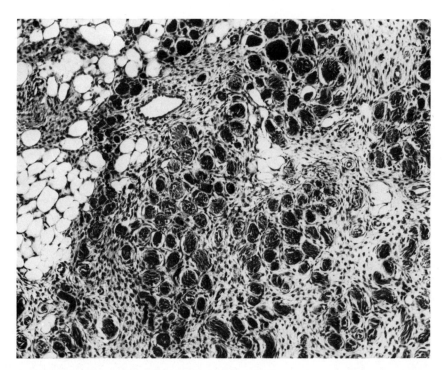

FIG. 11-30. Infantile fibromatosis, diffuse type, removed from the trapezius muscle of a 5½-month-old girl. The absence of digital malformations helps to distinguish it from an early nonossifying stage of fibrodysplasia ossificans progressiva. (×70.)

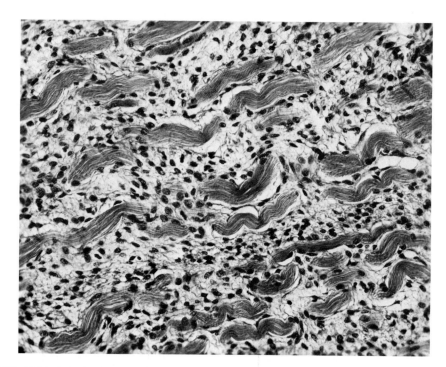

FIG. 11-31. Infantile fibromatosis, diffuse type. Note separation of striated muscle fibers by primitive fibroblasts showing little variation in size and shape. The diffuse type is chiefly seen in children between birth and 1 year of age. (×250.)

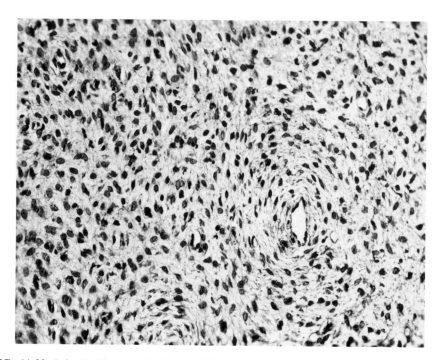

FIG. 11-32. Infantile fibromatosis. Sheets of immature fibroblasts within a myxoid background (diffuse fibromatosis). (× 160.)

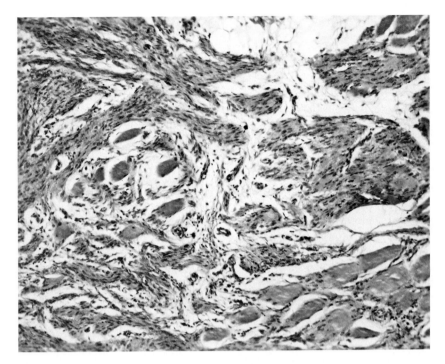

FIG. 11-33. Infantile fibromatosis showing a more cellular picture and greater amounts of collagen than in Figs. 11-30 and 11-31. This type prevails in children between 1 and 3 years of age. (×100.)

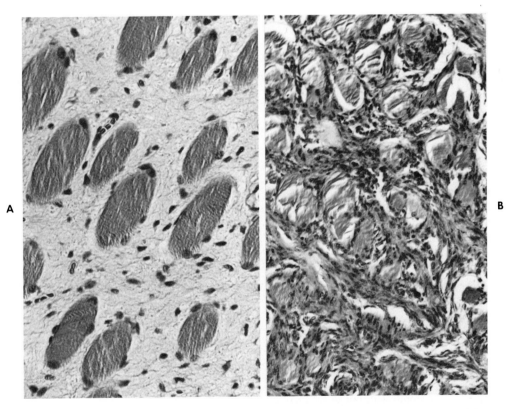

FIG. 11-34. Infantile fibromatosis. Diffuse (A) and fibrosing (B) types in different portions of the same tumor. (A and B, ×125.)

confusion with early stages of *calcifying aponeurotic fibroma* and *fibrodysplasia ossificans progressiva*. The former lesion is characterized by its location in the palmar and plantar regions, and the latter by the association of the lesion with bilateral malformations and shortenings (microdactylia) of fingers and toes.

Perhaps the most difficult problem in differential diagnosis is the separation of the more cellular variants of fibromatosis from *infantile fibrosarcoma*. This difficulty is expressed in terms such as "aggressive fibromatosis," "differentiated fibrosarcoma," and "fibrosarcoma-like fibromatosis."[168,192] In our experience, distinction is usually feasible if one pays attention to the infiltrative growth pattern of fibromatosis and its variation in the degree of cellularity, often with alternating cellular and more collagenous areas and foci of residual muscle tissue and fat. Yet in some cases reliable distinction between fibromatosis and fibrosarcoma may be very difficult, if not impossible. Tumors that are highly cellular, exhibit considerable mitotic activity, and grow in a rapidly expanding, destructive manner are probably best classified as infantile fibrosarcomas. Transitions from fibromatosis to fibrosarcoma have not been clearly established, and the recorded metastasizing cases of fibromatosis may actually be examples of infantile fibrosarcoma.[188] There is still no agreement as to whether or not the relative number and distribution of nucleolar organizer regions (AgNORs) is a prognostically useful indicator in distinguishing infantile fibromatosis from infantile fibrosarcoma.[169,174,186]

Discussion

Although the tumor does not metastasize, it may reach a large size, tends to recur locally when inadequately excised, and continues to grow in a progressive, infiltrative manner in one third to one half of cases. Encroachment on joints and entrapment of vessels and nerves may cause complications, especially when the tumor is located in the regions of the head and neck, the axilla, and the popliteal fossa. In the individual case, however, neither the location nor the morphological picture seems to permit an accurate prediction of the clinical course. Schmidt et al.[186] pointed out the presence of a larger number of undifferentiated mesenchymal cells and slitlike blood vessels in tumors that behaved more aggressively.

Complete excision with ample margins, the treatment of choice, is often extremely difficult and in some cases may be impossible without disfigurement or dysfunction. So far there is little information as to whether or not the tumor responds to radiotherapy, the preferred therapy for recurrent adult forms of fibromatosis.

The cause of the lesion is not clear. As in other forms of this disease, trauma has been implicated, but so far there is no proof that trauma plays a significant role in histogenesis. Unlike many other fibrous lesions, increased familial incidence has not been observed in this type of fibromatosis.

CALCIFYING APONEUROTIC FIBROMA

Although calcifying aponeurotic fibroma affects a much wider age range than other forms of juvenile fibromatosis and may occur in young adults, it is included here because it chiefly affects children and adolescents between birth and 16 years of age. It was first described as *juvenile aponeurotic fibroma* by Keasbey[201] in 1953, who pointed out its characteristic histological picture, its predilection for the palm and fingers of the hand, and its propensity to recur after local excision. Later, in view of the wide age range of patients, the term juvenile aponeurotic fibroma was changed to *aponeurotic fibroma*[202] and *calcifying aponeurotic fibroma*.[199] Since Keasbey's report, approximately 80 cases have been recorded in the literature.

Clinical findings

A slowly growing painless mass in the hands or feet of several months' or even years' duration is the usual presenting complaint. In most cases the mass is poorly circumscribed and causes neither discomfort nor limitation of movement. Lesions that have been present for several years are often more sharply defined and are distinctly nodular on palpation.

The age range is much wider than suggested by Keasbey's[201] first report. However, most cases seen in our consultation over the past 30 years occurred in children: the median age in our series was 12 years; the youngest patient was a 3-year-old boy, and the oldest was a 28-year-old woman. There is an even greater age range in the literature,[197,202,211] including a lesion that was present at birth and one that was removed from the wrist of a 64-year-old patient.[197] In our series there is a significant preponderance of males (70%), but in Keasbey's first series, four of the six cases were girls. There is no record of any increased familial incidence.[195]

The two principal sites of the growth are the hands and the feet. In our series, 77% of cases affected the hands and 13% the feet. In the hand, most lesions occurred in the palm or the fingers; in the foot, most were in the plantar or ankle region, with only one occurring in the toes. Isolated examples of the tumor have been observed at other sites, including the forearm, supraclavicular region, elbow, and popliteal fossa.[196,209,212] They are often attached to the aponeurosis, tendons, or fascia but may also be found as an isolated nodule within these structures. Thus, Moskovich and Posner[206] observed calcifying aponeurotic fibroma in the pollicis longus tendon, and Rios-Dalenz et al.[207] one in the fascia of the lumbar region of a 16-year-old boy. Another unusual presentation was reported by Adeyemi-Doro and Olude[194]: a 14-year-old boy with a large calcifying aponeurotic fibroma on the dorsum of the left hand. Multiple lesions are rare.[198]

Preoperative radiographic examination reveals a faint mass with calcific stippling, especially in the more heavily calcified examples of the tumor.

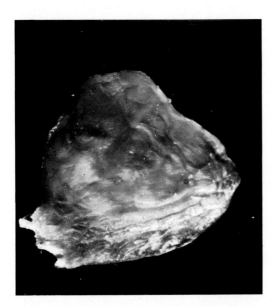

FIG. 11-35. Calcifying aponeurotic fibroma arising in the palmar aponeurosis of a 6-year-old boy.

Gross findings

The appearance of the gross specimen does not permit an accurate diagnosis. It usually consists of an ill-defined, firm or rubbery, gray-white nodule or mass rarely measuring more than 3 cm in greatest diameter. Often small punctate calcific areas give a gritty sensation when cut. Because there are no sharp boundaries, portions of the surrounding fat, skeletal muscle, and fibrous tissue frequently merge with tumor tissue (Fig. 11-35).

Microscopic findings

The histological picture varies little from case to case and consists of a fibrous growth that extends with multiple processes into the surrounding tissue and has more centrally located foci of calcification and cartilage formation. The growth varies in cellularity and is composed of plump fibroblasts with round or ovoid nuclei and indistinctly outlined cytoplasm separated by a densely collagenous stroma. Despite the focal cellularity of the lesion, mitotic figures are scarce. Not infrequently the fibrous growth is attached to tendon or aponeurosis and encircles blood vessels and nerves. Unlike other forms of fibromatosis there is often a peculiar linear or palisaded arrangement of the fibroblasts, especially near the areas of calcification.

Focal calcification is invariably present, except in those lesions that occur in infants or small children. The calcifications are usually of small size, have a bandlike configuration, and in about one third of cases are associated with cartilage cells and a matrix rich in sulfated mucopolysaccharides. Occasionally, giant cells are found along the calcified areas. Ossification occurs but is rare. Kindblom[203]

suggested that the calcification takes place in entrapped, degenerated, or necrotic portions of the aponeurosis rather than in viable portions of the fibrous growth. Calcification and cartilage formation are much more pronounced in lesions removed from older children and young adults. Whether this is a result of longer duration of the lesion or endocrine factors is not clear (Figs. 11-36 to 11-43).

Differential diagnosis

The differential diagnosis differs slightly from case to case, depending on the age of the patient at the time the lesion is excised. In infants and small children, when there is still little or no calcification, clear distinction from infantile or juvenile forms of fibromatosis may be difficult. But, in general, a correct diagnosis can be made if attention is paid to the plump appearance of the fibroblasts, their association with dense and often hyalinized collagen, and the characteristic location of the lesion in the fingers or palm of the hand.

Palmar and plantar fibromatoses, rare in children, can be distinguished by their nodular appearance (without the characteristic ramifications into the surrounding fatty tissue and voluntary muscle) and the absence of calcification or chondroid differentiation. Malignant spindle cell tumors, such as monophasic fibrous-type synovial sarcoma, may be mistaken for aponeurotic fibroma with a prominent spindle cell pattern.

In older patients distinction of the growth from a soft part chondroma may cause considerable problems, especially because both juvenile aponeurotic fibroma and soft part chondroma share the same location and are most common in the hands. Chondroma, however, usually occurs in the fingers of adult patients and, microscopically, displays less fibrous tissue, is lobulated, and undergoes calcification in a diffuse rather than a focal or linear manner.

Ultrastructural findings

According to Iwasaki et al.,[199,200] calcifying aponeurotic fibroma shows a biphasic pattern consisting of fibroblasts and occasional myofibroblasts and cartilage cells, with a well-developed granular endoplasmic reticulum, a prominent Golgi complex, and multiple microvilli. The cells are surrounded by a prominent intercellular matrix containing fine fibrils and spherical granules.

Prognosis and treatment

At least half of the cases of calcifying aponeurotic fibroma recur locally, but recurrence is more common in infants and children than in adults. In fact, it appears that in most cases the growth activity of the tumor slows down with advancing age of the patient. We have never encountered malignant transformation of calcifying aponeurotic fibroma in the AFIP material, but such a case has been seen in consultation by one of us (SWW), and another, a fibrosarcoma arising in a calcifying aponeurotic fibroma, has

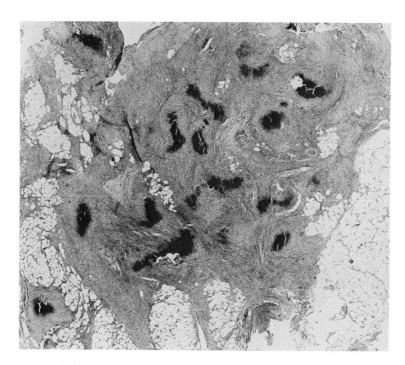

FIG. 11-36. Calcifying aponeurotic fibroma in the palm of a 1-year-old boy. Note poor circumscription of the lesion and multiple short bands of calcification within the proliferated fibrous tissue. (×10.)

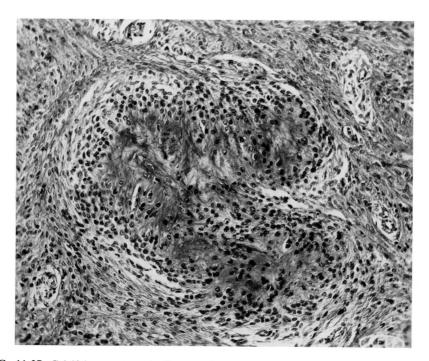

FIG. 11-37. Calcifying aponeurotic fibroma with early focal calcification in the palm of a 15-year-old boy. (Masson-trichrome stain; ×160.)

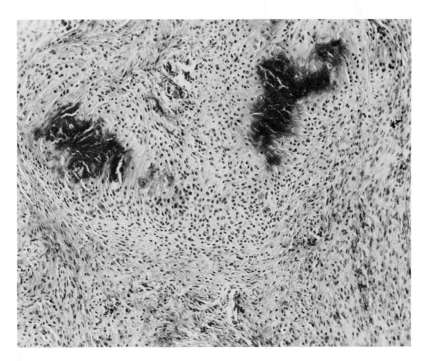

FIG. 11-38. Calcifying aponeurotic fibroma showing hyalinization of the fibrous tissue in the vicinity of heavily calcified areas. (×130.)

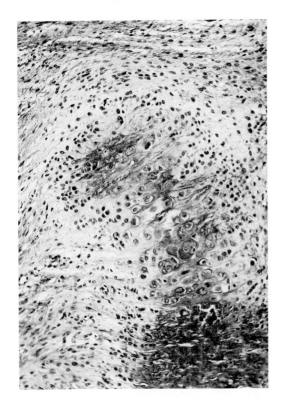

FIG. 11-39. Calcifying aponeurotic fibroma. Focus of calcification and cartilage formation. (×120.)

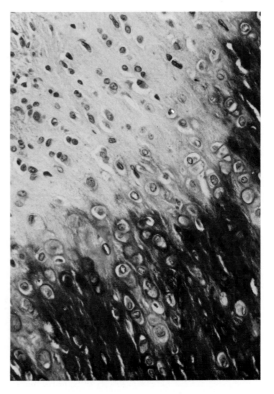

FIG. 11-40. Calcifying aponeurotic fibroma. Cartilaginous metaplasia within area of calcification. (×250.)

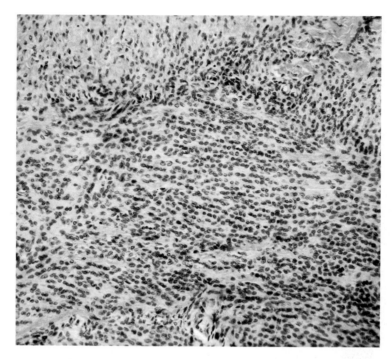

FIG. 11-41. Calcifying aponeurotic fibroma. Peripheral fibrous portion showing characteristic arrangement of fibroblasts in parallel cords. (×100.)

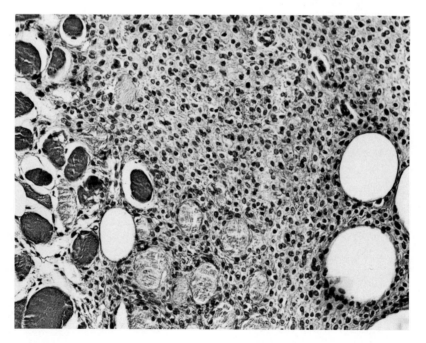

FIG. 11-42. Fibrous portion of calcifying aponeurotic fibroma with infiltration of muscle tissue and subcutaneous fat. (×160.)

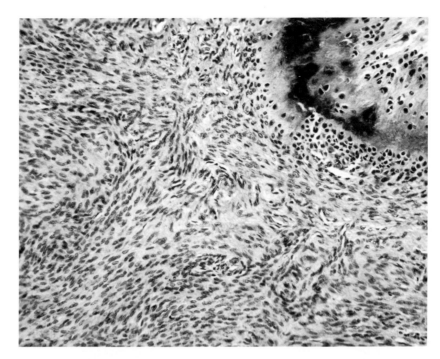

FIG. 11-43. Calcifying aponeurotic fibroma. Cellular fibrous portion resembling fibrosarcoma. (×160.)

been reported in the literature.[204] In the latter case the tumor metastasized to lung and bone 5 years after its second excision.

Surgical management should be conservative in all tumors showing the typical picture of calcifying aponeurotic fibroma. In fact, excision and reexcision, if necessary, appear to be preferable to radical or mutilating surgical procedures. Radical surgical therapy, of course, is required in those very rare cases that display evidence of malignant transformation.

Discussion

There seem to be two phases in the development of this tumor: (1) an initial phase, which is more common in infants and small children, in which the tumor grows diffusely and bears a close resemblance to infantile fibromatosis; and (2) a late phase, in which the tumor is more compact and nodular and shows a more prominent degree of calcification and cartilage formation. Indeed, in some of the latter cases, calcification and cartilage formation may be so prominent that it may be difficult to decide whether a given tumor is a calcifying aponeurotic fibroma or a calcifying chondroma. For this reason, Lichtenstein and Goldman[197,205] suggested the term *cartilage analogue of fibromatosis* for the lesion.

CONGENITAL AND ACQUIRED MUSCULAR FIBROSIS

This process was first defined as an entity by Hnevkovsky[220] in 1961 as *progressive fibrosis of the vastus intermedius muscle in children*. Since 1961 numerous examples of this condition have been published in the literature; most affected the quadriceps muscle,[213,215,216,219,226] but a number of cases have also been reported in the gluteus[214,224,225] and the deltoid.[217,218] Both congenital and acquired lesions of this type have been described.

Clinical findings

Although the onset of the lesion usually dates back to the first year of life, it develops slowly and usually does not become apparent before the second or third year. It manifests as a progressive painless mass or cordlike induration in muscle that is poorly circumscribed and may occur on one or both sides. Shortening and contracture of the muscle lead to various functional disturbances, depending on the extent of fibrosis and the muscle involved. Concomitant dimpling or depressions of the overlying skin are observed occasionally; they are most likely a result of fatty atrophy and extension of the fibrosing process into the adjacent fascia and subcutaneous fat.

The fibrosing process is most commonly encountered in

the quadriceps muscle, where it usually affects the distal portion of the intermedius and vastus lateralis. It severely limits the range of active and passive flexion in the knee joint and causes not only an abnormal gait but also difficulties in squatting and sitting straight. In such cases the patella is usually elevated or, less frequently, is dislocated laterally in order to achieve better flexion. Involvement of the gluteus muscle may lead to excessive abduction and external rotation of the leg in a seated position and a waddling gait. Napiontek and Ruszkowski[223] report paralytic footdrop after intramuscular injection and gluteal fibrosis with equinovarus or equinus deformity. Involvement of the deltoid may cause abduction contracture of the shoulder and lateral elevation of the arms.

Pathological findings

Grossly, the involved muscle shows patchy, firm, scarlike gray or gray-yellow areas, which consist microscopi-

cally of a conglomerate of collagenous fibrous tissue, residual partly degenerated, atrophic muscle fibers, and replacement of atrophic muscle by mature fat. Often the fibrosis extends into the muscle fascia or aponeurosis and even into the subcutaneous fat. There is no evidence of foreign body reaction or inflammation.

Discussion

Different concepts have been put forward as to the most likely cause of the fibrosing process, including (1) congenital muscular dysplasia, (2) a lesion similar to fibromatosis colli, and (3) muscular fibrosis secondary to intramuscular injections. The last of these concepts is supported in the majority of cases by a history of severe illness during infancy and treatment with multiple injections of antibiotics or other medications into the affected muscle.[222,224] There may be, however, a predisposing factor because muscular fibrosis and contraction occur only in a small minority of

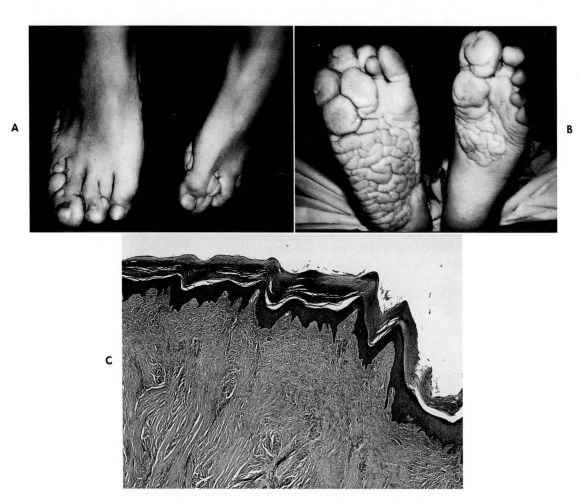

FIG. 11-44. Bilateral cerebriform (gyriform) fibrous proliferation of toes (A) and plantar surfaces (B), a process that may occur alone or in conjunction with lipomatous and hemangiomatous tumors and various skeletal changes, including scoliosis, multiple exostoses, and craniofacial asymmetry (Proteus syndrome). C, Microscopically, the lesions show extensive dermal fibrosis with acanthosis and hyperkeratosis of the overlying epithelium. (×160.)

infants who receive this type of therapy. At least, this is suggested by the observation of scarred puncture marks in the skin of some of the patients,[219] and of keloidlike changes in wound healing.[224] Yet there are also some reports of muscle fibrosis in children who are said to have had the lesions since birth and have had no history of intramuscular injections.[221] There is no clear hereditary pattern, but the condition was observed in four pairs of siblings[225] and in identical twins.[213,215]

Fibrosis and contractures of deltoid muscle in adults have also been reported following intramuscular injection of penicillin and pentazocine, respectively. In fact, in one of our cases, repeated injections of pentazocine (Talwin) led to bilateral fibrosis and contracture of the deltoid muscle and abduction of both arms. In order to regain a normal range of function, tenotomy rather than physical therapy or other conservative measures is the treatment of choice.

CEREBRIFORM FIBROUS PROLIFERATION (PROTEUS SYNDROME)

This entity is included here because the cerebriform or gyriform fibrous proliferation of the volar surfaces may be mistaken for fibromatosis. These changes, however, are an important feature of Proteus syndrome. They may occur alone or, and more commonly, in conjunction with a complex group of lesions involving the skin, the soft tissue, and the skeleton. The syndrome was first described in 1983[234] and was named after a Greek ocean deity, Proteus (the poly-

morphous) because of the broad range of its features. In retrospect, the "elephant man" (Joseph Merrick) seems to have suffered from this disease rather than from neurofibromatosis.[228,232]

The cerebriform fibrous changes affect the plantar and to a lesser degree the palmar surfaces and are often associated with unilateral or bilateral macrodactyly or hypertrophy of long bones (partial gigantism). Grossly, there is marked thickening of the skin in the volar areas, resulting in a coarse cerebriform or gyriform pattern. Microscopically, the plantar and palmar lesions consist of dense fibrosis involving both the dermis and subcutis, with hyperkeratosis of the overlying skin (Fig. 11-44).[231,233]

Other features characteristic of the disease include a variety of lipomatous and hemangiomatous tumors, epidermal nevi, and various skeletal changes such as scoliosis, exostoses, and craniofacial asymmetry. The lipomatous proliferations may be present in the subcutis but may also affect the abdomen, pelvis, and mesentery. There may also be neural changes such as hydrocephaly and argyria (lissencephaly).[229,230] There is no evidence of parental consanguinity or occurrence in more than one sibling, and a somatic mutation seems to be the most likely cause.

CALCIFYING FIBROUS PSEUDOTUMOR

This term has been used to describe a peculiar fibrous tumor that occurs both in children and young adults, and clinically and radiologically may mimic fibromatosis. It is

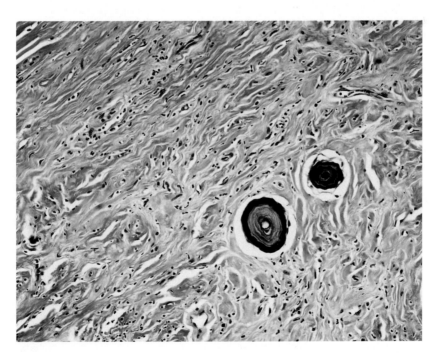

FIG. 11-45. Calcifying fibrous pseudotumor chiefly composed of a uniform, dense collagenous matrix with psammomatous calcifications and scattered inflammatory cells. (×160.)

a slowly growing, firm, highly collagenous tumor composed of thick birefringent bundles of collagen, scarce fibrocytelike spindle cells, psammomatous and dystrophic calcifications, lymphoid aggregates, and a lymphoplasmacytic infiltrate (Fig. 11-45).

Rosenthal and Abdul-Karim[236] were the first to report this lesion in the subcutis of two children, a 2-year-old and an 11-year-old girl. Fetsch et al.[235] described 10 similar cases in children and young adults, ranging from 1 to 33 years of age (median, 18.5 years). The majority of the lesions occurred in the extremities. Five of six patients who were followed up were well without recurrence; in one, the tumor recurred after 7 years and was reexcised after 10 years without further complications.

The lesion seems to be a specific entity, but it is not clear whether this is a true neoplasm or a late sclerosing phase of an inflammatory pseudotumor. Unlike amyloid tumor (amyloidoma) the lesion is devoid of giant cells or demonstrable amyloid.

REFERENCES

General

1. Allen PW: The fibromatoses: a clinicopathologic classification based on 140 cases. *Am J Surg Pathol* 1:255, 1977.
2. Chung EB: Pitfalls in diagnosing benign soft tissue tumors in infancy and childhood, in *Pathology annual*, part 2, vol. 20, Appleton-Century-Crofts, 1985, pp. 323-386.
3. Coffin CM, Dehner LP: Fibroblastic-myofibroblastic tumors in children and adolescents: a clinicopathologic study of 108 examples in 103 patients. *Pediatr Pathol* 11:569, 1991.
4. Conley J, Healey WV, Stout AP: Fibromatosis of the head and neck. *Am J Surg* 112:609, 1966.
5. Dehner LP, Askin FB: Tumors of fibrous tissue origin in childhood: a clinicopathologic study of cutaneous and soft tissue neoplasms in 66 children. *Cancer* 38:888, 1976.
6. Enjoji M, Iwasaki H, Yoshida I: Benign tumors and tumorlike lesions of soft tissues in infancy and childhood: histopathological and statistical study of 1,020 cases. *Fukuoka Acta Med* 67:234, 1976.
7. Enzinger FM: Fibrous tumors of infancy, in *Tumor of bone and soft tissues*. Chicago, 1965, Year Book Medical Publishers, pp. 375-396.
8. Rosenberg HS, Stenback WA, Spjut HJ: The fibromatoses of infancy and childhood. *Perspect Pediatr Pathol* 4:269, 1978.
9. Stout AP: Juvenile fibromatoses. *Cancer* 7:953, 1954.
10. Unnik AM: Fibromatoses bij kinderen. *Ned Tijdachr Geneeskd* 119:232, 1975.

Fibrous hamartoma of infancy

11. Aberer E, Mainitz M, Entacher U, et al: Fibrous hamartoma of infancy: infantile subcutaneous myofibroblastoma. *Dermatologica* 176:46, 1988.
12. Enzinger FM: Fibrous hamartoma of infancy. *Cancer* 18:241, 1965.
13. Fletcher CD, Powell G, van Noorden S, et al: Fibrous hamartoma of infancy: a histochemical and immunohistochemical study. *Histopathology* 12:65, 1988.
14. Greco MA, Schinella RA, Vuletin JC: Fibrous hamartoma of infancy: an ultrastructural study. *Hum Pathol* 15:717, 1984.
15. Groisman G, Kerner H: A case of fibrous hamartoma of infancy in the scrotum, including immunohistochemical findings. *J Urol* 144:340, 1990.
16. Groisman G, Lichtig C: Fibrous hamartoma of infancy: an immunohistochemical and ultrastructural study. *Hum Pathol* 22:914, 1991.
17. Harris CJ, Das S, Vogt PJ: Fibrous hamartoma of infancy in the scrotum. *J Urol* 127:781, 1982.
18. Iwasaki H, Enjoji M: Fibrous hamartoma of infancy: report of two cases. *Jpn J Cancer Clin* 20:216, 1974.
19. King DF, Barr RJ, Hirose FM: Fibrous hamartoma of infancy. *J Dermatol Surg Oncol* 5:482, 1979.
20. Mitchell ML, Di Sant'Agnese PA, Gerber JE: Fibrous hamartoma of infancy. *Hum Pathol* 13:586, 1982.
21. Paller AS, Gonzalez-Crussi F, Sherman JO: Fibrous hamartoma of infancy: eight additional cases and a review of the literature. *Arch Dermatol* 125:88, 1989.
22. Reye RDK: Considerations of certain subdermal "fibromatous tumors" of infancy. *J Pathol* 72:149, 1956.
23. Ritchie EL, Gonzalez-Crussi F, Zaontz MR: Fibrous hamartoma of infancy masquerading as a rhabdomyosarcoma of the spermatic cord. *J Urol* 140:800, 1988.
24. Robbins LB, Hoffman S, Kahn S: Fibrous hamartoma of infancy: case report. *Plast Reconstr Surg* 46:197, 1970.

Infantile digital fibromatosis

25. Ahlqvist J, Pohjanpelto P, Hjelt L, et al: Recurring digital fibrous tumor of childhood. I. Clinical and morphological aspects of a case. *Acta Pathol Microbiol Scand* 70:291, 1967.
26. Allen PW: recurring digital fibrous tumours of childhood. *Pathology* 4:215, 1972.
27. Arundell FD: Proceedings: recurring digital fibrous tumor of childhood, case 1. *Arch Dermatol* 111:1372, 1975.
28. Battifora H, Hines JR: Recurrent digital fibromas of childhood: an electron microscope study. *Cancer* 27:1530, 1971.
29. Bean SF: Infantile digital fibroma (letter to the editor). *Arch Dermatol Syphil* 100:124, 1969.
30. Beckett JH, Jacobs AH: Recurring digital fibrous tumors of childhood: a review. *Pediatrics* 59:401, 1977.
31. Bhawan J, Bacchetta C, Joris I, et al: A myofibroblastic tumor: infantile digital fibroma (recurrent digital fibrous tumor of childhood). *Am J Pathol* 94:19, 1979.
32. Bloem JJ, Vuzevski VD, Huffstadt AJC: Recurring digital fibroma of infancy. *J Bone Joint Surg* 56B:746, 1974.
33. Bonerandi JJ, Follana J, Migozzi B, et al: Fibromatose digitale infantile. Étude anatomoclinique et ultra-structurale. *Ann Dermatol Syphil* 103:161, 1976.
34. Burry AF, Kerr JFR, Pope JH: Recurring digital fibrous tumors of childhood: an electron microscopic and virological study. *Pathology* 2:287, 1970.
35. Cachaza JA, Caballero JJL, Fernandez JA, et al: Endocervical polyp with pseudosarcomatous pattern and cytoplasmic inclusions: an electron microscopic study. *Am J Clin Pathol* 85:633, 1986.
36. Canioni D, Richard S, Rambaud C, et al: Lingual localization of an inclusion body fibromatosis (Reye's tumor). *Pathol Res Pract* 187:886, 1991.
37. Choi KC, Hashimoto K, Setoyama M, et al: Infantile digital fibromatosis: immunohistochemical and immunoelectron microscopic studies. *J Cutan Pathol* 17:225, 1990.
38. Enzinger FM: Dermal fibromatosis, in *Tumors of bone and soft tissue*. Chicago, 1965, Year Book Medical Publishers, pp 375-396.
39. Faraggiana T, Churg J, Strauss L, et al: Ultrastructural histochemistry of infantile digital fibromatosis. *Ultrastruct Pathol* 2:241, 1981.

40. Frank A: Ein Fall von angeborenen Fibromen am Finger nebst Bei-traegen zur Kasuistic der Fingertumoren. *Wien Klin Rundschau* 22:659, 1908.

41. Fringes B, Thais H, Bohm N, et al: Identification of actin microfil-aments in the intracytoplasmic inclusions present in recurring infan-tile digital fibromatosis (Reye tumor). *Pediatr Pathol* 6:311, 1986.

42. Grunnet N, Genner J, Mogensen B, et al: Recurring digital fibrous tumour of childhood: case report and survey. *Acta Pathol Microbiol Scand* 81A:167, 1973.

43. Ishii N, Matsui K, Ichiyama S, et al: A case of infantile digital fi-bromatosis showing spontaneous regression. *Br J Dermatol* 121:129, 1989.

44. Iwasaki H, Kikuchi M, Mori R, et al: Infantile digital fibromatosis: ultrastructural, histochemical and tissue culture observations. *Can-cer* 46:2238, 1980.

45. Iwasaki H, Kikuchi M, Ohtsuki I, et al: Infantile digital fibromato-sis: identification of actin filaments in cytoplasmic inclusions by heavy meromyosin binding. *Cancer* 52:1653, 1983.

46. Iwasaki H, Tsuneyoshi M, Enjoji M: Infantile digital fibromatosis: histopathological and electron microscopic study with a review of the literature. *Acta Pathol Jpn* 24:717, 1974.

47. Jaschke E, Wohlfarth B: Rezidivierende Digitalfibrome im Kindes-alter. *Z Haut Geschlechtskr* 48:317, 1973.

48. Jensen AR, Martin LW, Longino LA: Digital neurofibrosarcoma in infancy. *J Pediatr* 51:566, 1957.

49. Kanamori M, Hashimoto K, Tanaka H, et al: SH abundant body in infantile digital fibromatosis: a histochemical study of distribution on sulfhydryl groups. *J Dermatol* 17:559, 1990.

50. Kapiloff B, Prior T: Fibromatosis in children. *Plast Reconstr Surg* 10:276, 1952.

51. Kawabata H, Masada K, Aoki Y, et al: Infantile digital fibromato-sis after web construction in syndactyly. *J Hand Surg* 11A:741, 1986.

52. McKenzie AW, Innes FLF, Rack JM, et al: Digital fibrous swell-ings in children. *Br J Dermatol* 83:446, 1970.

53. Miyamoto T, Mihara M, Hagari Y, et al: Posttraumatic occurrence of infantile digital fibromatosis: a histologic and electron microscopic study. *Arch Dermatol* 122:915, 1986.

54. Mortimer G, Gibson AAM: Recurring digital fibroma. *J Clin Pathol* 35:849, 1982.

55. Mukai M, Torikata C, Iri H, et al: Immunohistochemical identifica-tion of aggregated actin filaments in formalin-fixed, paraffin-embedded sections. I. A study of infantile digital fibromatosis by a new pretreatment. *Am J Surg Pathol* 16:110, 1992.

56. Mukai M, Torikata C, Iri H, et al: Infantile digital fibromatosis: an electron microscopic and immunohistochemical study. *Acta Pathol Jpn* 36:1605, 1986.

57. Navas-Palacios JJ, Conde-Zurita JM: Inclusion body myofibroblasts other than those seen in recurring digital fibroma of childhood. *Ul-trastruct Pathol* 7:109, 1984.

58. Pohjanpelto P, Ahlqvist J, Hurme K, et al: Recurring digital fibrous tumor of childhood. II. Isolation of a cell transforming agent. *Acta Pathol Microbiol Scand* 70:297, 1967.

59. Poppen NK, Niebauer JJ: Recurring digital fibrous tumors of child-hood. *J Hand Surg* 2:253, 1977.

60. Prior JT, Sisson BJ: Dermal and fascial fibromatosis. *Ann Surg* 139:453, 1954.

61. Purdy LJ, Colby TV: Infantile digital fibromatosis occurring outside the digit. *Am J Surg Pathol* 8:787, 1984.

62. Reye RDK: Recurring digital fibrous tumors of childhood. *Arch Pathol* 80:228, 1965.

63. Sakurane K: A case of fibroma durum multiplex on the tip of the fingers and toes of an infant. *Jpn J Dermatol* 24:8, 1924.

64. Stiller D, Katenkamp D: Morphogenesis of intracytoplasmic dense (inclusion) bodies in a recurring digital fibrous tumor of childhood: light and electron-microscopic investigations. *Virchows Arch (Pathol Anat)* 367:73, 1975.

65. Stout AP: Juvenile fibromatoses. *Cancer* 7:953, 1954.

66. Yun K: Infantile digital fibromatosis: Immunohistochemical and ul-trastructural observations of cytoplasmic inclusions. *Cancer* 61:500, 1988.

67. Zina AM, Rampini E, Fulcheri E, et al: Recurrent digital fibroma-tosis of childhood: an ultrastructural and immunohistochemical study of two cases. *Am J Dermatopathol* 8:22, 1986.

Myofibroma and myofibromatosis

68. Altemani AM, Amstalden EI, Martins FJ: Congenital generalized fi-bromatosis causing spinal cord compression. *Hum Pathol* 16:1063, 1985.

69. Baer JW, Radkowski MA: Congenital multiple fibromatosis: case re-port with review of the world literature. *Am J Roentgenol* 118:200, 1973.

70. Baird PA, Worth AJ: Congenital generalized fibromatosis: an auto-somal recessive condition. *Clin Genet* 9:488, 1976.

71. Bartlett RC, Otis RD, Laakso AO: Multiple congenital neoplasms of soft tissues: report of four cases in one family. *Cancer* 14:913, 1961.

72. Beatty EC Jr: Congenital generalized fibromatosis in infancy. *AMA J Dis Child* 103:620, 1962.

73. Benjamin SP, Mercer RD, Hawk WA: Myofibroblastic contraction in spontaneous regression of multiple congenital mesenchymal hamartomas. *Cancer* 40:2343, 1977.

74. Boman F, Foliguet B, Metaizeau JP, et al: Myofibromatosis in chil-dren: histopathologic and ultrastructural study of a localized form with a spontaneously regressive course. *Ann Pathol* 4:211, 1984.

75. Bracko M, Cindro L, Golouh R: Familial occurrence of infantile my-ofibromatosis. *Cancer* 69:1294, 1992.

76. Brill PW, Yandow DR, Langer LO, et al: Congenital generalized fibromatosis: case report and literature review. *Pediatr Radiol* 12:269, 1982.

77. Briselli MF, Soule EH, Gilchrist GS: Congenital fibromatosis: re-port of 18 cases of solitary and 4 cases of multiple tumors. *Mayo Clin Proc* 55:554, 1980.

78. Chang WW, Griffith KM: Solitary intestinal fibromatosis: a rare cause of intestinal obstruction in neonate and infant. *J Pediatr Surg* 26:1406, 1991.

79. Chung EB, Enzinger FM: Infantile myofibromatosis: a review of 59 cases with localized and generalized involvement. *Cancer* 48:1807, 1981.

80. Daimaru Y, Hashimoto H, Enjoji M: Myofibromatosis in adults (adult counterpart of infantile myofibromatosis). *Am J Surg Pathol* 13:859, 1989.

81. Dictor M, Elner A, Andersson T, et al: Myofibromatosislike heman-giopericytoma metastasizing as differentiated vascular smooth mus-cle and myosarcoma: myopericytes as a subset of "myofibroblasts." *Am J Surg Pathol* 16:1239, 1992.

82. Dimmick JE, Wood WS: Congenital multiple fibromatosis. *Am J Dermatopathol* 5:289, 1983.

83. Enzinger FM: Fibrous tumors of infancy, in *Tumors of bone and soft tissue*. Chicago, 1965, Year Book Medical Publishers, p 392.

84. Fletcher CD, Achu P, Van Noorden S, et al: Infantile myofibroma-tosis: a light microscopic, histochemical and immunohistochemical study suggesting true smooth muscle differentiation. *Histopathology* 11:245, 1987.

85. Hasegawa T, Hirose T, Seki K, et al: Solitary infantile myofibro-matosis of bone: an immunohistochemical and ultrastructural study. *Am J Surg Pathol* 17:308, 1993.

86. Heiple KG, Perrin E, Aikawa M: Congenital generalized fibroma-tosis: a case limited to osseous lesions. *J Bone Joint Surg* 54A:663, 1972.

87. Hogan SF, Salassa JR: Recurrent adult myofibromatosis: a case re-port. *Am J Clin Pathol* 97:810, 1992.

88. Hower J, Gobel FJ, Ruttner JR, et al: Familiäre kongenitale generalisierte Fibromatose bei zwei Halbschwestern. *Schweiz Med Wschft* 101:1381, 1971.

89. Inwards CY, Unni KK, Beabout JW, et al: Solitary congenital fibromatosis (infantile myofibromatosis) of bone. *Am J Surg Pathol* 15:935, 1991.

90. Jennings T, Duray PH, Collins FS, et al: Infantile myofibromatosis: evidence for an autosomal-dominant disorder. *Am J Surg Pathol* 8:529, 1984.

91. Kennedy S, Yunis E, Smith S, et al: Morphologic and molecular analysis of congenital myofibromatosis and fibromatosis. *Modern Pathol* 3:4P, 1990.

92. Kindblom LG, Angervall L: Congenital solitary fibromatosis of the skeleton: case report of a variant of congenital generalized fibromatosis. *Cancer* 41:636, 1978.

93. Kindblom LG, Termen G, Save-Soderbergh J, et al: Congenital solitary fibromatosis of soft tissues, a variant of congenital generalized fibromatosis: two case reports. *Acta Pathol Microbiol Scand* 85A:640, 1977.

94. Liew SH, Haynes HM: Localized form of congenital generalized fibromatosis: a report of three cases with myofibroblasts. *Pathology* 13:257, 1981.

95. Lin JJ, Svoboda DJ: Multiple congenital mesenchymal tumors: multiple vascular leiomyomas in several organs of a newborn. *Cancer* 28:1046, 1971.

96. Mande R, Hennequet A, Loubry P, et al: Fibromatose congenitale diffuse du nouveau-ne a evolution regressive. *Ann Pediatr* 12:692, 1965.

97. Moore JB, Waldenmaier N, Potchen EJ: Congenital generalized fibromatosis: a new management strategy provided by magnetic resonance imaging. *Am J Dis Child* 141:714, 1987.

98. Morettin LB, Mueller E, Schreiber M: Generalized hamartomatosis (congenital generalized fibromatosis). *Am J Roentgenol Radium Ther Nucl Med* 114:722, 1972.

99. Plaschkes J: Congenital fibromatosis: localized and generalized forms. *J Pediatr Surg* 9:95, 1974.

100. Roggli VL, Kim HS, Hawkins E: Congenital generalized fibromatosis with visceral involvement: a case report. *Cancer* 45:954, 1980.

101. Schaffzin EA, Chung SMK, Kaye R: Congenital generalized fibromatosis with complete spontaneous regressions. *J Bone Joint Surg* 54A:657, 1972.

102. Shnitka TK, Asp DM, Horner HR: Congenital generalized fibromatosis. *Cancer* 11:627, 1958.

103. Smith KJ, Skelton HG, Barrett TL, et al: Cutaneous myofibroma. *Modern Pathol* 2:603, 1989.

104. Speight PM, Dayan D, Fletcher CD: Adult and infantile myofibromatosis: a report of three cases affecting the oral cavity. *J Oral Pathol Med* 20:380, 1991.

105. Spraker MK, Stack C, Esterly NB: Congenital generalized fibromatosis: a review of the literature and report of a case associated with porencephaly, hemiatrophy, and cutis marmorata telangiectatica congenita. *J Am Acad Dermatol* 10:365, 1984.

106. Stenzel P, Fitterer S: Gastrointestinal multicentric infantile myofibromatosis: characteristic histology on rectal biopsy. *Am J Gastroenterol* 84:1115, 1989.

107. Teng P, Warden MJ, Cohn WL: Congenital generalized fibromatosis (renal and skeletal) with complete spontaneous regression. *J Pediatr* 62:748, 1963.

108. Walts AE, Asch M, Raj C: Solitary lesion of congenital fibromatosis: a rare cause of neonatal intestinal obstruction. *Am J Surg Pathol* 6:255, 1982.

109. Williams JO, Schrum D: Congenital fibrosarcoma: report of a case in a newborn infant. *AMA Arch Pathol* 51:548, 1951.

110. Wolfe JT III, Cooper PH: Solitary cutaneous "infantile" myofibroma in a 49-year-old woman. *Hum Pathol* 21:562, 1990.

Juvenile hyalin fibromatosis

111. Bedford CD, Sills JA, Sommelet-Olive D, et al: Juvenile hyaline fibromatosis: a report of two severe cases. *J Pediatr* 119:404, 1991.

112. Castro DJ, Hoover L, Lufkin RB, et al: Multicentric fibromatosis of familial inheritance. *Arch Pathol Lab Med* 111:867, 1987.

113. Drescher E, Woyke S, Markiewicz C, et al: Juvenile fibromatosis in siblings (fibromatosis hyalinica multiplex juvenilis). *J Pediatr Surg* 2:427, 1967.

114. Enjoji M, Kato N, Kamikozuru K, et al: Juvenile fibromatosis of the scalp in siblings. *Acta Med Univ Kagoshima* 10:145, 1968.

115. Fayad MN, Yacoub A, Salman S, et al: Juvenile hyaline fibromatosis: two new patients and review of the literature. *Am J Med Genet* 26:123, 1987.

116. Finlay AY, Ferguson SD, Holt PJA: Juvenile hyaline fibromatosis. *Br J Dermatol* 108:609, 1983.

117. Iwata S, Horiuchi R, Maeda H, et al: Systemic hyalinosis or juvenile hyaline fibromatosis: ultrastructural and biochemical study. *Arch Dermatol Res* 267:115, 1980.

118. Kitano Y: Juvenile hyalin fibromatosis. *Arch Dermatol* 112:86, 1976.

119. Kitano Y, Horiki M, Aoki T, et al: Two cases of juvenile hyalin fibromatosis: some histological, electron microscopic, and tissue culture observations. *Arch Dermatol* 106:877, 1972.

120. Mayer-da-Silva A, Poiares-Baptista A, Guerra-Rodrigo F, et al: Juvenile hyaline fibromatosis. A histologic and histochemical study. *Arch Pathol Lab Med* 112:928, 1988.

121. Murray J: On three peculiar cases of molluscum fibrosum in children. *Med Chir Trans* 38:235, 1873.

122. O'Neill DB, Kasser JR: Juvenile hyaline fibromatosis: a case report and review of musculoskeletal manifestations. *J Bone Joint Surg* 71A:941, 1989.

123. Puretic S, Puretic B, Fiser-Herman M: A unique form of mesenchymal dysplasia. *Br J Dermatol* 74:8, 1962.

124. Quintal D, Jackson R: Juvenile hyaline fibromatosis. A 15-year follow-up. *Arch Dermatol* 121:1062, 1985.

125. Remberger K, Krieg T, Kunze D, et al: Fibromatosis hyalinica multiplex (juvenile hyaline fibromatosis): light microscopic, electron microscopic, immunohistochemical and biochemical findings. *Cancer* 56:614, 1985.

126. Török E, Jellinek K, Schneider F, et al: Juvenile hyaline fibromatose. *Akt Dermatol* 10:6, 1984.

127. Wang NS, Knaack T: Fibromatosis hyalinica multiplex juvenilis. *Ultrastruct Pathol* 3:153, 1982.

128. Whitfield A, Robinson AH: A further report of a remarkable series of cases of molluscum fibrosum in children. *Med Chir Trans* 86:293, 1903.

129. Winchester P, Grossman H, Lim WN, et al: A new acid mucopolysaccharidosis with skeletal deformities simulating rheumatoid arthritis. *Am J Roentgenol* 106:121, 1969.

130. Woyke S, Domagala W, Markiewicz D: A 19-year follow-up of multiple juvenile fibromatosis. *J Pediatr Surg* 19:302, 1984.

131. Woyke S, Domagala W, Olszewski W: Ultrastructure of a fibromatosis hyalinica multiplex juvenilis. *Cancer* 26:1157, 1970.

Gingival fibromatosis

132. Angelopoulos AP, Goaz P: Incidence of diphenylhydantoin gingival hyperplasia. *Oral Surg Oral Med Oral Pathol* 34:898, 1972.

133. Bakaeen G, Scully C: Hereditary gingival fibromatosis in a family with the Zimmermann-Laband syndrome. *J Oral Pathol Med* 20:457, 1991.

134. Cuestas-Carnero R, Bornancini CA: Hereditary gingival fibromatosis associated with hypertrichosis: report of five cases in one family. *J Oral Maxillofac Surg* 46:415, 1988.

135. Dreyer WP, Thomas CJ: Diphenylhydantoinate-induced hyperplasia of the masticatory mucosa in an edentulous epileptic patient. *Oral Surg Oral Med Oral Pathol* 45:701, 1978.

136. Emerson TG: Hereditary gingival hyperplasia: a familial pedigree of four generations. *Oral Surg Oral Med Oral Pathol* 19:1, 1965.

137. Gould AR, Escobar VH: Symmetrical gingival fibromatosis. *Oral Surg Oral Med Oral Pathol* 51:62, 1981.

138. Heath C: Two cases of hypertrophy of the gums and alveoli treated by operation. *Trans Odont Soc Great Britain* 11:18, 1878.

139. Henefer EP, Kay LA: Congenital idiopathic gingival fibromatosis in the deciduous dentition. *Oral Surg Oral Med Oral Pathol* 24:65, 1967.

140. Laband PF, Habib G, Humphreys GS: Hereditary gingival fibromatosis: report of an affected family with associated splenomegaly and skeletal and soft tissue abnormalities. *Oral Surg Oral Med Oral Pathol* 17:339, 1964.

141. Ramon Y, Berman W, Bubis JJ: Gingival fibromatosis combined with cherubism. *Oral Surg Oral Med Oral Pathol* 24:435, 1967.

142. Savara BS, Suher T, Everett FG, et al: Hereditary gingival fibrosis: study of a family. *J Periodontol* 25:12, 1954.

143. Takagi M, Yamamoto H, Mega H, et al: Heterogeneity in the gingival fibromatoses. *Cancer* 68:2202, 1991.

144. Weski H: Elephantiasis gingivae hereditaria. *Dtsch Monatsschft Zahnh* 38:557, 1920.

145. Zegarelli EV, Kutcher AH, Lichtenthal R: Idiopathic gingival fibromatosis: report of 20 cases. *Am J Digest Dis* 8:782, 1962.

Fibromatosis colli

146. Armstrong D, Pickrell K, Fetter B, et al: Torticollis: analysis of 271 cases. *Plast Reconstr Surg* 35:14, 1965.

147. Binder H, Eng GD, Gaiser JF, et al: Congenital muscular torticollis: results of conservative management with long-term follow-up in 85 cases. *Arch Phys Med Rehabil* 68:222, 1987.

148. Bredenkamp JK, Hoover LA, Berke GS, et al: Congenital muscular torticollis: a spectrum of disease. *Arch Otolaryngol Head Neck Surg* 116:212, 1990.

149. Brown JB, McDowell F: Wry-neck facial distortion prevented by resection of fibrosed sternomastoid muscle in infancy and childhood. *Ann Surg* 131:721, 1950.

150. Brown JB, McDowell F, Fryer MP: Facial distortion in wryneck prevented by early resection of fibrosed sternocleidomastoid muscle. *Plast Reconstr Surg* 5:301, 1950.

151. Campbell CJ, Pedra G: Sternomastoid tumor in an identical twin. *J Bone Joint Surg* 38A:350, 1956.

152. Canale ST, Griffin DW, Hubbard CN: Congenital muscular torticollis: a long-term follow-up. *J Bone Joint Surg* 64A:810, 1982.

153. Chandler FA, Altenberg A: "Congenital" muscular torticollis. *JAMA* 125:476, 1944.

154. Coventry MB, Harris LE, Bianco AJ Jr, et al: Congenital muscular torticollis (wry neck). *Postgrad Med* 28:383, 1960.

155. Enzinger FM: Fibrous tumors of infancy. In *Tumors of bone and soft tissue*. Chicago, 1965, Year Book Medical Publishers.

156. Gonzales J, Ljung BM, Guerry T, et al: Congenital torticollis: evaluation by fine-needle aspiration biopsy. *Laryngoscope* 99:651, 1989.

157. Gruhn J, Hurwitt ES: Fibrous sternomastoid tumor of infancy. *Pediatrics* 8:522, 1951.

158. Karki E: Problems of etiology, prevention and treatment of juvenile muscular torticollis. *Beitr Orthop Traumatol* 23:701, 1976.

159. Lawrence WT, Azizkhan RG: Congenital muscular torticollis: a spectrum of pathology. *Ann Plast Surg* 23:523, 1989.

160. MacDonald D: Sternomastoid tumor and muscular torticollis. *J Bone Joint Surg* 51B:432, 1969.

161. Middleton DS: Pathology of congenital torticollis. *Br J Surg* 18:188, 1930.

162. Morrison DL, MacEwen GD: Congenital muscular torticollis: observations regarding clinical findings, associated conditions, and results of treatment. *J Pediatr Orthop* 2:500, 1982.

163. Radtke J: Fibromatosis colli: A benign tumor of the neck in diagnosis and therapy. *Dtsch Z Mund Kiefer Gesichtschir* 15:248, 1991.

164. Reske W: Muscular torticollis and results of treatment. *Arch Orthop Unfallchir* 53:297, 1961.

165. Suzuki S, Yamamuro T, Fujita A: The aetiological relationship between congenital torticollis and obstetrical paralysis. *Int Orthop* 8:175,1984.

166. Thompson F, McManus S, Colville J: Familial congenital muscular torticollis: case report and review of the literature. *Clin Orthop Rel Res* 202:193, 1986.

167. Wakeley PE, Price WG, Frable WJ: Sternomastoid tumor of infancy (fibromatosis colli): diagnosis by aspiration cytology. *Modern Pathol* 2:378, 1989.

Infantile (desmoid-type) fibromatosis

168. Allen PW: The fibromatoses: a clinicopathologic classification based on 140 cases. *Am J Surg Pathol* 1:255, 1977.

169. Boman F, Peters J, Ragge N, et al: Infrequent mutation of the p53 gene in fibrous tumors of infancy and childhood. *Diagn Mol Pathol* 2:14, 1993.

170. Carr RJ, Zaki GA, Leader MB, et al: Infantile fibromatosis with involvement of the mandible. *Br J Oral Maxillofac Surg* 30:257, 1992.

171. Connoly NK: Juvenile fibromatosis: a case report showing invasion of bone. *Arch Dis Child* 36:171, 1961.

172. Dehner LP, Askin FB: Tumors of fibrous tissue origin in childhood: a clinicopathologic study of cutaneous and soft tissue neoplasms in 66 children. *Cancer* 38:888, 1976.

173. Eady JL, Lundquist JE, Grant RE, et al: Congenital bowing of the ulna and aggressive fibromatosis. *J Natl Med Assoc* 83:978, 1991.

174. Egan M, Raafat F, Crocker J, et al: Nucleolar organiser regions in fibrous proliferations of childhood and infantile fibrosarcoma. *J Clin Pathol* 41:31, 1988.

175. Enzinger FM: Fibrous tumors of infancy. In *Tumors of bone and soft tissue*. Chicago, 1965, Year Book Medical Publishers, pp 375-396.

176. Fievez M, Mandard AM: Les fibromatoses de l'enfant: a propos de 22 cas. *Ann Anat Pathol (Paris)* 11:83, 1966.

177. Fisker AV, Philipsen HP: Desmoplastic fibroma of the jaw bones. *Int J Oral Surg* 5:285, 1978.

178. Fleischmajer R, Nedwich A, Reeves JR: Juvenile fibromatoses. *Arch Dermatol* 107:574, 1973.

179. Fromowitz FB, Hurst LC, Nathan J, et al: Infantile (desmoid type) fibromatosis with extensive ossification. *Am J Surg Pathol* 11:66, 1987.

180. Hidayat AA, Font RL: Juvenile fibromatosis of the periorbital region and eyelid: a clinicopathologic study of six cases. *Arch Ophthalmol* 98:280, 1980.

181. Levkoff H, Gonzalez G, Neher L: Congenital diffuse fibromatosis: a case report. *Pediatrics* 35:331, 1965.

182. Melrose JR, Abrams AM: Juvenile fibromatosis affecting the jaws: report of three cases. *Oral Surg Oral Med Oral Pathol* 49:317, 1980.

183. Peede LF Jr, Epker BN: Aggressive juvenile fibromatosis involving the mandible: surgical excision with immediate reconstruction. *Oral Surg Oral Med Oral Pathol* 43:651, 1977.

184. Rodu B, Weathers DR, Campbell WG Jr: Aggressive fibromatosis involving the paramandibular soft tissues: a study with the aid of electron microscopy. *Oral Surg Oral Med Oral Pathol* 52:395, 1981.

185. Rosenberg HS, Stenback WA, Spjut HJ: The fibromatoses of infancy and childhood. *Perspect Pediatr Pathol* 4:269,1978.

186. Schmidt D, Klinge P, Leuschner I, et al: Infantile desmoid-type fibromatosis: morphological features correlate with biological behaviour. *J Pathol* 164:315, 1991.

187. Shah AC, Katz RL: Infantile aggressive fibromatosis of the base of the tongue. *Otolaryngol Head Neck Surg* 98:346, 1988.

188. Shankwiler RA, Athey PA, Lamki N: Aggressive infantile fibromatosis: pulmonary metatastases documented by plain film and computed tomography. *Clin Imaging* 13:127, 1989.
189. Stout AP: Juvenile fibromatoses. *Cancer* 7:953, 1954.
190. Tagawa T, Ohse S, Hirano Y, et al: Aggressive infantile fibromatosis of the submandibular region. *Int J Oral Maxillofac Surg* 18:264, 1989.
191. Takagi M, Ishikawa G: Fibrous tumor of infancy: report of a case originating in the oral cavity. *J Oral Pathol* 2:293, 1973.
192. Thompson DH, Khan A, Gonzalez C, et al: Juvenile aggressive fibromatosis: report of three cases and review of the literature. *Ear Nose Throat J* 70:462, 1991.
193. Wilkins SA, Waldron CA, Mathews WH, et al: Aggressive fibromatosis of head and neck. *Am J Surg* 130:412, 1975.

Calcifying aponeurotic fibroma

194. Adeyemi-Doro HO, Olude O: Juvenile aponeurotic fibroma. *J Hand Surg* 10B:127, 1985.
195. Allen PW, Enzinger FM: Juvenile aponeurotic fibroma. *Cancer* 26:857, 1970.
196. Aprin H, Schwartz G, Lipper S: Juvenile nodular aponeurotic fibroma in the area of the knee joint. *Clin Orthop* 190:257, 1984.
197. Goldman RL: The cartilage analogue of fibromatosis (aponeurotic fibroma): further observations based on seven new cases. *Cancer* 26:1325, 1970.
198. Hassel B: Calcifying aponeurotic fibroma: a case of multiple primary tumours: case report. *Scand J Plast Reconstr Hand Surg* 26:115, 1992.
199. Iwasaki H, Enjoji M: Calcifying aponeurotic fibroma. *Fukuoka Acta Med* 64:52, 1973.
200. Iwasaki H, Kikuchi M, Eimoto T, et al: Juvenile aponeurotic fibroma: an ultrastructural study. *Ultrastruct Pathol* 4:75, 1983.
201. Keasbey LE: Juvenile aponeurotic fibroma (calcifying fibroma): a distinctive tumor arising in the palms and soles of young children. *Cancer* 6:338, 1953.
202. Keasbey LE, Fanselau HA: The aponeurotic fibroma. *Clin Orthop* 19:115, 1961.
203. Kindblom LG: Juvenilt aponeurotiskt fibrom: Kort översikt över fibrosa tumörer hos barn; jämte en fallbeskrivning. *Opuscula Medica* 15:295, 1970.
204. Lafferty KA, Nelson LE, Demuth RJ, et al: Juvenile aponeurotic fibroma with disseminated fibrosarcoma. *J Hand Surg* 11A:737, 1986.
205. Lichtenstein L, Goldman RL: The cartilage analogue of fibromatosis: a reinterpretation of the condition called "juvenile aponeurotic fibroma." *Cancer* 17:810, 1964.
206. Moskovich R, Posner MA: Intratendinous aponeurotic fibroma. *J Hand Surg* 13A:563, 1988.
207. Rios-Dalenz JL, Kim JS, McDowell FW: The so-called "juvenile aponeurotic fibroma." *Am J Clin Pathol* 44:632, 1965.
208. Shapiro L: Infantile digital fibromatosis and aponeurotic fibroma: case reports of two rare pseudosarcomas and review of the literature. *Arch Dermatol* 99:37, 1969.
209. Specht EE, Konkin LA: Juvenile aponeurotic fibroma: the cartilage analogue of fibromatosis. *JAMA* 234:626, 1975.
210. Stewart JB, Enzinger FM: Case for diagnosis: juvenile aponeurotic fibroma. *Military Med* 136:493, 1971.
211. Stout AP: Juvenile fibromatoses. *Cancer* 7:953, 1954.
212. Yee DY, Mott RC, Nixon BP: Calcifying aponeurotic fibroma. *J Foot Surg* 30:279, 1991.

Congenital and acquired muscular fibrosis

213. Chiu SS, Furuya K, Arai T, et al: Congenital contracture of the quadriceps muscle: four case reports in identical twins. *J Bone Joint Surg* 56A:1054, 1974.
214. Duran-Sacristan H, Sanchez-Barba A, Lopez-Duran Stern L, et al: Fibrosis of the gluteal muscles: report of three cases. *J Bone Joint Surg* 56A:1510, 1974.
215. Fairbank TJ, Barrett AM: Vastus intermedius contracture in early childhood: case report in identical twins. *J Bone Joint Surg* 43B:326, 1961.
216. Gammie WFP, Taylor JH, Urich H: Contracture of the vastus intermedius in children (a report of two cases). *J Bone Joint Surg* 45B:370, 1963.
217. Goodfellow JW, Nade S: Flexion contracture of the shoulder joint from fibrosis of the anterior part of the deltoid muscle. *J Bone Joint Surg* 51B:356, 1969.
218. Groves RJ, Goldner JL: Contracture of the deltoid muscle in the adult after intramuscular injections. *J Bone Joint Surg* 56A:817, 1974.
219. Gunn DR: Contracture of the quadriceps muscle: a discussion on the etiology and relationship to recurrent dislocation of the patella. *J Bone Joint Surg* 46B:492, 1964.
220. Hnevkovsky O: Progressive fibrosis of the vastus intermedius muscle in children. *J Bone Joint Surg* 43B:318, 1961.
221. Karlen A: Congenital fibrosis of the vastus intermedius muscle. *J Bone Joint Surg* 46B:488, 1964.
222. Mukherjee PK, Das AK: Injection fibrosis in the quadriceps femoris muscle in children. *J Bone Joint Surg* 62A:453, 1980.
223. Napiontek M, Ruszkowski K: Paralytic foot drop and gluteal fibrosis after intramuscular injections. *J Bone Joint Surg* 75B:83, 1993.
224. Peiro A, Fernandez CI, Gomar F: Gluteal fibrosis. *J Bone Joint Surg* 57A:987, 1975.
225. Shen YSH: Abduction contracture of the hip in children. *J Bone Joint Surg* 57B:463, 1975.
226. Williams PF: Quadriceps contracture. *J Bone Joint Surg* 50B:278, 1968.

Cerebriform fibromatosis (Proteus syndrome)

227. Botella-Estrada R, Alegre V, Sanmartin O, et al: Isolated plantar cerebriform collagenoma (letter). *Arch Dermatol* 127:1589, 1991.
228. Clark RD, Donnai D, Rogers J, et al: Proteus syndrome: an expanded phenotype. *Am J Med Genet* 27:99, 1987.
229. Costa T, Fitch N, Azouz EM: Proteus syndrome: report of two cases with pelvic lipomatosis. *Pediatrics* 76:984, 1985.
230. McCall S, Ramzy MI, Cure JK, et al: Encephalocraniocutaneous lipomatosis and the Proteus syndrome: distinct entities with overlapping manifestations. *Am J Med Genet* 43:662, 1992.
231. Samlaska CP, Levin SW, James WD, et al: Proteus syndrome. *Arch Dermatol* 125:1109, 1989.
232. Tibbles JAR, Cohen MM Jr: The Proteus syndrome: the Elephant Man diagnosed. *Br Med J* 293:683, 1986.
233. Viljoen DL, Saxe N, Temple-Camp C: Cutaneous manifestations of the Proteus syndrome. *Pediatric Dermatol* 5:14, 1988.
234. Wiedemann HR, Burgio GR, Aldenhoff P, et al: The Proteus syndrome: partial gigantism of the hands and/or feet, nevi, hemihypertrophy, subcutaneous tumors, macrocephaly or other skull anomalies and possible accelerated growth and visceral affections. *Eur J Pediatr* 140:5, 1983.

Calcifying fibrous pseudotumor

235. Fetsch JF, Montgomery EA, Meis JM: Calcifying fibrous pseudotumor. *Am J Surg Pathol* 17:502, 1993.
236. Rosenthal NS, Abdul-Karim FW: Childhood fibrous tumor with psammoma bodies: clinicopathologic features in two cases. *Arch Pathol Lab Med* 112:798, 1988.

CHAPTER 12

FIBROSARCOMA

Although fibrosarcoma is still best defined as a "malignant tumor of fibroblasts that shows no other evidence of cellular differentiation and is capable of recurrence and metastasis," the exact criteria for its diagnosis and, hence, our concept of its incidence in the general population have changed considerably over the years.

In earlier studies of soft tissue neoplasms this tumor was undoubtedly overdiagnosed. A diagnosis of fibrosarcoma was frequently made for virtually any richly cellular, collagen-forming spindle cell tumor, including malignant fibrous histiocytoma, monophasic fibrous-type synovial sarcoma, malignant peripheral nerve sheath tumor (malignant schwannoma, neurofibrosarcoma), and a host of other sarcomatous and pseudosarcomatous processes. During the past 30 years, however, pathologists have become much more selective in making this diagnosis, and, as a result, fibrosarcoma has become a relatively rare entity.

This trend is well illustrated in two classic surveys originating from the Mayo Clinic: in 1936 Meyerding et al.[34] reported that 65% of their reviewed soft tissue sarcomas were fibrosarcomas; in 1974 Pritchard et al.,[45] after revising the diagnoses in 113 of 330 cases, classified only 12% of 2310 soft tissue sarcomas as fibrosarcomas. Among their cases fibrosarcomas ranked third in frequency, following liposarcoma (21%) and rhabdomyosarcoma (19%). In the AFIP material, fibrosarcoma ranks even lower and is less common than liposarcoma, malignant fibrous histiocytoma, rhabdomyosarcoma, and synovial sarcoma.

On closer scrutiny several factors are probably responsible for the apparent decline in the incidence of fibrosarcoma. One is the recognition of malignant fibrous histiocytoma as a specific tumor type. Another is the segregation of fibromatosis (desmoid tumor) as a specific entity, intermediate in its behavior between a benign fibrous proliferation and a fibrosarcoma. Still another is the recognition of nodular fasciitis and other predominantly fibroblastic lesions as benign reactive processes curable by local excision. Moreover, advances in diagnosis and immunohistochemistry made it possible in recent years to separate fibrosarcoma from malignant peripheral nerve sheath tumors (malignant schwannoma), synovial sarcoma, and fibrous mesothelioma, and to distinguish it from spindle cell carcinoma and malignant melanoma. Immunohistochemical markers for cytokeratin and S-100 protein have become valuable tools for distinguishing and clearly identifying these tumors. Yet, despite much progress in this area, differential diagnosis of the various spindle cell tumors still remains a difficult, challenging, and sometimes inextricable problem, especially where only a small biopsy specimen is available for microscopic examination.

Therefore it is not surprising that, despite numerous articles on the subject of fibrosarcoma, especially in the earlier literature, there is still very little reliable information available on this subject. Many of the reported data clearly defy comparison and are of doubtful value for the assessment of the tumor's clinical behavior. Quite obviously there is an urgent need for more uniform diagnostic criteria, since even the most diligently gathered data are only as good as the underlying histological diagnoses.

Clinical findings

Like most other sarcomas, fibrosarcoma causes no characteristic symptoms and is difficult to diagnose clinically. It usually presents as a solitary palpable mass, ranging in size from 3 to 8 cm in greatest diameter and rarely becoming larger than 10 cm. In general, it is slow growing and in the initial phase causes pain only in about one third of cases. In fact, pain is encountered more commonly with synovial sarcoma and malignant peripheral nerve sheath tumor (malignant schwannoma) than with fibrosarcoma.

The skin overlying the tumor is generally intact. Ulceration of the skin may be seen in superficially located neoplasms that grow rapidly or have been traumatized; it may also occur following biopsy or attempted local excision. Such tumors, particularly when clinically neglected, may form large fungating masses in the areas of ulceration. In our experience the clinical duration of symptoms varies greatly and ranges from as little as a few weeks to as long as 20 years. Pritchard et al.[45] reported an average preoperative duration of 3 years and 4 months.

Table 12-1. Anatomical locations of fibrosarcoma (AFIP, 695 cases)

Anatomical location	No. patients	Percent
Lower extremities	313	45
Upper extremities	195	28
Trunk	118	17
Head, neck	69	10
TOTAL	695	100

Fibrosarcoma may occur at any age but is most common between the ages of 30 and 55 years. In the AFIP cases—excluding fibrosarcomas occurring in infants and children—the median age is 45 years, with two minor peaks in the early thirties and the mid-fifties. The median age is slightly higher in reported cases diagnosed before 1955, presumably because of the inclusion of malignant fibrous histiocytomas. The average age given in the literature is comparable to our data and ranges from 39.4[40] to 45 years.[49] The information as to sex incidence varies little; most reviewers describe a slightly higher incidence in men than in women. For instance, in the Scott et al. 1989 series[49] of 132 cases, 61% were men.

The tumor may occur anywhere in the body where fibrous tissue is found. According to our observations, it is most common in the region of the thigh and knee, followed in frequency by the trunk and distal portions of the extremities, especially the forearms and the lower legs. Fibrosarcoma in the region of the head and neck is rare, but such cases have been described in the nasal cavity, paranasal sinuses, and nasopharynx.[17,24,31] There are also reports of this tumor in the breast and thyroid gland[1,28] (Table 12-1).

Fibrosarcoma involves foremost deeper structures, where it tends to originate from the intramuscular and intermuscular fibrous tissue, fascial envelopes, aponeuroses, and tendons. Deeply situated tumors may even encircle bone and cause roentgenographically demonstrable periosteal and cortical thickenings, but in such cases distinction from parosteal sarcoma may be difficult. Other roentgenographic findings, in addition to a soft tissue mass, include occasional foci of calcification and ossification. Calcification, however, is much more common with synovial sarcoma than with fibrosarcoma. Yaghmai[65] described the angiographic features of this tumor. Fibrosarcomas arising from the subcutis—excluding fibrosarcoma arising in dermatofibrosarcoma protuberans—are rare, and tend to arise in tissues damaged by radiation, heat, or scarring.

There is no record of systemic changes associated with the disease, except for weight loss in patients with tumors of large size and long standing and in cases where tumors have widely metastasized. Hypoglycemia has been reported, presumably as the result of increased peripheral utilization of glycogen.[40]

Gross findings

Generally the excised tumor consists of a solitary, soft to firm, fleshy, rounded or lobulated mass, which is gray-white to tan-yellow and measures between 3 and 8 cm in greatest diameter (Figs. 12-1 and 12-2). Most of the smaller tumors tend to be well circumscribed and frequently are partly or completely encapsulated. Tumors of larger size, however, are less well defined; they often extend with multiple processes into the surrounding tissues or grow in a diffusely invasive or destructive manner. The frequent circumscription of smaller fibrosarcomas may be misleading and may result in an erroneous benign diagnosis and inadequate therapy.

Microscopic findings

Although there are minor variations in the histological picture, most fibrosarcomas have in common a rather uniform fasciculated growth pattern consisting of fusiform or spindle-shaped cells that vary little in size and shape, have a scanty amount of cytoplasm with indistinct borders, and are separated by interwoven collagen fibers arranged in a parallel fashion. In fact, the amount and orientation of the intervening collagen fibers seem to largely determine the shape of the tumor cells and reflect the degree of cellular differentiation. Mitotic activity varies, but caution should be exercised in making a diagnosis of fibrosarcoma in the absence of mitotic figures. Multinucleated giant cells or giant cells of bizarre size and shape are rarely a distinctive feature of this tumor.

There are no sharply defined morphological subdivisions as, for example, in liposarcoma and rhabdomyosarcoma, and histological grading of fibrosarcomas is mainly based on the degree of cellularity, cellular maturity, mitotic figures, amount of collagen produced by the tumor cells, and necrosis.

Well-differentiated fibrosarcomas are marked by the uniform, orderly appearance of the spindle cells, lack of nuclear hyperchromatism, and variable amounts of collagen (Fig. 12-3). In some cases the cells are oriented in curving or interlacing fascicles, forming the classic herringbone pattern (Figs. 12-4 to 12-6). In others the cells are separated by thick, wirelike collagen fibers that may be hyalinized (Figs. 12-7 and 12-8). Related to the latter is also a rare type of fibrosarcoma marked by more rounded cells with small nuclei and clear cytoplasm that are surrounded, individually or in groups or cords, by dense and often hyalinized collagen fibers (*sclerosing epithelioid fibrosarcoma*) (Fig. 12-9, *A* and *B*).

Poorly differentiated fibrosarcomas are characterized by closely packed, less well oriented tumor cells that are of small size, are more ovoid or rounded, and are associated with less collagen. The fascicular, or herringbone pattern is less distinct, mitotic figures are numerous, and there are areas of necrosis or hemorrhage (Figs. 12-10 to 12-12). The

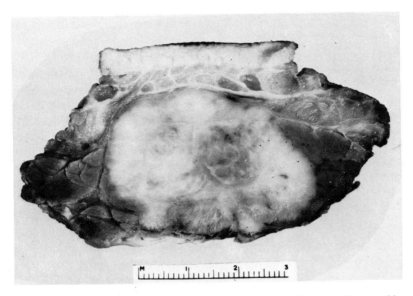

FIG. 12-1. Fibrosarcoma involving the musculature of the shoulder in a 63-year-old man.

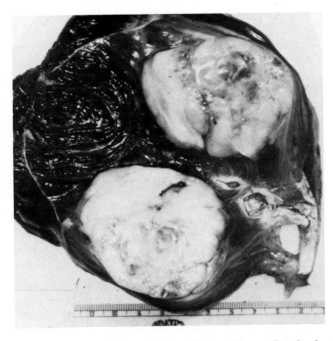

FIG. 12-2. Fibrosarcoma of the posterior thigh in a 37-year-old man. Despite the circumscription of the lesion and treatment by wide local excision, the tumor metastasized to the lung.

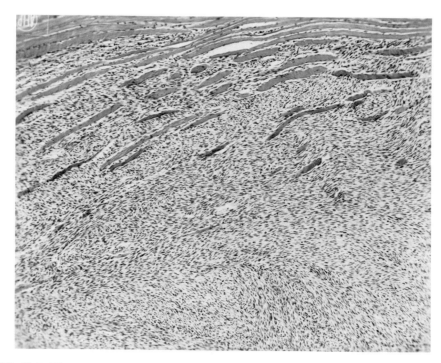

FIG. 12-3. Fibrosarcoma invading muscle tissue. Note orderly arrangement of spindle cells and lack of cellular pleomorphism. (×160.)

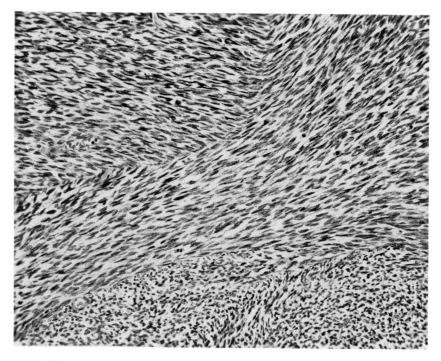

FIG. 12-4. Fibrosarcoma consisting of uniform spindle cells showing little variation in size and shape and a distinct fascicular pattern. (×160.)

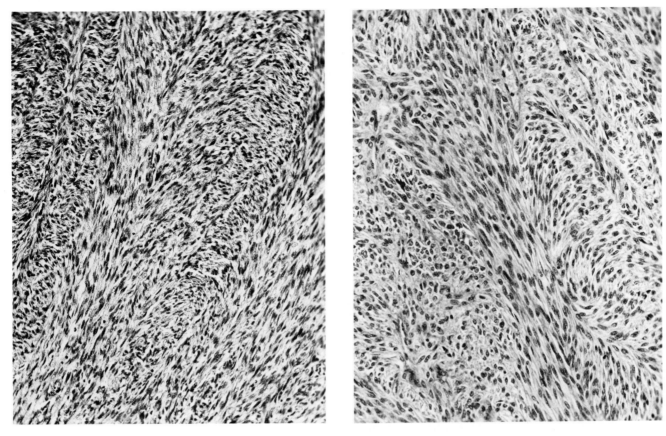

FIG. 12-5. Fibrosarcoma showing arrangement of the fibroblasts in distinct intersecting fascicles ("herringbone" pattern). (×130.)

FIG. 12-6. Another fibrosarcoma displaying the great uniformity of the tumor cells and the characteristic fascicular pattern. (×100.)

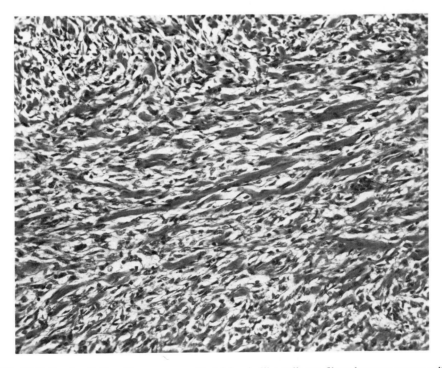

FIG. 12-7. Postirradiation fibrosarcoma with thick wirelike collagen fibers between tumor cells. (×160.)

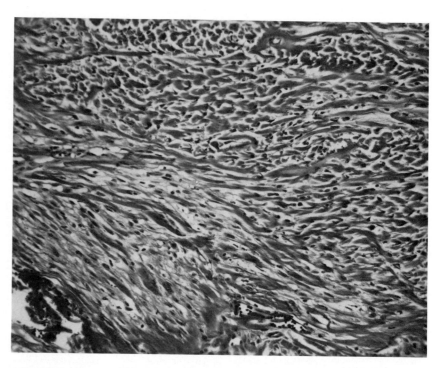

FIG. 12-8. Another well-differentiated fibrosarcoma with large amounts of birefringent collagen. Osseous metaplasia is seen occasionally in these tumors. (×160.)

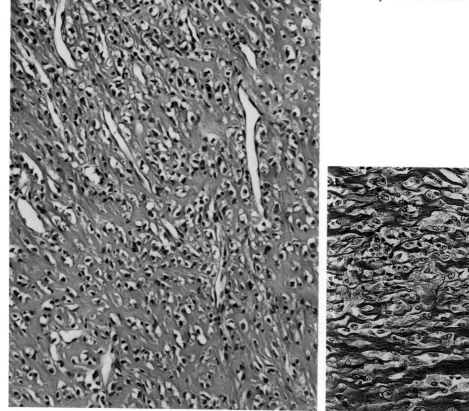

A

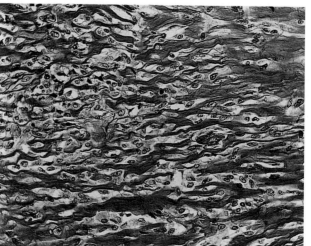

B

FIG. 12-9. A, Sclerosing epithelioid fibrosarcoma characterized by abundant hyalinized collagen between small rounded tumor cells with clear cytoplasm. (×160.) **B,** Another example of sclerosing epithelioid fibrosarcoma. (×210.)

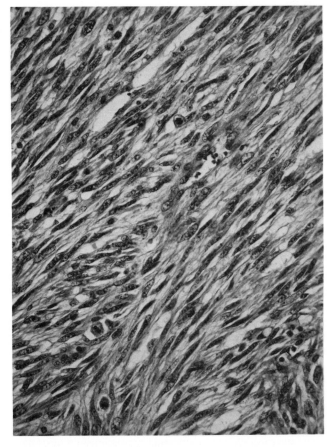

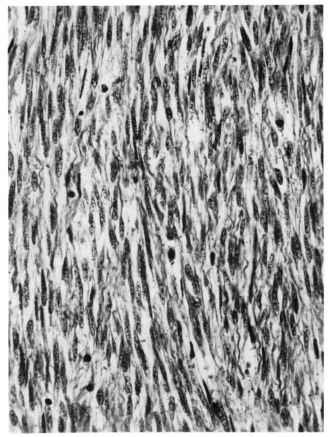

FIG. 12-10. Fibrosarcoma showing a lesser degree of differentiation with a more irregular cellular pattern and numerous mitotic figures. (×100.)

FIG. 12-11. Poorly differentiated fibrosarcoma displaying a high degree of cellularity with only small amounts of interstitial collagen. (×395.)

cells show some variation in size and shape, but marked cellular pleomorphism is more suggestive of malignant fibrous histiocytoma than fibrosarcoma. In some cases distinction of poorly differentiated fibrosarcoma from poorly differentiated synovial sarcoma or malignant peripheral nerve sheath tumors (malignant schwannoma) may be exceedingly difficult or even impossible, especially without the help of immunostaining or electron microscopy.

Secondary features are common: well-differentiated fibrosarcomas, which are rich in mature collagen, may focally show osseous or, less frequently, cartilaginous metaplasia. They may also contain accumulations of interstitial mucoid material (*myxofibrosarcoma*) (Figs. 12-13 and 12-14). In fact, the fibrosarcoma-like tumor described by Evans[14,15] as *"low grade fibromyxoid sarcoma"* probably belongs in this group. It is marked by alternating dense fibrous and myxoid areas or a whorled growth pattern, sometimes with a prominent capillary pattern. It does not show the cellular pleomorphism of myxoid malignant fibrous his-

tiocytoma. Despite its "deceptively benign appearance," its low cellularity, and its low mitotic rate, it is capable of metastasis, usually after multiple recurrences.

Myxoid changes, of course, may also be seen in fibrosarcoma-like synovial sarcomas, malignant peripheral nerve sheath tumors (malignant schwannoma), and malignant fibrous histiocytoma (myxoid MFH). There are also cases of fibrosarcoma in which portions of the tumor mimic fibroma or fibromatosis (desmoid tumor) (Fig. 12-15).

Reticulin preparations reveal in most cases a dense meshwork of collagen fibers between the individual cellular elements (Fig. 12-16). The cells are immunoreactive for vimentin but do not stain for cytokeratin or epithelial membrane antigen (EMA). The lack of cytokeratin reactivity aids in distinction from monophasic fibrous-type synovial sarcoma and malignant fibrous mesothelioma. Negative immunostaining for S-100 protein separates fibrosarcoma from spindle cell or desmoplastic malignant melanoma but not necessarily from malignant peripheral nerve sheath tumor.

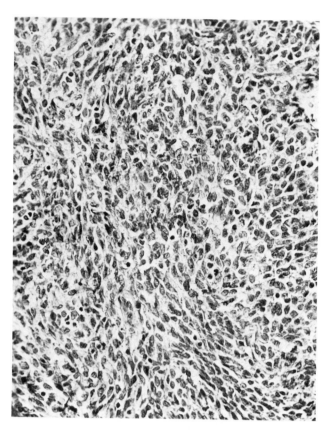

FIG. 12-12. Poorly differentiated fibrosarcoma with focal round cell pattern. (×210.)

Electron microscopic findings

As might be anticipated from the description of the light microscopic features, the tumors are largely composed of elongated fibroblast-like cells having irregularly outlined or indented nuclei, infrequent nucleoli, and prominent rough endoplasmic reticulum, which is often dilated and contains granular or amorphous material. Similar cells contain, in addition, intracytoplasmic bundles of microfilaments measuring up to 60 nm in diameter, focal condensations or dense bodies, and sometimes basal laminae, features characteristic of myofibroblasts.[8,56] Infrequently there are also scattered, round, histiocyte-like cells with multiple processes and a small number of lysosomes. The extracellular spaces contain a varying number of collagen fibers.

Differential diagnosis

It is often difficult to distinguish fibrosarcomas from other spindle cell tumors, and in many instances only careful examination of multiple sections and special stains, as well as immunohistochemical and ultrastructural studies, will permit a correct diagnosis. *Benign processes* likely to be mistaken for fibrosarcomas range from nodular fasciitis and proliferative fasciitis to fibrous histiocytoma and fibromatosis. *Malignant neoplasms* considered in the differential diagnosis are much more numerous and include foremost malignant peripheral nerve sheath tumor, malignant fibrous histiocytoma, and synovial sarcoma. Other tumors that tend to simulate fibrosarcoma are malignant fibrous me-

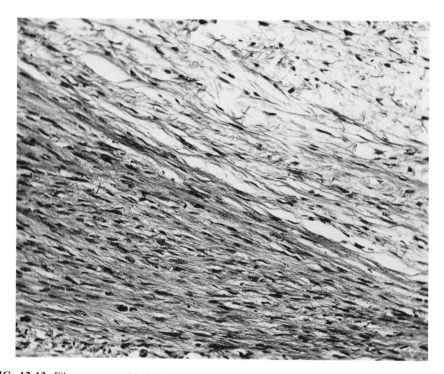

FIG. 12-13. Fibrosarcoma with focal myxoid change removed from the scapular region of a 37-year-old woman. (×130.)

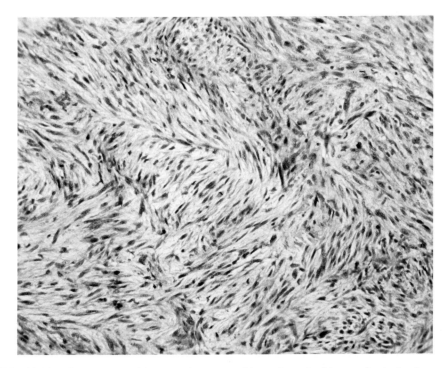

FIG. 12-14. Fibrosarcoma with a prominent myxoid matrix and without a fasciculated growth pattern. (×160.)

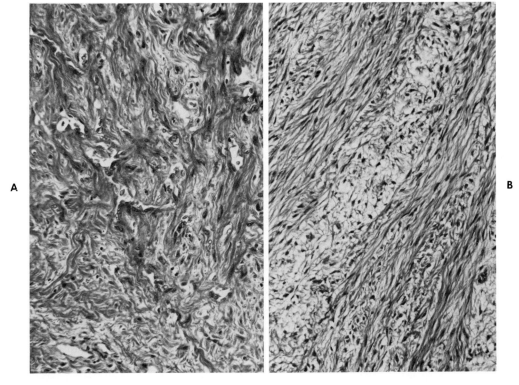

FIG. 12-15. Well-differentiated fibrosarcoma of the buttock. **A,** Richly collagenous fibroma-like areas. (×160.) **B,** Well-differentiated fascicular portions. (×160.)

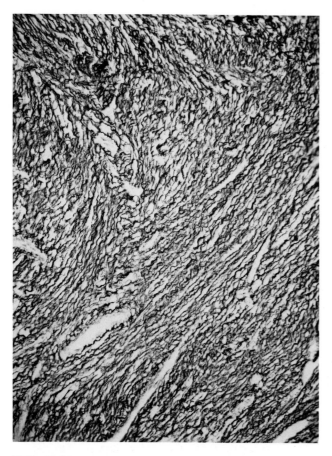

FIG. 12-16. Reticulin preparation of fibrosarcoma displaying well-oriented reticulin fibers separating fibroblasts. (×160.)

sothelioma, clear cell sarcoma, epithelioid sarcoma, dermatofibrosarcoma protuberans, desmoplastic leiomyosarcoma, and even spindle cell forms of rhabdomyosarcoma, liposarcoma, malignant melanoma, and carcinoma. Because the differential diagnosis of most of these tumors is discussed elsewhere, the following comments are limited to those lesions most frequently confused with fibrosarcoma.

Nodular fasciitis, a peculiar reactive fibroblastic proliferation that grows rapidly and is marked by its cellularity and immature cellular appearance, differs from fibrosarcoma by its smaller size and microscopically by its more irregular growth pattern; characteristically, its cells are arranged in short bundles but never in long, sweeping fascicles, or a herringbone pattern, as in fibrosarcoma. Moreover, there is usually a prominent myxoid matrix and scattered chronic inflammatory cells.

Fibrous histiocytoma (dermatofibroma) may also show a distinct spindle cell pattern but never exhibits the cellular polarity and distinct fascicular arrangement of fibrosarcoma. In fact, the cells are often arranged in a storiform pattern and there are interspersed collagen fibers at the periphery. In addition to the spindle cells, there are histiocyte-like cells, siderophages, and xanthoma cells, and occasionally multinucleated giant cells. In most cases fibrous histiocytoma is situated in the dermis or subcutis and, unlike fibrosarcoma and malignant fibrous histiocytoma, is very rare in deeper tissues. Mitotic figures are present in fibrous histiocytoma (and nodular fasciitis), but the presence of atypical mitotic figures lends strong support to the diagnosis of fibrosarcoma.

Musculoaponeurotic fibromatosis (desmoid tumor) may show a growth pattern similar to that of fibrosarcoma, but it is less cellular and contains more collagen. The cells are uniform and vesicular, with little chromatin and one or two minute nucleoli. Mitotic figures are rare, and the finding of more than one mitotic figure per high-power field in such a tumor should raise suspicion of fibrosarcoma. Since on rare occasions features of fibromatosis and fibrosarcoma are found together in the same neoplasm, careful sampling of the tumor is mandatory for a reliable diagnosis. Clinical considerations are of little help in the distinction of fibromatosis and fibrosarcoma because both tumors may occur at the same location and in patients of similar age.

Transitions between *dermatofibrosarcoma protuberans* and fibrosarcoma are fairly common and may herald a more aggressive clinical course.[10,23,64]

Malignant fibrous histiocytoma has been included in many of the earlier reports of poorly differentiated or pleomorphic fibrosarcomas. Clinically, malignant fibrous histiocytoma is principally a tumor of elderly persons, with a peak in the seventh decade; microscopically, it can be recognized by its storiform pattern and the presence of multinucleated bizarre giant cells, often having eosinophilic cytoplasm and containing delicate droplets of lipid material. Siderophages and xanthoma cells are also common features that assist in diagnosis. Transitions between malignant fibrous histiocytoma and fibrosarcoma do occur, but on closer examination most malignant spindle cell tumors with abundant hyalinized, intensely eosinophilic collagen turn out to be variants of malignant fibrous histiocytoma.

Malignant peripheral nerve sheath tumor (MPNST) may display areas that are virtually indistinguishable from fibrosarcoma, but in most of these cases specific features can be found that point toward a tumor of neural origin. These include not only a greater proportion of long, slender spindle cells and a less conspicuous fascicular pattern but also perivascular cuffing and arrangement of the tumor cells in distinct whorls or palisades. In addition, there is a more prominent myxoid matrix, and there are often transitions between malignant and benign neurofibroma-like areas. Cartilaginous metaplasia is also more frequent than in fibrosarcoma or any other noncartilaginous neoplasm. S-100 protein reactivity is demonstrable in one third to one half of malignant peripheral nerve sheath tumors (and spindle cell chondrosarcomas) and, of course, is negative in fibrosarcoma.[35]

There are also clinical differences: a high percentage of malignant peripheral nerve sheath tumors arise either from a large nerve or a neurofibroma or are associated with the manifestations of von Recklinghausen's disease. The latter neoplasms are rarely encountered in patients younger than 35 years of age. Also, fibrosarcoma-like forms of *synovial sarcoma, clear cell sarcoma,* and *poorly differentiated chondrosarcoma* may cause problems in diagnosis.[35] (See Chapters 29, 32, and 35.)

Survival

Many different criteria have been employed in the diagnosis of fibrosarcoma, and therefore it is not surprising that reported survival rates vary considerably, especially in earlier descriptions of the tumor. In more recent reports, however, the 5-year survival rates are more uniform and range from 39% in the Scott et al[49] series to 54.4% in the Mackenzie[30] series. These data differ considerably from those of Castro et al's.[5] who reported a 5-year survival rate of 70% and a 10-year rate of 60%. In the latter series, however, it is not clear whether fibromatoses were included as grade I fibrosarcomas. The survival rate seems to be closely related to the histological grade of the tumor. Scott et al.[49] report a 5-year survival rate of 58% for grade 1 or 2, 34% for grade 3, and 21% for grade 4 tumors. In this series there was also a close relationship between AJC grade and length of survival.

Recurrence

As with survival rates, recurrence rates of the tumor are markedly affected by the selection of cases. Recurrence, always an indicator of the inadequacy of the primary surgical attempt, is usually noted within the first year following surgery, but it may be delayed as long as 20 years; it is encountered in about half of cases and depends largely on the choice and mode of the initial therapy. Mackenzie[30] noted recurrence in 93 (48%) of 190 cases, and Pritchard et al.[45] in 113 (57%) of 199 cases. In the Scott et al.[49] study, the 5-year cumulative probability of local recurrence was 79% in tumors with inadequate surgical margins and 18% in tumors treated by wide or radical excision. Although recurrence may increase the risk of metastasis, a more significant predictor of metastasis seems to be the histological type and the degree of differentiation, especially since it appears that in many cases metastatic spread takes place prior to the initial therapy.

Metastasis

Metastasis of fibrosarcoma occurs almost exclusively by way of the bloodstream. The lung is the principal metastatic site, followed by the skeleton, especially the vertebrae and skull. The occurrence of a second tumor must be considered evidence of metastasis because there is no convincing record of multicentric fibrosarcomas. The majority of metastases are noted within the first 2 years after diagnosis, and in our material the time interval between first therapy and metastasis ranged from a few months to 11 years. But distant metastasis may occur as late as 22 years after surgery. Therefore a 5-year follow-up period is too short, and "5-year cure rates" are misleading.

Lymph node metastasis is rare, occurring in 0.5%[45] to 8%[52] of cases; the relative incidence is, of course, influenced by the number of autopsy cases in the reported material, for lymph nodes tend to be more often involved in the terminal phase of the disease. Therefore it seems regional lymph node excision is not a necessary part of the initial therapeutic regimen.

Factors influencing behavior

There is little evidence that duration of the tumor, size, and location play significant roles in determining its clinical behavior. Phelan and Nigogosyan[42] stated that "tumors of short duration and small size were just as lethal as those of long duration and large dimensions." Others[55] concur that "neither size nor anatomical location of the tumor had any significant effect upon the survival." Undoubtedly the general rule that deep-seated sarcomas pursue a more aggressive clinical course than superficial sarcomas applies equally to fibrosarcoma.

There is, however, a good relationship between the degree of differentiation and survival. This was clearly established as early as 1939 by Broders et al.[3] who demonstrated close parallels between prognosis and histological character. Their work has been amply confirmed by most authors who attempted to correlate histological grade and prognosis.[5,27,31,40,42] Mackenzie,[30] employing a three-grade classification, reported 5-year survival rates for 82.2% in grade 1, 55% in grade 2, and 35.5% in grade 3 tumors. Scott et al.,[49] using a four-grade classification, noted 34% survival for grades 1 or 2, 34% for grade 3, and 21% for grade 4. It is evident from these data and our cases that prognosis in regard to recurrence and metastasis is least favorable in tumors that are richly cellular, have more than two mitotic figures per high-power field, contain little collagen, and show evidence of necrosis. A second and equally important factor in determining prognosis is the type of therapy. Bizer[2] reported a 5-year survival rate of 30% in patients treated by local excision and 78% in patients treated by radical excision. Likewise, Scott et al.[49] found a 29% 5-year survival rate for the group treated with inadequate margins and a 40% rate for those treated with adequate margins. The incidence of recurrence was even more closely related to the extent of surgery. It was 79% in the group with inadequate margins and only 18% in patients treated with wide or marginal excision. In this series, however, there was no clear relationship between the extent of surgery and metastasis.

Treatment

Although opinions as to the best type of therapy vary slightly, surgical management is generally considered the treatment of choice. Once the diagnosis of fibrosarcoma is established by biopsy, the tumor should be promptly excised with a wide margin of normal tissue, the size of the margin depending on the degree of circumscription and cellular differentiation. Because tumors in the extremities are prone to extend proximally along the neurovascular bundle, a wider proximal than distal margin is advisable. As with other sarcomas, enucleation or shelling out of the tumor invites recurrent growth because this procedure does not take into account the frequent presence of small satellite nodules around the main tumor mass. When adequate margins cannot be obtained, as is often the case with tumors situated near large vessels, nerves, or joints, amputation or excision with supplementary radiotherapy is mandatory. Lymph node metastasis is a rare event, and removal of regional lymph nodes is generally unnecessary, unless there is strong clinical evidence of lymph node involvement.

There is still no agreement regarding the benefits of radiotherapy in the treatment of fibrosarcoma. Some reviewers recommend it only as a palliative measure for recurrent tumors of large size that cannot be adequately excised. But the majority believe that radiotherapy has a definite place in the management of this tumor, although the exact response in the individual case is difficult to predict.[63] Adjunctive systemic chemotherapy is indicated in high-grade fibrosarcomas, since in these tumors subclinical or microscopic metastases may exist at the time of the initial surgery.[59]

Discussion

There is little evidence that heredity plays a significant role in the development of fibrosarcoma. Among several hundred examples of fibrosarcoma at the AFIP, there is only a single instance of a tumor that occurred in two generations, father and son, of the same family, but only in one of the two tumors was histological material available for examination. We were unable to find a similar case in the literature, but Pritchard et al.[43] reported the occurrence of sarcomas of various types, including fibrosarcoma in a mother and her three children. The authors also mentioned that 19% of patients with fibrosarcoma in their series had a positive history of cancer.

Considering the prominent role of fibroblasts in posttraumatic repair, it is not surprising that trauma has been implicated repeatedly as a possible and even likely causative factor. Stout,[53] for example, reported 36 cases of fibrosarcoma arising in scar tissue (*cicatricial fibrosarcoma*) or at the site of a former injury. One patient had suffered an injury at age 9 years and developed a fibrosarcoma in the scar at age 35 years; it recurred when the patient was 65 years old. The patient was well and free of recurrence at age 91 years. Ivins et al.[27] noted a history of preceding trauma in 19 of 78 cases of fibrosarcoma but concluded that "only in one an etiologic significance was remotely possible." In our material we are aware of only four cases of fibrosarcoma that clearly arose at the site of a previous injury; the injuries include a shrapnel wound, a fracture, a chain saw injury, and an old incision. Still another case, similar to the one described by Denham and Dingley and others,[9,36,58] arose in a draining sinus of long duration. Heller and Sieber[25] observed the appearance of a fibrosarcoma in the right thigh, 4 months after a sledgehammer injury at the same site. Both Melzner[33] and Stout[53] described a fibrosarcoma that developed in a healed shotgun wound in close vicinity to the bullet; in both cases the tumor made its first clinical appearance after a latent period of 11 years.

Evaluation of the significance of these cases is difficult. In some of them trauma may be a contributing factor, but in others trauma may merely serve to alert the patient or the physician to the presence of the disease and may be an incidental finding rather than a tumor-provoking factor. To our knowledge, there is also no evidence of any increase in the number of fibrosarcomas in veterans of World War I or II or in the large number of persons who have suffered severe soft tissue injuries in agricultural or automobile accidents.

Factors other than trauma have also been implicated to induce or contribute to the development of fibrosarcoma; Burns et al.,[4] for instance, observed such a tumor arising in a 31-year-old man 10 years after a plastic repair of a lacerated femoral artery with a Teflon-Dacron prosthesis. Herrmann et al.[26] have described similar findings. Other fibrosarcomas were described at the site of a total knee joint replacement with cobalt chrome alloy[12] and following penicillin-sesame oil injection.[20]

POSTRADIATION FIBROSARCOMA

There is clearly a higher incidence of fibrosarcoma in patients who have been exposed to radiation than in the general population, but the total number of these tumors is very small compared with the large number of patients at risk. At the AFIP, malignant fibrous histiocytoma is by far the most common postradiation sarcoma, but we have also encountered fibrosarcomas following radiotherapy for carcinoma of the breast, cervix, and uterus and for embryonal carcinoma, seminoma, retinoblastoma, Wilms' tumor, and Hodgkin's disease.[29] In the literature there are also numerous reports in which a fibrosarcoma or fibrosarcoma-like tumor originated at the site of therapeutic radiation for various benign[7,21,41,51] and malignant* neoplasms, as well as for nonneoplastic disorders such as psoriasis and hypertrichosis.[52]

---

*References 1, 11, 18, 38, 41, 46, 48, 51, 61, 62.

The lag period between radiation and tumor development is of significance in the evaluation of these cases. In most cases the latency period is between 4 and 15 years. Tumors appearing after a latency period of less than 2 years are unlikely to be radiation induced. In our series the latent period ranged from 8 to 15 years, with a median of 10 years; patients treated with megavoltage radiation had a shorter latency period. Pettit et al.[41] described a fibrosarcoma in a 54-year-old woman that first appeared 27 years after radiotherapy for goiter. In this case, as well as in many other cases of radiation-induced fibrosarcoma, evidence of radiation damage such as fibrosis, often with atypical fibroblasts, intimal proliferation and atrophy, and necrosis of fat and muscle tissue, was noted in the nonneoplastic tissue adjacent to the sarcoma.[29] Opinions vary as to the significance of the radiation dose for tumor development, and both small and large doses have been implicated as being more likely to produce radiation-related neoplasms.

FIBROSARCOMA ARISING IN BURN SCARS

Although less common than postradiation fibrosarcoma, occasional fibrosarcomas arise in scars formed at sites of thermal injury. Nearly all of the affected patients suffered extensive burns as children and developed tumors after an interval of 30 or more years. At the AFIP there is one case in which a fibrosarcoma of the back developed 40 years after the patient sustained a third-degree burn as a 5-year-old child. Another patient suffered a severe burn at age 12 years and developed a fibrosarcoma at age 56, 44 years later. Fleming and Rezek[16] and Pack and Ariel[40] reported similar cases. The latent period in the former case (a 54-year-old man who had fallen into a bonfire at age 5 years) was 49 years; in the latter case (a 53-year-old man who suffered severe burns at age 6 years) was 47 years. This compares well with the 30- to 40-year latent period of carcinomas arising in burn scars (Marjolin's ulcer).[19] Wilson and Brunschwig[62] described the case of a 15-year-old girl who developed a fibrosarcoma 5 years after an extensive burn involving the right neck and cheek and after radiation of the resulting cicatricial contractures and keloids. Because carcinomas are more common than sarcomas as a late sequence of thermal injury, the possibility of a desmoplastic or spindle cell carcinoma should be ruled out before rendering a diagnosis of postradiation fibrosarcoma.

CONGENITAL AND INFANTILE FIBROSARCOMA

Fibrosarcoma in newborns, infants, and small children bears a close resemblance to adult fibrosarcoma, but it must be considered a separate entity because of its markedly different clinical behavior. It must also be distinguished from richly cellular but benign forms of infantile fibromatosis and especially from other types of childhood sarcoma, such as spindle cell embryonal rhabdomyosarcoma, that behave more aggressively, are prone to metastasize and require

more radical therapy. Fibrosarcomas in older children behave similarly to those occurring in adults.

Congenital or infantile fibrosarcoma is relatively rare, but over the past decades about 200 cases have been reported in the literature. Andersen,[67] who reported in 1951 her experience with various tumors of infancy and childhood, found 5 fibrosarcomas among 24 soft tissue sarcomas in her series of 175 malignant tumors; Stout,[96] reviewing the literature on this subject, was able to collect 31 cases. He added 11 cases of his own that developed in patients 5 years old or younger, including 4 that were present at birth. Additional cases were reported in the literature.*

Clinical findings

The principal manifestation of the disease is a nontender or painless swelling or mass that ranges in size from as small as 1 cm to as large as 20 cm. The mass may grow rapidly, and one tumor in our cases was reported to have "doubled its size within a period of 2½ weeks." In the majority of cases, the mass becomes evident during the first year of life. Among the 53 cases of our series[71] it was

---

*References 69, 71, 82-84, 89, 90, 93, 94, 98.

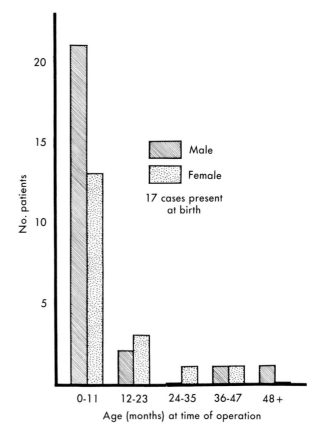

FIG. 12-17. Age distribution of 53 cases of infantile fibrosarcoma. (From Chung EB, Enzinger FM: *Cancer* 38:730, 1976.)

present at birth in 20 cases and appeared during the first 3 months of life in 27 cases. The patients' ages ranged from newborn to 4 years (Fig. 12-17). Males slightly predominated. The principal sites of the mass are the extremities, especially the regions of the foot, ankle, and lower leg and the hand, wrist, and forearm (Figs. 12-18 and 12-19). The trunk, head, and neck regions are less commonly involved.[70,97]

Roentgenographic examination may show, in addition to a soft tissue mass, cortical thickening, bending deformities, and, rarely, extensive destruction of the underlying bone (Figs. 12-20 to 12-22).

Gross findings

The tumors vary considerably in size when first detected. Some measure only a few centimeters; others are extremely

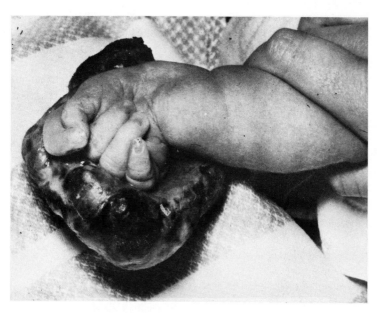

FIG. 12-18. Congenital fibrosarcoma, back of hand.

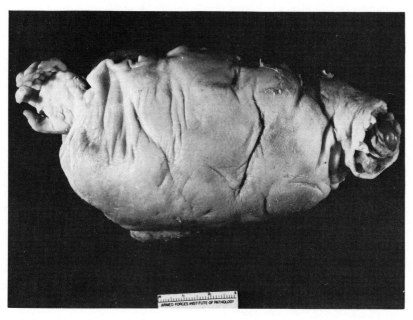

FIG. 12-19. Massive congenital fibrosarcoma occupying the entire forearm and portions of the upper arm in a stillborn boy.

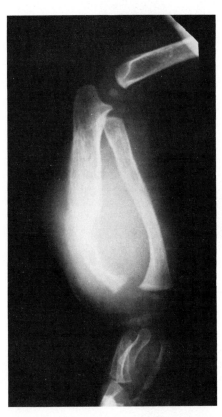

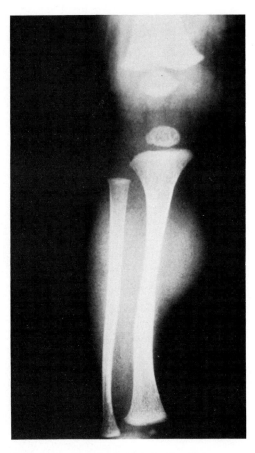

FIG. 12-20. Roentgenograph of infantile fibrosarcoma with marked bending deformity of radius. The lesion occurred in the forearm of a 1-year-old girl.

FIG. 12-21. Roentgenograph of infantile fibrosarcoma of the lower right leg in a 3-month-old girl.

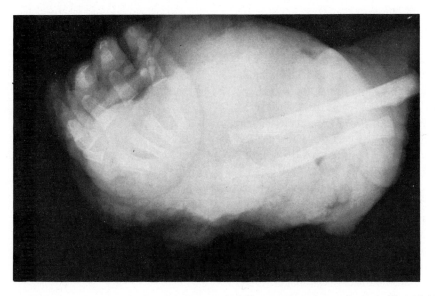

FIG. 12-22. Roentgenograph of massive congenital fibrosarcoma of arm shown in Fig. 12-19.

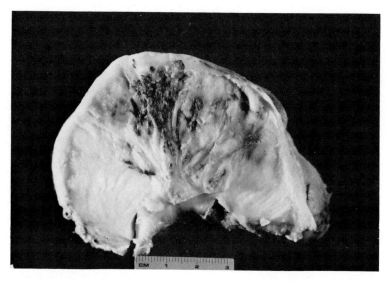

FIG. 12-23. Infantile fibrosarcoma of the right shoulder in a 1-month-old boy, showing marked interstitial hemorrhage.

large and may replace the entire distal portion of the involved limb. They are usually poorly circumscribed and have a gray-white or pale pink cut surface. Tumors of large size may be markedly distorted by central necrosis or hemorrhage (Fig. 12-23).

Microscopic findings

Characteristically, the tumors are composed of sheets of small, uniform, solidly packed, spindle-shaped cells separated by variable amounts of interstitial collagen. Tumors with abundant collagen, that is, tumors having a prominent reticulin pattern, tend to be more fasciculated and often approach the picture of adult fibrosarcoma (Figs. 12-24 to 12-26). Tumors with minimal amounts of collagen, on the other hand, show a lesser degree of cellular polarity and consist of small, more rounded immature-appearing cells showing only focal evidence of fibroblastic differentiation. Judging from our material, the more differentiated tumors, consisting of uniform spindle cells with ill-defined cytoplasm and little nuclear pleomorphism, are more common. Dahl et al.[72] distinguished between "medullary" and "desmoplastic" types of infantile fibrosarcoma (Figs. 12-27 to 12-29).

As in adult fibrosarcoma, multinucleated giant cells are rare. Mitotic figures, however, are fairly common; yet their number varies from tumor to tumor and even in different portions of the same neoplasm. Scattered chronic inflammatory cells, particularly lymphocytes, are another common and sometimes striking feature that helps to distinguish infantile from adult fibrosarcoma. Richly vascular areas and areas of hemorrhage occur not infrequently and may simulate angiosarcoma and especially hemangiopericytoma. The

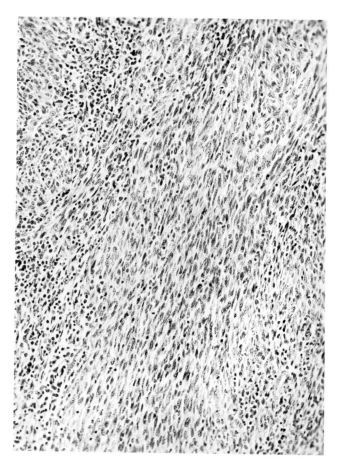

FIG. 12-24. Infantile fibrosarcoma composed of uniform well-oriented fibroblasts and scattered round cells. ($\times$145.)

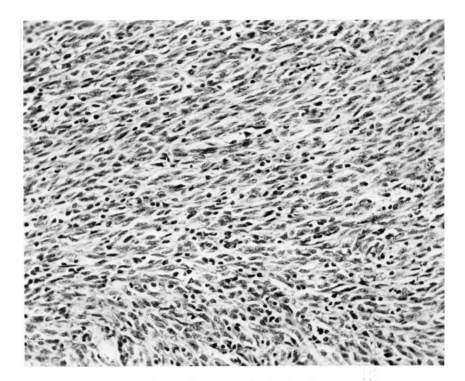

FIG. 12-25. Characteristic microscopic picture of infantile fibrosarcoma showing immature-appearing fibroblasts associated with small round cells, probably lymphocytes. The tumor occurred in the supraclavicular region of a 10-month-old girl. (×225.)

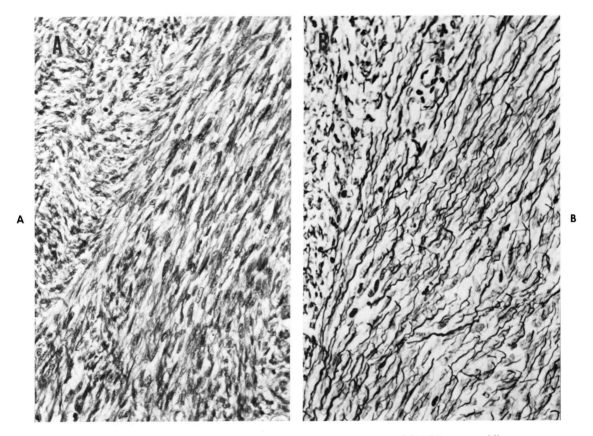

FIG. 12-26. Infantile fibrosarcoma showing fascicular arrangement of fibroblasts resembling an adult fibrosarcoma **(A)** and moderate number of reticulin fibers in parallel arrangements **(B)**. **(A,** ×225; **B,** ×260.)

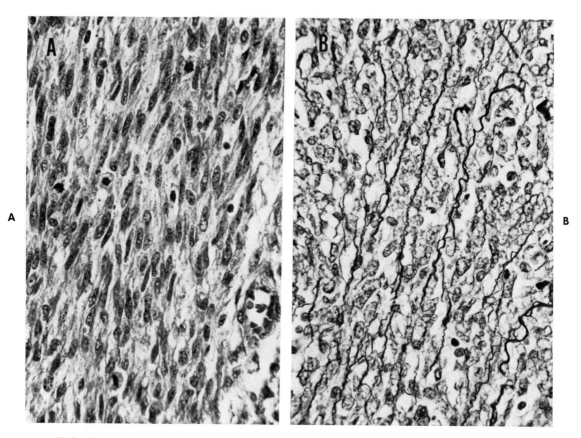

FIG. 12-27. Infantile fibrosarcoma of the right groin in a 3-month-old girl, showing poorly differentiated tumor cells with numerous mitotic figures (**A**) and a small number of reticulin fibers (**B**). (**A** and **B**, ×395.)

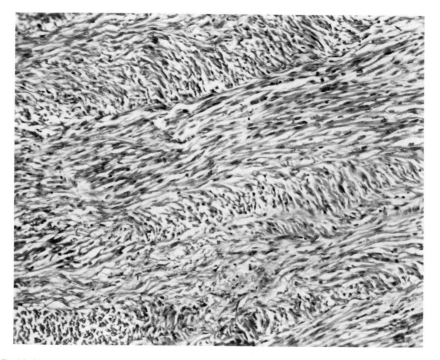

FIG. 12-28. Well-differentiated infantile fibrosarcoma with large amounts of interstitial collagen. (×130.)

spindle cells of infantile fibrosarcoma stain positively for vimentin but are negative for desmin, S-100 protein, and factor VIII.[100]

Electron microscopic findings

Ultrastructural examination[72,73,79] reveals fibroblast-like cells with large irregular nuclei, one or two nucleoli, free ribosomes, a well-developed Golgi complex, and a prominent, often dilated endoplasmic reticulum. Mitochondria and lysosomes are rare. The extracellular space contains scattered collagen fibers and abundant electron-dense material. Gonzalez-Crussi.[79] distinguished type I and type II tumor cells, the second type having a greater structural complexity.

Differential diagnosis

The microscopic picture may be confused with that of other mesenchymal neoplasms, but in most cases the uniformity of the spindle-shaped tumor cells, the solid growth pattern, and the fascicular arrangement, as well as the lack of any other form of cellular differentiation, will permit a reliable diagnosis. In doubtful cases, reticulin preparations should be obtained in order to demonstrate the capacity of the tumor cells to produce collagen. The solid growth pattern and the absence of rhabdomyoblasts and intracellular glycogen will help to rule out *embryonal*, or *spindle cells*, *rhabdomyosarcoma,* the most common malignant soft tissue sarcoma of infants and young children.

Infantile fibrosarcoma showing a marked degree of vascularity may raise the question of infantile *hemangiopericytoma*, a tumor usually marked by a distinct lobulated arrangement and more regularly distributed, dilated vascular channels, which often form a branching, or "staghorn," pattern. In some cases clear distinction may be difficult and may mandate examination of multiple sections from different portions of the tumor.

As mentioned in the previous chapter, cellular forms of *infantile fibromatosis* and fibrosarcoma may exhibit a very similar histological picture, and in some instances it may be extremely difficult to draw a sharp line between these two tumors. In fact, at the AFIP we have encountered cases in which the primary tumor showed the appearance and growth pattern of fibromatosis, whereas the recurrent tumor was much more cellular and virtually indistinguishable from fibrosarcoma. On the other hand, we have also observed tumors with a fibrosarcoma-like picture in the primary neoplasm and a fibromatosis-like appearance in the recurrence. In view of this it seems preferable to classify questionable or borderline lesions as infantile fibrosarcoma rather than as "aggressive fibromatosis" (Fig. 12-29). Perhaps, as suggested by Egan et al.,[75] the large number of nucleolar organizer regions (AgNORs) in infantile fibrosarcoma will facilitate distinction of this tumor from fibromatosis and other benign fibrous proliferations of childhood.

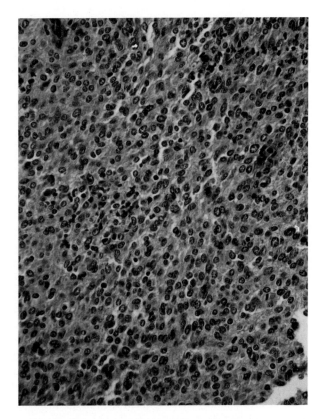

FIG. 12-29. Infantile fibrosarcoma involving the foot of a 3-month-old infant, with a prominent round cell pattern. (×250.)

Another peculiar tumor that enters into the differential diagnosis is a neoplasm reported by Lundgren et al.[85] as *"infantile rhabdomyofibrosarcoma."* This tumor, which was observed in three children 13 months to 3 years of age, shows the features of a spindle cell rhabdomyosarcoma and desmoplastic portions reminiscent of infantile fibrosarcoma. Its cells express vimentin, smooth muscle actin, and desmin but not myoglobin, and ultrastructurally they display the features of rhabdomyoblasts, with oriented thick and thin filaments, fibroblasts, and myofibroblasts. The exact nature of this tumor is still not clear. It may be, as suggested by the authors, an intermediate form between an infantile fibrosarcoma and a spindle cell rhabdomyosarcoma, but it seems more likely that the tumor is merely a richly desmoplastic form of spindle cell rhabdomyosarcoma.

Discussion

Compared with adult fibrosarcoma, the clinical course of infantile fibrosarcoma is a most favorable one. For example, the 5-year survival rate in our series was 84%. Only 4 (8%) of the 48 patients who were followed up died of metastatic disease, and one was living following lobectomy for metastatic tumor. Eight additional patients developed recurrence during the course of the disease; one had recurrences

5 and 17 years after the initial surgical procedure. The recurrent and nonrecurrent groups showed no demonstrable differences in regard to tumor site, age at onset, and size of tumor; in particular, recurrence was equally common among congenital and noncongenital cases. The initial therapy, however, was more radical in those cases that neither recurred nor metastasized.[71] In a similar series of 37 fibrosarcomas with follow-up occurring in infants and children between birth and 15 years of age, 6 (16%) died of metastatic disease and one was alive with metastasis. Three of the seven patients with metastasis were younger than 4 years at the time of treatment.[93]

There also was no difference in the histological picture that would permit a reliable prediction of the clinical course in the individual case. Neither the degree of cellularity and number of mitotic figures nor the extent of hemorrhage or necrosis correlated well with the clinical behavior. We were also unable to confirm the findings of Dahl et al.[72,73] that the more primitive, or "medullary," tumors carried a more favorable prognosis than the more collagenous "desmoplastic" type. Likewise, Soule and Pritchard[94] were unable to relate microscopic type and behavior. Salloum et al.[91] noted that two of the 10 cases that metastasized showed transitions toward malignant fibrous histiocytoma. There are also reports of incompletely excised infantile fibrosarcomas that have not recurred or metastasized after 3 years[100] and of an untreated tumor in a 2-year-old boy that regressed spontaneously over a period of 7 months.[86]

Despite rapid growth and a high degree of cellularity, most infantile fibrosarcomas are cured by wide local excision. Amputation may become necessary if the extent or large size of the tumor precludes surgical therapy.[81]

The value of radiotherapy or chemotherapy is difficult to assess because these forms of therapy have been used only in selected cases.[81] In view of the generally favorable clinical course, it appears that adjuvant radiotherapy and chemotherapy should be reserved for those examples of infantile fibrosarcoma that are unresectable or have recurred or metastasized.[88]

There is no evidence of increased familial incidence, but chromosome analysis revealed a nonrandom gain of extra chromosomes, +8, +11, +17, and +20,[68,73,74,87,95] and an abnormal karyotype, 48, XY, 11, and 20.[66] Another cytometric study of a congenital fibrosarcoma reports partial deletion of the short arm of chromosome 17.[80]

INFLAMMATORY FIBROSARCOMA OF THE MESENTERY AND RETROPERITONEUM

Inflammatory fibrosarcoma of the mesentery and retroperitoneum,[108] a lesion that has also been described as *inflammatory myofibroblastic tumor*[104] and *inflammatory pseudotumor*,[103,105] is a tumor of intermediate or low-grade malignancy, separate from infantile and adult fibrosarcoma. "Myxoid hamartoma," a richly myxoid, richly vascularized, infantile spindle cell tumor of the omentum and mes-

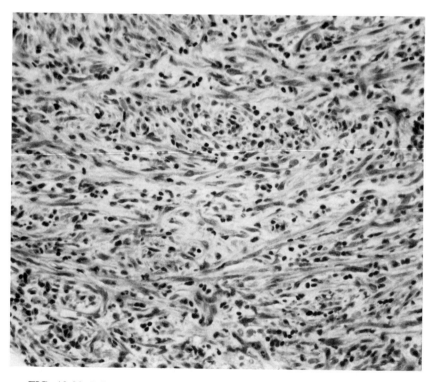

FIG. 12-30. Inflammatory fibrosarcoma that metastasized to the brain. (×160.)

entery, reported by Gonzalez-Crussi et al.[106] in 1983, is most likely a variant of this entity.

The process develops chiefly in the omentum and mesentery of children and young adults but also occurs in older patients. In our series[108] the age range was 2 months to 74 years, with a median age of 8.5 years. The lesion usually presents as a solitary or multinodular mass in the mesentery, retroperitoneum, and omentum that compresses intraabdominal structures and, in some cases, infiltrates the intestinal wall. It measures between 2 and 15 cm in diameter, but even larger examples have been recorded. The tumor is frequently associated with fever, weight loss, and anemia, and rarely with thrombocytosis and hyperglobulinemia.[103]

Microscopically, it consists of a mixture of loosely arranged spindle cells, mainly fibroblasts and myofibroblasts, with oval to elongated nuclei and prominent nucleoli. Frequently, there are also interspersed large cells with large inclusion-like nucleoli or histiocytoid cells resembling ganglion cells or myofibroblasts. The surrounding stroma contains numerous inflammatory cells, especially plasma cells, and is marked by varying degrees of fibrosis, hyalinization, and foci of calcification. Less commonly there is a myxoid background with a delicate vascular pattern. In our series the proliferated spindle cells stained for vimentin and actin and in 10 of 13 cases for keratin, possibly because of the frequent location of the tumor in the submesothelial region (Fig. 12-30).

Although many of the reported cases have done well,[103,113] the prognosis must be guarded, especially if the lesion occurs in older children and young adults. In our series of 27 cases,[108] the lesion recurred in 10 patients, with multiple recurrence in three patients and metastasis to the lung in two patients and the brain in one patient. Five patients died of the disease, and four of them were older than 10 years of age. Although evaluation of additional cases will be necessary for proper evaluation of this rare tumor, the presence of secondary pulmonary and cerebral lesions among our cases seems to support inflammatory fibrosarcoma over a multifocal reactive process.

A morphologically similar lesion, consisting of a loosely textured proliferation of plump spindle cells without nuclear pleomorphism and increased mitotic activity, occurs occasionally as a spontaneous or postoperative growth in the urinary bladder, vagina, or prostate.[102,109,110] The spindle cells stain for vimentin and smooth muscle actin and occasionally for desmin, cytokeratin, and epithelial membrane antigen; under the electron microscope they have the characteristics of fibroblasts and myofibroblasts. The lesion occurs mainly in adults but has also been observed in children.[112] The plasmacytic infiltrate is less prominent than in inflammatory fibrosarcoma of the mesentery and retroperitoneum. Although the lesion grows in an infiltrative manner and may be confused with a botryoid-type embryonal rhabdomyosarcoma or a myxoid leiomyosarcoma, prognosis in regard to recurrence and metastasis is excellent.

REFERENCES
Adult-type fibrosarcoma

1. Adam YG, Reif R: Radiation-induced fibrosarcoma following treatment for breast cancer. *Surgery* 81:421, 1977.
2. Bizer LS: Fibrosarcoma: report of 64 cases. *Am J Surg* 121:586, 1971.
3. Broders AC, Hargrave R, Meyerding HW: Pathological features of soft tissue fibrosarcoma, with special reference to the grading of its malignancy. *Surg Gynecol Obstet* 69:267, 1939.
4. Burns WA, Kanhouwa S, Tillman L, et al: Fibrosarcoma occurring at the site of a plastic vascular graft. *Cancer* 29:66, 1972.
5. Castro EB, Hajdu SI, Fortner JG: Surgical therapy of fibrosarcoma of the extremities. *Arch Surg* 107:284, 1973.
6. Cayley FE, Bijapur HI: Fibrosarcoma occurring in draining sinus. *J Bone Joint Surg* 45A:384, 1963.
7. Chen KTK, Bauer FW: Sarcomatous transformation of nasopharyngeal angiofibroma. *Cancer* 49:369, 1982.
8. Crocker DJ, Murad TM: Ultrastructure of fibrosarcoma in a male breast. *Cancer* 23:891, 1969.
9. Denham RH, Dingley F: Fibrosarcoma occurring in a draining sinus. *J Bone Joint Surg* 45A:384, 1963.
10. Ding J, Hashimoto H, Enjoji M: Dermatofibrosarcoma protuberans with fibrosarcoma areas: a clinicopathologic study of nine cases and a comparison with allied tumors. *Cancer* 64:721, 1989.
11. Donaldson I: Fibrosarcoma in a previously irradiated larynx. *J Laryngol Otol* 92:425, 1978.
12. Eckstein FS, Vogel U, Mohr W: Fibrosarcoma in association with a total knee joint prosthesis. *Virchows Arch (Pathol Anat)* 421:175, 1992.
13. Escalona-Zapata J: Tumors of the soft tissue: cytology and growth pattern of fibrosarcomas and related tumors. *Pathologica* 73:119, 1981.
14. Evans HL: Low-grade fibromyxoid sarcoma: a report of twelve cases. *Am J Surg Pathol* 17:595, 1993.
15. Evans HL: Low-grade fibromyxoid sarcoma: a report of two metastasizing neoplasms having a deceptively benign appearance. *Am J Clin Pathol* 88:615, 1987.
16. Fleming RM, Rezek PR: Sarcoma developing in an old burn scar. *Am J Surg* 54:457, 1941.
17. Fu YS, Perzin KH: Nonepithelial tumors of the nasal cavity, paranasal sinuses, and nasopharynx. VI. Fibrous tissue tumors (fibroma, fibromatosis, fibrosarcoma). *Cancer* 37:2912, 1976.
18. Gane NF, Lindup R: Radiation-induced fibrosarcoma. *Br J Cancer* 24:705, 1970.
19. Giblin T, Pickrell K, Pitts W, et al: Malignant degeneration in burn scars: Marjolin's ulcer. *Ann Surg* 162:291, 1965.
20. Goldenberg IS: Penicillin in sesame oil and fibrosarcoma: a report of two cases. *Cancer* 7:905, 1954.
21. Gray GR: Fibrosarcoma: A complication of interstitial radiation therapy for benign hemangioma occurring after 18 years. *Br J Radiol* 47:60, 1974.
22. Grier HE, Perez-Atayde AR, Weinstein HJ: Chemotherapy for inoperable infantile fibrosarcoma. *Cancer* 56:1507, 1985.

23. Grouls V, Hienz HA: Dermatofibrosarcoma protuberans: Übergang in ein Fibrosarkom. *Z Hautkr* 60:1690, 1985.

24. Heffner DK, Gnepp DR: Sinonasal fibrosarcomas, malignant schwannomas, and "Triton" tumors: a clinicopathologic study of 67 cases. *Cancer* 70:1089, 1992.

25. Heller EL, Sieber WK: Fibrosarcoma: a clinical and pathological study of 60 cases. *Surgery* 27:539, 1950.

26. Herrmann JB, Kanhouwa S, Kelley RJ, et al: Fibrosarcoma of the thigh associated with a prosthetic vascular graft. *N Engl J Med* 284:91, 1971.

27. Ivins JC, Dockerty MB, Ghormley RK: Fibrosarcoma of the soft tissues of the extremities: a review of 78 cases. *Surgery* 28:495, 1950.

28. Jones MW, Norris HJ, Wargotz ES, et al: Fibrosarcoma-malignant fibrous histiocytoma of the breast: a clinicopathological study of 32 cases. *Am J Surg Pathol* 16:667, 1992.

29. Laskin WB, Silverman TA, Enzinger FM: Post radiation soft tissue sarcomas. *Cancer* 62:2330, 1988.

30. Mackenzie DH: Fibroma: A dangerous diagnosis: a review of 205 cases of fibrosarcoma of soft tissues. *Br J Surg* 51:607, 1964.

31. Mark RJ, Sercarz JA, Tran L, et al: Fibrosarcoma of the head and neck: the UCLA experience. *Arch Otolaryngol Head Neck Surg* 117:396, 1991.

32. McLeak CJ, Papaionnau AN: Nonpancreatic tumors associated with hypoglycemia. *Arch Surg* 93:1019, 1966.

33. Melzner E: Über Sarkomentstehung nach Kriegsverletzung. *Arch Klin Chir* 147:153, 1927.

34. Meyerding HW, Broders AC, Hargrave RL: Clinical aspects of fibrosarcoma of the soft tissues of the extremities. *Surg Gynecol Obstet* 62:1010, 1936.

35. Mirra JM, Marcove R: Fibrosarcomatous differentiation of primary and secondary chondrosarcoma: review of five cases. *J Bone Joint Surg* 56A:285, 1974.

36. Morris JM: Fibrosarcoma within a sinus tract of chronic draining osteomyelitis. *J Bone Joint Surg* 46:853, 1964.

37. Ninane J, Gosseye S, Panteon E, et al: Congenital fibrosarcoma: preoperative chemotherapy and conservative surgery. *Cancer* 58:1400, 1986.

38. Oberman HA, Oneal RM: Fibrosarcoma of the chest wall following resection and irradiation of carcinoma of the breast. *Am J Clin Pathol* 53:407, 1970.

39. O'Neil MB Jr, et al: Radiation induced soft tissue fibrosarcoma: surgical therapy and salvage. *Ann Thorac Surg* 33:624, 1982.

40. Pack GT, Ariel IM: Fibrosarcoma of the soft somatic tissues: a clinical and pathologic study. *Surgery* 31:443, 1952.

41. Pettit VD, Chamness JT, Ackerman LV: Fibromatosis and fibrosarcoma following irradiation therapy. *Cancer* 7:149, 1954.

42. Phelan JT, Nigogosyan G: Fibrosarcoma of superficial soft-tissue origin. *Arch Surg* 86:276, 1963.

43. Pritchard DJ, Sim FH, Ivins JC: Fibrosarcoma of bone and soft tissues of the trunk and extremities. *Orthop Clin North Am* 8:869, 1977.

44. Pritchard DJ, Sim FH, Ivins JC, et al: Fibrosarcoma of bone and soft tissues of the trunk and extremities. In Moore TM, ed: *Symposium on tumors of the musculoskeletal system*, Philadelphia, 1977, WB Saunders, p 869.

45. Pritchard DJ, Soule EH, Taylor WF, et al: Fibrosarcoma: a clinicopathologic and statistical study of 199 tumors of the soft tissues of the extremities and trunk. *Cancer* 33:888, 1974.

46. Rachmaninoff N, McDonald JR, Cook JC: Sarcoma-like tumors of the skin following irradiation. *Am J Clin Pathol* 36:427, 1961.

47. Reade PC, Radden BG: Oral fibrosarcoma. *Oral Surg Oral Med Oral Pathol* 22:217, 1966.

48. Schwartz EE, Rothstein JD: Fibrosarcoma following radiation therapy. *JAMA* 203:296, 1968.

49. Scott SM, Reiman HM, Pritchard DJ, et al: Soft tissue fibrosarcoma: a clinicopathologic study of 132 cases. *Cancer* 64:925, 1989.

50. Sessions DG, Ogura JH: Fibrosarcoma of the head and neck. *Ann Otol* 84:439, 1974.

51. Soule EH, Scanlon PW: Fibrosarcoma arising in an extraabdominal desmoid tumor: report of a case. *Proc Staff Meetings Mayo Clin* 37:443, 1962.

52. Stout AP: The fibromatoses and fibrosarcoma. *Bull Hosp Joint Dis* 12:126, 1951.

53. Stout AP: Fibrosarcoma: the malignant tumor of fibroblasts. *Cancer* 1:30, 1948.

54. Stout AP: Fibrosarcoma of head and neck. *Am J Surg* 114:564, 1967.

55. Swain RE, Sessions DG, Ogura JH: Fibrosarcoma of the head and neck: a clinical analysis of 40 cases. *Ann Otol* 83:439, 1974.

56. Vasudev KS, Harris M: A sarcoma of myofibroblasts: an ultrastructural study. *Arch Pathol* 102:185, 1978.

57. Warren S, Sommer GN Jr: Fibrosarcoma of soft parts with special reference to recurrence and metastasis. *Arch Surg* 33:425, 1936.

58. Waugh W: Fibrosarcoma occurring in a chronic bone sinus. *J Bone Joint Surg* 34B:642, 1952.

59. Weiss SW: Proliferative fibroblastic lesions: from hyperplasia to neoplasia. *Am J Surg Pathol* 10:14, 1986.

60. Werf-Messing B van der, Unnik JA van: Fibrosarcoma of the soft tissues: a clinicopathologic study. *Cancer* 18:1113, 1965.

61. Wiklund TA, Blomquist CP, Raety J, et al: Postirradiation sarcoma: analysis of a nationwide cancer registry material. *Cancer* 68:524, 1991.

62. Wilson H, Brunschwig A: Irradiation sarcoma. *Surgery* 2:607, 1937.

63. Windeyer B, Dische S, Mansfield CM: The place of radiotherapy in the management of fibrosarcoma of the soft tissue. *Clin Radiol* 17:32, 1966.

64. Wrotnowski U, Cooper PH, Shmookler BM: Fibrosarcomatous change in dermatofibrosarcoma protuberans. *Am J Surg Pathol* 12:287, 1988.

65. Yaghmai I: Angiographic features of fibromas and fibrosarcomas. *Radiology* 124:57, 1977.

Congenital and infantile fibrosarcoma

66. Adam LR, Davison EV, Malcolm AJ, et al: Cytogenetic analysis of a congenital fibrosarcoma. *Cancer Genet Cytogenet* 52:37, 1991.

67. Andersen DH: Tumors of infancy and childhood: A survey of those seen in the pathology laboratory of the Babies Hospital during the years 1935-1950. *Cancer* 4:890, 1951.

68. Argyle JC, Tomlinson GE, Stewart D, et al: Ultrastructural, immunocytochemical, and cytogenetic characterization of a large congenital fibrosarcoma. *Arch Pathol Lab Med* 116:972, 1992.

69. Balsaver AM, Butler JJ, Martin RG: Congenital fibrosarcoma. *Cancer* 20:1607, 1967.

70. Bang G, Baardsen R, Gilhuus-Moe O: Infantile fibrosarcoma in the mandible: case report. *J Oral Pathol Med* 18:339, 1989.

71. Chung EB, Enzinger FM: Infantile fibrosarcoma. *Cancer* 38:729, 1976.

72. Dahl I, Angervall L, Save-Soderbergh J: Atypical fibroblastic tumors in early infancy. *Acta Pathol Microbiol Scand* 81A:224, 1973.

73. Dahl I, Save-Soderbergh J, Angervall L: Fibrosarcoma in early infancy. *Pathol Europ* 8:193, 1973.

74. Dal Cin P, Brock P, Casteels-Yan Daele M, et al: Cytogenetic characterization of congenital or infantile fibrosarcoma. *Eur J Pediatr* 150(8):579, 1991.

75. Egan MJ, Raafat F, Crocker J, et al: Nucleolar organiser regions in fibrous proliferations of childhood and infantile fibrosarcoma. *J Clin Pathol* 41:31, 1988.

76. Enzinger FM: Fibrous tumors of infancy. In *Tumors of bone and soft tissue: Eighth Annual Conference on Cancer 1963, M.D. Anderson Hospital*. Chicago, 1965, Year Book Medical Publishers Inc., p 375.

77. Exelby PR: Fibrosarcoma in children. *Clin Bull* 1:97, 1971.
78. Exelby PR, Knapper WH, Huvos AG, et al: Soft-tissue fibrosarcoma in children. *J Pediatr Surg* 8:415, 1973.
79. Gonzalez-Crussi F: Ultrastructure of congenital fibrosarcoma. *Cancer* 26:1289, 1970.
80. Gorman PA, Malone M, Pritchard J, et al: Deletion of part of the short arm of chromosome 17 in a congenital fibrosarcoma. *Cancer Genet Cytogenet* 48:193, 1990.
81. Grier HE, Perez-Atayde AR, Weinstein HJ: Chemotherapy for inoperable infantile fibrosarcoma. *Cancer* 56:1507, 1985.
82. Grubb RL, Dehner LP: Congenital fibrosarcoma of the thoracolumbar region. *J Pediatr Surg* 9:785, 1974.
83. Hays DM, Mirabal VQ, Karlan MS, et al: Fibrosarcoma in infants and children. *J Pediatr Surg* 5:176, 1970.
84. Iwasaki H, Enjoji M: Infantile and adult fibrosarcoma. *Acta Pathol Jpn* 29:377, 1979.
85. Lundgren L, Angervall L, Stenman G, et al: Infantile rhabdomyofibrosarcoma: a high-grade sarcoma distinguishable from infantile fibrosarcoma and rhabdomyosarcoma. *Hum Pathol* 24:785, 1993.
86. Madden NP, Spicer RD, Allibone EB, et al: Spontaneous regression of neonatal fibrosarcoma. *Br J Cancer Suppl* 18:572, 1992.
87. Mandahl N, Heim S, Rydholm A, et al: Nonrandom numerical chromosome aberrations (+8, +11, +17, +20) in infantile fibrosarcoma. *Cancer Genet Cytogenet* 40:137, 1989.
88. Ninane J, Gosseye S, Panteon E, et al: Congenital fibrosarcoma: preoperative chemotherapy and conservative surgery. *Cancer* 58:1400, 1986.
89. Pack GT, Ariel IM: Sarcomas of the soft somatic tissues in infants and children. *Surg Gynecol Obstet* 98:675, 1954.
90. Pritchard DJ, Soule EH: Fibrosarcoma of the soft tissues of the extremities and limb girdles in children. *J Bone Joint Surg* 57A:1026, 1975.
91. Salloum E, Caillaud JM, Flamant F, et al: Poor prognosis infantile fibrosarcoma with pathologic features of malignant fibrous histiocytoma after local recurrence. *Med Pediatr Oncol* 18:295, 1990.
92. Siegal A, Horowitz A: Aggressive fibromatosis—infantile fibrosarcoma: difficulty of diagnostic and prognostic evaluation. *Clin Pediatr* 17:517, 1978.
93. Soule EH, Mahour GH, Mills SD, et al: Soft tissue sarcomas of infants and children: a clinicopathologic study of 135 cases. *Mayo Clin Proc* 43:313, 1968.
94. Soule EH, Pritchard DJ: Fibrosarcoma in infants and children: a review of 110 cases. *Cancer* 40:1711, 1977.
95. Speleman F, Dahl I, Cin P, De Potter K, et al: Cytogenetic investigation of a case of congenital fibrosarcoma. *Cancer Genet Cytogenet* 39:21, 1989.
96. Stout AP: Fibrosarcoma in infants and children. *Cancer* 15:1028, 1962.
97. Unmat S, Nasser JG: Fibrosarcoma of the infratemporal fossa in childhood: a challenging problem. *J Otolaryngol* 21:441, 1992.
98. Vinik M, Altman DH: Congenital malignant tumors. *Cancer* 19:967, 1966.
99. Wee A, Pho RW, Ong LB: Infantile fibrosarcoma: report of cases. *Arch Pathol Lab Med* 103:236, 1979.
100. Wilson MB, Stanley W, Sens D, et al: Infantile fibrosarcoma—a misnomer? *Pediatr Pathol* 10:901, 1990.
101. Wood DK, Das Gupta TK: Soft tissue sarcomas in infancy and childhood. *J Surg Oncol* 5:387, 1973.

Inflammatory fibrosarcoma

102. Coyne JD, Wilson G, Sandhu D, et al: Inflammatory pseudotumor of the urinary bladder. *Histopathology* 18:261, 1991.
103. Day DL, Sane S, Dehner LP: Inflammatory pseudotumor of the mesentery and small intestine. *Pediatr Radiol* 16:210, 1986.
104. Dehner LP: Extrapulmonary inflammatory myofibroblastic tumor: the inflammatory pseudotumor as another expression of the fibrohistiocytic complex (abstract). *Lab Invest* 54:15A, 1986.
105. Dehner LP, Kaye V, Levitt C, et al: Cellular inflammatory pseudotumor in young individuals: a lesion distinguishable from fibrous histiocytoma or myosarcoma? *Lab Invest* 44:14A, 1981.
106. Gonzalez-Crussi F, de Mello DE, Sotelo-Avila C: Omental-mesenteric myxoid hamartomas: infantile lesions simulating malignant tumors. *Am J Surg Pathol* 7:567, 1983.
107. Jones EC, Clement PB, Young RH: Inflammatory pseudotumor of the urinary bladder. *Am J Surg Pathol* 17:264, 1993.
108. Meis JM, Enzinger FM: Inflammatory fibrosarcoma of the mesentery and retroperitoneum: a tumor closely simulating inflammatory pseudotumor. *Am J Surg Pathol* 15:1146, 1991.
109. Nochomovitz LE, Orenstein JM: Inflammatory pseudotumor of the urinary bladder: possible relationship to nodular fasciitis. *Am J Surg Pathol* 9:366, 1985.
110. Proppe KH, Scully RE, Rosai J: Postoperative spindle cell nodules of genitourinary tract resembling sarcomas: a report of 8 cases. *Am J Surg Pathol* 8:101, 1984.
111. Ro JY, Ayala AG, Ordonez NG, et al: Pseudosarcomatous fibromyxoid tumor of the urinary bladder. *Am J Clin Pathol* 86:583, 1986.
112. Saavedra JA, Manivel JC, Essenfeld H, et al: Pseudosarcomatous myofibroblastic proliferation in the urinary bladder of children. *Cancer* 66:1234, 1990.
113. Tang TT, Segura AD, Oechler HW, et al: Inflammatory myofibrohistiocytic proliferation simulating sarcoma in children. *Cancer* 65:1626, 1990.

CHAPTER 13

BENIGN FIBROHISTIOCYTIC TUMORS

The so-called benign fibrohistiocytic tumors are a diverse group of lesions that have in common certain morphological features, but they differ significantly in pathogenesis and biological nature. *Xanthoma* is a "pseudotumor" usually arising in response to disturbances in serum lipids. *Fibrous histiocytoma* may represent a true neoplasm possessing a definite growth potential but a limited capacity for aggressive behavior. Between these extremes are lesions of an indeterminate nature, as exemplified by *juvenile xanthogranuloma*. Although morphologically juvenile xanthogranuloma resembles a tumor, it usually regresses with time, thereby raising the question of its proper position in the spectrum between hyperplasia and neoplasia. The present classification represents a practical rather than a conceptual approach aimed at defining differences among several histologically similar lesions.

In the past, fibrohistiocytic tumors were so named to imply their origin from a tissue histiocyte that could assume fibroblastic properties. Recently the histiocytic origin has been questioned, and in the case of the malignant fibrous histiocytoma, fibroblastic origin has been proposed (see Chapter 15). For that reason, use of the term *fibrohistiocytic* is descriptive and merely denotes a lesion composed of cells that resemble normal histiocytes and fibroblasts.

FIBROUS HISTIOCYTOMA

Fibrous histiocytoma is a benign tumor composed of a mixture of fibroblastic and histiocytic cells that are often arranged in a cartwheel or storiform pattern and accompanied by varying numbers of inflammatory cells, foam cells, and siderophages. Most commonly this tumor occurs in the dermis and superficial subcutis, but it is also found in deep soft tissue and sporadically in parenchymal organs. When located in the skin, fibrous histiocytoma has also been referred to as *dermatofibroma*,[24,32] *histiocytoma cutis*,[8,35] *nodular subepidermal fibrosis*,[26,28] and *sclerosing hemangioma*.[11,21] Although many of these terms are now obsolete, some authors continue to subdivide cutaneous fibrous histiocytomas into dermatofibroma and histiocytoma,[32] the

former being characterized by large amounts of collagen and the latter by numerous phagocytic cells containing lipid and hemosiderin. Such a sharp distinction is not always possible because of the intrinsic variability of a given tumor, and when similar tumors are encountered in deep soft tissue, the use of some of these terms is obviously inappropriate. Therefore we have adopted a simplified approach and use the term *cutaneous fibrous histiocytoma* to refer to all superficial tumors of the skin regardless of appearance. Similar lesions involving the subcutis or deep structures only will be referred to simply as *fibrous histiocytoma*.

Clinical findings

Cutaneous fibrous histiocytoma is a solitary, slowly growing nodule that usually makes its appearance during early or mid-adult life. Although any part of the skin surface may be affected, it is most common on the extremities.[20] Roughly one third of these tumors are multiple and present metachronously. Synchronous development can occur in the setting of immunosuppression.[30]

Cutaneous fibrous histiocytomas are elevated or pedunculated lesions measuring a few millimeters to a few centimeters in diameter (Fig. 13-1). They impart a red or red-brown color to the overlying skin, but occasionally they appear blue or black as a result of excessive deposits of hemosiderin. Such lesions may be confused clinically with malignant melanoma. The presence of a central dimple on lateral compression is regarded as a useful clinical sign in distinguishing it from melanoma.[16]

Deeply situated fibrous histiocytomas are less common than cutaneous ones. The relative incidence is difficult to determine because the latter are less likely to be subjected to biopsy or excised than the former. In a study by Fletcher,[17] only 3 cases of fibrous histiocytoma involving skeletal muscle were culled from over 1000 fibrohistiocytic tumors. Like their cutaneous counterparts, they present as painless masses, usually on an extremity. Although they develop at any age, the majority occur between the ages of 20 and 40 years. They tend to be larger than the cutaneous tumors. Nearly half of these tumors are 5 cm or greater

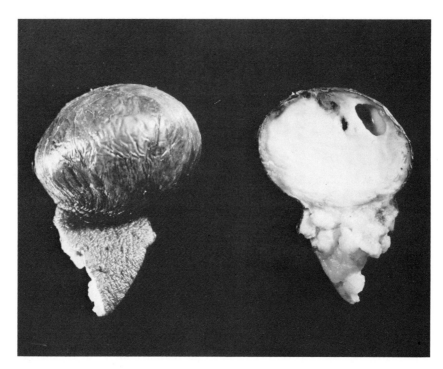

FIG. 13-1. Gross appearance of a pedunculated cutaneous fibrous histiocytoma. The light color of the lesion is a result of the presence of large amounts of lipid. Focal cystification is also present.

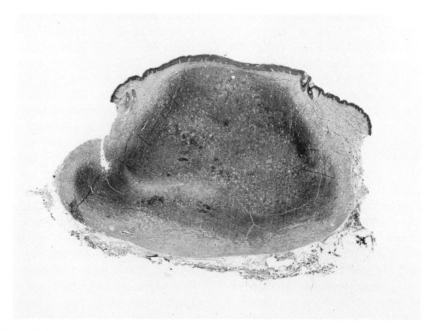

FIG. 13-2. Low-power view of a cutaneous fibrous histiocytoma. The lesion is confined to the dermis and has a smooth bulging deep margin. Hyperplasia of the epidermis, a characteristic feature of this group of tumors, is present in this specimen. (×6.)

when excised, compared with the majority of cutaneous fibrous histiocytomas, which are less than 3 cm in our experience. Grossly, they are circumscribed yellow or white masses, which may have focal areas of hemorrhage.

Microscopic findings

Cutaneous fibrous histiocytoma consists of a nodular cellular proliferation involving dermis and occasionally subcutis (Fig. 13-2). Its margins are not sharply defined, and the overlying epidermis frequently shows some degree of hyperplasia including acanthosis or elongation and widening of the rete pegs.[23] The presence of a rim of normal dermis between epidermis and tumor is variable. Most cutaneous fibrous histiocytomas consist of short intersecting fascicles of fibroblastic cells. The fascicles usually form a loose crisscross or vague storiform pattern (Fig. 13-3). Oc-

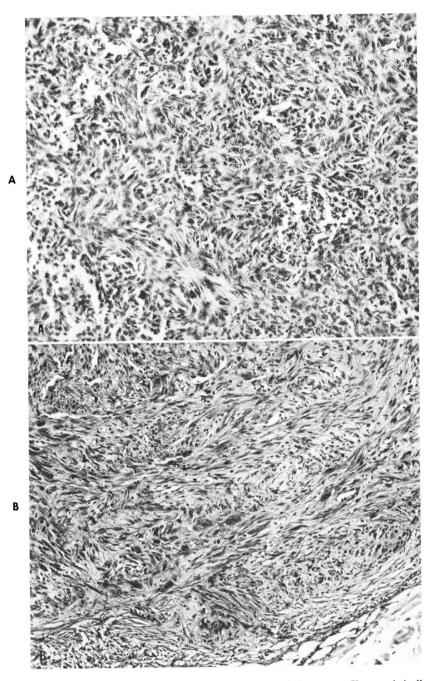

FIG. 13-3. Variable growth pattern of a cutaneous fibrous histiocytoma. Characteristically, most are composed of spindle cells arranged in a vague storiform (**A**) or fascicular (**B**) pattern. (**A**, ×165; **B**, ×100.)

casional rounded "histiocytic" cells accompany the spindle cells, but rarely do they predominate. Multinucleated giant cells of the foreign body or Touton type are a typical feature of this form of fibrous histiocytoma and often contain phagocytosed lipid and hemosiderin (Fig. 13-4). Inflammatory cells, particularly lymphocytes and xanthoma cells, are scattered randomly throughout the tumors but vary greatly

in number (Fig. 13-4). The stroma consists of a delicate collagen network surrounding individual cells. In a small number of cases, the vessels and stroma exhibit a striking hyalinization, a feature that has led to use of the misnomer *sclerosing hemangioma* (Fig. 13-5). This term conveyed the earlier belief that the cells of these tumors were derived from endothelium that was pinched off from obliterated ves-

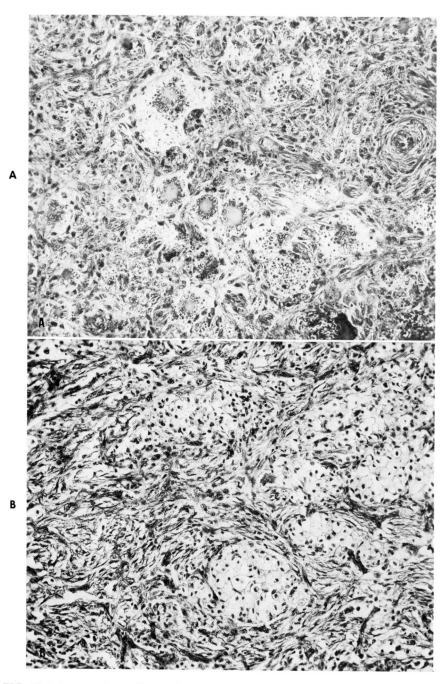

FIG. 13-4. Touton giant cells containing lipid and hemosiderin (**A**) and xanthoma cells (**B**) are common features of cutaneous fibrous histiocytomas. (**A** and **B**, ×160.)

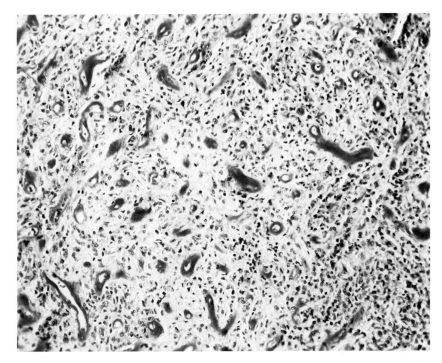

FIG. 13-5. Cutaneous fibrous histiocytoma with hyalinization of the vessels. Such lesions have been referred to in the past as *sclerosing hemangiomas*. (×160.)

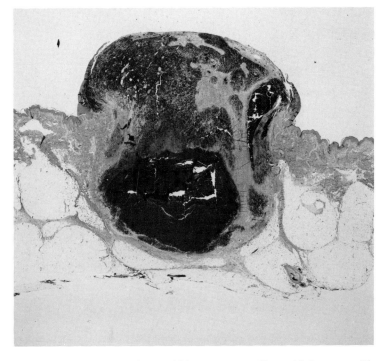

FIG. 13-6. Prominent cystic hemorrhage within a cutaneous fibrous histiocytoma. These tumors may be confused with a hemangioma or an angiomatoid form of fibrous histiocytoma. (×6.)

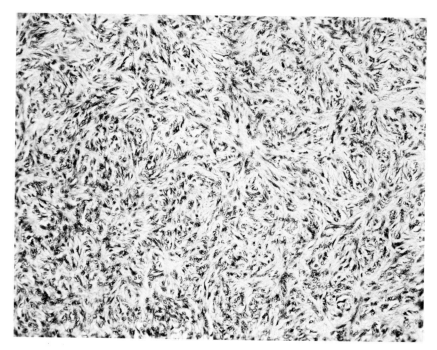

FIG. 13-7. Fibrous histiocytoma of soft tissue. In contrast to cutaneous fibrous histiocytomas, these have a more distinct storiform pattern but lack the variety of secondary elements such as xanthoma cells and siderophages. (×160.)

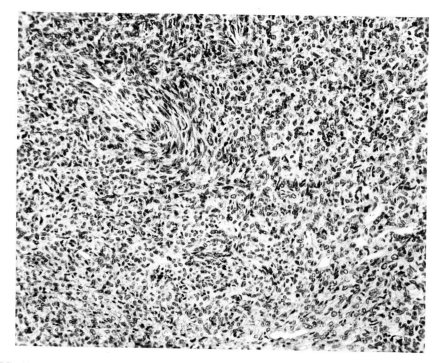

FIG. 13-8. Fibrous histiocytoma of soft tissue composed of rounded histiocyte-like cells. (×130.)

sels.[21] Cystic areas of hemorrhage are common (Fig. 13-6) and, where prominent, result in large accumulations of hemosiderin within the tumor cells.

Deep fibrous histiocytomas are similar to their cutaneous counterparts. However, they usually have a more prominent storiform pattern and fewer secondary elements such as xanthoma cells (Figs. 13-7 and 13-8). The stroma often undergoes myxoid change (Fig. 13-9) or hyalinization (Fig. 13-10). In unusual cases, dense bundles of collagen (amianthoid fibers) or even metaplastic osteoid may be detected. Not infrequently, deep fibrous histiocytomas blend with areas indistinguishable from a benign hemangiopericytoma (Figs. 13-11 and 13-12). This combination of hemangiopericytic and fibrohistiocytic areas is particularly characteristic of fibrous histiocytomas of the orbit. Rarely these tumors resemble a giant cell tumor of tendon sheath and consist principally of osteoclastic giant cells set among a background of rounded mononuclear cells (Fig. 13-13).

The benign nature of fibrous histiocytoma is usually apparent histologically. The cells are well differentiated and possess little pleomorphism or mitotic activity. The occasional pleomorphic cells with hyperchromatic nuclei and eosinophilic cytoplasm (Fig. 13-14), referred to by some as "monster cells," seem to be a degenerative phenomenon and do not affect the prognosis adversely.[10] However, the presence of both pleomorphism and mitotic activity should suggest malignancy. This problem is fortunately not common and is more often encountered in the evaluation of deep rather than superficial fibrous histiocytomas. A small subset of fibrous histiocytomas is characterized by somewhat longer, cellular fascicles of spindled cells bereft of other cellular elements. We have referred to these as *cellular fibrous histiocytomas*. Although benign, these lesions may have a higher local recurrence rate.

Histochemical, immunohistochemical, and electron microscopic studies have contributed little to the practical diagnosis of these tumors, but they have extended the observations made by conventional microscopy. Lysosomal (acid phosphatase, nonspecific esterase) and oxidative (succinate dehydrogenase) enzymes can be consistently demonstrated within these tumors[26,32] but are present in greater quantities in the cells resembling histiocytes rather than fibroblasts. This is in keeping with the prevalence of these enzymes in normal histiocytes. Between one fourth and three

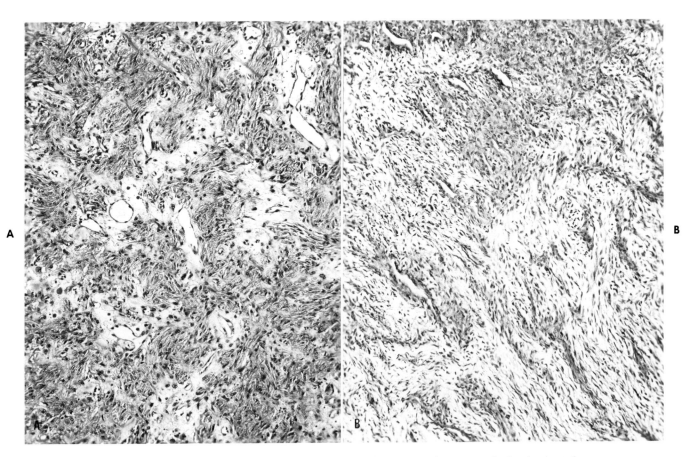

FIG. 13-9. Myxoid change of the stroma is a relatively common phenomenon in deeply situated fibrous histiocytoma and may be of a focal (**A**) or diffuse (**B**) nature. (**A** and **B**, ×100.)

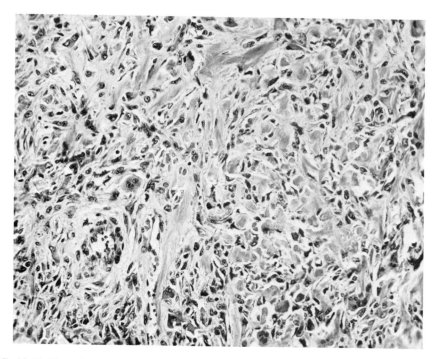

FIG. 13-10. Extensive hyalinization occurring within a fibrous histiocytoma of soft tissue. In such cases, the diagnosis may not be apparent unless more typical cellular areas can be identified. (×180.)

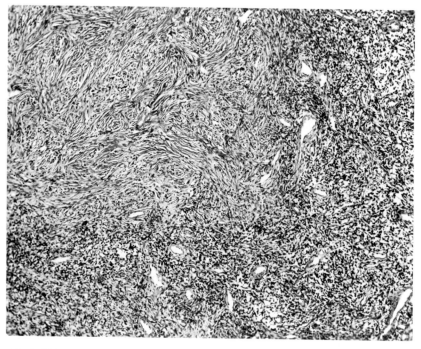

FIG. 13-11. Fibrous histiocytoma of soft tissue merging with areas indistinguishable from a benign hemangiopericytoma *(bottom right)*. (×60.)

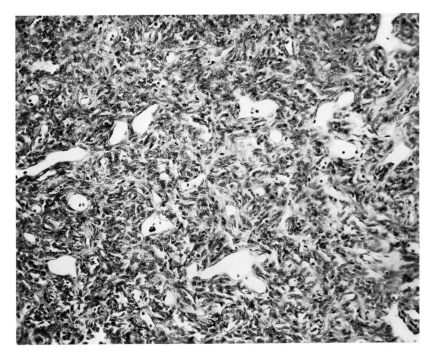

FIG. 13-12. Hemangiopericytoma-like area occurring within a fibrous histiocytoma of soft tissue. (×160.)

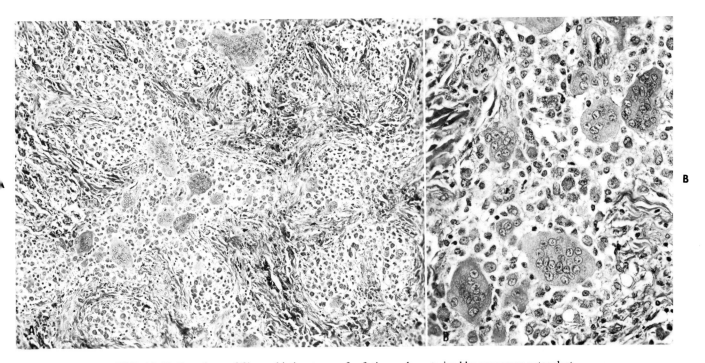

FIG. 13-13. Rare form of fibrous histiocytoma of soft tissue characterized by numerous osteoclast-type giant cells. These tumors closely resemble the giant cell tumor of tendon sheath. (**A,** ×100; **B,** ×250.)

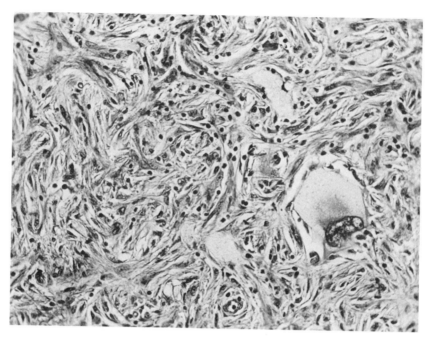

FIG. 13-14. Pleomorphic cell within an otherwise benign fibrous histiocytoma of the skin. These cells resemble those of reticulohistiocytoma and have abundant eosinophilic cytoplasm and no mitotic figures. (×245.)

fourths of cutaneous fibrous histiocytomas contain immunoreactive alpha-1-antitrypsin. Although this finding has been used to support histiocytic origin, the specificity of these proteolytic enzymes as markers of histiocytic differentiation has been questioned (see Chapter 8). Most recently, factor XIIIa[33] has been demonstrated within a significant portion of cells within fibrous histiocytoma, leading some to conclude these are tumors of dermal dendrocytes.[12]

Electron microscopic studies have shown a spectrum of cell types within these tumors. Cells resembling fibroblasts represent one end of the spectrum.[15] They contain organized lamellae of rough endoplasmic reticulum but few or no lipid droplets and no phagolysosomes.[15,29] Depending on the functional state of these cells, they may acquire features of myofibroblasts.[1,4,7] The other end of the spectrum is represented by rounded cells resembling histiocytes with numerous cell processes, mitochondria, and phagolysosomes.[15] Transitions between the histiocytic and fibroblastic cells have been documented[15] and have led to conflicting views as to whether the tumor is properly considered of histiocytic or fibroblastic origin. Only one ultrastructural study has suggested the tumor is of vascular origin because of the presence of Weibel-Palade bodies,[11] which are tubular organelles characteristic of endothelium.[6] However, in this study the vast majority of stromal cells did not contain this marker, and other studies have failed to confirm the presence of these bodies within any tumor cells.

Differential diagnosis

Fibrous histiocytomas are most frequently confused with other benign lesions, notably nodular fasciitis, neurofibroma, or leiomyoma. Although nodular fasciitis may display a storiform pattern, it is distinguished from fibrous histiocytoma by its loosely arranged bundles of fibroblasts. Cellular areas containing proliferating fibroblasts alternate with loose myxoid zones containing extravasated red cells and inflammatory cells. The vasculature in fasciitis is seldom as orderly or as uniform as that of fibrous histiocytoma. Finally, because most cases of fasciitis are excised during the period of active growth, they usually manifest much more mitotic activity than a fibrous histiocytoma of comparable cellularity. The distinction between a fibrous histiocytoma and a neurofibroma is usually not difficult. The cells of a neurofibroma have a more uniform orientation in bundles, distinctive serpentine nuclei characteristic of Schwann cells, and thick, wavy collagen bundles. Additional features of neural differentiation may include organoid structures reminiscent of sensory receptors or vague nuclear palisading. The usual lack of any storiform pattern or significant inflammation in the neurofibroma further underscores the difference between the two tumors. Sclerotic forms of leiomyoma may resemble a fibrous histiocytoma. However, smooth muscle tumors have a more distinct fascicular growth pattern. Their blunt-ended nuclei are plumper, and the cytoplasm typically has longitudinal striations corresponding to the presence of myofilamentous material, which can be accentuated with PTAH or Masson staining.

The most important diagnostic distinction is the separation of this tumor from aggressive forms of fibrohistiocytic neoplasms including dermatofibrosarcoma protuberans and malignant fibrous histiocytoma. Like fibrous histiocytoma, dermatofibrosarcoma protuberans occurs in the dermis and subcutis, but is more apt to show extensive subcutaneous involvement than benign fibrous histiocytoma. It is also characterized by a more uniform cellular population and lacks giant cells, inflammatory cells, and xanthomatous elements. Its fascicles, composed of slender attenuated cells, are longer and arranged in a distinct storiform pattern, unlike the short curlicue fascicles of fibrous histiocytoma. Its margins are infiltrative in contrast to the better defined margins of fibrous histiocytoma. Immunostaining reveals distinct differences in the cellular composition of these tumors as well. Fibrous histiocytomas contain a significant population of factor XIIIa−positive cells, although it has been debated whether these cells represent a population of neoplastic cells or a peculiar infiltrate that accompanies the tumor. In contrast, dermatofibrosarcoma protuberans contains only scattered factor XIIIa−positive cells, but in striking contrast to benign fibrous histiocytoma, expresses CD34 in a significant portion of neoplastic cells. The combination of these two stains, in our experience, has proved to be highly reliable in separating these two lesions, which often cause diagnostic problems, particularly when only a superficial biopsy specimen is available for review.

The difference between benign and frankly malignant fibrous histiocytomas is usually obvious because the latter is a pleomorphic, deeply situated tumor with numerous typical and atypical mitotic figures and prominent areas of hemorrhage and necrosis. Less obvious, however, is the difference between this tumor and the angiomatoid form of fibrous histiocytoma. The latter is a tumor of childhood characterized by sheets of histiocytic cells interrupted by cystic areas of hemorrhage. They are surrounded by a dense cuff of lymphocytes and plasma cells but almost never possess giant cells and xanthoma cells like the fibrous histiocytoma.

Discussion

Fibrous histiocytomas in general are considered benign tumors. In one large series, fewer than 5% of cutaneous fibrous histiocytomas recurred following local excision.[32] In our unpublished experience, the overall recurrence rate of cutaneous and soft tissue fibrous histiocytomas is approximately 10% following conservative therapy. However, those located in deep soft tissue have a recurrence rate that is somewhat higher and is reflective of the larger size and incompleteness of surgical excisions. In this regard, Franquemont et al.[19] reported a recurrence rate of nearly 50% for fibrous histiocytomas (8 cases) that extended into the subcutis or grew in a multinodular fashion, or both, and

Font and Kidayat[18] commented that 57% of orbital fibrous histiocytomas with infiltrative margins or hypercellular zones, or both, recurred compared with 31% of those without those features. Nonetheless, histological features play a disappointingly small role in predicting the biological behavior of these neoplasms. The presence of certain atypical histological features, including necrosis, marked cellularity, occasional atypical giant cells,[10] and mitotic activity, does not correlate well with clinical recurrence. Intravascular growth, reported in exceptional cases, has not been associated with aggressive behavior.[17,31] In one instance we have observed metastasis from a benign fibrous histiocytoma that lacked all of the foregoing features. Another instance of metastasis from a "benign fibrous histiocytoma" of the bronchus has been documented.[22]

The most controversial aspect of this tumor is its histogenesis. Although a reactive process (nodular subepidermal fibrosis)[28] is no longer a tenable concept, the lesion has been variably interpreted as a histiocytic or fibroblastic tumor. The presence of lysosomal and proteolytic enzymes within these tumors[13,25,26] and the phagocytic activity of the tumor following colloidal iron injection[35] have been interpreted as evidence favoring histiocytic origin. The predominantly fibroblastic appearance of the cells ultrastructurally[29] and the lack of a histiocytic marker (Langerhans' granules)[24] have been used in support of fibroblastic origin. Cell marker studies in malignant fibrous histiocytomas currently support a fibroblastic origin for this tumor (see Chapter 15). However, comparable studies have not been carried out on benign fibrous histiocytomas.

JUVENILE XANTHOGRANULOMA

Juvenile xanthogranuloma is a regressing or stabilizing fibrohistiocytic tumor usually occurring during infancy and characterized by one or more cutaneous nodules and less often by additional lesions in deep soft tissue or organs.[39,44,54,59,65] It has also been referred to as *congenital xanthoma multiplex*[38] or *nevoxanthoendothelioma*.[55] However, since these lesions are distinct from ordinary xanthomas and have no relationship to endothelial cells, the term *juvenile xanthogranuloma* has been used for the past 3 decades for these lesions. Recently Tahan et al.[64] suggested that the term should be changed to *xanthogranuloma*, since between 15% and 30% of these lesions occur in individuals older than 20 years of age. Use of this term alone, we feel, could be problematic since *xanthogranuloma* has been used for a variety of tumorous and reactive conditions that vary in their pathogenesis.

Clinical findings and gross appearance

This disease may occur exclusively as a cutaneous lesion or a disease affecting deep soft tissue or parenchymal organs. In the more common cutaneous form, one or more nodules develop shortly after birth, although approximately one fifth of the patients may have lesions at birth. Two thirds of patients develop the lesions by age 6 months. However, depending on the series, between 10% and 40% of patients develop the lesions after the age of 20 years.[42,62,64] There is no underlying lipid abnormality in the disease and no well-established familial incidence, although rare reports have documented the disease in parent and offspring. A finding of uncertain significance is the association of this disease with neurofibromatosis[51,54,58] and urticaria pigmentosa.[43]

About half of the lesions develop on the head and neck, followed by the trunk and extremities. They measure from a few millimeters to a few centimeters in diameter. The early lesions are red papules (Fig. 13-15), while the older lesions are brown or yellow. Following a limited period of growth, most nodules spontaneously regress, leaving a depressed, sometimes hyperpigmented area of skin. In patients with numerous skin nodules the tumors may appear in crops. Older lesions begin to regress as newer ones emerge so that lesions of various ages may be present. Although most lesions subside by adolescence, those lesions

that develop after the age of 20 years may persist in a stable form.[42]

In the less common form of the disease, cutaneous lesions may be accompanied by similar lesions in other sites such as the eye,[61] lung,[53,54] epicardium,[44,59,65] oral cavity,[52] and testis.[49] In a large series of referral cases, 5% of juvenile xanthogranulomas occurred in deep soft tissue (usually skeletal muscle) or parenchymal organs.[49] In such patients the presenting symptoms are often referable to the extracutaneous tumor, while the skin lesions may be overlooked or appear later. The eye is the most common extracutaneous site, and patients may present with anterior chamber hemorrhage and glaucoma. An unusual presentation was that of profound cyanosis in a 3-month-old child with a tumor of the epicardium.[44,59,65]

Microscopic findings

The cutaneous lesions consist of sheets of histiocytes involving the dermis and extending to, but not invading, the flattened epidermis (Fig. 13-16). The infiltrate closely apposes adnexal structures and extends into the subcutis.

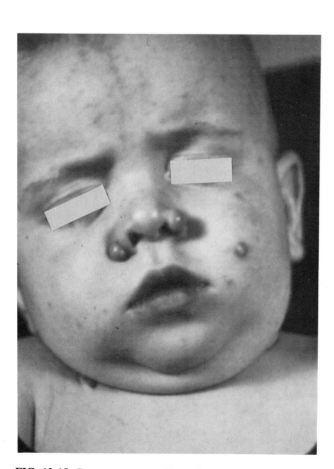

FIG. 13-15. Gross appearance of juvenile xanthogranuloma showing typical elevated red lesions that have a tendency to be multiple.

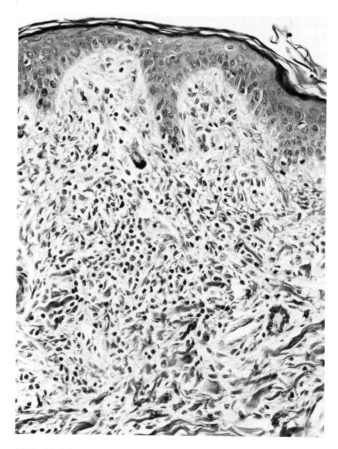

FIG. 13-16. Juvenile xanthogranuloma involving superficial dermis and extending to the epidermal junction. (×100.)

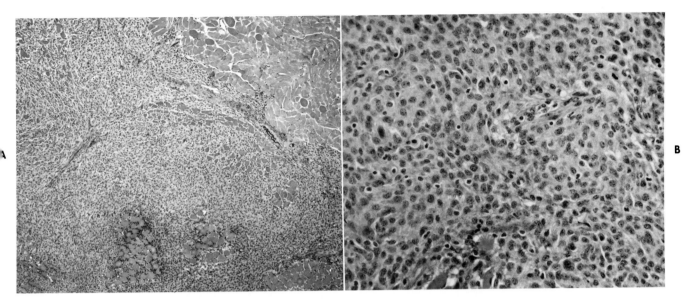

FIG. 13-17. Juvenile xanthogranuloma involving muscle. Lesion has a nodular circumscribed appearance (**A**) but blends with or infiltrates muscle fibers at its periphery (**B**). (**A**, ×4; **B**, ×180.)

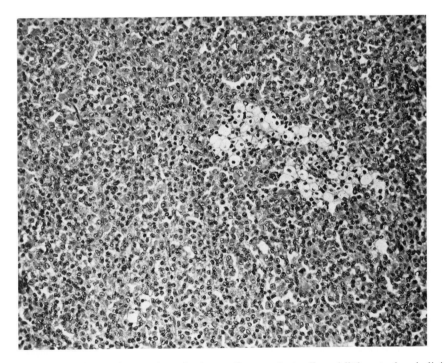

FIG. 13-18. Juvenile xanthogranuloma having no Touton giant cells and little cytoplasmic lipid. (×160.)

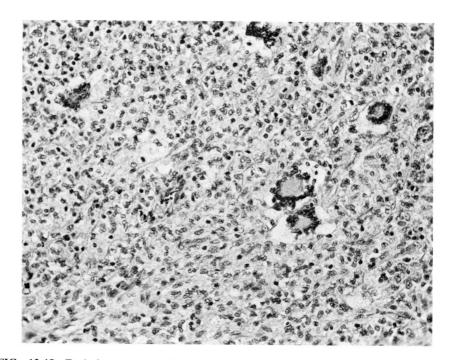

FIG. 13-19. Typical appearance of juvenile xanthogranuloma consisting of sheets of well-differentiated histiocytes punctuated with occasional Touton giant cells. The histiocytes in this case have a foamy appearance as a result of the presence of large amounts of cytoplasmic lipid. (×210.)

Deeply situated juvenile xanthogranulomas appear circumscribed but blend with or infiltrate skeletal muscle at their periphery (Fig. 13-17). In both forms of the disease the histiocytes are well differentiated and exhibit little pleomorphism and only rare mitoses. The cytoplasm varies, depending on the amount of lipid present. Early lesions have little lipid; hence, the cells have a homogeneous amphophilic or eosinophilic cytoplasm (Fig. 13-18). In older lesions the cells have a finely vacuolated or even xanthomatous cytoplasm (Figs. 13-19 and 13-20, *A*).[2] Giant cells, including Touton giant cells, are typical of this lesion (Fig. 13-19) but may vary considerably in number from area to area or from lesion to lesion. Usually a modest number of inflammatory cells are present, consisting of both acute and chronic inflammatory cells, especially eosinophils. Longstanding or regressive lesions eventually develop an interstitial fibrosis and even a vague storiform pattern (Fig. 13-20, *B*) so that they may resemble the more conventional fibrous histiocytoma seen in adults.

Electron microscopic studies show that the cells have characteristics of histiocytes.[45,46] They have numerous pseudopodia, lipid droplets, and lysosomes. Lipid, however, is not present to any extent within vessel walls,[45] in contrast to certain types of eruptive xanthomas. Langerhans' granules, tubular organelles associated with forms of histiocytosis X,[3] have not been demonstrated.[46]

The cells also express alpha-1-antitrypsin and alpha-1-antichymotrypsin.[62]

Differential diagnosis

Juvenile xanthogranuloma must be differentiated from forms of histiocytosis X involving skin. Juvenile xanthogranuloma does not generally invade the epidermis and shows greater cellular cohesion and fewer eosinophils than histiocytosis X. Touton giant cells, a feature of juvenile xanthogranuloma, are typically absent in histiocytosis. However, when they are scarce, distinction of the two diseases may be difficult. In these situations, ultrastructural studies documenting the presence or absence of Langerhans' granules can be helpful. Our preliminary experience and that of others[62] suggests that inasmuch as cells of histiocytosis X consistently express S-100 protein and the cells of juvenile xanthogranuloma do not, this antigen may serve as a reliable discriminant. Usually juvenile xanthogranuloma can be easily distinguished from xanthomas histologically because the latter contain a more uniform population of foamy cells and lack Touton giant cells and acute inflammation. Moreover, xanthomas associated with hypercholesterolemia often have large extracellular cholesterol deposits. The greater uniformity of juvenile xanthogranuloma, the usual lack of a storiform pattern, and the distinctive clinical setting distinguish it from solitary fibrous histiocytoma of adults.

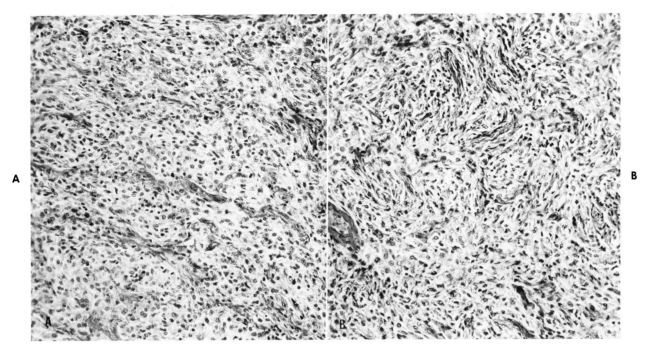

FIG. 13-20. Well-established juvenile xanthogranuloma showing xanthomatous change of the histiocytes in some areas (**A**) and interstitial fibrosis in others (**B**). The latter areas closely resemble the adult form of fibrous histiocytoma. (**A** and **B**, ×160.)

Discussion

The prognosis in this disease is excellent. The skin lesions usually regress or at least stabilize with time, and even large deeply located tumors pursue a favorable course. One patient with a large epicardial tumor was alive 13 months following excision.[44,59,65] Another child with skin lesions of juvenile xanthogranuloma proved on biopsy and pulmonary nodules presumed to be juvenile xanthogranulomas was well with no therapy at 4 years of age.[54] Therefore, conservative therapy is indicated. Only one patient died with the disease and had lesions of the lung and testes at autopsy;[49] however, death was due to other causes.[47] Radiotherapy has been employed for lesions in inaccessible locations such as the eye.[44]

Although the exact nature of this disease is unsettled, theories concerning its histogenesis have undergone considerable revision since the early description by McDonagh in 1912.[55] He coined the term *nevoxanthoendothelioma* because he believed that the tumor emanated from the vascular endothelium and that the Touton giant cells were actually small vessels with diminished or obliterated lumina. Others failed to confirm the continuity of the tumor cells and the endothelium and suggested the term *juvenile xanthogranuloma*.[49] This term not only underscores the histiocytic properties of the lipid-filled tumor cells, but also separates this disease from other xanthomatous lesions of childhood. Unlike the usual forms of pediatric xanthomas, juvenile xanthogranulomas occur at a younger age and are not associated with lipid abnormalities. Although it has been suggested that juvenile xanthogranuloma represents a limited or abortive form of histiocytosis X, current evidence suggests that they are different diseases. In addition to the light microscopic differences enumerated earlier, the consistent absence of Langerhans' granules, common to all three forms of histiocytosis X, suggests a different disease process. Moreover, even in cases of juvenile xanthogranuloma with deep-seated lesions, the prognosis is favorable.

The question remains as to whether these lesions represent a true neoplasm or an unusual reactive process. The involutional nature of the disease, although not completely excluding a neoplasm with limited growth potential, argues for a reactive process. It has been suggested that the disease may represent a response to viral infection. Circumstantial evidence for this idea is derived from an unusual case of juvenile xanthogranuloma occurring in a parotid gland showing the presence of cytomegalovirus.[39] Although this appears to be a unique case, there are parallel situations in animals. Localized histiocytic "tumors" may be induced experimentally[57,63] or occur spontaneously[40] in monkeys following viral infection. These lesions grow for a limited period and then regress. They are characterized by a proliferation of histiocytes and occasionally have a storiform pattern.[63] The viral etiology of juvenile xanthogranuloma at present remains speculative.

RETICULOHISTIOCYTOMA

Reticulohistiocytoma is a distinctive but rare lesion of adult life consisting of nodules of eosinophilic histiocytes, often showing multinucleation. These lesions may occur in two clinical settings: either as a nodular dermatosis *(reticulohistiocytoma, reticulohistiocytic granuloma)*[79,84] or as part of a systemic disease characterized by mucocutaneous nodules, destructive arthritis, and constitutional symptoms *(multicentric reticulohistiocytosis, lipoid dermatoarthritis).*[67-71,82,84,85]

Clinical findings

In the localized or cutaneous form of the disease, reticulohistiocytoma develops as a slowly growing, usually solitary nodule on the upper portion of the body. Most patients are adults, and fewer than one fifth have multiple tumors.[84] These lesions pursue a benign or self-limiting course. In one study,[84] 22 of 27 patients with follow-up information were cured by simple excision; 2 patients developed a recurrence, and 3 had a nodule elsewhere. Several patients with multiple nodules noted spontaneous regression of a lesion.

In contrast to the cutaneous disease, multicentric reticulohistiocytosis is a systemic and occasionally paraneoplastic disease, characterized by a myriad of symptoms including progressive symmetrical, erosive arthritis, episodes of pyrexia, and weight loss. Multiple cutaneous and mucosal nodules follow the arthritis within a period of months to years, although occasionally the skin lesions initiate the disease. The disease may be associated with a number of other conditions including tuberculosis, diabetes, Sjögren's syndrome, hypothyroidism, Wegener's granulomatosis, and polyarteritis.[66,81,86] In addition, malignancies of various types (carcinomas of colon, breast, lung, ovary, and cervix; sarcoma; and lymphoma) develop in about 30% of patients,[66,75,90] and in one dramatic case, the constitutional symptoms regressed when the underlying neoplasm was treated.[79] Despite the fact that the various lipid materials accumulate within lesional cells, no consistent or specific serum lipid abnormality has been identified in the disease. The disease is usually marked by a waxing and waning course over a period of several years, eventually leaving most patients with a disfiguring, crippling arthritis most severely affecting the distal interphalangeal joint and bearing some similarity to rheumatoid arthritis.

Gross appearance

The cutaneous lesions in both forms of the disease are similar. They are small nodules ranging in size from a few millimeters to a few centimeters in diameter and having a red, brown, or yellow hue. Occasionally the surface epithelium is crusted or ulcerated.

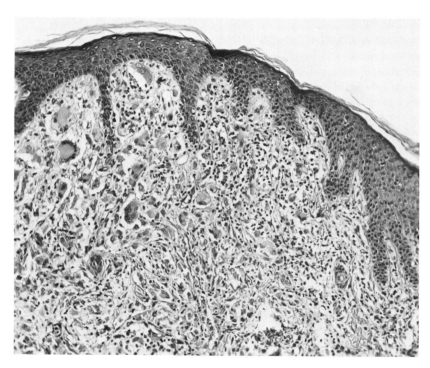

FIG. 13-21. Reticulohistiocytoma of the localized type involving skin. The lesions consist of eosinophilic histiocytes that often display multinucleation. (×160.)

Microscopic findings

The cutaneous lesions consist of circumscribed collections of histiocytes either confined to the dermis or extending to the epidermis and subcutis (Fig. 13-21). Delicate reticulin fibers are present around individual cells, and occasionally acute and chronic inflammatory cells may be present.

The characteristic cell of the lesion is a large multinucleated histiocyte having a glassy eosinophilic cytoplasm. Occasionally the histiocytes exhibit some degree of spindling. Considerable variation in cell size and degree of multinucleation is expressed such that some lesions may contain only a few multinucleated giant cells. Usually the histiocytes are well differentiated (Fig. 13-22, A), but occasionally they show moderate or even marked pleomorphism (Fig. 13-22, B). Mitotic figures are few in number or absent altogether. The staining reactions of the histiocytes are variable. In most cases they stain strongly with Sudan black B fat stain, oil red O, and PAS after diastase digestion and are believed to contain a mixture of phospholipid, mucoprotein or glycoprotein, and neutral fat.[66] The cells possess an enzymatic and immunophenotypic profile of phagocytic histiocytes that includes acid phosphatase, alpha naphthyl butyrate esterase, and lysozyme.[76] By electron microscopy the histiocytes have numerous lipid droplets and a dilated rough endoplasmic reticulum filled with granular material.[70] Langerhans' granules, tubular structures present in certain normal[5] and neoplastic[3] histiocytes, are usually not identified in multicentric reticulohistiocytosis,[76,78,94] although there have been some reports to the contrary.[70,73]

In the systemic form of the disease, similar histiocytic infiltrations are present in multiple organs including synovium, bone, lymph nodes, and endocardium. However, they may differ from the skin lesions in the number of multinucleated giant cells present and in the intensity of various staining reactions of the histiocytes.

Usually the disseminated form of the disease poses few diagnostic problems for the pathologist because evaluation of the skin lesions is aided immeasurably by the clinical history and, in some cases, by a confirmatory biopsy of synovium or other tissue. Isolated cutaneous lesions having some degree of pleomorphism must be distinguished from superficial forms of malignant fibrous histiocytoma (malignant giant cell tumor of soft parts) or even malignant epithelial lesions such as melanoma. In contrast to superficial forms of malignant fibrous histiocytoma, these tumors are smaller and have fewer mitotic figures, less prominent spin-

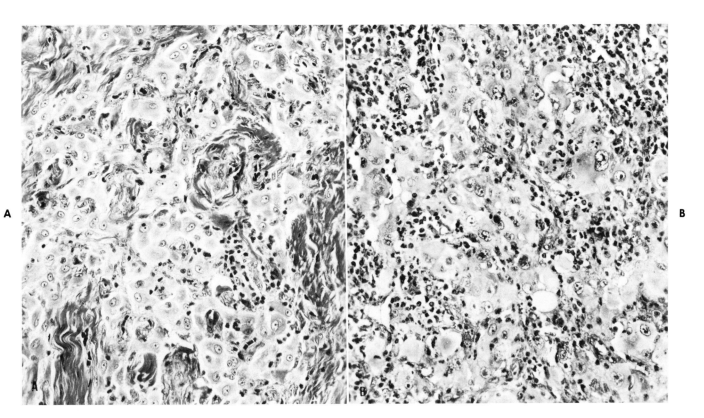

FIG. 13-22. Two cases of the localized form of reticulohistiocytoma. In one case the histiocytes have minimal pleomorphism (**A**); whereas in the other this feature is rather striking (**B**). (**A** and **B**, ×250.)

dling, and no necrosis. Unlike melanoma there is no junctional activity, more interstitial collagen, and a less distinct organoid growth pattern. The frequent accompaniment of acute inflammatory cells and numerous multinucleated cells also aids in the distinction.

Discussion

The etiology of these two conditions remains obscure, and it is likely that solitary cutaneous reticulohistiocytoma is unrelated to multicentric reticulohistiocytosis. Since a disproportionately large number of patients with multicentric reticulohistiocytosis have associated malignancies or other systemic disease, some have suggested that the disease is a reflection of an altered immune state. It furthermore appears that the histiocytes within these lesions possess the ability to secrete a wide variety of substances that may be responsible for many of the manifestations of the disease.[78,80,88] Beta-interleukin-1 and platelet-derived growth factor-B, both of which promote synovial proliferation, can be identified immunohistochemically within the histiocytes.[80] Urokinase is elevated in synovial tissue and could, by activation of collagenase, account for the destruction of articular tissue. Although in the past there was little or no therapy for the disease, a number of reports have attested to improvement of the condition with the use of chemotherapeutic agents, including alkylating agents.[72,74,77]

XANTHOMA

Xanthoma is a localized collection of tissue histiocytes containing lipid. It is not a true tumor but rather a reactive histiocyte proliferation, often occurring in response to alterations in serum lipids. Xanthomas may occur in all of the five subtypes[98] of essential hyperlipidemia, in disease states associated with a secondary hyperlipidemia (e.g., primary biliary cirrhosis, diabetes mellitus), and occasionally in the normolipemic state. Usually xanthomas occur in the skin and subcutis,[91,95,107,108] but occasionally they involve deep soft tissue such as tendon (xanthoma of tendon sheath)[94,97,99,100,106] or synovium.[96]

Clinical findings and gross appearance

Cutaneous xanthomas are designated according to gross appearance and clinical presentation (Table 13-1). *Eruptive xanthomas* are small yellow papules with a predilection for the gluteal surfaces. They occur in diseases associated with an increase in triglycerides and therefore are seen in types I, III, IV, and V hyperlipidemia and contain a high triglyceride content. *Tuberous xanthomas,* large plaquelike lesions of the subcutis, are usually located on the buttocks, elbows, knees, and fingers and are seen in types II and III hyperlipidemia. *Plane xanthomas* occur in skin folds such as the palmar creases and are characteristic of type III hyperlipidemia or type II associated with primary biliary cirrhosis. Occasionally they also occur in normolipemic persons, and in this setting they have a high association with reticuloendothelial malignancies.[105,117] *Xanthelasmas* are xanthomas of the eyelid and usually are observed in normolipemic persons,[2] although they also occur in type II and III hyperlipidemia. The last three types of xanthomas contain large amounts of cholesterol and its esters, which may be demonstrated under polarized light in fresh tissue as birefringent crystals.

Deep xanthomas occur most frequently in tendon[94,97,99,100,106] or synovium[96] and rarely bone.[102,113] The majority of tendinous xanthomas probably occur in the setting of hypercholesterolemia associated with either type II

Table 13-1. Comparison of clinical types of xanthomas

Type	Association with hyperlipidemia	Location	Histological appearance
Eruptive xanthoma	Types I, III, IV, and V	Predilection for buttocks	Sheets of nonfoamy and foamy histiocytes
Tuberous xanthoma	Tyeps II and III	Subcutis of elbow, buttocks, knees, and fingers	Sheets of xanthomatous histiocytes; large extracellular cholesterol deposits; significant fibrosis, modest inflammation
Tendinous xanthoma	Types II and III; rarely type IV; also associated with cerebrotendinous xanthomatosis	Tendons of hands and feet; Achilles tendon	Similar to tuberous xanthoma
Xanthelasma	Types II and III and normolipemic persons	Eyelids	Sheets of foamy histiocytes; little fibrosis and inflammation
Plane xanthoma	Type II (primary biliary cirrhosis), III, and normolipemic persons	Skin creases, particularly of palms	Sheets of foamy histiocytes; little fibrosis and inflammation

or III hyperlipidemia[97] and rarely in patients with a type IV pattern.[116] Usually the severity of the xanthomas is roughly proportional to the severity and duration of the increased cholesterol levels. A rare inherited disease known as *cerebrotendinous xanthomatosis* is now also recognized as a cause of bilateral xanthomas occurring exclusively in the Achilles tendon.[103,104,114] This disease, probably inherited as an autosomal recessive trait, is characterized by dementia, ataxia, cataracts, and tendinous xanthomas. The disease is a result of defective bile acid synthesis and deposition of cholesterol in the central and peripheral nerve myelin.

Most tendinous xanthomas present as painless, slowly growing masses that produce few symptoms unless joint function is compromised. The lesions may be solitary or multiple and occur in sites subjected to minor trauma such as the finger, wrist, and ankle. They are usually a few centimeters in diameter, although extremely large lesions in excess of 20 cm have been reported in the Achilles tendon (Fig. 13-23). Xanthomas may be either circumscribed or diffuse and are firmly attached to tendon but not to overlying skin. On cut section they have a variegated color ranging from yellow to brown to white, depending on the amount of lipid, hemorrhage, and fibrosis present from area to area (Fig. 13-24). Like tuberous and plane xanthomas, they also have a high cholesterol content.

Microscopic findings

The various types of xanthomas differ in histological appearance. Eruptive xanthoma, which represents an acute and evanescent lesion, contains a large proportion of nonfoamy histiocytes in addition to occasional foam cells and inflammatory cells. Tuberous xanthomas and tendinous xanthomas are essentially identical to each other (Figs. 13-25 and 13-27). Although in their early stages they may contain some nonfoamy histiocytes, the typical appearance is that of sheets of foamy histiocytes interspersed with occasional inflammatory cells (Fig. 13-26). The histiocytes are bland with small pyknotic nuclei. Some cells contain fine granules of hemosiderin. Collections of extracellular cholesterol (cholesterol clefts) flanked by giant cells are conspicuous (Fig. 13-26). Varying amounts of fibrosis may be present but are most marked in long-standing lesions. Both the plane xanthoma and xanthelasma are also characterized by sheets of xanthoma cells, but they rarely exhibit the degree of fibrosis present in the foregoing two lesions.[2] Ultrastructurally, xanthoma cells of all of these lesions are similar and contain numerous clear vacuoles, presumably representing cholesterol or its esters.[90,119] Eruptive xanthomas, in addition, have fat within vessel walls[110] as well as tissue macrophages.

Discussion

Cutaneous xanthomas usually present few problems in diagnosis or management. The superficial location, gross ap-

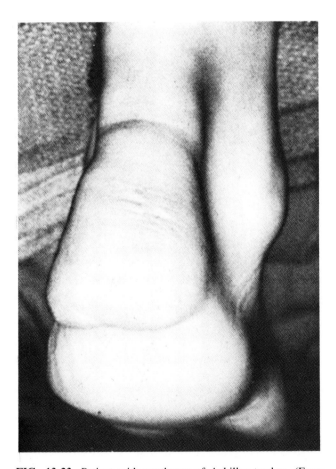

FIG. 13-23. Patient with xanthoma of Achilles tendon. (From Fahey JJ, Stark HH, Donovan WF, et al: *J Bone Joint Surg* 55A:1197, 1973.)

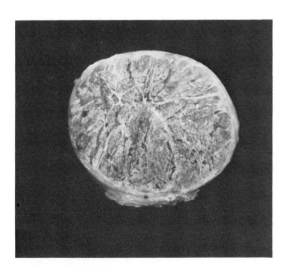

FIG. 13-24. Xanthoma of Achilles tendon cut in cross-section. White bands correspond to residual tendinous tissue that has been spread apart by xanthomatous infiltration.

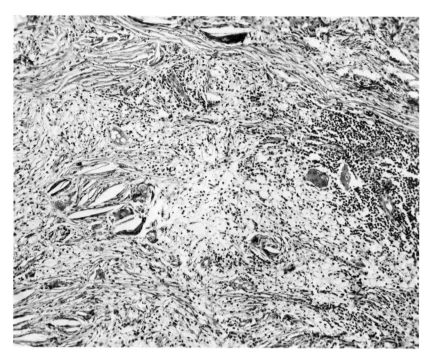

FIG. 13-25. Tuberous xanthoma of leg consisting of xanthoma cells admixed with inflammatory cells and giant cells surrounding cholesterol-containing clefts. (×100.)

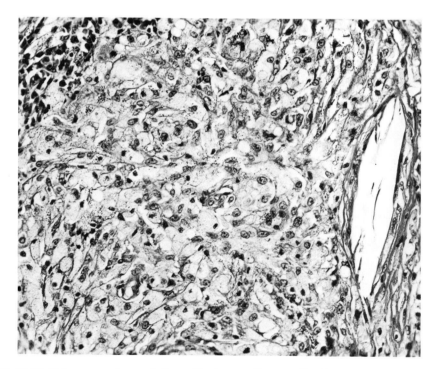

FIG. 13-26. Tuberous xanthoma of elbow. Xanthoma cells are well differentiated, and many contain dustlike granules of hemosiderin in addition to lipid. (×250.)

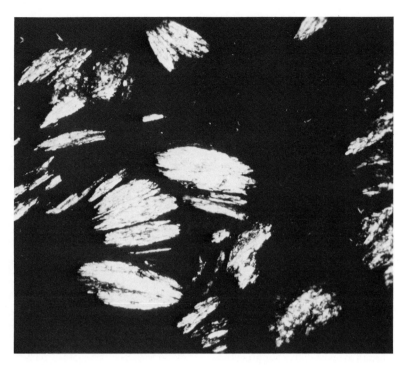

FIG. 13-27. Frozen section of xanthoma viewed under polarized light to illustrate numerous birefringent cholesterol crystals. (×25.)

pearance, and associated clinical findings leave little doubt as to the diagnosis. Xanthomas of tendon sheath may be more problematic. The deep location and slow but persistent growth occasionally raise the question of sarcoma. When a biopsy is done, such lesions should be adequately sampled because giant cell tumors of tendon sheath, diffuse villonodular synovitis, or sarcomas with xanthomatous change may focally resemble this lesion. The diagnosis of xanthoma of tendon sheath should always be considered in a patient with hypercholesterolemia, especially if the lesions are multiple.

Because of the nonneoplastic nature of these lesions, conservative therapy is generally recommended. In fact, xanthelasmas and tuberous xanthomas have regressed on medical therapy alone,[93,109] although months or years may be required before tangible benefits may be appreciated. Soft tissue radiographs may be helpful in the serial assessment of tendinous xanthomas under treatment.[101] Surgery, including excision with tendon reconstruction[118] or even amputation,[94] has been reserved only for large or symptomatic xanthomas. Surgically treated xanthomas may slowly recur, although generally reoperation is not necessary.[97] Radiation has also been employed as therapy for these lesions, but there are few data to support its efficacy. Long-term treatment of cerebrotendinous xanthomatosis with chenodeoxycholic acid has resulted in improvement of some of the neurological symptoms, but has not affected the tendinous xanthomas.[92]

Although xanthomas were formerly considered neoplastic, their association with hyperlipidemic states leaves little doubt that they are reactive lesions. Current evidence suggests that the lipid within them is derived from blood.[110,111,115] It has been demonstrated experimentally that serum lipoproteins leave the vascular compartment, traverse small vessels, and enter the macrophages of soft tissue.[111] This series of events can be confirmed ultrastructurally by the sequential finding of lipoprotein between endothelium and basement membrane and finally in the pericytes. Once ingested into macrophages, the lipoprotein is degraded to lipid, and the lipid is released to the extracellular space. The fibrosis characteristic of mature or long-standing xanthomas is believed to be related to the fibrogenic properties of extracellular cholesterol.[89] Although xanthomas can potentially occur at any soft tissue site, the localization stimulus seems directly related to the vascular permeability, since agents that increase permeability (e.g., histamine) can accelerate xanthoma formation at a given site.[111] Likewise, minor trauma or injury that results in histamine release also accelerates xanthoma formation.[112] This observation provides an explanation for the common occurrence of such lesions in the tendons of the hands and feet.

ATYPICAL FIBROXANTHOMA

Atypical fibroxanthoma is a pleomorphic spindle cell tumor that occurs principally on the actinic-damaged skin of the head and neck area of elderly persons. Conventionally it has been classified among the benign fibrohistiocytic tumors because of its almost uniformly excellent prognosis following conservative therapy. The tumor is, however, histologically indistinguishable from pleomorphic forms of malignant fibrous histiocytoma. For this reason, it seems best regarded conceptually as a superficial form of that tumor and is discussed in greater detail in Chapter 15. Both its small size and superficial location probably account for the benign clinical course.

RETROPERITONEAL XANTHOGRANULOMA

In 1935, Oberling described several patients with large retroperitoneal tumors consisting predominantly of xanthoma and inflammatory cells. Because of the polymorphic population of cells in these lesions, he believed they did not represent malignant tumors but rather variants of Hand-Schüller-Christian disease. The persistence of the term *retroperitoneal xanthogranuloma* has conveyed the general impression that such lesions are benign. However, in a critical review by Kahn of cases with adequate follow-up information, it has been shown that almost three fourths of patients either died of the tumor or were alive with persistent recurrent disease, and one fourth of the cases had metastatic disease at autopsy (see Chapter 15). There is little doubt now that the majority of retroperitoneal xanthogranulomas are malignant neoplasms and are probably best classified among the malignant fibrohistiocytic tumors. They are, therefore, discussed more fully in Chapter 15. Although there may be exceptional cases of "benign retroperitoneal xanthogranuloma," this diagnosis should be made with extreme caution. It should be considered only in cases that have been carefully sampled and display little or no atypia of the constituent cells.

MISCELLANEOUS HISTIOCYTIC REACTIONS RESEMBLING NEOPLASM

Histiocytic reactions may be difficult to distinguish from neoplasms when they are localized lesions with few inflammatory cells. In these cases it is necessary to obtain detailed clinical data, perform special staining procedures for microorganisms, and examine the specimen under polarized light for foreign material before rendering a diagnosis. Even under the best of circumstances, the etiology of only a small number of histiocytic reactions is determined. Some of the more distinctive ones are discussed in this section.

Infectious disease

Both gram-positive and gram-negative bacteria can induce inflammatory changes quite similar to those of xanthogranuloma. The lesions are composed of sheets of foamy histiocytes set against a mixed background of inflammatory cells. They differ from a neoplastic xanthogranuloma by the presence of focal abscesses and numerous microorganisms within the histiocytes. We have seen several cases of

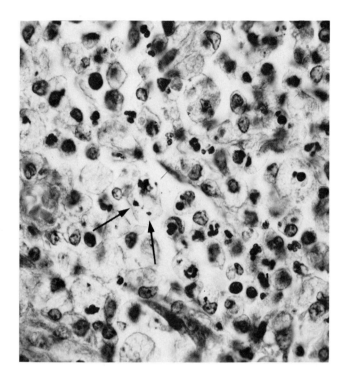

FIG. 13-28. Xanthogranulomatous inflammation secondary to chronic staphylococcal infection. Lesion presented as a large retroperitoneal mass. Brown and Hopps stain demonstrates presence of intracellular gram-positive cocci *(arrows)*. (×630.)

chronic staphylococcal infection with this appearance (Fig. 13-28), and we are aware of a similar lesion of the retroperitoneum secondary to *Arizona hinshawii,* a gram-negative bacillus.[128]

Histoid leprosy, a rare form of lepromatous leprosy described by Wade[135] in 1963, grossly and microscopically resembles fibrous histiocytoma (Fig. 13-29). Unlike the usual type of lepromatous leprosy, which spreads in an infiltrative manner, this develops as an expansile nodule of the subcutis and dermis. The cells resemble fibroblasts rather than histiocytes and are often arranged in a storiform pattern. Although the similarity of this disease to a true fibrous histiocytoma is striking, numerous intracellular acid-fast bacilli can be demonstrated with special stains (Fite-Feraco). Because this form of leprosy occurs in patients with long-standing lepromatous leprosy treated with sulfones, it has been suggested that these lesions occur as a result of the emergence of sulfone-resistant bacilli.

Malacoplakia

Malacoplakia is a rare inflammatory disease believed to represent an unusual host response to infection with a variety of organisms, including *Escherichia coli, Klebsiella,* and acid-fast bacilli, which results in the formation of yellow plaquelike lesions on the mucosal surface of affected organs.[122] The disease typically develops within the geni-

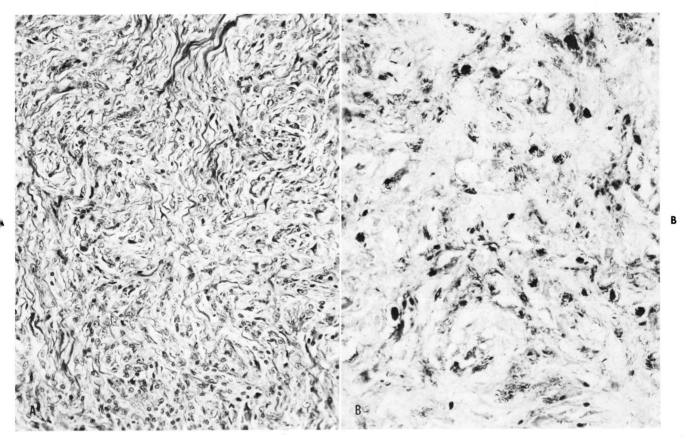

FIG. 13-29. **A,** Histoid leprosy having a pattern similar to a fibrous histiocytoma. (×250.) **B,** Fite-Feraco stain demonstrates numerous intracellular acid-fast bacilli. (×400.)

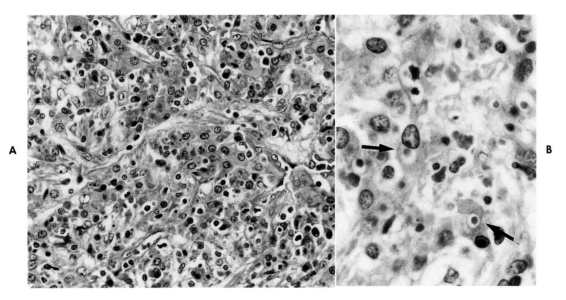

FIG. 13-30. **A,** Malacoplakia of retroperitoneum with solid sheets of histiocytes admixed with inflammatory cells. (×160.) **B,** High-power view showing Michaelis-Gutmann bodies within occasional cells *(arrows)*. (×400.)

316

tourinary tract, particularly the bladder, although it may affect the soft tissues of the retroperitoneum as well. It is characterized by sheets of pale, slightly granular, or vacuolated histiocytes (von Hansemann's cells) containing PAS-positive, diastase-resistant inclusions within the cytoplasm (Fig. 13-30). Lymphocytes, plasma cells, and neutrophils are typically abundant. The distinctive Michaelis-Gutmann bodies, small calcospherites that consist of a mixture of organic and inorganic materials including calcium and phosphate, can be identified within the histiocytes as well as extracellularly. Electron microscopic studies show that the von Hansemann histiocytes contain numerous phagolysosomes, occasional bacterial forms, and lamellated crystalline bodies representing the early stage of Michaelis-Gutmann bodies.[124]

Silica reaction

Although the usual response to silica in soft tissue is a localized foreign body reaction, exuberant reactions to the material simulate a fibrohistiocytic neoplasm (Figs. 13-30 and 13-31). In our experience this latter form of soft tissue

silicosis is probably related to the presence of large amounts of silica and seems to be principally an iatrogenic disease occurring secondary to the now obsolete injection therapy of hernia.[5,136] Clinically, these lesions present as slowly enlarging tumorous masses, usually in the inguinal region or abdominal wall. Typically they occur many years after the injection of silica so that the causal relationship of the injection is minimized or overlooked. Grossly, the lesions are ill-defined, gray-yellow masses with a gritty consistency on cutting. They consist of sheets of histiocytes with a clear or amphophilic cytoplasm (Fig. 13-31). Although usually well-differentiated, the histiocytes occasionally display moderate pleomorphism. Mitotic figures are rare. PAS-positive, diastase-resistant bodies may be present within the histiocytes and probably represent large phagolysosomes, organelles involved in the intracellular storage of silica. Numerous silica crystals can be identified under polarized light. A striking feature of the lesion is the large amount of fibrosis. The collagen varies from delicate interstitial or perivascular fibers in the early stages to broad bands and finally mats or large nodules. The presence of silica, ex-

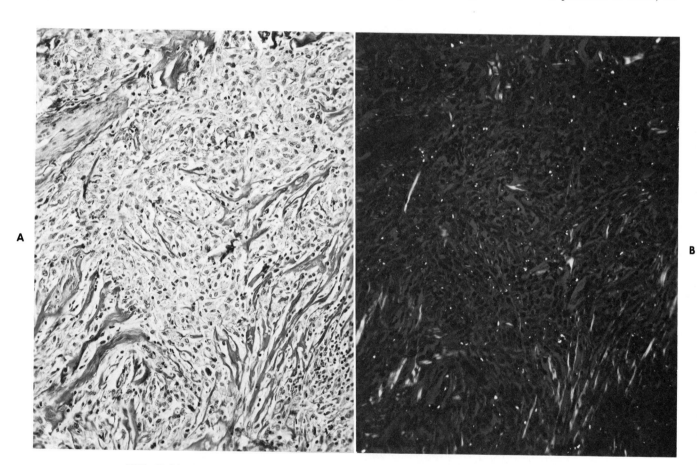

FIG. 13-31. A, Silica reaction occurring in inguinal region. The lesion is made up of sheets of well-differentiated histiocytes interlaced with fibrous bands. (×160.) **B,** Under polarized light, numerous small silica crystals can be identified both intracellularly and extracellularly. (×160.) (From Weiss SW, Enzinger FM, Johnson FB: *Cancer* 42:2738, 1978.)

tensive fibrosis, scarcity of mitotic figures, and poorly developed vasculature all serve to distinguish these lesions from benign or malignant fibrous histiocytomas.

Polyvinylpyrrolidone granuloma

Polyvinylpyrrolidone (PVP) is a polymer of vinylpyrrolidone, which was used notably as a plasma expander during wartime and until recently was utilized in various intravenous preparations in Asia. It has been marketed under various names including Plasgen, Periston, Plasmagel, Biseko, Blutogen, and Subplasm. Because of its hydroscopic properties it has also been used as a retardant in various injectable medicines (hormones, antihypertensives, and local anesthetics), as a clarifier in fruit juices, and as a resin in hair sprays.[137] The molecular weight of PVP varies depending on its chain length (MW 10,000 to 200,000). Low-molecular-weight PVP is filtered by the glomerulus and cleared by the kidney, whereas higher-molecular-weight PVP (MW 50,000 or greater) is retained indefinitely by the body and is stored throughout the reticuloendothelial system. The common appearance of PVP disease as seen following the intravenous injection of the substance is that of blue-gray histiocytes lining the sinusoids of the liver, spleen, and lymph nodes. A second form of PVP disease presumably occurs following the inhalation of the substance from hair spray.[129] The alveolar walls are thickened and macrophages fill the alveolar spaces. An uncommon form of PVP disease is a localized pseudotumor,[121,127,132] presumably caused by local injection of the material. Cases reported in the literature have documented PVP pseudotumors secondary to the anesthetic Depot-Impletol[126] and vasopressin.[132]

Histologically these lesions are composed of numerous histiocytes that are massively engorged with PVP (Figs. 13-32 and 13-33). The material appears either glassy blue or blue-gray in sections stained with hematoxylin-eosin. The histiocytes form sheets or small clusters within a matrix containing copious amounts of foreign material. Giant cells are occasionally present and may be very helpful in suggesting the diagnosis of a foreign body reaction. Another feature suggesting a reactive process is the manner in which the histiocytes "percolate" around the adnexal structures, nerves, and vessels. Typically there are few, if any, inflammatory cells and no necrosis.

The tinctoral properties of PVP have been well documented and serve to distinguish this lesion from other myxoid lesions (Table 13-2).[129] PVP characteristically does not stain with alcian blue and, therefore, stains differently from all myxoid tumors of soft tissue such as liposarcoma, chondrosarcoma, and chordoma. It does not stain blue with Giemsa stain and should therefore not be confused with the syndrome of sea-blue histiocytes. PVP is carminophilic, and recognition of this fact should be kept in mind, as occasional cases of PVP granuloma have been mistaken for

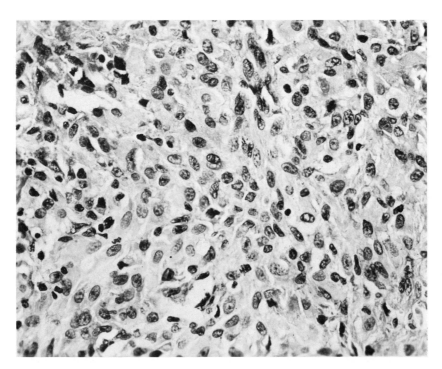

FIG. 13-32. Silica reaction of inguinal region showing well-differentiated histiocytes with no mitotic activity. (×390.) (From Weiss SW, Enzinger FM, Johnson FB: *Cancer* 42:2738, 1978.)

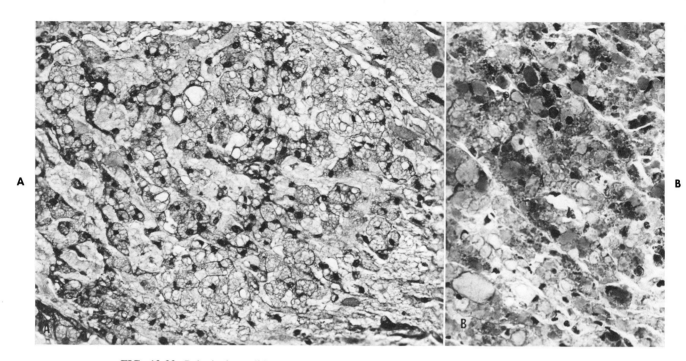

FIG. 13-33. Polyvinylpyrrolidone (PVP) granuloma. **A,** Clusters of bubbly histiocytes are suspended in pools of basophilic-appearing PVP. (×250.) **B,** Material stains brilliantly with Congo red. (×400.)

Table 13-2. Staining reactions of PVP

Positive	Negative
Congo red	PAS
Sirius red	Alcian blue
Mucicarmine	
Colloidal iron	

infiltrating carcinomas of the signet-ring type.[129] The best stains for demonstrating the cytoplasmic material are Congo red or Sirius red. Ultrastructurally the material is contained in large membrane-limited vacuoles believed to be distended lysosomes. Dense bodies, probably composed of ferritin, are condensed at the periphery of the vacuoles.

Granular cell reaction

Collections of histiocytes with granular eosinophilic cytoplasm occasionally accumulate at the site of surgical trauma.[134] These peculiar histiocytic reactions bear a close similarity to granular cell tumor but can usually be differentiated from the foregoing by the fact that the nuclei in these reactions are rather small and inconspicuous and the granules are large and coarsely textured (Fig. 13-35). Furthermore, the cells often surround nodules of granuloamorphous debris similar to the cytoplasmic granular material

(Fig. 13-36). Sobel et al.[134] point out that the staining reactions serve to distinguish the two lesions. The ceroid-lipofuscin substance in these histiocyte reactions is usually acid-fast and autofluorescent as compared with that of the granular cell tumor.

Extranodal (soft tissue) Rosai-Dorfman disease

Since the original description by Rosai and Dorfman in 1972[133] of sinus histiocytosis with massive lymphadenopathy (SHML), it has been recognized that this disease may occur in extranodal sites, often without any involvement of lymph nodes. Approximately 10% of all cases of Rosai-Dorfman disease are associated with soft tissue involvement, and in some cases, this may represent the sole manifestation of the disorder.[125,131] However, the actual incidence of associated lymphadenopathy in patients having soft tissue lesions depends greatly on the bias of the study. In the study by Foucar et al.[125] the majority had lymphadenopathy, whereas in the study by Montgomery et al.[131] only a minority did (4 of 23). The former study was based on a referral of all cases to the National SHML Registry at Yale University, whereas the latter represented referral cases to the Soft Tissue Registry of the Armed Forces Institute of Pathology. Patients with soft tissue Rosai-Dorfman disease tend to be older than those with lymph node-based disease. Microscopically these lesions consist of sheets or syncytia of large pale histiocytes with large,

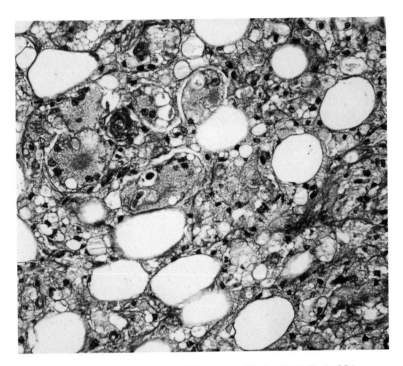

FIG. 13-34. Multinucleated histiocytes filled with PVP. (×25.)

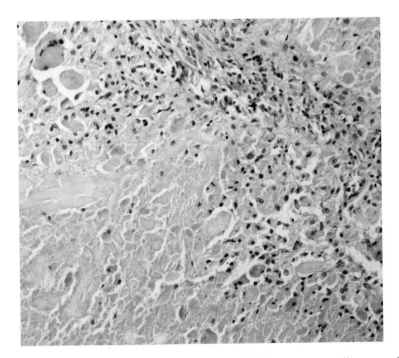

FIG. 13-35. Granular cell reaction illustrating fringe of histiocytes surrounding core of granuloamorphous material. (×60.)

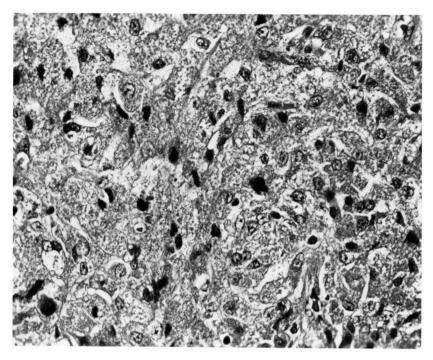

FIG. 13-36. Histiocytic reaction with "granular cell" features occurring at site of previous surgery. (×400.)

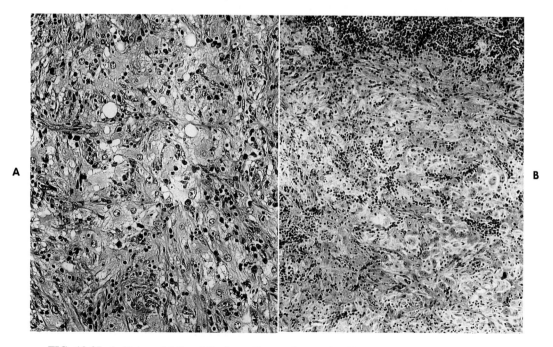

FIG. 13-37. A, Extranodal Rosai-Dorfman disease characterized by sheets of pale histiocytes with voluminous cytoplasm. **B,** High-power view illustrating mild nuclear atypia and emperipolesis. (**A,** × 200; **B,** × 600.)

round, vesicular nuclei having some degree of nuclear atypia (Fig. 13-37). Mitotic figures are usually difficult to detect or are absent altogether. The cytoplasm of the histiocytes may contain lymphocytes (emperipolesis), although this is seldom as striking as in the lesions of lymph nodes. Microabscesses, when present, suggest the possibility of an infectious process. The feature that tends to complicate the diagnosis of these unusual lesions is the presence of fibrosis, which distorts the sheetlike growth pattern, creating instead a storiform pattern. Predictably, the latter pattern, in association with atypical histiocytes, is often construed as evidence that one is dealing with a fibrohistiocytic tumor. The histiocytes of Rosai-Dorfman disease strongly express S-100 protein in virtually all cases and often a number of other histiocytic antigens. The presence of S-100 protein is useful in discriminating these lesions from malignant fibrous histiocytomas as well as histiocytic proliferations of infectious etiology. Obviously this antigen will not discriminate examples of soft tissue Rosai-Dorfman disease from Langerhans' cell histiocytosis, although usually the cytological differences between the proliferating histiocytes in the two conditions and the differences in the inflammatory cells accompanying them readily permit this distinction. The data, to present, suggest that the prognosis of soft tissue Rosai-Dorfman disease is good overall. Most patients with isolated soft tissue masses appeared well following surgery, although some developed persistent or recurrent disease.

REFERENCES
General

1. Gabbiani G, Ryan GB, Majno G: Presence of modified fibroblasts in granulation tissue and their possible role in wound contraction. *Experimentia* 27:549, 1971.
2. Lever WF, Schaumburg-Lever G: *Histopathology of the skin,* ed 5, Philadelphia, 1975, JB Lippincott.
3. Shamoto M: Langerhans' cell granule in Letterer-Siwe disease. *Cancer* 26:1102, 1970.
4. Taxy JB: Juvenile nasopharyngeal angiofibroma: an ultrastructural study. *Cancer* 39:1044, 1977.
5. Vernon ML, Fountain L, Krebs HM, et al: Birbeck granules (Langerhans' cell granules) in human lymph nodes. *Am J Clin Pathol* 160:771, 1973.
6. Weibel ER, Palade GE: New cytoplasmic components in arterial endothelia. *J Cell Biol* 23:101, 1964.
7. Wirman JA: Nodular fasciitis: an ultrastructural study. *Cancer* 38:2378, 1976.

Fibrous histiocytoma

8. Arnold HL, Tilden IL: Histiocytoma cutis: a variant of xanthoma. *Arch Dermatol Syph* 47:498, 1943.
9. Bates HR, Buis LJ, Johns TNP: Endobronchial histiocytoma. *Chest* 69:705, 1976.
10. Beham A, Fletcher CD: Atypical "pseudosarcomatous" variant of cutaneous benign fibrous histiocytoma: report of eight cases. *Histopathology* 17:167, 1990.
11. Carstens PHB, Schrodt GR: Ultrastructure of sclerosing hemangioma. *Am J Pathol* 77:377, 1974.
12. Cerio R, Spaull J, Wilson Jones E: Histiocytoma cutis: a tumour of dermal dendrocytes (dermal dendrocytoma). *Br J Dermatol* 120:197, 1989.
13. du Boulay CEH: Demonstration of alpha-1-antitrypsin and alpha-1-antichymotrypsin in fibrous histiocytomas using immunoperoxidase technique. *Am J Surg Pathol* 6:559, 1982.
14. Faludi JE, Kenyon K, Green WR: Fibrous histiocytoma of the corneoscleral limbus. *Am J Ophthalmol* 80:619, 1975.
15. Fine G, Morales MD, Pardo V: Ultrastructure of histiocytomas (abstract). *Am J Clin Pathol* 67:214, 1977.
16. Fitzpatrick TB, Gilchrest BA: Dimple sign to differentiate benign from malignant pigmented cutaneous lesions. *N Engl J Med* 296:1518, 1977.
17. Fletcher CD: Benign fibrous histiocytoma of subcutaneous and deep soft tissue: a clinicopathologic analysis of 21 cases. *Am J Surg Pathol* 14:801, 1990.
18. Font RL, Kidayat AA: Fibrous histiocytoma of the orbit: a clinicopathologic study of 150 cases. *Hum Pathol* 13:199, 1982.
19. Franquemont DW, Cooper PH, Shmookler BM, et al: Benign fibrous histiocytoma of the skin with potential for local recurrence: a tumor to be distinguished from dermatofibroma. *Mod Pathol* 3:58, 1990.
20. Gonzalez S, Duarte I: Benign fibrous histiocytoma of the skin: a morphologic study of 290 cases. *Pathol Res Pract* 174:379, 1982.
21. Gross RE, Wolbach SB: Sclerosing hemangiomas: their relationship to dermatofibroma, histiocytoma, xanthoma, and certain pigmented lesions of the skin. *Am J Pathol* 19:533, 1943.
22. Hakimi M, Pai R, Fine G, et al: Fibrous histiocytoma of the trachea. *Chest* 68:367, 1975.
23. Halpryn JH, Allen AC: Epidermal changes associated with sclerosing hemangiomas. *Arch Dermatol* 80:160, 1959.
24. Katenkamp D, Stiller D: Cellular composition of the so-called dermatofibroma (histiocytoma cutis). *Virchows Arch (Pathol Anat)* 367:325, 1975.
25. Kindblom LG, Jacobsen GK, Jacobsen M: Immunohistochemical investigation of tumours of supposed fibroblastic-histiocytic origin. *Hum Pathol* 13:834, 1982.
26. Klaus SN, Winkelmann RK: The enzyme histochemistry of nodular subepidermal fibrosis. *Br J Dermatol* 78:398, 1966.
27. Meister P, Konrad E, Krauss F: Fibrous histiocytoma: a histological and statistical analysis of 155 cases. *Pathol Res Pract* 162:361, 1978.
28. Michelson HE: Nodular subepidermal fibrosis. *Arch Dermatol Syph* 27:812, 1933.
29. Mihatsch-Konz B, Schaumburg-Lever G, Lever WR: Ultrastructure of dermatofibroma. *Arch Derm Forsch* 246:181, 1973.
30. Newman DM, Walter JB: Multiple dermatofibromas in patients with systemic lupus erythematosus on immunosuppressive therapy. *N Engl J Med* 289:842, 1973.
31. Nguyen G-K, Johnson ES: Invasive benign histiocytoma. *Am J Surg Pathol* 11:487, 1987.
32. Niemi KM: The benign fibrohistiocytic tumours of the skin. *Acta Dermatoven* 50(suppl 63):1, 1970.
33. Reid MB, Bray C, Gear JD, et al: Immunohistochemical demonstration of factors XIIIa and XIIIs in reactive and neoplastic fibroblastic fibrohistiocytic lesions. *Histopathology* 10:1171, 1986,
34. Rice DH, Batsakis JG, Headington JT, et al: Fibrous histiocytomas of the nose and paranasal sinuses. *Arch Otolaryngol* 100:398, 1974.

35. Senear FE, Caro MR: Histiocytoma cutis. *Arch Dermatol Syph* 33:209, 1936.

36. Smith NM, Davies JB, Shrimankar JS, et al: Deep fibrous histiocytoma with giant cells and bone metaplasia. *Histopathology* 17:365, 1990.

37. Soini Y, Miettinen M: Alpha 1-antichymotrypsin and lysozyme: their limited significance in fibrohistiocytic tumors. *Am J Clin Pathol* 91:515, 1989.

Juvenile xanthogranuloma

38. Adamson HG: Society intelligence: the dermatologic society of London. *Br J Dermatol* 17:222, 1905.

39. Balfour H, Speicher C: Juvenile xanthogranuloma associated with cytomegalovirus infection. *Am J Med* 50:380, 1971.

40. Bearcroft WBC, Jamieson MF: An outbreak of subcutaneous tumours in rhesus monkeys. *Nature (Lond)* 182:195, 1958.

41. Berson SK, Issroff SW, Kotton B, et al: Juvenile xanthogranuloma. *S Afr Med J* 46:565, 1972.

42. Cohen BA, Hood A: Xanthogranuloma: report on clinical and histologic findings in 64 patients. *Pediatr Dermatol* 6:262, 1989.

43. DeVillex RL, Limmer BL: Juvenile xanthogranuloma and urticaria pigmentosa. *Arch Dermatol* 111:365, 1975.

44. Eller JL: Roentgen therapy for visceral juvenile xanthogranuloma, including a case with involvement of the heart. *Am J Roentgenol* 95:52, 1965.

45. Esterly NB, Sahihi T, Medenica M: Juvenile xanthogranuloma: an atypical case with a study of ultrastructure. *Arch Dermatol* 105:99, 1972.

46. Gonzalez-Crussi F, Campbell RJ: Juvenile xanthogranuloma: ultrastructural study. *Arch Pathol* 89:65, 1970.

47. Helwig EB: Histiocytic and fibrocytic disorders. In Graham JH, Johnson WC, Helwig EG, editors: *Dermal pathology,* New York, 1972, Harper & Row.

48. Helwig EB: Personal communication, 1978.

49. Helwig EB, Hackney VC: Juvenile xanthogranuloma (nevoxanthoendothelioma). *Am J Pathol* 30:625, 1954.

50. Janney CG, Hurt MA, Santa Cruz DJ: Deep juvenile xanthogranuloma: subcutaneous and intramuscular forms. *Am J Surg Pathol* 15:150, 1991.

51. Jensen NE: Naevoxanthoendothelioma and neurofibromatosis. *Br J Dermatol* 85:326, 1971.

52. Kjaerheim A, Stokke T: Juvenile xanthogranuloma of the oral cavity. *Oral Surg Oral Med Oral Pathol* 38:414, 1974.

53. Lamb JH, Lain ES: Nevo-xantho-endothelioma. *South Med J* 30:585, 1937.

54. Lottsfeldt F, Good R: Juvenile xanthogranuloma with pulmonary lesions: a case report. *Pediatrics* 33:233, 1964.

55. McDonagh JER: A contribution to our knowledge of the naevoxanthoendotheliomata. *Br J Dermatol* 24:85, 1912.

56. Newell GB, Stone OJ, Mullins JF: Juvenile xanthogranuloma and neurofibromatosis. *Arch Dermatol* 107:262, 1973.

57. Niven JSF, Armstrong JA, Andrewes CH: Subcutaneous "growths" in monkeys produced by a poxvirus. *J Pathol Bacteriol* 81:1, 1961.

58. Nomland R: Nevoxantho-endothelioma: a benign xanthomatous disease of infants and children. *J Invest Dermatol* 22:207, 1954.

59. Pois AJ, Johnson LA: Multiple congenital xanthogranuloma of skin and heart: report of a case. *Dis Chest* 50:325, 1966.

60. Senear FE, Caro MR: Nevo-xantho-endothelioma or juvenile xanthoma. *Arch Dermatol Syph (Chicago)* 34:195, 1936.

61. Smith ME, Sanders TE, Bresnick GH: Juvenile xanthogranuloma of the ciliary body in an adult. *Arch Ophthalmol* 81:813, 1969.

62. Sonoda T, Hashimoto H, Enjoji M: Juvenile xanthogranuloma: clinicopathologic analysis and immunohistochemical study of 57 patients. *Cancer* 56:2280, 1985.

63. Sproul EE, Metzgar RS, Grace JT Jr: The pathogenesis of Yaba virus-induced histiocytomas in primates. *Cancer Res* 23:671, 1963.

64. Tahan SR, Pastel-Levy C, Bhan AK, et al: Juvenile xanthogranuloma: clinical and pathologic characterization. *Arch Pathol Lab Med* 113:1057, 1989.

65. Webster SB, Reister HC, Harman LE: Juvenile xanthogranuloma with extra-cutaneous lesions: a case report and review of the literature. *Arch Dermatol* 93:71, 1966.

Reticulohistiocytoma

66. Barrow MV, Holubar K: Multicentric reticulohistiocytosis. *Medicine* 48:287, 1969.

67. Conaghan P, Miller M, Dowling JP, et al: A unique presentation of multicentric reticulohistiocytosis in pregnancy. *Arthritis Rheum* 36:269, 1993.

68. Davies BT, Wood SR: The so-called reticulohistiocytoma of the skin: a comparison of two distinct types. *Br J Dermatol* 67:205, 1955.

69. Davies NEJ, Roenigk HH, Hawk WA, et al: Multicentric reticulohistiocytosis: report of a case with histochemical studies. *Arch Dermatol* 97:543, 1968.

70. Ehrlich GE, Young I, Nosheny SZ, et al: Multicentric reticulohistiocytosis (lipoid dermatoarthritis). *Am J Med* 52:830, 1972.

71. Flam M, Ryan SC, Mah-poy GL, et al: Multicentric reticulohistiocytosis: report of a case with atypical features and electron microscopic study of skin lesions. *Am J Med* 52:841, 1972.

72. Ginsburg WW, O'Duffy JD, Morris JL, et al: Multicentric reticulohistiocytosis: response to alkylating agents in six patients. *Ann Intern Med* 11:384, 1989.

73. Hashimoto K, Pritzker MS: Electron microscopic study of reticulohistiocytoma. *Arch Dermatol* 107:263, 1973.

74. Kenik JG, Fok F, Huerter CJ, et al: Multicentric reticulohistiocytosis in a patient with malignant melanoma: a response to cyclophosphamide and a unique cutaneous feature. *Arthritis Rheum* 33:1047, 1990.

75. Kuramoto Y, Iizawa O, Matsunaga J: Development of Ki-1 lymphoma in a child suffering from multicentric reticulohistiocytosis. *Acta Dermatol Venereol* 71:448, 1991.

76. Kuwabara H, Uda H, Tanaka S: Multicentric reticulohistiocytosis: report of a case with electron microscopic studies. *Acta Pathol Jpn* 42:130, 1992.

77. Lambert CM, Nuki G: Multicentric reticulohistiocytosis with arthritis and cardiac infiltration: regression following treatment for underlying malignancy. *Ann Rheum Dis* 51:815, 1992.

78. Lotti T, Santucci M, Casigliani R, et al: Multicentric reticulohistiocytosis: report of three cases with evaluation of tissue proteinase activity. *Am J Dermatopathol* 10:497, 1988.

79. Montgomery H, Polley HF, Pugh DG: Reticulohistiocytoma (reticulohistiocytic granuloma). *Arch Dermatol* 77:61, 1958.

80. Nakajima Y, Sato K, Morita H, et al: Severe progressive erosive arthritis in multicentric reticulohistiocytosis: possible involvement of cytokines in synovial proliferation. *J Rheumatol* 19:1643, 1992.

81. Oliver GF, Umbert I, Winkelmann RK, et al: Reticulohistiocytoma cutis: review of 15 cases and an association with systemic vasculitis in two cases. *Clin Exp Dermatol* 15:1, 1990.

82. Orkin M, Goltz RW, Good RA, et al: A study of multicentric reticulohistiocytosis. *Arch Dermatol* 89:640, 1964.

83. Perrin C, Lacour JP, Michiels JF, et al: Multicentric reticulohistiocytosis: immunohistochemical and ultrastructural study: a pathology of dendritic cell lineage. *Am J Dermatopathol* 14:418, 1992.

84. Purvis WE, Helwig EB: Reticulohistiocytic granuloma ("reticulohistiocytoma") of the skin. *Am J Clin Pathol* 24:1005, 1954.

85. Salisbury JR, Hall PAS, Williams HC, et al: Multicentric reticulohistiocytosis. *Am J Surg Pathol* 14:687, 1990.

86. Shiokawa S, Shingu M, Nishimura M, et al: Multicentric reticulohistiocytosis associated with subclinical Sjögren's syndrome. *Clin Rheumatol* 10:201, 1991.

87. Taylor DR: Multicentric reticulohistiocytosis. *Arch Dermatol* 113:330, 1977.
88. Zagala A, Guyot A, Bensa JC, et al: Multicentric reticulohistiocytomas: a case with enhanced interleukin-1, prostaglandin E2, and interleukin-2 secretion. *J Rheumatol* 15:136, 1988.

Xanthoma

89. Adams CWM, Bayliss LB, Ibrahim MZM, et al: Phospholipids in atherosclerosis: the modification of the cholesterol granuloma by phospholipid. *J Pathol Bacteriol* 86:43, 1963.
90. Anderson DR: Ultrastructure of xanthelasma. *Arch Ophthalmol* 81:692, 1969.
91. Beerman H: Lipid diseases as manifested in the skin. *Med Clin North Am* 35:433, 1951.
92. Berginer VM, Salen G, Shefer S: Long-term treatment of cerebrotendinous xanthomatosis with chenodeoxycholic acid. *N Engl J Med* 311:1649, 1984.
93. Buxtorf JC, Beaumont V, Jacotot B, et al: Regression de xanthomes et medicaments hypolipidemiants. *Atherosclerosis* 19:1, 1974.
94. Cristol DS, Gill AB: Xanthoma of tendon sheath. *JAMA* 122:1013, 1943.
95. Crocker AC: Skin xanthomas in childhood. *Pediatrics* 8:573, 1951.
96. DeSanto DA, Wilson PD: Xanthomatous tumors of joints. *J Bone Joint Surg* 21:531, 1939.
97. Fahey JJ, Stark HH, Donovan WF, et al: Xanthoma of the Achilles tendon: seven cases with familial hyperbetalipoproteinemia. *J Bone Joint Surg* 55A:1197, 1973.
98. Fredrickson DS, Lees RS: A system for phenotyping hyperlipoproteinemia. *Circulation* 31:321, 1965.
99. Friedman MS: Xanthoma of the Achilles tendon. *J Bone Joint Surg* 29:760, 1947.
100. Galloway JDB, Broders AC, Ghormley RK: Xanthoma of tendon sheaths and synovial membranes: a clinical and pathologic study. *Arch Surg* 40:485, 1940.
101. Gattereau A, Davignon J, Levesque HP: Roentgenological evaluation of Achilles-tendon xanthomatosis. *Lancet* 2:705, 1971.
102. Hamilton WC, Ramsey PL, Hanson SM, et al: Osseous xanthoma and multiple hand tumors as a complication of hyperlipidemia. *J Bone Joint Surg* 57A:551, 1975.
103. Hughes JD, Meriwether TW: Familial pseudohypertrophy of tendoachillis with multisystem disease. *South Med J* 64:311, 1971.
104. Kearns WP, Wood WS: Cerebrotendinous xanthomatosis. *Arch Ophthalmol* 94:148, 1976.
105. Lynch PJ, Winkelmann RK: Generalized plane xanthoma and systemic disease. *Arch Dermatol* 93:639, 1966.
106. McWhorter JE, Weeks C: Multiple xanthoma of the tendons. *Surg Gynecol Obstet* 40:199, 1925.
107. Montgomery H: Cutaneous xanthomatosis. *Ann Intern Med* 13:671, 1939.
108. Montgomery H, Osterberg AE: Xanthomatosis: correlation of clinical histopathologic and chemical studies of cutaneous xanthoma. *Arch Dermatol Syph (Chicago)* 37:373, 1938.
109. Palmer AJ, Blacket R: Regression of xanthomata of the eyelids with modified fat diet. *Lancet* 1:67, 1972.
110. Parker F, Odland GF: Electron microscopic similarities between experimental xanthoma and human eruptive xanthomas. *J Invest Dermatol* 52:136, 1969.
111. Parker F, Odland GF: Experimental xanthoma: a correlative biochemical, histologic, histochemical, and electron microscopic study. *Am J Pathol* 53:537, 1968.
112. Scott PJ, Winterbourn CC: Low density lipoprotein accumulation in actively growing xanthomas. *J Atheroscler Res* 7:207, 1967.
113. Siegelman SS, Schlossberg I, Becker NH, et al: Hyperlipoproteinemia with skeletal lesions. *Clin Orthop* 87:228, 1972.
114. Sloan HR, Frederickson DS: Rare familial diseases with neutral lipid storage: Wolman's disease, cholesterol ester storage disease, and cerebrotendinous xanthomatosis. In Stanbury JB, Wyngaarden JB, Frederickson DS, editors: *Metabolic basis of inherited disease*, ed 3, New York, 1972, McGraw-Hill Inc.
115. Walton KW, Thomas C, Dunkerley DJ: The pathogenesis of xanthomata. *J Pathol* 109:271, 1973.
116. Wilkes LL: Tendon xanthoma in type IV hyperlipoproteinemia. *South Med J* 70:254, 1977.
117. Wilson DE, Flowers CM, Hershgold EJ, et al: Multiple myeloma, cryoglobulinemia, and xanthomatosis: distinct clinical and biochemical syndromes in two patients. *Am J Med* 59:721, 1975.
118. Young F, Harris CT: Complete excision and reconstruction of both Achilles tendons for giant cell xanthoma. *Surg Gynecol Obstet* 61:662, 1935.
119. Zemel H, Deeken J, Asel N, et al: The ultrastructural features of normolipemic plane xanthoma. *Arch Pathol* 89:111, 1970.

Miscellaneous histiocytic reactions mimicking tumor

120. Bergman M, Flance IJ, Cruz PT, et al: Thesaurosis due to inhalation of hair spray: report of twelve new cases including three autopsies. *N Engl J Med* 266:750, 1962.
121. Bubis JJ, Cohen S, Dinbar J, et al: Storage of polyvinylpyrrolidone mimicking a congenital mucolipid storage disease in a patient with Munchhausen's syndrome. *Isr J Med Sci* 11:999, 1975.
122. Damjanov I, Katz SM: Malakoplakia. *Pathol Annu* 16:103, 1981.
123. Eisen RN, Buckley PJ, Rosai J: Immunophenotypic characterization of sinus histiocytomas with massive lymphadenopathy (Rosai-Dorfman disease). *Semin Diagn Pathol* 7:74, 1990.
124. Font RL, Bersani TA, Eagle RC: Malakoplakia of the eyelid: clinical, histopathologic and ultrastructural characteristics. *Ophthalmology* 95:61, 1988.
125. Foucar E, Rosai J, Dorman RF: Sinus histiocytosis with massive lymphadenopathy (Rosai-Dorfman disease): review of the entity. *Semin Diagn Pathol* 7:19, 1990.
126. Gille J, Brandau H: Fremdkorpergranulation in der Brusdruse nach Injektion eines polyvinylpyrrolidonhaltigen Praparats. Eine Fallbeobactung. *Geburtsch Frauen Heilk* 35:799, 1975.
127. Hizawa K, Inaba H, Nakanishi S, et al: Subcutaneous pseudosarcomatous polyvinylpyrrolidone granuloma. *Am J Surg Pathol* 8:393, 1984.
128. Keren DF, Rawlings W, Murray HW, et al: *Arizona hinshawii* osteomyelitis with antecedent enteric fever and sepsis: a case report and review of the literature. *Ann J Med* 60:577, 1976.
129. Kuo TT, Hsueh S: Mucicarminophilic histiocytosis: a polyvinylpyrrolidone (PVP) storage disease simulating signet ring carcinoma. *Am J Surg Pathol* 8:419, 1984.
130. Mansfield RE: Histoid leprosy. *Arch Pathol* 87:580, 1969.
131. Montgomery EA, Meis JM, Frizzera G: Rosai-Dorfman disease of soft tissue. *Am J Surg Pathol* 16:122, 1992.
132. Reske-Nielsen E, Bojsen-Moller M, Vetner M, et al: Polyvinylpyrrolidone-storage disease: light and microscopical, ultrastructural, and chemical verification. *Acta Pathol Microbiol Scand* 84A:397, 1976.
133. Rosai J, Dorfman RF: Sinus histiocytosis with massive lymphadenopathy: a pseudolymphomatous benign disorder: analysis of 34 cases. *Cancer* 30:1174, 1972.
134. Sobel H, Arvin E, Marquet E, et al: Reactive granular cells in sites of trauma: a cytochemical and ultrastructural study. *Am J Clin Pathol* 61:223, 1974.
135. Wade HW: Histoid variety of lepromatous leprosy. *Int J Leprosy* 31:129, 1963.
136. Weiss SW, Enzinger FM, Johnson FB: Silica reaction simulating fibrous histiocytoma. *Cancer* 42:2738, 1978.
137. Wessel W, Schoog M, Winkler E: Polyvinylpyrrolidone (PVP): its diagnostic, therapeutic, and technical application and consequences thereof. *Arzneim Forsch (Drug Res)* 21:1468, 1971.

CHAPTER 14

FIBROHISTIOCYTIC TUMORS OF INTERMEDIATE MALIGNANCY

Although formerly, fibrohistiocytic tumors of intermediate malignancy were represented primarily by dermatofibrosarcoma protuberans, a number of recently described tumors seem also to fit well within this general category of neoplasms. These include giant cell fibroblastoma, plexiform fibrohistiocytic tumor, and angiomatoid (malignant) fibrous histiocytoma. All have a significant risk of local recurrence but little or no risk of distant metastasis, making it appropriate to separate them from both benign and conventional (high-grade) malignant fibrous histiocytoma.

DERMATOFIBROSARCOMA PROTUBERANS

Dermatofibrosarcoma protuberans, first described in 1924 by Darier and Ferrand[20] as "progressive and recurring dermatofibroma," is a nodular cutaneous tumor characterized by a prominent storiform pattern. Over the years it has been considered a fibroblastic, histiocytic, and neural tumor, and to date there is no consensus concerning its histogenesis. It bears an unmistakable histological similarity to benign fibrous histiocytoma, and on this basis it, along with its pigmented counterpart (Bednař tumor), is tentatively classified with the fibrohistiocytic neoplasms. In contrast to fibrous histiocytoma, dermatofibrosarcoma protuberans grows in a more infiltrative fashion, possesses a greater capacity for local recurrence, and, in unusual instances, metastasizes. Distant metastasis, however, is usually a late event.

Clinical findings

Dermatofibrosarcoma protuberans typically presents during early or mid-adult life as a nodular cutaneous mass. It seldom occurs in children,[55] and only rare reports have documented the tumor during childhood or at birth.[21,22,55,74,91] Males are affected more frequently than females. Although these tumors may occur at almost any site, they are most frequent on the trunk and proximal extremities (Table 14-1). Antecedent trauma, reported in about 10% to 20% of cases, is probably coincidental.[72,74,92] However, several striking cases reporting origin of this tumor in a previous burn or surgical scar raise the question of a causal relationship.[40,57,87] Other interesting features of the disease include association with acanthosis nigricans,[58] chronic arsenic exposure,[86] acrodermatitis enteropathica,[85] regression following topical administration of a wild plant,[40] and rapid enlargement during pregnancy.[92] The first two cases, however, are not well documented and must be interpreted accordingly.

In most cases this tumor is characterized by slow but persistent growth over a long period, often several years. The clinical and gross appearances then are determined to a great extent by the stage of the disease. The initial manifestation is usually the development of a firm, plaquelike lesion of the skin, often having a surrounding red to blue discoloration.[92] These lesions have been compared with the morphea of scleroderma or morphea-like basal cell carcinoma.[43] Rarely the lesions appear as an area of atrophy.[4] Less often, multiple small subcutaneous nodules may appear initially rather than a plaque. The plaque may either grow slowly or remain stationary for a variable period, eventually entering a more rapid growth phase and giving rise to one or more nodules. Thus, only in the fully developed lesion is the typical "protuberant" appearance manifested. Neglected tumors may achieve enormous proportions and have multiple satellite nodules. However, despite

Table 14-1. Anatomical distribution of dermatofibrosarcoma protuberans (AFIP, 1960-1979)

Anatomical location	No. cases	Percent
Head and neck	124	14.5
Upper extremity	155	18.2
Trunk	404	47.4
Lower extremity	170	19.9
TOTAL	853	100.0

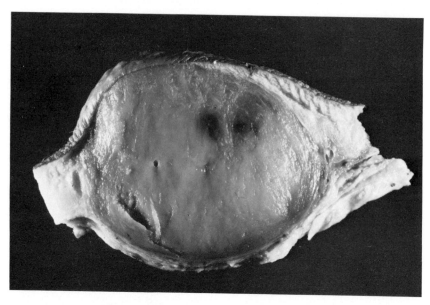

FIG. 14-1. Typical dermatofibrosarcoma protuberans involving dermis and subcutis in a nodular fashion.

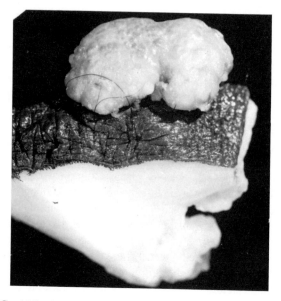

FIG. 14-2. Small dermatofibrosarcoma displaying protuberant growth.

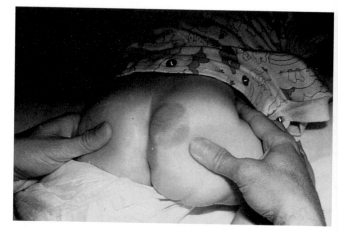

FIG. 14-3. Dermatofibrosarcoma protuberans from buttock of young child. Lesion had a reddish color.

the large size of many of these tumors, the patients appear surprisingly well and lack signs of cachexia associated with malignancies.

Gross findings

Biopsy of the majority of tumors is done in the nodular stage; therefore, the specimen consists of a solitary, protuberant, gray-white mass involving subcutis and skin (Figs. 14-1 to 14-3). The average size at surgery is approximately 5 cm.[92] Multiple discrete masses are usually not seen in the original tumor but are more characteristic of recurrent lesions (Fig. 14-4).[92] The skin overlying these tumors is taut or even ulcerated. Skeletal muscle extension is uncommon except in large or recurrent lesions. In our experience, this tumor may rarely be confined to the subcutis and lack dermal involvement altogether. Occasionally areas of the tumor have a translucent or gelatinous appearance corresponding microscopically to myxoid change. Hemorrhage and cystic change are sometimes seen in these tumors, but necrosis, a common feature of malignant fibrous histiocytoma, is rare.

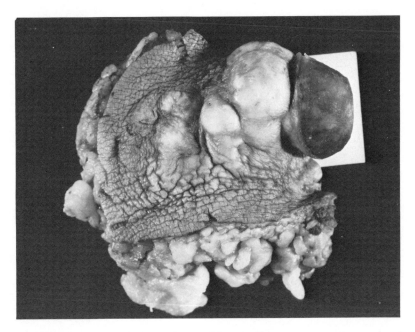

FIG. 14-4. Gross appearance of advanced case of dermatofibrosarcoma protuberans showing multiple nodules of tumor.

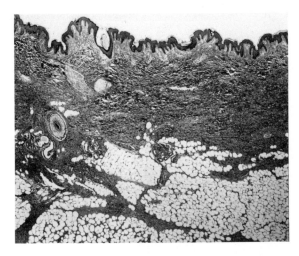

FIG. 14-5. Plaque form of dermatofibrosarcoma protuberans illustrating expansion of interface between dermis and subcutis as well as extension into subcutaneous fat. (×60.)

Microscopic findings

Despite the apparent gross circumscription of these lesions, the tumor diffusely infiltrates the dermis and subcutis (Fig. 14-5). The tumor may reach the epidermis or leave an uninvolved zone of dermis just beneath the epidermis. In either event, the overlying epidermis does not usually display the hyperplasia that characterizes some cases of cutaneous fibrous histiocytoma (dermatofibroma).[92] The peripheral portions of the tumor have a deceptively bland appearance due in part to the marked attenuation of the cells at their advancing edge. This is especially true in superficial areas, where the spread of slender cells between preexisting collagen is easily mistaken for cutaneous fibrous histiocytoma (dermatofibroma) (Fig. 14-6, *A*). In the deep regions the tumor spreads along connective tissue septa and between adnexae (Fig. 14-7) or intricately interdigitates with lobules of subcutaneous fat, creating a lacelike or honeycomb effect (Fig. 14-6, *B*).

The central or main portion of the tumor is composed of a uniform population of slender fibroblasts arranged in a distinct, often monotonous storiform pattern around an inconspicuous vasculature (Fig. 14-8). There is usually little nuclear pleomorphism and only low to moderate mitotic activity. Secondary elements such as giant cells, xanthoma cells, and inflammatory elements are few in number or absent altogether. In this respect, dermatofibrosarcoma protuberans displays remarkable uniformity compared with other fibrohistiocytic neoplasms. Although most tumors are characterized by these highly ordered cellular areas, occasional tumors may contain myxoid areas (Fig. 14-9). These myxoid areas were initially believed to be a feature of recurrent lesions,[92] but recent reports indicate they may also be seen in the primary tumor.[29] Myxoid areas are characterized by the interstitial accumulation of ground substance material. As myxoid change of the stroma becomes more pronounced, the storiform pattern becomes less distinct, while the vascular pattern becomes more apparent. By virtue of these features, such tumors can resemble myxoid liposarcoma (Fig. 14-9, *B*). Giant cells, similar to those in

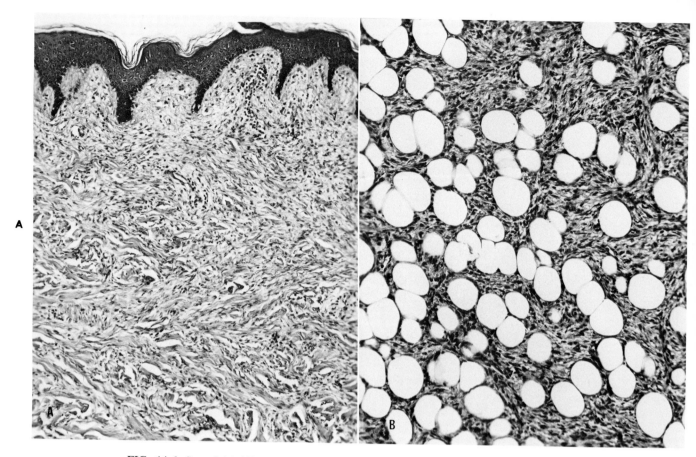

FIG. 14-6. Superficial (**A**) and deep extensions (**B**) of a dermatofibrosarcoma protuberans. The spread of the tumor between preexisting collagen of the dermis may simulate the appearance of a cutaneous fibrous histiocytoma (**A**). At the deep margin, the tumor intricately interdigitates with normal fat (**B**). (**A** and **B**, ×100.)

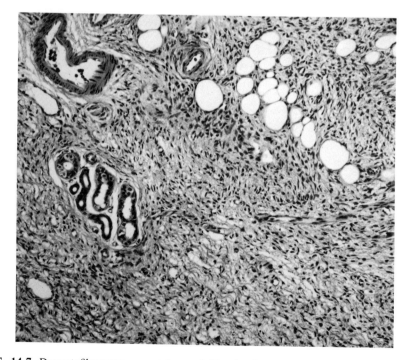

FIG. 14-7. Dermatofibrosarcoma protuberans infiltrating between adnexal structures. (×160.)

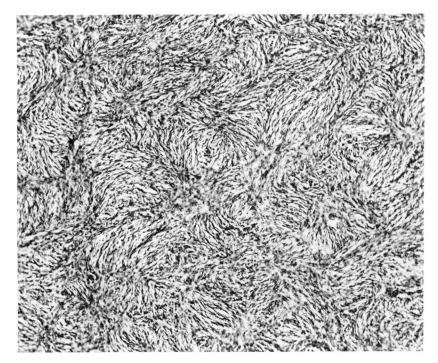

FIG. 14-8. Slender spindle cells arranged in a distinct storiform pattern characterize the majority of these tumors. (×180.)

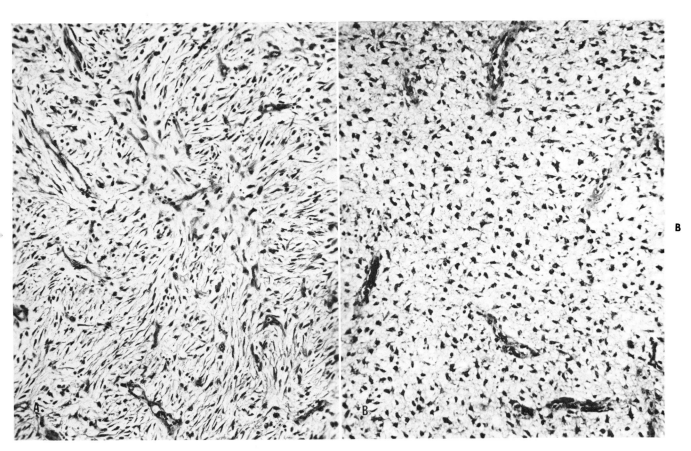

FIG. 14-9. A, Myxoid change within a dermatofibrosarcoma protuberans. (×160.) **B,** When myxoid change is quite prominent, the storiform pattern may be lacking altogether, and the tumor may resemble a myxoid liposarcoma. (×160.)

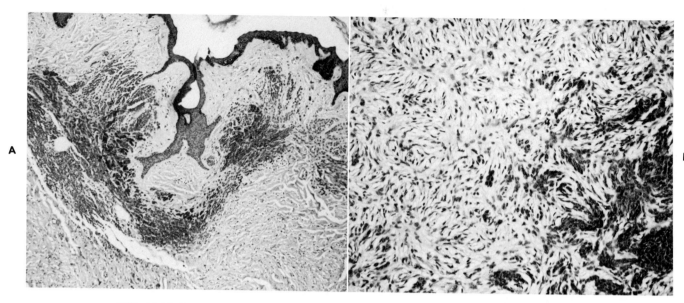

FIG. 14-10. Intradermal nevus (**A**) showing transition to a dermatofibrosarcoma protuberans (**B**). (**A**, ×25; **B**, ×250.)

giant cell fibroblastoma, can be identified in a small percentage of otherwise typical dermatofibrosarcomas. In one unique case we have reviewed, a dermatofibrosarcoma was associated with or arose from an intradermal nevus (Fig. 14-10).

Infrequently dermatofibrosarcoma protuberans contains areas that are indistinguishable from fibrosarcoma (Fig. 14-11). These areas consist of dense fascicles of cells usually, but not always, containing more pleomorphism and mitotic activity. In exceptional instances, dermatofibrosarcoma protuberans may even contain areas resembling malignant fibrous histiocytoma (Fig. 14-12).[67] Fibrosarcomatous areas are more commonly encountered in recurrent lesions (Fig. 14-11). The significance of this change has been the subject of several recent studies.[8,23,99] It has been our policy to designate dermatofibrosarcoma protuberans with only focal microscopic areas of malignancy as "dermatofibrosarcoma protuberans." However, when malignant areas are more prevalent (greater than 10%), it seems reasonable to regard the tumors as sarcomas, which possess a higher metastatic potential than the ordinary dermatofibrosarcoma protuberans. Such areas, in our opinion, can be recognized by a fascicular growth pattern at low power and usually by a plumper cell with more atypia. Mitotic figures are not necessarily elevated in these areas, however.

Metastatic deposits from this tumor occur most commonly in the lung and secondly in regional lymph nodes, where they may resemble the parent tumor or may appear more pleomorphic like a fibrosarcoma (Fig. 14-13). In one unique case, the regional lymph node metastases from a dermatofibrosarcoma were likened to Hodgkin's disease.[28,59] However, this case is most unusual in that the terminal course in the patient was marked by massive cervical, supraclavicular, and anterior thoracic lymphadenopathy, findings highly unusual for dermatofibrosarcoma but quite characteristic of Hodgkin's disease. Because no autopsy was performed, the possibility of Hodgkin's disease, as pointed out by the authors themselves, is not completely excluded.

Electron microscopic and immunohistochemical findings

Electron microscopic and histochemical observations of this tumor have led to conflicting observations and opinions concerning its histogenesis. Some have interpreted the tumor as fibroblastic because of the prevalence of fusiform cells containing organized lamellae of rough endoplasmic reticulum (Fig. 14-14).[33,61] Others believe the tumor is histiocytic. This theory is based not only on the finding of occasional cells within the tumor that resemble histiocytes, but also on the "histiocytic" features of tumor cells grown in tissue culture[68,71,101] and the presence of histiocytic enzymes within the cells.[44,101] However, others,[29] including ourselves, have not confirmed these findings. Two ultrastructural studies have proposed neural differentiation.[3,35] Both studies describe fibroblastic cells with certain modifications indicating a close relationship to perineurium. These cells have convoluted nuclei, elaborate cell processes, moderate numbers of desmosomes, and incomplete basal laminae around cells. All of these features are regarded as more characteristic of cells showing schwannian, rather than fibroblastic, differentiation. Most recently, the finding of

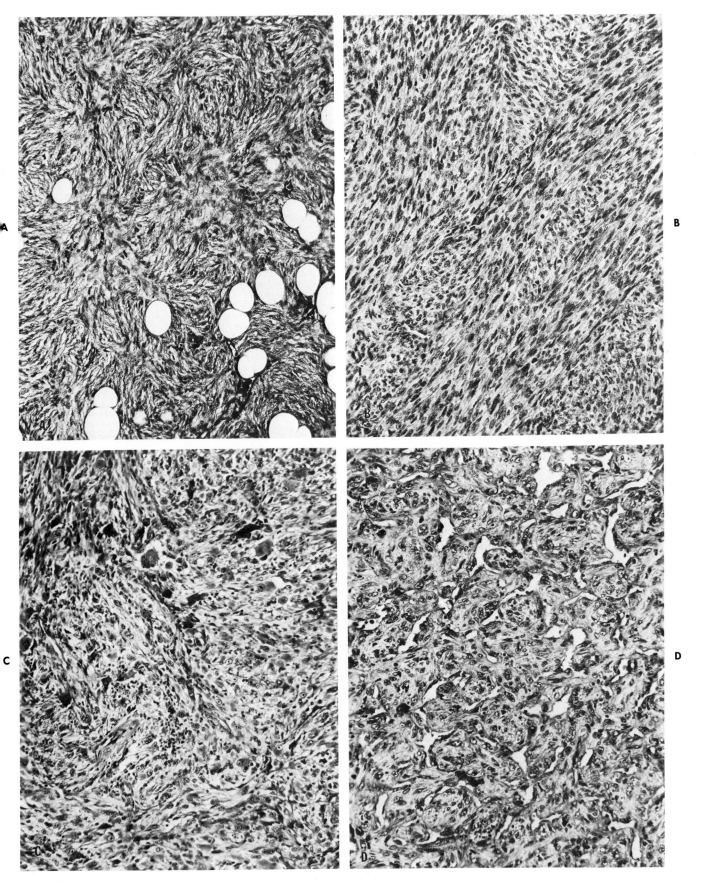

FIG. 14-11. Recurrent dermatofibrosarcoma protuberans of parotid region showing areas of malignant degeneration. **A,** Original tumor had typical appearance of dermatofibrosarcoma protuberans. Recurrences had an appearance of fibrosarcoma (**B**) or malignant fibrous histiocytoma (**C**). **D,** Occasional areas had a striking pericytoma pattern. (**A** to **D,** ×160.)

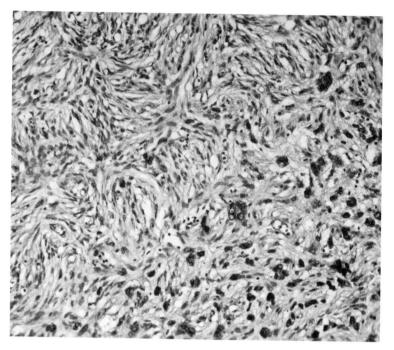

FIG. 14-12. Dermatofibrosarcoma showing transition *(lower right)* to malignant fibrous histiocytoma. (×250.)

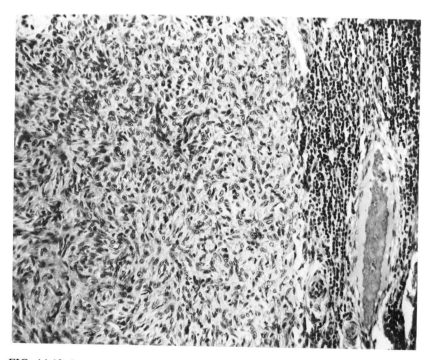

FIG. 14-13. Lymph node metastasis from a dermatofibrosarcoma protuberans. (×160.)

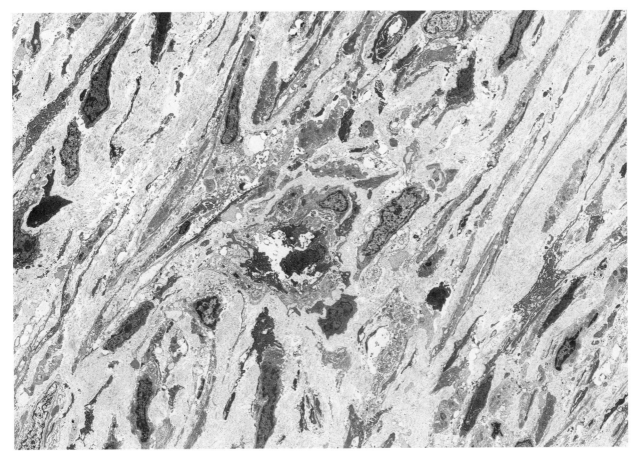

FIG. 14-14. Electron micrograph of a dermatofibrosarcoma protuberans showing center of a storiform area occupied by a small vessel. Fibroblast-like cells spin out from vessel and have numerous slender processes that may join each other by means of specialized cell contacts. (From Taxy JB, Battifora H: The electron microscope in the study and diagnosis of soft tissue tumors. In Trump BF, Jones RT, editors: *Diagnostic electron microscopy*, New York, 1980, John Wiley & Sons).

CD34 within dermatofibrosarcoma has been interpreted as suggestive evidence of a form of neural differentiation.[117] This antigen is not expressed by normal fibroblasts or within fibroblastic lesions but is present in some nerve sheath cells and nerve sheath tumors.

Cytogenetic analysis

A few cases of dermatofibrosarcoma have been studied cytogenetically. The most consistent finding has been the presence of a ring chromosome.[16,51,90] Although the significance of this finding is not clear, mesenchymal tumors that have a ring chromosome as a sole finding are generally benign or low-grade tumors.

Differential diagnosis

The most common problem in differential diagnosis is the distinction of this tumor from other fibrohistiocytic neoplasms. In general, dermatofibrosarcoma protuberans has a more uniform appearance and smaller cells and displays a more distinct storiform pattern with fewer secondary elements (giant cells, inflammatory cells) than either a benign or malignant fibrous histiocytoma. The distinction between benign fibrous histiocytoma and dermatofibrosarcoma occasionally proves difficult when only the superficial portion of the dermatofibrosarcoma is present in a biopsy specimen, because these areas may appear so well differentiated. Under these circumstances, knowledge of the size and configuration of the lesion in question suggests the diagnosis, and biopsy of a deeper portion confirms it. In addition, since CD34 is almost consistently expressed by dermatofibrosarcoma and rarely by benign fibrous histiocytoma, this is an extremely useful antigen in analyzing this problem.[117] Malignant fibrous histiocytoma is not often confused with this tumor, because it is characterized by far more pleomorphism, mitotic activity, and necrosis. Moreover, its typical deep location in muscle and more rapid growth are at variance with the indolent course of this tumor. Rarely one may encounter dermatofibrosarcoma protuberans with areas of malignant fibrous histiocytoma (see Fig. 14-11). As indicated earlier, when such areas represent more than just a microscopic focus, it seems preferable to regard these tumors as fully malignant sarcomas.

A second common problem is the confusion of this tumor with benign neural tumors; specifically, a diffuse form of neurofibroma. This is most likely to occur when dermatofibrosarcoma is in the plaque stage or when a biopsy is done on only the periphery of the tumor. However, neurofibroma usually contains tactoid structures or other features of neural differentiation, and it lacks the highly cellular areas with mitotic figures that characterize the central portion of a dermatofibrosarcoma. The presence of S-100 protein in virtually all neurofibromas and its absence in dermatofibrosarcoma is an additional contrasting point.

Finally, highly myxoid forms of dermatofibrosarcoma may resemble myxoid liposarcomas by virtue of the prominent vasculature and bland stellate or fusiform cells. However, the superficial location, gross configuration, and especially the complete absence of lipoblasts should raise serious questions concerning the diagnosis of liposarcoma. In such cases additional sampling of the tumor or review of the original material in a recurrent lesion may reveal the diagnostic cellular areas.

Discussion

Unlike the benign fibrous histiocytoma that it resembles, dermatofibrosarcoma protuberans is a locally aggressive neoplasm that recurs in up to half of patients.[57,92] The high recurrence rate in part reflects the extensive infiltration of the tumor compared with fibrous histiocytoma and the failure to appreciate this phenomenon at the time of surgery. It is clear that prompt wide local excision of this lesion can markedly alter the recurrence rate, as reflected by the lower rates of 20.5%,[72] 33%,[17] and 1.75%[74] in patients given primary therapy at large centers. The risk of local recurrence, furthermore, correlates well with the extent of the wide excision. If the margin of excision is 3 cm or more, the recurrence rate is 20%, compared with 41% if the margin is 2 cm or less.[78] If local recurrence develops, it is usually within 3 years of the initial surgery,[57] but recurrences after several years have been reported, attesting to the need for long-term follow-up care. In patients who develop multiple recurrences, progressively shorter intervals between successive recurrences have been noted.[92]

Despite the locally aggressive behavior, this tumor infrequently metastasizes and, therefore, should be clearly separated from conventional sarcomas. The incidence of metastasis is difficult to assess because of the bias introduced in selectively reporting metastasizing tumors. In one

large study of 115 patients, no metastases were observed,[98] whereas in two other studies, 5 of 86 patients[57] and 4 of 96 patients[74] developed metastases. In the latter study the follow-up period was 15 years. Thus long-term follow-up may indicate higher metastatic rates than previously accepted. Of the 471 patients reported in the literature, 16 (3.4%) have developed metastatic disease.[74] About three fourths of patients with metastases have hematogenous spread to the lung, and one fourth have lymphatic spread to regional lymph nodes. Metastases to other sites such as the brain, the bones, and the heart have also been documented.

Although some have suggested that the presence of fibrosarcomatous areas within dermatofibrosarcoma protuberans is accompanied by a higher local recurrence rate and, thus, a more aggressive course, the status and adequacy of surgical excisions in these cases is not made clear in these reports.[23] Connelly and Evans[18] have reported no difference in the local recurrence rate or in time to recurrence compared with conventional dermatofibrosarcoma protuberans. Recurrences in their patients depended solely on the adequacy of surgical excision. They did, however, report that two of their six patients with fibrosarcomatous areas developed metastatic disease, a risk that would appear to be greater than for ordinary dermatofibrosarcoma protuberans.[18] Nonetheless, it is quite difficult to predict which tumors will metastasize. Although some of the metastasizing cases reported in the literature have displayed fibrosarcomatous change,[64] others have not.[1,43] This latter group may display few features that would distinguish them from nonmetastasizing lesions. In one study, it was noted that three out of five metastasizing tumors had a high mitotic rate. Because one nonmetastasizing lesion had also had a comparable mitotic rate, this feature is not completely reliable.[57] Metastasizing lesions, however, share some common clinical features; they are almost always recurrent lesions, and there is usually an interval of several years between diagnosis and metastasis.

Ideally, therapy should consist of wide local excision initially. In some cases it may be admissible to perform less surgery. Such cases would include those in which an initial excision would necessarily dictate amputation or other mutilating procedures. This temporizing approach can be justified on the grounds that the risk of metastatic disease is negligible and the patient may enjoy a long disease-free period before a possible recurrence. Obviously a conservative approach cannot be justified in cases where local recurrence of an incompletely excised lesion would seriously jeopardize a vital structure. The low incidence of regional lymph node metastasis and the negative findings in a small series of blind lymph node dissections do not warrant routine node dissections. Resection of isolated pulmonary metastases has been advocated because of the overall low-grade behavior of the tumor.[1] There is little data to support the value of radiotherapy.[17,92] Limited experience using Mohs' chemosurgery in resecting these lesions has been reported.[77]

The histogenesis of this tumor is still controversial. Traditionally, the prominent storiform pattern and the overall similarity to benign and malignant fibrous histiocytomas have been used as presumptive evidence for including this tumor with the other fibrohistiocytic tumors. Nonetheless, there is some evidence that the progenitor cell may be more closely related to a fibroblast or a fibroblast showing partial schwannian differentiation. This is supported by recent ultrastructural studies showing cells with Schwann cell features.[3,35] Even more recently, the finding of CD34 expression in this tumor, an antigen which is expressed by some cells of the endoneurium and some nerve sheath tumors, has prompted us to suggest that this may represent an unusual variant of a nerve sheath tumor.[117]

BEDNAŘ TUMOR (PIGMENTED DERMATOFIBROSARCOMA PROTUBERANS, STORIFORM NEUROFIBROMA)

In 1957 Bednař[9] described a group of nine cutaneous tumors characterized by indolent growth and a prominent storiform pattern, and in four cases by the presence of melanin pigment. He regarded these tumors as variants of neurofibroma *(storiform neurofibroma)*; he cited as evidence the presence of similar areas within neural nevi[8] and the presence of melanin. In our practice, we have reserved the term *Bednař tumor* for those tumors that resemble dermatofibrosarcoma protuberans but which, in addition, possess melanin pigment. These tumors are uncommon[9,24,26,30] as evidenced by the fact that Bednař gleaned only four cases

from among 100,000 biopsy specimens; in our cases, these tumors account for fewer than 5% of all cases of dermatofibrosarcoma protuberans. Although, as suggested by Bednař, these tumors may represent neural lesions, their nonpigmented portions are virtually identical to dermatofibrosarcoma protuberans. Moreover, their clinical and gross features are also similar. The majority are slowly growing cutaneous masses that extend to the epidermis and advance into the deep subcutis. The number of melanin-bearing cells varies greatly within these tumors. In some, large numbers of melanin-containing cells cause a black discoloration of the tumor (Fig. 14-15), whereas in others, melanin is so sparse as to be appreciated only microscopically. These cells are scattered irregularly throughout the tumor (Fig. 14-16). Their tentacle-like processes emanating from a central nucleus-containing zone give them a characteristic bipolar or multipolar shape, depending on the plane of section (Fig. 14-16, *B*). Melanin stains with conventional methods including Fontana's stain and Warthin-Starry (pH 3.2) stain and ultrastructurally consists of mature membrane-bounded melanosomes. Electron microscopic studies reveal that most areas are made up of slender fibroblastic cells arranged in a delicate collagen matrix (Fig. 14-17), although other areas have cells more suggestive of Schwann cell differentiation (Fig. 14-18). The cells have numerous interlocking processes elaborately invested with basal laminae. Mature and immature melanosomes can be identified within the tumor cells. We have suggested this indicates that the tumor synthesizes rather than phagocytoses melanin (Fig. 14-19), although others have suggested that the tumor is simply colonized by melanin-bearing cells.[30] On the other

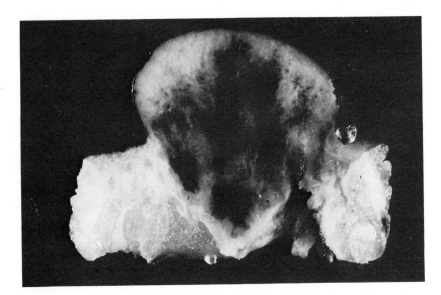

FIG. 14-15. Bednař tumor. Gross appearance of tumor is identical to the conventional dermatofibrosarcoma protuberans, but substance of tumor is flecked with melanin pigment.

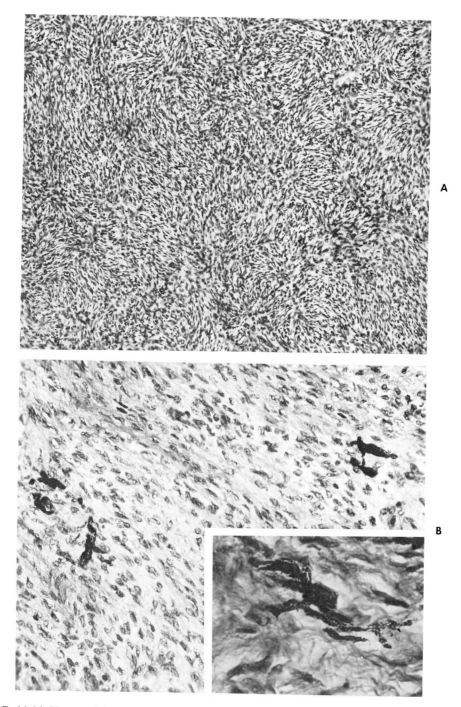

FIG. 14-16. Pigmented dermatofibrosarcoma protuberans (Bednař tumor). **A,** Some areas are identical to the conventional dermatofibrosarcoma protuberans. (×100.) **B,** Others have numerous melanin-bearing cells with thin dendritic processes *(inset).* (×250; inset ×630.)

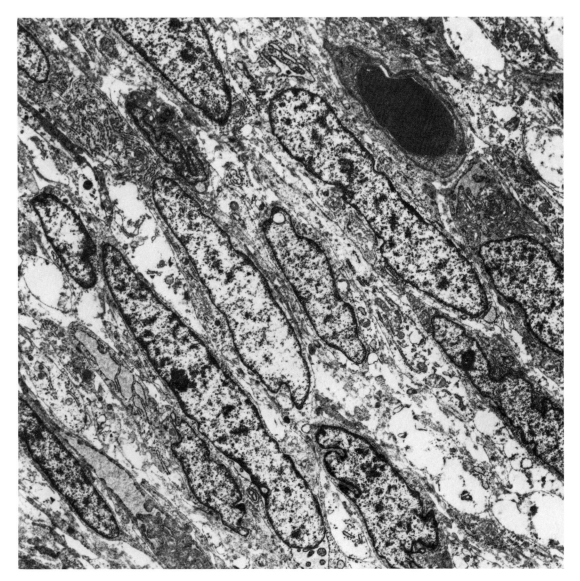

FIG. 14-17. Predominant cells within Bednař tumor have features of fibroblasts. (×5700.) (From Dupree SB, Langloss JM, Weiss SW: *Am J Surg Pathol* 9:630, 1985.)

hand, we have not been able to identify S-100 protein[63] (an acidic protein present in certain neural tumors[25,31,65,66]) within Bednař tumors or their nonpigmented counterparts.

Owing to the paucity of cases, it is difficult to assess the biological behavior of this tumor. Of the four cases reported by Bednař, none recurred. One of our nine cases with follow-up information recurred.[26] However, judging from the infiltrative growth and the overall similarity to conventional dermatofibrosarcoma, the biological behavior is probably comparable. There is one report in the literature of a Bednař tumor with pulmonary metastasis.[71]

GIANT CELL FIBROBLASTOMA

Giant cell fibroblastoma was first described in 1982 in abstract form by Shmookler and Enzinger. It is a clinically and morphologically distinctive lesion that occurs almost exclusively in children, and it has a number of similarities to dermatofibrosarcoma protuberans. This would suggest that it is, in effect, a juvenile analogue of the latter.[116]

Clinical findings

Giant cell fibroblastoma develops as a painless nodule or mass in the dermis or subcutis, with a predilection for the

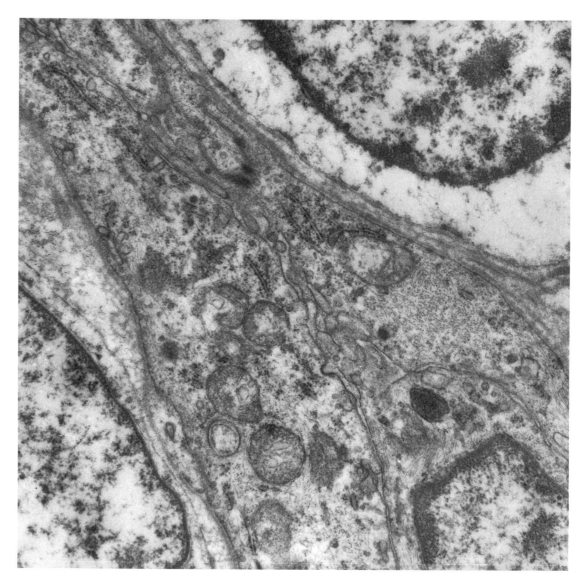

FIG. 14-18. Schwann cell–like areas of Bednař tumor where cells have interlacing processes, junctions, and basal lamina. (×24,800.) (From Dupree WB, Langloss JM, Weiss SW: *Am J Surg Pathol* 9:630, 1985.)

back of the thigh, inguinal region, and chest wall. It affects predominantly infants and children but is encountered infrequently in adults. In our experience, about two thirds of children were younger than 5 years of age when brought to medical attention, and the median age was 3 years. Infrequent cases have been recorded in adults.[105,110] About two thirds of patients are male and one third are female.

Pathologic findings

Grossly the lesions consist of gray to yellow mucoid masses that are poorly circumscribed and measure between 1 and 8 cm. They are composed of loosely arranged, wavy spindle cells with a moderate degree of nuclear pleomor-

phism that infiltrate the deep dermis and subcutis and encircle adnexal structures in a fashion similar to dermatofibrosarcoma protuberans (Figs. 14-20 to 14-23). The tumors vary in their cellularity from those approximating the cellularity of dermatofibrosarcoma protuberans (Fig. 14-22) to those that are hypocellular with a myxoid or hyaline stroma (Fig. 14-23). The characteristic feature of the tumor, however, is the peculiar pseudovascular spaces, which seem to reflect a loss of cellular cohesion. Large and irregular in shape, the pseudovascular spaces are lined by a discontinuous row of multinucleated cells that represent variants of the basic proliferating tumor cell (Fig. 14-24). Although these cells appear to contain multiple overlapping nuclei by

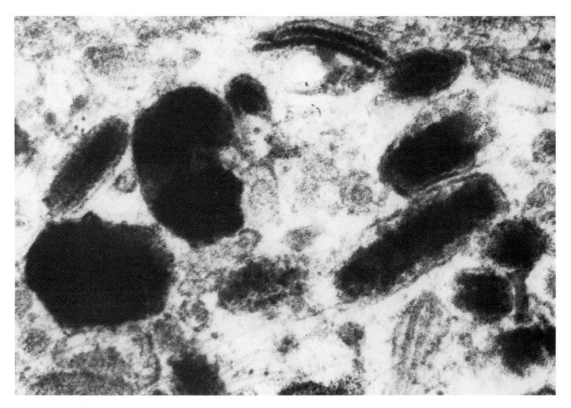

FIG. 14-19. Mature and immature melanosomes within a Bednař tumor. (×93,900.) (From Dupree WB, Langloss JM, Weiss SW: *Am J Surg Pathol* 9:630, 1985.)

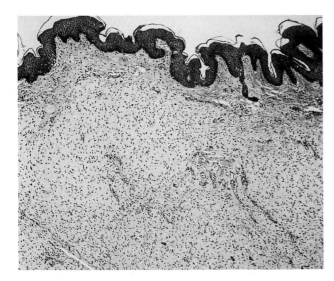

FIG. 14-20. Giant cell fibroblastoma showing involvement of dermis with abutment of epidermis. (×60.)

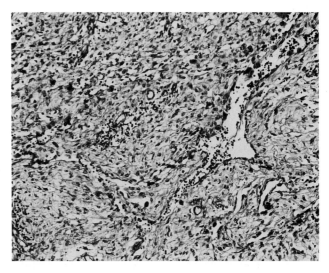

FIG. 14-21. Giant cell fibroblastoma showing solid areas interrupted by angiectatic areas lined by giant cells. (×100.)

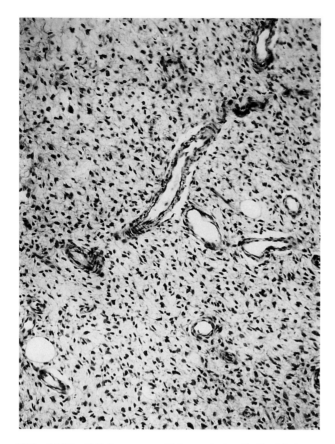

FIG. 14-22. Cellular areas within a giant cell fibroblastoma. (×160.)

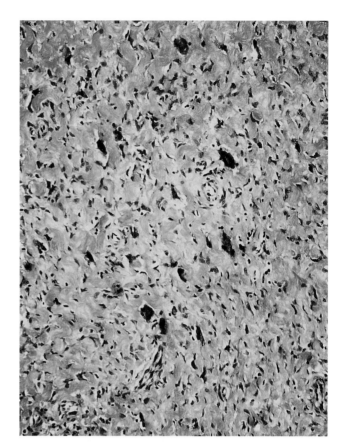

FIG. 14-23. Hypocellular hyalinized zones within giant cell fibroblastoma. (×160.)

light microscopy, they actually represent multiple sausage-like lobations of a single nucleus when studied ultrastructurally.[116] Immunohistochemical studies indicate that these tumors express vimentin but lack S-100 protein and vascular markers.[110] Some giant cell fibroblastomas express CD34, a feature they share with dermatofibrosarcoma protuberans.[117]

Differential diagnosis

In our experience, about 40% of giant cell fibroblastomas are misdiagnosed as sarcoma.[117] Because of the myxoid areas and hyperchromatic giant cells, there is a tendency to assume they represent examples of myxoid liposarcoma or myxoid malignant fibrous histiocytoma occurring in an unusually young individual. Important clues to diagnosis include superficial location, lack of an intricate vasculature, and presence of hyperchromatic cells, which lie preferentially along the pseudovascular spaces.

Discussion

There have been approximately 50 cases of giant cell fibroblastoma reported in the literature. Recurrences have developed in about one half of cases, but metastases have not

been reported to date. Treatment of these tumors ideally is wide local excision. If less therapy is contemplated, conscientious follow-up care is advisable to document and treat recurrences.

Authors have continually speculated about the lineage of these tumors, some suggesting a fibrohistiocytic origin and others a fibroblastic origin.[109] Ultrastructurally, the cells, replete with rough endoplasmic reticulum, seem to resemble fibroblasts most closely. However, the recent finding of CD34 within these lesions raises some question as to whether these could represent an unusual nerve sheath tumor.[117] Regardless of the lineage, the preponderance of evidence closely links this tumor with dermatofibrosarcoma protuberans. Both occur in superficial soft tissues, with a strong predilection for the abdominal wall, back, and groin. Even more compelling is the observation that hybrid tumors occur. For example, occasional dermatofibrosarcomas of adults contain giant cells or foci similar to those of giant cell fibroblastoma,[106] and, less frequently, otherwise typical giant cell fibroblastomas of childhood contain areas of dermatofibrosarcoma protuberans.[113] There have also been a number of recorded instances in which either dermatofibrosarcoma protuberans or giant cell fibroblastoma has re-

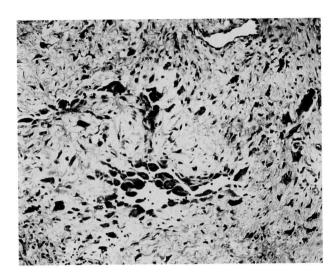

FIG. 14-24. Pseudovascular spaces lined by discontinuous layer of giant cells in a giant cell fibroblastoma. (×250.)

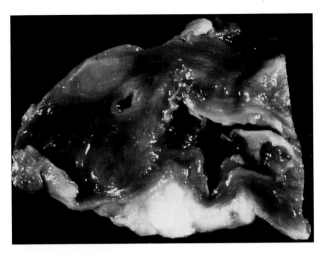

FIG. 14-25. Gross specimen of angiomatoid fibrous histiocytoma. Note cystic spaces.

curred and recapitulated the pattern of the other tumor in the recurrence.[103,104,108]

ANGIOMATOID FIBROUS HISTIOCYTOMA

Previously termed *angiomatoid malignant fibrous histiocytoma*,[120] this distinctive tumor of children and young adults has been renamed *angiomatoid fibrous histiocytoma* by the World Health Organization Committee for the Classification of Soft Tissue Tumors, to reflect the relative rarity of metastasis and the overall excellent clinical course.

Clinical findings

Angiomatoid fibrous histiocytoma is a tumor that occurs primarily in children and young adults and is, therefore, rarely encountered over the age of 40 years. It develops as a slowly growing nodular, multinodular, or cystic mass of the hypodermis or subcutis. Most occur on the extremities. Local symptoms such as pain and tenderness are uncommon, but systemic symptoms such as anemia, pyrexia, and weight loss are occasionally encountered and suggest the production of cytokines by the neoplasm.

Gross and microscopic findings

The tumors are firm, circumscribed lesions that usually measure a few centimeters in diameter and vary in color from gray-tan to red-brown, depending on the amount of hemosiderin present. One of the most characteristic features is the presence of irregular blood-filled cystic spaces best appreciated on cross-section (Fig. 14-25). This feature may be so striking as to give the impression of hematoma, hemangioma, or a thrombosed vessel.

These lesions are characterized by three features: irregular solid masses of histiocyte-like cells, cystic areas of hemorrhage, and chronic inflammation. In general, the solid masses of histiocyte-like cells interspersed with areas of hemorrhage occupy the central portion of the tumor, while the inflammatory cells form a dense peripheral cuff that blends with the surrounding pseudocapsule (Figs. 14-26 and 14-27).

The histiocyte-like cells are usually quite uniform; they have a round or oval nucleus and a faintly staining eosinophilic cytoplasm often containing finely particulate hemosiderin. In most instances the cells are quite bland, such that some may be confused with the histiocytes of granulomas. However, in about one fifth of cases there may be significant nuclear atypia or hyperchromatic giant cells, a feature that does not correlate with more aggressive behavior.[118] In a small number of cases, myxoid change may develop within the tumor. Lipid and especially hemosiderin are present within the cells, but xanthoma cells are usually absent. Multifocal hemorrhage is a striking feature in all cases and results in the formation of irregular cystic spaces (Fig. 14-28). Although these spaces resemble vascular spaces, they are not lined by endothelium but rather by flattened tumor cells. Small vessels may be present at the periphery of the nodules, but they do not seem to be the major components of these tumors. Inflammatory cells consist of a mixture of lymphocytes and plasma cells. Germinal center formation is occasionally observed, a feature that suggests lymph node metastasis, especially if the tumor is a recurrent one. The resemblance to a lymph node is further heightened by the thick pseudocapsule, a structure often interpreted as a lymph node capsule. However, unlike a true lymph node, there are no subcapsular or medullary sinuses, and germinal center formation occurs randomly around the tumor, without a predilection for the subcapsu-

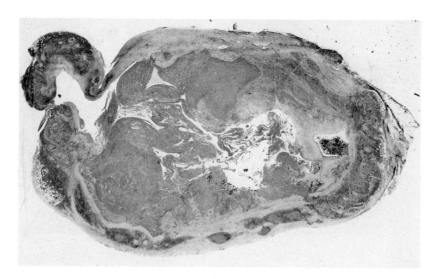

FIG. 14-26. Angiomatoid fibrous histiocytoma showing partially cystic tumor mass surrounded by a dense fibrous pseudocapsule and prominent lymphoid cuff. (×5.) (From Enzinger FM: *Cancer* 44:2147, 1979.)

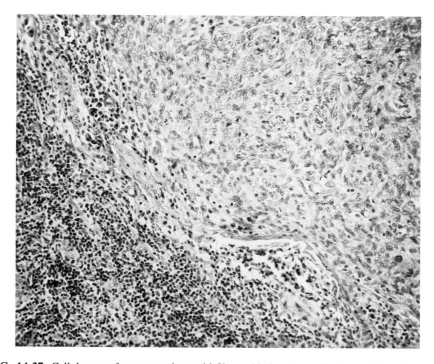

FIG. 14-27. Cellular area from an angiomatoid fibrous histiocytoma. Histiocyte-like cells are arranged in solid sheets. Lymphoid infiltrate surrounds tumor nodule. (×160.) (From Enzinger FM: *Cancer* 44:2147, 1979.)

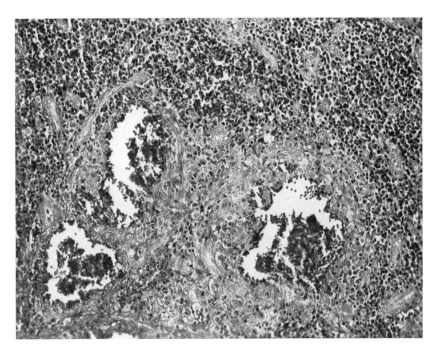

FIG. 14-28. Cystic area of angiomatoid fibrous histiocytoma. Hemorrhagic spaces simulate vascular spaces but are lined by several layers of tumor cells rather than normal endothelium. (×160.)

lar zone. Differentiation of these tumors from hemorrhagic fibrous histiocytomas is discussed in Chapter 13.

Discussion

Angiomatoid fibrous histiocytoma was originally believed to be a reasonably aggressive neoplasm, based on follow-up of a small number of cases ascertained retrospectively.[120] Evaluation of a large number of cases diagnosed accurately and treated adequately indicates that the tumor has a relatively good prognosis, however.[118] Of over 100 patients evaluated, only 20% developed local recurrence and less than 1% (one patient) developed distant metastatic disease. A number of factors can be correlated with the risk of local recurrence. These include infiltrating margins, location on the head and neck, or involvement of skeletal muscle as opposed to subcutis.[118] Complete surgical excision without adjuvant therapy is the appropriate approach for these low-grade tumors.

Since the original description of this tumor in 1979, a number of views have been espoused concerning the line of differentiation. Early views endorsing the belief that these lesions were endothelial[126] are unsupported by immunohistochemical data showing that the lesions do not express any of the well-known vascular markers.[118,121,124] Although the lesions have a decidedly histiocytic appearance and show ample evidence of phagocytosis of hemosiderin, immunohistochemical analysis of histiocytic antigens has likewise been disappointing.[118] The tumors do not express

muramidase, L-1, or Leu-M. About half of cases express CD68 (KP-1),[118] probably because of acquisition of this antigen in cells that are phagocytic and possess a high density of phagolysosomes. An intriguing, but not yet fully understood, observation is the finding of desmin in occasional cases.[118,121] Although this finding has been construed as evidence of myoid differentiation,[121] the presence of this antigen in occasional tumors that are clearly not myoid urges a conservative interpretation of this finding at present.

PLEXIFORM FIBROHISTIOCYTIC TUMOR
Clinical findings

Plexiform fibrohistiocytic tumor is the most recently described of the fibrohistiocytic tumors of intermediate malignancy.[129] Like giant cell fibroblastoma and angiomatoid fibrous histiocytoma, it occurs almost exclusively in children and young adults and is rarely encountered after the age of 30 years. It typically presents as a slowly growing mass of the deep dermis and subcutaneous tissues. In our experience, the most common location is the upper extremity (63%), followed by the lower extremity (14%).

Gross and microscopic findings

The lesions are relatively small (1 to 3 cm) ill-defined masses having a gray-white trabecular appearance. In its most typical form, accounting for about 40% of cases, the lesion contains a mixture of two components: a differentiated fibroblastic component and a round cell histiocytic

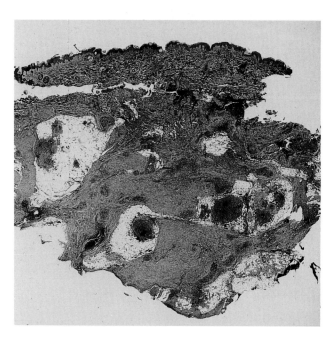

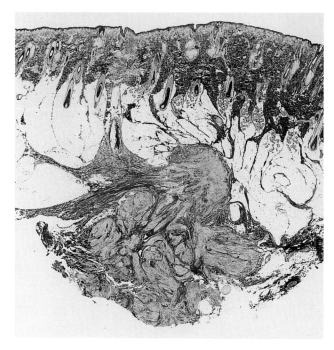

FIG. 14-29. Plexiform fibrohistiocytic tumor showing multiple nodules involving subcutis. (×5.)

FIG. 14-30. Plexiform fibrohistiocytic tumor showing ramifying fascicles of tumor in the subcutis. (×5.)

component containing multinucleated giant cells. At low power one is impressed by the numerous tiny cellular nodules that occupy the dermis and subcutaneous tissue (Figs. 14-29 and 14-30). These nodules are composed of nests of histiocytic cells that often contain multinucleated, osteoclast-like giant cells and occasionally undergo focal hemorrhage (Figs. 14-31 to 14-35). The cells within these nodules are very well differentiated and do not display atypia or significant levels of mitotic activity. These nodules, in turn, are circumscribed by short fascicles of fibroblastic cells (Fig. 14-30) that intersect slightly or ramify within the soft tissue, creating a plexiform growth pattern. The fascicles of spindled cells to some extent resemble fibromatosis, except that the cells are usually plumper and the fascicles shorter than those of fibromatosis. In the less typical case, the two components described above may not be equally represented. For example, in a minority of cases the nodules of giant cells may be rare or absent, and only short intersecting fascicles of plump spindled cells are seen (Fig. 14-33). In other cases there may be a blending between the nodules and the fascicles, and the cells within these two zones may appear to be in an intermediate stage between fibroblasts and histiocytes (Fig. 14-34). In rare cases, which probably represent part of the same spectrum, nodules of histiocytes and giant cells will infiltrate the soft tissue without a fibroblastic component. Such lesions will initially suggest the diagnosis of giant cell tumor of tendon sheath, except for the pattern of growth and the location.

Immunohistochemically the cells within these tumors express smooth muscle actin, suggesting myofibroblastic differentiation. Curiously the rounded cells within the nodules express CD68,[131] a panhistiocyte marker, but not other histiocyte-associated markers, including lysozyme, HLA-DR, and L-1. Ultrastructural studies have identified cells with features of histiocytes as well as myofibroblasts.[128] Cytogenetic analysis has been carried out in one case.[132]

Differential diagnosis

A variety of benign diagnoses that include granuloma, fibrous hamartoma, fibrous histiocytoma, giant cell tumor, and fibromatosis are entertained in these cases. The most important distinctions are those that will materially affect the management of the patient. It is essential to distinguish the lesion from an infectious granulomatous process. In the typical case the presence of the associated fibroblastic cuffing of the histiocytic nodules is usually sufficient to suggest an alternative diagnosis. However, in those tumors that are predominantly histiocytic, the important observations include the fact that these tumors do not have a surrounding inflammatory infiltrate nor do the histiocytic nodules undergo central necrosis. Predominantly fibroblastic forms of plexiform fibrohistiocytic tumor may resemble fibromatosis; however, in fibromatosis, the fascicles are wider, longer, and composed of more slender fibroblastic cells.

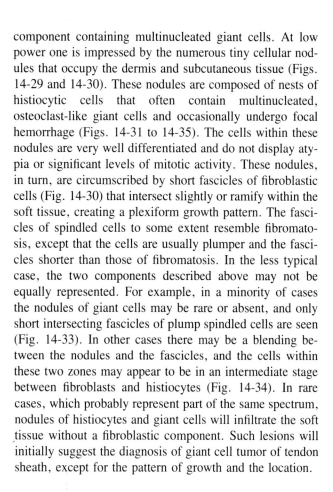

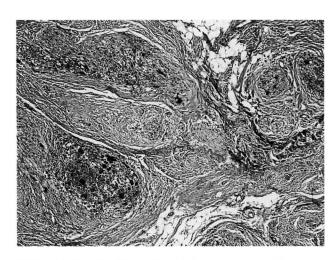

FIG. 14-31. Plexiform fibrohistiocytic tumor illustrating histiocyte-like nodule circumscribed by fascicles of fibroblasts. (×100.)

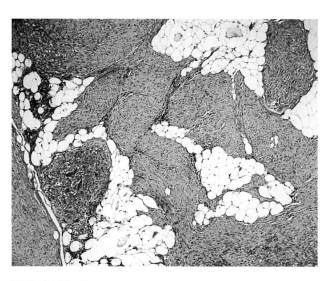

FIG. 14-32. Tumor illustrating histiocyte-like nodule circumscribed by fascicles of fibroblasts. (×100.)

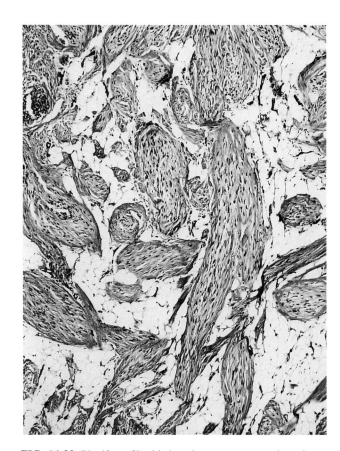

FIG. 14-33. Plexiform fibrohistiocytic tumor composed nearly exclusively of short, ramifying fascicles of fibroblasts without nodules of histiocytes. (×160.)

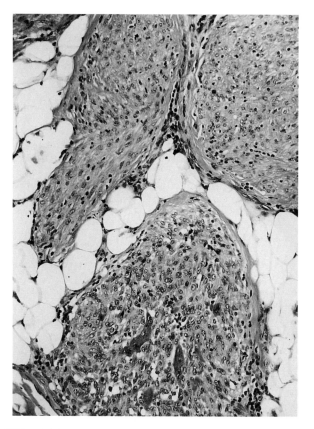

FIG. 14-34. Plexiform fibrohistiocytic tumor showing a subtle blending of the rounded histiocytic component with the fibroblastic component. (×250.)

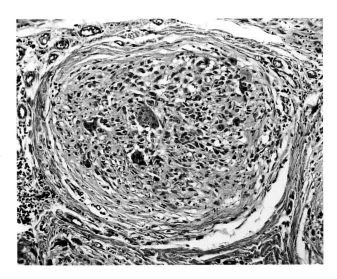

FIG. 14-35. Plexiform fibrohistiocytic tumor showing high-power view of histiocyte-like cells comprising tumor nodules. Center of nodule contains osteoclast-like giant cells. (×250.)

Discussion

Based on the original series of 65 cases, these tumors appear to be low-grade neoplasms that frequently recur (40%) within 1 to 2 years of the original diagnosis.[129] In addition, Enzinger and Zhang reported lymph node metastasis in two of the 32 patients with follow-up information. Both of these patients developed recurrence; within 9 to 36 months the lymph node metastasis ensued. One of these two patients was alive and well following radical excision of the lymph node metastasis and chemotherapy, whereas the other was lost to follow-up. Unfortunately, no histological parameters (e.g., mitotic activity, vascular invasion) have been correlated with aggressive behavior. Ideally these lesions should be completely, if not widely, excised. It does not seem appropriate to commit the patient to adjuvant therapy based on the limited risk of regional lymph node disease.

REFERENCES
Dermatofibrosarcoma protuberans and Bednař tumor

1. Adams JT, Salzstein SL: Metastasizing dermatofibrosarcoma protuberans. *Am Surg* 29:879, 1963.
2. Albini A, Krieg T, Schmoeckel C, et al: Dermatofibrosarcoma protuberans: Altered collagen metabolism in cell culture. *J Invest Dermatol* 85:381, 1985.
3. Alguacil-Garcia A, Unni KK, Goellner JR: Histogenesis of dermatofibrosarcoma protuberans. An ultrastructural study. *Am J Clin Pathol* 69:427, 1978.
4. Ashack RJ, Tejada E, Parker C, et al: A localized atrophic plaque on the back: dermatofibrosarcoma protuberans (DFSP) (atrophic variant). *Arch Dermatol* 128:1549, 1990.
5. Aubock L: Zur Ultrastruktur fibröser und histiocytärer Hauttumoren (Dermatofibrom, Dermatofibrosarcoma protuberans, Fibroxanthom und Histiocytom). *Virchows Arch (Pathol Anat)* 368:253, 1975.
6. Banjerjee SS, Harris M, Eyden BP, et al: Granular cell variant of dermatofibrosarcoma protuberans. *Histopathology* 17:375, 1990.
7. Barnhill DR, Boling R, Nobles W, et al: Vulvar dermatofibrosarcoma protuberans. *Gynecol Oncol* 30:149, 1988.
8. Bednař B: Storiform neurofibroma in core of naevocellular naevi. *J Pathol* 101:199, 1970.
9. Bednař B: Storiform neurofibromas of the skin, pigmented and nonpigmented. *Cancer* 10:368, 1957.
10. Bezecny R: Lungenmetastasen beim Dermatofibrosarcoma protuberans. *Arch Dermatol u Syphil* 169:347, 1933.
11. Binkley GW: Dermatofibrosarcoma protuberans. Report of six cases. *Arch Dermatol* 40:578, 1939.
12. Bock JE, Andreasson B, Thorn A, et al: Dermatofibrosarcoma protuberans of the vulva. *Gynecol Oncol* 20:129, 1985.
13. Bonnabeau RC, Stoughton WB, Armanious AW, et al: Dermatofibrosarcoma protuberans: report of a case with pulmonary metastasis and multiple intrathoracic recurrences. *Oncology* 29:1, 1974.
14. Borrie P: Dermatofibrosarcoma protuberans. *Br J Surg* 39:452, 1952.
15. Brenner W, Schaefler K, Chhabra H, et al: Dermatofibrosarcoma protuberans metastatic to a regional lymph node. *Cancer* 36:1897, 1975.
16. Bridge JA, Neff JR, Sandberg AA: Cytogenetic analysis of dermatofibrosarcoma protuberans. *Cancer Genet Cytogenet* 49:199, 1990.
17. Burkhardt BR, Soule EH, Winkelmann RK: Dermatofibrosarcoma protuberans: study of 56 cases. *Am J Surg* 111:638, 1966.
18. Connelly JH, Evans HL: Dermatofibrosarcoma protuberans: a clinicopathologic review with emphasis on fibrosarcomatous areas. *Am J Surg Pathol* 16:921, 1992.
19. Costa OG: Progressive recurrent dermatofibroma (Darier-Ferrand). *Arch Dermatol* 54:432, 1946.
20. Darier J, Ferrand M: Dermatofibromas progressifs et recidivants ou fibrosarcomes de la peau. *Ann Dermatol Syph* 5:545, 1924.
21. David MMV, Preaux J: Dermatofibrosarcome de Darier-Ferrand chez l'enfant. *Bull Soc Franc Derm Syph* 75:187, 1968.
22. Degos R, Mouly R, Civatte J, et al: Dermatofibro-sarcome de Darier-Ferrand, datant de 70 ans, opere au stade ultime de tumeur monstrueuse. *Bull Soc Franc Derm Syph* 74:190, 1967.
23. Ding JA, Enjoji M: Dermatofibrosarcoma protuberans with fibrosarcomatous areas: a clinicopathologic study of nine cases and a comparison with allied tumors. *Cancer* 64:7212, 1989.
24. Ding JA, Hashimoto H, Sugimoto T, et al: Bednař tumor (pigmented dermatofibrosarcoma protuberans). An analysis of six cases. *Acta Pathol Jpn* 40:744, 1990.
25. Dohan FC, Kornblith PL, Wellum GR: S-100 protein and 2′, 3′-cyclic nucleotide 3′ phosphohydrololase in human brain tumors. *Acta Neuropathol* (Berl) 40:123, 1977.
26. Dupree WB, Langloss JM, Weiss SW: Pigmented dermatofibrosarcoma protuberans (Bednař tumor): A pathologic, ultrastructural, and immunohistochemical study. *Am J Surg Pathol* 9:630, 1985.
27. Fettich J: Dermatofibrosarcoma protuberans with periosteal reaction. *Acta Dermatol Venerol* 36:158, 1956.
28. Fisher ER, Hellstrom HR: Dermatofibrosarcoma with metastases simulating Hodgkin's disease and reticulum cell sarcoma. *Cancer* 19:1165, 1966.
29. Fletcher CDM, Evans BJ, Macartney JC, et al: Dermatofibrosarcoma protuberans: a clinicopathological and immunohistochemical study with a review of the literature. *Histopathology* 9:921, 1985.

30. Fletcher CD, Theaker JM, Flanagan A, et al: Pigmented dermatofibrosarcoma protuberans (Bednař tumour): melanocytic colonization or neuroectodermal differentiation? A clinicopathological and immunohistochemical study. *Histopathology* 13:631, 1988.

31. Gaynor R, Irie R, Morton D, et al: S-100 protein: A marker for human malignant melanomas. *Lancet* 1:869, 1981.

32. Gentele H: Malignant fibroblastic tumors of the skin: clinical and pathological-anatomical studies of 129 cases of malignant fibroblastic tumors of the cutaneous and subcutaneous tissue observed at radiumhemmet during period 1927-1947. *Acta Dermatol Venerol* 31(suppl 27):1, 1951.

33. Gutierrez G, Ospina JE, de Baez NE, et al: Dermatofibrosarcoma protuberans. *Int J Dermatol* 23:396, 1984.

34. Hagedorn M, Thomas C, von Kannen W: Dermatofibrosarcoma protuberans mit Ubergang in ein sogenanntes Fibrosarkom. *Dermatologica* 149:84, 1974.

35. Hashimoto K, Brownstein MH, Jakobiec FA: Dermatofibrosarcoma protuberans. *Arch Dermatol* 110:874, 1974.

36. Hertlber AE: Fibrosarcomatous tumors of the skin of the trunk. *Ann Surg* 84:489, 1926.

37. Hess KA, Hanke CW, Estes NC, et al: Chemosurgical reports: myxoid dermatofibrosarcoma protuberans. *J Dermatol Surg Oncol* 11:268, 1985.

38. Hoffert PW: Dermatofibrosarcoma protuberans: a review of the literature and presentation of three cases. *Surgery* 31:705, 1952.

39. Hoffmann E: Uber das knollentreibende Fibrosarkom der Haut (Dermatofibrosarkoma protuberans). *Dermat Ztschr* 43:1, 1925.

40. Holm J: Dermatofibrosarcoma protuberans: report of a case with review of the literature. *Acta Chir Scand* 134:303, 1968.

41. Ishii T, Koide O: An autopsy case of metastasizing protuberant dermatofibrosarcoma. *Acta Pathol Jpn* 25:503, 1975.

42. Junaid TA, Ani AN, Ejeckam GC: Dermatofibrosarcoma protuberans in the parotid gland: a case report. *Br J Oral Surg* 12:298, 1975.

43. Kahn LB, Saxe N, Gordon W: Dermatofibrosarcoma protuberans with lymph node and pulmonary metastases. *Arch Dermatol* 114:599, 1978.

44. Kindblom LG, Jacobsen GK, Jacobsen M: Immunohistochemical investigations of tumors of supposed fibroblastic-histiocytic origin. *Hum Pathol* 13:834, 1982.

45. Lambert WC, Aggress R, Figge DC, et al: Dermatofibrosarcoma protuberans of the vulva. *Gynecol Oncol* 16:288, 1983.

46. Lautier R, Wolff HH, Jones RE: An immunohistochemical study of dermatofibrosarcoma protuberans supports its fibroblastic character and contradicts neuroectodermal or histiocytic components. *Am J Dermatopathol* 12:25, 1990.

47. Leake JF, Buscema J, Cho KR, et al: Dermatofibrosarcoma protuberans of the vulva. *Gynecol Oncol* 41:245, 1991.

48. Longhin S: Considerations sur le diagnostic histopathologique et sur le traitement du dermatofibrome de Darier-Ferrand. *Ann Dermatol Syph (Paris)* 94:159, 1967.

49. Lopes JM, Paiva ME: Dermatofibrosarcoma protuberans: A histological and ultrastructural study of 11 cases with emphasis on the study of recurrences and histogenesis. *Pathol Res Pract* 187:806, 1991.

50. Manalan SS, Cohen IK, Theogaraj SD: Dermatofibrosarcoma protuberans or keloid—a warning. *Plast Reconstr Surg* 54:96, 1974.

51. Mandahl N, Heim S, Willen H, et al: Supernumerary ring chromosome as the sole cytogenetic abnormality in a dermatofibrosarcoma protuberans. *Cancer Genet Cytogenet* 49:273, 1990.

52. Marks LB, Suit HD, Rosenberg AE, et al: Dermatofibrosarcoma protuberans treated with radiation therapy. *Int J Radiat Oncol Biol Phys* 17:379, 1989.

53. McGregor JK: Dermatofibrosarcoma protuberans. *Am J Surg* 99:97, 1960.

54. McGregor JK: Role of surgery in the management of dermatofibrosarcoma protuberans. *Ann Surg* 154:255, 1961.

55. McKee PH, Fletcher CD: Dermatofibrosarcoma protuberans presenting in infancy and childhood. *J Cutan Pathol* 18:241, 1991.

56. McLeiland J, Chu T: Dermatofibrosarcoma protuberans arising in a BCG vaccination scar. *Arch Dermatol* 124:496, 1988.

57. McPeak CJ, Cruz T, Nicastri AD: Dermatofibrosarcoma protuberans: an analysis of 86 cases—five with metastasis. *Ann Surg* 166(suppl 12):803, 1967.

58. Melezer M, Dvorszky C: Acanthosis nigricans bei Dermatofibrosarcoma protuberans mit multiplen Hautmetastasen. *Haurtazt* 8:54, 1957.

59. Mendoza CB, Gerwig WH, Watne AL: Dermatofibrosarcoma protuberans with metastases treated with methotrexate. *Am J Surg* 120:119, 1970.

60. Miyamoto Y, Morimatsu M, Nakashima T: Pigmented storiform neurofibroma. *Acta Pathol Jpn* 34:821, 1984.

61. Michelson HE: Dermatofibrosarcoma protuberans. *Surgery* 31:705, 1952.

62. Michelson HE: Dermatofibrosarcoma protuberans (Darier Hoffman). *Arch Dermatol* 25:1127, 1932.

63. Moore BW: A soluble protein characteristic of the nervous system. *Biochem Biophys Res Commun* 19:739, 1965.

64. Mopper C, Pinkus H: Dermatofibrosarcoma protuberans. Report of two cases. *Am J Clin Pathol* 20:171, 1950.

65. Nakajma T, Watanabe S, Sato Y, et al: Immunohistochemical demonstration of S100 protein in human malignant melanoma and pigmented nevi. *Gan* 72:335, 1981.

66. Nakazato Y, Ishizeki J, Takahashi KN, et al: Immunohistochemical localization of S100 protein in granular cell myoblastoma. *Cancer* 49:1624, 1982.

67. O'Dowd J, Laidler P: Progression of dermatofibrosarcoma protuberans to malignant fibrous histiocytoma: report of a case with implications for tumour histogenesis. *Hum Pathol* 19:368, 1988.

68. Oku T, Takigawa M, Fukamizu H, et al: Tissue cultures of benign and malignant fibrous histiocytomas: SEM observations. *J Cutan Pathol* 11:534, 1984.

69. Onoda N, Tsutsumi Y, Kakudo K, et al: Pigmented dermatofibrosarcoma protuberans (Bednař tumor). An autopsy case with systemic metastasis. *Acta Pathol Jpn* 40:935, 1990.

70. Ozawa A, Niizuma K, Onkido M, et al: Pigmented dermatofibrosarcoma protuberans: an analysis of six cases. *Acta Pathol Jpn* 40:935, 1990.

71. Ozzello L, Hamels J: The histiocytic nature of dermatofibrosarcoma protuberans: tissue culture and electron microscopic study. *Am J Clin Pathol* 65:136, 1976.

72. Pack GT, Tabah EJ: Dermatofibrosarcoma protuberans. *Arch Surg* 62:391, 1951.

73. Petkov I, Andreev VC: Dermatofibrosarcoma protuberans in seltener Lokalisation. *Hautarzt* 23:508, 1972.

74. Petoin DS, Verola O, Banzet P, et al: Dermatofibrosarcome de Darier et Ferrand: Etude de 96 cas sur 15 ans. *Chirurgie* 111:132, 1985.

75. Phelan JT, Juardo J: Dermatofibrosarcoma protuberans. *Am J Surg* 106:943, 1963.

76. Przybora LA, Wojnerowicz C: Malignancy of dermatofibrosarcoma protuberans and report of two cases with lymph gland metastases. *Oncology* 12:236, 1959.

77. Robinson JK: Dermatofibrosarcoma protuberans resected by Mohs' surgery (chemosurgery): a 5-year prospective study. *J Am Acad Dermatol* 12:1093, 1985.

78. Roses DF, Valensi Q, Latrenta G, et al: Surgical treatment of dermatofibrosarcoma protuberans. *Surg Gynecol Obstet* 162:449, 1986.

79. Rutgers EJ, Kroon BB, Albus-Lutter CE, et al: Dermatofibrosar-

coma protuberans: treatment and prognosis. *Eur J Surg Oncol* 18:241, 1992.

80. Sauter LS, DeFeo CP: Dermatofibrosarcoma protuberans of the face. *Arch Dermatol* 104:671, 1971.

81. Schiff BL, Tye MJ, Kern AB, et al: Dermatofibrosarcoma protuberans: review of the literature and report of four cases. *Am J Surg* 99:301, 1960.

82. Sciacchitano G: Sopra un caso di fibrosarcoma cutaneo con metastasi pulmonari. *Tumori* 9:427, 1935.

83. Senear FE, Andrews E, Willis DA: Progressive and recurrent dermatofibrosarcoma. *Arch Dermatol* 17:821, 1928.

84. Shaw MH: A case of dermatofibrosarcoma protuberans. *Br J Plast Surg* 8:257, 1955.

85. Shelley WB: Malignant melanoma and dermatofibrosarcoma in a 60-year-old patient with lifelong acrodermatitis enteropathica. *J Am Acad Dermatol* 6:63, 1982.

86. Shneidman D, Belizaire R: Arsenic exposure followed by the development of dermatofibrosarcoma protuberans. *Cancer* 58:1585, 1986.

87. Simstein NL, Tuthill RJ, Sperber EE, et al: Dermatofibrosarcoma protuberans: case reports and review of literature. *South Med J* 70:487, 1977.

88. Smola MG, Soyer HP, Scharnagl E: Surgical treatment of dermatofibrosarcoma protuberans: a retrospective study of 20 cases with review of the literature. *Eur J Surg Oncol* 17:44, 1991.

89. Srivastava VK, Bhargava KS: Dermatofibrosarcoma protuberans. *Indian J Cancer* 9:257, 1972.

90. Stephenson CF, Berger CS, Leong SP, et al: Ring chromosome in a dermatofibrosarcoma protuberans. *Cancer Genet Cytogenet* 58:52, 1992.

91. Talib VH, Sultana Z, Patil SK, et al: Dermatofibrosarcoma protuberans: report of four cases with review of literature. *Indian J Cancer* 11:200, 1974.

92. Taylor HB, Helwig EB: Dermatofibrosarcoma protuberans: a study of 115 cases. *Cancer* 15:717, 1962.

93. Tremblay M, Bonenfant J-L, Cliche J: Le dermatofibrosarcome protuberant: Etude clinico-pathologique de trente cas avee'ultrastructure de deux cas. *Union Med Can* 99:871, 1970.

94. Tsuneyoshi M, Enjoji M: Bednař tumor (pigmented dermatofibrosarcoma protuberans): an analysis of six cases. *Acta Pathol Jpn* 40:744, 1990.

95. Virmani P: Dermatofibrosarcoma protuberans. *Br J Surg* 49:435, 1962.

96. Weber L, Meigel WN: Nature of collagen in dermatofibrosarcoma protuberans. *Arch Dermatol Res* 265:55, 1979.

97. Whalen WP: Dermatofibrosarcoma protuberans. *Plast Reconstr Surg* 31:461, 1963.

98. Wooldridge WE: Dermatofibrosarcoma protuberans: a tumor too lightly considered. *Arch Dermatol* 75:132, 1957.

99. Wrotnowski U, Cooper PH, Shmookler BM: Fibrosarcomatous change in dermatofibrosarcoma protuberans. *Am J Surg Pathol* 12:287, 1988.

100. Yaffee HS: Pseudosarcomatous dermatofibroma. *Br J Dermatol* 89 (suppl 9):651, 1973.

101. Yosida H, Matsui K, Hashimoto K, et al: Dermatofibrosarcoma protuberans and its tissue culture study: ultrastructural, enzyme, histochemical, and immunological study. *Acta Pathol Jpn* 32:83, 1982.

Giant cell fibroblastoma

102. Abdul-Karim FW, Evans HL, Silva EG: Giant cell fibroblastoma: a report of three cases. *Am J Clin Pathol* 83:165, 1985.

103. Alguacil-Garcia A: Giant cell fibroblastoma recurring as a dermatofibrosarcoma protuberans. *Am J Surg Pathol* 15:798, 1991.

104. Allen PW, Zwi J: Giant cell fibroblastoma transforming into dermatofibrosarcoma protuberans (letter). *Am J Surg Pathol* 15:1127, 1992.

105. Barr RJ, Young EM, Liao SY: Giant cell fibroblastoma: an immunohistochemical study. *J Cutan Pathol* 13:301, 1986.

106. Beham A, Fletcher DC: Dermatofibrosarcoma protuberans with areas resembling giant cell fibroblastoma: report of two cases. *Histopathology* 17:165, 1990.

107. Chou P, Gonzalez-Crussi F, Mangkornkanok M: Giant cell fibroblastoma. *Cancer* 63:756, 1989.

108. Coyne J, Kaftan SM, Craig, RD: Dermatofibrosarcoma protuberans recurring as a giant cell fibroblastoma. *Histopathology* 21:184, 1992.

109. Dymock RB, Allen PW, Stirling JW, et al: Giant cell fibroblastoma: a distinctive recurrent tumor of childhood. *Am J Surg Pathol* 11:263, 1987.

110. Fletcher CD: Giant cell fibroblastoma of soft tissue: a clinicopathologic and immunohistochemical study. *Histopathology* 13:499, 1988.

111. Hirose T, Sasaki M, Shintaku M: Giant cell fibroblastoma. *Acta Pathol Jpn* 40:540, 1990.

112. Kanai Y, Mukai M, Sugiura H, et al: Giant cell fibroblastoma: a case report and immunohistochemical comparison with ten cases of dermatofibrosarcoma protuberans. *Acta Pathol Jpn* 41:552, 1991.

113. Michal M, Zamecnik M: Giant cell fibroblastoma with a dermatofibrosarcoma protuberans component. *Am J Dermatopathol* 14:549, 1992.

114. Nair R, Kane SV, Borges A, et al: Giant cell fibroblastoma. *J Surg Oncol* 53:136, 1993.

115. Rosen LB, Amazon K, Weitzner J, et al: Giant cell fibroblastoma: a report of a case and review of the literature. *Am J Dermatopathol* 11:242, 1989.

116. Shmookler BM, Enzinger FM, Weiss SW: Giant cell fibroblastoma: a juvenile form of dermatofibrosarcoma protuberans. *Cancer* 15:2154, 1989.

117. Weiss SW, Nickoloff BJ: CD34 is expressed by a distinctive cell population in peripheral nerve, nerve sheath tumors, and related lesions. *Am J Surg Pathol* 17:1039, 1993.

Angiomatoid fibrous histiocytoma

118. Costa MJ, Weiss SW: Angiomatoid malignant fibrous histiocytoma: a follow-up study of 108 cases with evaluation of possible histologic predictors of outcome. *Am J Surg Pathol* 14:1126, 1990.

119. El-Naggar AK, Ro JY, Ayala AG, et al: Angiomatoid malignant fibrous histiocytoma: flow cytometric DNA analysis of six cases. *Surg Oncol* 40:201, 1989.

120. Enzinger FM: Angiomatoid malignant fibrous histiocytoma: a distinct fibrohistiocytic tumor of children and young adults simulating a vascular neoplasm. *Cancer* 44:2147, 1979.

121. Fletcher CD: Angiomatoid "malignant fibrous histiocytoma": an immunohistochemical study indicative of myoid differentiation. *Hum Pathol* 22:563, 1991.

122. Kay S: Angiomatoid malignant fibrous histiocytoma: report of two cases with ultrastructural observations of one case. *Arch Pathol Lab Med* 109:934, 1985.

123. Leu HJK, Makek M: Angiomatoid malignant fibrous histiocytoma. *Arch Pathol Lab Med* 110:2010, 1977.

124. Pettinato G, Manivel JC, De Rosa G, et al: Angiomatoid malignant fibrous histiocytoma: cytologic, immunohistochemical, ultrastructural, and flow cytometric study of 20 cases. *Mod Pathol* 3:479, 1990.

125. Smith ME, Costa MJ, Weiss SW: Evaluation of CD68 and other histiocytic antigens in angiomatoid malignant fibrous histiocytoma. *Am J Surg Pathol* 15:757, 1991.

126. Sun CC Jr, Toker C, Breitenecker R: An ultrastructural study of angiomatoid fibrous histiocytoma. *Cancer* 40:2103, 1982.

127. Wegmann W, Heitz PU: Angiomatoid malignant fibrous histiocytoma: evidence for the histiocytic origin of tumor cells. *Virchows Arch (Pathol Anat)* 406:59, 1985.

Plexiform fibrohistiocytic tumor

128. Angervall L, Kindsblom LG, Lindholm K, et al: Plexiform fibro-histiocytic tumor: report of a case involving preoperative aspiration cytology and immunohistochemical and ultrastructural analysis of surgical specimens. *Pathol Res Pract* 188:350, 1992.

129. Enzinger FM, Zhang RY: Plexiform fibrohistiocytic tumor presenting in children and young adults: An analysis of 65 cases. *Am J Surg Pathol* 12:818, 1988.

130. Giard F, Bonneau R, Raymond GP: Plexiform fibrohistiocytic tumor. *Dermatologica* 183:290, 1991.

131. Hollowood K, Holley MP, Fletcher CD: Plexiform fibrohistiocytic tumour: clinicopathological, immunohistochemical and ultrastructural analysis in favour of a myofibroblastic lesion. *Histopathology* 19:503, 1991.

132. Smith S, Fletcher CD, Smith MA, et al: Cytogenetic analysis of a plexiform fibrohistiocytic tumor. *Cancer Genet Cytogenet* 48:31, 1990.

CHAPTER 15

MALIGNANT FIBROHISTIOCYTIC TUMORS

The term *malignant fibrous histiocytoma* was first introduced in 1963 to refer to a group of soft tissue tumors characterized by a storiform or cartwheel-like growth pattern. Although the tumors initially described by Ozzello et al.[107] and later by O'Brien and Stout[105] had a predominantly fibroblastic appearance, it was postulated that they were derived from histiocytes that could assume the appearance and function of fibroblasts ("facultative fibroblasts"). This theory was based principally on tissue culture studies of tumor explants[107] in which the cultured tumor cells initially resembled histiocytes and exhibited ameboid movement and phagocytosis. Later the cells assumed bipolar shapes resembling fibroblasts. The versatility of the histiocyte became an accepted means of explaining the bimodal population of cells often encountered in these tumors. The large number of earlier ultrastructural studies has both endorsed and refuted the histiocytic origin of these tumors, while at the same time raising fundamental questions concerning structure and function.

The advent of immunohistochemistry and the accessibility of numerous monoclonal antibodies directed against various structural proteins of specific cell types have answered some questions and also raised new ones. The debate as to whether malignant fibrous histiocytoma represents a true histiocytic neoplasm has largely subsided. Most studies have failed to confirm monocyte and macrophage differentiation, but rather have established a closer phenotypic link with the fibroblast. The more contentious issue has been whether malignant fibrous histiocytoma represents a homogenous entity or a collection of sarcomas of diverse type in which subtle differentiation has been overlooked. Clearly the extent to which this represents a homogenous versus a heterogeneous entity will depend, in part, on the degree of sampling and the number of ancillary studies a pathologist is willing to devote to a given case, as well as his or her definitional criteria for making alternative diagnoses. A recent large retrospective study of tumors diagnosed as pleomorphic sarcoma indicated that approximately one fourth actually fulfilled current diagnostic criteria for malignant fi-

brous histiocytoma.[53] Undoubtedly, "interlopers" will be found within the category of malignant fibrous histiocytoma from time to time; however, this is still a useful category of tumors, provided a modicum of care is taken in establishing the diagnosis. Specific issues related to diagnostic criteria are discussed later in the chapter. There is little pressing need to change the term *malignant fibrous histiocytoma*, even though it is a taxonomically inaccurate term, because it is well accepted in the clinical literature and it implies a pleomorphic high-grade sarcoma, usually of adults, lacking specific light microscopic features of differentiation apart from collagen production.

The ambiguity concerning the behavior of these tumors expressed in the early work of O'Brien and Stout has been clarified by several large clinical studies[33,78,108,132,134] indicating the malignant nature of the lesions and the fact that prognosis can be related to various factors, including size, depth, location, and clinical stage.

The spectrum of malignant fibrohistiocytic tumors includes atypical fibroxanthoma, a cutaneous form that carries an excellent prognosis because of its small size and superficiality, as well as the conventional or more deeply situated malignant fibrous histiocytoma, which is divided into several subtypes (storiform-pleomorphic, myxoid, giant cell, and inflammatory). Angiomatoid malignant fibrous histiocytoma, a distinctive tumor of childhood, which was formerly classified with the conventional malignant fibrous histiocytomas of adults, has been grouped with the fibrohistiocytic tumors of intermediate malignancy (see Chapter 14) because of its excellent rate of survival.

Although malignant fibrous histiocytoma has been defined classically as a soft tissue sarcoma, it may arise from supporting structures of various organs. Indeed, it has recently been described in bone* as well as other organs.† In these sites its incidence, biological potential, and diagnostic criteria are not fully defined and are beyond the scope of this chapter.

---

*References 42, 51, 52, 64, 95, 99, 101, 122.
†References 35, 40, 44, 57, 60, 83, 123.

ATYPICAL FIBROXANTHOMA

Atypical fibroxanthoma is a pleomorphic tumor that usually occurs on actinic-damaged skin of the elderly. It has been referred to in the past as *pseudosarcoma of the skin*,[8,25] *paradoxical fibrosarcoma*,[4] *pseudosarcomatous dermatofibroma*,[17] and *pseudosarcomatous reticulohistiocytoma*.[10] It is histologically indistinguishable from pleomorphic forms of malignant fibrous histiocytoma. From a conceptual point of view we regard it as a superficial form of that tumor, which, by virtue of its superficial location, almost invariably pursues a benign course. However, from a practical point of view we have retained the term *atypical fibroxanthoma* to separate it from deep forms of malignant fibrous histiocytoma, which require more radical therapy and carry a less favorable prognosis. Unfortunately the term *atypical fibroxanthoma* has also been loosely used to refer to borderline or even malignant-appearing fibrohistiocytic tumors not occurring in the skin.[3,16] The nonrestrictive use of this term, however, is confusing and should be discouraged.

Clinical findings

Atypical fibroxanthoma occurs in two clinical settings.[9] In the more common form of the disease the lesion presents on the exposed surface of the head and neck, particularly the nose, cheek, and ear. Elderly persons are afflicted with this form of the disease. In the less common form, which accounts for about one fourth of cases, the tumor occurs on the limbs and trunk of young persons. Both forms of the disease are characterized by a solitary nodule or ulcer that produces few symptoms aside from bleeding; it is often present several months before biopsy.

Solar radiation probably represents a predisposing factor in the pathogenesis of this disease. This is supported by the common occurrence of the tumor on actinic-damaged skin and its frequent association with other actinic-related lesions (e.g., basal cell carcinoma, squamous carcinoma). Occupational and therapeutic irradiation may also be etiological factors, but this is less well documented. The incidence of previous irradiation varies from less than 5%[9] in some series to over 50%[12] in others. In most instances the latent period between the previous irradiation and the appearance of the atypical fibroxanthoma is more than 10 years and, thus, well in keeping with the accepted interval for a radiation-induced tumor. Indeed, many early reports of sarcoma-like lesions of skin following irradiation are probably examples of atypical fibroxanthoma.[19]

Gross appearance

Grossly, the lesions are solitary nodules or ulcers usually measuring less than 2 cm in diameter (Figs. 15-1 and 15-2). Their appearance is not distinctive, and for this reason a variety of preoperative diagnoses are considered, including basal cell carcinoma, squamous carcinoma, pyogenic granuloma, and sebaceous cyst.[9]

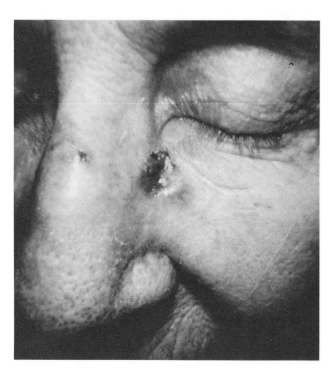

FIG. 15-1. Ulcerating atypical fibroxanthoma from nose of 80-year-old woman. Grossly, tumor resembled a basal cell carcinoma. (From Fretzin DF, Helwig EB: *Cancer* 31:1541, 1973.)

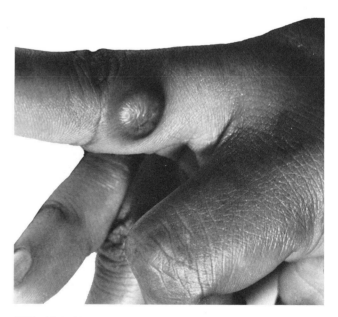

FIG. 15-2. Nodular atypical fibroxanthoma from finger of 36-year-old woman. Atypical fibroxanthomas in young patients typically occur on the extremities in contrast to those in elderly patients, which are located on sun-exposed or actinic-damaged surfaces. (From Fretzin DF, Helwig EB: *Cancer* 31:1541, 1973.)

Microscopic findings

These tumors are expansile dermal nodules that may abut the epidermis, causing pressure atrophy or ulceration. Alternatively, a *grenz* zone of uninvolved dermis may be present (Fig. 15-3). The tumor compresses the skin appendages laterally and extends into the subcutis. However, by definition, the tumor does not extensively involve the subcutis, nor does it invade deeper structures such as fascia or muscle. Areas adjacent to these lesions may display solar elastosis, vascular dilatation, and capillary proliferation.

Histologically these tumors resemble pleomorphic forms of malignant fibrous histiocytoma. They are characterized by bizarre cells arranged in a haphazard or vague fascicular pattern (Fig. 15-4). Rarely is a storiform pattern evident. The cells are spindle shaped or rounded and exhibit multinucleation, pleomorphism, and numerous typical and atypical mitotic figures. The cells occasionally possess small droplets of neutral fat as well as PAS-positive, diastase-resistant material, two features probably reflecting in part degenerative changes. Occasional inflammatory cells may be present. Rarely foci of osteoid may be noted.[5] Necrosis, a common feature of malignant fibrous histiocytoma, is rare and, if present in significant degree, should raise serious question as to the diagnosis of atypical fibroxanthoma (see discussion).

Overall the ultrastructural features of this tumor are quite similar to those of malignant fibrous histiocytoma. Cells possessing characteristics of fibroblasts,[2] myofibroblasts,[24] and histiocytes[1,2] have been reported. Although Langerhans' granules have been reported,[1] this finding should be questioned in view of the fact that Langerhans' cells can secondarily populate these lesions.[20] In no cases of atypical fibroxanthoma have there been prominent intercellular junctions, tonofibrils, or other features specifically suggesting epithelial differentiation. Therefore, electron microscopy has confirmed the light microscopic impression that atypical fibroxanthoma is a mesenchymal lesion rather than a spindled carcinoma or melanoma.

Differential diagnosis

The most common problem in differential diagnosis is distinguishing atypical fibroxanthoma from spindled carcinoma or melanoma. Although in general atypical fibroxanthoma is more pleomorphic, we have seen many cases of both primary and metastatic epithelial neoplasms that have exactly mimicked atypical fibroxanthoma in areas. Therefore there is no substitute for extensively sampling a given tumor, particularly when a presumptive atypical fibroxanthoma presents in an unusual setting. The tumor should be examined to make certain there is neither junctional activity nor focal epithelial differentiation. In addition to the obvious value of mucin and melanin stains, immunostains for cytokeratin and S-100 protein are extremely helpful and, in some cases, mandatory for excluding the other diag-

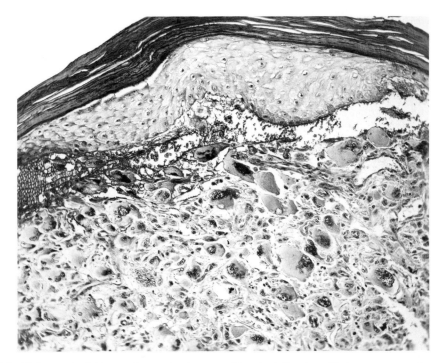

FIG. 15-3. Atypical fibroxanthoma abutting on epidermis. Dilated capillaries are commonly seen adjacent to the tumor. In this case dilatation of subepidermal vessels leads to apparent separation of epidermis from underlying tumor, a common phenomenon in these lesions. (×130.)

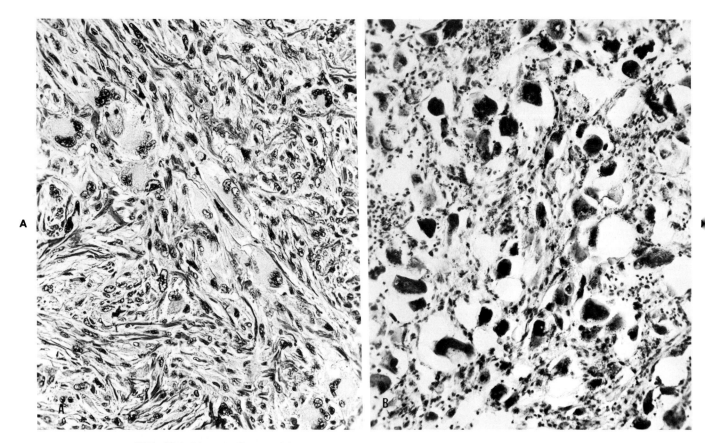

FIG. 15-4. Bizarre cells comprising atypical fibroxanthoma vary from plump spindled cells (**A**) to large rounded cells (**B**). Pleomorphism is marked, and mitotic figures are common. Occasional inflammatory cells may be scattered throughout the tumor, and in some, intracytoplasmic hemosiderin deposits (**B**) obscure cytoplasmic detail. (**A**, ×130; **B**, ×110.)

noses. Care must be exerted in interpreting S-100 protein stains in this tumor. Langerhans' histiocytes, which express S-100 protein, may be present within atypical fibroxanthomas and should not be interpreted as evidence that the lesion is a neuroectodermal tumor, specifically a melanoma. In this regard incorporation of melanoma-associated antigen (HMB-45) into the diagnostic armamentarium can be useful. Generally, distinguishing squamous carcinomas from atypical fibroxanthomas is not difficult provided immunostains are performed that will detect high-molecular-weight cytokeratins.

Atypical fibroxanthoma must also be separated from other mesenchymal tumors, most commonly malignant fibrous histiocytoma. Because we currently regard atypical fibroxanthoma as a superficial or even an early form of malignant fibrous histiocytoma, the distinction of the two is, to some extent, arbitrary. The more selective one is in making the diagnosis of atypical fibroxanthoma, the better the resultant behavior. In our opinion, if a tumor extensively involves the subcutis, penetrates fascia and muscle, or displays necrosis or vascular invasion, it should be diagnosed as malignant fibrous histiocytoma, since such tumors run a

definite risk of recurrence and metastasis. Thus tumors reported recently by Helwig and May[11] as atypical fibroxanthoma with metastases would have been designated by us as malignant fibrous histiocytoma, since the majority displayed deep invasion, necrosis, or vascular invasion.

Atypical fibroxanthoma is sometimes mistaken for leiomyosarcoma; however, leiomyosarcomas have distinct fascicles containing cells with characteristic blunt-ended nuclei. Cytoplasmic glycogen is often abundant. Trichrome stains, furthermore, demonstrate distinct longitudinal striations corresponding ultrastructurally to myofilamentous material dispersed throughout the cytoplasm. From a practical point of view, the distinction of dermal (primary) leiomyosarcoma and atypical fibroxanthoma may simply be an act of discipline because of the similarity in therapy and prognosis. However, leiomyosarcoma (particularly of the retroperitoneum) may rarely present as a cutaneous metastasis.

Discussion

Although this tumor is histologically indistinguishable from some forms of malignant fibrous histiocytoma, it deserves a special designation because of its almost uniformly excellent prognosis following conservative therapy. In the largest series in the literature, only 9 patients out of 140 developed recurrence, and none developed metastasis.[9] It is now recognized that in exceptional instances this tumor does metastasize. One such case, characterized by vascular invasion, was mentioned by Fretzin and Helwig[9] but was not included in their series. A second case was reported by Jacobs et al.[13] Although this tumor located on the nose was histologically very typical, it recurred, involved the nasal cartilage, and ultimately metastasized to a cervical lymph node. We have also seen similar cases in which an apparent atypical fibroxanthoma progressed to malignant fibrous histiocytoma and eventually metastasized. As mentioned above, the lesions reported by Helwig and May[11] as metastatic atypical fibroxanthoma, in our opinion, would have been better classified as superficial forms of malignant fibrous histiocytoma. In view of the rarity of metastases, conservative therapy is initially indicated. However, when atypical fibroxanthoma recurs as a large deeply situated mass, it should be considered malignant fibrous histiocytoma and must be treated accordingly.

Despite the widespread use of the term *atypical fibroxanthoma,* some have suggested it is not an entity but rather a heterogenous group of mesenchymal and epithelial lesions arising in a common clinical setting.[1] This view has been proposed to explain the ultrastructural variations within this group of tumors, in particular the presence of Langerhans' granules.[1] Because the diagnosis of atypical fibroxanthoma is, to some extent, an exclusionary one, it is inevitable that certain cases may be misdiagnosed. However, by thoroughly sampling such tumors and by selectively applying electron microscopy and immunohistochemistry in ambiguous cases, we believe that heterogeneity will be minimal and that the term will refer to a relatively homogenous group of superficial fibrohistiocytic neoplasms.

MALIGNANT FIBROUS HISTIOCYTOMA

Malignant fibrous histiocytoma is the most common soft tissue sarcoma of late adult life.[134] This tumor manifests a broad range of histological appearances; for this reason we have found it necessary to divide it into the following subtypes:[47-49,132]

1. Storiform-pleomorphic
2. Myxoid (myxofibrosarcoma)
3. Giant cell (malignant giant cell tumor of soft parts)
4. Inflammatory (xanthosarcoma, malignant xanthogranuloma)

Most malignant fibrous histiocytomas are cellular neoplasms having a mixture of storiform and pleomorphic areas; they have been descriptively termed the *storiform-pleomorphic* type. Depending on the relative proportions of these areas, the tumor may appear well differentiated and resemble dermatofibrosarcoma protuberans or may appear highly anaplastic. This subtype serves as the prototype for much of our thinking concerning the behavior of this group of neoplasms. The *myxoid* type, which accounts for roughly one fourth of malignant fibrous histiocytomas, is the second most common type.[132,135] It is characterized by prominent myxoid change of the stroma and also contains cellular areas indistinguishable from the foregoing type. It is separated from the storiform-pleomorphic type not only because of its distinctive appearance but also because of its better prognosis. The last two types are less common. The *giant* cell type (malignant giant cell tumor of soft parts)[58] contains numerous osteoclast-type giant cells, while the *inflammatory* type is characterized by a predominance of xanthoma cells and acute inflammatory cells. The latter group has also been called malignant *xanthogranuloma, xanthosarcoma,*[71,72,75] and *inflammatory fibrous histiocytoma.*[77,84] Although formerly grouped with malignant fibrohistiocytic tumors, angiomatoid fibrous histiocytoma has been reclassified as a fibrohistiocytic tumor of intermediate grade.

Clinical findings

The clinical features of the various subtypes are similar and are considered together (Table 15-1). Malignant fibrous histiocytoma is characteristically a tumor of late adult life,

Table 15-1. Comparison of various subtypes of malignant fibrous histiocytoma

Clinicopathological characteristics	Storiform-pleomorphic (200 cases)[134]	Myxoid (80 cases)[133]	Giant cell (32 cases)[58]	Inflammatory
Peak age	Seventh decade	Seventh decade	Late adulthood	Late adulthood
Common location	Skeletal muscle of extremities, followed by retroperitoneum	Skeletal muscle of extremities, followed by retroperitoneum	Skeletal muscle of extremities	Retroperitoneum, followed by extremities
Gross appearance	Multinodular white-gray mass	Multinodular translucent or gelatinous gray mass	Multinodular mass with prominent hemorrhage	Bulky white-yellow mass
Recurrence rate	44%	66%	~50%	Approximately one half[55]
Metastatic rate	42%	23%	~50%	Approximately one third[55]

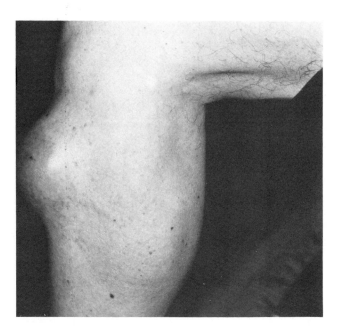

FIG. 15-5. Malignant fibrous histiocytoma of lower leg of a 62-year-old man. (From Guccion JG, Enzinger FM: *Cancer* 29:1518, 1972.)

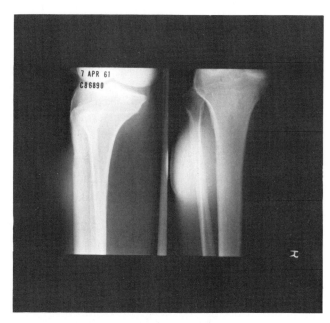

FIG. 15-6. Radiograph showing a malignant fibrous histiocytoma of the lower leg (same case as Fig. 15-5). Ill-defined soft tissue mass has eroded portion of tibial cortex.

with the majority of cases occurring in persons between the ages of 50 and 70 years.[134] Tumors in children having the same histological features as the adult forms of malignant fibrous histiocytoma are rare, and this diagnosis should always be made with caution in patients under 20 years of age. Approximately two thirds of malignant fibrous histiocytomas occur in men, and whites are affected more often than blacks or Asians. The tumor occurs most frequently on the lower extremity (Figs. 15-5 and 15-6), especially the thigh, followed by the upper extremity and retroperitoneum. A notable exception is inflammatory malignant fibrous histiocytoma, which is most often located in the retroperitoneum; relatively few are found in the extremities.

When on an extremity, the tumor presents as a painless enlarging mass usually of several months' duration. However, the duration is greatly influenced by the growth rate. For instance, we have seen several examples of slowly growing myxoid tumors in which 2 years or more have elapsed before the patients sought medical attention,[135] while rapid acceleration of the growth rate can prompt the patient to seek medical attention quickly. As with other sarcomas, acceleration of the growth rate has been observed during pregnancy.[135] In contrast to patients with extremity lesions, patients with retroperitoneal tumors develop constitutional symptoms including anorexia, malaise, weight loss, and signs of increasing abdominal pressure.[134]

Occasionally fever and leukocytosis with neutrophilia or eosinophilia may dominate the clinical presentation of this disease. This unusual constellation of symptoms has been

documented in the inflammatory type of malignant fibrous histiocytoma,[84] although we have seen it occur in other types as well. Both eosinophil chemotactic factor[66] and eosinophilopoietic activity[116] have been detected in tumor extracts of malignant fibrous histiocytoma. The symptoms usually remit following removal of the tumor. Rarely hypoglycemia may occur in association with this disease.[84,134] The mechanism of this abnormality is not clearly defined, but in one of our cases there was some evidence of secretion of an insulin-like substance by the tumor.[134] Malignant fibrous histiocytoma rarely presents as a metastatic tumor without a clinically evident primary lesion[134]; however, a small percentage of patients will present with synchronous primary and metastatic disease.[113] A number of cytogenetic abnormalities have been identified within malignant fibrous histiocytomas, but none has proved to be a consistent finding.[37,106,114]

Etiological factors

Like atypical fibroxanthoma there is excellent circumstantial evidence that some of these tumors are radiation induced. We have seen cases of malignant fibrous histiocytoma following irradiation of breast carcinoma, retinoblastoma, Hodgkin's disease, and multiple myeloma.[134] In each instance malignant fibrous histiocytoma occurred within the irradiated area after an appropriately long interval of several years. Similar reports have been mentioned in the literature.[30,57] In fact, it seems likely that some cases of postirradiation pleomorphic sarcoma are actually malignant fi-

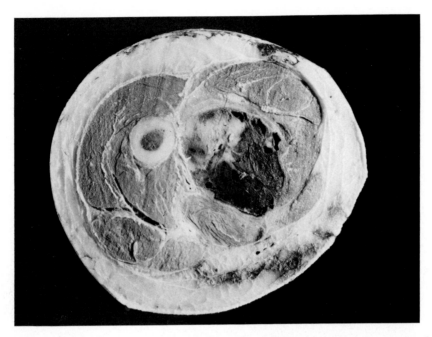

FIG. 15-7. Transverse section through a thigh amputation specimen showing the common location of these tumors in deep skeletal muscle. Tumor is represented by partially hemorrhagic mass adjacent to the femur. (From Guccion JG, Enzinger FM: *Cancer* 29:1518, 1972.)

brous histiocytomas. Aside from these sporadic iatrogenic tumors, there are few data on etiological factors in this disease. About 10% of patients with malignant fibrous histiocytoma have had or subsequently develop a second neoplasm. This does not seem statistically meaningful in view of the older age of these patients in general and the accepted risk of a second neoplasm complicating the course of a first. Several instances of malignant fibrous histiocytoma have occurred in patients exposed to phenoxyacids, although a direct causal relationship has not been established.[50] The tumor has also been reported in a patient with Lynch II syndrome.[38] The tumor has been induced in experimental animals with tea extracts[74] and with macrophages transformed with SV40 virus.[138] Intraosseous malignant fibrous histiocytomas have occurred in preexisting bone infarcts[95,98,99] and within bone at the site of shrapnel injury.[90]

Gross findings

Typically the lesions are solitary multilobulated fleshy masses between 5 and 10 cm in diameter when first detected, although retroperitoneal lesions are much larger than lesions in the extremities.[108] About two thirds of these tumors are located within skeletal muscle (Fig. 15-7), while fewer than 10% are confined exclusively to the subcutis. Tumors located adjacent to bone may induce mild degrees of periosteal reaction or cortical erosion, which can be detected radiographically (see Fig. 15-6). Although malignant fibrous histiocytoma has a circumscribed appearance

grossly, it often spreads for a considerable distance along fascial planes or between muscle fibers microscopically (Figs. 15-8 and 15-9); this accounts for its high rate of local recurrence.

On cut section most tumors are gray to white (Fig. 15-10), but this may be modified by an abundance of one or more elements. For example, the inflammatory form of malignant fibrous histiocytoma *(malignant xanthogranuloma, xanthosarcoma)* may have a yellow color because of the predominance of xanthoma cells, while hemorrhagic tumors appear brown. Myxoid malignant fibrous histiocytoma typically has a translucent mucoid appearance (see Figs. 15-22 and 15-23) and, in this respect, cannot be distinguished grossly from other myxoid sarcomas such as myxoid liposarcoma. In contrast to less aggressive fibrohistiocytic tumors, hemorrhage and necrosis are common features of this tumor. In fact about 5% of malignant fibrous histiocytomas undergo such extensive hemorrhage that they present clinically as fluctuant masses and are diagnosed as cystic hematomas.[134] Nonetheless, residual tumor cells can be identified microscopically in the wall of such "cysts," leaving no doubt as to the correct diagnosis.

Malignant fibrous histiocytoma: storiform-pleomorphic type

Microscopically, this form of malignant fibrous histiocytoma has a highly variable morphological pattern[134] and shows frequent transitions from storiform to pleomorphic

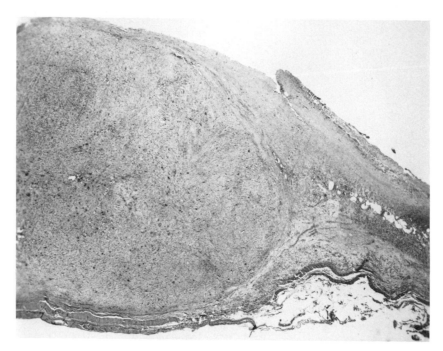

FIG. 15-8. Malignant fibrous histiocytoma arising in superficial fascia and extending along this structure. (×15.)

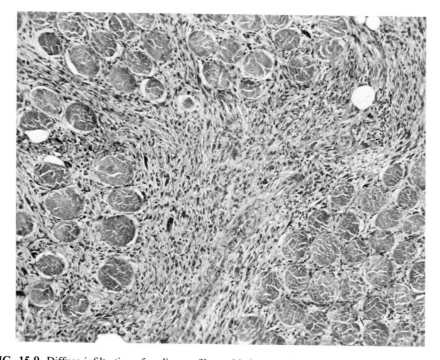

FIG. 15-9. Diffuse infiltration of malignant fibrous histiocytoma between individual skeletal muscle fibers accounts for high rate of local recurrence following limited excisions. (×100.)

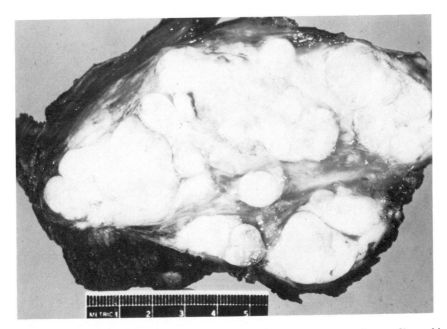

FIG. 15-10. Multinodular gray-white mass is typical appearance of most malignant fibrous histiocytomas. (From Weiss SW, Enzinger FM: *Cancer* 41:2250, 1978.)

areas (Fig. 15-11). In its classic form the tumor consists of plump spindled cells arranged in short fascicles in a cartwheel or storiform pattern around slitlike vessels. The spindle cells are well differentiated and resemble fibroblasts. Although such tumors resemble dermatofibrosarcoma protuberans, they differ by a less distinctive storiform pattern and by the presence of occasional plump histiocytic cells, numerous typical and atypical mitotic figures, and secondary elements, including xanthoma cells and modest numbers of chronic inflammatory cells. Although this pattern of malignant fibrous histiocytoma is easily recognized, it is seldom seen throughout the entire tumor. Instead, most tumors have a combination of storiform and pleomorphic areas, with an emphasis on the latter. Least often tumors have a fascicular growth pattern and resemble fibrosarcomas, except for scattered giant cells. In contrast to the storiform areas, pleomorphic areas contain plumper fibroblastic cells and greater numbers of rounded histiocytic cells arranged haphazardly without any particular orientation to vessels. Pleomorphism and mitotic activity are usually more prominent. A characteristic feature of these areas is the presence of large numbers of giant cells with multiple hyperchromatic irregular nuclei. The intense eosinophilia of these giant cells often suggests cells showing myoblastic differentiation, but they consistently lack myofibrils, as demonstrated by special stains (Fig. 15-12). Although small droplets of neutral fat and PAS-positive, diastase-resistant droplets may be seen in mononuclear cells in this tumor, they are especially prominent in the giant cells and probably reflect degenerative changes.

Both the stroma and secondary elements vary considerably within both the storiform and pleomorphic areas. Usually the stroma consists of delicate collagen fibrils encircling individual cells. Occasionally the collagenization becomes marked and widely separates cells (Fig. 15-13). Focal myxoid change is also a common phenomenon and consists of localized collections of hyaluronidase-sensitive acid mucopolysaccharide. When this change becomes especially prominent, the tumors are classified as myxoid variants of malignant fibrous histiocytoma. Rarely the stroma contains metaplastic osteoid or chondroid. We have even seen one case in which mature lamellar bone with marrow elements was present within a very pleomorphic malignant fibrous histiocytoma.

The vasculature, although quite elaborate, is seldom appreciated with routine hematoxylin-eosin staining but is better demonstrated by PAS or reticulin preparations. Sometimes the vessels become dilated, and the close apposition of the tumor cells to their walls simulate the pattern of hemangiopericytoma (Fig. 15-14).

Modest numbers of lymphocytes or plasma cells characterize the majority of these tumors. In about one fifth of cases, inflammatory cells are quite numerous, usually with a predominance of either acute or chronic inflammatory cells rather than equal mixtures of both. The inflammatory cells are scattered throughout a tumor with some predilection for the periphery of the lesion and the immediate perivascular zones (Figs. 15-15 and 15-16). Occasionally the intermingling of bizarre histiocytic cells and lymphocytes at the periphery may closely simulate lymphoma, par-

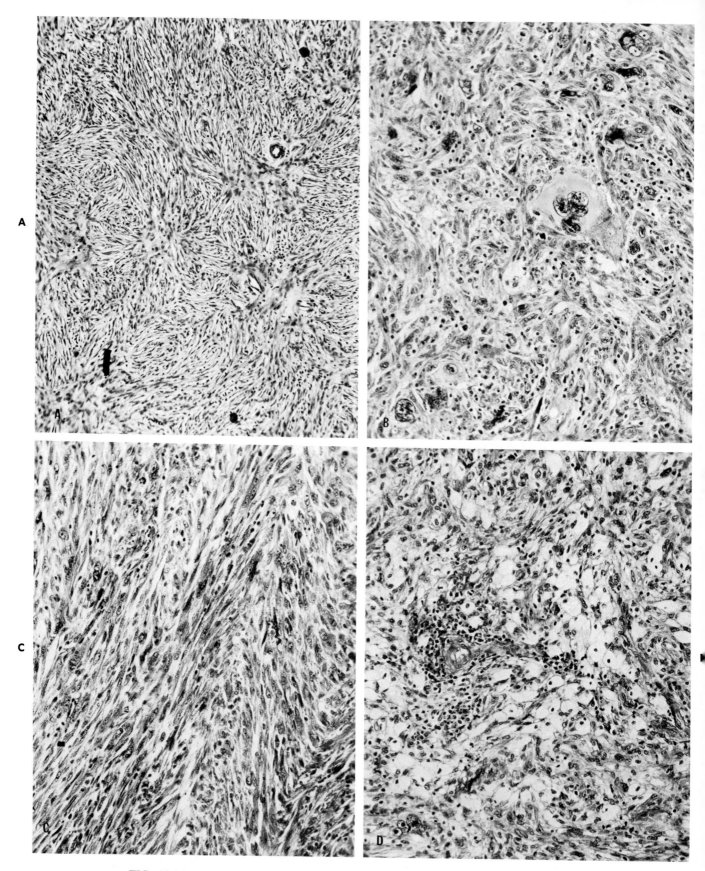

FIG. 15-11. Malignant fibrous histiocytoma showing the wide range of histological patterns all within the same tumor. Some areas have a distinct storiform pattern (**A**), while other areas are more pleomorphic (**B**) or have a fascicular pattern (**C**). Foci of xanthoma cells and inflammatory cells are commonly present (**D**). (**A**, × 90; **B**, × 180; **C**, × 165; **D**, ×165.) (From Weiss SW, Enzinger FM: *Cancer* 41:2250, 1978.)

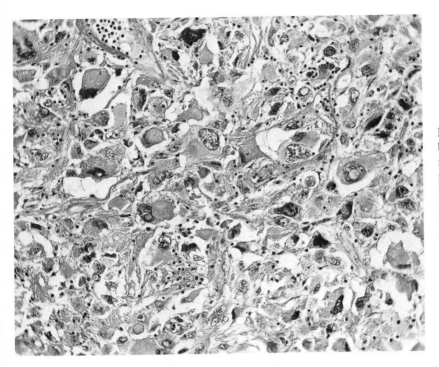

FIG. 15-12. Pleomorphic area of malignant fibrous histiocytoma consisting of sheets of bizarre cells with abundant eosinophilic cytoplasm. Tumors having such areas have often been diagnosed as pleomorphic rhabdomyosarcoma or even anaplastic carcinoma. (×145.) (From Weiss SW, Enzinger FM. *Cancer* 41:2250, 1978.)

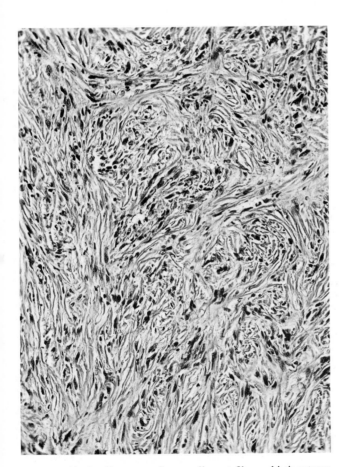

FIG. 15-13. Storiform area from malignant fibrous histiocytoma showing marked hyalinization resulting in wide separation of tumor cells. (×165.) (From Weiss SW, Enzinger FM: *Cancer* 41:3350, 1978.)

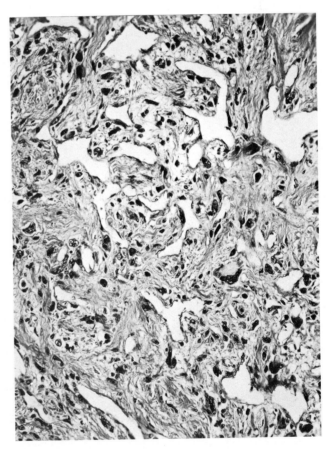

FIG. 15-14. Dilated vessels flanked by tumor cells simulating the pattern of a hemangiopericytoma within a malignant fibrous histiocytoma. (×160.) (From Weiss SW, Enzinger FM: *Cancer* 41:2250, 1978.)

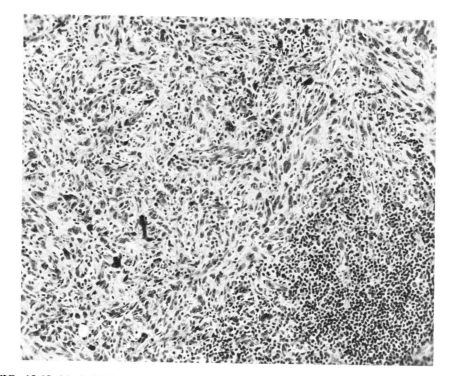

FIG. 15-15. Marked inflammatory response within or around a malignant fibrous histiocytoma may create some resemblance to a malignant lymphoma. (×165.) (From Weiss SW, Enzinger FM: *Cancer* 41:2250, 1978.)

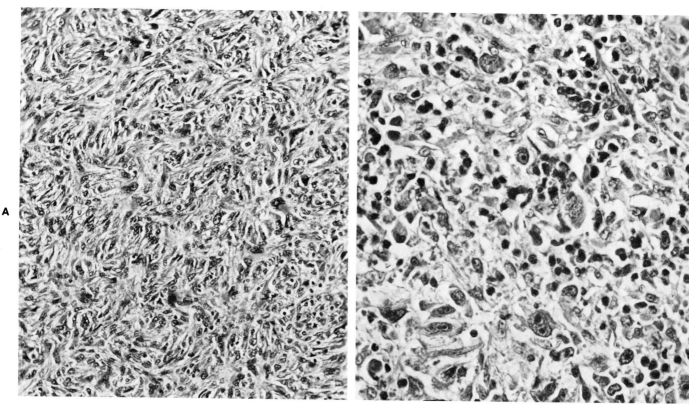

FIG. 15-16. Malignant fibrous histiocytoma showing distinct storiform areas (**A**) adjacent to areas lacking such a pattern but having inflammation (**B**). The latter areas (**B**) with histiocyte-like cells intermingled with chronic inflammatory cells resemble lymphoma. (**A,** ×180; **B,** ×395.) (From Weiss SW, Enzinger FM: *Cancer* 41:2250, 1978.)

ticularly Hodgkin's disease. The significance and mechanism of a prominent inflammatory component in these tumors is not clear, but possibly relates to cytokine production by the tumor cells. In our experience, there is some evidence that such tumors have a slightly better prognosis than comparable tumors with little or no inflammation.[135]

Metastatic deposits from malignant fibrous histiocytoma involve organs in a nodular fashion. In rare instances metastatic lesions to lymph nodes are diffuse and consist of nests of cells scattered throughout a lymph node, thereby resembling lymphoma. However, usually adjacent nodes can be found with the more typical solid pattern of involvement. Metastatic lesions in general resemble the original tumor, although they are less likely to manifest a storiform pattern.

Immunohistochemical findings. The role of immunohistochemistry in the diagnosis of malignant fibrous histiocytoma has traditionally been an ancillary one, primarily serving as a means of excluding other pleomorphic tumors such as anaplastic carcinoma and sarcoma that may bear a resemblance to malignant fibrous histiocytoma. Thus the diagnosis of malignant fibrous histiocytoma continues to presuppose excellent sampling and evaluation of hematoxylin- and eosin-stained sections. Yet despite the limited diagnostic applications of immunohistochemistry, they have provided ample evidence that these tumors are not derived from cells of monocyte or macrophage lineage[36,110,111,137] (Table 15-2) but rather from fibroblasts. Although several workers earlier suggested that the presence of two histiocytic enzymes, alpha-1-antitrypsin and alpha-1-antichymotrypsin, within these tumors supported their histiocytic origin,[81,93,100] it has been shown that these enzymes are present inconsistently and that they

Table 15-2. Enzymatic and immunohistochemical characteristics of malignant fibrous histiocytoma compared with normal histiocytes

Immunohistochemical markers	Malignant fibrous histiocytoma	Histiocyte
Lysozyme[113,137]	Some +	+
A1-AT[113,137]	Some +	+
Acid phosphatase[137]	Some +	+
Alpha-naphthyl butyrate esterase[137]	—	+
Leu-M3[137]	—	+
Leu-3[137]	—	+
T-200[137]	—	+
OK-M1[112]	—	Most +
HLA-DR[113,137]	Some +	+
Fibroblast associated antigen[112]	+	—

may be present within sarcomas of diverse types as well as carcinomas, possibly as a result of endocytosis from plasma.[110] More reliable histiocytic markers such as Leu-3 and Leu-M3 have not been identified in these tumors.[137] Likewise, CD68, a panhistiocytic marker detected by monoclonal antibody KP-1, cannot be identified within these tumors in our experience, despite one recent report to the contrary.[34] Moreover, cells of malignant fibrous histiocytoma do not express T-200 (CD45), a leukocyte common antigen.[137] Although malignant fibrous histiocytomas express HLA-DR, a major histocompatibility antigen present on most histiocytes,[111] this substance is not specific for histiocytes and is also present on endothelial cells and on certain types of stimulated fibroblasts.[137] Two studies have documented the fact that fibroblast-associated antigens can also be identified on the surface of cells of malignant fibrous histiocytoma[67,110] and laminin intracytoplasmically.[117,118] Mutant p53 can be detected immunohistochemically in about 30% of cases, although the significance of this finding in terms of prognosis is not clear.[120]

With the widespread use of monoclonal antibodies a number of interesting questions have been raised regarding the diagnostic criteria for this neoplasm. It has been repeatedly observed that tumors that qualify by light microscopy as malignant fibrous histiocytomas may express a number of intermediate filaments such as keratin, desmin, and neurofilament protein.[61,88,91,96,112] Under these circumstances the immunoreactivity is usually focal. Initially such findings were dismissed as technical artifacts or unusual patterns of cross-reactivity. It is clear, however, that true expression of some intermediate filaments, specifically keratin, occurs in malignant fibrous histiocytoma[112,133] and that the incidence of this immunoreactivity increases as the sensitivity of the method is enhanced.[91] This has been confirmed by immunoblotting[112] studies and by the fact that immunostaining can be reproduced on a given tumor by a number of different antibody preparations. Moreover, recognition that normal mesenchymal cells may express certain types of keratin seems to have paved the way toward a growing acceptance that their neoplastic counterparts may also do so. The issue then becomes whether minor patterns of immunoreactivity within an otherwise typical malignant fibrous histiocytoma should be considered as sufficient evidence of specific differentiation and, accordingly, alter the diagnosis. We have adopted the approach that focal immunostaining for substances such as keratin and desmin in otherwise typical malignant fibrous histiocytomas is not sufficient in itself to alter the diagnosis but should be corroborated by other light microscopic or ultrastructural features. On the other hand, diffuse, intense immunoreactivity for one of these antigens is more likely reflective of specific differentiation. For example, rare desmin-positive cells within malignant fibrous histiocytoma can probably be ascribed to focal myofibroblastic differentiation, whereas

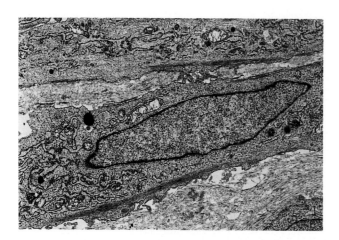

FIG. 15-17. Electron micrograph showing fibroblast-like cells comprising malignant fibrous histiocytoma. Cells are elongated with numerous profiles of rough endoplasmic reticulum. Actin-like filaments are often clustered beneath the cytoplasmic membrane. (×17,000.) (Courtesy Dr. Bruce Mackay, M.D. Anderson Cancer Hospital.)

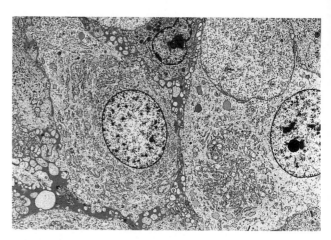

FIG. 15-18. Electron micrograph of malignant cells having histiocyte-like features. They contain numerous phagolysosomes within cytoplasm. (×6300.) (Courtesy Dr. Bruce Mackay, M.D. Anderson Cancer Hospital.)

large areas of desmin immunoreactivity are more likely indicative of pleomorphic rhabdomyosarcoma or leiomyosarcoma masquerading as malignant fibrous histiocytoma. In ambiguous situations, one can take solace in the fact that the choice between two or more forms of pleomorphic sarcoma is an academic one and will not, in current therapy protocols, alter the fundamental approach to the patient. Obviously, however, the distinction between anaplastic carcinoma and pleomorphic sarcoma is usually a therapeutically important distinction that materially affects the management of the patient.

Ultrastructural findings. With widespread use of immunohistochemistry, electron microscopic studies have assumed a diminished role in the diagnosis of malignant fibrous histiocytoma. Moreover, as pointed out by Taxy and Battifora,[126,127] electron microscopy is a "confirmatory procedure" that is best applied when the differential diagnosis has been narrowed down by light microscopy. The limited role of electron microscopy reflects the fact that there are no ultrastructural features that are ultimately specific for malignant fibrous histiocytoma, and cells with similar characteristics can be found in other tumors.[59,62,85,86] Thus electron microscopy is used principally to establish the absence of certain organelles that would indicate a higher order of differentiation. Three cell types can be identified within the tumors[28,54,65]: a fibroblastic cell with elongated nuclei, prominent nucleoli, and abundant lamellae of rough endoplasmic reticulum (Fig. 15-17).[28,54,127] Some of these cells manifest nuclear clefting and contain wispy actinlike filaments beneath the cytoplasmic membrane[41] and resemble "myofibroblasts" seen in a variety of conditions. Rounded cells, compared with "histiocytes," contain oval or lobated nuclei, cytoplasmic processes, a prominent Golgi

zone, and numerous lysosomes, phagosomes, and lipid droplets (Fig. 15-18).[28,54,127] Langerhans' granules, structures present in certain alleged histiocytic tumors, are almost always absent. Occasionally filamentous material may be present in a perinuclear location. Primitive mesenchymal cells having a narrow rim of cytoplasm largely devoid of organelles except for free ribosomes are present in small numbers.[28,54]

Differential diagnosis. The most common and difficult problem in differential diagnosis is the distinction of this form of malignant fibrous histiocytoma from other malignant neoplasms showing a comparable degree of cellular pleomorphism. Pleomorphic liposarcoma, in particular, may show areas that closely simulate malignant fibrous histiocytoma. It usually lacks a distinct whorled or storiform pattern, contains less stromal collagen, and, most importantly, shows evidence of specific cellular differentiation (i.e., lipoblasts of typical form and structure). Intracellular fat in varying amounts is generally present in both tumors, but the lipid in malignant fibrous histiocytoma is more finely dispersed or irregularly distributed and as a rule does not displace or indent the nucleus as in typical lipoblasts. Intracellular lipid, of course, may also be encountered in various other mesenchymal neoplasms, especially in areas of cellular degeneration and at the margin of the tumor where it has infiltrated the surrounding normal fat (Fig. 15-19). Rarely have we encountered sarcomas showing areas of "dedifferentiation" that exactly mimic malignant fibrous histiocytomas. These tumors have included liposarcoma, extraosseous osteosarcoma, chondrosarcoma (Fig. 15-20), malignant schwannoma, and leiomyosarcoma. By convention, however, we have classified such tumors by the area showing the more specific form of differentiation.

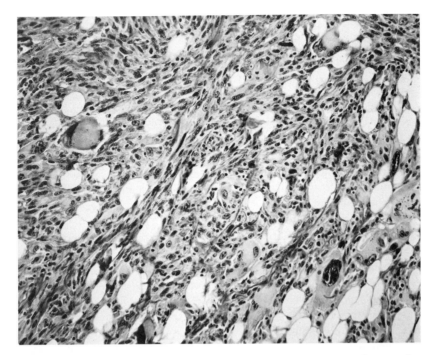

FIG. 15-19. Malignant fibrous histiocytoma infiltrating fat. Residual normal fat as well as nonspecific accumulation of lipid within tumor cells may lead to confusion with pleomorphic forms of liposarcoma. (×80.)

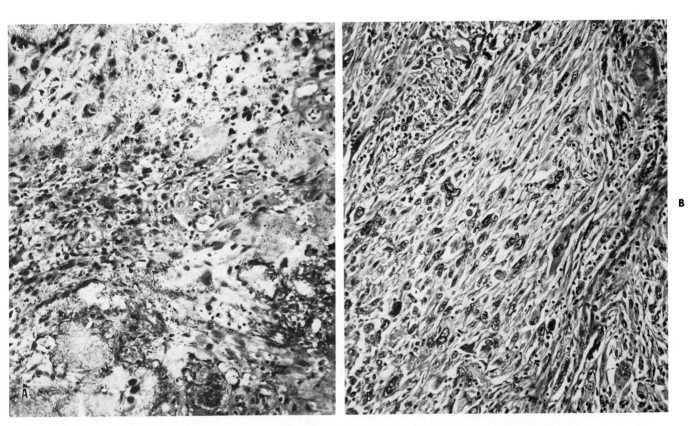

FIG. 15-20. Chondrosarcoma with dedifferentiated areas. Soft tissue tumor of foot that contained chondroid areas (**A**) in addition to pleomorphic spindled areas (**B**) resembling malignant fibrous histiocytoma. Pleomorphic tumors such as this underscore the need for careful sampling. (**A** and **B**, ×160.)

Distinction from pleomorphic rhabdomyosarcoma may also cause difficulties. Traditionally the deeply eosinophilic giant cells of malignant fibrous histiocytoma were considered to be rhabdomyoblasts; consequently many cases of malignant fibrous histiocytoma were classified and reported as pleomorphic rhabdomyosarcoma. In our experience, pleomorphic rhabdomyosarcoma in adult patients is a rare tumor, and most tumors so diagnosed are actually examples of malignant fibrous histiocytoma. In contrast to malignant fibrous histiocytoma, pleomorphic rhabdomyosarcoma usually is composed of cells that have more uniformly and deeply eosinophilic cytoplasm, display more cell-to-cell molding, and usually have less interstitial collagenization. The presence of longitudinal striations in some of these cells is not sufficient evidence of rhabdomyoblastic differentiation. By electron microscopy, longitudinal striations correspond to cells containing actinlike filaments, organelles now known to be present in a variety of neoplastic mesenchymal and epithelial cells. Therefore the diagnosis of adult or pleomorphic rhabdomyosarcoma should be restricted to those rare sarcomas showing cross-striations by light microscopy, typical thin (6 to 8 nm) and thick (12 to 15 nm) filaments or Z-band material ultrastructurally, or specific

muscle protein (e.g., myoglobin or desmin) by immunohistochemistry. As mentioned above, however, focal or weak desmin immunoreactivity is probably not sufficient by itself to warrant a diagnosis of myosarcoma, since myofibroblasts may express this antigen.

Distinction between malignant fibrous histiocytoma and pleomorphic carcinoma may also pose a difficult problem for the pathologist. This is especially true in pleomorphic forms of malignant fibrous histiocytoma composed chiefly of haphazardly arranged round or polygonal cells without a storiform pattern. Such pleomorphic tumors, therefore, when occurring in visceral organs or in patients known to have an epithelial malignancy, should be carefully sampled for evidence of epithelial differentiation (Fig. 15-21). Stains for mucin and glycogen, and immunostains for cytokeratin may prove helpful. As noted above, however, keratin may be expressed in a small percentage of malignant fibrous histiocytomas, but almost invariably manifests as focal, weak staining. Electron microscopy may also aid in the distinction by detecting minor degrees of epithelial differentiation not readily apparent by light microscopy, such as numerous large intercellular junctions or tonofibrils. In most cases of malignant fibrous histiocytoma, distinction from benign

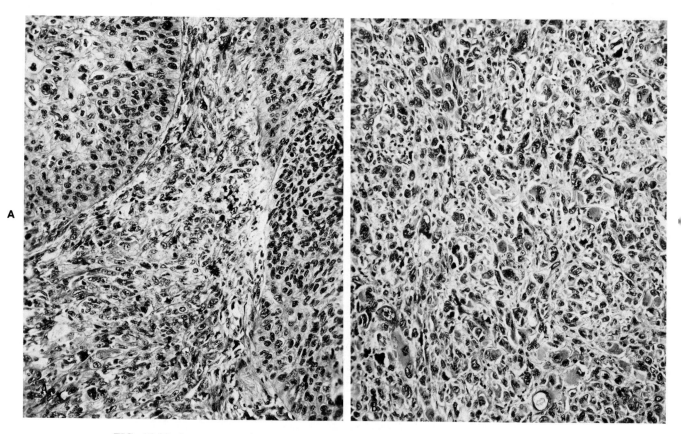

FIG. 15-21. Squamous carcinoma of the esophagus (**A**) with dedifferentiated areas (**B**) resembling a malignant fibrous histiocytoma. (**A** and **B**, ×160.)

fibrous histiocytoma or dermatofibrosarcoma protuberans is not difficult, because the latter two usually have conspicuous storiform patterns and lack pleomorphic cells and necrosis. Occasional tumors may have borderline histological features. As pointed out in Chapter 13, when such lesions are large and deeply situated, they should be regarded as potentially malignant. Likewise, the distinction between malignant fibrous histiocytoma and atypical fibroxanthoma is principally one of size and clinical extent, as discussed previously in this chapter.

Rarely, malignant fibrous histiocytoma may resemble Hodgkin's disease. This resemblance occurs most often in tumors in which histiocyte-like cells intermingle with chronic inflammatory cells. The extranodal location and the finding of cohesive groups of spindle cells usually aid in the distinction. In exceptional instances when metastatic malignant fibrous histiocytoma involves a lymph node diffusely, the resemblance to Hodgkin's disease may be so striking that a histological distinction is not possible without employing immunostains for markers such as Leu-M1, which identify Reed-Sternberg cells but not cells of malignant fibrous histiocytoma. Because malignant fibrous histiocytoma rarely presents as lymphadenopathy without a known primary soft tissue mass, clinical information is quite helpful.

Discussion. Since the original description of malignant fibrous histiocytoma in the early 1960s there has been a gradual, yet diametric, change in our views of this tumor. This tumor is no longer believed to show histiocytic differentiation but rather fibroblastic differentiation, and it has come to represent the prototype of the high-grade pleomorphic sarcoma of adult life. An emerging question, however, has been whether the tumor exists at all or whether it represents a potpourri of various mesenchymal and nonmesenchymal tumors having certain superficial similarities.[43] To be sure, failure to examine a tumor fully may result in the inclusion of other lesions within this group. The recent study by Fletcher[53] analyzing 159 cases that had been diagnosed as pleomorphic sarcoma over more than a 30-year period at his hospital addresses this issue. He indicates that only about 100 would actually qualify as malignant fibrous histiocytoma by current light microscopic criteria. Careful analysis of the entire group by means of extensive tissue sampling, immunohistochemistry, or electron microscopy indicated that 42 would continue to meet the diagnostic criteria of malignant fibrous histiocytoma (in large part these criteria are defined as the absence of differentiation). Thus, this study indicates that slightly less than half of cases that might be diagnosed by pathologists as malignant fibrous histiocytoma would continue to fulfill the criteria when extensively studied. This figure will obviously vary depending on the experience of the pathologist making the initial diagnosis. Based on this study and our own experience, we feel that the diagnosis continues to serve a useful purpose

in identifying an undifferentiated pleomorphic sarcoma, although in time it may become intellectually more forthright to consider a change in nomenclature.

This tumor is a fully malignant sarcoma, although previous large retrospective studies indicating a local recurrence rate and metastatic rate of nearly one half have been superceded by more recent studies from large cancer centers indicating far lower rates, probably because of more immediate efficacious therapy. In a review of 78 deeply situated malignant fibrous histiocytomas of the extremities reported by Bertoni et al.,[33] 37.5% of patients receiving initial therapy at the hospital developed local recurrence within one to 28 months following therapy. Recurrences were directly related to adequacy of the surgical therapy, with a recurrence rate of nil following adequate wide excision or amputation, and recurrence rates between 50% and 84% following inadequate local excisions. The overall 5-year survival rate was 36%. Pezzi et al.,[108] from the M.D. Anderson Cancer Hospital, reported a 25% local recurrence rate, a metastatic rate of 34%, and an overall survival rate of 50%, including those patients dying of other causes. Most metastases occur in the lung (90%) followed by bone (8%) and liver (1%). Regional lymph node metastasis, formerly believed to be common, is quite uncommon. In our series of 20 regional lymph node dissections or biopsies,[134] seven samples (35%) contained tumor, but this figure is falsely high because it represents a preselected group of patients. The true incidence of regional lymph node metastases lies closer to 12%, the overall incidence of lymph node metastases in our series. The incidence of lymph node metastases, in the experience of Bertoni et al.[33] and Kearney et al.,[78] was 4% and 17%, respectively.

The factors that seem to consistently correlate with metastasis or survival, or both, are depth, tumor size, and grade. In general, the more superficial a tumor, the better the prognosis. For example, fewer than 10% of tumors confined entirely to the subcutis without fascial involvement metastasize.[134] In this respect they are analogous to atypical fibroxanthoma. Tumors involving the subcutis and fascia metastasize in 27% of cases, while those in skeletal muscle metastasize in 43%.[134] Tumor size can be correlated with survival rates.[108,113] Tumors smaller than 5 cm have a 5-year survival rate of 82%, 5 to 10 cm 68%, and larger than 10 cm 51%. Although histological grade determines survival as well, one must remember that the majority of malignant fibrous histiocytomas are grade III or IV, and thus it has been difficult to collect a group large enough to analyze grade as an independent variable. In the experience of Pezzi et al.,[108] intermediate-grade lesions (grade II) were accompanied by an 80% 5-year survival rate, compared with a 60% survival rate for high-grade (grade III) lesions.[108] Distal tumors, in the experience of some, also have had a better prognosis than proximal ones. Vascular invasion, tumor necrosis,[32] and local recurrence may also

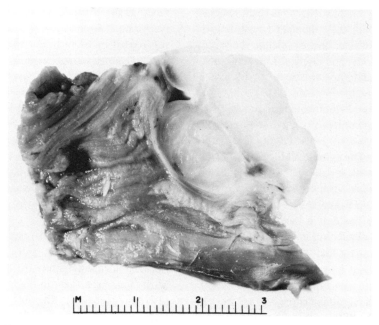

FIG. 15-22. Myxoid malignant fibrous histiocytoma involving skeletal muscle. Tumor has translucent appearance as a result of the admixture of cellular and myoxoid zones. (From Weiss SW, Enzinger FM: *Cancer* 39:1672, 1977.)

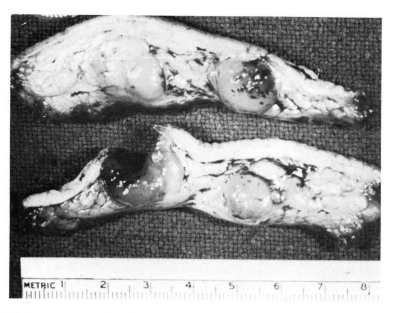

FIG. 15-23. Recurrent myxoid malignant fibrous histiocytoma involving the subcutis. In contrast to the tumor in Fig. 15-22, the tumor is almost entirely myxoid and hence has a distinctly gelatinous appearance. (From Weiss SW, Enzinger FM: *Cancer* 39:1672, 1977.)

affect outcome adversely.[113]

A number of recent studies suggest in a preliminary fashion that aneuploidy,[109] nuclear shape factor,[32] and heat shock protein 27 (HSP-27)[128] may provide prognostic information. HSP-27 is one of a family of stress proteins that appear in all types of normal cells following certain types of stress injury. It has been identified within breast carcinoma and is associated with chemoresistance and poor prognosis. Identified within approximately 50% of malignant fibrous histiocytomas by immunohistochemistry, it seems to portend an improved prognosis. Analysis of proliferating antigens in these tumors correlates with mitotic rate and nuclear grade but does not provide prognostic information with respect to survival over and above histological grade.[139]

Malignant fibrous histiocytoma: myxoid type

This form of malignant fibrous histiocytoma is characterized by myxoid areas in association with cellular areas indistinguishable from ordinary malignant fibrous histiocytoma (Figs. 15-22 to 15-24).[135] Although the proportion of myxoid and cellular areas can vary within these tumors, at least half of the tumor should appear myxoid before it is designated a "myxoid variant."

The myxoid areas appear either as small foci blending with the adjacent cellular areas or as large areas abutting on cellular areas with little transition (Fig. 15-25). In the extreme case an entire nodule of a tumor may appear myx-

oid, while an adjacent one may be cellular. Qualitatively the myxoid zones are similar to the cellular zones; they differ principally in the interstitial accumulation of hyaluronidase-sensitive acid mucopolysaccharide. As a result the storiform pattern becomes less evident, while the vasculature becomes more prominent (Figs. 15-26 and 15-27). The vessels typically form arcs along which tumor cells and inflammatory cells condense. Less often the vessels are extremely delicate and assume an intricate plexiform pattern similar to that of myxoid liposarcoma (Fig. 15-27).

As in the cellular areas, the cells within the myxoid zones show a spectrum of differentiation from well-differentiated fibroblasts to cells showing pleomorphism, mitotic activity, and multinucleation. Highly myxoid tumors with a predominance of the former cells may be bland enough to be confused with myxoma or nodular fasciitis. Such tumors have sometimes been designated myxofibrosarcoma.[82,89] Occasionally cells within the myxoid zones contain coarse cytoplasmic vacuoles, thereby resembling lipoblasts (Fig. 15-28). However, unlike lipoblasts these vacuoles contain acid mucin rather than neutral fat. A number of ultrastructural studies of this tumor have been performed[62,63,82,86,89] documenting cells with characteristics of fibroblasts[82,89] that are embedded in an electron-dense filamentous matrix (Fig. 15-29). The vacuolization of the cells is caused by dilatation of the endoplasmic reticulum as well as by the formation of "pseudocanaliculi" by delicate cytoplasmic processes.[86]

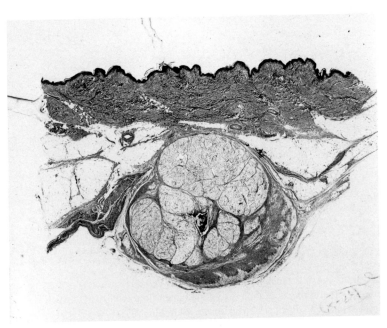

FIG. 15-24. Myxoid malignant fibrous histiocytoma of the deep subcutis. Note the majority of the tumor is myxoid, but in areas it abruptly changes into a more cellular tumor. (×4.) (From Weiss SW, Enzinger FM: *Cancer* 39:1672, 1977.)

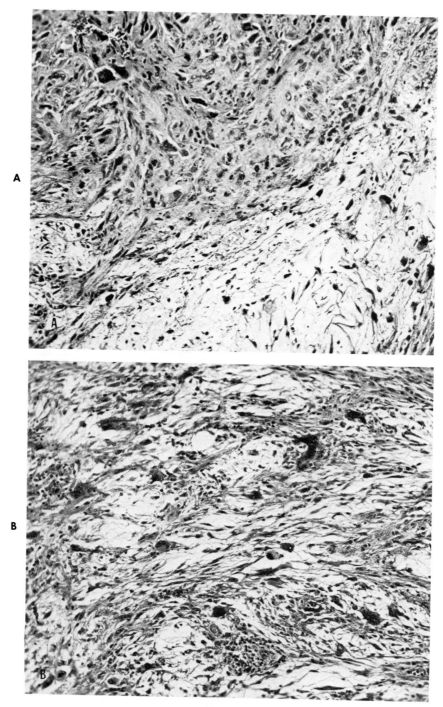

FIG. 15-25. Broad myxoid zones may abut sharply on cellular areas **(A)** or may be scattered on small microscopic foci throughout the myxoid malignant fibrous histiocytoma **(B)**. (A, ×110; **B,** ×130.) (From Weiss SW, Enzinger FM: *Cancer* 39:1672, 1977.)

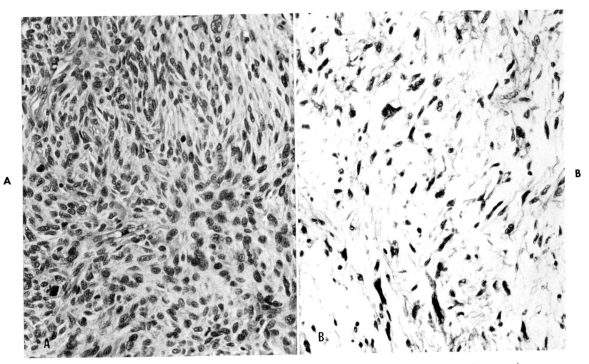

FIG. 15-26. Myxoid malignant fibrous histiocytoma showing cellular area with prominent storiform pattern (**A**) and myxoid area where the storiform pattern is absent (**B**). (**A** and **B**, ×195.) (From Weiss SW, Enzinger FM: *Cancer* 39:1672, 1977.)

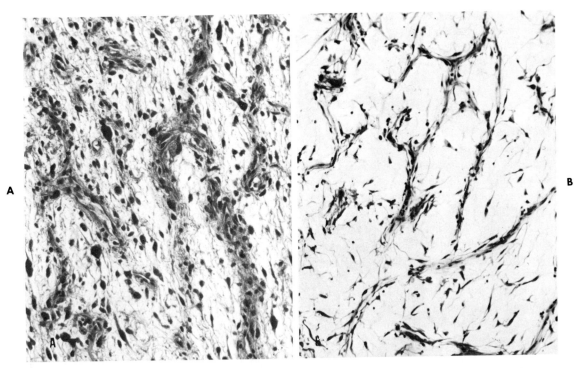

FIG. 15-27. The vasculature in the myxoid zones of these tumors becomes more prominent and typically consists of curvilinear vessels along which the tumor cells are anchored (**A**). Less commonly the vessels are exceedingly delicate and intricate and mimic the vasculature of a myxoid liposarcoma (**B**). (**A**, ×195; **B**, ×210.) (From Weiss SW, Enzinger FM: *Cancer* 39:1672, 1977.)

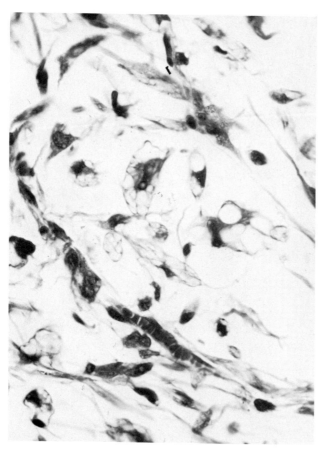

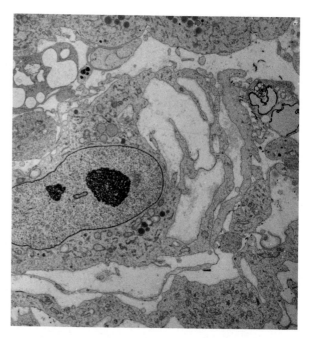

FIG. 15-29. Electron micrograph of a myxoid malignant fibrous histiocytoma. Cells are surrounded by abundant ground substance. Vacuolation of cells is caused by numerous invaginations of cytoplasmic membrane with trapping of ground substance around nucleus and also by dilatation of endoplasmic reticulum. (Courtesy Dr. Bruce Mackay.)

FIG. 15-28. Vacuolated lipoblast-like cells within myxoid malignant fibrous histiocytoma. Unlike lipoblasts, however, the vacuoles are more irregular and contain acid mucopolysaccharide rather than neutral fat. (×530.) (From Weiss SW, Enzinger FM: *Cancer* 39:1672, 1977.)

Differential diagnosis. The most important aspect of differential diagnosis is the clear distinction of this lesion from benign myxoid lesions such as nodular fasciitis and myxoma. Although nodular fasciitis may have focal myxoid change, it lacks the extensive orderly vasculature, bizarre cells, and atypical mitotic figures seen in myxoid malignant fibrous histiocytoma. Myxomas also lack the extensive vasculature of the malignant fibrous histiocytoma and usually have small cells with minimal atypia and few, if any, mitotic figures.

The sarcoma most nearly resembling this tumor is liposarcoma. Although myxoid liposarcoma resembles this tumor grossly, it consists of a more uniform population of small spindle cells embedded in a clear matrix with a delicate plexiform vasculature. Bizarre cells are absent, and mitotic figures are infrequent. Lipoblasts are usually present. Pleomorphic liposarcoma, on the other hand, does have bizarre cells similar to myxoid malignant fibrous histiocytoma, but it has a cellular rather than a myxoid background, is more uniform in appearance, and also contains lipoblasts.

Discussion. The myxoid form of malignant fibrous histiocytoma is distinguished primarily because of its better prognosis compared with the storiform-pleomorphic type.[133] Although this tumor recurs in almost two thirds of cases, it metastasizes in only about one fourth of cases. The indolent course of this tumor is, furthermore, underscored by the longer interval between the time of diagnosis and metastasis. Thus we have adopted the approach that malignant fibrous histiocytomas that are predominantly (greater than 50%) myxoid are classified as grade II, in contrast to the vast majority of malignant fibrous histiocytomas, which are classified as grade III. Despite its improved prognosis, the myxoid form of malignant fibrous histiocytoma should be treated by wide local excision or amputation. All previous comments concerning metastatic sites, therapy, and prognostic criteria for the storiform-pleomorphic type are equally applicable to this type. The significance of myxoid change within these tumors is not entirely clear. It is unlikely that it is a degenerative feature because other features of degeneration are lacking. Viewed simplistically it might be regarded as an area in which the cells multiply more slowly but produce abundant mucoid matrix as a form of differentiation. This would explain the better prognosis

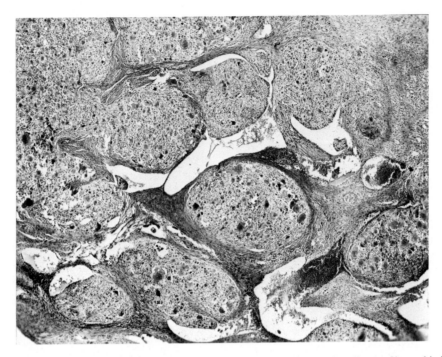

FIG. 15-30. Characteristic multinodular pattern of the giant cell type of malignant fibrous histiocytoma. (×38.) (From Guccion JG, Enzinger FM: *Cancer* 29:1518, 1972.)

most myxoid tumors have over their cellular counterparts (e.g., myxoid liposarcoma, myxoid chondrosarcoma).

Malignant fibrous histiocytoma: giant cell type

This type of malignant fibrous histiocytoma, also termed malignant giant cell tumor of soft parts,[58] is a multinodular tumor composed of a mixture of histiocytes, fibroblasts, and osteoclast-type giant cells. Dense fibrous bands containing vessels encircle the nodules of tumor, while secondary hemorrhage and necrosis are commonly present within them (Fig. 15-30). As in other fibrohistiocytic tumors, the relative amounts of the three cell types vary. Most tumors contain all three cell types arranged randomly, with some tendency for the fibroblasts to aggregate at the periphery of a nodule (Fig. 15-31). The fibroblasts and histiocytes are similar to those in other malignant fibrous histiocytomas. They display pleomorphism and mitotic activity and often contain ingested material such as lipid and hemosiderin. The hallmark of this tumor is the giant cell. Although these cells resemble normal osteoclasts, they are usually not found in association with osteoid but are rather intimately associated with histiocytic cells, suggesting that they arise by fusion or amitotic division of these mononuclear precursors. The giant cells have voluminous eosinophilic cytoplasm with numerous small uniform nuclei. Phagocytic vacuoles and asteroid bodies are occasionally present.

In approximately half of cases, focal osteoid or mature bone is present (Fig. 15-32). This material is usually located at the periphery of a tumor nodule and appears to be produced by neoplastic cells. In view of this feature the question can legitimately be raised as to whether this tumor is one of bone-forming mesenchyme. Ultrastructural studies have presented divergent views on this point. One study documented the same spectrum of cell types as have been seen in other forms of malignant fibrous histiocytoma and have regarded it as a variant thereof.[29] Another study described a population of cells with features of primitive osteoblasts or chondroblasts[129] and matrix material similar to osteoid.

In our experience a small number of giant cell tumors of soft parts may be composed of relatively bland rounded cells lacking the usual level of atypia and mitotic activity expected in a malignant tumor. Although the follow-up of such tumors is limited, we have usually designated such lesions as low-grade forms of malignant giant cell tumor of soft parts.

We believe for the most part this tumor has more in common with other forms of malignant fibrous histiocytoma. On occasion the neoplastic cells acquire some of the properties of osteoblasts or chondroblasts. As long as osteoid is relatively focal, we classify these tumors as giant cell forms of malignant fibrous histiocytoma. When osteoid is promi-

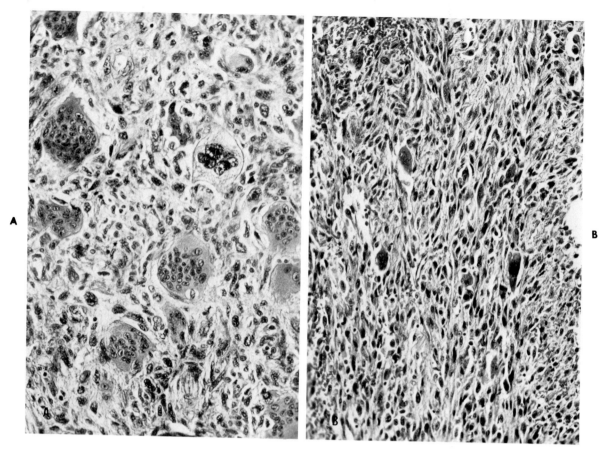

FIG. 15-31. Proliferation of mononuclear histiocyte-like cells and osteoclast-type giant cells typify the giant cell type of malignant fibrous histiocytoma (**A**). Intermixed with these areas and often occurring at the periphery of tumor nodules are spindled areas more closely resembling the conventional malignant fibrous histiocytoma (**B**). (**A**, ×200; **B**, ×150.)

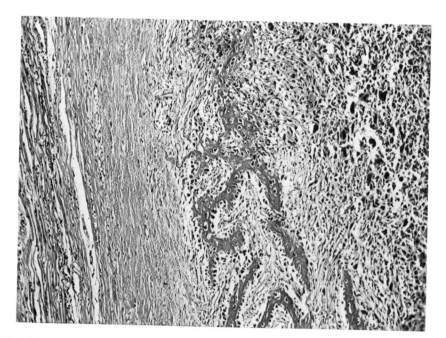

FIG. 15-32. Metaplastic bone is occasionally present in the giant cell type of malignant fibrous histiocytoma and is typically located at the periphery of the tumor nodule. (Hematoxylin-eosin; ×45.)

nent, a diagnosis of extraosseous osteosarcoma seems justified. This approach implies a close histogenetic relationship of the two tumors.

Differential diagnosis. The distinctive appearance of this neoplasm usually causes few problems in diagnosis. Deeply situated tumors may raise the question of a giant cell tumor of bone involving soft tissue. This tumor, however, has a degree of multinodularity not generally encountered in giant cell tumors of bone and does not create major osseous defects as would be expected in a bone tumor.

Discussion. Although there is considerably less data concerning this form of malignant fibrous histiocytoma compared with that of the foregoing types, the original study of 32 cases[58] indicates the same general tendencies as discussed previously. Superficial tumors involving either subcutis or fascia have a much better prognosis than deeply situated tumors. Two thirds of superficial tumors recur, but only about one sixth metastasize. On the other hand, about 40% of deep tumors recur and about half metastasize, a proportion that is roughly comparable to the ordinary forms of malignant fibrous histiocytoma. This tumor should also be treated by prompt radical surgery.

Malignant fibrous histiocytoma: inflammatory type

One of the earliest complete descriptions of this tumor was that of Oberling[104] in 1935. He presented three cases of his own and three from the literature[45,102,103] under the name "retroperitoneal xanthogranuloma." These tumors were bulky infiltrating retroperitoneal masses that contained a polymorphic population of xanthoma cells and inflammatory cells. Despite his astute observations, Oberling concluded that these lesions were not malignant tumors but were variants of Hand-Schüller-Christian disease, a view subsequently endorsed by others.[130] Unfortunately since Oberling's early description, the term *xanthogranuloma* has been applied inappropriately to a variety of retroperitoneal lesions characterized by xanthoma cells. These processes probably have included conditions such as retroperitoneal fibrosis, xanthogranulomatous pyelonephritis, and nonspecific inflammatory conditions. Thus it is not surprising that "retroperitoneal xanthogranuloma" has remained an elusive diagnostic and biological concept for the pathologist and clinician. The heterogeneity of such lesions probably accounts in part for the earlier belief that they were not only benign but also nonneoplastic.[26]

However, it is clear that lesions similar to Oberling's occasionally occur outside the retroperitoneum, that rarely they do metastasize, and that they frequently contain a fibroblastic element similar to other forms of malignant fibrous histiocytoma. In fact, lesions comparable to Oberling's have been reported under the rubric of *inflammatory fibrous histiocytoma.*[84] We have modified this term to *inflammatory malignant fibrous histiocytoma* to emphasize the aggressive nature of the tumor. In some respects this term fails to convey fully the difference between this tumor and the other forms of malignant fibrous histiocytoma.

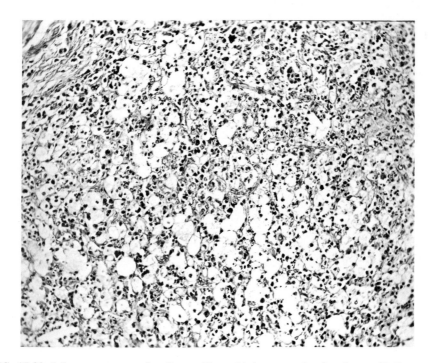

FIG. 15-33. Inflammatory type of malignant fibrous histiocytoma showing sheets of inflammatory cells and xanthoma cells. (× 165.)

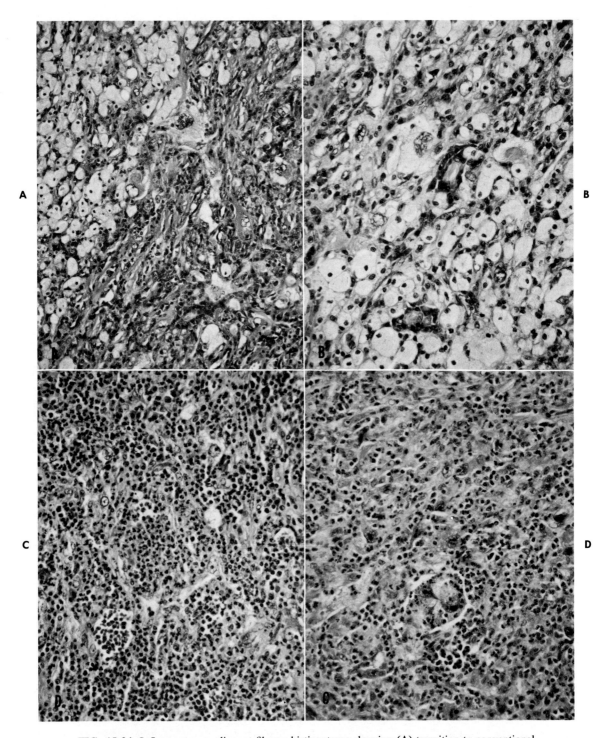

FIG. 15-34. Inflammatory malignant fibrous histiocytoma showing **(A)** transition to conventional spindle cell areas, **(B)** sheets of benign and malignant xanthoma cells, **(C)** xanthoma cells with phagocytosed acute inflammatory cells, and **(D)** sheets of inflammatory cells with only occasional tumor cells. Areas portrayed in **C** and **D** are apt to be confused with Hodgkin's disease. (**A,** ×160; **B-D,** ×250.)

Although acute inflammatory cells are striking, so too are xanthoma cells, and it is the latter that conveys upon this tumor its almost invariable yellow color. Analysis of tumor extracts has documented eosinophilic and neutrophilic chemotactic activity, along with myelopoietic activity, suggesting that production of specific cytokines by the tumor could explain all of the unusual associated blood manifestations.[66,116,124] Histologically the tumor is composed of inflammatory cells set in a stroma of amorphous hyaline material with little collagen (Figs. 15-33 and 15-34). The majority of histiocytes appear xanthomatous because of the prominent cytoplasmic lipid. However, occasional cells having little lipid resemble the histiocytic cells seen in other forms of malignant fibrous histiocytoma. Although it is almost always possible to identify xanthoma cells having significant atypia and mitotic activity, large areas of bland xanthoma cells with pyknotic nuclei may also be present and make the diagnosis difficult, especially in biopsy specimens. Multinucleated histiocytes and xanthoma cells are quite common and also vary in appearance from benign to malignant forms.

The inflammatory component is characteristically prominent and usually consists of a mixture of acute and chronic inflammatory cells with a marked emphasis on the former. Both benign histiocytes and tumor cells may display striking phagocytosis of the inflammatory cells. However, we have also seen cases in which chronic inflammatory cells predominated or in which the inflammatory component was minimal. A delicate vasculature is sometimes appreciated throughout the tumor, creating a superficial resemblance to granulation tissue. Frequent transitions can be seen to spindled areas having a fascicular or even a storiform growth pattern. These areas resemble the more typical malignant fibrous histiocytoma and are, therefore, of great help in establishing a diagnosis. Metastases from this tumor usually resemble the parent lesion; where metastases are different, they usually appear to be less xanthomatous and more fibroblastic.

Differential diagnosis. The differential diagnosis consists primarily in separating this tumor from nonneoplastic xanthomatous processes. Although xanthogranulomatous pyelonephritis may involve the retroperitoneal soft tissue, it first and foremost affects the kidneys and is accompanied by the usual constellation of symptoms of urinary tract infection. Xanthogranulomatous inflammatory processes may also be seen in other settings,[80,97] some of which are related to infectious agents.[80] Thus culture of these lesions and bacterial stains are mandatory. Ultimately the distinction of this tumor from xanthogranulomatous inflammation

rests on the documentation of atypia or mitotic activity in the xanthoma cells or fibroblastic areas resembling the usual form of malignant fibrous histiocytoma. Therefore careful sampling of large xanthomatous lesions, especially in the retroperitoneum, is of the utmost importance.

The malignant tumor most often confused with inflammatory malignant fibrous histiocytoma is lymphoma. Small biopsies or peripheral sampling of large tumors may result in a close intermingling of rounded histiocyte-like cells with inflammatory cells simulating the pattern of lymphoma. Although the clinical symptoms of fever and leukemoid reaction, which occasionally characterize inflammatory malignant fibrous histiocytoma, are rare in lymphoma, it is often necessary to perform a number of immunostaining procedures to establish the diagnosis. Negative immunostaining for both leukocyte common antigen and Leu-M1 provides circumstantial evidence for inflammatory malignant fibrous histiocytoma as opposed to lymphoma.

Discussion. In the past it has been difficult to characterize the behavior of these tumors because of the uncertainty of diagnosis in some cases or the limited follow-up information in others. However, in a review of 29 acceptable cases from the literature,[72] approximately half of the patients had persistent or recurrent disease, while about one third developed distant metastases in such sites as the liver, the lung, and the lymph nodes. The aggressive nature of the tumor is corroborated by another report of seven cases[84] in which virtually all patients suffered severe effects of local disease and four eventually developed metastases. Although it is obvious that these lesions are malignant, it is not clear to what extent they should be regarded as comparable to the other forms of malignant fibrous histiocytoma. It might be expected that the prominent inflammatory component would confer on such lesions an improved prognosis. This hypothesis is suggested by our experience with other forms of malignant fibrous histiocytoma (discussed previously in this chapter) and is supported by the slightly lower metastatic rate of this subtype compared with the storiform-pleomorphic subtype. However, the deep location of most of these tumors, the surgical inaccessibility, and the therapeutic delays resulting from diagnostic errors all adversely affect the prognosis of these cases. As a result, it has thus far not been possible to find properly matched groups for comparison.

Radical surgery is indicated for these tumors. Radiotherapy and chemotherapy have generally been used as adjunctive or palliative measures. In a case reported by Kyriakos and Kempson,[84] reduction of the tumor was noted following a single high dose of nitrogen mustard.

REFERENCES
Atypical fibroxanthoma

1. Alguacil-Garcia A, Unni KK, Goellner JR, et al: Atypical fibroxanthoma of the skin. *Cancer* 40:1471, 1977.

2. Barr RJ, Wuerker RB, Graham JH: Ultrastructure of atypical fibroxanthoma. *Cancer* 40:736, 1977.

3. Berschadsky M, Gianetti CO, David A: Atypical fibroxanthoma in the pharynx. *Plast Reconstr Surg* 52:443, 1973.

4. Bourne RB: Paradoxical fibrosarcoma of the skin (pseudosarcoma): a review of 13 cases. *Med J Aust* 50:504, 1963.

5. Chen KTK: Atypical fibroxanthoma of the skin with osteoid production. *Arch Dermatol* 116:113, 1980.

6. Dahl L: Atypical fibroxanthoma of the skin. A clinicopathological study of 57 cases. *Acta Pathol Microbiol Scand* 84:183, 1976.

7. Evans HL, Smith JL: Spindle cell squamous carcinoma and sarcoma-like tumors of the skin: a comparative study of 38 cases. *Cancer* 45:2687, 1980.

8. Finlay-Jones LR, Nicoll P, ten Seldam REJ: Pseudosarcoma of the skin. *Pathology* 3:215, 1971.

9. Fretzin DF, Helwig EB: Atypical fibroxanthoma of the skin. *Cancer* 31:1541, 1973.

10. Gordon HW: Pseudosarcomatous reticulohistiocytoma: a report of four cases. *Arch Dermatol* 90:319, 1964.

11. Helwig EB, May D: Atypical fibroxanthoma of the skin with metastases. *Cancer* 57:368, 1986.

12. Hudson AW, Winkelmann RK: Atypical fibroxanthoma of the skin: a reappraisal of 19 cases in which the original diagnosis was spindle-cell squamous carcinoma. *Cancer* 29:413, 1972.

13. Jacobs DS, Edwards WD, Ye RC: Metastatic atypical fibroxanthoma of the skin. *Cancer* 35:457, 1975.

14. Kempson RL, McGavran MH: Atypical fibroxanthomas of the skin. *Cancer* 17:1463, 1964.

15. Kroe DJ, Pitcock JA: Atypical fibroxanthoma of the skin: report of 10 cases. *Am J Clin Pathol* 51:487, 1969.

16. Lesica A, Harwood TR, Yokoo H: Atypical fibroxanthoma of the ethmoid sinus. *Arch Otolaryngol* 101:506, 1975.

17. Levan NE, Hirsch P, Kwong MQ: Pseudosarcomatous dermatofibroma. *Arch Dermatol* 88:908, 1963.

18. Mandard AM, Herline P, Chasle J, et al: Cutaneous pseudosarcomas: electron microscopic study of three tumors. *J Submicrosc Cytol Pathol* 10:441, 1978.

19. Rachmaninoff N, McDonald JR, Cook JC: Sarcoma-like tumors of the skin following irradiation. *Am J Clin Pathol* 36:427, 1961.

20. Ricci A, Cartun RW, Zakowski MF: Atypical fibroxanthoma: a study of 14 cases emphasizing the presence of Langerhans' histiocytes with implications for differential diagnosis by antibody panels. *Am J Surg Pathol* 12:591, 1988.

21. Rippey JJ, Craig MB: Atypical fibroxanthoma of the skin. *S Afr Med J* 47:326, 1973.

22. Starink TM, Hausman R, Van Delden L, et al: Atypical fibroxanthoma of the skin: presentation of five cases and review of the literature. *Br J Dermatol* 97:167, 1977.

23. Vargas-Cortes F, Winkelmann RK, Soule EH: Atypical fibroxanthomas of the skin: further observations with 19 additional cases. *Mayo Clin Proc* 48:211, 1973.

24. Weedon D, Kerr JFR: Atypical fibroxanthoma of the skin: an electron microscopic study. *Pathology* 7:173, 1975.

25. Woyke S, Momagala W, Olszewski W, et al: Pseudosarcoma of the skin: an electron microscopic study and comparison with the fine structure of the spindle cell variant of squamous carcinoma. *Cancer* 33:970, 1974.

Malignant fibrous histiocytoma

26. Ackerman LV: *Tumors of the retroperitoneum, mesentery and peritoneum.* Washington, DC, 1954, AFIP Fascicle.

27. Alcott DL, McCort J: Retroperitoneal xanthogranuloma. *Cancer Sem* 5:187, 1959.

28. Alguacil-Garcia A, Unni KK, Goellner JR: Malignant fibrous histiocytoma: an ultrastructural study of six cases. *Am J Clin Pathol* 69:121, 1978.

29. Alguacil-Garcia A, Unni KK, Goellner JR: Malignant giant cell tumor of soft parts: ultrastructural study of four cases. *Cancer* 40:244, 1977.

30. Angervall L, Johnsson S, Kindblom LG, et al: Primary malignant fibrous histiocytoma of bone after radiation. *Acta Pathol Microbiol Scand* 87(A)6:437, 1979.

31. Asirwatham JE, Pickren JW: Inflammatory fibrous histiocytoma: case report. *Cancer* 41:1467, 1978.

32. Becker RL Jr, Venzon D, Lack EE, et al: Cytometry and morphometry of malignant fibrous histiocytoma of the extremities: prediction of metastasis and mortality. *Am J Surg Pathol* 15:957, 1991.

33. Bertoni F, Capanna R, Biagini R, et al: Malignant fibrous histiocytoma of soft tissue: an analysis of 78 cases located and deeply seated in the extremities. *Cancer* 56:356, 1985.

34. Binder SW, Said JW, Shintaku IP, et al: A histiocyte-specific marker in the diagnosis of malignant fibrous histiocytoma: use of monoclonal antibody KP-1 (CD68). *Am J Clin Pathol* 97:759, 1992.

35. Bonfiglio TA, Patten SF, Woodworth FE: Fibroxanthosarcoma of the uterine cervix: cytopathologic and histopathologic manifestations. *Acta Cytol (Balt)* 20:501, 1976.

36. Brecher ME, Franklin WA: Absence of mononuclear phagocyte antigens in malignant fibrous histiocytoma. *Am J Clin Pathol* 86:344, 1986.

37. Bridge JA, Sanger WG, Shaffer B, et al: Cytogenetic findings in malignant fibrous histiocytoma. *Cancer Genet Cytogenet* 29:97, 1987.

38. Buckley C, Thomas V, Cros J, et al: Cancer family syndrome associated with multiple malignant melanomas and a malignant fibrous histiocytoma. *Br J Dermatol* 126:83, 1992.

39. Burgdorf WHC, Duray P, Rosai J: Immunohistochemical identification of lysozyme in cutaneous lesions of alleged histiocytic nature. *Am J Clin Pathol* 75:162, 1981.

40. Canalis RF, Green M, Konrad HR, et al: Malignant fibrous xanthoma of the larynx. *Arch Otolaryngol* 101:135, 1975.

41. Churg AM, Kahn LB: Myofibroblasts and related cells in malignant fibrous and fibrohistiocytic tumors. *Hum Pathol* 8:205, 1977.

42. Dahlin DC, Unni KK, Matsuno T: Malignant (fibrous) histiocytoma of bone—fact or fancy? *Cancer* 39:1508, 1977.

43. Dehner LP: Malignant fibrous histiocytoma: nonspecific morphologic pattern, specific pathologic entity, or both? (editorial). *Arch Pathol Lab Med* 112:236, 1988.

44. Delgado-Partida P, Rodrigues-Trujillo F: Fibrosarcoma (malignant fibroxanthoma) involving conjunctiva and ciliary body. *Am J Ophthalmol* 74:479, 1972.

45. Dietrich A: Über ein Fibroxanthosarkom mit eigenartiger Ausbreitung. *Virchows Arch (Pathol Anat)* 212:119, 1913.

46. duBoulay CEH: Demonstration of alpha-1-antitrypsin and alpha-1-antichymotrypsin in fibrous histiocytomas using immunoperoxidase technique. *Am J Surg Pathol* 6:559, 1982.

47. Enjoji M, Hashimoto H, Iwasaki H: Malignant fibrous histiocytoma: a clinicopathologic study of 130 cases. *Acta Pathol Jpn* 30:727, 1980.

48. Enzinger FM: Malignant fibrous histiocytoma 20 years after Stout. *Am J Surg Pathol* 10(suppl 1):43, 1986.

49. Enzinger FM: Recent developments in the classification of soft tissue sarcomas. In: *Management of primary bone and soft tissue sarcomas.* Chicago, 1977, Year Book Medical Publishers.

50. Eriksson M, Hardell L, Berg NO, et al: Soft tissue sarcomas and exposure to chemical substances: a case referent study. *Br J Indust Med* 38:27, 1981.

51. Feldman F, Lattes R: Primary malignant fibrous histiocytoma (fibrous xanthoma) of bone. *Skeletal Radiol* 1:145, 1977.

52. Feldman F, Norman D: Intra- and extraosseous malignant histiocytoma (malignant fibrous xanthoma). *Radiology* 104:497, 1972.

53. Fletcher CD: Pleomorphic malignant fibrous histiocytoma: fact or fiction? A critical reappraisal based on 159 tumors diagnosed as pleomorphic sarcoma. *Am J Surg Pathol* 16:213, 1992.

54. Fu Y-S, Gabbiani G, Kaye GI, et al: Malignant soft tissue tumors of probable histiocytic origin (malignant fibrous histiocytoma): general considerations and electron microscopic and tissue culture studies. *Cancer* 35:176, 1975.

55. Fukuda T, Tsuneyoshi M, Enjoji M: Malignant fibrous histiocytoma of soft parts: an ultrastructural quantitative study. *Ultrastruct Pathol* 12:117, 1988.

56. Genberg M, Mark J, Hakelius L, et al: Origin and relationship between different cell types in malignant fibrous histiocytoma. *Am J Pathol* 135:1185, 1989.

57. Gonzalez-Vitale JC, Slavin RE, McQueen DJ: Radiation-induced intracranial malignant fibrous histiocytoma. *Cancer* 37:2960, 1976.

58. Guccion JG, Enzinger FM: Malignant giant cell tumor of soft parts: an analysis of 32 cases. *Cancer* 29:1518, 1972.

59. Hayashi Y, Kikuchi-Tada A, Jitsukawa K, et al: Myofibroblasts in malignant fibrous histiocytoma: histochemical, immunohistochemical, ultrastructural and tissue culture studies. *Clin Exp Dermatol* 13:402, 1988.

60. Hensley GT, Friedrich EG: Malignant fibroxanthoma: a sarcoma of the vulva. *Am J Obstet Gynecol* 116:289, 1973.

61. Hirose T, Kudo E, Hasegawa T, et al: Expression of intermediate filaments in malignant fibrous histiocytomas. *Hum Pathol* 20:871, 1989.

62. Hirose T, Sano T, Hizawa K: Ultrastructural study of the myxoid area of malignant fibrous histiocytomas. *Ultrastruct Pathol* 12:621, 1988.

63. Huang WL, Ordonez NG, Mackay B: Myxoid malignant fibrous histiocytoma with erythrophagocytosis. *Ultrastruct Pathol* 13:315, 1989.

64. Huvos AG: Primary malignant fibrous histiocytoma of bone: clinicopathologic study of 18 patients. *N Y State J Med* 76:552, 1976.

65. Inada O, Yumoto T, Furuse K, et al: Ultrastructural features of malignant fibrous histiocytoma. *Acta Pathol Jpn* 26:491, 1976.

66. Isoda M, Yasumoto S: Eosinophil chemotactic factor derived from a malignant fibrous histiocytoma. *Clin Exp Dermatol* 11:253, 1986.

67. Iwasaki H, Isayama T, Johzaki H, et al: Malignant fibrous histiocytoma: evidence of perivascular mesenchymal cell origin immunocytochemical studies with monoclonal anti-MFH antibodies. *Am J Pathol* 128:528, 1987.

68. Iwasaki H, Isayama T, Ohjimi Y, et al: Malignant fibrous histiocytoma: a tumor of facultative histiocytes showing mesenchymal differentiation in cultured cell lines. *Cancer* 69:437, 1992.

69. Iwasaki H, Yoshitake K, Ohjimi Y, et al: Malignant fibrous histiocytoma: proliferative compartment and heterogeneity of "histiocytic" cells. *Am J Surg Pathol* 16:735, 1992.

70. Jabi M, Jeans D, Dardick I: Ultrastructural heterogeneity in malignant fibrous histiocytoma of soft tissue. *Ultrastruct Pathol* 11:583, 1987.

71. Kahn LB: Retroperitoneal xanthogranuloma and xanthosarcoma. *S Afr Med J* 46:1767, 1972.

72. Kahn LB: Retroperitoneal xanthogranuloma and xanthosarcoma (malignant fibrous xanthoma). *Cancer* 31:411, 1973.

73. Kanzaki T, Kitajima S, Suzomori K: Biological behavior of cloned cells of human malignant fibrous histiocytoma in vivo and in vitro. *Cancer Res* 51:2133, 1991.

74. Kapadia GJ, Paul BD, Chung EB, et al: Carcinogenicity of Camelia sinesis (tea) and some tannin-containing fold medicinal herbs administered subcutaneously in rats. *J Natl Cancer Inst* 57:207, 1976.

75. Kaplan G, Sarino EF: Malignant fibrohistiocytoma (fibroxanthoma): case report. *Radiology* 100:155, 1971.

76. Kato T, Takeya M, Takagi K, et al: Chemically induced transplantable malignant fibrous histiocytoma of the rat: analyses with immunohistochemistry, immunoelectron microscopy and [3H] thymidine autoradiography. *Lab Invest* 62:635, 1990.

77. Kay S: Inflammatory fibrous histiocytoma (?xanthogranuloma): report of two cases with ultrastructural observations in one. *Am J Surg Pathol* 2:313, 1978.

78. Kearney MM, Soule EH, Ivins JC: Malignant fibrous histiocytoma: a retrospective study of 167 cases. *Cancer* 45:167, 1980.

79. Kempson RL, Kyriakos M: Fibroxanthosarcoma of the soft tissue: a type of malignant fibrous histiocytoma. *Cancer* 29:961, 1972.

80. Keren DF, Rawlings W, Murray HW, et al: Arizona hinshawii osteomyelitis with antecedent enteric fever and sepsis. *Am J Med* 60:577, 1976.

81. Kindblom LG, Jacobsen GK, Jacobsen M: Immunohistochemical investigations of tumours of supposed fibroblastic-histiocytic origin. *Hum Pathol* 13:834, 1982.

82. Kindblom LG, Merck C, Svendsen P: Myxofibrosarcoma: a pathological-anatomical, microangiopathic and angiographic correlative study of eight cases. *Br J Radiol* 50:876, 1977.

83. Klugo RC, Farah RN, Cerny JC: Renal malignant histiocytoma. *J Urol* 112:727, 1974.

84. Kyriakos M, Kempson RL: Inflammatory fibrous histiocytoma: an aggressive and lethal lesion. *Cancer* 37:1584, 1976.

85. Lagace R: The ultrastructural spectrum of malignant fibrous histiocytoma. *Ultrastruct Pathol* 11:153, 1987.

86. Lagace R, Delage C, Seemayer TA: Myxoid variant of malignant fibrous histiocytoma: ultrastructural observations. *Cancer* 43:526, 1979.

87. Laskin WB, Conklin RC, Enzinger FM: Malignant fibrous histiocytoma associated with hyperlipoproteinemia. *Am J Surg Pathol* 12:727, 1988.

88. Lawson CW, Fisher C, Gatter KC: An immunohistochemical study of differentiation in malignant fibrous histiocytoma. *Histopathology* 11:375, 1987.

89. Leak LV, Caulfield JB, Burke JF, et al: Electron microscopic studies on a human fibromyxosarcoma. *Cancer Res* 27:261, 1967.

90. Lindeman G, McKay MJ, Taubman KL, et al: Malignant fibrous histiocytoma developing in bone 44 years after shrapnel trauma. *Cancer* 66:2229, 1990.

91. Litzky LA, Brooks JJ: Cytokeratin immunoreactivity in malignant fibrous histiocytoma and spindle cell tumors: comparison between frozen and paraffin-embedded tissues. *Mod Pathol* 5:30, 1992.

92. Mandahl N, Heim S, Willen H, et al: Characteristic karyotypic anomalies identify subtypes of malignant fibrous histiocytoma. *Genes Chromosom Cancer* 1:9, 1989.

93. Meister P, Nathrath W: Immunohistochemical markers of histiocytic tumors. *Hum Pathol* 11:300, 1980.

94. Merkow LP, Frich JC, Sliekin M, et al: Ultrastructure of a fibroxanthosarcoma (malignant fibroxanthoma). *Cancer* 28:372, 1971.

95. Michael RH, Dorfman HD: Malignant fibrous histiocytoma associated with bone infarcts. *Clin Orthop* 118:180, 1976.

96. Miettinen M, Soini Y: Malignant fibrous histiocytoma: heterogeneous patterns of intermediate filament proteins by immunohistochemistry. *Arch Pathol Lab Med* 113:1363, 1989.

97. Minkowitz S, Friedman F, Henniger G: Xanthogranuloma of the ovary. *Arch Pathol* 80:209, 1965.

98. Mirra JM, Bullough PG, Marcove RC, et al: Malignant fibrous histiocytoma and osteosarcoma in association with bone infarcts. *J Bone Joint Surg* 56A:932, 1974.

99. Mirra JM, Gold RH, Marafiote R: Malignant (fibrous) histiocytoma arising in association with a bone infarct in sickle cell disease: coincidence or cause-and-effect? *Cancer* 39:186, 1977.

100. Nemes Z, Thomazy V: Factor XIIIa and the classic histiocytic markers in malignant fibrous histiocytoma: a comparative immunohistochemical study. *Hum Pathol* 19:822, 1988.

101. Newland RC, Harrison MA, Wright RG: Fibroxanthosarcoma of bone. *Pathology* 7:203, 1975.

102. Noel R, Michel-Bechet R: Xanthome perirenal intratesticulaire droit et sarcome fusocellulaire perirenal gauche. *Ann Anat Pathol* 10:215, 1933.

103. Nothen: Ein Fall von Fibroxanthosarcom. *Zeitsch f Pathol* 23:471, 1920.

104. Oberling C: Retroperitoneal xanthogranuloma. *Am J Cancer* 23:477, 1935.

105. O'Brien JE, Stout AP: Malignant fibrous xanthomas. *Cancer* 17:1445, 1964.

106. Orndal C, Mandahl N, Carlen B, et al: Near-haploid clones in a malignant fibrous histiocytoma. *Cancer Genet Cytogenet* 60:147, 1992.

107. Ozzello L, Stout AP, Murray MR: Cultural characteristics of malignant histiocytomas and fibrous xanthomas. *Cancer* 16:331, 1963.

108. Pezzi CM, Rawlings MS Jr, Esgro JJ, et al: Prognostic factors in 227 patients with malignant fibrous histiocytoma. *Cancer* 69:2098, 1992.

109. Radio SJ, Wooldridge TN, Linder J: Flow cytometric DNA analysis of malignant fibrous histiocytoma and related fibrohistiocytic tumors. *Hum Pathol* 19:74, 1988.

110. Roholl PJ, Kleyne J, Elbers J, et al: Characterization of tumour cells in malignant fibrous histiocytomas and other soft tissue tumours in comparison with malignant histiocytes. I. Immunohistochemical study on paraffin sections. *J Pathol* 147:87, 1985.

111. Roholl PJM, Kleyne J, Van Unnik JAM: Characterization of tumour cells in malignant fibrous histiocytomas and other soft tissue tumors, in comparison with malignant histiocytes. II. Immunoperoxidase study on cryostat sections. *Am J Pathol* 121:269, 1985.

112. Roholl PJ, Prinsen I, Rademakers LP, et al: Two cell lines with epithelial cell-like characteristics established from malignant fibrous histiocytomas. *Cancer* 68:1963, 1991.

113. Rooser B, Willen H, Gustafson P, et al: Malignant fibrous histiocytoma of soft tissue: a population-based epidemiologic and prognostic study of 137 patients. *Cancer* 67:499, 1991.

114. Rydholm A, Mandahl N, Heim S, et al: Malignant fibrous histiocytomas with a 19p+ marker chromosome have increased relapse rate. *Genes Chromosom Cancer* 2:296, 1990.

115. Rydholm A, Syk I: Malignant fibrous histiocytoma of soft tissue: correlation between clinical variables and histologic malignancy grade. *Cancer* 57:2323, 1986.

116. Serke S, Brenner M, Zimmerman R, et al: Malignant fibrous histiocytoma associated with peripheral blood eosinophilia: in vitro studies demonstrating tumor-derived eosinophilopoietic activity. *Oncology* 43:230, 1986.

117. Soini Y, Autio-Harmainen H: Tumor cells of malignant fibrous histiocytomas express mRNA for laminin. *Am J Pathol* 139:1061, 1991.

118. Soini Y, Autio-Harmainen H, Miettinen M: Immunoreactivity for laminin and type IV collagen in malignant and benign fibrous histiocytoma. *J Pathol* 158:223, 1989.

119. Soini Y, Miettinen M: Immunohistochemistry of markers of histiomonocytic cells in malignant fibrous histiocytomas: a monoclonal antibody study. *Pathol Res Pract* 186:759, 1990.

120. Soini Y, Vahakangas K, Nuorva K, et al: p53 immunohistochemistry in malignant fibrous histiocytomas and other mesenchymal tumours. *J Pathol* 168:29, 1992.

121. Soule EH, Enriquez P: Atypical fibrous histiocytoma, malignant fibrous histiocytoma, malignant histiocytoma and epithelioid sarcoma. *Cancer* 30:128, 1972.

122. Spanier SS, Enneking WF, Enriquez P: Primary malignant fibrous histiocytoma of bone. *Cancer* 36:2084, 1975.

123. Spector GJ, Pgura JH: Malignant fibrous histiocytoma of the maxilla. *Arch Otolaryngol* 99:385, 1974.

124. Takahashi K, Kimura Y, Naito M, et al: Inflammatory fibrous histiocytoma presenting leukemoid reaction. *Pathol Res Pract* 184:498, 1989.

125. Takeya M, Yoshimura T, Leonard EJ, et al: Production of monocyte chemoattractant protein-1 by malignant fibrous histiocytoma: relation to the origin of histiocyte-like cells. *Exp Mol Pathol* 54:61, 1991.

126. Taxy JB, Battifora H: The electron microscope in the study and diagnosis of soft tissue tumors. In Trump BF, Jones RT, editors: *Diagnostic electron microscopy,* vol 3, New York, 1980, John Wiley & Sons.

127. Taxy JB, Battifora H: Malignant fibrous histiocytoma: a clinicopathologic and ultrastructural study. *Cancer* 40:254, 1977.

128. Tetu B, Lacasse B, Bouchard HL, et al: Prognostic influence of HSP-27 expression in malignant fibrous histiocytoma: a clinicopathological and immunohistochemical study. *Cancer Res* 52:2325, 1992.

129. van Haelst UJGM, de Haas van Dorsser AH: Giant cell tumor of soft parts: an ultrastructural study. *Virchows Arch (Pathol Anat)* 371:199, 1976.

130. Waller JI, Hellwig CA, Barbosa E: Retroperitoneal xanthogranuloma associated with visceral eosinophilic granuloma. *Cancer* 10:388, 1957.

131. Wasserman TH, Stuard ID: Malignant fibrous histiocytoma with widespread metastases: autopsy study. *Cancer* 33:141, 1974.

132. Weiss SW: Malignant fibrous histiocytoma: a reaffirmation. *Am J Surg Pathol* 6:773, 1982.

133. Weiss SW, Bratthauer GL, Morris PA: Postirradiation malignant fibrous histiocytoma expressing cytokeratin: implications for the immunodiagnosis of sarcomas. *Am J Surg Pathol* 12:554, 1988.

134. Weiss SW, Enzinger FM: Malignant fibrous histiocytoma: an analysis of 200 cases. *Cancer* 41:2250, 1978.

135. Weiss SW, Enzinger FM: Myxoid variant of malignant fibrous histiocytoma. *Cancer* 39:1672, 1977.

136. Wolff K: The Langerhans cell. *Curr Probl Dermatol* 4:79, 1972.

137. Wood GS, Beckstead JH, Turner RR, et al: Malignant fibrous histiocytoma tumor cells resemble fibroblasts. *Am J Surg Pathol* 10:323, 1986.

138. Yumoto T, Morimoto K: Experimental approach to fibrous histiocytoma. *Acta Pathol Jpn* 30:767, 1980.

139. Zehr RJ, Bauer TW, Marks KE, et al: Ki-67 and grading of malignant fibrous histiocytomas. *Cancer* 66:1984, 1990.

CHAPTER 16

BENIGN LIPOMATOUS TUMORS

ADIPOSE TISSUE
Structure

Although adipose tissue has been the subject of intensive investigation in recent years, its significance and multiple functions are not always fully appreciated. Fat serves not only as one of the principal and most readily available sources of energy in the body, but it also functions as a barrier for the conservation of heat and as mechanical protection of the underlying tissues against physical injury.

Two basic forms of adipose tissue can be distinguished: *white fat,* which is chiefly deposited in the subcutaneous tissue, mediastinum, abdomen, and retroperitoneum; and *brown fat,* which is largely restricted to the interscapular region, neck, mediastinum, axillae, and retroperitoneum, especially the perirenal region. Brown fat is much more conspicuous in rodents and hibernating animals than in humans. In humans it is found mainly in infants and children; in adults it is much less conspicuous and, in addition to the regions of the neck and mediastinum, is found mainly around the kidneys, adrenals, and aorta. The principal function of brown fat is heat production.[4]

Differentiated *white fat* consists of spherical or polygonal cells in which most of the cytoplasm has been replaced by a single large lipid droplet, leaving only a narrow rim of cytoplasm at the periphery. The eccentrically placed nucleus is flattened and is crescent shaped on cross section; not infrequently it contains one small lipid invagination (Lochkern). The white fat cells (lipocytes) measure up to 120 µ in diameter. Like any metabolically active tissue, white fat is highly vascularized, a feature that is much more evident in atrophic than in normal fat. In the subcutis and to a lesser extent in deeper tissues, the fat cells are arranged in distinct lobules separated by a thin membrane of fibrous connective tissue. The lobular architecture of white fat is most prominent in areas subjected to pressure and probably has a cushioning effect.[8-11]

Brown fat plays an insignificant role in humans. Its cells are smaller in size, measuring 25 to 40 µ in diameter, are round or polygonal, and contain a greater amount of cytoplasm that stains deeply eosinophilic with hematoxylin-eosin preparation. The cells are mostly multivacuolated, with distinctly granular cytoplasm between the individual lipid droplets. Intermixed with these cells are nonvacuolated, purely granular cells and cells with a single large lipid vacuole, resembling lipocytes. The nuclei are rounded and situated in a central position; however, the nucleus may be displaced to the periphery in cells with large lipid vacuoles as in white fat. The cells are arranged in distinct lobular aggregates and are intimately associated with a prominent vascular network and numerous nerves (Fig. 16-1). There are apparent transitions between brown and white fat in both humans and animals, but brown fat can be clearly identified under the electron microscope by the prominence of mitochondria and the richly vascular pattern. Brown fat is increased in cachectic and chronic hypoxemic states and in patients with pheochromocytoma and increased plasma catecholamines.

Prenatal development

White fat makes its first appearance at a relatively late stage of development and is rarely encountered before the third or fourth month of intrauterine life. In its earliest stages, after 10 to 14 weeks' gestation, it consists merely of delicate branching capillaries that are surrounded by an adventitial "cloud" of undifferentiated spindle- or stellate-shaped mesenchymal cells closely resembling fibroblasts (preadipocytes). At later stages (14 to 24 weeks' gestation), small oil-red-O positive and sudanophilic lipid droplets appear in these cells, gradually converting them to rounded or spherical, multivacuolated lipoblasts (Figs. 16-2 and 16-3). Intracellular glycogen is usually present at this stage of development. The multiple lipid droplets then fuse to a single vacuole and displace the nucleus marginally and form the mature fat cell or lipocyte. Small aggregates of lipocytes form small lobules, which make their first appearance in the regions of the face, neck, and breast. The lobules

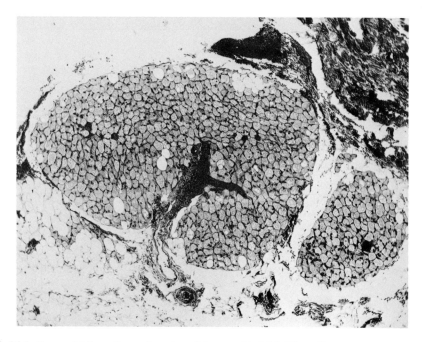

FIG. 16-1. Brown fat from the neck region of 1-year-old child. The cells are arranged in lobular aggregates and have distinctly granular appearance. (×55.)

multiply and enlarge, and by the end of the fifth month a continuous subcutaneous layer of fat is formed in the extremities.[7]

The circumscribed complex of branching capillaries and maturing preadipocytes and fat cells was described by Wasserman[12] as the "primitive fat organ." Because mature fat has no proliferative capacity,[1] "the primitive fat organ" is the main source of mature adipose tissue. However, later in life fat may also be formed in a similar manner from the ubiquitous stores of primitive perivascular mesenchyme.

Ultrastructure

According to Napolitano's[5,6] classic description, the ultrastructure of adipose tissue cells in the earliest stage of development closely resembles that of fibroblasts: the cells are spindle shaped, have slender cytoplasmic extensions, and contain small spherical mitochondria and abundant highly organized endoplasmic reticulum. At later stages of development the endoplasmic reticulum becomes less conspicuous, and one or more inclusions of nonmembrane-bound lipid make their appearance in the cytoplasm, usually adjacent to the nucleus. There are also irregular, smooth-surfaced, membrane-limited vesicles, a rather poorly developed Golgi apparatus, and, in close association with the lipid inclusions, glycogen granules. An amorphous basal lamina sets the cells apart from the surrounding collagen and occasional nonmyelinated nerves; the basal lamina is present in all stages of cellular differentiation and helps to distinguish preadipocytes from fibroblasts.

Continued accumulation of cytoplasm and increasing amounts of intracellular lipid lead to more rounded cells, which are characterized by a large, centrally located lipid droplet, a thin rim of cytoplasm, and a peripherally placed, flattened or crescent-shaped nucleus. There is a membrane separating the central lipid inclusion from the surrounding cytoplasm. This "signet ring" stage of cellular development represents the lipocyte of mature adipose tissue.

The brown fat cell shows for the most part similar ultrastructural features,[3,366] but it is usually smaller and can be recognized by numerous lipid inclusions of small size and mitochondria that are both more numerous and more complex in structure. There are also scattered ribosomes, variable amounts of glycogen, and a poorly developed endoplasmic reticulum. The profusion of mitochondria and the rich vascularity are responsible for the typical reddish brown color of brown fat. The ultrastructural features do not support the concept that brown fat is merely an arrested stage in the development of white fat.

CLASSIFICATION OF BENIGN LIPOMATOUS TUMORS

It is widely assumed that benign lipomatous tumors represent a common group of neoplasms that cause few complaints or complications and hardly ever any difficulties in diagnosis. This may be largely true for the ordinary subcutaneous lipoma, but this does not take into account the great variety of benign tumors and tumorlike lesions of adipose tissue that are well defined but often have received little attention in the medical literature.

The bulk of benign lipomatous tumors may be grouped

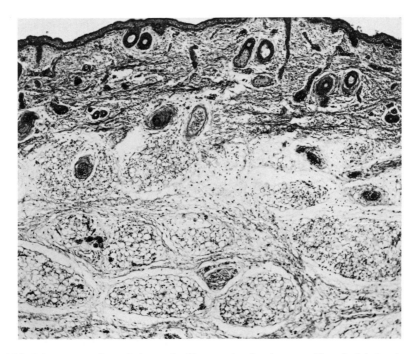

FIG. 16-2. Subcutaneous fat at sixth month of intrauterine development. Note the lobulated growth, the "primitive fat organs" of Wassermann. (×55.)

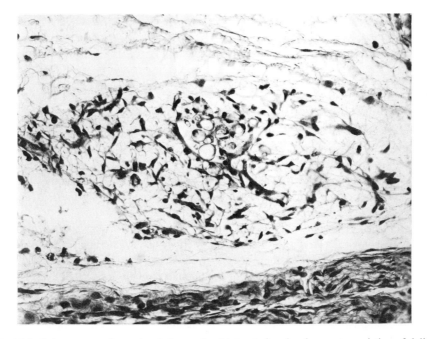

FIG. 16-3. Subcutaneous fat at the sixth month of intrauterine development consisting of delicate branching capillaries surrounded by a "cloud" of spindle and stellate-shaped mesenchymal cells gradually being transformed into lipoblasts. (×250.)

into five categories, each of which may be further divided into several subdivisions:

1. *Lipoma,* a tumor that is composed of mature fat and represents by far the most common mesenchymal neoplasm. It may be single or multiple and may occur as a superficial (subcutaneous) or deep-seated tumor.

2. *Variants of lipoma* that are much less common and differ from ordinary lipoma by a characteristic microscopic picture and specific clinical setting. This group is chiefly represented by angiolipoma, myolipoma, angiomyolipoma, myelolipoma, chondroid lipoma, spindle cell and pleomorphic lipoma, and benign lipoblastoma. "Atypical lipoma" is a term applied to superficial forms of well-differentiated liposarcoma. It is discussed in the chapter on liposarcoma (see Chapter 17).

3. *Heterotopic lipomas, neoplasms or hamartomatous lesions* that arise from or are intimately associated with specific tissue other than adipose tissue. The main subdivisions of this group are angiomyolipoma, intramuscular and intermuscular lipoma, lipoma of tendon sheath, neural fibrolipoma with and without macrodactyly (fibrolipomatous hamartoma), and lumbosacral lipoma.

4. *Infiltrating or diffuse neoplastic or nonneoplastic proliferations of mature fat* that may cause compression of vital structures or may be confused with well-differentiated liposarcoma. This group is composed of six separate entities: diffuse lipomatosis, pelvic lipomatosis, symmetrical lipomatosis (Madelung's disease), adiposis dolorosa (Dercum's disease), steroid lipomatosis, and nevus lipomatosus.

5. *Hibernoma,* the benign tumor of brown fat.

In describing the various entities, we have made no attempt to distinguish between true neoplasms, hamartomatous processes, and localized overgrowth of fat, for this is largely speculative and of little practical consequence.

LIPOMA

Solitary lipomas, consisting entirely of mature fat, have stirred little interest in the past and have been largely ignored in the literature. This continued neglect is not surprising, considering that most lipomas grow insidiously and cause few problems other than those of a localized mass. Many lipomas remain unrecorded or are brought to the attention of a physician only if they reach a large size or cause cosmetic problems or complications because of their anatomical site. As a consequence, the reported incidence of lipoma is probably much lower than the actual incidence. But even if we consider only the recorded data, lipomas outnumber other benign or malignant soft tissue tumors by a considerable margin and doubtlessly represent the most common soft tissue tumor. This is true for the solitary subcutaneous lipoma as well as lipomas in general, regardless of histological type.

Age and sex incidence

Lipoma is rare during the first 2 decades of life and usually makes its appearance when fat begins to accumulate in inactive individuals. Most become apparent in patients between ages 40 and 60 years and, when unexcised, persist for the remainder of life; they hardly increase in size after the initial growth period. Statistics as to sex incidence vary, but most report a higher incidence in men.[35,37] There seems to be no difference in regard to race, and in the United States whites and blacks are affected in proportion to their distribution in the general population.

Localization

Two types of solitary lipomas can be distinguished. *Subcutaneous* or *superficial lipomas* are most common in the regions of the upper back and neck, shoulder, and abdomen, followed in frequency by the proximal portions of the extremities, chiefly the upper arms, buttocks, and upper thigh. They are seldom encountered in the face, hands, lower legs, and feet.[15,25,31,35,87]

Deep lipomas are rare in comparison. They are often detected at a relatively late stage of development, and consequently the average size tends to be larger than that of cutaneous lipomas. Numerous sites may be involved. When in the extremities they often arise from the subfascial tissues of the hands and feet, where they have often been mistaken for ganglion cysts.* They may also arise from juxta-articular regions or the periosteum (*parosteal lipoma),†* sometimes causing nerve compression, erosion of bone, or focal cortical hyperostosis. There may also be secondary bone and cartilage formation within the tumor or association with congenital skeletal anomalies.[26,32,36,51] Deep lipomas in the region of the head occur chiefly in the forehead and scalp;[23] those in the trunk are found principally in the thorax and mediastinum,‡ chest wall and pleura,[67,77] pelvis and retroperitoneum,[53,69,81] and paratesticular region.[45]

In the gastrointestinal tract, lipomas are mainly found in the submucosa and subserosa of the small and large intestines, and are mostly an incidental finding at autopsy.[42,78] They are solitary or multiple, and present as a sessile or pedunculated mass; sometimes they are associated with ulceration and bleeding, intussusception, Crohn's disease, or malignancies.[66,80]

Deep or subfascial lipomas tend to be less well circumscribed than superficial ones, and their contours are usually determined by the spaces they occupy. Intrathoracic lipomas, for instance, may extend from the upper mediastinum, neck, or subpleural region (*cervicomediastinal lipoma*) into the subcutis of the chest wall, sometimes assuming an hourglass configuration (*transmural lipoma*).

*References 44, 46-49, 52, 59, 70, 71, 73.
†References 21, 55, 62, 68, 75, 79.
‡References 50, 56, 58, 60, 61, 63, 65, 72.

Deep-seated lipomas of the hand or wrist form irregular masses with multiple processes beneath fascia or aponeurosis; they may attain a large size and, on rare occasions, may extend from the palm to the dorsal surface of the hand. These tumors must be distinguished from lipomas growing within the tendon sheath (endovaginal lipomas) and lipomas involving major nerves in the regions of the hand and wrist (neural fibrolipomas), lesions that usually occur in younger patients.

There are also rare lipoma-like fatty proliferations in the region of the umbilicus and inguinal ring (hernial lipoma) that may be associated with direct or indirect hernias or merely simulate a hernia clinically. A similar overgrowth of fat arising from surgical scars has been termed incisional lipoma.

Clinical findings

The usual clinical history of lipoma is that of an asymptomatic, slow-growing, round or discoid mass having a soft or doughy consistency. The fact that the mass hardens after application of ice has been used by some clinicians as a diagnostic criterion. There is usually good mobility, and there is dimpling of the skin on movement. Pain is rare in ordinary lipomas, and when it occurs, it is a late symptom generally confined to angiolipomas or lipomas of large size

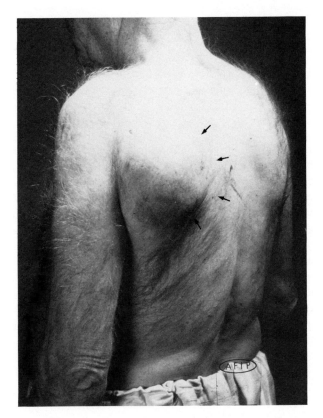

FIG. 16-4. Large lipoma (arrows) of the left shoulder region in a 65-year-old man.

that compress peripheral nerves. Rarely nerve compression leads to sensory and motor disturbances and carpal or tarsal tunnel syndrome.[73] Lipomas are more common in obese persons and often increase in size during a period of rapid weight gain. In contrast, severe weight loss in cachectic patients or during periods of prolonged starvation rarely affects the size of lipoma, suggesting that the fatty tissue of lipomas (or liposarcomas) is largely unavailable for the general metabolism.

Deep or subfascial lipomas may cause a variety of symptoms, depending upon their site and size. The symptoms range from a feeling of fullness and discomfort on motion and, rarely, restriction of movement with lipomas of the hand to dyspnea or palpitation with mediastinal tumors. Distinction of large lipomas of the retroperitoneum from well-differentiated liposarcomas may be exceedingly difficult on the basis of clinical presentation. In fact, most of the huge retroperitoneal lipomas described in the earlier literature represent well-differentiated liposarcomas rather than lipomas.

Roentgenographs are most helpful in diagnosis; lipomas present as globular radiolucent masses clearly outlined by the greater density of the surrounding tissue. On CT scan and MRI, lipomas have the appearance of subcutaneous fat and, like fat, have a much more uniform density than liposarcomas. MRI does not permit separation from old hematomas.[64]

Gross findings

Subcutaneous lipoma usually manifests as a soft, well-circumscribed, thinly encapsulated, rounded mass varying in size from a few millimeters to 5 cm or more (median, 3 cm); lipomas larger than 10 cm are rare (Fig. 16-4). On cross section lipoma is pale yellow to orange and has a uniform greasy surface and an irregular lobular pattern (Fig. 16-5, A). Lipomas of deeper structures vary much more in shape, but they also tend to be well delineated from the surrounding tissues by a thin capsule. Focal discoloration caused by hemorrhage or fat necrosis occurs, but it is much less common than in liposarcoma.

Chemical analysis of normal adipose tissue and lipomas revealed quantitative rather than qualitative differences, such as increased lipoprotein lipase, indicating merely greater lipid synthesis and triglyceride accumulation than mobilization.[2,37]

Microscopic findings

Lipomas differ little in microscopic appearance from the surrounding fat. Like fat they are composed of mature fat cells, but the cells vary slightly in size and shape and are somewhat larger, measuring up to 200 μ in diameter (Fig. 16-5, B). The nuclei are fairly uniform, but the presence of a rare cell with a hyperchromatic nucleus is still compatible with a benign diagnosis. Subcutaneous lipomas are usually thinly encapsulated and have distinct lobular pat-

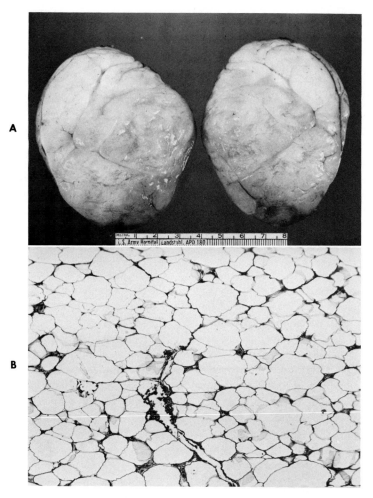

FIG. 16-5. **A,** Lipoma of the thigh showing a distinct multilobular pattern. **B,** Lipoma consisting throughout of mature fat cells showing only slight variation in cellular size and shape. (×100.)

terns. Deep-seated lipomas possess a more irregular configuration, largely depending on the site of origin. All are well vascularized, but under normal conditions the vascular network is compressed by the distended lipocytes and is not clearly discernible. The rich vascularity of these tumors, however, becomes clearly apparent in atrophic lipomas in which the markedly reduced volume of the lipocytes reveals the intricate vascular network within the interstitial spaces (Fig. 16-6, *B*).

Lipomas are occasionally altered by the admixture of other mesenchymal elements that form an intrinsic part of the tumor. The most common of these is fibrous connective tissue, which is often hyalinized and may or may not be associated with the capsule or the fibrous septa. Lipomas with these features are often classified as *fibrolipomas* (Fig. 16-7). *Myxolipomas* are lipomas in which portions of the tumor are replaced by mucoid substances that stain well with alcian blue and are removed or depolymerized by prior

treatment of the sections with testicular hyaluronidase (Figs. 16-6 and 16-8). Distinction of these tumors from *myxomas* and *myxoid liposarcomas* may be difficult. In general, however, the presence of transitional zones between fat and myxoid areas helps to rule out myxoma, and the absence of lipoblasts and a plexiform capillary pattern militates against myxoid liposarcoma.[123] Atypical vacuolated cells containing mucoid material are occasionally seen in myxolipoma, but unlike neoplastic lipoblasts, these cells lack hyperchromatic nuclei and distinctly outlined lipid droplets within the cytoplasm. Like normal fat cells, the cytoplasmic rim of the fat cells of lipoma is immunoreactive for S-100 protein.[19]

Cartilaginous or osseous metaplasia *(chondrolipoma, osteolipoma)* is rare and is mainly encountered in lipomas of large size and long standing.[28] Some pathologists prefer to classify these variants of lipoma as *benign mesenchymomas. Myolipoma,* a lipoma with a distinct smooth muscle

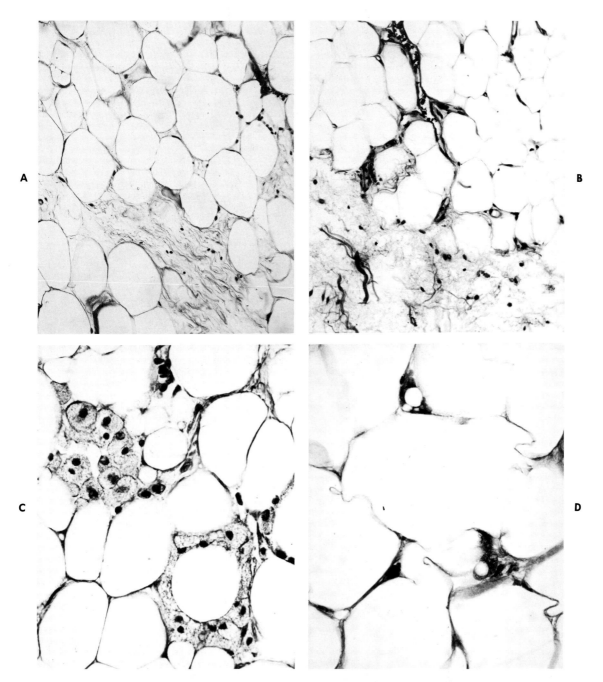

FIG. 16-6. Lipoma with early edema and fibrosis **(A)**, myxoid change **(B)**, macrophages **(C)**, vacuolated nucleus (Lochkern), a common feature of both mature fat and lipomas that has been confused for evidence of lipoblastic activity **(D)**. **(A,** ×160; **B,** ×145; **C,** ×350; **D,** ×400.)

component, and *chondroid lipoma,* a tumor displaying features of both chondrolipoma and hibernoma, are discussed below as separate entities.

Secondary changes occur occasionally as the result of impaired blood supply or traumatic injury. Prolonged ischemia may lead to infarction, hemorrhage, and calcification[33] and

may terminate in cystlike changes. Similarly, infection or trauma may cause fat necrosis and local liquefaction of fat, a process that is marked by phagocytic activity and formation of lipid cysts. Characteristically, nests of foamy macrophages are found in the intercellular spaces or around lipocytes that have been ruptured or traumatized (Fig. 16-6,

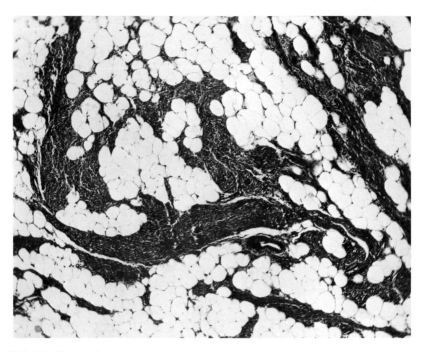

FIG. 16-7. Fibrolipoma showing replacement of fatty tissue by dense trabeculae and septa of richly collagenous fibrous connective tissue. (Trichrome stain; ×160.)

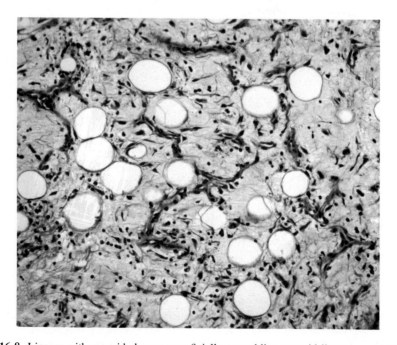

FIG. 16-8. Lipoma with myxoid change superficially resembling myxoid liposarcoma. (×160.)

C). This process is sometimes accompanied by multinucleated giant cells and scattered inflammatory elements, chiefly lymphocytes or plasma cells. As in lipogranuloma, hyaline fibrosis and calcification may become prominent features in late stages of this process. Rarely there is a nodular pattern caused by encapsulation of the necrotic lobules of fat.

Ultrastructure

Like normal white fat, lipomas are composed of mature lipocytes with a single centrally positioned large lipid vacuole and peripherally placed cytoplasm and nucleus. The cytoplasm consists of smooth membrane-bound vesicles, ribosomes, and round or oval mitochondria, together with small amounts of glycogen, rough endoplasmic reticulum, and an inconspicuous Golgi apparatus. The nuclei display peripheral condensation of chromatin and prominent nucleoli. There are also numerous pinocytotic vesicles and a well-developed basal lamina.[18,22] Small spindle cells with occasional lipid vacuoles are often situated along the interstitial capillaries; these are probably potential precursors of adipocytes (preadipocytes).[37]

Behavior and treatment

Lipomas are benign. They may recur locally, but following local excision the recurrence rate is less than 5% of all tumors.[13,43] Malignant changes in a lipoma are exceedingly rare, and only a few examples have been reported in the literature. It is likely, however, that some of these are pleomorphic lipomas, and others are well-differentiated liposarcomas in which the malignant characteristics were absent or missed when the tumor was first examined. Deep lipomas have a greater tendency to recur, presumably because of the greater difficulty of complete surgical removal.

Etiological factors

Aside from the relatively small number of patients in whom an increased familial incidence of lipomas can be demonstrated, very little is known about the pathogenesis of these tumors. Certainly lipomas are more common in obese than in slender persons and, perhaps as a consequence, are more frequently encountered in patients older than 45 years. An increased incidence of lipomas is also claimed for diabetic patients and patients with elevation of serum cholesterol. It is doubtful, however, whether the stated association of lipoma with rheumatoid arthritis or with a family history of cancer is more than a mere coincidence.[37]

Trauma or radiation may lead to overgrowth of fat indistinguishable from a lipoma. In particular, such lesions, often exceeding 10 cm in diameter, have been observed to develop secondary to blunt, bruising injuries, often preceded by a large hematoma.[16,27,30,34]

Chromosomal abnormalities demonstrated in lipoma include translocation of t(3;12)(q27;q13) and t(3;12)(q28;q14), rearrangement of band 12q14, and ring chromosomes.[20,38,41,89,95]

MULTIPLE LIPOMAS

Approximately 5% to 8% of all patients with lipomas have multiple tumors that grossly and microscopically are indistinguishable from solitary lipomas.[82] The term "lipomatosis" has been used to describe this lesion, but we prefer to use this name for a diffuse neoplastic proliferation of fat.

Multiple lipomas vary in number from a few to several hundred lesions and occur predominantly in the upper half of the body, with a predilection for the back, shoulder, and upper arms (Fig. 16-9). Not infrequently the lipomas are arranged in a symmetrical distribution, with a slight predilection for the extensor surfaces of the extremities. They are about three times as common in men as in women.[37] Most have their onset during the fifth and sixth decades; occasional lesions appear as early as puberty. Hyperlipidemia with high serum levels of cholesterol was reported in some cases.[76,92] Local excision and suction lipectomy have been recommended as the treatment of choice.[54]

There is a definite hereditary trait in about one third of patients with this condition (*familial multiple lipomas*).[93] For instance, in one of our cases multiple lipomas were observed in members of the same family during three successive generations. In most reports both males and females are affected, suggesting simple dominant inheritance.[37,93,96,98]

There is no evidence of any chemical differences in the composition of solitary and multiple lipomas.[2] Associated hypercholesterolemia, however, was noted repeatedly.[92,98] Increased incidence of multiple lipomas is also reported in diabetic patients at the site of insulin injections,[40] in patients with psoriasis and arthritis,[86] and during pregnancy.[85] According to our material, coronary infarction is slightly more common in patients with solitary or multiple lipomas, but this may be related to the age incidence and male predominance of these tumors.

The question of a relationship between multiple lipomas and neurofibromatosis has been raised repeatedly in the literature, but to our knowledge there is no convincing proof of this association, including Alsberg's[83] much quoted case of "neurolipoma." In fact, we have never observed solitary or multiple lipomas in a patient with neurofibromatosis, nor are we aware of such a case in the medical literature.

There are several syndromes with multiple lipomatous lesions: *Bannayan-Zonana syndrome* is characterized by the congenital association of multiple lipomas (including lipomatosis of the thoracic and abdominal cavity in some cases), hemangiomas, and macrocephaly.[84,90,94,100] *Cowden's syndrome* consists of multiple lipomas and hemangiomas associated with goiter and lichenoid, papular, and

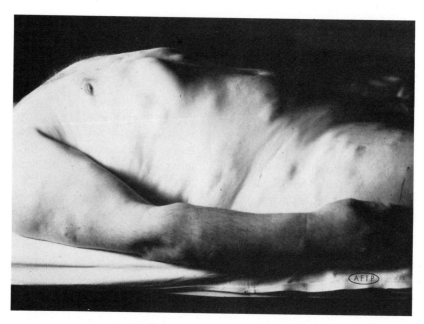

FIG. 16-9. Patient with multiple lipomata affecting the arm, trunk, and thigh.

papillomatous lesions of skin and mucosae.[99] *Fröhlich's syndrome* is defined by multiple lipomas, obesity, and sexual infantilism. *Proteus syndrome* is marked by multiple lipomatous lesions, including pelvic lipomatosis, fibroplasia of the feet and hands, skeletal hypertrophy, exostoses and scoliosis, and various pigmented lesions of the skin.[295]

ANGIOLIPOMA

Angiolipoma occurs chiefly as a subcutaneous nodule in young adults, often making its first appearance when the patient is in the late teens or early twenties; it is rare in children and, unlike solitary or multiple subcutaneous lipomas, in patients older than 50 years. The forearm is by far the most common single site, and almost two thirds of all angiolipomas are found in this location. Next in frequency are the trunk and the upper arm. Like all lipomas it seldom occurs in the face, scalp, hands, and feet.[103,112] Spinal angiolipoma is a specific entity that should be distinguished from cutaneous angiolipoma.[109]

Multiple angiolipomas are much more common than solitary ones and are found in about two out of three patients with angiolipoma.[105,107] Sometimes there are numerous lesions in the same patient.[102] Belcher et al.,[101] for example, reported a 31-year-old male patient who developed no fewer than 204 angiolipomas in a 15-year period.

Characteristically, angiolipomas are tender to painful, often only on touch or palpation, particularly so during the initial growth period; frequently pain becomes less severe or ceases entirely when the tumor reaches its final size, which is rarely more than 2 cm. There seems to be no correlation between the degree of vascularity and the occurrence or intensity of pain. Nor is the pain intensified by heat, cold, or venous occlusion. Increased familial incidence has been recorded, but, as in ordinary lipomas, familial incidence does not exceed 5% of all cases. Trauma has been implicated as a possible contributing or causative factor.[111]

At operation angiolipomas are always located in the subcutis, where they present as encapsulated yellow nodules having a more or less pronounced reddish tinge. Under the microscope these nodules consist of mature fat cells separated by a branching network of small vessels (Figs. 16-10 and 16-11); the proportion of fatty tissue and vascular channels varies, but usually the vascularity is slightly more prominent in the subcapsular areas. Late forms of this tumor frequently undergo perivascular and interstitial fibrosis (Fig. 16-12). Characteristically, the vascular channels contain fibrin thrombi, a feature that is absent in ordinary lipomas[95] (Fig. 16-13). Dixon and McGregor[104] demonstrated fluorescein-labeled antihuman fibrinogen in the thrombi and, to a lesser degree, in the surrounding endothelial cells.

Ultrastructurally, angiolipoma consists of adipocytes and interspersed vascular structures lined by elongated endothelial cells with irregular fingerlike extensions, basal lamina, and long tight junctions, and surrounded by pericytes. Compared with normal endothelium, Weibel-Palade bodies are scarce. The fibrin thrombi are associated with disrupted endothelial cells. There is no evidence of systemic coagulopathy.[104]

Hypercellular angiolipomas (Fig. 16-14), composed almost entirely of vascular channels, should not be confused

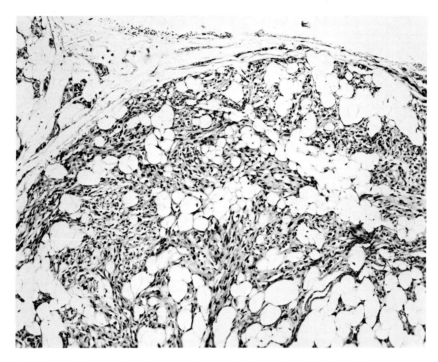

FIG. 16-10. Angiolipoma showing sharp circumscription and proliferation of numerous vascular channels of uniformly small caliber. (×100.)

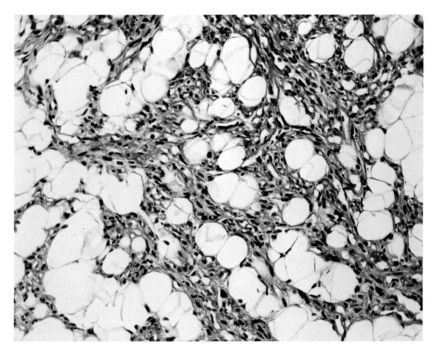

FIG. 16-11. Angiolipoma consisting of a mixture of mature fat cells and narrow vascular channels. (×210.)

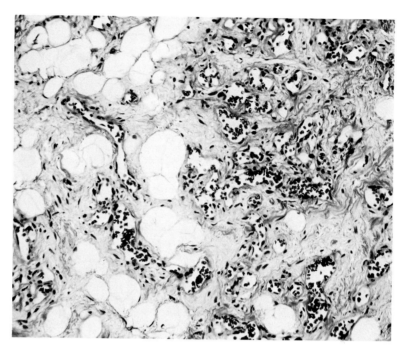

FIG. 16-12. Angiolipoma with prominent perivascular fibrosis. (×160.)

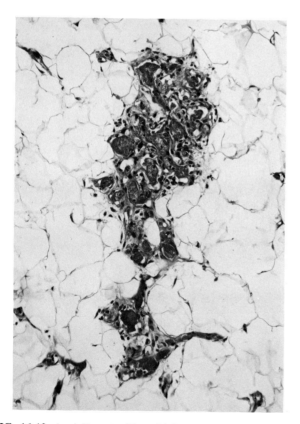

FIG. 16-13. Angiolipoma with multiple microthrombi, a characteristic feature of this tumor. (×160.)

with *Kaposi's sarcoma* or *angiosarcoma*. In general, a correct diagnosis should not be too difficult if attention is paid to the encapsulation of the lesion and especially to the presence of microthrombi in some of the vessels, as well as the small size, multiplicity, and subcutaneous location of the lesion. These features will also help in separating the tumor from *intramuscular hemangioma* having an unusually prominent fatty component, a tumor that has also been reported under the name of *cellular* or *infiltrating angiolipoma*.[106,108,110]

Angiolipomas are benign. There is no evidence that these lesions ever undergo malignant transformation.

MYOLIPOMA

This is a very rare variant of lipoma marked by the proliferation of fat and smooth muscle tissue. It occurs in adults, but there seems to be no preference for any particular site. It is found both in the subcutis and in deeper tissues, including the abdominal cavity and the retroperitoneum. Seven of the reported nine cases[135] were larger than 10 cm, the largest, a tumor of the pelvis, being 26 cm in greatest diameter. Myolipoma is usually well circumscribed, and microscopically consists of mature adipose tissue and interspersed smooth muscle bundles. The smooth muscle elements stain well with Masson trichrome preparation and are immunoreactive for smooth muscle actin and desmin (Figs. 16-15 and 16-16). Because of its large size and frequent deep location, the tumor may be confused with sarcoma, but neither the adipose tissue nor the smooth mus-

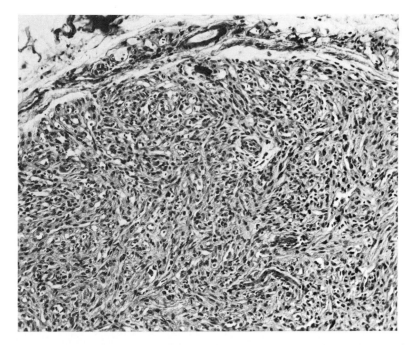

FIG. 16-14. Cellular angiolipoma in which the fatty component is replaced almost entirely by vascular component. Lesions of this type have been mistaken for Kaposi's sarcoma or spindle cell angiosarcoma. (×100.)

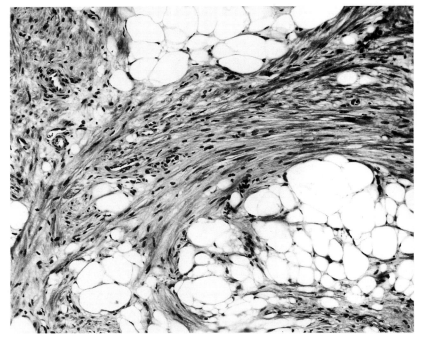

FIG. 16-15. Myolipoma showing mixture of elongated eosinophilic smooth muscle cells and adipocytes. (×165.)

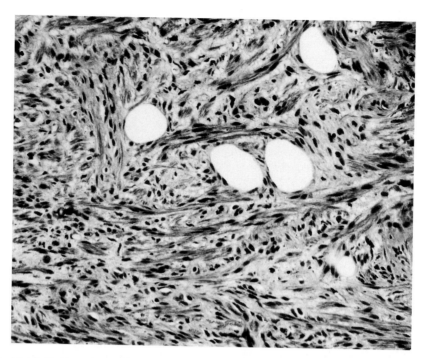

FIG. 16-16. Portion of myolipoma showing only a few mature fat cells among the proliferated smooth muscle cells. (×165.)

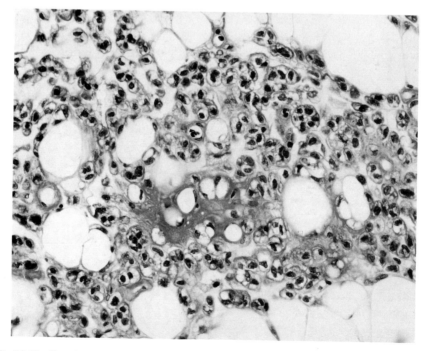

FIG. 16-17. Chondroid lipoma showing vacuolated cells associated with mature fat cells and focal hyalinization. (×210.)

cle component shows nuclear atypism or increased mitotic activity. Tumors of similar appearance in the retroperitoneum and the uterus were described as "angiomyolipoma," "fibrolipomyoma," and "lipoleiomyoma."[127-129,132]

CHONDROID LIPOMA

This is a rare fatty tumor that has been confused with liposarcoma and chondrosarcoma. A typical example of this tumor was previously reported as "extraskeletal chondroma with lipoblast-like cells."[119] In our series of 20 cases,[134] this tumor occurred foremost in the upper and lower limbs of adult patients (median age, 36 years) and presented in the subcutis or muscle as a well-demarcated yellow mass (median size, 4 cm).

Microscopically, chondroid lipoma has a lobular pattern and consists of strands and nests of round or polygonal eosinophilic cells, many with lipid vacuoles closely simulating lipoblasts. The surrounding stroma consists of a mixture of mature fat, myxoid and chondroid material, and partly hyalinized fibrous tissue (Fig. 16-17). The multivacuolated cells contain neutral fat and glycogen. They stain positively with ORO and PAS stains and are positive for vimentin and S-100 protein. The exact nature of this tumor is still uncertain; since it shows features of both lipoma and hibernoma, an ultrastructural study will be needed to resolve the question of histogenesis. Despite its cellular atypism, the lesion seems to be benign, and there were no recurrences or metastases.

SPINDLE CELL LIPOMA

This is a histologically distinct type of lipoma that is characterized by replacement of mature fat by collagen-forming spindle cells. Despite its cellularity it is a benign lesion that is readily cured by local excision. Clinically and morphologically, it is related to pleomorphic lipoma.

Spindle cell lipoma has a typical clinical setting; it occurs mainly in male patients between 45 and 65 years of age and is found chiefly in the regions of the posterior neck and shoulder (Fig.16-18).[118,121,126,133,136] Unusual sites are the oral cavity, orbit, and extremities.[116,125,130,133] Younger individuals and women are not exempt, and occasional examples of the tumor may also occur at other sites. We have never encountered this tumor, however, in adolescents or children. Like ordinary lipoma it manifests as a solitary, circumscribed or encapsulated, painless, firm nodule in the deep subcutis that is slow growing and often has been present for several years. Multiple lesions are very rare, but one of us (SWW) has encountered several such cases, including one with over a hundred lesions and another in which four members of one family, all males, had multiple spindle cell lipomas.

Grossly, the nodule resembles a lipoma except for gray-white gelatinous foci, representing the areas of spindle cell proliferation. The lesions average in size between 3 and 5

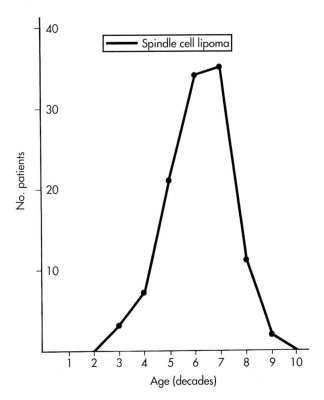

FIG. 16-18. Age distribution of 114 patients with spindle cell lipoma, ranging from 25 to 89 years, with a median age of 56 years. Of these patients, 91% were males.

cm. Microscopically, the tumor varies in appearance: most are composed of a mixture of mature fat cells and uniform spindle cells that are closely associated with a mucoid matrix and a varying number of birefringent collagen fibers; some show mostly the features of lipoma, with only a portion of the lesion being replaced by the typical mixture of spindle cells and lipocytes (Fig. 16-19). The spindle cells tend to be well aligned, and generally there is little cellular pleomorphism (Figs. 16-20 to 16-21); transitional forms between spindle cell and pleomorphic lipoma do occur, however (see Fig.16-28). Occasionally lipocytes are rare or absent, and the spindle cells dominate the histological picture (Figs. 16-22 and 16-23). There are also highly myxoid tumors with relatively few spindle cells that may be confused with myxoma. In most cases the vascular pattern is inconspicuous and consists of a few thick-walled vessels of small or intermediate size. Extensive vascularization, reminiscent of a myxoid liposarcoma or even a vascular tumor, is occasionally observed[139] (Fig. 16-24). Immunostaining of the spindle cell varies. Some are positive for vimentin and S-100 protein, but they are not immunoreactive for laminin and are negative for monocyte/macrophage antigen (MAC-387).[117]

The exact nature of the spindle cells is still uncertain,

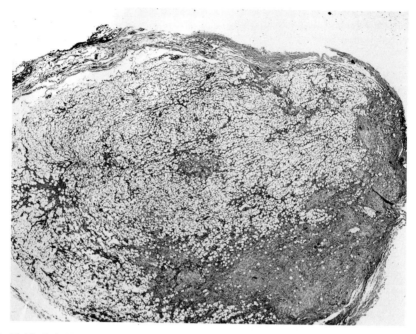

FIG. 16-19. Spindle cell lipoma. Note circumscription of the lesion and irregular distribution of the spindle cell areas. (×5.)

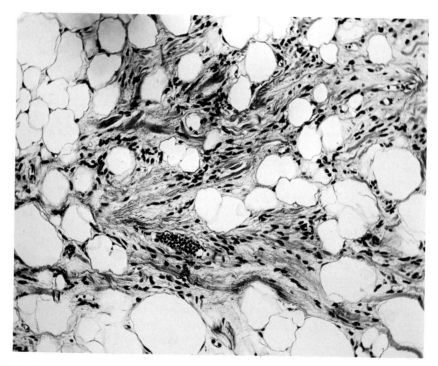

FIG. 16-20. Spindle cell lipoma showing an equal mixture of mature fat cells and uniform spindle cells. The spindle cells are associated with a mucoid matrix and bundles of collagen. (×140.)

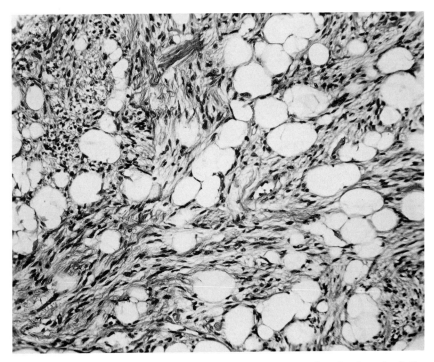

FIG. 16-21. Spindle cell lipoma. Most of the lesion consists of small well-oriented spindle cells showing no evidence of cellular pleomorphism. (×160.)

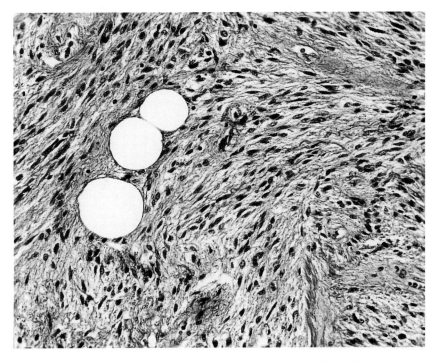

FIG. 16-22. Spindle cell lipoma showing proliferation of uniform, collagen-forming spindle cells with interspersed mature fat cells. (×165.)

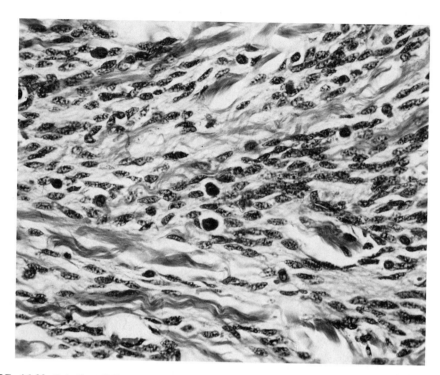

FIG. 16-23. Spindle cell lipoma composed almost entirely of spindle cells accompanied by bundles of mature collagen and scattered mast cells. Fat cells were present in other portions of the lesion. (×400.)

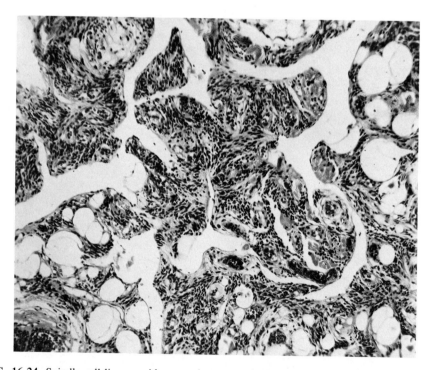

FIG. 16-24. Spindle cell lipoma with a prominent vascular pattern, a feature that is occasionally encountered in lesions of long duration and may be mistaken for evidence of vascular origin. (×110.)

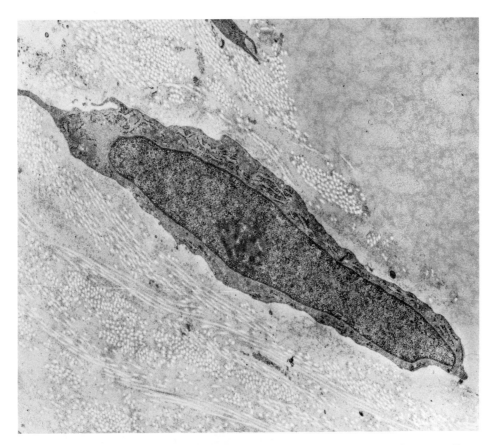

FIG. 16-25. Electron micrograph of spindle cell lipoma. Note the close resemblance to a fibroblast and the presence of collagen fibrils in the extracellular space. (×12,500.)

especially since it is difficult to distinguish early fibroblasts and prelipoblasts under the electron microscope[122] (Fig. 16-25). It is likely that the spindle cells originate from primitive mesenchymal cells, especially since the spindle cells lack a basal lamina and produce considerable amounts of collagen.[113,117,131] Bolen and Thorning[118] suggested that the spindle cells are analogous to the stellate mesenchymal cells of the primitive fat lobule.

Clear distinction from *liposarcoma* with a predominantly spindle cell pattern is essential for diagnosis and usually can be readily accomplished if attention is paid to the uniformity of the spindle cells, their association with mature collagen fibers, and the absence of lipoblasts. In support of a benign diagnosis are also the superficial location and circumscription of the tumor as well as its characteristic predilection for patients older than 50 years.

Spindle cell lipoma, as the name indicates, is a benign lesion, and local excision usually effects lasting relief.

PLEOMORPHIC LIPOMA

The term *pleomorphic lipoma* has been applied to a neoplasm that closely simulates a pleomorphic or sclerosing liposarcoma but most likely represents a benign, exceedingly

pleomorphic variant of spindle cell lipoma.[115,120,121,137,138] Spindle cell and pleomorphic lipomas have been included by some reviewers[114,124] among the "atypical lipomas," but we feel that both of these lesions, on clinical and microscopical examination, are sufficiently characteristic to justify consideration as distinct entities (see Chapter 17).

Like spindle cell lipoma, pleomorphic lipoma occurs as a circumscribed subcutaneous mass in the neck and shoulder region of men older than 45 years. It differs, however, from this lesion by the presence of scattered bizarre giant cells, frequently having a concentric "floretlike" arrangement of multiple hyperchromatic nuclei about the deeply eosinophilic cytoplasm and, in most instances, considerable amounts of interstitial collagen (Figs. 16-26 and 16-27). The latter feature together with the typical clinical setting and a clinical history of the lesion having been present for several years are the main criteria for diagnosis. As in spindle cell lipoma, the pleomorphic changes may occupy the entire growth or only part of it. Transitional forms between spindle cell and pleomorphic lipomas are not uncommon (Fig. 16-28).

Differential diagnosis from *sclerosing liposarcoma* may be difficult but usually can be accomplished on the basis of

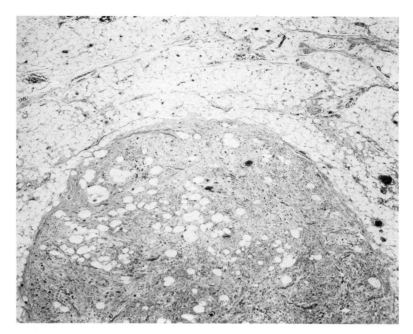

FIG. 16-26. Pleomorphic lipoma showing distinct localization of the pleomorphic portion of the tumor. This benign lesion may be mistaken for liposarcoma arising in a lipoma. (×4.)

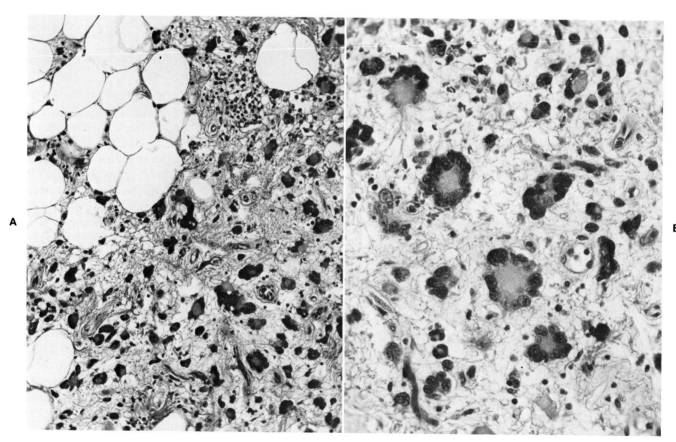

FIG. 16-27. Pleomorphic lipoma. A, Mixture of mature fat cells, multinucleated giant cells, chronic inflammatory elements, and a loosely textured fibrous stroma. (×145.) B, Characteristic floretlike giant cells with multiple peripherally placed nuclei and abundant cytoplasm that stains deeply eosinophilic with the hematoxylin-eosin preparation. (×300.)

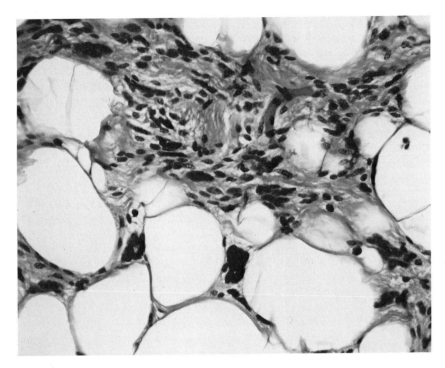

FIG. 16-28. Tumor showing transition between spindle cell lipoma and pleomorphic lipoma. Both tumors chiefly occur in the subcutis of the shoulder and neck region of men 45 years or older. They are rare in women and in other portions of the body. (×360.)

the typical setting of the lesion in the shoulder, head, and neck region, its location in the subcutis, and its circumscription. "Floret cells" are not specific of pleomorphic lipoma; they are occasionally also seen in sclerosing liposarcoma. Despite the bizarre cellular features and the occasional presence of lipoblast-like cells with atypical mitotic figures, the prognosis is excellent, and local excision is nearly always adequate for cure.

BENIGN LIPOBLASTOMA AND LIPOBLASTOMATOSIS

These names refer, respectively, to the circumscribed and the diffuse forms of the same tumor that represents a peculiar variant of lipoma and lipomatosis occurring almost exclusively during the years of infancy and early childhood. These lesions differ from lipoma and lipomatosis by their cellular immaturity and their close resemblance to the myxoid form of liposarcoma.

Lipoblastomatosis was named by Vellios et al.[152] in 1958, who reported an infiltrating lipoblastoma in the regions of the anterior chest wall, axilla, and supraclavicular region of an 8-month-old girl. The tumor had not recurred after 30 months. Earlier, Van Meurs[151] reported a similar tumor as "embryonic lipoma." He was able to demonstrate with repeated biopsies its transformation to a common lipoma.

Lipoblastoma is a tumor of infancy and usually is noted during the first 3 years of life and occasionally at birth. Sporadic examples were also described in older children.[147,149] In our series,[142,145] it occurred twice as frequently in boys as in girls and affected chiefly the upper and lower extremities as a painless nodule or mass (Fig. 16-29). Less commonly other sites, such as the head and neck area, trunk, mediastinum, mesentery, and retroperitoneum, are involved.[142,144,146,150] Circumscribed lesions (benign lipoblastoma) are confined to the subcutis; diffuse forms (diffuse lipoblastomatosis) tend to infiltrate not only the subcutis but also the underlying muscle tissue. CT scans do not permit separation from lipoma or liposarcoma.[64]

On section lipoblastoma is more pale staining than the ordinary lipoma, and its cut surfaces are distinctly myxoid or gelatinous (Fig. 16-30). Under the microscope, it consists of irregular small lobules of immature fat cells separated by connective tissue septa of varying thickness and mesenchymal areas having a loose myxoid appearance[142,148] (Figs. 16-31 to 16-33). The individual lobules are composed of lipoblasts in different stages of development, ranging from primitive, stellate, and spindle-shaped mesenchymal cells (preadipocytes) to lipoblasts approaching the univacuolar "signet ring" picture of a mature fat cell. The degree of cellular differentiation may be the same throughout the tumor or may vary in different tumor lobules. There are also occasional examples in which the cells are more rounded and finely vacuolated with intracellular eosinophilic granules, resembling the cells of brown fat.[143] Characteristically, the lipoblasts are surrounded by mucinous material, the amount of which is inversely proportional to the degree of cellular differentiation. The cellular composition is the same regardless of whether the tumor is circumscribed or diffuse. Diffuse tumors *(diffuse lipoblastomatosis),* however, show a less pronounced lobular pattern and usually contain an admixture of residual muscle fibers similar to intramuscular lipoma. Cases with sheets of primitive mesenchymal cells or broad fibrous septa may be mistaken for infantile fibromatosis (Fig. 16-34). Cellular maturation of lipoblastoma has been observed with multiple biopsies[151] (Fig. 16-35).

Ultrastructural studies disclose a variable picture. As in normal developing fat, the cells display a wide morphological spectrum ranging from immature mesenchymal cells and preadipocytes to multivacuolar lipoblasts and univacuolar lipocytes. The lipoblasts contain numerous vesicles, round to oval mitochondria, and well-developed Golgi membranes. Pinocytotic vesicles are abundant along the

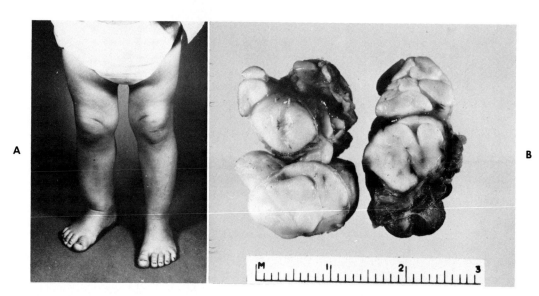

FIG. 16-29. Lipoblastoma of right lower leg of 2-year-old boy. Clinical **(A)** and multilobular gross appearance **(B).**

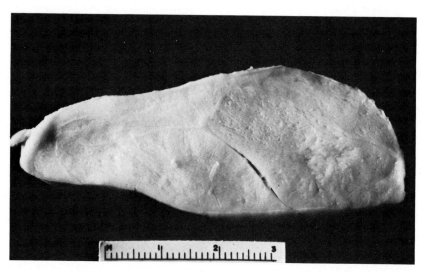

FIG. 16-30. Lipoblastoma of retroperitoneum of 6-month-old girl. Note characteristic multilobular pattern and glistening cut surface.

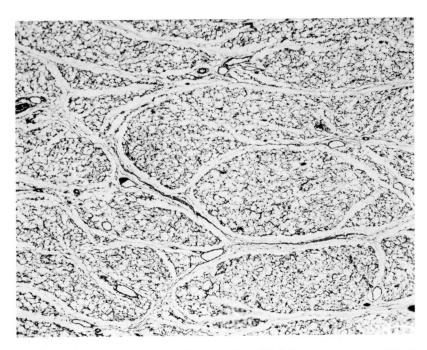

FIG. 16-31. Lipoblastoma showing the characteristic multilobular pattern and considerable uniformity in the degree of cellular differentiation. (×50.)

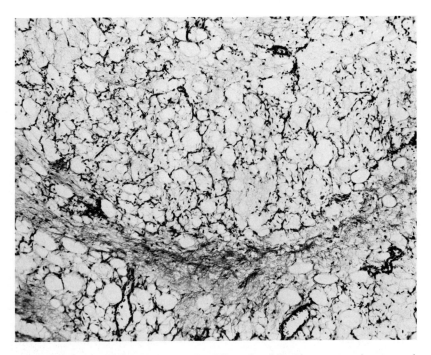

FIG. 16-32. Lipoblastoma composed of partly differentiated lipoblasts, a prominent vascular pattern, and abundant mucoid matrix. The absence of cells with hyperchromatic nuclei is characteristic of this lesion. (×80.)

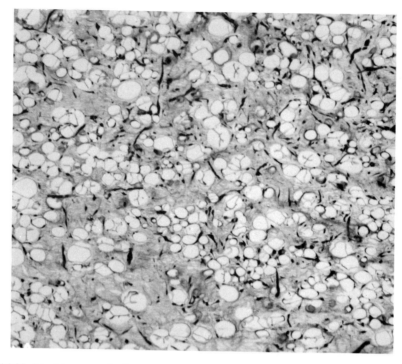

FIG. 16-33. Lipoblastoma of a 2-year-old child composed of lipoblasts and a prominent mucoid matrix. (×160.)

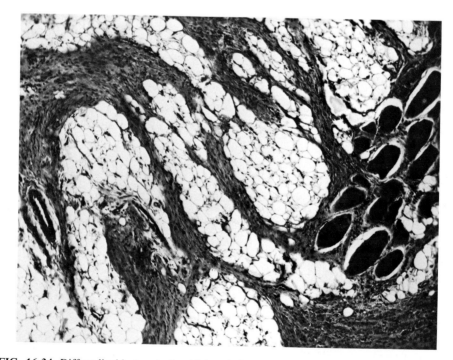

FIG. 16-34. Diffuse lipoblastomatosis with broad fibrous septa involving striated muscle. (×80.)

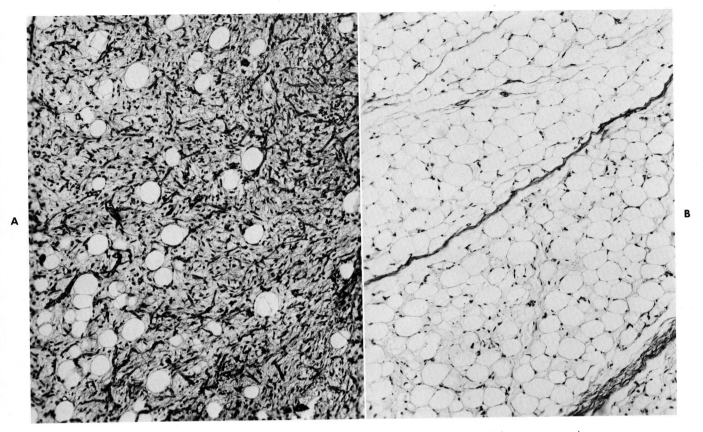

FIG. 16-35. Lipoblastoma showing progressive maturation of the tumor cells in two consecutive biopsy specimens taken 1 year apart. (**A** and **B**, ×100.)

plasma membrane. Stellate mesenchymal cells with prominent rough endoplasmic reticulum (RER) may be present in the peripheral portions of the lobules.[141] The extracellular matrix contains fibrillar material and collagen fibers.[140,146]

Prognosis is excellent. Recurrence is rare and as a rule affects patients with the diffuse rather than the circumscribed type. Therefore wide local excision of the diffuse or infiltrating type of lipoblastomatosis is well advised.

ANGIOMYOLIPOMA

The term *angiomyolipoma* should be reserved for a specific hamartomatous lesion arising in one or both kidneys as a solitary or multicentric mass; rarely the mass is a pedunculated growth or presents as a satellite nodule outside the renal capsule (Fig. 16-36). Multiple and bilateral lesions are less common than solitary ones and are more often encountered in patients with tuberous sclerosis.[185]

Angiomyolipoma occurs more commonly in women than men, with a median age of 46 years. In about two thirds of cases it causes symptoms such as abdominal or flank pain, hematuria, or chills and fever. Less commonly it is asymptomatic and is discovered as an incidental finding at operation for some unrelated cause or at autopsy. Rarely, sudden and severe flank pain and shock is caused by rupture of the tumor and massive perirenal or retroperitoneal hemorrhage.[153,173,183,184,200] Rare instances of associated hypertension have been recorded.[167,170]

Approximately one third of patients with angiomyolipoma present with manifestations of the tuberous sclerosis complex, ranging from hyperpigmented spots, shagreen patches, periungual fibromas, and angiofibromas to renal cysts, cardiac rhabdomyoma, and gliosis and calcification of the cerebral cortex with mental deficiency.[169,174,179,192,197] There are also rare cases in which the tumor is associated with lymphangiomyoma and lymphangiomyomatosis of the lung,[181,185,190] renal cell carcinoma,[178,183,197] and neurofibromatosis.[196] de Jong et al.[165] reported trisomy 7 in a patient with angiomyolipoma.

CT scan and MRI reveal a fatty mass with intermixed soft tissue densities, except in those cases in which absence of fat or hemorrhage obscures the radiological findings.[156,159,195] Ultrasonography seems to be less reliable, and does not always permit ruling out renal cell carcinoma,

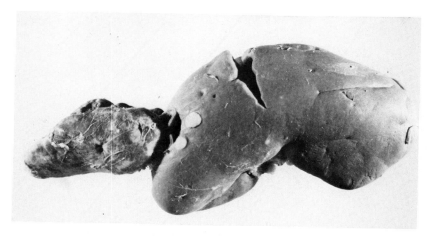

FIG. 16-36. Angiomyolipoma of the left kidney manifesting as a pedunculated mass. Unlike this lesion, most angiomyolipomas are located in the kidney or are attached to the kidney with a broad base.

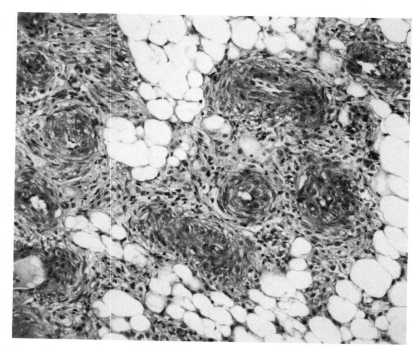

FIG. 16-37. Angiomyolipoma showing the basic components of the tumor; mature adipose tissue and smooth muscle surrounding thick-walled, medium-sized vascular channels. (×160.)

especially in the absence of a significant fatty component.[175] Aspiration or needle biopsy has been successfully employed for confirmation of diagnosis.[171,187]

Grossly the tumor presents as a yellow to gray mass, varying in size from a few cm to 20 cm or more (average, 9 cm). Very large examples may become attached to the diaphragm or liver.[176,180] Focal hemorrhage is present in

about half of cases. Nearly always the tumor is well delineated from the surrounding renal parenchyma.

Microscopically, angiomyolipoma is composed of three different tissue components that vary greatly in distribution: (1) mature adipose tissue showing some variations in cellular size and nuclear appearance; (2) convolutes of thick-walled blood vessels with little or abnormal elastica and fre-

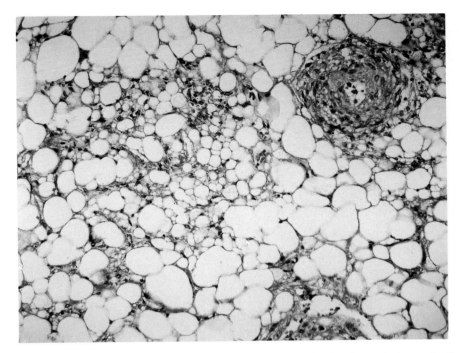

FIG. 16-38. Angiomyolipoma exhibiting considerable variation in the size and shape of adipocytes, a feature that should not be mistaken for liposarcoma. (×160.)

quent hyalinization of the media; and (3) irregularly arranged sheets and interlacing bundles of smooth muscle often having a prominent perivascular arrangement (Figs. 16-37 to 16-39). In some cases the smooth muscle element displays a striking degree of cellular pleomorphism, with hyperchromatic nuclei, occasional multinucleated giant cells, and foci of necrosis (Fig. 16-40). Additionally, there may be epithelioid smooth muscle cells containing spherical granules and dense PAS-positive needle-shaped or rhomboid crystals that are similar to those in juxtaglomerular tumors but do not stain for renin.[186,203] Immunohistochemically, the large cells of angiomyolipoma and lymphangiomyoma (lymphangiomyomatosis) are not only immunoreactive for actin and desmin but also, and unlike other smooth muscle tumors, are positive for melanoma-associated antigen as defined by HMB-45, suggesting a close histogenetic relationship between these tumors.[163] Because of this staining reaction, a possible linkage to the clear cell or "sugar" tumor of the lung has also been suggested.[189] Ultrastructurally many of the muscle cells contain myofilaments, glycogen particles, and electron-dense granules, some with transverse striations, similar to melanosomes.[188,202]

Although the histological appearance of the tumor is characteristic and should not cause any difficulties in diagnosis, it is sometimes mistaken for *liposarcoma* or *leiomyosarcoma* because of its large size, focal cellularity, cellular

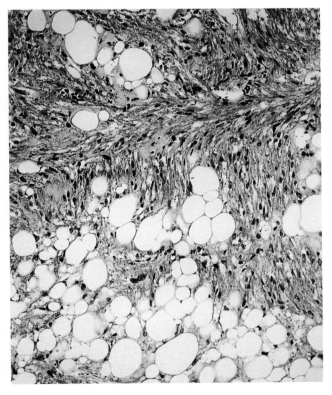

FIG. 16-39. Angiomyolipoma displaying moderate pleomorphism of the fatty and smooth muscle components. (×160.)

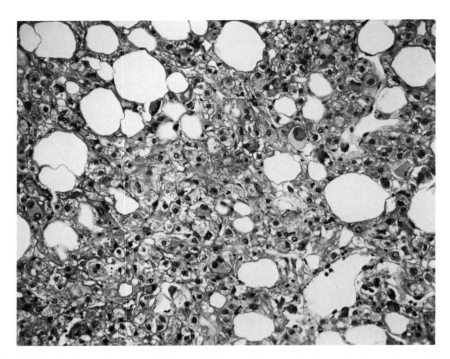

FIG. 16-40. Angiomyolipoma exhibiting striking variation in the size and shape of smooth muscle elements, a feature that has been mistaken for evidence of malignancy. (×160.)

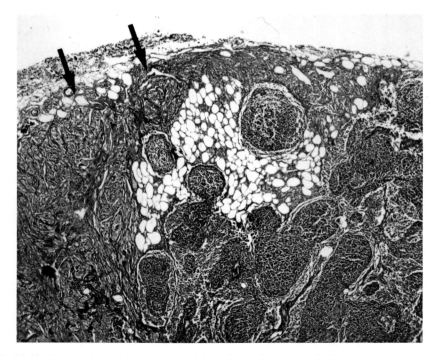

FIG. 16-41. Retroperitoneal lymph node with angiomyolipomatous infiltrate *(arrows)*, a rare and benign feature of this condition. (×40.)

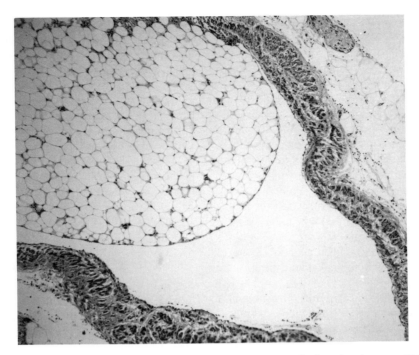

FIG. 16-42. Intravascular growth in an angiomyolipoma, a rare finding that is compatible with benign behavior. (×160.)

pleomorphism, and the occasional growth of the tumor in lymph nodes (Fig. 16-41). Yet despite these atypical features, nearly all angiomyolipomas seem to pursue a benign clinical course. In fact, there is no evidence that the presence of regional or systemic lymph node involvement, perirenal satellite tumors, or angiomyolipomatous growth in other organs reflects malignant potential.*

Extrarenal sites of angiomyolipoma include the liver and very rarely the mediastinum, spleen, and spermatic cord.[162,172,177,191,202] However, the subcutaneous angiomyolipoma of the ear, reported by Argenyi et al.[155] seems to be a vascular hamartoma.

Malignant transformation, if it ever occurs, must be exceedingly rare. Cellular pleomorphism and intravascular growth have been interpreted as evidence of malignancy,[157,182,199] but marked cellular pleomorphism is not uncommon in angiomyolipoma, and intravascular growth may be found in perfectly benign tumors, as illustrated in one of our cases (Fig. 16-42). There are, however, three reports of leiomyosarcomatous transformation of pleomorphic angiomyolipomas, with subsequent metastasis. In one described by Lowe et al.,[182] multiple sarcomatous lesions were found in various organs 18 months after removal of a pleomorphic renal angiomyolipoma. In another case re-

ported by Ferry et al.[168] the patient developed multiple pulmonary lesions that were diagnosed by fine-needle biopsy as metastatic angiomyolipoma. The third case, an "angiolipomyosarcoma" reported by Hartveit and Hallerbraker,[176] is most likely a bilateral angiomyolipoma in which the pleomorphic tumor in the opposite kidney was interpreted as a metastasis.

Angiomyolipoma grows very slowly and is adequately treated by partial nephrectomy. Asymptomatic tumors of small size may merely require careful follow-up; total nephrectomy, however, may become necessary in very large tumors. There also are cases that were successfully treated by therapeutic embolization.[166,194,198,201]

MYELOLIPOMA

Although myelolipoma, a tumorlike growth of mature fat and bone marrow elements, is most common in the adrenal glands,* it also occurs as an isolated soft tissue mass, especially in the pelvic region, in patients without hepatosplenomegaly and without any evidence of hematopoietic disorders.[205,209,220] It must be distinguished from *extramedullary hematopoietic tumors* that are more often multiple than solitary, are frequently associated with splenomegaly and hepatomegaly, and are secondary to severe

---

*References 154, 158, 160, 161, 164, 183, 197.

*References 204, 207, 212, 214, 216, 217, 219.

anemia (thalassemia, hereditary spherocytosis), various myeloproliferative diseases, myelosclerosis, and skeletal disorders.[206,211,215]

Myelolipomas are very rare in young patients, and most are encountered in persons older than 40 years. Smaller tumors tend to be asymptomatic and often are detected as incidental findings during surgery for some unrelated disease or at autopsy. Larger tumors may cause abdominal pain, constipation, or nausea. The nature and histogenesis of this lesion are not wholly clear, although the condition is more likely to represent a hamartoma than a true neoplasm derived from misplaced hematopoietic cells.

Roentgenographically, myelolipoma presents as a well-circumscribed radiolucent mass, usually in the pelvis or retroperitoneum. When occurring in the adrenal gland, it causes inferior renal displacement on intravenous urography. It is avascular on arteriography and echodense on ultrasonography.[222]

Grossly, myelolipoma shows the features of a lipoma, but when the myeloid elements prevail, the tumor assumes a more grayish or grayish red appearance. The lesion rarely measures more than 5 cm in diameter, but a few very large

tumors are on record. Damjanov et al.,[208] for example, reported a myelolipoma that arose in an ectopic adrenal gland and measured 15 cm in diameter. Microscopically, the lesion is composed of a mixture of bone marrow elements and lipocytes in varying proportions (Fig. 16-43).

Adrenal myelolipomas may be secondary to prolonged stress and excessive stimulation with adrenocorticotropic hormones, and they may be associated with endocrine disorders such as hermaphrodism, Cushing's disease, Addison's disease, or obesity of uncertain etiology.[204,213] Escuin et al.[210] reported an angiomyelolipoma associated with bilateral adrenocortical hyperplasia and hypertension. Selye and Stone[221] produced adrenal myelolipomas in rats by injection of crude adrenocorticotropic hormone and testosterone.

INTRAMUSCULAR AND INTERMUSCULAR LIPOMA

This is a relatively common condition that frequently causes concern to both clinicians and pathologists because of its frequent large size, its deep location, and its infiltrative growth. Intramuscular lipomas outnumber intermuscular lipomas by a considerable margin, but many involve both muscular and intermuscular tissues.[223,224,226] The condition has also been described in the literature as *infiltrating lipoma*.[225,227,230]

The tumor arises at all ages, but the majority occur in adults between 30 and 60 years of age. Occasionally it is encountered in children.[229] In such cases distinction from diffuse lipomatosis and lipoblastomatosis may be difficult.

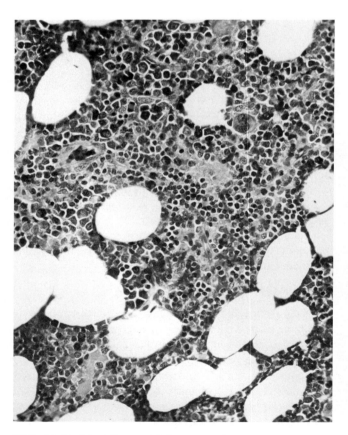

FIG. 16-43. Myelolipoma of the retroperitoneum in a 58-year-old woman showing a mixture of mature fat cells and bone marrow elements. (×250.)

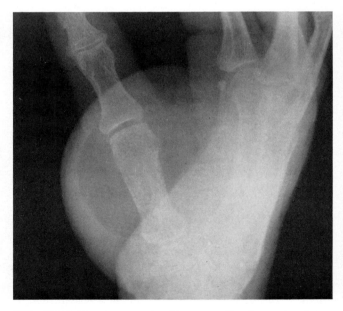

FIG. 16-44. Roentgenograph of intramuscular lipoma involving the muscles of the thenar eminence. Note sharply circumscribed radiolucent mass surrounded by a rim of muscle tissue.

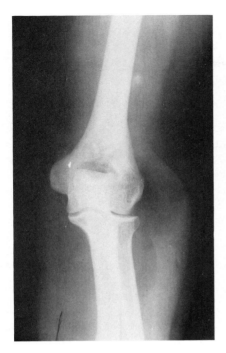

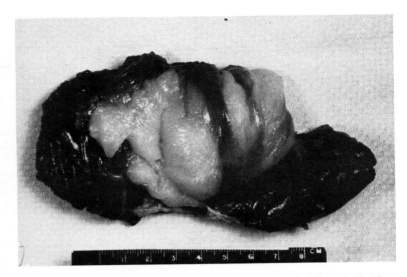

FIG. 16-46. Gross picture of tumor shown in Fig. 16-45. Note replacement of muscle tissue by mature fat.

FIG. 16-45. Roentgenograph of a poorly circumscribed intramuscular lipoma involving the brachioradial muscle of the left arm in a 38-year-old man.

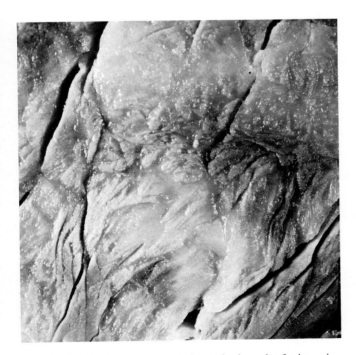

FIG. 16-47. Partial replacement of muscle tissue by fat in an intramuscular lipoma of the calf in a 22-year-old man.

There is general agreement that males are more often afflicted than females and that the most important sites are the large muscles of the extremities, especially those of the thigh, shoulder, and upper arm. Most tumors are slow growing and painless and often become apparent only during muscle contraction when the tumor is converted into a firm spherical mass. Sometimes movement causes aching or pain, but pain is rarely severe. The size varies considerably and ranges from minute lesions to tumors measuring 20 cm or more in diameter. Occasional examples were found on routine radiological examination because intramuscular lipomas, like other forms of lipoma, are radiolucent and are readily demonstrated roentgenographically (Figs. 16-44 and 16-45). Microangiographically, intramuscular lipoma is much less vascular than the surrounding muscle tissue.[228]

Cross-sections of the intramuscular lipoma reveal gradual replacement of the muscle tissue by fat that may extend beyond the muscle fascia into the intermuscular connective tissue spaces (Figs. 16-46 and 16-47). On longitudinal section it often assumes a striated appearance caused by the proliferation of fat cells between muscle fibers.

Microscopic examination reveals lipocytes that infiltrate muscle in a diffuse manner. The entrapped muscle fibers usually show few changes other than various degrees of muscular atrophy (Figs. 16-48 to 16-50). Characteristically, the lipocytes are mature, and there are no lipoblasts or cells with atypical nuclei as in *well-differentiated liposarcoma*. Nonetheless, careful sampling of these tumors is mandatory because portions of well-differentiated, intramuscular liposarcoma may be indistinguishable from those of intramuscular lipoma. In *diffuse lipoblastomatosis and lipoma-*

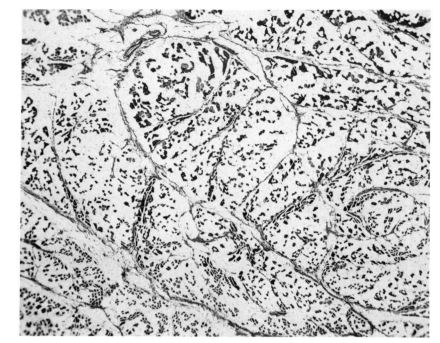

FIG. 16-48. Low-power photomicrograph of intramuscular lipoma that has diffusely infiltrated striated muscle tissue. Intramuscular liposarcomas usually display a much more irregular growth pattern, with massive destruction of muscle tissue. (×25.)

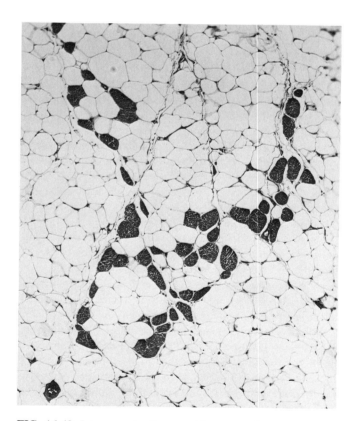

FIG. 16-49. Intramuscular lipoma with entrapped striated muscle fibers in cross-section. There is some atrophy of the fat cells, but there are no lipoblasts or cells with hyperchromatic nuclei as in well-differentiated liposarcoma. (×70.)

tosis, lesions that occur mostly in infants and children, subcutis *and* muscle are affected, and generally more than one muscle is involved. In some *intramuscular hemangiomas,* "ex vacuo" growth of fat may simulate the picture of an intramuscular lipoma, and such cases have been misinterpreted as "angiolipoma."[191]

The prospect of cure is excellent if the tumor is completely removed. In the AFIP series, 85% of patients remained well following the initial excision, and in 15% the tumor recurred.[226] In the reported cases the recurrence rate varied from as little as 3%[228] to 62.5%,[225] probably depending on the completeness of the excision and doubtlessly also on the criteria employed for diagnosis and distinction from well-differentiated intramuscular liposarcoma.

LIPOMA OF TENDON SHEATHS AND JOINTS

Among these very rare lesions there are two types: (1) solid fatty masses extending along tendons for varying distances and (2) *lipoma-like* lesions consisting chiefly of hypertrophic synovial villi distended by fat, most commonly seen in the region of the knee joint *(lipoma arborescens).* When occurring within tendon sheaths, these lesions have been described as *endovaginal* tumors, in distinction to *epivaginal* tumors (e.g., deep lipomas arising outside the tendon sheath).

According to Sullivan et al.,[237] lipoma of tendon sheath occurs with about equal frequency in both sexes, chiefly in young persons between 15 and 35 years, and affects the wrist and hand and, less commonly, the ankle and foot.

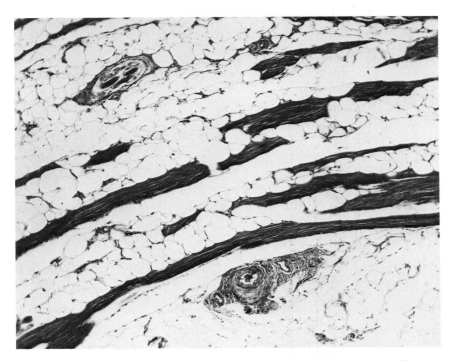

FIG. 16-50. Intramuscular lipoma with striated muscle fibers in longitudinal section. Note complete absence of cellular atypism. (×60.)

About half are bilateral and show a symmetrical distribution. Occasionally they involve both the hands and feet of the same individual. At the time the patient seeks treatment most of the lesions have been present for several years, and many cause pain that may be rather severe in character. Rupture of a tendon secondary to lipoma of tendon sheath has been reported. As in other types of lipoma, radiological examination will show a mass of lesser density than the surrounding tissue and, therefore, may be helpful in diagnosis.[233,236,240]

Lipoma of joints *(lipoma arborescens)* is more common than lipoma of tendon sheath and occurs mainly in the region of the knee joint, including the suprapatellar pouch.[235,238,239] Grossly and microscopically, both lesions consist either of mature fibrofatty tissue or thickened, grapelike or fingerlike villi infiltrated by fat and lined by synovium (Figs. 16-51 and 16-52). Lipoma arborescens is probably a reactive process; it is mostly found in older patients with joint trauma, meniscal lesions, or chronic synovitis and arthritis. It is likely that some of the symmetrical lipoma arborescens-like lesions of tendon sheath are also reactive hyperplastic lesions associated with various forms of chronic tenosynovitis. Traumatic proliferation of fatty tissue in the retropatellar portion of the knee joint is sometimes referred to as *Hoffa's disease*.[234]

LUMBOSACRAL LIPOMA

Lumbosacral lipoma is another curious type of lipomatous growth that deserves recognition because of its close relationship to the spinal cord and its coverings. It is characterized by a diffuse proliferation of mature fat overlying the lower portion of the spine in the lumbosacral region. The lesion is always associated with spina bifida or a similar laminar defect (lipomyeloschisis), and there is a stalk-like connection (tethered cord) between the fatty growth and a portion of the spinal cord that often also harbors an intradural or extradural lipoma. The stalk may cause traction and ischemia. Lipomas extending from the middle to one side are more likely to contain a meningocele or a myelocele.[245,246] According to Rickwood et al.,[251] its overall incidence is slightly less than 1 in 10,000 live births.

Clinically, lumbosacral lipoma tends to be asymptomatic initially and often is noted only because of the presence of a large soft tissue mass or because of a sinus, skin tag, hemangioma, or excessive hair associated with a soft swelling in the lumbosacral region. Later, in about two thirds of cases, progressive myelopathy or radiculopathy causes motor or sensory disturbances in the lower legs, bladder, or bowel.[249,250]

The lesion affects females almost twice as often as males and is encountered chiefly in infants or children between birth and 10 years of age. Occasional cases in adults have

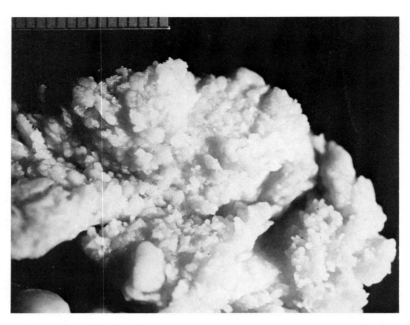

FIG. 16-51. "Lipoma arborescens," a reactive, lipoma-like lesion caused by overgrowth of fat within hypertrophied synovial villi.

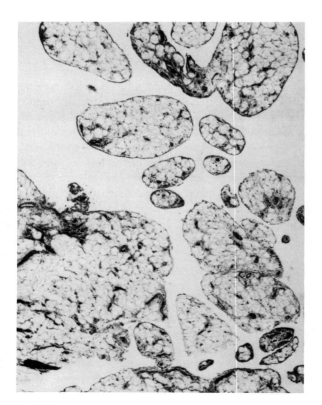

FIG. 16-52. Cross-section of synovial villi in "lipoma arborescens" showing stromal deposition of mature fat. (×40.)

been reported[242,247,248]; Loeser and Lewin[247] describe such a case in a 34-year-old man who complained of weakness of 4 or 5 years' duration in both legs, associated with a spina bifida at L4-5 and an intradural filling defect. In the series of Lassman and James,[246] all 19 patients had evidence of spina bifida, and 9 had evidence of progressive neuropathy. The authors also found 26 cases of lumbosacral lipoma among 100 cases of occult spina bifida.

Sonography, CT scan, or MRI is essential for diagnosis and for planning therapy; these procedures show not only the exact position of the cord and its relationship to the lipoma but also the association of the mass with spina bifida or some degree of sacral dysgenesis; on myelography there is frequently blockage of the spinal canal.[244,252,253]

At operation the lipomatous growth is usually unencapsulated and consists of lobulated adipose tissue microscopically indistinguishable from lipoma. In some cases vascular proliferation and smooth muscle tissue are present in addition to the adipocytes. Rarely islets of neuroglia, ependyma-lined tubular structures, and primitive renal tissue are found near the spinal defect.[241]

Surgical exploration—laminectomy and division of the stalk and the fibrous bands forming at the upper margin of the spinal defect—should be performed as early as possible, preferably prior to the onset of neurological symptoms. This, however, does not prevent the development of leg paralysis and neurogenic bladder in all cases.[251]

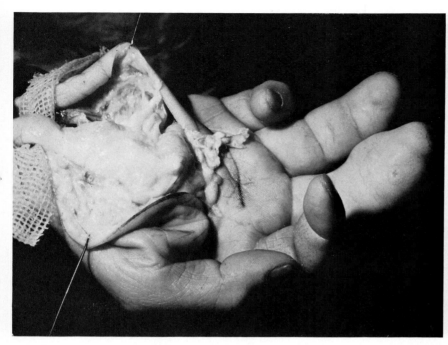
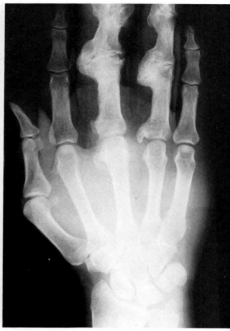

FIG. 16-53. Neural fibrolipoma in a 39-year-old man. The deformities of the fingers and hand have been present for many years, beginning in early childhood and allegedly following a crush injury at age 2. **A,** Gross picture showing deformities of the fingers and hand and proliferation of fatty tissue along median nerve. **B,** Roentgenograph displaying chronic osteoarthritis and fusion of joints.

NEURAL FIBROLIPOMA (LIPOFIBROMATOUS HAMARTOMA OF NERVES)

This is a tumorlike lipomatous process that involves principally the volar aspects of the hands, wrist, and forearm of young persons; it usually manifests as a soft slowly growing mass consisting of proliferating fibrofatty tissue surrounding and infiltrating major nerves and their branches.[257,258] Other terms applied to this condition are *lipofibromatous hamartoma of nerves*[259] and *neurolipomatosis*.[82]

About one third of neural fibrolipomas are associated with overgrowth of bone and macrodactyly.[255,260] For example, in our series of 26 cases,[264] 7 were associated with macrodactyly. Lesions of this type have also been described as *macrodystrophia lipomatosa*,[256] but it seems preferable to refer to them as *neural fibrolipoma with macrodactyly* (Fig. 16-53).

Almost always the lesion is seen during the first 3 decades of life, usually because of increasing pain, tenderness, diminished sensation, or paresthesias associated with a gradually enlarging mass causing compression neuropathy. There may also be some loss of strength. Growth is usually slow and in most patients has been noted for many years. Lesions present at birth or infancy outnumber by far those recognized later in childhood or adult life. Males are more often involved than females, and the left hand is more often affected than the right. There may be a genetic disposition, but there is no history of any hereditary disorders. The onset is linked to trauma in some cases. Carpal tunnel syndrome is a late complication in some lesions.[261]

At operation neural fibrolipoma presents as a soft, gray-yellow, fusiform, sausage-shaped mass that has diffusely infiltrated and replaced portions of a large nerve and its branches. The median nerve is affected in the great majority of cases. Very rarely, the lesion is also found in other nerves, such as the ulnar nerve or the nerves of the toes.[264] Under the microscope, the lesion consists of fibrofatty tissue that has surrounded and infiltrated the nerve trunk and has grown along the epineurium and perineurium (Figs. 16-54 and 16-55). Prolonged duration and compression of nerves by the fatty tissue result in neural degeneration and atrophy, which accounts for the usual late appearance of symptoms. Masses of fibrofatty tissue may also be found outside the involved nerves, unattached to either the overlying skin or neighboring tendons and indistinguishable from a deep-seated lipoma. There is also marked thicken-

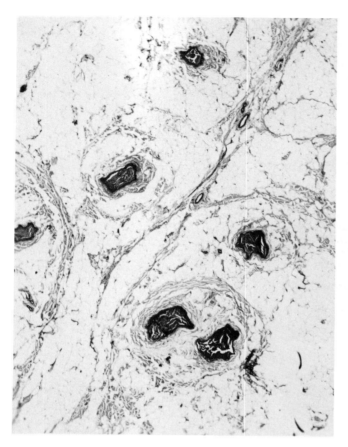

FIG. 16-54. Neural fibrolipoma (fibrolipomatous hamartoma of nerves) showing fat tissue surrounding and splaying apart peripheral nerves. (×25.)

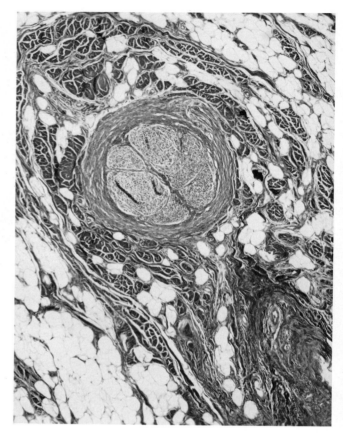

FIG. 16-55. Neural fibrolipoma (fibrolipomatous hamartoma of nerves) showing fibrosis of nerve sheath and perineural fibrofatty growth. (×60.)

ing of the perineurium and the perivascular fibrous tissue. The diffuse infiltrative character of the lesion separates it from localized and circumscribed lipomas of nerves occurring elsewhere in the body, including lipomas originating in the spinal canal.[243] Unlike *neuromas* and *neurofibromas,* there is atrophy rather than proliferation of neural elements. Clear distinction from *diffuse lipomatosis with overgrowth of bone* is not always possible, but diffuse lipomatosis is primarily a lesion of the subcutis and muscle and only secondarily affects nerves.

There is no effective therapy for neural fibrolipoma. Complete excision of the fibrofatty growth is contraindicated because it may cause severe sensory or motor disturbances. If necessary, biopsy of a small cutaneous nerve will establish the diagnosis.[263] Pain and sensory loss may be partially or completely relieved by division of the transverse carpal ligament and decompression of the median nerve.[254,262]

DIFFUSE LIPOMATOSIS

Diffuse lipomatosis may be defined as an extremely rare, diffuse overgrowth of mature adipose tissue that usually affects large portions of an extremity or the trunk. Although it simulates liposarcoma by its size and aggressive growth, it is indistinguishable from lipoma microscopically. Like lipoma it consists entirely of adult-type fat, and despite its frequent rapid enlargement, there is no evidence of lipoblastic activity or cellular pleomorphism.

The condition is not limited to the panniculus, and in nearly all cases subcutis and muscle are diffusely involved. Many lesions are associated with osseous hypertrophy, leading to macrodactyly or giantism of a digit or limb[267,271,274,276] (Fig. 16-56), but unlike perineural fibrolipoma, there is no involvement of nerves and the process is not limited to the extremities. Association with lipomas or angiomas in other portions of the body is by no means rare. In addition to the extremities and the trunk the lesion

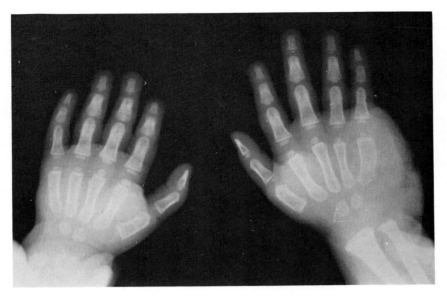

FIG. 16-56. Diffuse lipomatosis of right hand with slight overgrowth of phalangeal bones.

also occurs in the head and neck, intestinal tract, abdominal cavity, and pelvis.[269] Hoskins et al.[268] reported a patient with mediastinal lipomatosis causing a "sabre sheath" trachea. There are also reports of symmetrical lipomatosis of the hands[266] and diffuse lipomatosis of the leg following poliomyelitis.[270] Most cases have their onset during the first 2 years of life, but we and others have also observed typical examples of this tumor in adolescents and adults[272,273,275,277] (Fig. 16-57).

Differential diagnosis may be difficult. *Intramuscular lipoma* may exhibit a similar microscopic picture, but this tumor is always confined to muscle or intermuscular tissue spaces and usually contains a greater number of entrapped muscle fibers. *Diffuse angiomatosis* may be accompanied by considerable fatty and osseous overgrowth, but it is always recognizable by its more pronounced vascular pattern. *Well-differentiated liposarcoma* is usually less of a problem if the tumor is carefully sampled for evidence of lipoblastic activity and cellular pleomorphism. Distinction is also facilitated by the age of the patient. Liposarcomas are extremely rare during infancy, and virtually all lipoblastic tumors occurring during this period represent examples of benign lipoblastoma or lipoblastomatosis.

Diffuse lipomatosis tends to recur, often repeatedly over a period of many years. It may reach a large size and in rare instances may cause severe impairment of function, necessitating drastic surgery.

SYMMETRICAL LIPOMATOSIS

Symmetrical lipomatosis is a rare and fascinating disease that has also been described under the ep-

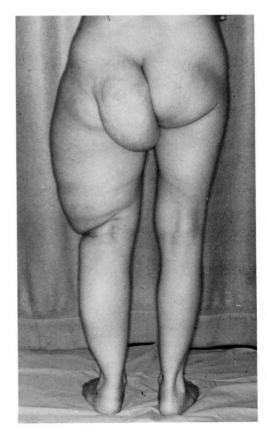

FIG. 16-57. Diffuse lipomatosis confined mainly to left buttock and thigh.

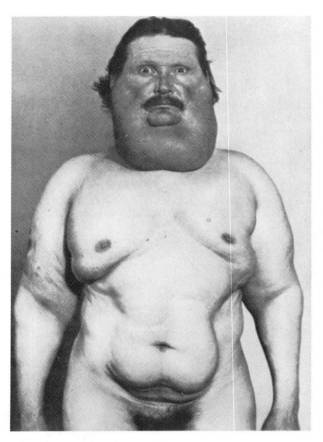

FIG. 16-58. Symmetric lipomatosis (Madelung's disease). (From Saalfeld E, Saalfeld U: *Klinik der gutartigen Tumoren;* Handbuch der Haut und Geschlechtskrankheiten, Geschwuelste der Haut, Berlin, 1932, Julius Springer.)

onyms of *Madelung's disease* or *Launois-Bensaude syndrome.*[284,285,288-290] Patients with this condition suffer from massive symmetrical deposition of mature fat in the region of the neck, so that the head appears to be pushed forward by a hump that has been likened to a horse collar or doughnut-shaped ring *(lipoma annulare colli)* (Fig. 16-58).

The disease affects almost exclusively middle-aged men, often with a background of excessive alcohol intake or liver disease.[279] The fatty deposits grow insidiously, frequently over many years, and, in contrast to Dercum's disease (adiposis dolorosa), are nontender and painless. They are chiefly located bilaterally in the region of the neck but also may involve the cheeks, breast, upper arm, and axilla. The distal portions of the forearm and leg remain unaffected. There may also be sensory and autonomic neuropathies with trophic disturbances.[281,283] Chalk et al.[280] report coexisting neuropathy in four of seven siblings who had no history of alcohol abuse or serum lipid abnormalities.

The fatty deposits are poorly circumscribed and affect both the subcutis and deep soft tissue spaces, frequently ex-

tending in tonguelike projections between the cervical and thoracic muscles. Massive deposits in the deep portion of the neck, larynx, and mediastinum may cause dysphagia, stridor, and respiratory embarrassment.[286] or progressive vena caval compression.[281] As a rule, patients with this condition are not particularly obese, a fact that adds to the striking appearance of the fatty deposits in the neck. Grossly and microscopically, the accumulated fat is indistinguishable from mature fat, except for varying degrees of fibrosis and, rarely, calcification and ossification. Analysis of the fatty growth by Mueller et al.[287] revealed higher levels of acid mucopolysaccharides when compared with normal fat.

The exact cause of the condition remains obscure. Patients with this lesion may have diabetes, glucose intolerance, hyperlipidemia, or hyperuricemia—alone or in combination—and there may be an increased familial incidence.[280,287] It was also suggested that the increased synthesis of fat may be the result of damage or loss of sympathetic innervation or a defect in catecholamine-stimulated lipolysis.[281,283] Enzi[281] reported elevated lipoprotein lipase activity and plasma hyperalphalipoproteinemia. The same authors also described fatty infiltration of muscle in the supraclavicular, suprascapular, and deltoid region of female patients as "shoulder girdle lipomatosis."[282]

Although conservative surgery and liposuction have been used effectively in the treatment of the disease, this may not be necessary, since in some cases the deposited fat may recede with abstinence from alcohol and correction of nutritional deficiencies.[283]

Symmetrical lipomatosis must be distinguished from *adiposis dolorosa (Dercum's disease).*[291] This condition is marked by tender or painful, diffuse or nodular accumulation of subcutaneous fat, predominating in postmenopausal women and affecting primarily the regions of the pelvic girdle and the thigh. The lesion is associated with marked asthenia (e.g., loss of strength and fatigue with the least amount of effort), depression, and psychic disturbances. As in symmetrical lipomatosis, there is no evidence of any hormonal abnormality.

PELVIC LIPOMATOSIS

This entity, first described by Engels[297] in 1959, is characterized by an overgrowth of fat in the perirectal and perivesical regions, causing compression of the lower urinary tract and rectosigmoid colon. The lesion is probably more common than is implied by the relatively small number of cases so far described.[293,298-300,305-307]

The condition chiefly affects black men in the third and fourth decades of life. Women are rarely affected.[303,304] According to the 1991 review of the literature by Heyns[300] 67% of patients were black and 78% were between 20 and 60 years old. The only clinical complaints in the early

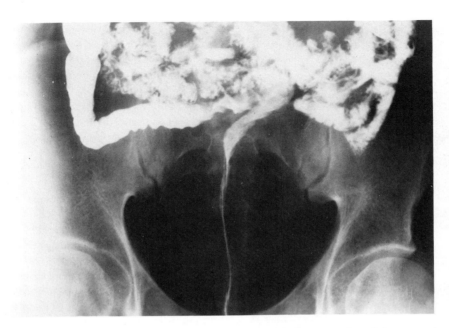

FIG. 16-59. Roentgenograph of pelvic lipomatosis with marked compression of the rectum by the accumulated radiolucent fat.

stages of the disease consist of mild perineal pain and increased urinary frequency. At later stages, patients often complain in addition of hematuria, constipation, nausea, lower abdominal pain, or backache of increasing severity and sometimes of edema of the lower extremities. Hypertension is present in about one third of patients. There also may be associated cystitis glandularis or follicularis, alone or in conjunction with carcinoma.[296,301,308]

Roentgenographically (excretory urogram and CT scan), the typical findings include a pear- or gourd-shaped urinary bladder with elevated base, a high-lying prostate gland, and straightening and tubular narrowing of the rectosigmoid as the result of extrinsic pressure by a radiolucent mass (Fig. 16-59). The mass may cause dilatation and media displacement of one or both ureters and occasionally unilateral or bilateral hydronephrosis. CT scans reveal a homogenous perivesical mass with linear densities, reflecting fibrous bands within the proliferated fatty tissue.[292,298]

Pelvic lipomatosis is the result of massive overgrowth of fat in the perivesical and perirectal portions of the pelvic retroperitoneum. The fatty growth is diffuse rather than nodular and consists entirely of mature fat indistinguishable grossly and microscopically from fatty tissue elsewhere in the body. Increased vascularity, fibrosis, and inflammatory changes may be present but are rare.

The cause of this overgrowth is unknown, but it appears that it is a hyperplastic rather than a neoplastic process that almost always is limited to the pelvic region. Cases with associated multiple lipomata[299] and manifestations of Proteus syndrome[295] have been reported, however. *Lipomatosis of the ileocecal region*—submucosal, polypoid fatty infiltration of the ileocecal valve[294]—and *renal replacement lipomatosis,* secondary to long-standing inflammation and calculi with severe atrophy and destruction of the renal parenchyma,[302] should not be confused with this lesion. The symmetrical diffuse growth helps to rule out liposarcoma.

Prediction of the clinical course is difficult in the individual case. Frequently, pelvic lipomatosis is a slowly progressive process that may cause vesicoureteric obstruction, hydronephosis, and uremia requiring surgical intervention, mainly urinary diversion and attempts toward excision of the accumulated fat.

STEROID LIPOMATOSIS

This term is used here to describe a benign, diffuse fatty overgrowth caused by prolonged stimulation by adrenocortical hormones. The condition may be endogenous, as in Cushing's disease and adrenal cortical hyperplasia, or the result of prolonged corticosteroid therapy or steroid immunosuppression in transplant patients. As in Cushing's disease the newly formed fat is unevenly distributed and tends to be concentrated in certain portions of the body. Thus in some cases the accumulation of fat is found mainly in the face (moon face), episternal region (dewlap),[317] or interscapular region (buffalo hump); in others it is limited to the mediastinum,[310,316,318,322,325] pericardium,[326] paraspinal region,[324] mesentery,[323,324] retroperitoneum,[313] or epidural space.[309,311,312,314,319] Depending on the location the

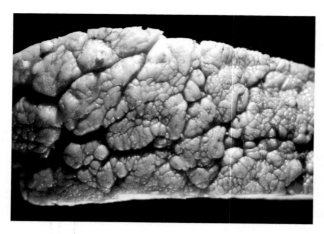

FIG. 16-60. Nevus lipomatosus cutaneous superficialis showing cerebriform, wrinkled skin. (×2.5.)

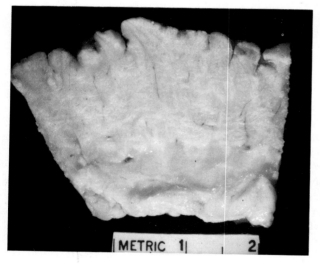

FIG. 16-61. Cross-section of nevus lipomatosus cutaneous superficialis showing characteristic dermal accumulation of fat. (×2.2.)

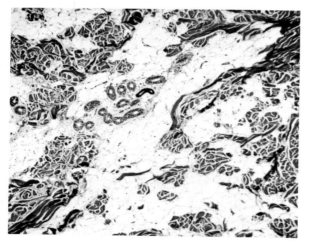

FIG. 16-62. Nevus lipomatosus cutaneous superficialis with separation of dermal collagen by mature fat. (×100.)

symptoms vary but are usually the result of compression within a confined space, such as compression of the trachea within the mediastinum or the spinal cord within the spinal canal.[320] In rare cases spinal compression may result in paraplegia.[315] CT scan and demonstration of increased serum and urine cortisol levels are essential for diagnosis.[321] Steroid lipomatosis tends to resolve when the steroid concentration is lowered.[324]

NEVUS LIPOMATOSUS CUTANEOUS SUPERFICIALIS

First described by Hoffman and Zurhelle in 1921,[333] this condition consists of multiple asymptomatic flesh-colored, yellow, or brown dermal nodules that are sessile, dome-shaped, or pedunculated. They tend to be arranged in a linear fashion along skin folds and often form confluent masses or plaques with a soft wrinkled or cerebriform surface (Figs. 16-60 and 16-61). There is no sex prevalence, and patients are otherwise in good health. The lesions are found principally in the regions of the flank, buttocks, and upper part of the posterior thigh. In most instances they are congenital or become apparent during the first 20 years of life. Solitary nodules of similar appearance are less common and may occur later in life and at other sites such as the head and neck region.[329,330,332,334-336,339]

Under the microscope the nodules are composed of aggregates of mature fat cells within the mid and upper dermis, sometimes with keratotic plugs, increased vascularity, and scattered lymphocytes, mast cells, and histiocytes (Fig. 16-62). Like other connective tissue nevi, the lesion should be considered a developmental anomaly or hamartomatous growth.

Another peculiar variant of this condition is marked by excessive symmetrical, circumferential folds of skin with underlying nevus lipomatosus that affects the neck, forearms, and lower legs and resolves spontaneously during childhood; it has been aptly described as *Michelin tire baby syndrome*.[328] The syndrome is inherited as an autosomal dominant trait and, according to Bass et al.[327] and others,[331,337] is characterized by deletion of chromosome 11. Association with smooth muscle hamartomas and multiple anomalies has been described.[338]

HIBERNOMA

The term *hibernoma*, coined by Gery[351] in 1914, is well established and should be retained even though not all hibernomas occur at the few sites in which brown fat is encountered in humans. Such terms as *lipoma of immature adipose tissue, lipoma of embryonic fat,* and *fetal lipoma* were also proposed by some authors because brown fat bears a close resemblance to early stages in the development of white fat.

Hibernomas occur chiefly in adults, but patients with hibernoma are on the average considerably younger than those with lipoma. In our unpublished series of 32 cases the median age was 26 years; the youngest was 18 years and the oldest 52 years. There is only one report of hibernoma in a small child,[347] and this case, a tumor of the mediastinum and neck in a 6-week-old infant, probably represents a variant of lipoblastomatosis simulating hibernoma.

In the AFIP series, as well the literature, the tumor predominates in the scapular and interscapular regions, mediastinum, and upper thorax,* but there are also a number of cases originating in the thigh and the popliteal fossa, sites normally devoid of brown fat.[348,359,367] Less common locations are the neck, chest wall, and retroperitoneum, as well as the axillary and inguinal regions.[345,357,360,361,365]

Clinically, hibernomas are slow-growing painless tumors that occur in the subcutis or rarely in muscle and are often noted for several years before they are excised.[355] They are usually well defined, soft, and mobile and range from 5 to 10 cm in diameter; hibernomas as large as 18 cm in diameter have been reported, however.[363] Their color varies from tan to a deep red-brown (Fig. 16-63).

Microscopically, hibernomas display a distinct lobular pattern and are composed of cells that show varying degrees of differentiation ranging from uniform, round to ovoid, granular eosinophilic cells with a distinct cellular membrane to multivacuolated cells with multiple, small oil-red-O positive lipid droplets and centrally placed nuclei. There are also intermixed univacuolar cells with one or

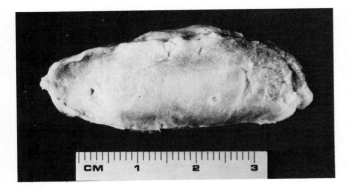

FIG. 16-63. Gross picture of hibernoma of the back in a 22-year-old man.

*References 340, 343, 344, 346, 350, 354, 356, 362, 364.

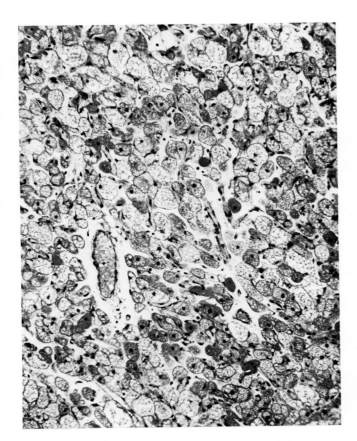

FIG. 16-64. Hibernoma composed of finely vacuolated or granular cells characteristic of brown fat. (×100.)

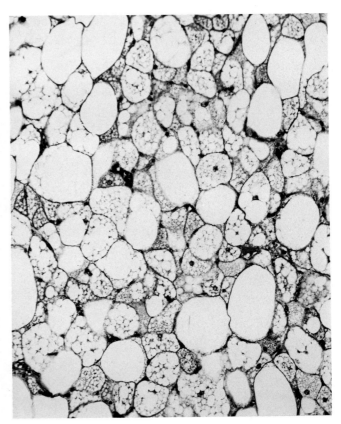

FIG. 16-65. Hibernoma showing gradual transition between brown and white fat cells. (×250.)

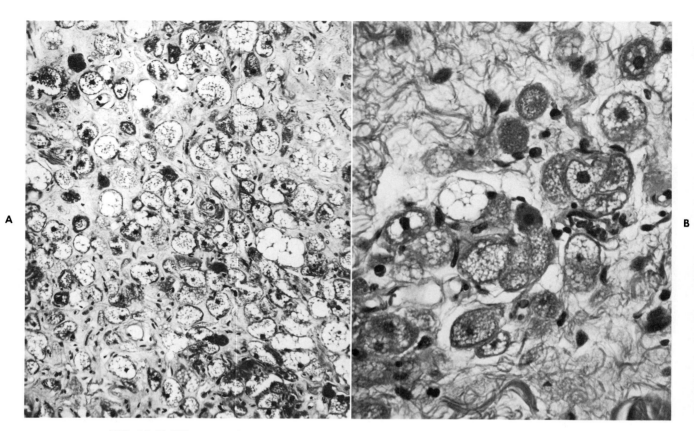

FIG. 16-66. Hibernoma with lipoblast-like cells **(A)** and extensive myxoid change **(B).** (A, ×160; B, × 250.)

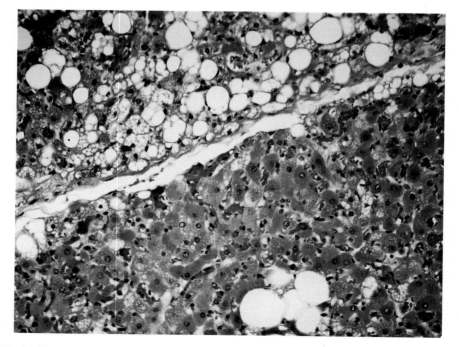

FIG. 16-67. Hibernoma showing lobular pattern with uniform granular eosinophilic cells and cells with multiple lipid vacuoles in different portions of the tumor. (×165.)

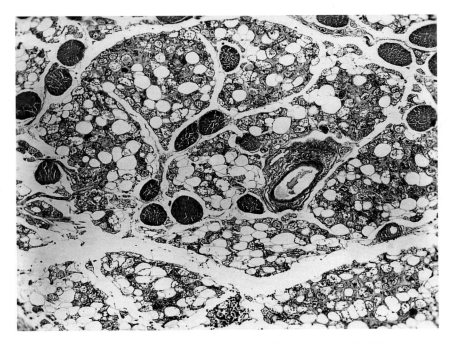

FIG. 16-68. Hibernoma infiltrating striated muscle tissue. (×40.)

more large lipid droplets and peripherally placed nuclei resembling lipocytes (Figs. 16-64, 16-66, and 16-67). In cases with numerous univacuolar cells, microscopic distinction from lipoma may be difficult (Fig. 16-65). Less commonly there are myxoid changes and infiltration of the underlying muscle tissue (Figs. 16-66 and 16-68). Fleishman and Schwartz[349] described diastase-resistant PAS-positive cytoplasmic masses at the periphery of hibernomas. The vascular supply is considerably more prominent in hibernoma than in lipoma, a fact that has been demonstrated angiographically by Angervall et al.[342] and others.[24,360,353] In fact, the distinctly brown color of hibernoma is due to the prominent vascularity and profusion of mitochondria in the tumor.

Ultrastructural studies[349,352,358,366] reveal multivacuolated and univacuolated cells packed with round to tubular mitochondria with parallel transverse cristae, a varying number of well-defined lipid droplets, and occasional lysosomes with a well-formed limiting membrane. In addition there are pinocytotic vesicles and a well-defined basal lamina. The nucleus contains uniformly distributed chromatin condensed under a well-defined nuclear membrane. The scarcity of rough endoplasmic reticulum and a prominent Golgi apparatus distinguish the cells from the preadipocytes of white fat. Allegra et al.[341] noted in perisinusoidal cells of a hibernoma "endoplasmacrine" lipid granule secretion, rows of pedunculated plasmalemmal granules, and periodic plasmalemmal densities, resembling secretory features present in the cortical cells of the adrenal gland.

The likelihood of confusion with other tumors is minimal. *Adult rhabdomyoma* is made up of similar eosinophilic cells, but its cells are larger and contain considerable amounts of glycogen and, on careful search, crystals and cross-striations. *Granular cell tumors* bear a superficial resemblance to hibernoma but are readily distinguished by the complete absence of intracellular oil red O positive lipid vacuoles. We are uncertain as to the existence of malignant hibernoma. We have encountered possible cases but have interpreted them microscopically as variants of round cell liposarcoma with multivacuolar eosinophilic lipoblasts. However, an accurate diagnosis of these cases would require ultrastructural studies.

REFERENCES
Adipose tissue: histology and ultrastructure

1. Cameron GR, Seneviratne RD: Growth and repair of adipose tissue. *J Pathol Bacteriol* 59:665, 1947.
2. Gellhorn A, Benjamin W: Lipid composition and metabolism of subcutaneous adipose tissue and lipoma of man. In *Handbook of physiology*, sec 5, Adipose tissue, Washington, DC, 1965, American Physiological Society, p 661.
3. Gieseking R: Elektronenoptische Befunde bei der Fettmobilisation und Fettassimilation im braunen Fettgewebe. *Zbl Allg Path* 103:561, 1961.

4. Heaton JM: The distribution of brown adipose tissue in the human. *J Anat* 112:35, 1972.

5. Napolitano L: The differentiation of white adipose tissue cells: an electron microscope study. *J Cell Biol* 18:663, 1963.

6. Napolitano L: The fine structure of adipose tissues. In *Handbook of physiology,* sec 5, Adipose tissue. Washington, DC, 1965, American Physiological Society, p 109.

7. Poissonet CM, La Velle M, Bordi AR: Growth and development of adipose tissue. *J Pediatr* 113:1, 1988.

8. Sigwart U, Tedeschi LG, Tedeschi CG: Factors in adipogenesis. *Hum Pathol* 1:399, 1970.

9. Tedeschi CG: Pathological anatomy of adipose tissue. In *Handbook of physiology,* sec 5, Adipose tissue, Washington, DC, 1965, American Physiological Society, p 141.

10. Wells HG: Adipose tissue: a neglected subject. *JAMA* 114:2117, 2284, 1940.

11. Wells HG: The fat metabolism of lipomas. *Arch Intern Med* 10:297, 1912.

12. Wasserman F: Die Fettorgane des Menschen: Entwicklung, Bau und systematische Stellung des sogenannten Fettgewebes. *Z Zellforsch Micr Anat* 3:235, 1926.

Lipoma

13. Adair FE, Pack GT, Farrier JH: Lipomas. *Am J Cancer* 16:1104, 1932.

14. Allen PW: *Tumors and proliferations of adipose tissue: a clinicopathologic approach,* New York, 1981, Masson Publishing, USA.

15. Bick EM: Lipomas of the extremities. *Ann Surg* 104:139, 1936.

16. Brasfield RD, Das Gupta TK: Soft tissue tumors: benign tumors of adipose tissue. *Cancer* 19:3, 1969.

17. Enjoji M, Iwasaki H, Yoshida I: Benign tumors and tumor-like lesions of soft tissues in infancy and childhood: histopathological and statistical study of 1020 cases. *Fukuoka Acta Medica* 67:234, 1976.

18. Fu YS, Parker FG, Kaye GI, et al: Ultrastructure of benign and malignant adipose tissue tumors. In Sommers SC, Rosen PP, editors: *Pathology annual,* part I, New York, 1980, Appleton-Century-Crofts, pp 67-89.

19. Hashimoto H, Daimaru Y, Enjoji M: S-100 protein distribution in liposarcoma: an immunoperoxidase study with special reference to the distinction of liposarcoma from myxoid malignant fibrous histiocytoma. *Virchows Arch (Pathol Anat)* 405:1, 1984.

20. Heim S, Mandahl N, Kristoffersson U, et al: Reciprocal translocation t(3;12)(q27;q13) in lipoma. *Cancer Genet Cytogenet* 23:301, 1986.

21. Kawashima A, Magid D, Fishman EK, et al: Parosteal ossifying lipoma: CT and MR findings. *J Comput Assist Tomogr* 17:147, 1993.

22. Kim YH, Reiner L: Ultrastructure of lipoma. *Cancer* 50:102, 1982.

23. Koopman RJ, van der Wey LP, van Rappard JH: Subfascial lipoma of the forehead. *Ned Tijdschr Geneeskd* 136:844, 1992.

24. Kransdorf MJ, Moser RP, Meis JM, et al: Fat-containing soft tissue masses of the extremities. *Radiographics* 11:81, 1991.

25. Leffert RD: Lipomas of the upper extremity. *J Bone Joint Surg* 54A:1262, 1972.

26. Lidor C, Lotem M, Hallel T: Parosteal lipoma of the proximal radius: a report of five cases. *J Hand Surg* 17A:1095, 1992.

27. Meggit BF: The battered buttock syndrome: a report of a group of traumatic lipomata. *Br J Surg* 59:165, 1972.

28. Murphy NG: Ossifying lipoma. *Br J Radiol* 47:97, 1974.

29. Myhre-Jensen O: A consecutive 7-year series of 1331 benign soft tissue tumors: clinicopathologic data: comparison with sarcomas. *Acta Orthop Scand* 52:287, 1981.

30. Penoff JH: Traumatic lipomas/pseudolipomas. *J Trauma* 22:63, 1982.

31. Phalen GS, Kendrik JI, Rodriguez JM: Lipomas of the upper extremity: a series of 15 tumors in the hand and wrist. *Am J Surg* 121:298, 1971.

32. Plaut GS, Salm R, Truscott DE: Three cases of ossifying lipoma. *J Pathol Bacteriol* 78:292, 1959.

33. Robson PN: A large calcified lipoma of the thigh. *J Bone Joint Surg* 32B:384, 1950.

34. Rozner L, Isaacs GW: The traumatic pseudolipoma. *N Z J Surg* 47:779, 1977.

35. Rydholm A, Berg NO: Size, site and clinical incidence of lipoma: factors in differential diagnosis of lipoma and sarcoma. *Acta Orthop Scand* 54:929, 1983.

36. Sauer JM, Ozonoff MB: Congenital bone anomalies associated with lipomas. *Skeletal Radiol* 13:276, 1985.

37. Solvonuk PF, Taylor GP, Hancock R, et al: Correlation of morphologic and biochemical observations in human lipomas. *Lab Invest* 51:469, 1984.

38. Sreekantaiah C, Leong SP, Davis JR: Intratumoral cytogenetic heterogeneity in a benign neoplasm. *Cancer* 67:3110, 1991.

39. Tedeschi CG, Lyon WH: Fat tissue growths. *Mt Sinai J Med* 24:1272, 1957.

40. Tranquada RE: Subcutaneous lipomas at sites of insulin injection. *Diabetes* 15:807, 1966.

41. Turc-Carel C, Dal Cin P, Boghosian L, et al: Cytogenetic studies of adipose tissue tumors. I. A benign lipoma with reciprocal translocation t(3;12)(q28;q14). *Cancer Genet Cytogenet* 23:283, 1986.

42. Weinberg T, Feldman M: Lipomas of the gastrointestinal tract. *Am J Clin Pathol* 25:272, 1955.

43. Wurlitzer F, Bedrossian C, Ayala A, et al: Problems of diagnosis and treating lipomas. *Ann Surg* 39:240, 1973.

Deep lipoma

44. Aldredge WM, Halpert B: Lipoma of the thenar. *Surgery* 24:853, 1948.

45. Ashby BS, MacGillivray JB: Paratesticular lipoma. *Br J Surg* 53:828, 1966.

46. Booher R: Lipoblastic tumors of the hands and feet: review of the literature and report of 33 cases. *J Bone Joint Surg* 47A:727, 1965.

47. Bosch TD, Bernhard WG: Lipoma of the palm. *Am J Clin Pathol* 20:262, 1950.

48. Campbell CS, Wulf RF: Lipoma producing a lesion of the deep branch of the radial nerve: a case report. *J Neurosurg* 11:310, 1954.

49. Carrol RE, Doyle JR: Lipoma of the hand. *J Bone Joint Surg* 49A:581, 1967.

50. Cicciarelli RE, Soule EH, McGoon DC: Lipoma and liposarcoma of the mediastinum: a report of 14 tumors including lipomas of the thymus. *J Thorac Cardiovasc Surg* 47:411, 1964.

51. Demos DC, Bruno E, Dobozi WR: Parosteal lipoma with enlarging osteochondroma. *Am J Roentgenol* 143:365, 1984.

52. Dertinger K: Über tiefsitzende Lipome. *Beitr Klin Chir* 38:76, 1903.

53. De Weerd JH, Dockerty MB: Lipomatous retroperitoneal tumors. *Am J Surg* 84:397, 1952.

54. Ersek RA, Lele E, Surak GS, et al: Hereditary progressive nodular lipomatosis: a report and selective review of a new syndrome [see comments]. *Ann Plast Surg* 23:450, 1989.

55. Fairbank HAT: A parosteal lipoma. *J Bone Joint Surg* 35B:589, 1953.

56. Graham EA, Wiese ER: Lipomas of the mediastinum. *Arch Surg* 16:380, 1928.

57. Greenberg SD, Isensee C, Gonzalez-Angulo A, et al: Infiltrating lipomas of the thigh. *Am J Clin Pathol* 39:66, 1963.

58. Hodge J, Aponte G, McLaughlin E: Primary mediastinal tumors. *J Thorac Surg* 37:730, 1959.

59. Hoehn JG, Farber HF: Massive lipoma of palm. *Ann Plast Surg* 11:431, 1984.

60. Johannson L, Soderlund S: Intrathoracic lipoma. *Acta Chir Scand* 126:558, 1963.

61. Keeley JL, Gumbiner SH, Guzauskus AC, et al: Mediastinal lipoma successful removal of a 1700 gram mass: case report and review of recent literature of intrathoracic lipomas. *J Thorac Surg* 25:316, 1953.

62. Kenin A, Levine J. Spinner M: Parosteal lipoma. *J Bone Joint Surg* 41A:1122, 1959.

63. Kleinhaus S, Ducharme JC: Mediastinal lipoma in children. *Surgery* 66:790, 1969.

64. Kransdorf MJ, Moser RP, Meis JM, et al: Fat containing soft tissue masses of the extremities. *Radiographics* 11:81, 1991.

65. Krause LG, Ross CA: Intrathoracic lipomas: a report of three cases and a review of the literature. *Arch Surg* 84:444, 1962.

66. Michowitz M, Lazebnik N, Lazebnik R: Lipoma of the colon: a report of 22 cases. *Am Surg* 51:449, 1985.

67. Millward S, Escott N, Masood K: The diagnosis of a pleural lipoma by CT and fine needle biopsy to avoid thoracotomy. *Can Assoc Radiol J* 39:57, 1988.

68. Moon N, Marmor L: Parosteal lipoma of the proximal part of the radius. *J Bone Joint Surg* 46A:608, 1964.

69. Mowat AP, Clark CG: Presacral lipomata. *Br J Surg* 49:230, 1961.

70. Oster LH, Blair WF, Steyers CM: Large lipomas in the deep palmar space. *J Hand Surg* 14A:700, 1989.

71. Paarlberg D, Linscheid RL, Soule EH: Lipomas of the hand: including a case of lipoblastomatosis in a child. *Mayo Clin Proc* 47:121, 1972.

72. Pachter MR, Lattes R: Mesenchymal tumors of the mediastinum. I. Tumors of fibrous tissue, adipose tissue, smooth muscle and striated muscle. *Cancer* 16:74, 1963.

73. Phalen GS, Kendrik JI, Rodriguez JM: Lipomas of the upper extremity, a series of 15 tumors in the hand and wrist and 6 tumors causing nerve compression. *Am J Surg* 121:298, 1971.

74. Regan JM, Bickle WH, Broders AC: Infiltrating benign lipomas of the extremities. *West J Surg* 54:87, 1946.

75. Rosen H: Parosteal lipoma. *Bull Hosp Joint Dis* 20:96, 1959.

76. Rubinstein A, Goor Y, Gazit E, et al: Non symmetric subcutaneous lipomatosis associated with familial combined hyperlipidaemia. *Br J Dermatol* 120:689, 1989.

77. Saini VK, Wahi PI: Hourglass transmural type of intrathoracic lipoma. *J Thorac Cardiovasc Surg* 47:600, 1964.

78. Schottenfeld LE: Lipomas of the gastrointestinal tract: with special reference to the small intestine, including the ileum: review of the literature and report of six cases. *Surgery* 14:47, 1943.

79. Schweitzer G: Parosteal lipoma of the radius: a case report. *S Afr Med J* 44:648, 1970.

80. Siegal A, Witz M: Gastrointestinal lipoma and malignancies. *J Surg Oncol* 47:170, 1991.

81. Von Wahlendorf ARL: Ueber retroperitoneale Lipome. *Arch Klin Chir* 115:751, 1921.

Multiple lipomas

82. Adair FE, Pack GT, Farrior JH: Lipomas. *Am J Cancer* 16:1104, 1932.

83. Alsberg A: Ueber Neurolipome, Inaugural Dissertation, Berlin, 1892, Gustav Schade.

84. Bannayan GA: Lipomatosis, angiomatosis, and macrocephalia: a previously undescribed congenital syndrome. *Arch Pathol* 92:1, 1971.

85. Benny PS, Macvicar J: Multiple lipomas in pregnancy. *Br Med J* 1:1679, 1979.

86. Buschke A, Mattissohn L: Symmetrische Lipomatosis (Uebersicht nebst Mitteilung von 2 Fällen, kombiniert mit Psoriasis and Arthritis). *Arch Dermatol* 120:537, 1914.

87. Grosshans EM: Subfascial lipoma of the forehead (letter). *J Am Acad Dermatol* 23:153, 1990.

88. Heim S, Mandahl N, Kristoffersson U, et al: Marker ring chromosome—a new cytogenetic abnormality characterizing lipogenic tumors? *Can Genet Cytogenet* 24:319, 1987.

89. Heim S, Mandahl N, Kristoffersson U, et al: Reciprocal translocation t(3;12)(q27;q13) in lipoma. *Can Genet Cytogenet* 23:301, 1986.

90. Higginbottom MC, Schultz P: The Bannayan syndrome: an autosomal dominant disorder consisting of macrocephaly, lipomas, hemangiomas, and risk for intracranial tumors. *Pediatrics* 69:632, 1982.

91. Humphrey AA, Kingsley PC: Familial multiple lipomas: report of a family. *Arch Dermatol* 37:30, 1938.

92. Kurzweg FT, Spencer R: Familial multiple lipomatosis. *Am J Surg* 82:726, 1951.

93. Leven D: Erblichkeit der multiplen Lipome. *Derm Wchschrft* 40:11, 1928.

94. Miles JH, Zonana J, McFarlane J, et al: Macrocephaly with hamartomas: Bannayan-Zonana syndrome. *Am J Med Genet* 19:225, 1984.

95. Sandberg AA, Turc-Carel C: The cytogenetics of solid tumor: relation to diagnosis, classification and pathology. *Cancer* 59:387, 1987.

96. Shanks JA, Paranchych W, Tuba J: Familial multiple lipomatosis. *Can Med Assoc J* 77:881, 1957.

97. Sreekantaiah C, Leong SP, Chu D, et al: Translocation (X;12)(q27;q14) in a lipoma. *Cancer Genet Cytogenet* 49:235, 1990.

98. Stephens FE, Isaacson A: Hereditary multiple lipomatosis. *J Heredity* 50:51, 1959.

99. Weary PE, Gorlin RJ, Gentry WC, et al: Multiple hamartoma syndrome (Cowden's disease). *Arch Dermatol* 106:682, 1972.

100. Zonana J, Rimoin DL, Davis DC: Macrocephaly with multiple lipomas and hemangiomas. *J Pediatr* 89:600, 1976.

Angiolipoma

101. Belcher RW, Czarnetzki BM, Carney JF, et al: Multiple (subcutaneous) angiolipomas: clinical, pathologic and pharmacologic studies. *Arch Dermatol* 110:583, 1974.

102. Bowen JT: Multiple subcutaneous hemangiomas, together with multiple lipomas, occurring in enormous numbers in an otherwise healthy, muscular subject. *Am J Med Sci* 144:189, 1912.

103. Campos GM, Grandini SA, Lopes RA: Angiolipoma of the cheek. *Int J Oral Surg* 9:486, 1980.

104. Dixon AY, McGregor DH: Angiolipomas: an ultrastructural and clinicopathological study. *Hum Pathol* 12:739, 1981.

105. Enjoji M, Tsuneyoshi M, Hashimoto H: Subcutaneous angiolipoma: a clinicopathologic observation. *Fukuoka Acta Medica* 67:82, 1976.

106. Harms D, Grebe W: Ueber das Vorkommen von Mikrothromben in Lipomen. *Virchows Arch (Pathol Anat)* 355:41, 1972.

107. Howard WR, Helwig EB: Angiolipoma. *Arch Dermatol* 82:924, 1960.

108. Hunt SJ, Santa Cruz DJ, Barr RJ: Cellular angiolipoma. *Am J Surg Pathol* 14:75, 1990.

109. Palkovic S, Wassmann H, Bonse R, et al: Angiolipoma of the spinal cord: magnetic resonance imaging and microsurgical management. *Surg Neurol* 29:243, 1988.

110. Pribyl C, Burke SW, Roberts JM, et al: Infiltrating angiolipoma or intramuscular hemangioma? A report of five cases. *J Pediatr Orthop* 6:172, 1986.

111. Rasanen O, Nohteri H, Dammert K: Angiolipoma and lipoma. *Acta Chir Scand* 133:461, 1974.

112. Reilly JS, Kelly DR, Royal SA: Angiolipoma of the parotid: case report and review. *Laryngoscope* 98:818, 1988.

Spindle cell and pleomorphic lipoma

113. Angervall L, Dahl I, Kindblom LG, et al: Spindle cell lipoma. *Acta Pathol Microbiol Scand* 84:477, 1976.

114. Azumi N, Curtis J, Kempson R, et al: Atypical and malignant neoplasms showing lipomatous differentiation: a study of 111 cases. *Am J Surg Pathol* 11:161, 1987.

115. Azzopardi JG, Iocco J, Salm R: Pleomorphic lipoma: a tumour simulating liposarcoma. *Histopathology* 7:511, 1983.

116. Bartley GB, Yeatts RP, Garrity JA, et al: Spindle cell lipoma of the orbit. *Am J Ophthalmol* 100:605, 1985.

117. Beham A, Schmid C, Hodl S, et al: Spindle cell and pleomorphic lipoma: an immunohistochemical study and histogenetic analysis. *J Pathol* 158:219, 1989.

118. Bolen JW, Thorning D: Spindle-cell lipoma: a clinical, light- and electron-microscopical study. *Am J Surg Pathol* 5:435, 1981.

119. Chan JK, Lee KC, Saw D: Extraskeletal chondroma with lipoblast-like cells. *Hum Pathol* 17:1285, 1986.

120. Digregorio F, Barr RJ, Fretzin DF: Pleomorphic lipoma: case reports and review of the literature. *J Dermatol Surg Oncol* 18:197, 1992.

121. Enzinger FM: Benign lipomatous tumors simulating a sarcoma. In *Management of primary bone and soft tissue tumors*, Chicago, 1977, Year Book Medical Publishers, p 11.

122. Enzinger FM, Harvey DA: Spindle cell lipoma. *Cancer* 36:1852, 1975.

123. Enzinger FM, Winslow DJ: Liposarcoma: a study of 103 cases. *Virchows Arch (Pathol Anat)* 335:367, 1962.

124. Evans HL, Soule EH, Winkelman RK: Atypical lipoma, atypical intramuscular lipoma and well differentiated liposarcoma. *Cancer* 43:574, 1979.

125. Fletcher CD, Martin-Bates E: Spindle cell lipoma: a clinicopathological study with some original observations. *Histopathology* 11:803, 1987.

126. Gorelkin L, Conrad-England R: Spindle cell lipoma: a benign variant with potential hazards of diagnostic misinterpretation. *South Med J* 71:1163, 1978.

127. Honore LH: Uterine fibrolipoleiomyoma: report of a case with discussion of histogenesis. *Am J Obstet Gynecol* 132:635, 1978.

128. Hruban RH, Bhagavan BS, Epstein JI: Massive retroperitoneal angiomyolipoma: a lesion that may be confused with well differentiated liposarcoma. *Am J Clin Pathol* 92:805, 1989.

129. Jacobs DS, Cohen H, Johnson JS: Lipoleiomyomas of the uterus. *Am J Clin Pathol* 44:45, 1965.

130. Johnson BL, Linn JG Jr: Spindle cell lipoma of the orbit. *Arch Ophthalmol* 97:133, 1979.

131. Kitano M, Enjoji M, Iwasaki H: Spindle cell lipoma—a clinicopathologic analysis of 12 cases. *Acta Pathol Jpn* 29:891, 1979.

132. Lehrman BJ, Nisenbaum HL, Glasser SA et al: Uterine myolipoma: magnetic resonance imaging, computed tomography, and ultrasound appearance. *J Ultrasound Med* 9:665, 1990.

133. McDaniel RK, Newland JR, Chiles DG: Intraoral spindle cell lipoma: case reported with correlated light and electron microscopy. *Oral Surg Oral Med Oral Pathol* 57:52, 1984.

134. Meis JM, Enzinger FM: Chondroid lipoma: a unique tumor simulating liposarcoma and myxoid chondrosarcoma. *Am J Surg Pathol* 17:1103, 1993.

135. Meis JM, Enzinger FM: Myolipoma of soft tissue. *Am J Surg Pathol* 15:121, 1991.

136. Meister P: Spindle cell lipoma: report of 2 cases and differential diagnosis. *Beitr Pathol* 161:376, 1977.

137. Muenchow T, Senitz D, Goertchen R: Pleomorphic lipoma. *Zbl Allg Path* 130:13, 1985.

138. Shmookler BM, Enzinger FM: Pleomorphic lipoma: a benign tumor simulating liposarcoma: a clinicopathologic analysis of 48 cases. *Cancer* 47:126, 1981.

139. Warkel RL, Rehme CG, Thompson WH: Vascular spindle cell lipoma. *J Cutan Pathol* 9:113, 1982.

Lipoblastoma and lipoblastomatosis

140. Alba-Greco M, Garcia RL, Vuletin JC: Benign lipoblastomatosis: ultrastructure and histogenesis. *Cancer* 45:511, 1980.

141. Bolen JW, Thorning D: Benign lipoblastoma and myxoid liposarcoma: a comparative light and electron-microscopic study. *Am J Surg Pathol* 4:163, 1980.

142. Chung EB, Enzinger FM: Benign lipoblastomatosis: an analysis of 35 cases. *Cancer* 32:482, 1973.

143. Cox RW: "Hibernoma": the lipoma of immature adipose tissue. *J Pathol Bacteriol* 68:511, 1954.

144. Enghardt MH, Warren RC: Congenital palpebral lipoblastoma: first report of a case. *Am J Dermatopathol* 12:408, 1990.

145. Enzinger FM: Benign lipomatous tumors simulating a sarcoma. In *Management of primary bone and soft tissue tumors*. Chicago, 1977, Year Book Medical Publishers.

146. Greco MA, Garcia RL, Vuletin JC: Benign lipoblastomatosis: ultrastructure and histogenesis. *Cancer* 45:511, 1980.

147. Jimenez JF: Lipoblastoma in infancy and childhood. *J Surg Oncol* 32:238, 1986.

148. Kauffman SL, Stout AP: Lipoblastic tumors in children. *Cancer* 12:912, 1959.

149. Mahour GH, Bryan BJ, Isaacs H: Lipoblastoma and lipoblastomatosis: a report of six cases. *Surgery* 104:577, 1988.

150. Stringel G, Shandling B, Mancer K, et al: Lipoblastoma in infants and children. *J Pediatr Surg* 17:277, 1982.

151. Van Meurs DP: The transformation of an embryonic lipoma to a common lipoma. *Br J Surg* 34:282, 1947.

152. Vellios F, Baez JM, Shumacker HB: Lipoblastomatosis: a tumor of fetal fat different from hibernoma: report of a case, with observations on the embryogenesis of human adipose tissue. *Am J Pathol* 34:1149, 1958.

Angiomyolipoma

153. Allen TD, Risk W: Renal angiomyolipoma. *J Urol* 94:203, 1965.

154. Ansari SJ, Stephenson RA, Mackay B: Angiomyolipoma of the kidney with lymph node involvement. *Ultrastruct Pathol* 15:531, 1991.

155. Argenyi ZB, Piette WW, Goeken JA: Cutaneous angiomyolipoma: a light microscopic, immunohistochemical and electron microscopic study. *Am J Dermatopathol* 13:497, 1991.

156. Back W, Heine M, Potempa D: Intravascular form of angiomyolipoma of the kidney: case report and review of the literature. *Pathologe* 13:212, 1992.

157. Berg JW: Angiolipomyosarcoma of kidney (malignant hamartomatous angiolipomyoma) in a case with solitary metastasis from bronchogenic carcinoma. *Cancer* 8:759, 1955.

158. Bloom DA, Scardino P, Ehrlich RM: The significance of lymph node involvement in renal angiomyolipoma. *J Urol* 128:1292, 1982.

159. Bosniak MA, Megibow AJ, Hulnick DH, et al: CT diagnosis of renal angiomyolipoma: the importance of detecting small amounts of fat. *AJR* 151:497, 1988.

160. Brecher ME, Gill WB, Straus FH: Angiomyolipoma with regional lymph node involvement and long-term follow-up study. *Hum Pathol* 17:962, 1986.

161. Busch FM, Bark CJ, Clyde HR: Benign renal angiomyolipoma with regional lymph node involvement. *J Urol* 116:715, 1976.

162. Castillenti TA, Bertin AP: Angiomyolipoma of the spermatic cord: case report and literature review. *J Urol* 142:1308, 1989.

163. Chan JKC, Tsang WYW, Tang MC, et al: Lymphangiomyomatosis and angiomyolipoma. *Modern Pathol* 6:5A, 1993.

164. Dao AH, Pinto AC, Kirchner FK, et al: Massive nodal involvement

in a case of renal angiomyolipoma. *Arch Pathol Lab Med* 108:612, 1984.

165. de Jong B, Castedo SM, Oosterhuis JW, et al: Trisomy 7 in a case of angiomyolipoma. *Cancer Genet Cytogenet* 34:219, 1988.

166. Edelman MA, Mitty HA, Dan SJ, et al: Angiomyolipoma: postembolization liquefaction and percutaneous drainage. *Urol Radiol* 12:145, 1990.

167. Farrow GM, Harrison EG Jr, Utz DC, et al: Renal angiomyolipoma: a clinicopathologic study of 32 cases. *Cancer* 22:564, 1968.

168. Ferry JA, Malt RA, Young RH: Renal angiomyolipoma with sarcomatous transformation and pulmonary metastases. *Am J Surg Pathol* 15:1083, 1991.

169. Fischer W: Die Nierentumoren bei der tuberösen Hirnsklerose. *Beitr Path* 50:235, 1911.

170. Futter NG, Collins WE: Renal angiomyolipoma causing hypertension. *Br J Urol* 46:485, 1974.

171. Glenthoj A, Partoft S: Ultrasound guided percutaneous aspiration biopsy of renal angiomyolipoma: report of two cases diagnosed by cytology. *Acta Cytol* 28:265, 1984.

172. Goodman ZD, Ishak KG: Angiomyolipomas of the liver. *Am J Surg Pathol* 8:745, 1984.

173. Hajdu SI, Foote FW Jr: Angiomyolipoma of the kidney: report of 27 cases and review of the literature. *J Urol* 102:396, 1969.

174. Harbitz A: Tuberöse Tumoren gleichzeitig mit Nierengeschwülsten (Myxo-Lipo-Sarkomen) und einer Hautkrankheit (Adenoma sebaceum). *Zentralbl Allg Pathol* 23:868, 1912.

175. Hartman DS, Goldman SM, Friedman AC, et al: Angiomyolipoma: ultrasonic-pathologic correlation. *Radiology* 139:451, 1981.

176. Hartveit F, Hallerbraker B: A report of three angiomyolipomata and one angiomyoliposarcoma. *Acta Pathol Microbiol Scand* 49:329, 1960.

177. Hulbert JC, Graf R: Involvement of the spleen by renal angiomyolipoma: metastasis or multicentricity. *J Urol* 130:328, 1983.

178. Kavaney PB, Fielding I: Angiomyolipoma and renal cell carcinoma in the same kidney. *Urology* 6:643, 1975.

179. Kirpicznik J: Ein Fall von tuberoeser Sclerose und gleichzeitigen multiplen Nierengeschwülsten. *Virchows Arch (Pathol Anat)* 201:358, 1910.

180. Kragel PJ, Toker C: Infiltrating recurrent renal angiomyolipoma with fatal outcome. *J Urol* 133:90, 1985.

181. Lack E, Dolan MF, Finisio J, et al: Pulmonary and extrapulmonary lymphangioleiomyomatosis: report of a case with bilateral renal angiomyolipomas: multifocal lymphangioleiomyomatosis and a glial polyp of the endocervix. *Am J Surg Pathol* 10:650, 1986.

182. Lowe BA, Brewer J, Houghton DC, et al: Malignant transformation of angiomyolipoma. *J Urol* 147:1356, 1992.

183. Malone MJ, Johnson PR, Jumper BM, et al: Renal angiomyolipoma: six case reports and literature review. *J Urol* 135:349, 1986.

184. McCullough LD, Scott R, Seybold HM: Renal angiomyolipoma (hamartoma). *J Urol* 105:32, 1971.

185. Monteforte WJ, Kohnen PW: Angiomyolipomas in a case of lymphangiomyomatosis syndrome: relationship to tuberous sclerosis. *Cancer* 34:317, 1974.

186. Mukai M, Torikata C, Iri H, et al: Crystalloids in angiomyolipoma: a previously unnoticed phenomenon of renal angiomyolipoma occurring at a high frequency. *Am J Surg Pathol* 16:1, 1992.

187. Nguyen GK: Aspiration biopsy cytology of renal angiomyolipoma. *Acta Cytol* 28:261, 1984.

188. Okada K, Yokoyama S, Nakayama I, et al: An electron microscopic study of hepatic angiomyolipoma. *Acta Pathol Jpn* 39:743, 1989.

189. Pea M, Bonetti F, Zamboni G, et al: Clear cell tumor and angiomyolipoma (letter). *Am J Surg Pathol* 15:199, 1991.

190. Pielsticker K, Kunze E, Stern G: Lymphangiomatose mit diffusem Befall der Lungen und multiplen Angiomyolipomen der Nieren. *Beitr Pathol* 147:189, 1972.

191. Pounder DJ: Hepatic angiomyolipoma. *Am J Surg Pathol* 6:667, 1982.

192. Price EB, Mostofi FK: Symptomatic angiomyolipoma of the kidney. *Cancer* 18:761, 1965.

193. Ro JY, Ayala AG, el-Naggar A, et al: Angiomyolipoma of kidney with lymph node involvement: DNA flow cytometric analysis. *Arch Pathol Lab Med* 114:65, 1990.

194. Sanchez FW, Vujic I, Ayres RI et al: Hemorrhagic renal angiomyolipoma: superselective renal arterial embolization for preservation of renal function. *Cardiovasc Intervent Radiol* 8:39, 1985.

195. Sherman JL, Hartman DS, Friedman AC, et al: Angiomyolipoma: computed tomographic-pathologic correlation of 17 cases. *Am J Roentgenol* 137:1221, 1981.

196. Stone NN, Atlas I, Kim US, et al: Renal angiomyolipoma associated with neurofibromatosis and primary carcinoid of mesentery. *Urology* 41:66, 1993.

197. Taylor RS, Joseph DB, Kohaut EC, et al: Renal angiomyolipoma associated with lymph node involvement and renal cell carcinoma in patients with tuberous sclerosis. *J Urol* 141:930, 1989.

198. Uchino A, Itoh K, Egashira K, et al: Therapeutic embolization of renal angiomyolipoma: case report and review of the literature. *Radiat Med* 5:191, 1987.

199. Umeyama T, Saitoh Y, Tomaru Y, et al: Bilateral renal angiomyolipoma associated with bilateral renal vein and inferior vena caval thrombi. *J Urol* 148:1885, 1992.

200. Vasko JS, Brockman SK, Bomar RL: Renal angiomyolipoma (hamartoma): review of the literature and report of spontaneous retroperitoneal hemorrhage. *Ann Surg* 161:715, 1965.

201. Watanabe T, Morimoto S, Shinka T, et al: Therapeutic embolization of renal angiomyolipoma: a case report. *Hinyokika Kiyo* 35:1183, 1989.

202. Weeks DA, Malott RL, Arnesen M, et al: Hepatic angiomyolipoma with striated granules and positivity with melanoma-specific antibody (HMB-45): a report of two cases. *Ultrastruct Pathol* 15:563, 1991.

203. Yum M, Ganguly A, Donohue JP: Juxtaglomerular cells in renal angiomyolipoma: ultrastructural observation. *Urology* 24:283, 1984.

Myelolipoma

204. Bennett BD, McKenna TJ, Hough AJ, et al: Adrenal myelolipoma associated with Cushing's disease. *Am J Clin Pathol* 73:443, 1980.

205. Benson PA, Janko AB: Pelvic myelolipoma (rare presacral tumor). *Am J Obstet Gynecol* 92:884, 1965.

206. Burrows S, Drake WM Jr, Singley TL: Large retroperitoneal myelolipoma associated with acute myelogenous leukemia. *Am J Clin Pathol* 52:733, 1969.

207. Chen KTK, Felix EL, Flam MS: Extraadrenal myelolipoma. *Am J Clin Pathol* 78:386, 1982.

208. Damjanov I, Katz SM, Catalano E, et al: Myelolipoma in a heterotopic adrenal gland: light and electron microscopic findings. *Cancer* 44:1350, 1979.

209. Dodge OG, Evans DMD: Haemopoiesis in a presacral fatty tumor (myelolipoma). *J Pathol Bacteriol* 72:313, 1956.

210. Escuin F, Gomez P, Martinez M, et al: Angiomyelolipoma associated with bilateral adrenocortical hyperplasia and hypertension. *J Urol* 133:655, 1985.

211. Fowler MR, Williams RB, Alba JM, et al: Extra-adrenal myelolipomas compared with extramedullary hematopoietic tumors: a case of presacral myelolipoma. *Am J Surg Pathol* 6:363, 1982.

212. Giffen HK: Myelolipoma of the adrenals: report of seven cases. *Am J Pathol* 23:613, 1947.

213. Hunter SB, Schemakewitz EH, Patterson C, et al: Extraadrenal myelolipoma: a report of two cases. *Am J Clin Pathol* 97:402, 1992.

214. Ishikawa H, Tachibana M, Hata M, et al: Myelolipoma of the adrenal gland. *J Urol* 126:777, 1981.

215. Knoblich R: Extramedullary hematopoiesis presenting as intrathoracic tumor. *Cancer* 13:462, 1960.

216. McDonnell W: Myelolipoma of adrenal. *Arch Pathol (Chicago)* 61:407, 1956.

217. Noble MJ, Montague DK, Levin HS: Myelolipoma: an unusual surgical lesion of the adrenal gland. *Cancer* 49:952, 1982.

218. Peters WM, Dixon MF, Williams NS: Angiomyelolipoma of the liver. *Histopathology* 7:99, 1983.

219. Plaut A: Myelolipoma in the adrenal cortex (myelo-adipose structures). *Am J Pathol* 34:487, 1958.

220. Saaleby ER: Heterotopia of bone marrow without apparent cause. *Am J Pathol* 1:69, 1925.

221. Selye H, Stone H: Hormonally induced transformation of adrenal into myeloid tissue. *Am J Pathol* 26:211, 1950.

222. Sutker B, Balthazar EJ, Fazzini E: Presacral myelolipoma: CT findings. *J Comput Assist Tomogr* 9:1128, 1985.

Intramuscular and intermuscular lipoma

223. Austin RM, Mack GR, Townsend CM, et al: Infiltrating (intramuscular) lipomas and angiolipomas. *Arch Surg* 115:281, 1980.

224. Behrend M: Intermuscular lipomas. Report of three cases. *Am J Surg* 7:857, 1929.

225. Dionne GP, Seemayer TA: Infiltrating lipomas and angiolipomas revisited. *Cancer* 33:732, 1974.

226. Enzinger FM: Benign lipomatous tumors simulating a sarcoma. In *Management of primary bone and soft tissue tumors*. Chicago, 1977, Year Book Medical Publishers.

227. Greenberg SD, Isensee C, Gonzalez-Angulo A, et al: Infiltrating lipomas of the thigh. *Am J Clin Pathol* 39:66, 1963.

228. Kindblom LG, Angervall L, Stener B, et al: Intermuscular and intramuscular lipomas and hibernomas: a clinical, roentgenologic, histologic and prognostic study of 46 cases. *Cancer* 33:754, 1974.

229. Kubota M, Nagasaki A, Ohgami H, et al: An infantile case of infiltrating lipoma in the buttock. *J Pediatr Surg* 26:230, 1991.

230. Regan JM, Bickle WH, Broders AC: Infiltrating benign lipomas of the extremities. *West J Surg* 54:87, 1946.

231. Seemayer TA, Dionne PG: Infiltrating lipomas of soft tissue. *Lab Invest* 30:304, 1974.

232. Stimpson N: Infiltrating angiolipomata of the skeletal muscle. *Br J Surg* 58:464, 1971.

Lipoma of tendon sheaths and joints

233. Charache H: Tumors of tendon sheaths. *Arch Surg* 44:1038, 1942.

234. Hoffa A: Zur Bedeutung des Fettgewebes für die Pathologie des Kniegelenks. *Dtsch Med Wochenschr* 30:337, 1904.

235. Martinez D, Millner PA, Coral A, et al: Case report 745: synovial lipoma arborescens. *Skeletal Radiol* 21:393, 1992.

236. Strauss A: Lipoma of the tendon sheaths: with report of a case and review of the literature. *Surg Gynecol Obstet* 35:161, 1922.

237. Sullivan CR, Dahlin DC, Bryan RS: Lipoma of the tendon sheath. *J Bone Joint Surg* 38A:1275, 1956.

238. Valdoni P: Lipoma arborescente sistemico delle guaine tendince della mano e del piede. *Chir de Organ d Movimento* 15:509, 1931.

239. Weitzman G: Lipoma arborescens of the knee: report of a case. *J Bone Joint Surg* 47A:1030, 1965.

240. White JR: Arborescent lipoma of tendon sheaths: a report of two cases. *Surg Gynecol Obstet* 38:489, 1924.

Lumbosacral and spinal lipoma

241. Alston SR, Fuller GN, Boyko OB, et al: Ectopic immature renal tissue in a lumbosacral lipoma: pathologic and radiologic findings. *Pediatr Neurosci* 15:100, 1989.

242. Balagura S: Late neurological dysfunction in adult lumbosacral lipoma with tethered cord. *Neurosurgery* 15:724, 1984.

243. Giuffre R: Intradural spinal lipoma: review of the literature (99 cases) and report of an additional case. *Acta Neurochir* 14:69, 1966.

244. Hageman G, Veiga-Pires JA, de Graaff R, et al: Lumbosacral lipoma investigated by conventional radiography, ultrasound and direct coronal mode CT-scanning. *Computertomographie* 2:92, 1982.

245. Kieck C, Villiers J: Subcutaneous lumbosacral lipomas. *S Afr Med J* 49:1563, 1975.

246. Lassman LP, James CCM: Lumbosacral lipomas: critical survey of 26 cases submitted to laminectomy. *J Neurol Neurosurg Psychol* 30:174, 1967.

247. Loeser JD, Lewin RD: Lumbosacral lipoma in an adult. *J Neurosurg* 29:405, 1968.

248. Maiuri F, Corriero G, Gallichio B, et al: Late neurological dysfunction in adult lumbosacral lipoma. *J Neurosurg Sci* 31:7, 1987.

249. Naidich TP, McLone DG, Mutluer S: A new understanding of dorsal dysraphism with lipoma (lipomyeloschisis). *Am J Roentgenol* 140:1065, 1983.

250. Pasternak JF, Volpe JJ: Lumbosacral lipoma with acute deterioration during infancy. *Pediatrics* 66:125, 1980.

251. Rickwood AMK, Hemalatha V, Zachary RB: Lipoma of the cauda equina (lumbosacral lipoma): a study of 74 cases operated in childhood. *Z Kinderchir* 27:159, 1979.

252. Taviere V, Brunelle F, Baraton J, et al: MRI study of lumbosacral lipoma in children. *Pediatr Radiol* 19:316, 1989.

253. Walker AE: Dilatation of the vertebral canal associated with congenital anomalies of the spinal cord. *Am J Roentgenol* 52:571, 1944.

Neural fibrolipoma

254. Barsky AJ: Macrodactyly. *J Bone Joint Surg* 49A:1255, 1967.

255. Erichsen B, Medgyesi S: Congenital lipoma imitating giantism of the toe. *Scand J Plast Reconstr Surg* 17:77, 1983.

256. Feriz H: Macrodystrophia lipomatosa progressiva. *Virchows Arch (Pathol Anat)* 260:308, 1926.

257. Friedlander HL, Rosenberg NJ, Graubard DJ: Intraneural lipoma of the median nerve. *J Bone Joint Surg* 51A:352, 1969.

258. Haverbush TJ, Kendrick JL, Nelson CL: Intraneural lipoma of the median nerve: report of two cases. *Cleve Clin Q* 37:145, 1970.

259. Johnson RJ, Bonfiglio M: Lipofibromatous hamartoma of the median nerve. *J Bone Joint Surg* 51A:984, 1969.

260. Minkowitz S, Minkowitz F: A morphological study of macrodactylism: a case report. *J Pathol Bacteriol* 90:323, 1965.

261. Morley GH: Intraneurolipoma of the median nerve and the carpal tunnel. *J Bone Joint Surg* 46B:734, 1964.

262. Paletta FX, Rybka FJ: Treatment of hamartomas of the median nerve. *Ann Surg* 176:217, 1972.

263. Patel ME, Silver JW, Lipton DE, et al: Lipofibroma of the median nerve in the palm and digits of the hand. *J Bone Joint Surg* 61A:393, 1979.

264. Silverman TA, Enzinger FM: Fibrolipomatous hamartoma of nerve: a clinicopathologic analysis of 26 cases. *Am J Surg Pathol* 9:7, 1985.

Diffuse lipomatosis

265. Bannayan GA: Lipomatosis, angiomatosis and macrocephalia: a previously undescribed congenital syndrome. *Arch Pathol* 92:1, 1971.

266. Findlay GH, Duvenage M: Acquired symmetric lipomatosis of the hands: a distal form of Madelung-Launois-Bensaude syndrome. *Clin Exp Dermatol* 14:58, 1989.

267. Greiss ME, Williams DH: Macrodystrophia lipomatosis in the foot: a case report and review of the literature. *Arch Orthop Trauma Surg* 110:220, 1991.

268. Hoskins MC, Evans RA, King SJ, et al: "Sabre sheath" trachea with mediastinal lipomatosis mimicking a mediastinal tumor. *Clin Radiol* 44:417, 1991.

269. Karademir M, Kocak M, Usal A, et al: A case of infiltrating lipomatosis with diffuse, symmetrical distribution. *Br J Clin Pract* 44:728, 1990.

270. Kindblom L, Moller-Nielson J: Diffuse lipomatosis of the leg after poliomyelitis. *Acta Pathol Microbiol Scand* 83:339, 1975.

271. Kleine-Natrop HE, Bellmann G, Seebacher C: Riesenwuchs eines Fingers bei angeborenem Lipoma. *Hautarzt* 19:432, 1968.

272. Lewis D, Geschickter CF: Diffuse lipoma of the right upper extremity. *Ann Surg* 102:154, 1935.

273. Lippit DH, Johnston JR: Diffuse lipomatosis of a lower extremity: report of case. *Bull Ayer Clinic Pa Hosp* 4:55, 1954.

274. McCarthy DM, Dorr CA, Mackintosh CE: Unilateral localized giantism of the extremities with lipomatosis, arthropathy and psoriasis. *J Bone Joint Surg* 51B:348, 1969.

275. Nixon HH, Scobie WG: Congenital lipomatosis: a report of four cases. *J Pediatr Surg* 6:742, 1971.

276. Oosthuizen SF, Barnetson J: Two cases of lipomatosis involving bone. *Br J Radiol* 20:426, 1947.

277. Schlicht D: Recurrent lipoblastomatosis in a child. *Med J Austr* 2:959, 1965.

Symmetrical lipomatosis

278. Basse P, Lohmann M, Hovgard C, et al: Multiple symmetric lipomatosis: combined surgical treatment and liposuction: case report. *Scand J Plast Reconstr Surg Hand Surg* 26:111, 1992.

279. Berlit P, Krause KH, Herold S: Lipomatosis symmetrica benigna und neurologische Komplikationen bei chronischen Alkoholismus. *Nervenarzt* 53:168, 1982.

280. Chalk CH, Mills KR, Jacobs JM, et al: Familial multiple symmetric lipomatosis with peripheral neuropathy. *Neurology* 40:1246, 1990.

281. Enzi G: Multiple symmetrical lipomatosis: an updated clinical report. *Medicine (Baltimore)* 63:56, 1984.

282. Enzi G, Carraro R, Alfieri P, et al: Shoulder girdle lipomatosis. *Ann Intern Med* 117:749, 1992.

283. Kodish ME, Alsever RN, Block MB: Benign symmetric lipomatosis: functional sympathetic denervation of adipose tissue and possible hypertrophy of brown fat. *Metabolism* 23:937, 1974.

284. Launois PE, Bensaude R: De l'adenolipomatose symétrique. *Soc Med Hosp Paris Bull Mem* 15:298, 1889.

285. Madelung OW: Ueber den Fetthals. *Arch Klin Chir* 37:106, 1888.

286. Morelli JA: Laryngeal involvement in benign symmetrical lipomatosis. *Arch Otolaryngol* 97:495, 1973.

287. Mueller MM, Fuchs H, Schwarzmeier JD, et al: Zur Biochemie der benignen symmetrischen Lipomatose (Adenolipomatose Launois-Bensaude, Madelung'sche Krankheit). *Wien Klin Wochenschr* 88:94, 1976.

288. Ross M, Goodman MM: Multiple symmetric lipomatosis (Launois-Bensaude syndrome). *Int J Dermatol* 31:80, 1992.

289. Schuler FA III, Graham JK, Horton CHE: Benign symmetrical lipomatosis (Madelung's disease). *Plast Reconstr Surg* 57:662, 1976.

290. Taylor LM, Beahrs OH, Fontana RS: Benign symmetric lipomatosis. *Mayo Clin Proc* 36:96, 1961.

291. Whol MG, Pastor N: Adiposis dolorosa (Dercum's disease). *JAMA* 110:1261, 1938.

Pelvic lipomatosis

292. Baath L, Nyman V, Aspetin P, et al: Computed tomography of pelvic lipomatosis: report of a case. *Acta Radiol* 27:311, 1986.

293. Becker JA, Weiss RM, Schiff M Jr, et al: Pelvic lipomatosis: a consideration in the diagnosis of intrapelvic neoplasms. *Arch Surg* 100:94, 1970.

294. Boquist L, Bergdahl L, Andersson A: Lipomatosis of the ileocecal valve. *Cancer* 29:136, 1972.

295. Costa T, Fitch N, Azouz EM: Proteus syndrome: report of two cases with pelvic lipomatosis. *Pediatrics* 76:984, 1985.

296. Duffis AW, Weinberg B, Diakoumakis EE: A case of cystitis glandularis with associated pelvic lipomatosis: ultrasound evaluation. *J Clin Ultrasound* 18:733, 1990.

297. Engels EP: Sigmoid colon and urinary bladder in high fixation: Roentgen changes simulating pelvic tumor. *Radiology* 72:419, 1959.

298. Fogg LB, Smyth JW: Pelvic lipomatosis: a condition simulating pelvic neoplasm. *Radiology* 90:558, 1968.

299. Grimmett GM, Hall MG, Aird CC, et al: Pelvic lipomatosis. *Am J Surg* 125:347, 1973.

300. Heyns CF: Pelvic lipomatosis: a review of its diagnosis and management. *J Urol* 146:267, 1991.

301. Heyns CF, De Kock ML, Kirsten PH, et al: Pelvic lipomatosis associated with cystitis glandularis and adenocarcinoma of the bladder. *J Urol* 145:364, 1991.

302. Honda H, McGuire CW, Barloon TJ, et al: Replacement lipomatosis of the kidney: CT features. *J Comput Assist Tomogr* 14:229, 1990.

303. Honecke K, Butz M: Pelvic lipomatosis in a female: diagnosis and initial therapy. *Urol Int* 46:93, 1991.

304. Joshi KK, Wise HA: Pelvic lipomatosis: 9-year follow-up in a woman. *J Urol* 129:1233, 1983.

305. Klein FA, Vernon-Smith MJ, Kasenetz I: Pelvic lipomatosis: 35 year experience. *J Urol* 139:998, 1988.

306. Lucey DT, Smith MJV: Pelvic lipomatosis. *J Urol* 105:341, 1971.

307. Mahlin MS, Dovitz BW: Perivesical lipomatosis. *J Urol* 100:720, 1968.

308. Yalla SV, Ivker M, Burros HM, et al: Cystitis glandularis with perivesical lipomatosis: Frequent association of two unusual proliferative conditions. *Urology* 5:383, 1975.

Steroid lipomatosis

309. Butcher DL, Sahn SA: Epidural lipomatosis, a complication of corticosteroid therapy. *Ann Intern Med* 90:60, 1979.

310. Drasin GF, Lynch T, Temes GP: Ectopic ACTH production and mediastinal lipomatosis. *Radiology* 127:610, 1978.

311. Fessler RG, Johnson DL, Brown FD, et al: Epidural lipomatosis in steroid treated patients. *Spine* 17:183, 1992.

312. George WE Jr, Wilmot M, Greenhouse A, et al: Medical management of steroid-induced epidural lipomatosis. *N Engl J Med* 308:316, 1983.

313. Gilsanz V, Brill PW, Wolf BS: Increased retroperitoneal fat: a sign of corticosteroid therapy. *Radiology* 123:147, 1977.

314. Haddad SF, Hitchon PW, Godersky JC: Idiopathic and glucocorticoid induced spinal epidural lipomatosis. *Neurosurg* 75:839, 1991.

315. Kaplan JG, Barasch E, Hirschfeld A, et al: Spinal epidural lipomatosis: a serious complication of iatrogenic Cushing's syndrome. *Neurology* 39:1031, 1989.

316. Koerner JH, Sun DC: Mediastinal lipomatosis secondary to steroid therapy. *Am J Roentgenol* 98:461, 1966.

317. Lugena GE, Bennet WM, Pierre RV: "Dewlap," a corticosteroid induced episternal fatty tumor. *N Engl J Med* 275:834, 1966.

318. Nemec J, Zamrazil V, Lavickova E, et al: Pseudotumoröse Vermehrung des mediastinalen Fettgewebes beim Morbus Cushing. *Fortschr Roentgenstr* 118:106, 1973.

319. Noel P, Pepersack T, Vanbinst A, et al: Spinal epidural lipomatosis in Cushing's syndrome secondary to adrenal tumor. *Neurology* 42:1250, 1992.

320. Perling LH, Laurent JP, Cheek WR: Epidural hibernoma as a complication of corticosteroid treatment. *J Neurosurg* 69:613, 1988.

321. Roy-Camille R, Mazel C, Husson JL, et al: Symptomatic spinal epidural lipomatosis induced by a long-term steroid treatment: review of the literature and report of two additional cases. *Spine* 16:1365, 1991.

322. Shuman BM: Mediastinal lipomatosis complicating steroid therapy of regional enteritis. *Gastroenterology* 61:244, 1971.

323. Siskind BN, Weiner FR, Frank M, et al: Steroid induced mesenteric lipomatosis. *Comput Radiol* 8:175, 1984.

324. Streiter ML, Schneider HJ, Proto AV: Steroid induced thoracic lipomatosis: paraspinal involvement. *Am J Roentgenol* 139:679, 1982.

325. Teates CD: Steroid induced mediastinal lipomatosis. *Radiology* 96:501, 1970.

326. Van de Putte LBA, Wagenaar JPM: Pericardiac lipomatosis in exogenous Cushing syndrome. *Thorax* 28:653, 1973.

Nevus lipomatosus cutaneous superficialis

327. Bass HN, Caldwell S, Brooks BS: Michelin tire baby syndrome: familial constriction bands during infancy and early childhood in four generations. *Am J Med Genet* 45:370, 1993.

328. Burgdorf WH, Doran CK, Worret WI: Folded skin with scarring: Michelin tire baby syndrome? *J Am Acad Dermatol* 7:90, 1982.

329. Chanoki M, Sugamoto I, Suzuki S, et al: Nevus lipomatosus cutaneous superficialis of the scalp. *Cutis* 43:143, 1989.

330. Dotz W, Prioleau PG: Nevus lipomatosus cutaneous superficialis: a light and electron microscopic study. *Arch Dermatol* 120:376, 1984.

331. Gardner EW, Miller HM, Lowney ED: Deletion of chromosome 11 in babies with Michelin tire syndrome. *Arch Dermatol* 116:622, 1980.

332. Hendricks WM, Limber GK: Nevus lipomatosus cutaneous superficialis. *Cutis* 29:183, 1982.

333. Hoffman E, Zurhelle E: Ueber einen Naevus lipomatosus cutaneous superficialis der linken Glutaealgegend. *Arch Dermatol* 130:327, 1921.

334. Lynch FW, Goltz RW: Nevus lipomatosus cutaneous superficialis (Hoffman-Zurhelle): presentation of a case and review of the literature. *Arch Dermatol* 78:479, 1958.

335. Mehregan AH, Tovafoghi V, Ghandchi A: Nevus lipomatosus cutaneous superficialis (Hoffman-Zurhelle). *J Cutan Pathol* 2:307, 1975.

336. Pursley TV: Nevus lipomatosus cutaneous superficialis. *Int J Dermatol* 22:430, 1983.

337. Ross CM: Generalized folded skin with underlying lipomatous nevus: the Michelin tire baby. *Arch Dermatol* 106:766, 1972.

338. Schnur RE, Herzberg AJ, Spinner N, et al: Variability in the Michelin tire syndrome: a child with multiple anomalies, smooth muscle hamartoma, and familial paracentric inversion of chromosome 7q. *J Am Acad Dermatol* 28:364, 1993.

339. Wilson-Jones E, Marks R, Pongshirun D: Naevus superficialis lipomatosus. *Br J Dermatol* 93:121, 1975.

Hibernoma

340. Ahn C, Harvey JC: Mediastinal hibernoma, a rare tumor. *Ann Thorac Surg* 50:828, 1990.

341. Allegra SR, Gmuer C, O'Leary GP Jr: Endocrine activity in a large hibernoma. *Hum Pathol* 14:1044, 1983.

342. Angervall L, Björntrop P, Stener B: The lipid composition of hibernomas as compared with that of lipoma and mouse brown fat. *Cancer Res* 25:408, 1965.

343. Angervall L, Nilsson L, Stener B: Microangiographic and histologic studies in two cases of hibernoma. *Cancer* 17:685, 1964.

344. Beetstra A, Quast WH: Intrathoracic hibernoma. *Arch Chir Neurol* 10:203, 1958.

345. Bonnell MF: Tumeur du creux de l'aisselle. *Bull Soc Anat Paris* 89:110, 1914.

346. Brines OA, Johnson MH: Hibernoma: a special fatty tumor (report of a case). *Am J Pathol* 25:467, 1949.

347. Cox RW: "Hibernoma": the lipoma of immature adipose tissue. *J Pathol Bacteriol* 68:511, 1954.

348. Fentiman IS, Davies EE, Ramsay GS: Hibernoma of the thigh. *Clin Oncol* 1:71, 1975.

349. Fleishman JS, Schwartz RA: Hibernoma: ultrastructural observations. *J Surg Oncol* 23:285, 1983.

350. Gaffney EF, Hargreaves HK, Semple E, et al: Hibernoma: distinctive light and electron microscopic features and relationship to brown adipose tissue. *Hum Pathol* 14:677, 1983.

351. Gery L: Discussions. *Bull Mem Soc Anat (Paris)* 89:111, 1914.

352. Gould VE, Jao W, Gould NS, et al: Electron microscopy of adipose tissue tumors: comparative features of hibernomas, myxoid and pleomorphic liposarcomas. *Pathobiol Annu* 9:339, 1979.

353. Hertzanu Y, Mendelsohn DB, Louridas G: CT findings in hibernoma of the thigh. *J Comput Assist Tomogr* 7:1109, 1983.

354. Inglis K: So-called interscapular gland and tumours arising therein. *J Anat* 61:452, 1927.

355. Kindblom G, Angervall L, Stener B, et al: Intermuscular and intramuscular lipomas and hibernomas. *Cancer* 33:754, 1974.

356. Kittle CF, Boley JO, Schafer PW: Resection of an intrathoracic "hibernoma." *J Thorac Surg* 19:830, 1950.

357. Lawson W, Biller HF: Cervical hibernoma. *Laryngoscope* 86:1258, 1976.

358. Levine GD: Hibernoma: an electron microscopic study. *Hum Pathol* 3:351, 1972.

359. Marline AF, Pike RF: Hibernoma of the thigh: a case report. *J Bone Joint Surg* 55A:406, 1973.

360. McLane RC, Meyer LC: Axillary hibernoma: review of the literature with report of a case examined angiographically. *Radiology* 127:673, 1978.

361. Mesara BW, Batsakis JG: Hibernoma of the neck. *Arch Otolaryngol (Chicago)* 85:199, 1967.

362. Miller JR, Dockerty MB: Interscapular hibernoma: report of a case with a brief review of the literature. *Calif Med* 77:38, 1952.

363. Pachaly L, Schürmann R, Martinez A: Bericht über zwei sogenannte Hibernome, Tumoren des braunen Fettgewebes. *Zentralbl Allg Pathol* 105:370, 1964.

364. Peabody JW, Ziskind J, Buechner HA, et al: Intrathoracic hibernoma, third reported case. *N Engl J Med* 249:329, 1953.

365. Rigor VU, Goldstone SE, Jones J, et al: Hibernoma: a case report and discussion of a rare tumor. *Cancer* 57:2207, 1986.

366. Seemayer TA, Knaack J, Wang NS, et al: On the ultrastructure of hibernoma. *Cancer* 36:1785, 1975.

367. Sieber WK, Heller EL: Hibernoma: unusual location in popliteal space. *Am J Clin Pathol* 22:977, 1952.

CHAPTER 17

LIPOSARCOMA

Liposarcoma is one of the most common soft tissue sarcomas of adult life. This is indicated not only by the more than three thousand liposarcomas in the accumulated Armed Forces Institute of Pathology (AFIP) cases, but also by the reported data in the literature. Among soft tissue sarcomas its incidence ranges from 9.8%[29] to 16%.[100] Moreland and McNamara[85] noted an incidence of 0.056% among benign and malignant neoplasms of all types, and Kindblom et al.[64] reported an annual incidence of 2.5 per million in Sweden.

Besides its high incidence among sarcomas, liposarcoma is remarkable because of its frequent large size, which is probably unsurpassed among tumors in general, and its variable histological picture ranging from well-differentiated lipoma-like and myxoid tumors to extremely cellular or pleomorphic neoplasms. In its more differentiated forms it reflects with astounding accuracy different stages in the development of normal fat. In its less well differentiated forms it may mimic other forms of sarcomas, and in some of these tumors a reliable diagnosis may not be possible in the absence of lipoblasts.

The clinical behavior of liposarcoma closely reflects the variable microscopic appearance: the well-differentiated forms are of low-grade malignancy and rarely metastasize (atypical lipoma); the poorly differentiated ones are often highly aggressive in behavior; they tend to recur and produce metastases in a high percentage of cases. For this reason, determination of the histological subtype and degree of differentiation is of utmost importance for prognosis and selection of the proper therapy. Diagnosis of liposarcoma without further qualification as to the exact histological type is meaningless and provides no clear information as to the likely behavior of the tumor.

CLINICAL FINDINGS
Age and sex incidence

Liposarcoma is primarily a tumor of adult life with a peak incidence of between 40 and 60 years. It is virtually unknown in infants and small children, but there seems to be no upper age limit, and liposarcomas have been observed repeatedly in octogenarians. In a review of 1067 liposarcomas accessioned at the AFIP during a 10-year period, the youngest patient was 8 months and the oldest 87 years. The median age was 53 years (Fig. 17-1). Other reports closely correspond with these data: Reszel et al.[97] reported a mean age of 50.2 years and Orson et al.[89] a mean age of 52.9 years. The average age depends to some extent on the anatomical distribution of the tumor. Thus individuals with liposarcoma in the retroperitoneum are on the average 5 to 10 years older than those with tumors in the extremities, presumably because liposarcomas of the retroperitoneum are detected and treated at a later stage of the disease. This may also be partly responsible for the fact that well-differentiated and pleomorphic liposarcomas occur in slightly older patients than liposarcomas of the myxoid and round cell types.[33]

As with many other soft tissue sarcomas, men are affected more often (from 55%[33,64] to 61%[97]), with the exception of a slightly higher proportion of women in retroperitoneal liposarcoma. There is no evidence that liposarcoma has a predilection for any particular race or geographical region.

Liposarcomas in children

Although most liposarcomas occur in patients older than 15 years, occasional examples do occur in younger patients, especially those between 10 and 15 years of age. Liposarcoma in infants and children younger than 10 years, however, is extremely rare, and nearly all lipoblastic tumors in this age group are examples of benign lipoblastoma or lipoblastomatosis.[16,108] Yet there are several reports of liposarcoma in children[48,68]; we have encountered unequivocal examples in an 8-month-old boy with a massive tumor in the scapular region and a 3-year-old girl with a tumor of the knee. The former had a tumor of the round cell type and the latter of the myxoid type. It is remarkable that both of these patients were well more than 2 years after the initial diagnosis. In fact, the youngest patient in our series of 17 childhood liposarcomas who died of the disease was an 11-year-old boy with myxoid liposarcoma of the right ax-

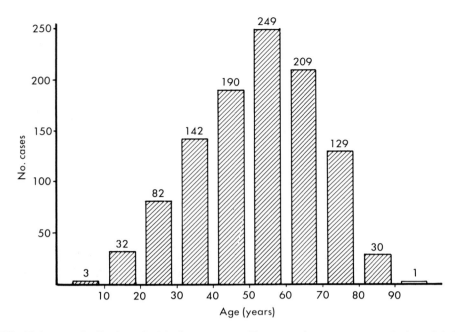

FIG. 17-1. Age distribution of 1067 liposarcomas. The tumor is most common during adult life and is rare in children, especially in those under 10 years of age.

illa that was treated by local excision and postoperative radiotherapy.[108] Many of the reported cases are poorly illustrated and difficult to evaluate.[59,70,92] Castleberry et al.[16] reviewed in 1984 the reported childhood liposarcomas.

Localization

Liposarcoma takes its origin from primitive mesenchymal cells rather than mature fat cells, and the presence of adipocytes is by no means a prerequisite for its development. In fact, liposarcomas are rare in the subcutaneous fat and the submucosa and subserosa of the intestinal tract, the two most common locations of lipoma; they are almost always encountered in deeper structures and often seem to arise from intermuscular fascial planes or similar deep-seated and richly vascular structures. Lipomas and lipomatoses do not seem to predispose to the development of liposarcoma.

The two major sites of liposarcoma are the extremities, particularly the thigh[30,54,94,111] and the retroperitoneum.* Other somewhat less common sites are the regions of the spermatic cord and scrotum (paratesticular liposarcoma),† chest wall and breast,[14,40,53,84] mediastinum,[57,81,95,128] omentum, and mesentery.[83,98,132] Liposarcomas in the breast may arise as primary tumors or in cystosarcoma phyllodes (Table 17-1).[6] Liposarcomas are least common in the head and neck, including the oral cavity, larynx, and orbit

*References 2, 25, 66, 67, 80, 122.
†References 11, 21, 22, 26, 52, 76, 79.

(Fig. 17-2),* the small and large intestines,[91] and the hands and feet.[103]

Most reports in the literature agree as to the prevalent sites of liposarcoma. The lower limb is the most common site in the series of Pack and Pierson (62%)[90] and Spittle et

*References 4, 55, 63, 73, 78, 102, 123.

Table 17-1. Anatomical locations of liposarcoma (AFIP, 1067 cases)

Anatomical location	No. cases	Percent
Head-neck	60	5.6
Neck (36), face (13)		
Scalp (4)		
Trunk	452	42.4
Retroperitoneum (198)		
Inguinal region (130)		
Back (29), chest (29)		
Upper extremities	113	10.6
Shoulder-axilla (44)		
Upper arm (44), forearm (19)		
Lower extremities	442	41.4
Thigh-knee (321)		
Buttock (62)		
Lower leg (49)		
TOTAL	1067	100.0

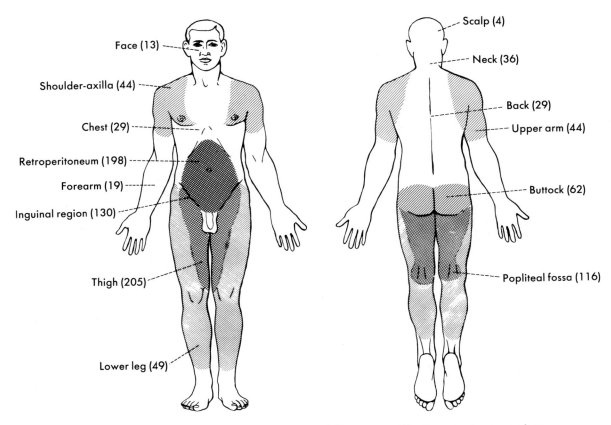

FIG. 17-2. Anatomical distribution of 1067 cases of liposarcoma. The three most common locations are the thigh, the retroperitoneum, and the inguinal region. Liposarcoma is rare in the hands and feet.

al. (68%)[111] Similarly, Reszel et al.[97] report that 123 (55%) of 222 liposarcomas of the extremities were located in the thigh. These tumors are usually deep seated and are found mainly in the quadriceps muscle and the popliteal fossa. For unknown reasons, the right side tends to be more commonly involved than the left.[33,111]

The *retroperitoneum* is the second most common site, with approximately 15% to 20% of liposarcomas. In this location they are usually larger than those in the thigh and sometimes may reach a very large size. When occurring in the renal region, they push the kidney forward and medially, or deflect and compress the ureter. In the pelvic region they occasionally extend through the inguinal canal or obturator foramen into the thigh or along the pararectal tissues into the perianal region. In fact, one of the latter tumors in our cases was clinically mistaken for hemorrhoids. Liposarcomas in the *spermatic and paratesticular region,* another common site, usually are well differentiated or myxoid tumors of long duration that may present as an inguinal or scrotal mass and be mistaken initially for an inguinal hernia or hydrocele.[79]

Clinical complaints

There is nothing characteristic about the clinical history. Nearly always the first manifestation of the disease is an insidiously growing, deep-seated, ill-defined mass that has usually reached a large size when the patient seeks treatment. Pain, tenderness, or functional disturbances occur in about 10% to 15% of cases, but these are usually late complaints associated with large tumors. Likewise, weight loss and emaciation are features that become evident late in the course of the disease; these signs occur despite the presence of large bulky tumors containing considerable amounts of lipid material. As with lipomas, the fat stored in liposarcomas is largely unavailable for the general metabolism.

Liposarcomas in the retroperitoneum are usually slow to be recognized. They cause gradual and diffuse abdominal enlargement, weight loss, or abdominal pain and sometimes, as the result of increased intraabdominal pressure, are associated with inguinal or femoral hernias or pitting edema in one or both lower extremities. Massive ascites is rare. Involvement of the intestinal tract may cause anorexia, vomiting, constipation, diarrhea, or painful defecation. Displacement and compression of the kidney or ureter, much more common events, may lead to hydronephrosis, pyelonephritis, and uremia. Evaluation of renal function is, therefore, mandatory with any primary or recurrent liposarcoma of the retroperitoneum. Pyrexia is seen occasionally and almost always is the result of kidney infection or tumor necrosis.

Data as to the clinical duration are often unreliable because of the silent growth and deep location of many liposarcomas. In the average case, however, the patient has been aware of an enlarging mass or swelling for several months; occasional examples of well-differentiated "lipoma-like" liposarcomas have been known to be present for 20 or more years. Several such examples are in our series as well as in the literature.[30,33]

Role of trauma

As with most soft tissue sarcomas, the significance of trauma for the development of liposarcoma is difficult to assess, particularly in view of the frequency with which bruises and minor trauma are sustained regularly by patients of all ages. More importantly, a definite history of trauma to the exact site of the tumor is extremely rare, and most investigators deny or are doubtful as to the existence of such a relationship.[97,117] Yet there are isolated cases in which such a possibility cannot be dismissed entirely. In most of these, trauma and a hematoma precede the onset of the tumor by about 1 year. For example, in one of our cases, a 33-year-old man developed a hematoma of the thigh after he hit his leg on a frame in a mill. Sixteen months later a myxoid liposarcoma was removed from the site of injury. Another patient, a 61-year-old man, stuck a butcher knife deep into his right lower leg. Following evacuation of a large hematoma, the patient was well for 1 year when a myxoid liposarcoma was diagnosed at the same site. Still another patient was injured by the fall of a boiler-stack. Twelve months later a nodule became apparent at the site of injury; on biopsy, it was diagnosed as a liposarcoma. There are further cases in our material and the literature in which a liposarcoma developed at the exact site of trauma.[33,90,124,138]

Postradiation liposarcoma is also extremely rare. There is only one such case in our series. It occurred in a 13-year-old girl who developed a liposarcoma in the left peri-

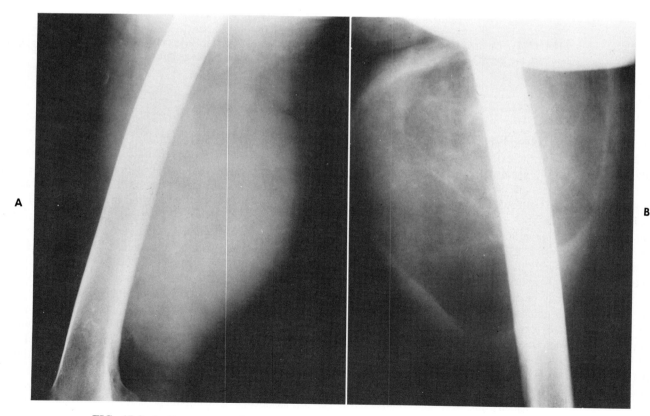

FIG. 17-3. A, Roentgenograph of a myxoid liposarcoma of the right posterior thigh. Note large size and marked radiopacity of the tumor. **B,** Well-differentiated, lipoma-like liposarcoma recognizable by its markedly reduced radiodensity compared with the surrounding soft tissues.

orbital and temporal region 12 years after radiation for ret-inoblastoma. There are also reports of liposarcomas that developed in the region of prior radiation for carcinoma of the mouth and carcinoma of the breast, respectively.[5,30] Conversely, Hodgkin's disease developed in one of our patients 8 years after radiotherapy (5000 rad) for a retroperitoneal liposarcoma.

Liposarcoma arising in preexisting lipoma

Liposarcoma arising in a preexisting lipoma is extremely rare. In fact, we have never encountered such a case, and there are only a few possible cases in the literature.[77,85,104,138] In their assessment it is well to keep in mind the structural variability of some liposarcomas, particularly the occasional coexistence of well-differentiated and poorly differentiated areas in the same tumor (dedifferentiated liposarcoma). Moreover, morphological variants of benign lipomas may demonstrate focal myxoid, spindle cell, and pleomorphic areas that are likely to be mistaken for an incipient sarcoma, especially when these changes coincide with a sudden spurt of growth. Yet there are some reports of well-circumscribed, subcutaneous liposarcoma that may have arisen in a lipoma.[101,116] Furthermore, there are rare cases in which a liposarcoma is associated with one or more lipomas occurring at other sites (see Fig. 17-10).[9] It is conceivable that some of these have arisen in a preexisting lipoma.[114,127]

RADIOGRAPHIC FINDINGS

The radiographic features of liposarcoma differ considerably and largely depend on the histological type and composition of the tumor: well-differentiated liposarcomas, like normal fat or lipoma, show a well-delineated radiolucency that can be clearly distinguished from the surrounding muscle tissue (Fig. 17-3). Myxoid, round cell, and pleomorphic liposarcomas, on the other hand, are usually less well defined and may stand out from normal tissues by their greater density (Fig. 17-4). Mixed types are common. If these contain well-differentiated portions, they can be positively identified by the coexistence of increased and decreased radiopacities. These changes, of course, are more readily apparent in x-ray films of the extremities than in those of the retroperitoneum. There are also occasional cases with radiopaque foci caused by calcification and ossification, especially in well-differentiated liposarcomas.

Angiographically, the degree of vascularity is directly related to the degree of radiopacity. Thus radiolucent tumors (e.g., well-differentiated liposarcomas) show relatively little vascularity, whereas the radiopaque myxoid, round cell, and pleomorphic forms are richly vascular (Fig. 17-5). CT scans and MRI have largely replaced angiograms in pinpointing the exact location, size, anatomical relationship, and density of the primary tumor and in planning effective surgical management (Fig. 17-6). They are also most valuable for the early detection of recurrent neoplasms, especially when the tumor is located in the retroperito-

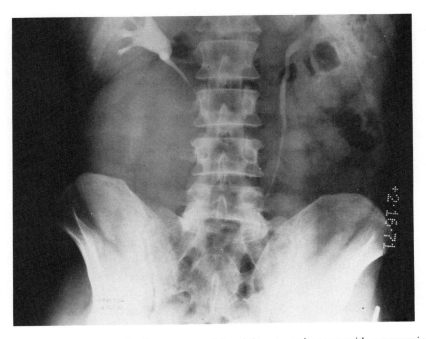

FIG. 17-4. Roentgenograph of a liposarcoma of the right retroperitoneum with compression and marked deviation of the right ureter.

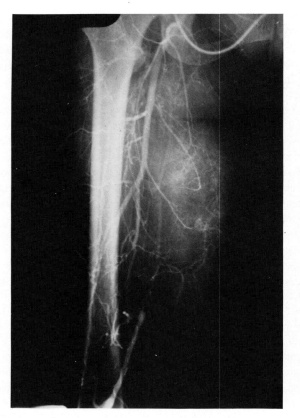

FIG. 17-5. Angiograph of well-differentiated sclerosing liposarcoma of the right thigh.

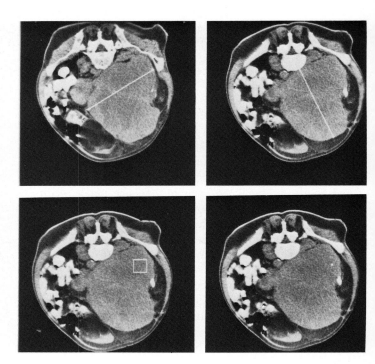

FIG. 17-6. CT scan of large retroperitoneal liposarcoma with displacement of intestines.

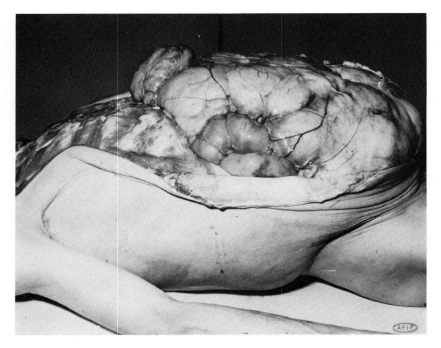

FIG. 17-7. Myxoid liposarcoma of enormous size arising in the retroperitoneum and filling the entire abdominal cavity. The tumor measured 39 cm in greatest diameter.

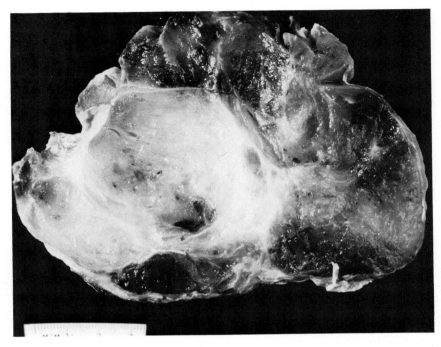

FIG. 17-8. Myxoid liposarcoma markedly distorted by areas of hemorrhage and fibrosis.

neum.[24,41,56,75,118] Juxtaposition of a well-differentiated lipomatous tumor and a nonlipomatous mass of tissue of nonspecific appearance may suggest a dedifferentiated liposarcoma[69] (see Chapter 3).

GROSS FINDINGS

Although most liposarcomas measure between 5 and 10 cm in greatest diameter, some reach a very large size, and examples measuring 15 cm or more in diameter are not particularly rare. Usually the largest examples are found in the retroperitoneum. One of these cases in the literature weighed 63 lb[132]; another among our cases measured 39 cm in greatest diameter and extended from the diaphragm to the pelvis (Fig. 17-7). There are also several examples of liposarcoma in the literature that weighed in excess of 50 lb. In fact, the retroperitoneal liposarcoma reported by Delamater[23] in the *Cleveland Medical Gazette* of 1859— probably unequalled by any reported neoplasm—is alleged to have weighed close to 200 lb at the time of the patient's death.

Liposarcomas tend to be well circumscribed or encapsulated and usually show a distinct lobulated pattern (Figs. 17-8 and 17-9). Not infrequently small lobules become separated from the main tumor mass and form satellite nodules, an important fact that must be kept in mind during surgical removal of the tumor. On section the appearance of the tumor varies considerably, depending on the histological type, including the relative amounts of mucinous

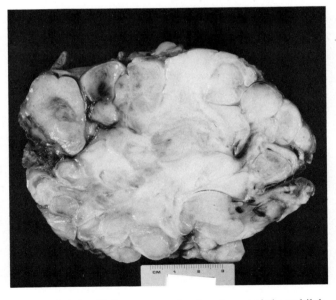

FIG. 17-9. Myxoid liposarcoma showing characteristic multilobular pattern.

and lipid material and the extent of fibrosis. Many have a myxoid or gelatinous appearance (Figs. 17-9 and 17-10), often with foci of hemorrhage (Fig. 17-8). Those with greater amounts of lipid material have a firmer consistency and are pale yellow to bright orange in color. Still others

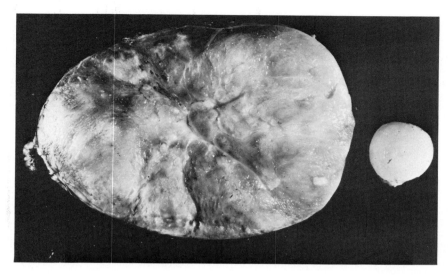

FIG. 17-10. Myxoid liposarcoma of the retroperitoneum and lipoma removed from another site in the same patient.

are white or gray-white as a result of extensive fibrosis. Less well-differentiated liposarcomas often display a brain-like quality and are distorted by areas of necrosis, hemorrhage, and cyst formation. Cartilage or bone is seen occasionally but, when it occurs, is more conspicuous in the microscopic preparations than in the gross specimen.

MICROSCOPIC FINDINGS
Histological classification

The classification of liposarcoma is greatly facilitated by its fairly uniform cellular picture, which generally varies little from tumor to tumor and even from primary tumor to recurrence and metastasis. Considerable changes in the histological picture, however, do occur in some instances during the course of the disease[110]; therefore careful sampling is mandatory in each case, because the degree of differentiation is still the most reliable yardstick in the prediction of clinical behavior and selection of the mode of therapy.

Over the years there have been many attempts at classi-

fication, all reflecting a combination of two basic histological aspects of the tumor: (1) the stage in the development of lipoblasts, judged by the relative amounts of lipid in the cells and mucinous material in the extracellular spaces; and (2) the overall degree of cellularity and cellular pleomorphism. None of the proposed classifications is all-inclusive or fully satisfactory. At the AFIP we have used a simplified classification that divides liposarcoma into five basic histological categories: (1) myxoid liposarcoma, (2) round cell liposarcoma, (3) well-differentiated liposarcoma (including atypical lipoma), (4) dedifferentiated liposarcoma, and (5) pleomorphic liposarcoma (see the accompanying box). About half of cases are of the myxoid type, followed in frequency by well-differentiated, dedifferentiated, round cell, and pleomorphic liposarcomas. In addition, there are mixed forms in about 5% to 10% of cases that display a combination of two or more histological types. The term *atypical lipoma* applies to well-differentiated forms of lipoma-like or sclerosing liposarcomas occurring in the subcutis.[7,13,35,37,62]

Myxoid liposarcoma

This is by far the most common type, accounting for 45% to 55% of all liposarcomas. As in fetal fat, the tumor is composed of three main tissue components: (1) proliferating lipoblasts in varying stages of differentiation, (2) a delicate plexiform capillary pattern, and (3) a myxoid matrix containing abundant nonsulfated glycosaminoglycans. These three components form an intimate relationship, with minor variations from tumor to tumor (Figs. 17-11 to 17-14).

In the most primitive form of myxoid liposarcoma, most of the proliferated cells cannot be clearly distinguished from primitive mesenchymal cells; in fact, such tumors have

---

Histological classification of liposarcoma

Well-differentiated liposarcoma
Lipoma-like
Inflammatory
Sclerosing

Myxoid liposarcoma
Round cell liposarcoma
Dedifferentiated liposarcoma
Pleomorphic liposarcoma

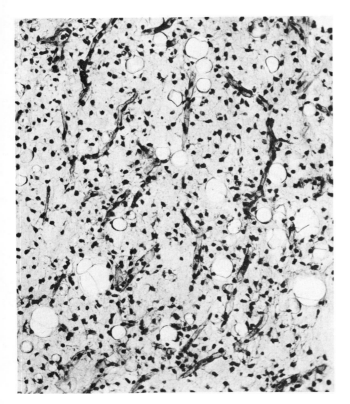

FIG. 17-11. Myxoid liposarcoma, consisting of lipoblasts in varying stages of differentiation, a prominent plexiform capillary pattern, and an abundance of myxoid material between vessels and tumor cells. (×250.)

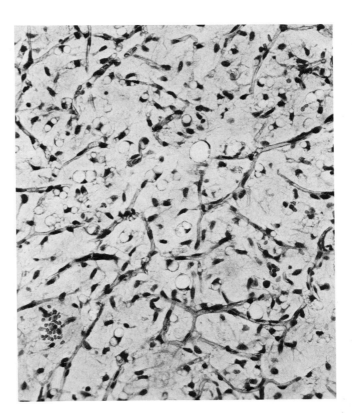

FIG. 17-12. Myxoid liposarcoma showing the close association between capillaries and differentiating lipoblasts having a "signet-ring" appearance. Note the uniform caliber of the vascular channels. (×250.)

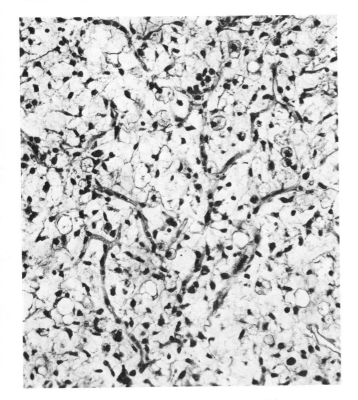

FIG. 17-13. Myxoid liposarcoma. Some of the lipoblasts are granular or multivacuolated and resemble the cells of brown fat.

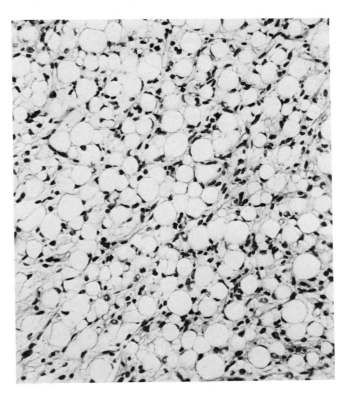

FIG. 17-14. Myxoid liposarcoma showing a considerable degree of cellular differentiation, with numerous lipoblasts, an indistinct vascular pattern, and only small amounts of intercellular mucoid material. (×250.)

been reported as malignant mesenchymoma (Fig. 17-15).[38,46] In the majority of cases, however, scattered lipoblasts, usually of the small "signet-ring" type, can be identified, especially at the margin of the tumor lobules (Fig. 17-16). With increasing lipid deposition, the multivacuolar lipoblasts turn into univacuolar or "signet-ring" cells closely resembling adult fat cells. If these changes are rather uniform, the problem of distinguishing myxoid from well-differentiated liposarcoma may arise (Fig. 17-14). Not infrequently there are interspersed spindle cells (Fig. 17-17) or small granular cells that recall the cellular appearance of brown fat (Fig. 17-18). Multinucleated lipoblasts or giant cells may be present, but are never as numerous as in pleomorphic liposarcoma. The paucity or complete absence of mitotic figures contrasts with the rapid growth of myxoid liposarcoma.

A maze of branching narrow thin-walled vessels of uniform size and caliber (5 to 15 μm in diameter) is one of the most distinct microscopic features (see Figs. 17-11 and 17-12). As a rule, the rich plexiform vascular network is most prominent in those tumors in which the cells retain their primitive character. It is less apparent in tumors that contain a large number of more differentiated lipoblasts. Occasionally, foci of telangiectatic vessels may closely imitate the pattern of hemangioma (Fig. 17-19). Tumors containing few lipoblasts and having a poorly developed vascular pattern may be mistaken for myxomas or myxosarcomas. The microangiographic features of these tumors were described and illustrated by Kindblom et al.[64]

The amount and distribution of the characteristic mucoid material vary; it is present primarily in extracellular compartments but also may be found within individual tumor cells. Frequently the extracellular mucoid material forms large pools, often creating a cribriform or lacelike pattern in the tumor (Fig. 17-20). The cellular condensation at the rim of these pools sometimes produces a pseudoacinar pattern (Fig. 17-21); in others the weak staining of the accumulated mucinous material and the endothelium-like arrangement of the surrounding tumor cells mimics a cystic lymphangioma or lymphangiosarcoma. Interstitial hemorrhage is common and may be so prominent that the tumor is confused with a vascular neoplasm or hematoma.

A peculiar subtype of myxoid liposarcoma consists almost entirely of loosely arranged fibroblast-like spindle cells oriented along a single plane and surrounded by a reticulin meshwork of varying density (Figs. 17-22 and 17-23). The uniformity of the spindle cells distinguishes this tumor from the more irregularly shaped and distributed cells of well-differentiated sclerosing liposarcoma.

Focal cartilaginous, leiomyomatous, or, very rarely, osseous metaplasia occurs in myxoid (and well-differentiated) liposarcoma, but these changes do not seem to alter significantly the clinical behavior. Therefore separate classification of these tumors as malignant mesenchymomas seems to be unwarranted.[36,119] Leiomyosarcomatous and rhabdomyosarcomatous components, alone and combined, have also been described in dedifferentiated liposarcomas.[121]

As in most liposarcomas, there is a lobular pattern, and

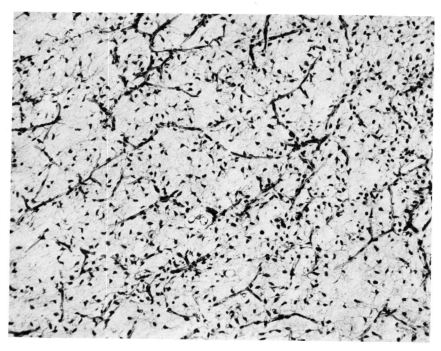

FIG. 17-15. Myxoid liposarcoma with only a few scattered lipoblasts but a typical vascular and myxoid pattern. Tumors of this type have been interpreted as malignant mesenchymoma. (×120.)

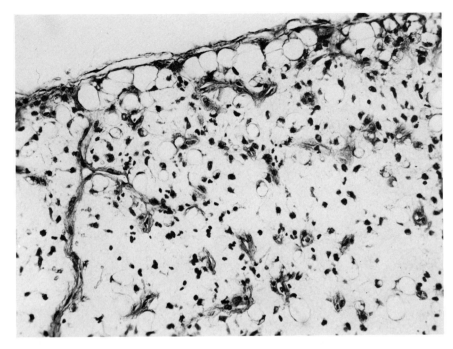

FIG. 17-16. Myxoid liposarcoma showing characteristic lipoblastic differentiation at the periphery. (× 250.)

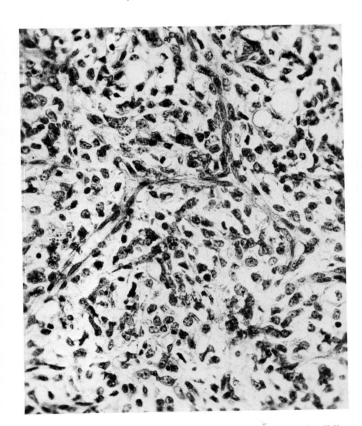

FIG. 17-17. Transitional form between myxoid and round cell liposarcoma consisting of numerous undifferentiated tumor cells in addition to scattered univacuolar lipoblasts. (×305.)

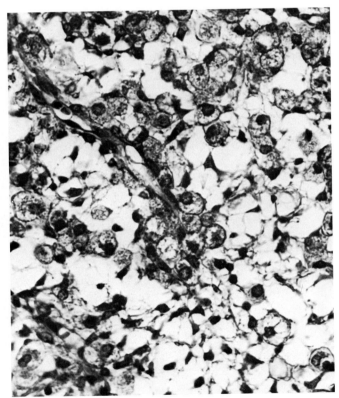

FIG. 17-18. Transitional form between myxoid and round cell liposarcoma with numerous rounded granular cells resembling brown fat. (×550.)

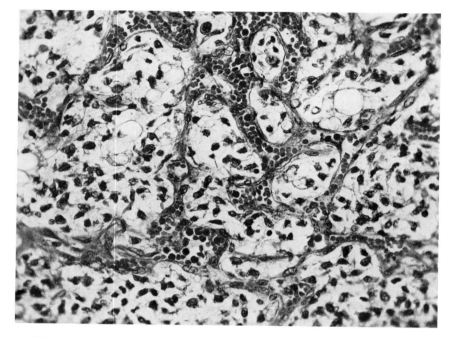

FIG. 17-19. Hemangioma-like vascular pattern in myxoid liposarcoma. (×305.)

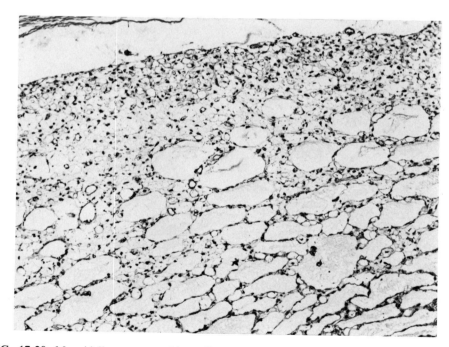

FIG. 17-20. Myxoid liposarcoma with pooling of myxoid material resulting in a cribriform or lacelike pattern. (×60.)

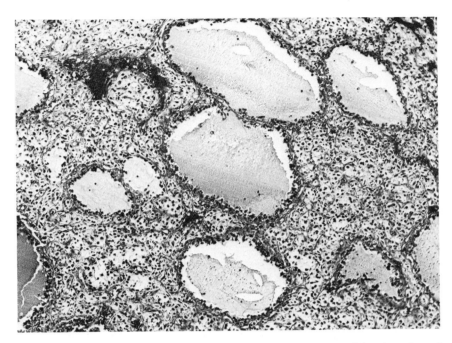

FIG. 17-21. Myxoid liposarcoma with focal pooling of the myxoid material and condensation of the tumor cells along the mucoid pools. (×75.)

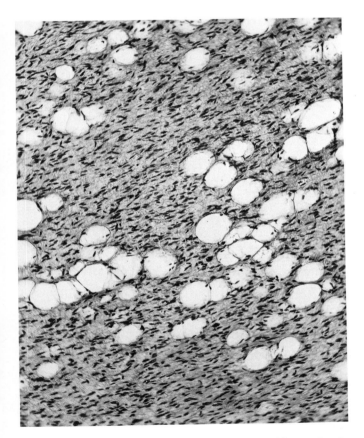

FIG. 17-22. Myxoid (spindle cell) liposarcoma with prominent spindling of the tumor cells and indistinct vascular pattern. (×80.)

the individual tumor lobules are enveloped by a thin fibrous membrane. As mentioned, this circumscription or encapsulation of the tumor and its lobules is more apparent than real, and not infrequently satellite or daughter nodules are sequestered in the vicinity of the main tumor mass (Figs. 17-24 and 17-25).

Round cell liposarcoma (poorly differentiated myxoid liposarcoma)

Although this type is closely related to myxoid liposarcoma and actually represents its poorly differentiated form, it deserves separate consideration because of its aggressive clinical course and its tendency to metastasize.

The main characteristic of this relatively rare tumor is an excessive proliferation of small, uniformly shaped, rounded cells with vesicular nuclei vaguely reminiscent of Ewing's sarcoma, malignant lymphoma, or some other small cell sarcoma. Intracellular lipid formation is rare, and there is little intercellular mucoid matrix. The vascular network is obscured by the vast number of proliferated tumor cells and is much less prominent than in the myxoid form (Figs. 17-26 to 17-29). Although in most cases the cells show no particular arrangement, they occasionally form branching cords and rows along abortive capillaries, resulting in a trabecular or adenoid pattern (Figs. 17-30 and 17-31). Transitions toward the myxoid type are common, and often constitute the only reliable diagnostic feature (see Figs. 17-17 and 17-18). There are also rare cases in which the primary tumor displays the features of myxoid liposar-

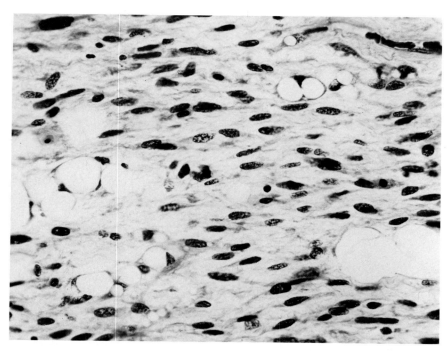

FIG. 17-23. Liposarcoma with prominent spindling and scattered lipoblasts. The presence of lipoblasts and variably sized spindle cells with hyperchromatic nuclei helps to distinguish this lesion from a spindle cell lipoma. (×250.)

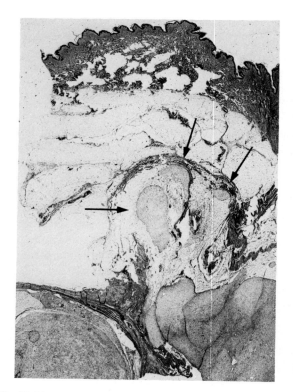

FIG. 17-24. Myxoid liposarcoma showing nests of tumor cells outside the main tumor mass *(arrows)*, a feature that emphasizes the need for wide local excision. (×45.)

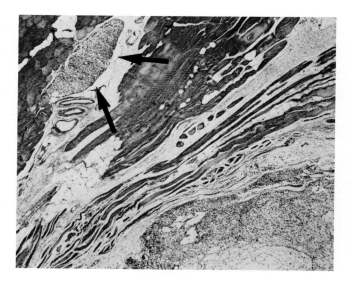

FIG. 17-25. Myxoid liposarcoma. Small nest of tumor cells *(arrows)* at some distance from the main tumor. (×25.)

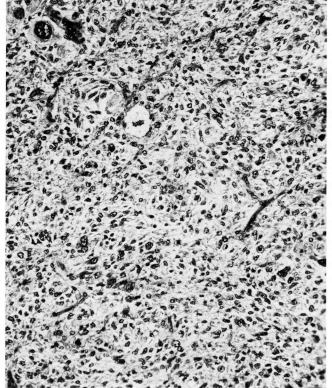

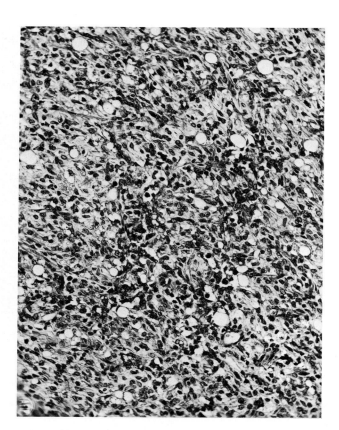

FIG. 17-26. Round cell liposarcoma with a single multivacuolated lipoblast and occasional cells with hyperchromatic muclei. (×165.)

FIG. 17-27. Round cell liposarcoma. The vascular pattern is obscured by the cellular proliferation, and there is only a scattering of lipoblasts identifying the tumor as a liposarcoma. (×160.)

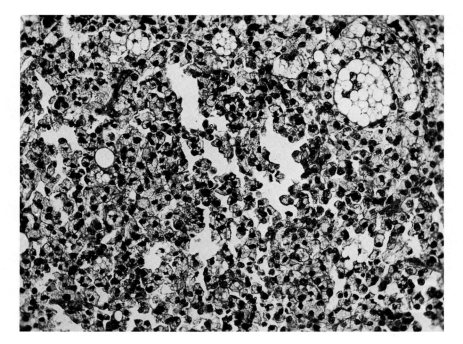

FIG. 17-28. Round cell liposarcoma with finely vacuolated or granular tumor cells resembling the cells of brown fat. Similar tumors have been interpreted as malignant hibernomas. (×180.)

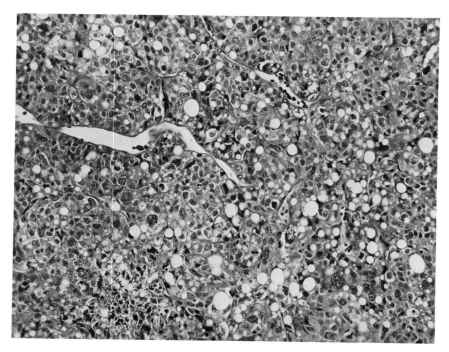

FIG. 17-29. Round cell liposarcoma with large epithelial-like tumor cells and an indistinct pericytoma pattern. (×250.)

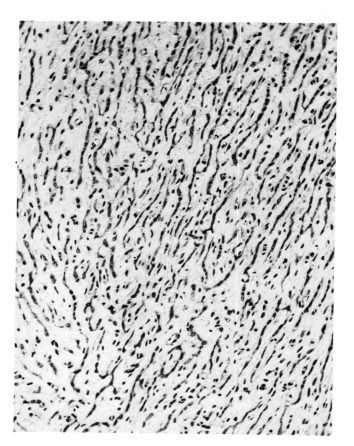

FIG. 17-30. Variant of round cell liposarcoma with cording of the undifferentiated tumor cells. (×180.)

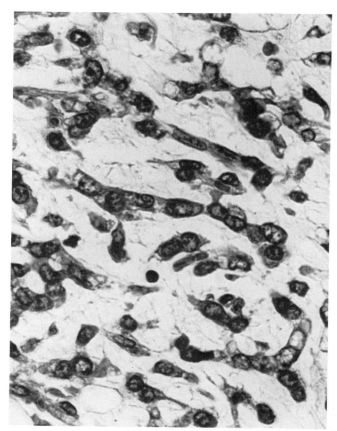

FIG. 17-31. Variant of round cell liposarcoma with branching cellular cords similar to those seen in Fig. 17-30. (×400.)

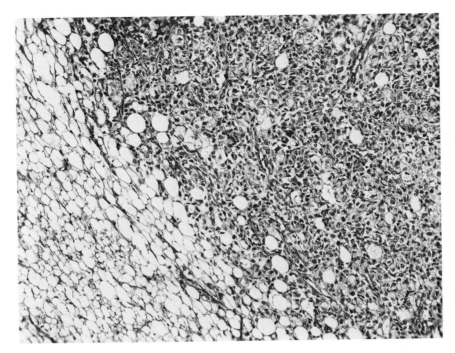

FIG. 17-32. Well-differentiated and round cell liposarcoma in different portions of the same tumor (mixed-type liposarcoma). (×100.)

coma and the round cell pattern is evident only in the recurrence or metastasis. Transitions toward the well-differentiated type are rare, however (Fig. 17-32). As in the myxoid form, mitotic figures are uncommon even in the most cellular examples of this tumor. There are also occasional variants of liposarcoma that are composed of large round cells with eosinophilic granular or multivacuolar cytoplasm intermediate between round cell liposarcoma and malignant hibernoma, a differential diagnosis that can only be resolved by examination with the electron microscope (see Fig. 17-28).

Well-differentiated liposarcoma

Histologically, three closely related subtypes of the well-differentiated liposarcoma can be distinguished: (1) well-differentiated "lipoma-like" liposarcoma, (2) well-differentiated inflammatory liposarcoma, and (3) well-differentiated sclerosing liposarcoma. Because well-differentiated liposarcomas are intrinsically tumors of low-grade malignancy that recur but do not metastasize, the terms *atypical lipoma* and *atypical intramuscular lipoma* have been introduced for the subcutaneous and muscular forms of well-differentiated liposarcoma.[7,37,62]

The *lipoma-like type of well-differentiated liposarcoma* is the most common form of this group. It closely simulates lipoma except for a scattering of lipoblasts with atypical, irregularly shaped, hyperchromatic nuclei and one or more lipid droplets in their cytoplasm. Small scattered nests of multivacuolated cells are another common feature. Frequently, the atypical cells or vacuolated lipoblasts are admixed with fibroblast-like spindle cells that are situated within narrow fibrous bands or septa surrounding irregularly sized lobules of fat. The associated lipoma-like areas consist of adult fat cells, often showing a slightly greater variation in size and shape than those of normal fat (Figs. 17-33 to 17-35). Rarely, there are irregular multinucleated giant cells indistinguishable from the "floret cells" of pleomorphic lipoma.

The *inflammatory type* is much less common than the lipoma-like type. It occurs mostly in the retroperitoneum and is marked by scattered lipoblasts or cells with one or more hyperchromatic nuclei and an inflammatory infiltrate consisting of a variable number of lymphocytes and plasma cells within a background of mature-appearing fat cells. Since lipoblasts and cells with atypical nuclei are often rare in this tumor, this type of liposarcoma is apt to be confused with lipoma or a lipogranulomatous process (Fig. 17-36).

The *sclerosing type* prevails in the groin and retroperitoneum, but may also be found in muscle and other deep tissues of the extremities. It consists of scattered atypical cells with hyperchromatic nuclei and occasional lipoblasts within a matrix in which lipomatous portions alternate with areas of dense fibrosis consisting of a meshwork of delicate eosinophilic collagen fibrils of varying density. Purely lipoma-

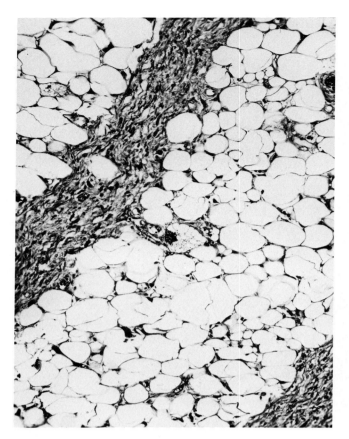

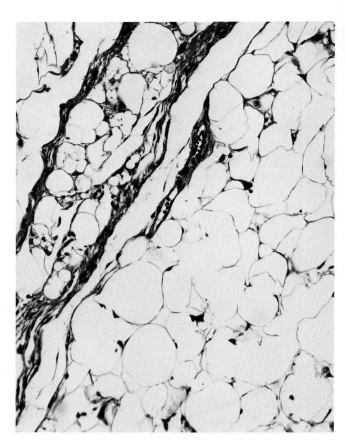

FIG. 17-33. Well-differentiated liposarcoma (atypical lipoma) of the anterior chest wall in a 66-year-old, composed of occasional lipoblasts and broad fibrous septa containing cells with atypical hyperchromatic nuclei—a characteristic feature of this tumor. (×160.)

FIG. 17-34. Well-differentiated liposarcoma (atypical lipoma). Note the slight variation in the size and shape of the fat cells and the aggregate of multivacuolar lipoblasts. (×160.)

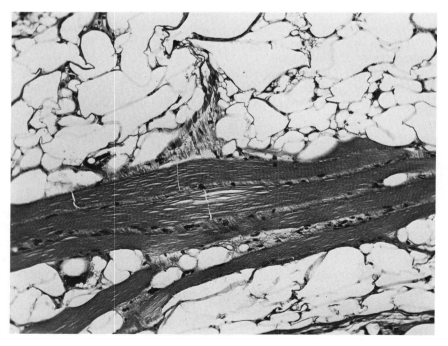

FIG. 17-35. Well-differentiated liposarcoma in the muscle of the left thigh. These tumors tend to infiltrate and replace striated muscle in a more irregular fashion than intramuscular lipoma. (×130.)

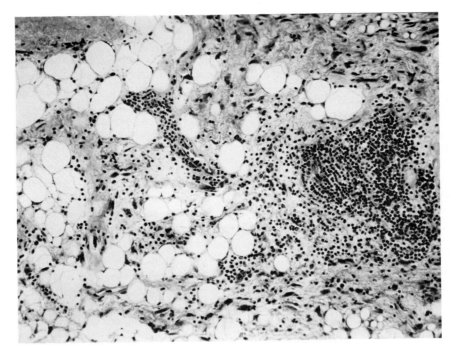

FIG. 17-36. Inflammatory type of well-differentiated liposarcoma of the retroperitoneum of a 61-year-old man. This neoplasm has been confused with an inflammatory process. (×160.)

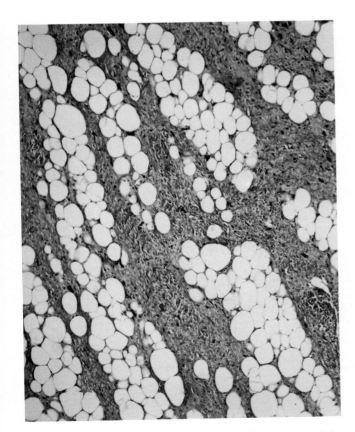

FIG. 17-37. Well-differentiated sclerosing liposarcoma of the right arm in a 75-year-old man. Note broad fibrous septa containing cells with atypical, hyperchromatic nuclei. (×100.)

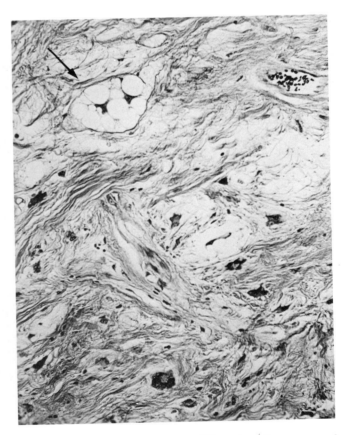

FIG. 17-38. Sclerosing type of well-differentiated liposarcoma of the retroperitoneum. Like other forms of well-differentiated liposarcoma, this tumor rarely metastasizes, but it may recur and cause complications by its large size. (×160.)

like and sclerosing areas may also be found in different portions of the same tumor (Figs. 17-37 and 17-38).

Atypical lipoma and well-differentiated liposarcoma

Well-differentiated liposarcomas have long been recognized as tumors of very low grade malignancy.[30,33] When located in the subcutis they rarely recur and are usually cured by local excision. When located in deep soft tissues, such as muscle of the extremities, retroperitoneum, and groin they may recur but never develop metastases. For these reasons, and in order to spare the patient a diagnosis of malignancy and unnecessary radical therapy, Kindblom et al.[62] and Evans et al.[37] proposed the term *atypical lipoma* for all tumors formerly classified as well-differentiated liposarcomas, with the exception of those occurring in the retroperitoneum. More recently, however, Evans,[35] on the basis of a 10-year follow-up study, suggested that the noncommittal term *atypical lipomatous tumor* be used in place of *atypical lipoma*.

Judging from our material, *atypical lipoma* is an appropriate and useful term, but this diagnosis should be made with caution, and only after careful sampling of the lesion in tumors of large size. In fact, it seems best to restrict its use to the subcutaneous form of this tumor, especially to those of small size with minimal atypical changes, and to retain the term *well-differentiated liposarcoma* for all well-differentiated liposarcomas that arise in deep soft tissues, including the musculature of the extremities, the groin, and the retroperitoneum. This approach is favored because of the potential of the deep-seated tumors to recur and, less commonly, to undergo dedifferentiation, often after persisting for many years. This is clearly evident from the studies of Weiss and Rao,[135] who noted not only recurrence in 43.5% (20 of 46) of well-differentiated liposarcomas in the muscles of the extremities and in 78.6% (11 of 14) of those in the groin, but also late dedifferentiation in three tumors arising in skeletal muscle and in four involving the groin. Likewise, dedifferentiation of highly differentiated liposarcomas in the muscles of the extremities was reported by Brooks and Connor[15] and others.[35,106] Therefore complete excision with small margins of surrounding tissues may be adequate for the subcutaneous tumors (atypical lipomas), but a wider surgical margin is required for the treatment of well-differentiated liposarcomas occurring in deep soft tis-

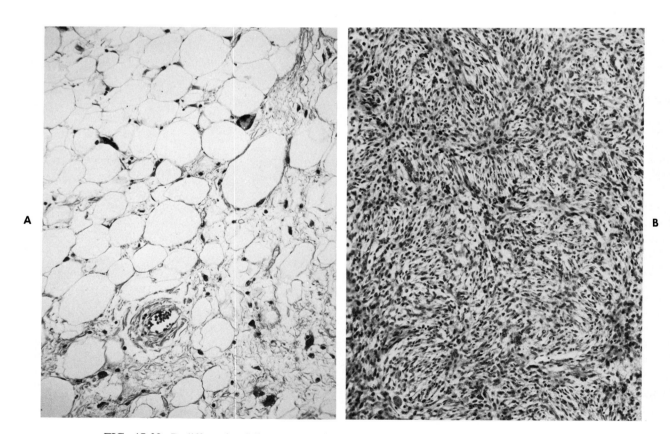

FIG. 17-39. Dedifferentiated liposarcoma of the retroperitoneum in a 50-year-old woman with well-differentiated lipoma-like portion in the primary tumor (**A**) and malignant fibrous histiocytoma-like pattern in the recurrent neoplasm (**B**). (**A** and **B**, ×160.)

sues, including those arising in the muscles of the extremities and the groin (Fig. 17-39).

Evans et al.[37] and Azumi et al.[7] included spindle cell and pleomorphic lipomas among the atypical lipomas in order to emphasize their benign clinical course. In our experience, however, based on review of a large number of cases, spindle cell and pleomorphic lipomas are closely related, clinically and morphologically well-defined entities. These tumors also have a characteristic clinical setting: they occur chiefly in the region of the shoulder or back in men older than 50 years, are confined to the subcutis, are well circumscribed and have no potential for dedifferentiation, recurrence, or metastasis. For these reasons spindle cell and pleomorphic lipomas are being discussed among the benign lipomatous tumors in Chapter 16.[8,31,32,109]

Dedifferentiated liposarcoma

Dedifferentiated liposarcoma—a term coined by Evans[34] in 1979 in analogy to dedifferentiated chondrosarcomas—is characterized by the coexistence of well-differentiated and poorly differentiated, nonlipogenic areas in portions of the same neoplasm or in the primary tumor and the recurrent tumor or metastasis. The interval between the primary appearances of the tumor and the dedifferentiated recurrence varies greatly and in most cases exceeds 5 years. In more than two thirds of cases the poorly differentiated component of the tumor resembles that of a malignant fibrous histiocytoma (Fig. 17-39), but occasionally it may show other forms of differentiation, including fibrosarcoma, leiomyosarcoma, or even rhabdomyosarcoma (Fig. 17-40)[121]; it may also be so poorly differentiated that it defies further classification (Fig. 17-41). The opposite, a poorly differentiated, malignant fibrous histiocytoma-like tumor that recurs as a well-differentiated liposarcoma, is much less common in our experience.

Dedifferentiated liposarcoma is encountered most often in the retroperitoneum and groin, but may also be encountered in the muscles of the extremities.[15,35] In fact, Weiss and Rao,[135] in a review of 92 well-differentiated liposarcomas (atypical lipomas) of the deep tissues, observed dedifferentiation in 12% (11 of 92) of the cases, including four each in the retroperitoneum and groin and three in the muscles of the extremities. Several (6 of 11) had dedifferentiated foci in the first recurrence, and some patients died of metastatic disease. The long interval between first diagnosis and dedifferentiation (mean, 7.9 years) suggested that dedifferentiation is more dependent on time than site and occurs in all locations with a high likelihood of clinical persistence of the disease. Similarly, Hashimoto and Enjoji[51] and others[15,35,64] observed dedifferentiation in well-differentiated liposarcomas that had recurred. Indeed, in three of these cases the tumor had been initially interpreted as an atypical lipoma.

As in dedifferentiated chondrosarcomas and osteosarcomas it is doubtful that differentiated cells ever undergo dedifferentiation and it is more likely that the poorly differentiated portions of these tumors are the result of an overgrowth of persisting undifferentiated mesenchymal elements or of mutagenesis with outgrowth of a new clone. Prior radiation may play a role in this process, but most patients with dedifferentiated liposarcoma give no history of having been exposed to radiation.[135]

Pleomorphic liposarcoma

This group includes two related although clearly distinguishable forms; both share a disorderly growth pattern and an extreme degree of cellular pleomorphism, including bizarre giant cells, but both differ in content of intracellular lipid material.

In the first form, which is by far the more common and amounts to about 5% to 10% of all liposarcomas, the most

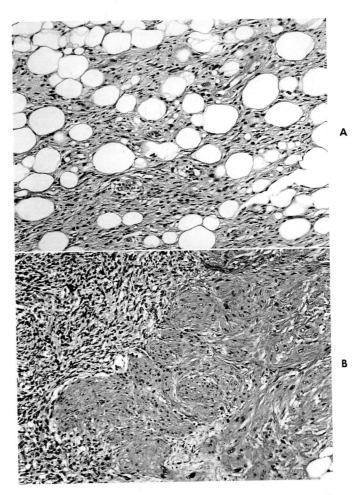

FIG. 17-40. Dedifferentiated liposarcoma showing both a well-differentiated spindle cell pattern **(A)**, poorly differentiated areas, and focal smooth muscle differentiation **(B)**. **(A** and **B**, ×165.)

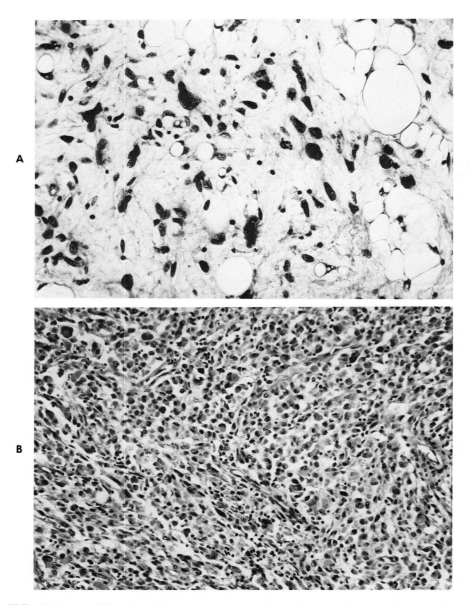

FIG. 17-41. Dedifferentiated liposarcoma of the right thigh in a 54-year-old man with well-differentiated and pleomorphic areas in one portion of the tumor **(A)** and poorly differentiated areas in another **(B)**. (A and B, ×160.)

characteristic feature is giant lipoblasts with bizarre, hyperchromatic, often scalloped nuclei, many of which have a deeply acidophilic cytoplasm reminiscent of giant cells found in pleomorphic rhabdomyosarcoma and malignant fibrous histiocytoma, tumors with which this form is often confused. Indeed, in the absence of characteristic univacuolar or multivacuolar lipoblasts, separation from malignant fibrous histiocytoma may be difficult if not impossible (Figs. 17-42 and 17-43). Eosinophilic hyaline globules, an occasional feature of giant cells, are most likely a nonspe-

cific degenerative feature that pleomorphic liposarcoma shares with other poorly differentiated neoplasms (Fig. 17-44).

The second form of pleomorphic liposarcoma is rare. It mainly consists of numerous haphazardly arranged giant cells containing multiple lipid droplets, which bestow on these cells a grape- or mulberry-like appearance. The giant cells have large irregular nuclei that may reach an enormous size and contain lobulated or lumped masses of chromatin (Fig. 17-45). Hemorrhage and necrosis are usually com-

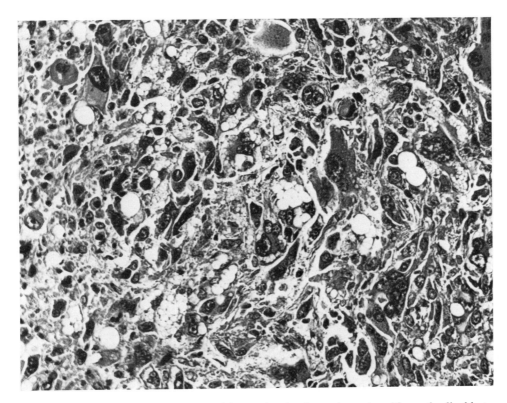

FIG. 17-42. Pleomorphic liposarcoma with occasional univacuolar and multivacuolar lipoblasts. Because of the large, deeply eosinophilic giant cells, many of these tumors are mistaken for pleomorphic rhabdomyosarcoma or malignant fibrous histiocytoma. (×180.)

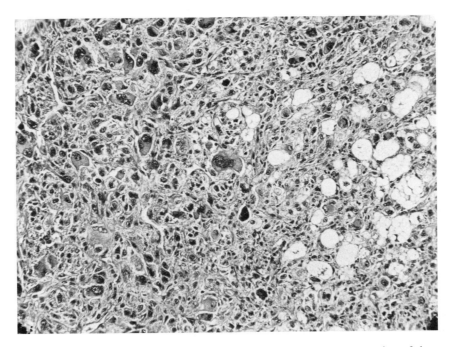

FIG. 17-43. Pleomorphic liposarcoma with clustering of lipoblasts in one portion of the tumor. (×150.)

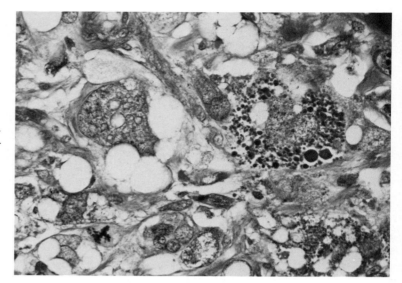

FIG. 17-44. Giant lipoblasts in pleomorphic liposarcoma. The hyaline globules in one of the tumor cells are a frequent but not specific feature of this tumor. (×400.)

mensurate with the degree of cellular pleomorphism. Mitotic activity is prominent, much more so than in other types of liposarcoma.

Electron microscopic findings

According to the studies of Lagace et al.[71] and others,* the cells of liposarcoma bear a close resemblance to different stages in the development of fat but show a much greater variability in cellular differentiation. They range in appearance from "primitive" spindle- or stellate-shaped mesenchymal cells with few and poorly developed organelles and an irregular basal lamina to intermediate cells with dilated rough endoplasmic reticulum resembling fibroblasts and more differentiated cells characteristic of lipoblasts. The lipoblasts possess one or more non–membrane-bound lipid droplets of variable size and density and little or no endoplasmic reticulum. The lipid droplets are associated with a moderate to large number of mitochondria and, in some of the cells, filamentous material, smooth membrane vesicles, and varying amounts of glycogen, usually situated near the lipid droplet. There are no desmosomes or other cellular attachments, but there are numerous pinocytotic vesicles and often a well-defined or discontinuous basal lamina. A Golgi apparatus and lysosomes are inconspicuous or scarce. The nuclei are large and deeply indented and are usually located at the periphery. Pleomorphic liposarcoma has a greater number of fibroblast- and myofibroblast-like cells, with a more irregular nucleus, and more prominent rough endoplasmic reticulum.[47,120] In most instances, lipoblasts, pericytes, and lipid-free primitive mesenchymal cells are closely related to capillaries and are surrounded by amor-

phic or granular material of low electron density intermixed with a variable number of collagen fibers. In contrast to lipoblasts, macrophages, when present, contain membrane-bound, phagocytized lipid material (Figs. 17-46 and 17-47).

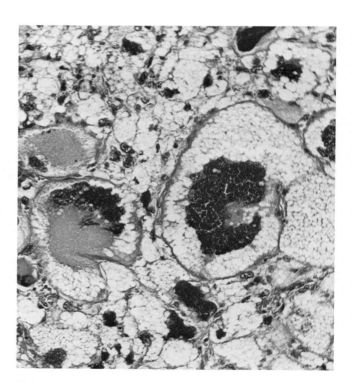

FIG. 17-45. Pleomorphic liposarcoma consisting almost entirely of bizarre lipoblasts with numerous lipid droplets in the cytoplasm and hyperchromatic nuclei. (×200.)

---

*References 10, 44, 47, 65, 74, 99, 125.

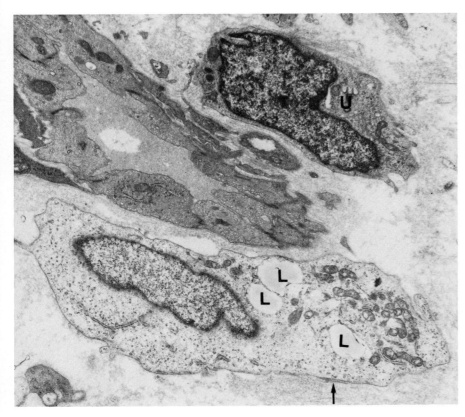

FIG. 17-46. Electron microscopic picture of myxoid liposarcoma. Capillary with associated undifferentiated mesenchymal cell *(U)* and lipoblasts with multiple non–membrane-bound lipid inclusions *(L)*. Note basal lamina at arrow. (From Taxy JB, Battifora H: The electron microscope in the study and diagnosis of soft tissue tumors. In Trump BF, Jones RT, editors: *Diagnostic electron microscopy,* New York, 1980, John Wiley & Sons.)

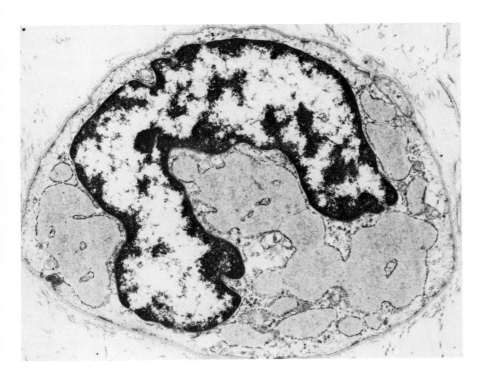

FIG. 17-47. Electron microscopic picture of undifferentiated mesenchymal cell in a case of myxoid liposarcoma. The dilated endoplasmic reticulum elaborates amorphous or granular proteinaceous material suggestive of mucopolysaccharides. The cell is surrounded by a continuous basal lamina. (From Taxy JB, Battifora H: The electron microscope in the study and diagnosis of soft tissue tumors. In Trump BF, Jones RT, editors: *Diagnostic electron microscopy,* New York, 1980, John Wiley & Sons.)

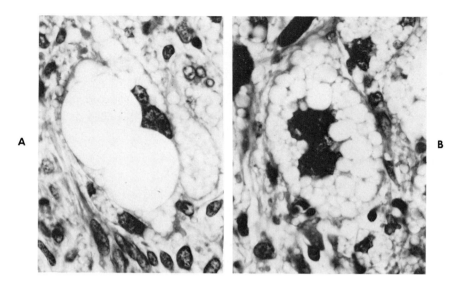

FIG. 17-48. Typical lipoblasts. **A,** Fusion of two lipid droplets and deformed and peripherally placed hyperchromatic nucleus. (×600.) **B,** Multiple introcytoplasmic lipid droplets causing scalloping of the centrally situated hyperchromatic nucleus. (×600.)

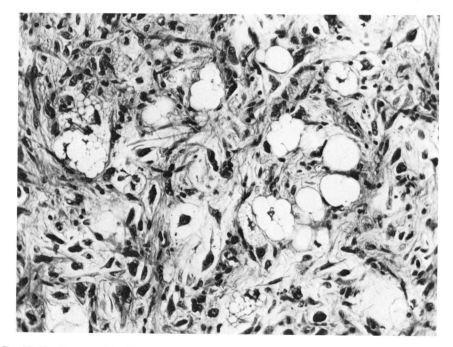

FIG. 17-49. Pleomorphic liposarcoma with multiple lipoblasts of characteristic appearance. (×200.)

Cytogenetics

Chromosome analysis has revealed a specific cytogenetic marker in myxoid liposarcoma, a reciprocal translocation of t(12;16)(q13;p11.2) and trisomy 8 as a nonrandom secondary change. This marker, however, is not a feature of well-differentiated and pleomorphic liposarcomas (see Chapter 5).*

DIFFERENTIAL DIAGNOSIS
Identification of lipoblasts

By far the most important problem facing the pathologist in the diagnosis of liposarcoma is the positive identification of lipoblasts and their distinction from other vacuolated cells commonly occurring in a variety of mesenchymal and epithelial neoplasms. As in developing fat, the lipoblasts of liposarcoma range from primitive mesenchymal cells containing only tiny lipid droplets in the cytoplasm to large "signet-ring" cells in which most of the cytoplasm is occupied by a single droplet of fat. More frequently, however, is an intermediate form that has a scanty amount of cytoplasm, multiple lipid droplets of varying size, and a single small nucleus located either in the center of the cell or its periphery. Characteristically, the lipid droplets in these cells are sharply defined, and cause compression and scalloping of the nucleus (Figs. 17-48 and 17-49). In general, the lipoblasts vary considerably in size and shape and may reach giant proportions with multiple large, irregular, hyperchromatic nuclei in pleomorphic liposarcoma. Small eosinophilic granular cells, resembling the cells of brown fat, are sometimes found in the round cell type of liposarcoma.

It must be emphasized that vacuolated cells are a common feature of a variety of sarcomas. They are particularly frequent in degenerating tumors (vacuolar degeneration) or in tumors containing large amounts of mucin or glycogen. These cells tend to have indistinct or more irregularly outlined vacuoles and rounded rather than indented or scalloped nuclei. Furthermore, lipoblast-like cells are also common in sarcomas invading fat.

Special stains and immunohistochemistry

As in other sarcomas, careful sampling of a given tumor may be of greater value for diagnosis than the preparation of multiple special stains. Stains for lipid, however, are sometimes useful in demonstrating the presence of intracellular lipid and in excluding other intracellular substances such as mucin or glycogen (Fig. 17-50). The importance of the lipid stain for the diagnosis of liposarcoma, however, should not be overemphasized, because lipid may be scarce in some liposarcomas (especially in liposarcomas of the round cell and pleomorphic types) and may be abundant in other and unrelated mesenchymal or epithelial neoplasms, even in those that are well preserved and show little evidence of degeneration or necrosis.

The mucinous matrix, characteristic of many liposarcomas, consists of non–protein-linked glycosaminoglycans

*References 87, 88, 105, 112, 113, 133.

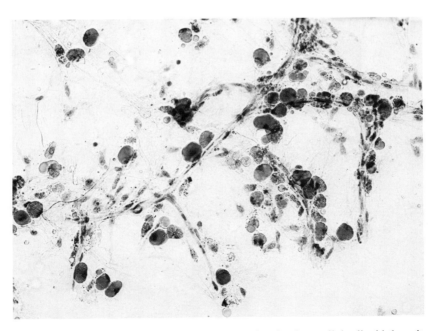

FIG. 17-50. Oil red 0 fat stain of myxoid liposarcoma showing intracellular lipoid deposits. Note close association between lipoblasts and capillaries. (×210.)

that stain well with alcian blue and the colloidal iron preparations, are metachromatic with the toluidine blue and the cresyl violet stains, and are weakly carminophilic with Meyer's mucicarmine stain. These stains are inhibited by depolymerization of the mucinous material by hyaluroni-

dase (Fig. 17-51). In contrast, sulfated glycosaminoglycans are resistant to hyaluronidase, a procedure that aids in the distinction of liposarcoma from myxoid chondrosarcoma and chordoma.[136]

Intracellular glycogen—diastase-sensitive, PAS-positive

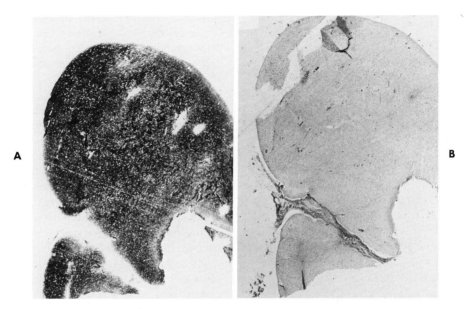

FIG. 17-51. Colloidal iron stain of myxoid liposarcoma. **A,** Prior to treatment with hyaluronidase. (×15.) **B,** After treatment with hyaluronidase and depolymerization of glycosaminoglycans. (×15.)

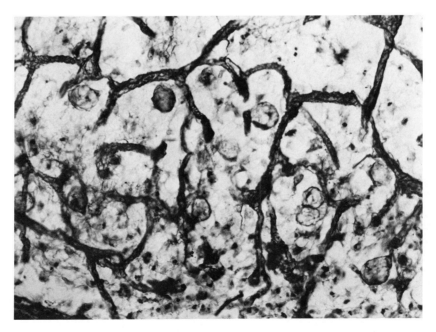

FIG. 17-52. Reticulin preparation of myxoid liposarcoma revealing dense reticulin network around capillaries and individual lipoblasts. (×260.)

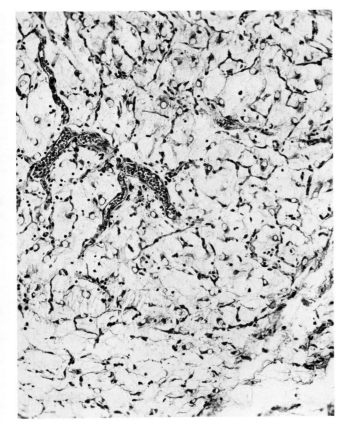

FIG. 17-53. Atrophy and myxoid change in a lipoma mimicking a myxoid liposarcoma. (×145.)

material—is demonstrable in some but not all liposarcomas. Reticulin preparations are of little diagnostic value but may bring out clearly the fibrillary reticulin meshwork that is wrapped about vascular channels and lipoblasts (Fig. 17-52).

Immunohistochemical preparations may help in differential diagnosis. Adipocytes and lipoblasts stain positively for vimentin and S-100 protein, but the stains vary in intensity, and poorly differentiated liposarcomas do not express these antigens. Hashimoto et al.[50] recommended the use of this stain for separating liposarcomas and malignant fibrous histiocytomas. Smooth muscle actin may also be demonstrated in some of the tumor cells.[20] It is present in all liposarcomas with benign and malignant smooth muscle differentiation.[36,121]

Nonneoplastic lesions simulating liposarcoma

A cause for occasional error in diagnosis is the presence of severe atrophic or myxoid change in the subcutaneous fat and other fatty deposits. This change is usually the result of mechanical trauma or other type of injury and is marked by atrophic lipocytes within a mucinous background (Fig. 17-53). Myxoid change in normal fat is particularly common in the region of the wrist, where it precedes or is associated with ganglion cysts. Similar changes without ganglion cysts occasionally may form tumorlike masses on the dorsum of the foot.

There is also a variety of inflammatory processes affecting normal fat in which the mixture of mature fat cells and

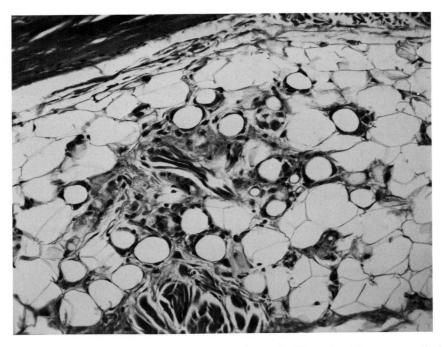

FIG. 17-54. Fat necrosis of subcutaneous fat simulating well-differentiated liposarcoma. (×160.)

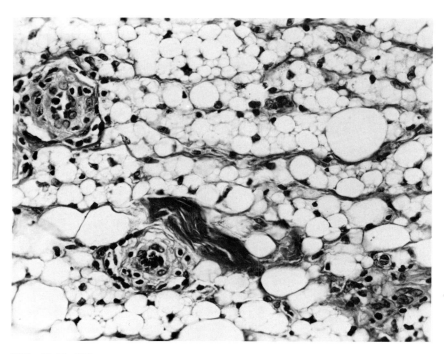

FIG. 17-55. Silicone granuloma bearing some resemblance to a liposarcoma. (×130.)

lipid-filled macrophages or xanthoma cells bears a superficial resemblance to a liposarcoma (Fig. 17-54). These lesions include not only cases of ordinary lipase-induced fat necrosis but also various forms of panniculitis or lipogranuloma that may form tumorlike masses in the subcutaneous fat or in the adipose tissue of the retroperitoneum, mesentery, or omentum (sclerosing mesenteritis, mesenteric panniculitis, sclerosing lipogranuloma). The lipid macrophages, the predominant cell of most of these lesions, differ from lipoblasts by the presence of granular or finely vacuolated cytoplasm and small centrally positioned nuclei, suggesting pyknosis. These cells are often arranged in small nests or as the lining of lipid cysts. They may be associated with multinucleated giant cells, inflammatory elements, and areas of fibrosis. Macrophages also can be identified by immunohistochemical means and ultrastructurally by the presence of multiple processes, lysosomes, and membrane-bound lipid vacuoles. The latter findings help in the distinction of liposarcoma from lesions caused by exogenous lipids or lipidlike material such as paraffin or silicone (Fig. 17-55).

Neoplasms simulating liposarcoma

Vacuolated cells that may be confused with lipoblasts are encountered in a variety of neoplasms. They may be seen in the marginal portion of malignant tumors that have invaded and phagocytized normal fat or in various mesenchymal and epithelial neoplasms that have been distorted by severe focal or diffuse vacuolar degeneration, often in association with areas of necrosis. It may also be caused by poor fixation of the tissue. Less frequently, lipoblasts are simulated by xanthoma cells, especially when these cells assume atypical characteristics, as in some forms of malignant fibrous histiocytoma, or by the accumulation of mucinous material, as in the physaliphorous cells of chordoma. Vacuolated cells may also be observed in embryonal rhabdomyosarcoma and Ewing's sarcoma, but these cells contain glycogen rather than fat. In addition, there exist rare lipomatous forms of meningioma,[58] balloon cell types of malignant melanoma, and vacuolated forms of malignant lymphoma ("signet-ring" lymphoma) that contain PAS-positive immunoglobulin. Ewing's sarcoma and malignant lymphoma may also be confused with round cell liposarcoma (Fig. 17-56).[49,61]

Intramuscular myxoma and the myxoid form of *malignant fibrous histiocytoma* are also apt to be mistaken for liposarcoma. Intramuscular myxoma, however, is marked by the complete absence of a vascular pattern and lipoblasts, whereas myxoid malignant fibrous histiocytoma may be distinguished by its cellular pleomorphism, absence of glycogen, lack of staining for S-100 protein, and presence of irregular vacuolated cells containing mucinous material rather than lipid.[50,127]

Aggressive angiomyxoma is chiefly located in the vulvar and paravaginal regions of young women of child-bearing age; the tumor lacks lipoblasts and displays a more coarsely

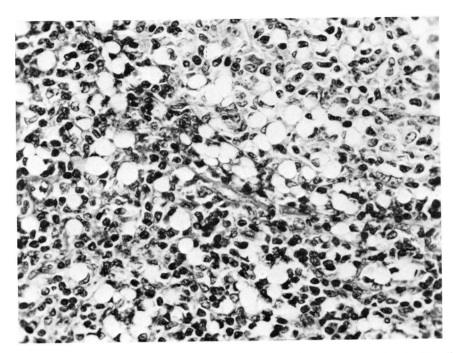

FIG. 17-56. Malignant lymphoma with "signet-ring" change that has been confused with a liposarcoma. (×440.)

vascular pattern than myxoid liposarcoma.[115] There is little cellular pleomorphism in *myxoid chondrosarcoma*, but this tumor can be clearly separated from liposarcoma by its distinctly multinodular pattern, the lacelike arrangement of its tumor cells, and the presence of a matrix rich in sulfated glycosaminoglycans (hyaluronidase-resistant sulfated mucopolysaccharides). Other benign and malignant neoplasms that may be confused with liposarcoma are listed in the accompanying box.

CLINICAL BEHAVIOR
Recurrence

Recurrence is common in deep-seated liposarcomas of all types. In these cases surgical removal of the tumor is often incomplete and tumor tissue is left behind, especially when satellite nodules are present about the main tumor mass, or when the tumor has infiltrated adjacent tissues and has grown along fascial planes. In most cases the recurrence becomes apparent within the first 6 months after the initial excision and shows a structure similar to that of the primary neoplasm. Less commonly the recurrent tumor assumes a different pattern or is much less well differentiated than the primary neoplasm (dedifferentiated liposarcoma). Recurrence may also be delayed for 5 or even 10 years following the initial therapy. In fact, we have encountered two cases of liposarcoma that recurred 30 and 31 years, respectively, after the initial excisions. As already

Neoplasms simulating liposarcoma

Benign neoplasms
Spindle cell lipoma
Pleomorphic lipoma
Lipoblastoma
Angiomyolipoma
Diffuse lipomatosis
Pelvic lipomatosis
Hibernoma
Intramuscular myxoma
Aggressive angiomyxoma
Nerve sheath myxoma
Juxtaarticular myxoma

Malignant neoplasms
Myxoid dermatofibrosarcoma protuberans
Malignant fibrous histiocytoma
Embryonal (botryoid) rhabdomyosarcoma
Myxoid chrondrosarcoma
Chordoma
"Signet-ring" lymphoma
Lipomatous meningioma
"Balloon cell" melanoma
Clear cell myeloma
Mucinous adenocarcinoma

emphasized, recurrence is very rare in well-differentiated, subcutaneous liposarcomas (atypical lipomas).

The reported recurrence rates vary slightly and depend largely on the location and accessibility of the tumor and the extent and completeness of the surgical excision. In our series,[33] 57% of the tumors recurred; in another series,[51] the recurrence rate was 46%. Liposarcomas in the retroperitoneum have a higher recurrence rate than those in the extremities, presumably because of the difficulty of complete excision. In fact, in one series[66] dealing exclusively with liposarcomas of the retroperitoneum, all 34 tumors recurred regardless of histological type. Massive recurrence in the retroperitoneum may cause complications or may even prove fatal as the result of tumor extension into the adjacent tissues and compression of the intestines or the ureter.

Although the overall recurrence rate seems to be influenced less by the histological type of the tumor than its location, the number of recurrences, for obvious reasons, is closely related to the length of survival. Multiple recurrences, therefore, are more common with the myxoid and well-differentiated types of liposarcoma. For example, one of our cases, a myxoid liposarcoma of the pelvic retroperitoneum, recurred 5 times in a 26-year period; another, a well-differentiated lipoma-like liposarcoma, recurred 7 times in an interval of 34 years. Ewing and Harrison[38] described a liposarcoma that recurred 10 times within 20 years. Evidently there is no assurance of cure even if the patient has been free of tumor for 5 or more years.

Metastasis

As in other kinds of mesenchymal tumors, the rate of metastasis is closely related to the type and degree of histological differentiation. The less differentiated, the more cellular, and the more pleomorphic a given liposarcoma, the more likely it is that it will metastasize. Apparently the incidence of metastasis is dependent to a lesser extent on the location and the size of the tumor and perhaps also on the mode of therapy.

In our review of liposarcomas[33] the rates of metastatis and mortality for myxoid and well-differentiated liposarcomas were much lower than those of the round cell, pleomorphic, and dedifferentiated types. A close correlation between tumor grade and metastasis was also reported by Chang et al.,[18] Reszel et al.,[97] and Enterline et al.[30] In Enterline's series 86% of poorly differentiated "nonmyxoid" liposarcomas metastasized.

The metastatic sites vary considerably: most poorly differentiated liposarcomas metastasize to the lung, other visceral organs, and bone. Myxoid liposarcomas, for unknown reasons, tend to produce secondary lesions on the serosal surfaces of the pleura, pericardium, and diaphragm, sometimes alone or in combination with metastasis to the viscera. Patients with these tumors may also develop another liposarcoma of similar appearance in the retroperitoneum or, less commonly, at other sites; these lesions have been interpreted as multicentric liposarcomas.

Lymph node metastasis is rare and is a feature of advanced disease; therefore, it is more commonly encountered in specimens obtained at autopsy. For this reason, regional lymph node excision has no place in the routine therapy of liposarcomas, except in those cases in which enlargement of regional lymph nodes is clearly evident.

The factors that affect the frequency and site of metastasis also affect the time interval between the appearance of the primary tumor and the metastasis. This interval may be as short as a few months in poorly differentiated liposarcomas but may reach many years in tumors of the myxoid type.[30] This is exemplified by one of our cases, a 32-year-old woman who had a myxoid liposarcoma of the right thigh that was widely excised. During the next 26 years it recurred 5 times; finally, 7 years after the last recurrence and hemipelvectomy, the tumor metastasized to the posterior mediastinum and the vertebral column when the patient was 65 years of age, 33 years after the initial therapy.

Metastasis versus multicentric liposarcoma

Drawing a sharp line between multicentric and metastatic liposarcomas is not only difficult but is often impossible. In favor of the existence of multicentric liposarcomas is the frequent occurrence of another liposarcoma at sites in which metastasis normally does not occur, as well as the long interval between the appearance of the first and second neoplasms. Evidence against this concept, however, is the frequent similarity in the histological pictures of these tumors and the fact that many so-called multicentric liposarcomas develop outright metastases to the lung or other visceral organs at a later stage of the disease.

In our cases almost 10% of the patients with primary liposarcomas of the thigh developed a second lesion in the retroperitoneum, with the second lesion making its appearance about 2 or more years after the tumor in the thigh was removed. Most of these tumors were liposarcomas of the myxoid type, and many of these patients developed visceral metastasis 1 or 2 years after appearance of the lesion in the retroperitoneum. There were also cases in which a second liposarcoma involved the opposite limb. One of these, a 35-year-old man with a liposarcoma of the *right* upper thigh, developed histologically similar tumors in the *left* lower thigh and chest wall 2 years after right hemipelvectomy. At autopsy, 1 year later, metastatic tumor was present in the lung, pancreas, and lumbar vertebrae as well as in the mediastinal and paraaortic lymph nodes. Reszel et al.[97] report five cases in which a second liposarcoma occurred in the opposite limb; one of these was noted after 7 years and two after 10 years. These authors claimed that "the late appearance of these tumors strongly suggests that they were liposarcomas of multicentric origin." Yet it is doubtful whether this long interval does indeed rule out a metastasis, since visceral metastasis has been observed as late as 10 or 15 years after the initial therapy, especially in liposarcomas of the myxoid type. Liposarcomas showing a similar setting have been reported by others.[1,30]

Survival rates

Although the survival rates reported in the earlier literature vary considerably, more recently published data on this subject are quite similar: the 5-year survival rates vary from 59%[89] and 64%[111] to 70%[107]; the 10-year survival rates range from 45%[89] to 50%[111] and 53%.[107] Hence, 14% to 17% of the patients die after the initial 5-year period. As mentioned, one major factor influencing the survival rate is the histological type of the tumor. For example, myxoid and well-differentiated liposarcomas have much more favorable 5-year survival rates than round cell and pleomorphic types. Chang et al.,[18] for instance, report a 5-year survival rate of 56% for pleomorphic, 88% for myxoid, and 100% for well-differentiated liposarcomas. Another significant factor affecting survival rates is the location of the tumor: for instance, in our series, the 5-year survival rate of patients with liposarcomas in the retroperitoneum was 39%; that of patients with tumors in the extremities was 71%.[33] Others report a 5-year survival rate of 41% for tumors of the retroperitoneum[66] and 60% for tumors of the paratesticular region.[11] These differences with regard to the

location of the tumor are even more remarkable with well-differentiated liposarcomas. Survival rates are excellent for patients with well-differentiated liposarcomas located in the subcutis (atypical lipoma) and skeletal muscle, but are less favorable when these tumors occur in the retroperitoneum (Fig. 17-57).[2,37] Even when well-differentiated liposarcomas occur in the retroperitoneum, death is caused by local extension rather than metastasis. Other related factors influencing survival rates are tumor size and completeness of surgical excision.[18]

Treatment

Although there is little precise information as to the effectiveness of the various types of therapy, wide or radical excision continues to be the treatment of choice for deep-seated liposarcomas. Treatment by simple enucleation or shelling out of the tumor should be discouraged, since doubtlessly this is the main cause of local recurrence and, in some instances, metastasis. Although many liposarcomas appear to be well circumscribed, their exact boundaries often cannot be determined macroscopically, and, in consequence, satellite nodules are frequently missed and left behind at the time of excision. In such cases examination of multiple frozen sections obtained at the time of the surgical procedure will ensure completeness of the excision. Amputation does not seem to have any major advantage

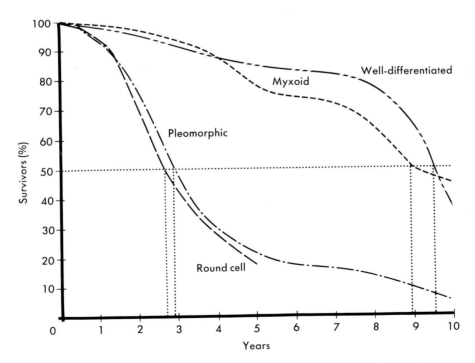

FIG. 17-57. Liposarcoma. Survival rates according to histological types (retroperitoneum and lower extremities combined). (From Enzinger FM, Winslow DJ: *Virchows Arch (Pathol Anat)* 335:367, 1962.)

over radical local excision, but in rare instances it may become necessary for technical reasons because of the bulk of the tumor or its involvement with large vessels or nerves. Fortunately, liposarcomas in the extremities tend to be smaller, more accessible, and hence more amenable to aggressive surgical therapy than those in the retroperitoneum. Complete local excision is appropriate for atypical lipomas (e.g., for well-differentiated lipoma-like liposarcomas arising in the subcutis).

According to Walaas and Kindblom[131] positive identification of liposarcoma is possible on the sole basis of fine-needle aspiration cytology if the clinical and radiographic parameters are carefully evaluated. In their series, 13 of 15 patients with liposarcoma were treated by radical removal without previous open biopsy.

Postoperative radiation is a valuable adjunct to surgical therapy,[28,82,93,107] especially for liposarcomas of the myxoid type[30,42] and those that were partially excised or unresectable. Adjunctive radiotherapy is not only capable of retarding further growth and delaying or preventing local recurrence, but it may obviate the need for amputation. Also, in selected cases preoperative radiotherapy may shrink the tumor and may render it resectable. Radiation, however, should not be used in preference to radical operation.[96] Metastatic lesions, when radiated, may respond strikingly,[126] but in advanced cases this mode of therapy is more likely to achieve palliation than cure (see Chapter 2).

There are still insufficient data on the efficacy of chemotherapy, and evaluation of this type of therapy will have to await further, better controlled follow-up studies.

REFERENCES

1. Ackerman LV: Multiple primary liposarcomas. *Am J Pathol* 20:789, 1944.
2. Adam YG, Oland J, Halevy A, et al: Primary retroperitoneal soft tissue sarcomas. *J Surg Oncol* 25:8, 1984.
3. Alho A, Eeg Larsen T: A case of multifocal liposarcoma? *Acta Orthop Scand* 63:98, 1992.
4. Allsbrook WC, Harmon JD, Congchitnan N, et al: Liposarcoma of the larynx. *Arch Pathol Lab Med* 109:294, 1985.
5. Arbabi L, Warhol MJ: Pleomorphic liposarcoma following radiotherapy for breast carcinoma. *Cancer* 49:878, 1982.
6. Austin RM, Dupree WB: Liposarcoma of the breast: a clinicopathologic study of 20 cases. *Hum Pathol* 17:906, 1986.
7. Azumi N, Curtis J, Kempson RL, et al: Atypical and malignant neoplasms showing lipomatous differentiation: a study of 111 cases. *Am J Surg Pathol* 11:161, 1987.
8. Azzopardi JG, Iocco J, Salm R: Pleomorphic lipoma: a tumour simulating liposarcoma. *Histopathology* 7:511, 1983.
9. Barkhof F, Melkert P, Meyer S, et al: Derangement of adipose tissue: a case report of multicentric retroperitoneal liposarcoma, retroperitoneal lipomatosis, and multiple subcutaneous lipomas. *Eur J Oncol* 17:547, 1991.
10. Battifora H, Nunez-Alonso C: Myxoid liposarcoma: study of 10 cases. *Ultrastruct Pathol* 1:157, 1980.
11. Bellinger MF, Gibbons MD, Koontz WW Jr, et al: Paratesticular liposarcoma. *Urology* 11:285, 1978.
12. Bolen JW, Thorning D: Benign lipoblastoma and myxoid liposarcoma. *Am J Surg Pathol* 4:163, 1980.
13. Bolen JW, Thorning D: Liposarcomas: a histogenetic approach to the classification of adipose tissue neoplasms. *Am J Surg Pathol* 8:3, 1984.
14. Breckenridge RL: Liposarcoma of the breast: report of a case. *Am J Clin Pathol* 24:954, 1954.
15. Brooks JJ, Connor AM: Atypical lipoma of the extremities and peripheral soft tissues with dedifferentiation: implications for management. *Surg Pathol* 3:169, 1990.
16. Castleberry RP, Kelly DR, Wilson ER, et al: Childhood liposarcoma: report of a case and review of the literature. *Cancer* 54:579, 1984.
17. Chang HR, Gaynor J, Tan C, et al: Multifactorial analysis of survival in primary extremity liposarcoma. *World J Surg* 14:610, 1990.
18. Chang HR, Hajdu SI, Collin C, et al: The prognostic value of histologic subtypes in primary extremity liposarcoma. *Cancer* 64:1514, 1989.
19. Cocchia D, Lauriola L, Stolfi VM, et al: S-100 antigen labels neoplastic cells in liposarcoma and cartilaginous tumours. *Virchows Arch (Pathol Anat)* 402:139, 1983.
20. Coindre JM, de Loynes B, Bui NB, et al: Dedifferentiated liposarcoma: a clinicopathologic study of 6 cases. *Ann Pathol* 12:20, 1992.
21. D'Abrera V, Burfitt-Williams W: A giant scrotal liposarcoma. *Med J Aust* 2:854, 1973.
22. Datta NS, Singh SM, Bapna BC: Liposarcoma of the spermatic cord: report of a case and review of the literature. *J Urol* 106:888, 1971.
23. Delamater J: Mammoth tumor. *Cleve Med Gaz* 1:31, 1859.
24. De Santos LA, Ginaldi S, Wallace S: Computed tomography in liposarcoma. *Cancer* 47:46, 1981.
25. DeWeerd JH, Dockerty MB: Lipomatous retroperitoneal tumors. *Am J Surg* 84:397, 1952.
26. Dimacopoulis DG: Paratesticular liposarcoma. *Br J Urol* 46:347, 1974.
27. Dreyfuss U, Ben-Arich JY, Hirschowitz B: Liposarcoma: Rare complication in neurofibromatosis: case report. *Plast Reconstr Surg* 61:287, 1978.
28. Edland RW: Liposarcoma: a retrospective study of 15 cases, a review of the literature, and a discussion of radiosensitivity. *Am J Roentgenol* 103:778, 1968.
29. Enjoji M, Hashimoto H: Diagnosis of soft tissue sarcomas. *Pathol Res Pract* 178:215, 1984.
30. Enterline HT, Culberson JD, Rochlin DB, et al: Liposarcoma: a clinical and pathological study of 53 cases. *Cancer* 13:932, 1960.
31. Enzinger FM: Benign lipomatous tumors simulating a sarcoma. In *Management of primary bone and soft tissue tumors*. MD Anderson Hospital and Tumor Institute. Chicago, 1977, Year Book Medical Publishers, p 11.
32. Enzinger FM, Harvey DA: Spindle cell lipoma. *Cancer* 36:23, 1975.
33. Enzinger FM, Winslow DJ: Liposarcoma: a study of 103 cases. *Virchows Arch (Pathol Anat)* 335:367, 1962.
34. Evans HL: Liposarcoma: a study of 55 cases with a reassessment of its classification. *Am J Surg Pathol* 3:507, 1979.
35. Evans HL: Liposarcomas and atypical lipomatous tumors: a study of 66 cases followed for a minimum of 10 years. *Surg Pathol* 1:41, 1988.
36. Evans HL: Smooth muscle in atypical lipomatous tumors: a report of three cases. *Am J Surg Pathol* 14:714, 1990.
37. Evans HL, Soule EH, Winkelman RK: Atypical lipoma, atypical intramuscular lipoma, and well differentiated retroperitoneal liposarcoma. *Cancer* 43:574, 1979.

38. Ewing MR, Harrison CV: Mesenchymoma. *Br J Surg* 44:408, 1957.

39. Fischer G, Altmannsberger M, Schauer A, et al: Klassifikation und biologisches Verhalten des Liposarkoms. *Verh Dtsch Ges Pathol* 65:440, 1981.

40. Fontanelle LJ, Radlauer DB: Liposarcoma of anterior chest wall. *Am Surg* 39:63, 1973.

41. Friedman AC, Hartman DS, Sherman J, et al: Computed tomography of abdominal fatty masses. *Radiology* 139:415, 1981.

42. Friedman M, Egan JW: Effect of irradiation on liposarcoma. *Acta Radiol* 54:225, 1960.

43. Frierson H, Cooper PH: Myxoid variant of dermatofibrosarcoma protuberans. *Am J Surg Pathol* 7:445, 1983.

44. Fu YS, Parker FG, Kaye GI, et al: Ultrastructure of benign and malignant adipose tissue tumors. *Pathol Annu* 15:67, 1980.

45. Georgiades DE, Alcalais DB, Karabela VG: Multicentric well-differentiated liposarcomas: a case report and a brief review of the literature. *Cancer* 24:1091, 1969.

46. Gilmour JR: A recurrent tumour of mesenchyme in an adult. *J Pathol Bacteriol* 55:495, 1943.

47. Gould VE, Wellington J, Gould NS: Electron microscopy of adipose tissue tumors: comparative features of hibernomas, myxoid and pleomorphic liposarcomas. *Pathobiol Annu* 9:339, 1979.

48. Hanada M, Tokuda R, Ohnishi Y, et al: Benign lipoblastoma and liposarcoma in children. *Acta Pathol Jpn* 36:605, 1986.

49. Hanna W, Kahn HJ, From L: Signet ring lymphoma of the skin: ultrastructural and immunohistochemical features. *J Am Acad Dermatol* 14:344, 1986.

50. Hashimoto H, Daimaru Y, Enjoji M: S-100 protein distribution in liposarcoma: an immunoperoxidase study with special reference to the distinction of liposarcoma from myxoid malignant fibrous histiocytoma. *Virchows Arch (Pathol Anat)* 405:1, 1984.

51. Hashimoto H, Enjoji M: Liposarcoma: a clinicopathologic subtyping of 52 cases. *Acta Pathol Jpn* 32:933, 1982.

52. Hausfield KF, Guiva AC: Liposarcoma of the spermatic cord: a case report. *Ohio State Med J* 64:1036, 1968.

53. Hummer CD, Burkart TJ: Liposarcoma of the breast: a case of bilateral involvement. *Am J Surg* 113:558, 1967.

54. Hutton I: Liposarcoma of the thigh. *Proc R Soc Med* 67:655, 1974.

55. Jakobiec FA, Rini F, Char D, et al: Primary liposarcoma of the orbit: problems in the diagnosis and management of five cases. *Ophthalmology* 96:180, 1989.

56. Jelinek JS, Kransdorf MJ, Schmookler BM, et al: Liposarcoma of the extremities: MR and CT findings in the histologic subtypes. *Radiology* 186:455, 1993.

57. Joske EA: Liposarcoma of mediastinum. *Med J Aust* 2:236, 1944.

58. Kasantikul V, Brown WJ: Lipomatous meningioma associated with cerebral vascular malformation. *J Surg Oncol* 26:35, 1984.

59. Kauffman SL, Stout AP: Lipoblastic tumors of children. *Cancer* 12:912, 1959.

60. Kenan S, Klein M, Lewis MM: Juxtacortical liposarcoma: a case report and review of the literature. *Clin Orthop* 243:225, 1989.

61. Kim H, Dorfman RF, Rappaport H: Signet ring cell lymphoma: a rare morphological and functional expression of nodular (follicular) lymphoma. *Am J Surg Pathol* 2:119, 1978.

62. Kindblom LG, Angervall L, Fassina AS: Atypical lipoma. *Acta Pathol Microbiol Scand* 90A:27, 1982.

63. Kindblom LG, Angervall L, Jarlstedt J: Liposarcoma of the neck: a clinicopathologic study of four cases. *Cancer* 42:774, 1978.

64. Kindblom LG, Angervall L, Svendsen P: Liposarcoma: a clinicopathologic, radiographic and prognostic study. *Acta Pathol Microbiol Scand* 253:1, 1975.

65. Kindblom LG, Säve-Söderbergh J: The ultrastructure of liposarcoma: a study of 10 cases. *Acta Pathol Microbiol Scand (A)* 87:109, 1979.

66. Kinne DW, Chu FCH, Huvos AG, et al: Treatment of primary and recurrent retroperitoneal liposarcoma: twenty-five-year experience at Memorial Hospital. *Cancer* 31:53, 1973.

67. Knapp RW, Campbell RJ: Huge retroperitoneal liposarcoma. *Am J Surg* 110:970, 1965.

68. Knowles CHR, Huggill PH: Liposarcoma: with report of a case in a child. *J Pathol Bacteriol* 68:235, 1954.

69. Kransdorf MJ, Meis JM, Jelinek JS: Dedifferentiated liposarcoma of the extremities: imaging findings in four patients. *AJR Am J Roentgenol* 161:127, 1993.

70. Kretschmer HL: Retroperitoneal lipo-fibro-sarcoma in a child. *J Urol* 43:61, 1940.

71. Lagace R, Jacob S, Seemayer TA: Myxoid liposarcoma: an electronmicroscopic study: biological and histogenic considerations. *Virchows Arch (Pathol Anat)* 384:159, 1979.

72. Lagrange JL, Despins P, Spielman M, et al: Cardiac metastases: case report on an isolated cardiac metastasis of a myxoid liposarcoma. *Cancer* 58:2333, 1986.

73. Lane CM, Wright JE, Garner A: Primary myxoid liposarcoma of the orbit. *Br J Ophthalmol* 72:912, 1988.

74. Lazarus SS, Trombetta LD: Ultrastructure and histochemical identification of sclerosing liposarcoma. *Histopathology* 5:223, 1981.

75. Lindahl S, Markhede G, Berlin O: Computed tomography of lipomatous and myxoid tumors. *Acta Radiol* 26:709, 1985.

76. Mackenzie I, Roberts GH: Liposarcoma of paratesticular origin: a case report. *Br J Urol* 46:467, 1974.

77. Mariotti A, Vertaccini N: A study of the pathogenesis of liposarcoma. *Arch Ital Patol Clin Tumori* 3:1456, 1959.

78. McCulloch TM, Makielski KH, McNutt MA: Head and neck liposarcoma: a histopathologic reevaluation of reported cases. *Arch Otolaryngol Head Neck Surg* 118:1045, 1992.

79. McFadden DW: Myxoid liposarcoma of the spermatic cord. *J Surg Oncol* 40:132, 1989.

80. McLaughlin CW Jr, Sharpe JC: Malignant fatty tumors of retroperitoneal region. *Am J Surg* 41:512, 1938.

81. McLean TR, Almassi GH, Hackbarth DA, et al: Mediastinal involvement by myxoid liposarcoma. *Ann Thorac Surg* 47:920, 1989.

82. McNeer GP, Cantin J, Chu F, et al: Effectiveness of radiation therapy in the management of sarcomas of soft somatic tissues. *Cancer* 22:391, 1968.

83. Menne FR, Birge RF: Primary liposarcoma of great omentum. *Arch Pathol* 22:823, 1936.

84. Menon M, Velthoven PM: Liposarcoma of the breast. *Arch Pathol* 98:370, 1974.

85. Moreland RB, McNamara WL: Liposarcoma: report of nine cases. *Arch Surg* 45:164, 1942.

86. O'Connor M, Snover DC: Liposarcoma: a review of factors influencing prognosis. *Am Surg* 49:379, 1983.

87. Ohjimi Y, Iwasaki H, Ishiguro M, et al: Myxoid liposarcoma with t(12;16)(q13;p11): possible usefulness of chromosome analysis in a poorly differentiated sarcoma. *Pathol Res Pract* 188:736, 1992.

88. Orndal C, Mandahl N, Rydholm A, et al: Chromosomal evolution and tumor progression in a myxoid liposarcoma. *Acta Orthop Scan* 61:99, 1990.

89. Orson GG, Sim FH, Reiman HM, et al: Liposarcoma of the musculoskeletal system. *Cancer* 60:1362, 1987.

90. Pack GT, Pierson JC: Liposarcoma: a study of 105 cases. *Surgery* 36:687, 1954.

91. Papadopoulos T, Kirchner T, Bergmann M, et al: Primary liposarcoma of the jejunum. *Pathol Res Pract* 186:803, 1990.

92. Peeples WJ, Hazra T: Retroperitoneal liposarcoma in a child. *Urology* 7:89, 1976.

93. Perry H, Chu FCH: Radiation therapy in the palliative management of a soft tissue sarcoma. *Cancer* 15:179, 1962.

94. Quinonez GE: Liposarcoma of the lower extremity: a review of 30 cases from the Ohio State University Hospital from 1955 to 1970. *Ohio State Med J* 68:942, 1972.

95. Razzuk MA, Urschel HC, Race GJ, et al: Liposarcoma of the mediastinum: case report and review of the literature. *J Thorac Cardiovasc Surg* 61:819, 1971.

96. Reitan JB, Kaalhus I, Brennhovd IO, et al: Prognostic factors in liposarcoma. *Cancer* 55:2482, 1985.

97. Reszel PA, Soule EH, Coventry MB: Liposarcoma of the extremities and limb girdles: a study of 222 cases. *J Bone Joint Surg* 48A:229, 1966.

98. Robb WAT: Liposarcoma of the greater omentum. *Br J Surg* 47:537, 1960.

99. Rossouw DJ, Cinti S, Dickersin GR: Liposarcoma: an ultrastructural study of 15 cases. *Am J Clin Pathol* 85:649, 1985.

100. Russell WO, Cohen J, Enzinger FM, et al: A clinical and pathological staging system for soft tissue sarcomas. *Cancer* 40:1562, 1977.

101. Sampson CC, Saunders EH, Green WE, et al: Liposarcoma developing in a lipoma. *Arch Pathol* 69:506, 1960.

102. Saunders JR, Jaques DA, Casterline PF, et al: Liposarcomas of the head and neck: a review of the literature and addition of four cases. *Cancer* 43:162, 1979.

103. Sawhney KK, McDonald MJ, Jaffe HW: Liposarcoma of the hand. *Am Surg* 41:117, 1975.

104. Schiller H: Lipomata in sarcomatous transformation. *Surg Gynecol Obstet* 27:218, 1918.

105. Schoenmaker HF, Kools PF, Kazmierczak B, et al: Isolation of a somatic cell hybrid retaining the der(16) t(12;16)(q13;p11.2) from a myxoid liposarcoma cell line. *Cytogenet Cell Genet* 62:159, 1993.

106. Shimoda T, Yamashita H, Furusato M, et al: Liposarcoma: a light and electron microscopic study with comments on their relation to malignant fibrous histiocytoma and angiosarcoma. *Acta Pathol Jpn* 30:779, 1980.

107. Shiu MH, Chu F, Castro EB, et al: Results of surgical and radiation therapy in the treatment of liposarcoma arising in an extremity. *Am J Roentgenol* 123:577, 1975.

108. Shmookler BM, Enzinger FM: Liposarcoma occurring in children: an analysis of 17 cases and review of the literature. *Cancer* 52:567, 1983.

109. Shmookler BM, Enzinger FM: Pleomorphic lipoma: a benign tumor simulating liposarcoma. *Cancer* 47:126, 1981.

110. Snover DC, Sumner HW, Dehner LP: Variability of histologic pattern in recurrent soft tissue sarcomas originally diagnosed as liposarcoma. *Cancer* 49:1005, 1982.

111. Spittle MF, Newton KA, Mackenzie DH: Liposarcoma: a review of 60 cases. *Br J Cancer* 24:696, 1971.

112. Sreekantaiah C, Karakousis CP, Leong SP, et al: Cytogenetic findings in liposarcoma correlate with histopathologic subtypes. *Cancer* 69:2484, 1992.

113. Sreekantaiah C, Karakousis CP, Leong SPL, et al: Trisomy 8 as a nonrandom secondary change in myxoid liposarcoma. *Cancer Genet Cytogenet* 51:195, 1991.

114. Starkloff GB, Saxton JA, Johnson RE: Liposarcoma of an extremity associated with multiple subcutaneous lipomas. *Ann Surg* 133:261, 1951.

115. Steeper TA, Rosai J: Aggressive angiomyxoma of the female pelvis and perineum: report of nine cases of a distinctive type of gynecologic soft tissue neoplasm. *Am J Surg Pathol* 7:463, 1983.

116. Sternberg SS: Liposarcoma arising within a subcutaneous lipoma. *Cancer* 5:975, 1952.

117. Stout AP: Liposarcoma, the malignant tumor of lipoblasts. *Ann Surg* 119:86, 1944.

118. Sundaram M, Baran G, Merenda G, et al: Myxoid liposarcoma: magnetic resonance imaging appearances with clinical and histological correlation. *Skeletal Radiol* 19:359, 1990.

119. Suster S, Wong TY, Moran CA: Sarcomas with combined features of liposarcoma and leiomyosarcoma: study of two cases of an unusual soft-tissue tumor showing dual lineage differentiation. *Am J Surg Pathol* 17:905, 1993.

120. Suzuki T: Ultrastructural characteristics of a pleomorphic liposarcoma: a possible involvement of myofibroblasts. *Acta Pathol Jpn* 37:843, 1987.

121. Tallini G, Erlandson RA, Brennan MF, et al: Divergent myosarcomatous differentiation in retroperitoneal liposarcoma. *Am J Surg Pathol* 17:546, 1993.

122. Tamaki I, Suzuki M, Sano K, et al: A case of huge retroperitoneal liposarcoma. *Jpn J Cancer Clin* 18:693, 1972.

123. Tanaka K, Hizawa K, Tonei M: Liposarcoma: a clinicopathological study of 136 cases based on the histologic subtyping in WHO. *Jpn J Cancer Clin* 20:1036, 1974.

124. Tanaka N, Chen WC: A case of angiolipomyxosarcoma arising from traumatic hematoma of the thigh. *Gann* 45:265, 1954.

125. Taxy JB, Battifora H: The electron microscope in the study and diagnosis of soft tissue tumors. In *Diagnostic electron microscopy*. New York, 1980, John Wiley & Sons Inc, p 147.

126. Tong ECK, Rubenfeld S: Cardiac metastasis from myxoid liposarcoma emphasizing its radiosensitivity. *Am J Roentgenol* 103:792, 1968.

127. Tsuneyoshi M, Hashimoto H, Enjoji M: Myxoid malignant fibrous histiocytoma versus myxoid liposarcoma: a comparative ultrastructural study. *Virchows Arch (Pathol Anat)* 400:187, 1983.

128. Uner R, Balim AI, Oktem K: Mediastinal liposarcoma: report of a case. *Chest* 43:103, 1963.

129. Virchow R: Ein Fall von bösartigen zum Theil in der Form des Neuroms auftretenden Fettgeschwülsten. *Virchows Arch (Pathol Anat)* 11:281, 1857.

130. Virchow R: Myxoma lipomatodes malignum. *Virchows Arch (Pathol Anat)* 32:545, 1865.

131. Walaas L, Kindblom LG: Lipomatous tumors: a correlative cytologic and histologic study of 27 tumors examined by fine needle aspiration cytology. *Hum Pathol* 16:6, 1985.

132. Waldeyer W: Grosses Lipo-Myxom des Mesenteriums mit sekundaeren sarcomatoesen Herden in der Leber und Lunge. *Virchows Arch (Pathol Anat)* 32:543, 1865.

133. Walter TA, Decker HJ, Leong SP, et al: A case of myxoid liposarcoma with translocation t(12;16) as the only abnormality. *Cancer Genet Cytogenet* 34:117, 1988.

134. Ward RM, Evans HL: Cystosarcoma phyllodes. *Cancer* 58:2282, 1986.

135. Weiss SW, Rao VK: Well differentiated liposarcoma (atypical lipoma) of deep soft tissue of the extremities, retroperitoneum and miscellaneous sites: a follow-up study of 92 cases with analysis of the incidence of "dedifferentiation." *Am J Surg Pathol* 16:1051, 1992.

136. Winslow DJ, Enzinger FM: Hyaluronidase-sensitive acid mucopolysaccharides in liposarcomas. *Am J Pathol* 37:497, 1960.

137. Witz M, Shapira Y, Dinbar A: Diagnosis and treatment of primary and recurrent retroperitoneal liposarcomas. *J Surg Oncol* 47:41, 1991.

138. Wright CJE: Liposarcoma arising in a simple lipoma. *J Pathol Bacteriol* 60:483, 1948.

CHAPTER 18

BENIGN TUMORS OF SMOOTH MUSCLE

To some extent the distribution of benign muscle tumors parallels the distribution of smooth muscle tissue within the body. Thus they tend to be relatively common in the genitourinary and gastrointestinal tracts, less frequent in the skin, and rare in deep soft tissue. In the experience of Farman,[1] based on 7748 leiomyomas, approximately 95% occurred within the female genital tract, and the remainder were scattered over various sites, including the skin (230 cases), gastrointestinal tract (67 cases), and bladder (5 cases). This study, based on surgical material, however, probably underestimates the large number of asymptomatic gastrointestinal and genitourinary lesions that are documented only in autopsy material. In general, soft tissue leiomyomas cause little morbidity; therefore there are few studies in the literature concerning their presentation, diagnosis, and therapy. For purposes of classification these tumors can be divided into several groups.

Cutaneous leiomyomas (leiomyoma cutis) are the most common group and are of two types. Those arising from the pilar arrector muscles of the skin are often multiple and associated with significant pain. Those arising from the network of muscle fibers that lie in the deep dermis of the scrotum (dartoic muscles), labia majora, and nipple are almost always solitary and are collectively referred to as *genital leiomyomas.* The second group of benign smooth muscle tumors are the *angiomyomas (vascular leiomyomas),* which are distinctive, painful, subcutaneous tumors composed of a conglomerate of thick-walled vessels associated with smooth muscle tissue. They differ from cutaneous leiomyomas in their anatomical distribution, predominantly subcutaneous location, and predilection for women. The *leiomyomas of deep soft tissue* comprise the third group of benign smooth muscle tumors. These tumors are much larger than their superficial counterparts, usually display a greater spectrum of histological changes, and must be clearly separated from leiomyosarcomas, which are statistically more common in deep soft tissue. Some deep leiomyomas probably arise from blood vessels, but their large size at the time of diagnosis makes it difficult to establish this point with certainty. *Leiomyomatosis peritonealis disseminata* and *intravenous leiomyomatosis* are also included, although they are not strictly soft tissue tumors. The first can be conceptualized as a diffuse metaplastic response of the peritoneal surfaces in which multiple smooth muscle nodules form. The second is a uterine tumor that extends into the uterine or pelvic veins. Both may be confused with metastatic leiomyosarcoma because of their unusual growth patterns. Lastly, a number of newly described lesions are discussed in this chapter *(palisaded myofibroblastoma, myofibroblastoma of breast, and angiomyofibroblastoma)* that are composed of modified smooth muscle cells.

STRUCTURE AND FUNCTION OF SMOOTH MUSCLE CELLS

Smooth muscle cells are widely distributed throughout the body and contribute to the wall of the gastrointestinal, genitourinary, and respiratory tracts. They constitute the muscles of the skin, erectile muscles of the nipple and scrotum, and iris of the eye. Their characteristic arrangements within these organs determine the net effect of contraction. For instance, the circumferential arrangement within blood vessels results in narrowing of the lumen during contraction, whereas the contraction of the longitudinal and circumferential muscle layers within the gastrointestinal tract causes the propulsive peristaltic wave.

Smooth muscle cells are fusiform in shape and possess centrally located cylindrical nuclei with rounded ends that develop deep indentations during contraction. The length of the muscle cell varies depending on the organ, achieving its greatest length in the gravid uterus, where it may measure as much as 0.5 mm. The cells are usually arranged in fascicles in which the nuclei are staggered so that the tapered end of one cell lies in close association with the thick nuclear region of an adjacent cell.

Typically there are no connective tissue cells between individual muscle fibers, although a delicate basal lamina and small connective tissue fibers, presumably synthesized by the muscle cells,[7] can be seen as a delicate PAS-positive rim around individual cells in light microscopic preparations.

Ultrastructurally, the cells are characterized by clusters of mitochondria, rough endoplasmic reticulum, and free ribosomes, which occupy the zone immediately adjacent to the nucleus. The remainder of the cytoplasm (sarcoplasm) is filled with myofilaments that are oriented parallel to the long axis of the cell.[4] There are three types of filaments within the cell. Thick myosin filaments (12 nm) are surrounded by seven to nine thin actin filaments (6 to 8 nm). Thick and thin filaments are aggregated into larger groups or units, which correspond by light microscopy to linear myofibrils. In addition to the contractile proteins, intermediate filaments, measuring 10 nm and forming part of the cytoskeleton, are centered around the dense bodies or plaques, which are believed to be the smooth muscle analogue of the Z-band. The plasma membrane is dotted with tiny pinocytotic vesicles, and overlying the surface of the cell is a delicate basal lamina. Although the basal lamina separates individual cells, limited areas exist between cells in which the substance is lacking and in which the plasma membranes lie in close proximity, separated by a space of about 2 nm. This area, known as a gap junction or nexus, may allow spread of electrical impulses between adjacent cells.

Smooth muscle cells display diversity in their content of contractile and intermediate filament proteins, depending on their location and function. It is useful to be aware of some of the regional variations in evaluating neoplasms. For example, the gamma isoform of muscle actin is present along with desmin in most smooth muscle cells, whereas in vascular smooth muscle the alpha isoform of muscle actin and vimentin predominate.

CUTANEOUS LEIOMYOMA (LEIOMYOMA CUTIS)

Superficial or cutaneous leiomyomas are of two types: those arising from the pilar arrector muscles of the skin may be solitary or multifocal, and are often associated with considerable pain and tenderness; the other form, the genital leiomyoma, arises from the diffuse network of muscle in the deep dermis of the genital zones (e.g., scrotum, nipple, areola, and vulva). In the scrotum they arise from the dartoic muscles (dartoic leiomyoma) and in the nipple from the muscularis mamillae and areolae. This form is nearly always solitary and rarely causes significant pain.

Leiomyoma of pilar arrector origin

Although formerly believed to be the more common form of cutaneous leiomyoma,[17,35] leiomyomas of pilar arrector origin are probably far less common than previously thought[39] and are probably outnumbered by those arising in genital sites. They may be solitary or multiple. Most develop during adolescence or early adult life, although occasional cases appearing at birth or early childhood are known. Some of these lesions occur on a familial basis,[12,17,22,37] possibly inherited as an autosomal dominant

trait.[22] The distribution of lesions among affected family members does not always follow a similar pattern.[12] Multiple cutaneous leiomyomas have also been associated with dermatitis herpetiformis and HLA-B8,[18] premature uterine leiomyomas,[16] increased erythropoietin activity,[15,36] and multiple endocrine adenomatosis (type I).[13] Typically the lesions develop as small discrete papules, which in the incipient stage can be palpated more readily than they can be seen. Eventually they form nodules that coalesce into a fine linear pattern following a dermatome distribution. The extensor surfaces of the extremities are most often affected. The lesions often produce significant amounts of pain that can be triggered by exposure to cold. In one unusual case reported by Fisher and Helwig,[17] the patient claimed strong emotions evoked pain in the lesions. It is not clear whether the pain produced by these tumors is the result of contraction of the muscle tissue or compression of nearby nerves by the tumors. Usually the tumors grow slowly over a period of years, with new lesions forming as older lesions stabilize. The slowly progressive nature of the disease probably accounts for the fact that patients often seek medical attention only after a number of years. The majority of pilar leiomyomas are 1 to 2 cm in diameter. They lie within the dermal connective tissue and are separated from the overlying atrophic epidermis by a *grenz* zone. The lesions are less well defined than the angiomyoma and blend in an irregular fashion with the surrounding dermal collagen and adjacent pilar muscle. The central portions of the lesions are usually devoid of connective tissue and consist exclusively of packets or bundles of smooth muscle fibers. They usually intersect in an orderly fashion and often create the impression of a hyperplasia or overgrowth of the pilar arrector muscle (Fig. 18-1, *A*). The cells resemble normal smooth muscle cells (Fig. 18-1, *B*), and myofibrils can be demonstrated rather easily with special stains such as the Masson trichrome stain, in which they appear as red linear streaks traversing the cytoplasm in a longitudinal fashion. In the phosphotungstic acid–hematoxylin (PTAH) stain they have a similar appearance but are blue-purple. Ultrastructurally, the cells have myofilaments, surface pinocytotic vesicles, and investing basal laminae.[24]

Diagnosis is rarely difficult in the typical case, particularly one with a characteristic history. Occasionally solitary forms of the disease are mistaken for other benign tumors such as the cutaneous fibrous histiocytoma (dermatofibroma). The cells within the fibrous histiocytoma are slender, less well ordered, and lack myofibrils. Secondary elements such as inflammatory cells, giant cells, and xanthoma cells, common to the cutaneous fibrous histiocytoma, are lacking in the cutaneous leiomyoma.

Although this is a benign disease that is not known to undergo malignant transformation, it nonetheless may be difficult to treat. The lesions are often so numerous that total surgical excision is not possible; furthermore, half of the

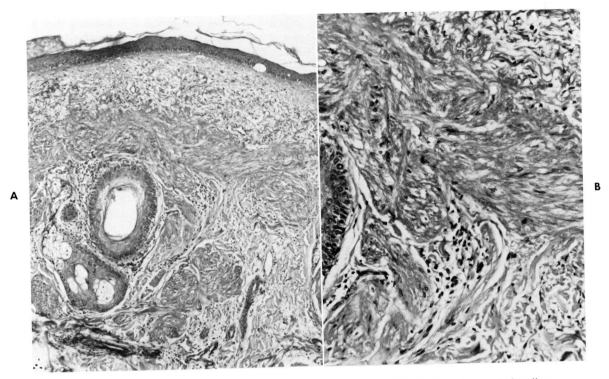

FIG. 18-1. **A,** Cutaneous leiomyoma of pilar arrector origin. (×25.) **B,** Smooth muscle bundles are closely associated with hair follicles and consist of well-differentiated, highly oriented cells. (×160.)

patients who undergo surgery develop recurrences or new lesions in the same area.[17] In a few patients pain may be so severe as to be incapacitating. Nitroglycerin has been used successfully to abort attacks,[16] and phenoxybenzamine along with hyoscine hydrobromide has been used to decrease pain.[11,36]

Genital leiomyomas

Earlier studies based on referred consultations suggested that genital leiomyomas were far less common than those of pilar arrecti origin.[17] Judging from recent hospital-based series, genital leiomyomas may outnumber pilar ones by a margin of 2 to 1.[39] Affected sites include the areola of the nipple, scrotum, labium, penis, and vulva. The tumors are small, seldom exceeding 2 cm, and pain is not a prominent symptom. Histologically, genital leiomyomas, with the exception of the nipple lesions, differ from pilar leiomyomas in that they tend to be more circumscribed, more cellular, and display a greater range of histologic appearances.[17,29] For example, Tavassoli and Norris,[33] in a review of 32 vulvar leiomyomas, noted myxoid change as well as epithelioid phenotype of the cells, features that are not encountered in pilar leiomyomas.

ANGIOMYOMA (VASCULAR LEIOMYOMA)

The angiomyoma is a solitary form of leiomyoma that usually occurs in the subcutis and is composed of numerous thick-walled vessels. In the early literature little attempt was made to separate these lesions from cutaneous leiomyomas, and both were collectively termed *tuberculum dolorosum* because of their pain-producing properties. Stout[35] later designated them *vascular leiomyomas* to contrast them with the cutaneous leiomyoma that possessed inconspicuous thin-walled vessels. These lesions account for about 5% of all benign soft tissue tumors[45] and one fourth[27] to one half[35] of all superficial leiomyomas. They occur more frequently in women,[42] except for those in the oral cavity, where the reverse is true.[44] Unlike cutaneous leiomyomas, these tumors develop later in life, usually between the fourth and sixth decade, as solitary lesions.[42,45] They occur preferentially on the extremities, particularly the lower leg. In the series reported by Hachisuga et al., 375 out of 562 occurred in the lower extremity, 125 on the upper extremity, 48 on the head, and 14 on the trunk.[45] The majority were less than 2 cm in diameter. Isolated cases of angiomyoma have been associated with paraproteinemia, myomas of the uterus, and astrocytoma.[40]

Affected patients complain most often of a small, slowly enlarging mass that is usually of several years' duration. Pain is a prominent feature in about half of the cases,[42] and in some cases it is exacerbated by pressure, change in temperature, pregnancy,[42,45] or menses.[40] The prevalence of pain has led some to suggest that these tumors are probably derived from arteriovenous anastomoses, similar to the glomus tumor.[43] They differ in appearance from the glomus tumor and are almost never encountered in a subungual location, however. The tumors are usually located in the subcutis and less often in the deep dermis, where they produce overlying elevations of the skin but without surface changes of the epidermis. Grossly, the tumors are circumscribed, glistening, white-gray nodules. Occasional cases may be blue or red, and rarely calcium flecks are visible grossly. The leiomyomas that visibly contract or writhe when touched or surgically manipulated are probably of this type.

Microscopically the tumors have a very characteristic appearance that varies little from case to case. They consist of a well-demarcated nodule of smooth muscle tissue punctuated with thick-walled vessels with partially patent lumina (Fig. 18-2). Typically the inner layers of smooth muscle of the vessel are arranged in an orderly circumferential fashion, while the outer layers spin or swirl away from the vessel, merging with the less well-ordered peripheral muscle fibers (Fig. 18-3, *A*). Areas of myxoid change (Fig. 18-3, *B*), hyalinization, calcification, and fat are seen. The vessels within these tumors are difficult to classify because they are not altogether typical of veins or arteries. Their thick walls and small lumina are reminiscent of arteries, but they consistently lack internal and external elastic laminae. A minority of angiomyomas may be made up of predomi-

nantly cavernous-type vessels, in the experience of Hachisuga et al.[45] Nerve fibers are usually difficult to demonstrate, but undoubtedly are present to account for the exquisite sensitivity of these lesions to manipulation. Rarely angiomyomas display degenerative nuclear atypia similar to that seen in symplastic leiomyomas.[41] The angiomyoma is a benign tumor, causing few problems apart from pain. Simple excision is adequate therapy. In the cases reported by Duhig and Ayer,[42] none developed recurrence following excision. Only two patients developed recurrence in the series of Hachisuga et al.,[45] although their follow-up data were incomplete.

LEIOMYOMA OF DEEP SOFT TISSUE

Compared with the foregoing tumors, leiomyomas of deep soft tissue are very uncommon, and only sporadic cases have been reported in the literature. Except for the childhood years, these lesions may occur at almost any age and seem to affect the sexes equally. Most are located in the deep muscle of the extremities or within the abdominal cavity or retroperitoneum. They tend to be much larger than those of the skin, probably because they produce few symptoms and are therefore discovered at a relatively late stage. Many are calcified; therefore they may be detected radiographically (Fig. 18-4), leading to diagnoses such as "calcifying neurilemoma," "synovial sarcoma," or "myositis ossificans." Others are highly vascular, giving the radiologist the impression of malignancy.[50] Grossly, they are well-circumscribed, gray-white lesions. Some may have a gelatinous appearance if significant myxoid change has occurred.

Histologically, these tumors are similar to their cutaneous counterparts, except that they are likely to undergo degenerative or regressive changes. Most are easily recognized as smooth muscle tumors because of the orderly pattern of intersecting fascicles of deeply acidophilic cells with blunt-ended nuclei without significant cellular pleomorphism and mitotic activity (Fig. 18-5). In occasional cases nuclear palisading (Fig. 18-6) and perinuclear vacuolization (Fig. 18-7) may be noted. Leiomyomas with nuclear palisading can be distinguished from neurilemomas in that the former tumor has significant amounts of cytoplasmic glycogen, cytoplasmic fuchsinophilia, and longitudinal striations (Fig. 18-8).

Some leiomyomas of soft tissue accumulate large amounts of myxoid ground substance between the cells, resulting in loss of the fascicular pattern. These tumors vaguely resemble the myxoid zones of nodular fasciitis or myxoma (Fig. 18-9) but can be distinguished from both by the cellular staining characteristics elaborated earlier. Mature fat may be seen in smooth muscle tumors of all types, including angiomyomas, intravenous leiomyomatosis, and deep leiomyomas. In the uterus these mixed lesions have been termed "lipoleiomyoma," whereas in deep soft tissue

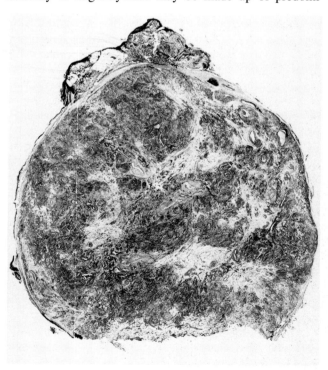

FIG. 18-2. Angiomyoma of subcutaneous tissue. Congeries of thick-walled vessels constitute a major portion of the lesion and blend with surrounding smooth muscle tissue and focal myxoid stroma. (Masson trichrome stain, ×8.)

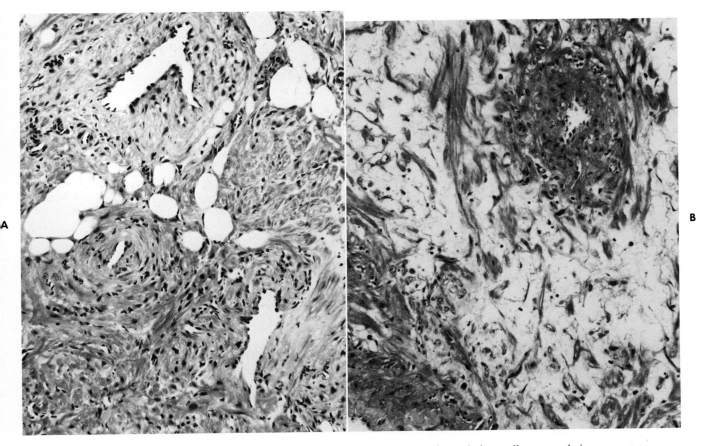

FIG. 18-3. Thick-walled vessel of angiomyoma. **A,** Inner layer of muscle is usually arranged circumferentially, while outer layer blends with less well-ordered smooth muscle tissue of tumors. (×250.) **B,** Focal myxoid change within angiomyoma. (×250.)

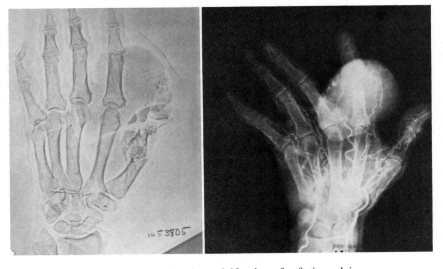

FIG. 18-4. Radiograph showing calcification of soft tissue leiomyoma.

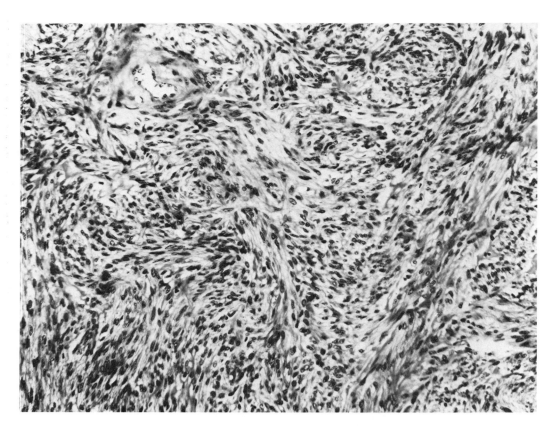

FIG. 18-5. Leiomyoma of deep soft tissue. Fascicles of smooth muscle tend to be less well-oriented and more cellular than in cutaneous leiomyomas. (×180.)

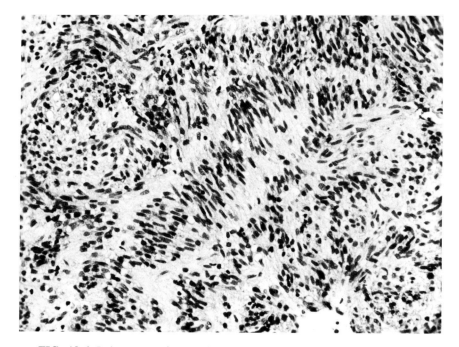

FIG. 18-6. Leiomyoma of stomach showing focal nuclear palisading. (×160.)

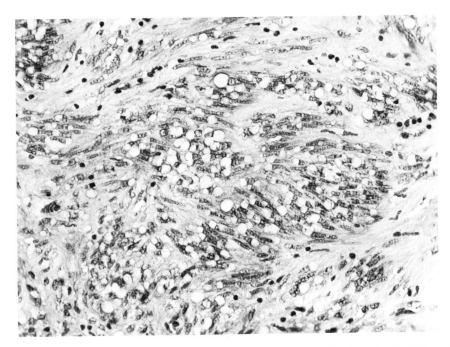

FIG. 18-7. Leiomyoma of stomach with prominent perinuclear vacuolization of cells. This feature may be present in benign and malignant smooth muscle tumors. (×180.)

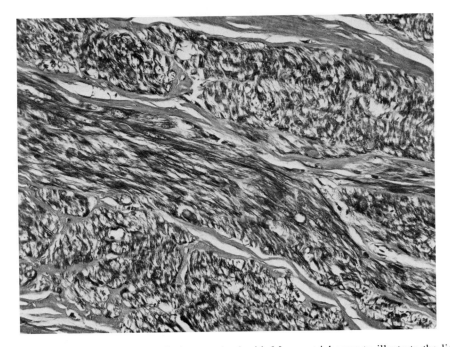

FIG. 18-8. Leiomyoma of deep soft tissue stained with Masson trichrome to illustrate the linear striations within the cytoplasm. (Masson trichrome stain, ×160.)

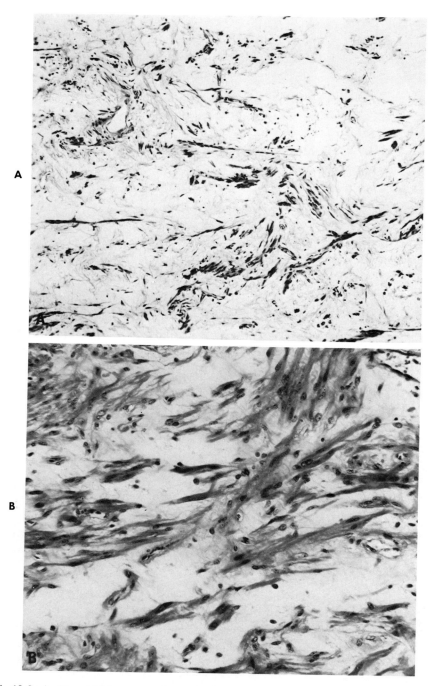

FIG. 18-9. **A,** Myxoid leiomyoma simulating the appearance of a myxoma. (×100.) **B,** In contrast to a myxoma, cells in this tumor are better oriented and more elongated and possess more cytoplasm. (×250.)

they have been referred to both as "lipoleiomyoma"[54] and "myolipoma"[52] (see Chapter 16), depending on the emphasis the authors have chosen to give to the two elements. Although some of these tumors seem to truly represent primary soft tissue tumors, others, particularly those in the pelvic regions, may well represent uterine leiomyomas that have undergone autoamputation or smooth muscle tumors arising from hormonally sensitive smooth muscle tissue of the parametrial region. The principal significance of these lesions is that the intermingling of wisps of smooth muscle cells between lobules of mature fat may suggest alternative diagnoses such as well-differentiated liposarcoma. Recognition that the spindled element consists of mature smooth muscle, rather than the atypical, hyperchromatic spindled cells of liposarcomas, is a critical observation to arriving at the correct diagnosis.

Another uncommon feature in leiomyomas is "clear cell change" (Fig. 18-10) of the cytoplasm. When this change is extreme, a variety of diagnoses may be entertained, including clear cell carcinoma, balloon cell melanoma, or adnexal tumor. Careful sampling to document typical smooth muscle cells is usually sufficient to establish the correct diagnosis. Immunostaining for desmin may also be helpful, since this protein is often demonstrable in benign smooth muscle tumors but not in malignant ones (see Chapter 19).

Regressive changes are quite common in large leiomyomas, particularly those of long duration. Most commonly these include fibrosis, calcification,[46,47,49,53] and in rare cases ossification. Calcium is usually laid down in distinct spherules reminiscent of psammoma bodies (Fig. 18-11); this sometimes invokes a surrounding giant cell reaction (Fig. 18-12).

Evaluation of malignancy in deeply situated smooth muscle tumors is difficult. Because leiomyosarcomas are more common in deep soft tissue than leiomyomas, it is mandatory that smooth muscle tumors in this location be carefully sampled. In general, mitotic activity is the principal criterion used to evaluate malignancy in these lesions and is discussed in detail in Chapter 19. It should be pointed out that in rare instances degenerative nuclear atypia occurs within leiomyomas. This phenomenon is analogous to the nuclear atypia in long-standing neurilemomas (ancient schwannoma). The nuclei are enlarged and hyperchromatic but are not associated with mitotic activity (Fig. 18-13). These tumors, moreover, are usually not highly cellular lesions and may even have large hyalinized areas. It is important that these rare examples of pleomorphic leiomyoma be distinguished from leiomyosarcomas, which are characterized not only by nuclear atypia but also by mitotic activity and areas of increased cellularity.

Although assessment of mitotic activity remains the cornerstone to determining malignancy in smooth muscle tumors of soft tissue, information regarding location in certain circumstances is invaluable as well. For example, an occasional problem in differential diagnosis arises when a differentiated, but mitotically active, smooth muscle tumor

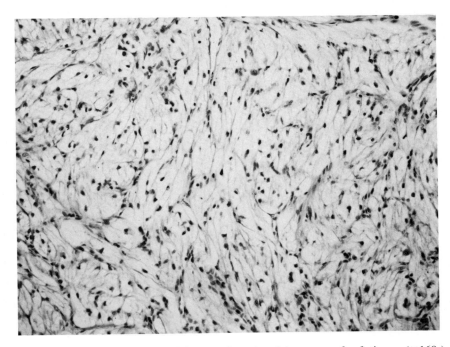

FIG. 18-10. Clear cell change of the cytoplasm in a leiomyoma of soft tissue. (×160.)

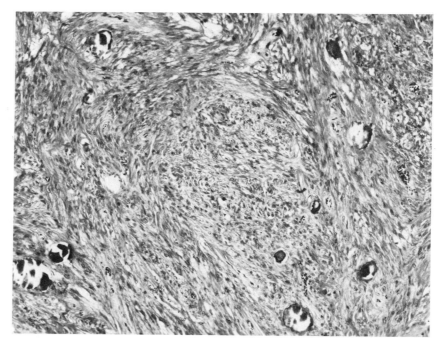

FIG. 18-11. Leiomyoma of deep soft tissue containing focal calcification resembling psammoma bodies. (×100.)

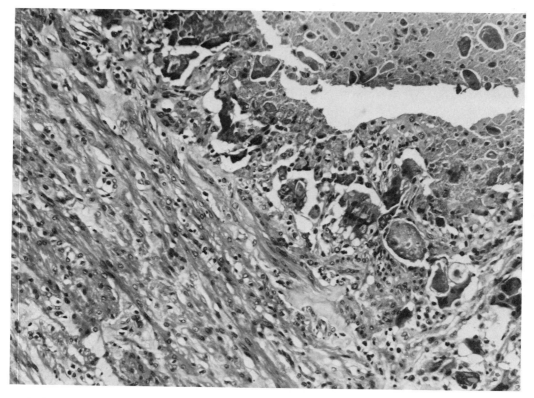

FIG. 18-12. Leiomyoma of deep soft tissue with extensive calcification and giant cell reaction simulating the appearance of tumoral calcinosis. (×200.)

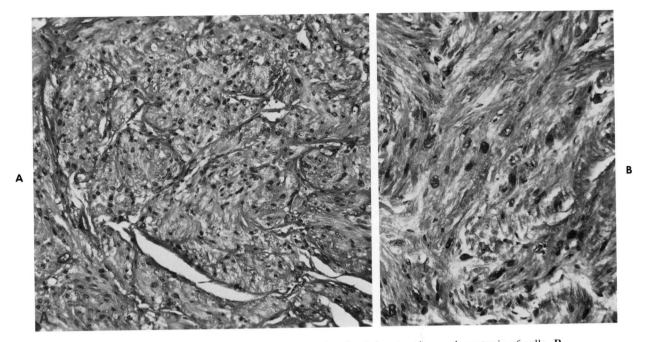

FIG. 18-13. A, Leiomyoma of soft tissue showing focal degenerative nuclear atypia of cells. B, Pleomorphic leiomyoma. (A, ×100; B, ×160.)

arises in the lower abdomen of a woman. Under these circumstances, it is essential to determine if the lesion bears any relationship to the uterus or other hormonally sensitive smooth muscle of the adnexa or parametrium. If so, it is more appropriate to employ the more conservative criteria of malignancy for uterine smooth muscle tumors. In rare instances we have even seen cases of uterine leiomyomas that extended through the sacral notch into the buttock and that, without the benefit of radiographic studies, would have been interpreted as a well-differentiated leiomyosarcoma because of low levels of mitotic activity.

True leiomyomas of soft tissue are benign lesions that require complete excision with a small cuff of surrounding normal tissue. Unfortunately there is little information in the literature regarding long-term prognosis.

INTRAVENOUS LEIOMYOMATOSIS

Intravenous leiomyomatosis is a rare condition in which gross nodules of benign smooth muscle tissue grow within the veins of the myometrium and occasionally extend for a variable distance into the uterine and hypogastric veins. In about 10% of patients cardiac symptoms may predominate due to the presence of tumor within the vena cava and heart. This condition may develop as a result of extensive vascular invasion by a leiomyoma or by de novo origin from the uterine veins.[61]

The lesion develops primarily in premenopausal middle-aged women, and prior pregnancy is noted in about half of the patients. The common presenting symptoms are abnormal vaginal bleeding and pelvic pain. In over half of the patients the uterus is enlarged. Grossly, the lesion is rather distinctive and is characterized by coiled masses within the myometrium and in some cases by serpiginous extensions of the process into the uterine veins of the broad ligament (Fig. 18-14). The masses have a rubbery texture and a pink to white-gray color similar to an ordinary uterine myoma. Histologically the smooth muscle proliferations in leiomyomatosis may show the same spectrum of changes as those in ordinary leiomyomas. The lesions may vary from highly cellular smooth muscle proliferations to less cellular ones marked by fibrosis, hydropic change, and perivascular hyalinization. A rather characteristic feature, however, is the presence of thick-walled vessels occurring within the plugs of intravascular smooth muscle tissue, creating a "vessel within a vessel" appearance. Unusual features in this condition include epithelioid change of the cells, fat, or endometrial glands in association with smooth muscle cells,[57] sex cord pattern,[81] and bizarre nuclear changes similar to those of symplastic leiomyoma.[57] Despite the intravascular location, the smooth muscle cells are quite well differentiated, showing in nearly all cases no or only modest degrees of nuclear hyperchromatism. Mitotic figures are rare, with an incidence well below that associated with borderline (5 to 9 mitoses per 10 HPF) or malignant (greater than or equal

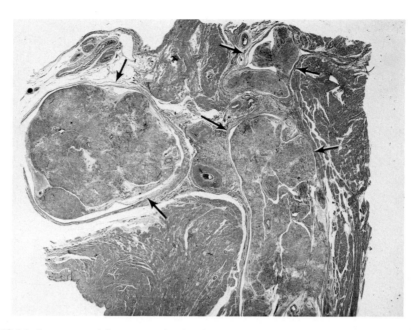

FIG. 18-14. Intravenous leiomyomatosis showing plugs of smooth muscle tissue within uterine veins *(arrows)*. (×60.) (Courtesy Dr. H.J. Norris.)

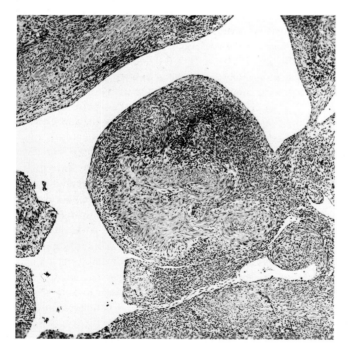

FIG. 18-15. Intravenous leiomyomatosis showing protrusion or early invasion of uterine leiomyoma into vascular lumen. This phenomenon represents the principal pathogenetic mechanism. (×100.) (Courtesy Dr. H.J. Norris.)

to 10 mitoses per 10 HPF) smooth muscle tumors of the uterus (see Chapter 19). Thus from a purely morphological point of view, that would be classified as "leiomyoma."

The pathogenesis of these tumors has been debated, but current evidence suggests that two mechanisms are operational.[61] In most cases there are associated uterine leiomyomas, supporting the notion that extensive angioinvasion by one or more myometrial tumors results in this condition (Fig. 18-15). In a few instances, however, the smooth muscle proliferation appears to be entirely intravascular, indicating direct origin from the venous walls (Fig. 18-16). In fact, as pointed out by Norris and Parmley,[61] women in general may be particularly susceptible to development of intravascular smooth muscle proliferations, as evidenced by the inordinately high incidence of leiomyosarcomas of the vena cava in women and the peculiar intimal changes of vessels that develop secondary to reproductive steroids.

Despite the intravascular location, the prognosis in most cases is quite good. About 70% of patients will be cured by hysterectomy, whereas the remaining 30% will have persistence or recurrence of disease.[56] Unfortunately recurrence rates have not correlated well with the presence of extrauterine extension noted at the time of the original surgery. In a small percentage of patients the disease may be fatal because of extension into the hepatic veins, the heart, and even the lungs.[56,61,62,65,66] Resection of these cardiac and caval extensions, if technically feasible, is compatible with prolonged survival.[54,56,65,66] Since some cases of in-

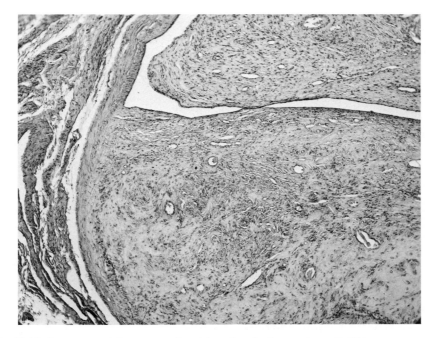

FIG. 18-16. Intravenous leiomyomatosis arising directly from vein wall. This represents a second, but apparently far less common, pathogenetic mechanism. (×35.) (From Norris HJ, Parmley TH. *Cancer* 36:2161, 1975.)

travenous leiomyomatosis possess steroid receptors,[59,67] it has been suggested that oophorectomy or estrogen antagonists should play a therapeutic role in those patients in whom tumor excision has been incomplete. It is likely that some cases of "benign metastasizing leiomyoma" of the lung evolve by way of "intravenous leiomyomatosis."[61] Others may evolve as a result of microscopic showers of tumor emboli occurring at the time of myomectomy, and still others may represent well-differentiated leiomyosarcomas in which the original tumor or the metastasis was misdiagnosed as a leiomyoma.[68]

The best name for this condition may be debatable, since the ability of a tumor to invade the bloodstream and grow in foreign tissue would satisfy a minimum definition of malignancy for some. On the other hand, the condition is compatible with long survival and differs histologically from the vast majority of leiomyosarcomas of venous origin. The latter are usually high-grade tumors composed of smooth muscle cells with easily recognized mitotic figures. They arise preferentially in the vena cava, particularly the upper portion, and usually carry a poor prognosis because of their unresectability (see Chapter 19).

LEIOMYOMATOSIS PERITONEALIS DISSEMINATA

Leiomyomatosis peritonealis disseminata is a rare condition in which multiple smooth muscle or smooth muscle–like nodules develop in a subperitoneal location throughout the abdominal cavity. The lesion occurs exclusively in women, usually during the child-bearing years. Most cases reported in the United States have been in African-American women. Over half have occurred in pregnant women. Others have occurred in women taking oral contraceptives, and one patient had a functioning ovarian tumor.[91] These observations, and the fact that the lesion regresses following pregnancy,[72] provide circumstantial evidence for the involvement of hormonal factors in the pathogenesis of the condition. The rarity of the condition suggests that other unknown factors must also be important. In most instances leiomyomatosis is discovered incidentally at the time of surgery for other medical or obstetric conditions, although vague abdominal pain is often an accompanying symptom. Grossly, the disease has an alarming appearance. The peritoneal surfaces, including the surfaces of the bowel, urinary bladder, and uterus, are studded with firm white-gray nodules of varying sizes. The smallest nodules may be only a few millimeters, whereas the largest are several centimeters in diameter (Fig. 18-17). Although the diffuseness of the process initially suggests an intraabdominal malignancy, the lesions lack hemorrhage and necrosis. Moreover, they do not violate the parenchyma of the affected organs, nor are they found in extraabdominal sites such as the lung or within lymph nodes. Leiomyomas of the uterus have been identified in some but not all

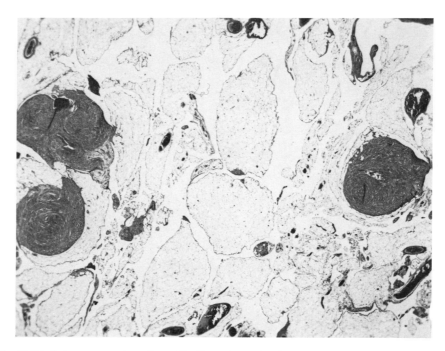

FIG. 18-17. Leiomyomatosis peritonealis disseminata showing numerous smooth muscle nodules of various sizes arising beneath the peritoneal surface and involving underlying fat. Early nodules are present as small microscopic foci. (×45.)

cases of leiomyomatosis, indicating that the lesions do not represent localized spread of an intrauterine lesion.

Microscopic findings

Although the term *leiomyomatosis* obviously indicates the similarity of this process to normal smooth muscle and to benign leiomyomas, reports in the literature, coupled with cases reviewed at the AFIP,[89] suggest that there is a range of histological changes perhaps not fully appreciated when the term was coined. In the classic case the earliest nodules develop as small microscopic foci of proliferating smooth muscle immediately subjacent to the peritoneum (Fig. 18-18, *A*). With progressive growth they may remain nodular or may, in addition, dissect through the underlying soft tissue in a more permeative fashion. Except for the unusual location and pattern of growth, the lesion is similar to the common leiomyoma. The slender cells are arranged in close compact fascicles oriented perpendicularly to each other, so that both transverse and longitudinal fascicles may be seen side by side (Fig. 18-18, *B*). The cells may show a minimal degree of nuclear pleomorphism that falls far short of a leiomyosarcoma. Mitotic figures may be seen, but they are rather infrequent. Bundles of longitudinally oriented myofibrils can be identified within the cells by means of conventional special stains (Masson trichrome stain). In some cases endometriosis has been present within the smooth muscle nodules.[77,79]

In a significant number of cases, however, the histological appearance of these subperitoneal nodules may be more fibroblastic or "myofibroblastic" (Fig. 18-19). Cases of this type have been described by Parmley et al.,[85] Winn et al.,[92] and Pieslor et al.[86] The proliferating cell is usually large, has a plump eosinophilic cytoplasm, and is usually not arranged in well-defined fascicles. Rounded decidual cells having an eosinophilic or foamy cytoplasm are usually scattered amidst the spindled cells, and at times it may be impossible to clearly delimit these cells from the spindled cells by light microscopy (Fig. 18-19, *A*). In these cases the cells lack distinct longitudinal striations as are seen in the foregoing type. In cases of regressing or regressed leiomyomatosis, hyalinization of the nodules is seen (Fig. 18-20). The one case in the literature allegedly representing lipomatous differentiation within the cells is dubious, judging from the photomicrographs.[78]

Ultrastructural findings

In view of the range of changes observed by light microscopy, it is not surprising that electron microscopy has produced such conflicting reports regarding the histogenesis of this condition. In the studies of Nogales et al.,[82] Kuo et al.,[79] and Goldberg et al.,[73] the majority of the cells resembled mature smooth muscle cells and possessed an investiture of basal lamina, surface-oriented pinocytotic vesicles, and abundant longitudinally oriented myofilaments.

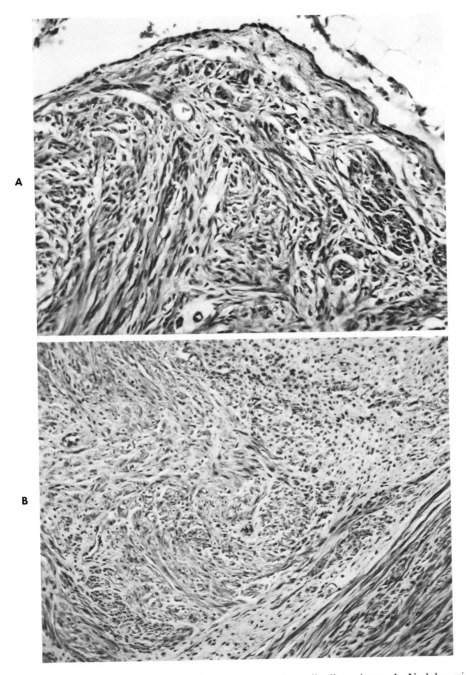

FIG. 18-18. Classic appearance of leiomyomatosis peritonealis disseminata. **A,** Nodules arise in subperitoneal location and consist of well-oriented fascicles of mature smooth muscle tissue **(B).** **(A** and **B,** ×160.)

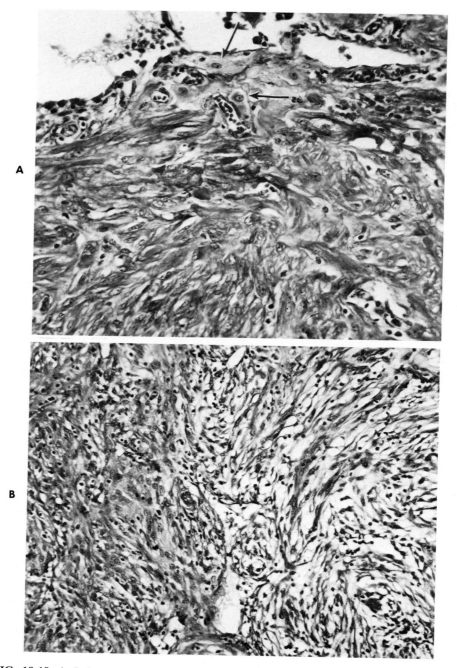

FIG. 18-19. A, Leiomyomatosis peritonealis disseminata associated with decidual cells *(arrows)* and having a more fibroblastic or myofibroblastic appearance **(B)** than is depicted in Fig. 18-17. (**A** and **B,** ×160.)

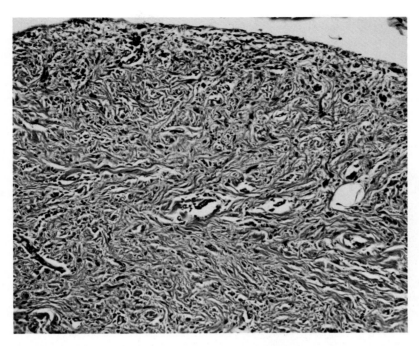

FIG. 18-20. End stage of leiomyomatosis peritonealis disseminata showing extensive interstitial fibrosis. (×100.)

On the other hand, Parmley et al.[85] and Winn et al.[92] believed the predominant cells were fibroblastic and, based on the close relationship with the decidual cells, suggested that leiomyomatosis is a reparative fibrosis occurring within a preexisting decidual reaction (fibrosing deciduosis). Others have documented a variety of cell types, including fibroblasts, myofibroblasts, and smooth muscle cells[86,89] and suggested a close interrelationship of all three.[89] The theory that leiomyomatosis represents a metaplasia or differentiation of pluripotential cells of the serosa or subserosal tissue along several closely related cell lines is supported by the experimental work of Fujii et al.[74] Estrogen administered to guinea pigs induces peritoneal nodules similar to those of leiomyomatosis peritonealis. These nodules are composed of fibroblasts and myofibroblasts in animals receiving estrogen only, whereas smooth muscle differentiation and decidualization occurs if estrogen and progesterone are administered.

Behavior and treatment

In view of the benign nature of this condition, no particular therapy is warranted once the diagnosis has been firmly secured. In fact, there seems to be some evidence that following pregnancy or removal of the estrogenic source, regression of the lesions occurs,[86] but with subsequent pregnancy, progression or recrudescence occurs.[80] The case reported by Aterman, et al.,[70] documents partial regression of lesions 5 months after the initial surgery and without any intervening therapy, and regression of another lesion within 12 weeks.[76] Recently, gonadotropin-releasing hormone antagonists (e.g., leuprolide acetate) have been used with some success in this disease.[75] There have been two cases purporting to show malignant degeneration of this condition. The case reported by Akkersdijk et al.[69] is scantily illustrated, and no autopsy was performed on the patient. On the other hand the case reported by Rubin et al.[87] is better documented and may well represent an example in which the patient succumbed to multiple intraabdominal tumors and skeletal metastasis.

PALISADED MYOFIBROBLASTOMA OF LYMPH NODE (INTRANODAL HEMORRHAGIC SPINDLE CELL TUMOR WITH AMIANTHOID FIBERS)

Reported simultaneously by Weiss et al.,[104] and Suster and Rosai,[103] the palisaded myofibroblastoma is a distinctive benign spindle cell tumor arising exclusively from the lymph nodes and bearing an unmistakable similarity to a neurilemoma. In fact, so striking is the resemblance that these lesions were originally regarded as neurilemomas of lymph node[99] and reported as such in the first two editions of this textbook. However, with the advent of immunohistochemistry it has become clear that the tumor is more closely related to a myofibroblast or modified smooth muscle cell. The tumor may develop at any age but typically presents as a localized swelling in the region of the groin. A few cases have been reported in submandibular lymph nodes,[93,98] and one of us (SWW) has reviewed one case, in consultation, from the mediastinal nodes. On cut section the tumors are gray-white, focally hemorrhagic masses that usually obscure the nodal landmarks (Fig. 18-21). On cut section it is usually possible to identify a rim of residual node at the periphery of the tumors. The tumors are com-

posed of differentiated spindled cells arranged in short intersecting or crisscrossed fascicles with vaguely palisaded nuclei focally (Fig. 18-22). In some areas the cells may form broad sheets having slitlike extracellular spaces containing erythrocytes similar to those of Kaposi's sarcoma. The cells usually possess little atypia and only a rare mitotic figure. The cells seem to represent an unusual myofibroblastic (or myoid) cell in that they strongly express actin and vimentin but not desmin. Linear striations, which are easily identified within conventional benign smooth muscle cells, cannot be demonstrated with Masson trichrome stain, although in many cases fuchsinophilic bodies, representing accumulations of actin, are prominent.

The most distinctive feature of the tumor is the amianthoid fibers or thick collagen mats that are nearly always present. These structures appear as broad eosinophilic bands, ellipses, or circular profiles, depending on the plane of section (Fig. 18-23). They contain a central collagen-rich zone surrounded by a paler collagen-poor zone containing actin and other materials extruded from nearby degenerating cells. Immunohistochemically, type I collagen can be identified throughout the amianthoid fibers, while type III collagen is localized peripherally.[102] Although the name "amianthoid" was used by Suster and Rosai for these distinctive bodies, it has recently been pointed out that these structures do not meet the strict definition of amianthoid fibers.[102] These should be thick collagen fibers measuring between 280 and 1000 nm, whereas the fibers within these structures have the width of normal collagen fibers. The mechanism of formation of these unusual bodies is not fully

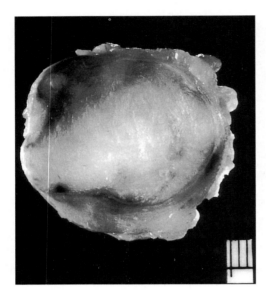

FIG. 18-21. Gross specimen of a palisaded myofibroblastoma. Note focal hemorrhages.

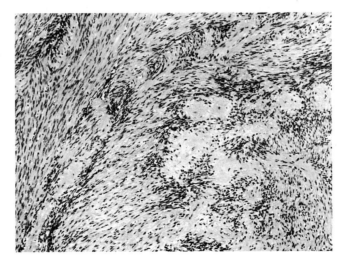

FIG. 18-22. Palisaded myofibroblastoma with vaguely palisaded fascicles of spindled cells. (×100.)

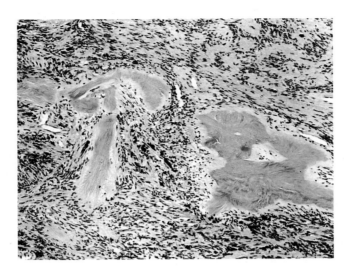

FIG. 18-23. Amianthoid fibers within a palisaded myofibroblastoma. Note central dark zone and lighter peripheral zone. (×100.)

clear. Some have suggested they represent a degenerative change occurring around vessels[103] to which the tumor cells and their contents become adherent.[95,104] These lesions appear to arise from modified smooth muscle cells that normally are found in lymph node capsule and stroma. The predilection of this tumor to occur within the groin probably reflects the relative frequency with which smooth muscle cells are found in this location relative to other lymph node chains.[104]

Of the cases reported in the literature all have behaved in a benign fashion, with no recurrences or metastases.[103,104] It is most important to recognize that this lesion represents a primary benign mesenchymal lesion and not a metastatic sarcoma. These tumors, however, are quite well differentiated and possess extremely low levels of mitotic activity in contrast to most metastatic sarcomas. Moreover, sarcomas infrequently metastasize to lymph nodes, and when they do so, it is usually an expression of disseminated disease and rarely an initial presentation.

MYOFIBROBLASTOMA OF THE BREAST

Myofibroblastoma of the breast is an uncommon but highly characteristic mesenchymal tumor that occurs most frequently in elderly men.[108] Of the 16 original cases reported by Wargotz et al.,[108] 11 were men and the average age was 63 years. The tumor develops as a discrete, well-marginated mass that does not intermingle with the surrounding breast tissue (Fig. 18-24). The tumors contain

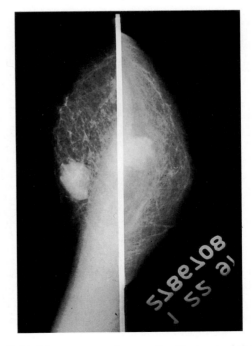

FIG. 18-24. Mammogram of a myofibroblastoma of the breast. Note sharp circumscription of lesion.

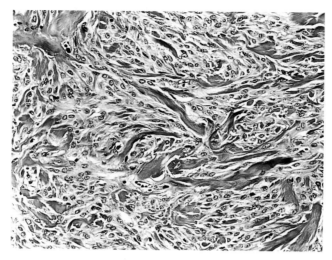

FIG. 18-25. Myofibroblastoma of the breast. (×250.)

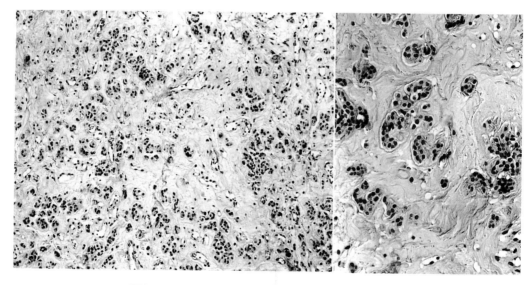

FIG. 18-26. Angiomyofibroblastoma of vulva. (×100.)

slender fibroblast-like spindled cells arranged in sheets or short packets that are separated by broad collagen bundles. Mast cells may be scattered throughout the lesions (Fig. 18-25). Rarely chondroid metaplasia is seen. On electron microscopy and immunohisochemistry the proliferating cells seem most closely related to myofibroblasts. They express desmin[107,108] and contain collections of actin filaments,

dense bodies, basal lamina, and surface-oriented pinocytotic vesicles.[106]

Once they become familiar with the pattern of this tumor, most pathologists have little difficulty in identifying it correctly. Those unfamiliar with this lesion have a tendency to regard it as a well-differentiated metaplastic carcinoma or sarcoma. Perhaps the most helpful feature seen

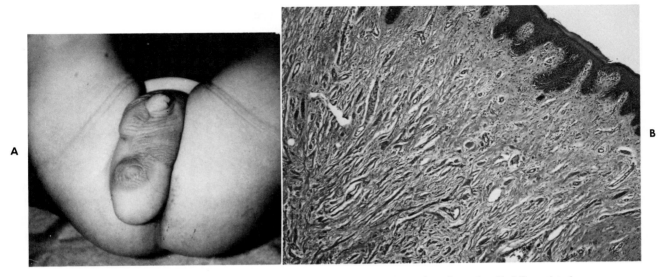

FIG. 18-27. Accessory scrotum in an infant (A). Microscopic section showed well-differentiated smooth fibers oriented perpendicular to skin surface (B). (×60.)

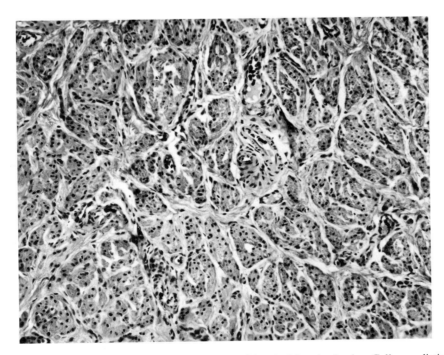

FIG. 18-28. Round ligament removed at the time of inguinal herniorrhaphy. Cells are distinctly rounded with small centrally placed nuclei. (×160.)

at low power is the impressive circumscription of this lesion compared to malignant spindle cell lesions of the breast. It is also helpful to note that the lesion does not insinuate itself within the substance of the breast, as one would see in carcinomas or stromal sarcomas. The presence of short fascicles of plump cells interrupted by collagen bundles is also at variance with fibromatosis, which consists of long, sweeping fascicles of attenuated fibroblastic cells.

These tumors are entirely benign. None of the original cases described by Wargotz et al.[108] developed either recurrences or metastases. Thus, once the correct diagnosis is established, simple excision is adequate.

ANGIOMYOFIBROBLASTOMA OF THE VULVA

Angiomyofibroblastoma is a distinctive tumor of the vulva,[109] which we believe is closely related to, if not identical to, an epithelioid leiomyoma. These tumors develop as slowly growing, marginated masses in the subcutaneous tissues of the vulva and are, therefore, diagnosed clinically as Bartholin's cyst. The tumors contain prominent, somewhat ectatic vessels surrounded by eosinophilic epithelioid smooth muscle cells, some of which blend or fan out from the muscular walls of the vessels. The cells may lie in small chains, cords, or singly within a matrix that varies from myxoid to hyaline (Fig. 18-26). Those tumors with a prominent hyaline matrix can be confused with the so-called angiomyxoma, another highly vascularized lesion of the lower gynecological tract. It is not unusual for the epithelioid cells to spindle and to resemble conventional smooth muscle cells at the periphery of the lesion. Immunohistochemically these cells express vimentin and desmin but not actin.

Although none of the original 10 cases reported by Fletcher et al.[109] recurred, we have encountered recurrences in our material. This appears to be more common where tumors are less sharply marginated and are therefore more difficult to excise completely.

MISCELLANEOUS LESIONS CONFUSED WITH LEIOMYOMAS

Although the diagnosis of leiomyoma is seldom difficult, occasionally hamartomatous or choristomatous deposits of smooth muscle tissue may suggest leiomyoma. Examples of this include accessory scrotal (Fig. 18-27) or areolar tissue. The clinical appearance and location of the lesions usually suggest the correct diagnosis. Round ligament, when removed incidentally in the repair of an inguinal hernia, may also be misinterpreted as a leiomyoma. Round ligament is composed of distinctive, closely packed, polygonal muscle cells with small, dark, centrally placed nuclei (Fig. 18-28).

REFERENCES
General

1. Farman AG: Benign smooth muscle tumors. *S Afr Med J* 48:1214, 1974.
2. Gallagher PJ: Blood vessels. In Sternberg SS, editor: *Histology for pathologists.* New York, 1992, Raven Press.
3. Harman JW, O'Hegarty MT, Byrnes CK: The ultrastructure of human smooth muscle. I. Studies of cell surface and connections in normal and achalasia esophageal smooth muscle. *Exp Mol Pathol* 1:204, 1962.
4. Hashimoto H, Komori A, Kosaka M, et al: Electron microscopic studies on smooth muscle of the human uterus. *J Jpn Obstet Gynecol Soc* 7:115, 1960.
5. Morales AR, Fine G, Pardo V, et al: The ultrastructure of smooth muscle tumors with a consideration of the possible relationship of glomangiomas, hemangiopericytomas, and cardiac myxomas. *Pathol Ann* 10:65, 1975.
6. Rosenbluth J: Smooth muscle: an ultrastructural basis for the dynamics of its contraction. *Science* 148:1337, 1965.
7. Ross R: The smooth muscle cell. II. Growth of smooth muscle in culture and formation of elastic fibers. *J Cell Biol* 50:172, 1971.
8. Scharch LW, Skalli O, Seemeyer TA, et al: Intermediate filament proteins and actin isoforms as markers for soft tissue tumour differentiation and origin. 1. Smooth muscle tumors. *Am J Pathol* 128:91, 1987.
9. Skalli O, Ropraz P, Trzeciak A, et al: A monoclonal antibody against alpha smooth muscle actin: a new probe for smooth muscle differentiation. *J Cell Biol* 103:2787, 1986.
10. Uehara Y, Campbell GR, Burnstock G: Cytoplasmic filaments in developing and adult vertebrate smooth muscle. *J Cell Biol* 50:484, 1971.

Cutaneous leiomyoma

11. Archer CB, Whittaker S, Greaves MW: Pharmacological modulation of cold-induced pain in cutaneous leiomyomata. *Br J Dermatol* 118:255, 1988.
12. Auckland G: Hereditary multiple leiomyoma of the skin. *Br J Dermatol* 79:63, 1967.
13. Burton JL, Hartog M: Multiple endocrine adenomatosis (Type I) with cutaneous leiomyomata and cysts of Moll. *Br J Dermatol* 97(suppl 15):75, 1977.
14. Christopherson WM: Solitary cutaneous and subcutaneous leiomyomas. *Arch Surg* 60:779, 1950.
15. Eldor A, Even-Paz Z, Polliak A: Erythrocytosis associated with multiple cutaneous leiomyomata: report of a case with demonstration of erythropoietic activity in the tumour. *Scand J Haematol* 16:245, 1976.
16. Engelke H, Christophers E: Leiomyomatosis cutis et uteri. *Acta Derm Venereol* 59(suppl 85):51, 1979.
17. Fisher WC, Helwig EB: Leiomyomas of the skin. *Arch Dermatol (Chicago)* 88:510, 1963.
18. Fox SR: Leiomyomatosis cutis. *N Engl J Med* 263:1248, 1960.
19. Grenier R, Rostas A, Wilkinson RD: Dermatitis herpetiformis and leiomyomas with HLA-B8, a marker of immune disease. *Can Med Assoc J* 115:882, 1976.
20. Jansen LH, Driessen FML: Leiomyoma cutis. *Br J Dermatol* 70:446, 1958.
21. Katenkamp D, Stiller D: Unusual leiomyoma of the vulva with fibroma-like pattern and pseudoelastin production. *Virchows Arch (Pathol Anat)* 388:361, 1980.
22. Kloepfer HW, Krafchuk J, Derbes V, et al: Hereditary multiple leiomyoma of the skin. *Am J Hum Genet* 10:48, 1958.

23. Libchke JH: Leiomyoma of the breast. *J Pathol* 98:89, 1969.

24. Mann PR: Leiomyoma cutis: an electron microscope study. *Br J Dermatol* 82:463, 1970.

25. Matsubara J, Miura K: Leiomyoma of the scrotum: a case report and review of the literature. *Jpn J Cancer Clin* 17:151,1971.

26. Merrill RG, Downs JR: Oral leiomyomas, report of two cases. *Oral Surg Oral Med Oral Pathol* 23:438, 1967.

27. Montgomery H, Winkelmann RK: Smooth muscle tumors of the skin. *Arch Dermatol* 79:32, 1959.

28. Nascimento AG, Karas M, Rosen PP, et al: Leiomyoma of the nipple. *Am J Surg Pathol* 3:151, 1979.

29. Newman PL, Fletcher CDM: Smooth muscle tumours of the external genitalia: clinicopathologic analysis of a series. *Histopathology* 8:523, 1991.

30. Ormsby OS: Leiomyomatosis cutis. *Arch Dermatol* 11:466, 1925.

31. Prabhakar BR, Davessar K, Chitkara NL, et al: Leiomyoma of the areolar region of the breast. *Ind J Cancer* 6:260, 1969.

32. Siegel GP, Gaffey TA: Solitary leiomyomas arising from the tunica dartos scrotis. *J Urol* 116:69, 1976.

33. Tavassoli FA, Norris HJ: Smooth muscle tumors of the vulva. *Obstet Gynaecol* 53: 213, 1979.

34. Stout AP: Leiomyoma of the oral cavity. *Am J Cancer* 34:31, 1938.

35. Stout AP: Solitary cutaneous and subcutaneous leiomyoma. *Am J Cancer* 24:435, 1937.

36. Venencie PY, Puissant A, Boffa GA, et al: Multiple cutaneous leiomyomata and erythrocytosis. *Br J Dermatol* 107:483,1982.

37. Verma KC, Chawdhry SD, Rathi KS: Cutaneous leiomyomata in two brothers. *Br J Dermatol* 90:351, 1973.

38. Williams ED, Celestin LR: The association of bronchial carcinoid and pluriglandular adenomatosis. *Thorax* 17:120, 1962.

39. Yokayama R, Hashimoto H, Daimaru Y, et al: Superficial leiomyomas: a clinicopathologic study of 34 cases. *Acta Pathol Jpn* 37:1415, 1987.

Angiomyoma (vascular leiomyoma)

40. Bardach H, Ebner H: Das Angioleiomyoma der Haut. *Hautarzt* 26:638, 1975.

41. Carla TG, Filotico R, Filotico M: Bizarre angiomyomas of superficial soft tissues. *Pathologica* 83:237, 1991.

42. Duhig JJ, Ayer JP: Vascular leiomyoma: a study of 61 cases. *Arch Pathol* 68:424, 1959.

43. Ekestrom S: Comparison between glomus tumour and angioleiomyoma. *Acta Pathol Microbiol Scand* 27:86, 1950.

44. Gutmann J, Cifuentes C, Balzarini MA, et al: Angiomyoma of the oral cavity. *Oral Surg Oral Med Oral Pathol* 38:269, 1974.

45. Hachisuga T, Hashimoto H, Enjoji M: Angioleiomyoma: a clinicopathologic reappraisal of 562 cases. *Cancer* 54:126,1984.

Leiomyoma of deep soft tissue

46. Bulmer JH: Smooth muscle tumors of the limbs. *J Bone Joint Surg* 49B: 52, 1967.

47. Cooperman B, McAllister FF, Smith FM: Recurrent calcified leiomyoma of the pelvis and gluteal regions complicated by pregnancy. *J Bone Joint Surg* 40A:1149, 1958.

48. Drew EJ: Large leiomyoma of upper extremity. *Am J Surg* 112:938, 1966.

49. Goodman AH, Briggs RC: Deep leiomyoma of an extremity. *J Bone Joint Surg* 47A:529, 1965.

50. Herrin K, Willen H, Rydholm A: Deep-seated soft tissue leiomyomas: report of four cases. *Skeletal Radiol* 19:363, 1990.

51. Ledesma-Medina J, Oh KS, Girdany BR: Calcification in childhood leiomyoma. *Radiology* 135:339, 1980.

52. Meis JM, Enzinger FM: Myolipoma of soft tissue. *Am J Surg Pathol* 15:121, 1991.

53. Ross LS, Eckstein MR, Hirschhorn R, et al: Calcified leiomyoma: an unusual cause of large soft-tissue calcification of calf in childhood. *NY State J Med* 83:747, 1983.

54. Scurry JP, Carey MP, Targett CS, et al: Soft tissue lipoleiomyoma. *Pathology* 23:360, 1991.

55. Smith JW, Danon A, Radgett D, et al: Leiomyomas of the lower extremity. *Orthopedics* 14:594, 1991.

Intravenous leiomyomatosis

56. Clement PH: Intravenous leiomyomatosis of the uterus. *Pathol Annu* 23:153, 1988.

57. Clement PH, Young RH, Scully, RE: Intravenous leiomyomatosis of the uterus: a clinicopathological analysis of 16 cases with unusual histologic features. *Am J Surg Pathol* 12:932, 1988.

58. Harper RS, Scully RE: Intravenous leiomyomatosis of the uterus. *Obstet Gynecol* 18:519, 1961.

59. Heinonen PK, Taina E, Nerdrum T, et al: Intravenous leiomyomatosis. *Ann Chir Gynaecol* 73:100, 1984.

60. Kawakami S, Sagoh T, Kumada H, et al: Intravenous leiomyomatosis of uterus: MR appearance. *J Comput Assist Tomogr* 15:686, 1991.

61. Norris HJ, Parmley TH: Mesenchymal tumors of the uterus. V. Intravenous leiomyomatosis: a clinical and pathologic study of 14 cases. *Cancer* 36:2164, 1975.

62. Ohmori T, Uraga N, Tavei R, et al: Intravenous leiomyomatosis: a case report emphasizing the vascular component. *Histopathology* 13:470, 1988.

63. Rotter AJ, Lundell CJ: MR of intravenous leiomyomatosis of the uterus extending into the inferior vena cava. *J Comput Assist Tomogr* 15:690, 1991.

64. Scharfenberg JC, Geary WL: Intravenous leiomyomatosis. *Obstet Gynecol* 43:909, 1974.

65. Shida T, Yoshimura M, Chihara H, et al: Intravenous leiomyomatosis of the pelvis and re-extension into the heart. *Ann Thorac Surg* 42:104, 1986.

66. Suginami H, Kaura R, Ochi H, et al: Intravenous leiomyomatosis with cardiac extension: successful surgical management and histopathologic study. *Obstet Gynecol* 76:527, 1990.

67. Tierney WM, Ehrlich CE, Bailey JC, et al: Intravenous leiomyomatosis of the uterus with extension into the heart. *Am J Med* 69:471, 1980.

68. Wolff M, Silva F, Kaye G: Pulmonary metastases (with admixed epithelial elements) from smooth muscle neoplasms: report of nine cases including three males. *Am J Surg Pathol* 3:325,1979.

Leiomyomatosis peritonealis disseminata

69. Akkersdijk GJ, Flu PK, Giard RW, et al: Malignant leiomyomatosis peritonealis disseminata. *Am J Obstet Gynecol* 163: 591, 1990.

70. Aterman K, Fraser GM, Lea RH: Disseminated peritoneal leiomyomatosis. *Virchows Arch (Pathol Anat)* 374:13, 1977.

71. Chen KT, Hendricks EJ, Freeburg B: Benign glandular inclusion of the peritoneum associated with leiomyomatosis peritonealis disseminata. *Diagn Gynecol Obstet* 4:41, 1982.

72. Crosland DB: Leiomyomatosis peritonealis disseminata: a case report. *Am J Obstet Gynecol* 117:179, 1973.

73. Goldberg MF, Hurt WG, Frable WJ: Leiomyomatosis peritonealis disseminata: report of a case and review of the literature. *Obstet Gynecol* 49:46, 1977.

74. Fujii S, Nakashima N, Okamura H, et al: Progesterone-induced smooth muscle–like cells in subperitoneal nodules produced by estrogen: experimental approach to leiomyomatosis peritonealis disseminata. *Am J Obstet Gynecol* 139:164, 1981.

75. Hales HA, Peterson CM, Jones KP, et al: Leiomyomatosis peritonealis disseminata treated with a gonadotropin-releasing hormone agonist: a case report. *Am J Obstet Gynecol* 167:515, 1992.

76. Hovnck van Papendrecht HPCM, Gratam S: Leiomyomatosis peritonealis disseminata. *Eur J Obstet Reprod Biol* 14:251, 1983.

77. Kaplan C, Bernirschke K, Johnson KC: Leiomyomatosis peritonealis disseminata with endometrium. *Obstet Gynecol* 55:119,1980.

78. Kitazawa S, Shiraishi N, Maeda S: Leiomyomatosis peritonealis disseminata with adipocytic differentiation. *Acta Obstet Gynecol Scand* 71:482, 1992.

79. Kuo T, London SN, Dinh TV: Endometriosis occurring in leiomyomatosis peritonealis disseminata: ultrastructural study and histogenetic consideration. *Am J Surg Pathol* 4:197, 1980.

80. Lim OW, Segal A, Ziel HK: Leiomyomatosis peritonealis disseminata associated with pregnancy. *Obstet Gynecol* 55:122,1980.

81. Ma KF, Chow LT: Sex cord–like pattern leiomyomatosis peritonealis disseminata: a hitherto undescribed feature. *Histopathology* 21:389, 1992.

82. Nogales FF, Matilla A, Carrascal E: Leiomyomatosis peritonealis disseminata: an ultrastructural study. *Am J Clin Pathol* 69:452, 1978.

83. Ober WB, Black MB: Neoplasms of subcoelomic mesenchyme. *Arch Pathol Lab Med* 59:698, 1955.

84. O'Sullivan BT: Leiomyomatosis peritonealis disseminata. *Aust N Z J Obstet Gynaecol* 18:94, 1978.

85. Parmley TH, Woodruff JD, Winn K, et al: Histogenesis of leiomyomatosis peritonealis disseminata (disseminated fibrosing deciduosis). *Obstet Gynecol* 46:511, 1975.

86. Pieslor PC, Orenstein JM, Hogan DL, et al: Ultrastructure of myofibroblasts and decidualized cells in leiomyomatosis peritonealis disseminata. *Am J Clin Pathol* 72:875, 1979.

87. Rubin SC, Wheeler JE, Mikuta JJ: Malignant leiomyomatosis peritonealis disseminata. *Obstet Gynecol* 68:126, 1986.

88. Taubert H-D, Wissner SE, Haskins AL: Leiomyomatosis peritonealis disseminata: an unusual complication of genital leiomyomata. *Obstet Gynecol* 25:561, 1965.

89. Tavassoli FA, Norris HJ: Peritoneal leiomyomatosis (leiomyomatosis peritonealis disseminata). *Int J Gynecol Pathol* 1:59, 1982.

90. Valente PT: Leiomyomatosis peritonealis disseminata: a report of two cases and review of the literature. *Arch Pathol Lab Med* 108:669, 1984.

91. Willson JR, Peale AR: Multiple peritoneal leiomyomas associated with a granulosa-cell tumor of the ovary. *Am J Obstet Gynecol* 64:204, 1952.

92. Winn KJ, Woodruff JD, Parmley TH: Electron microscopic studies of leiomyomatosis peritonealis disseminata. *Obstet Gynecol* 48:225, 1976.

Palisaded myofibroblastoma

93. Alguacil-Garcia A: Intranodal myofibroblastoma in a submandibular lymph node: a case report. *Am J Clin Pathol* 97:69, 1992.

94. Barbareschi M, Mariscotti C, Ferrero S, et al: Intranodal hemorrhagic spindle cell tumor: a benign Kaposi-like nodal tumor. *Histopathology* 17:93, 1990.

95. Bigotti G, Coli A, Mottolese M, et al: Selective location of palisaded myofibroblastoma with amianthoid fibres. *J Clin Pathol* 44:761, 1991.

96. Burns MK, Headington JT, Rasmussen JE: Palisaded myofibroblastoma simulating chronic primary lymphadenopathic Kaposi's sarcoma. *J Am Acad Dermatol* 25:566, 1991.

97. Deligdish L, Loewenthal M, Friedlaender E: Malignant neurilemoma (schwannoma) in the lymph nodes. *Int Surg* 49:226, 1968.

98. Fletcher CD, Stirling RW: Intranodal myofibroblastoma presenting in the submandibular region: evidence of a broader clinical and histological spectrum. *Histopathology* 16:287, 1990.

99. Katz D: Neurilemoma with calcerosiderotic nodules. *Israel J Med Sci* 10:1156, 1974.

100. Lee JY-Y, Abell E, Shevechek GJ: Solitary spindle cell tumor with myoid differentiation of lymph node. *Arch Pathol Lab Med* 113:547, 1989.

101. Michal M, Chlumska A, Povysilova V: Intranodal "amianthoid" myofibroblastoma: report of six cases with immunohisochemical and electron microscopical study. *Pathol Res Pract* 188:199, 1992.

102. Skalova A, Michal M, Chlumska A, et al: Collagen composition and ultrastructure of the so-called amianthoid fibres in palisaded myofibroblastoma: ultrastructural and immunohistochemical study. *J Pathol* 167:335, 1992.

103. Suster S, Rosai J: Intranodal hemorrhagic spindle-cell tumor with "amianthoid" fibers: report of six cases of a distinctive mesenchymal neoplasm of the inguinal region that simulates Kaposi's sarcoma. *Am J Surg Pathol* 13:347, 1989.

104. Weiss SW, Gnepp DR, Bratthauer GL: Palisaded myofibroblastoma: a benign mesenchymal tumor of lymph node. *Am J Surg Pathol* 13:341, 1989.

Myofibroblastoma of the breast

105. Amin MB, Gottlieb CA, Fitzmaurice M, et al: Fine-needle aspiration cytologic study of myofibroblastoma of the breast: immunohistochemical and ultrastructural findings. *Am J Clin Pathol* 99:593, 1993.

106. Begin LR: Myogenic stromal tumor of the male breast (so-called myofibroblastoma). *Ultrstruct Pathol* 15:613, 1991.

107. Lee AH, Sworn MJ, Theaker JM, et al: Myofibroblastoma of breast: immunohistochemical study. *Histopathology* 22:75, 1993.

108. Wargotz ES, Weiss SW, Norris HJ: Myofibroblastoma of the breast: sixteen cases of a distinctive benign mesenchymal tumor. *Am J Surg Pathol* 11:493, 1987.

Angiomyofibroblastoma

109. Fletcher CD, Tsang WY, Fisher C, et al: Angiomyofibroblastoma of the vulva: a benign neoplasm distinct from aggressive angiomyxoma. *Am J Surg Pathol* 16:373, 1992.

110. Hiruki T, Thomas MJ, Clement PB: Vulvar angiomyofibroblastoma. *Am J Surg Pathol* 17:423, 1993.

CHAPTER 19

LEIOMYOSARCOMA

Leiomyosarcomas account for between 5% and 10% of soft tissue sarcomas.[10,28,42] They are principally tumors of adult life, but they are far outnumbered by the more common adult sarcomas such as liposarcoma and malignant fibrous histiocytoma. Likewise, they are less common than leiomyosarcomas of uterine or gastrointestinal origin, and only some of the data gleaned from the collective experience with tumors in these two sites are directly applicable to the soft tissue counterpart. Few predisposing or etiological factors are recognized in this disease. In general, these tumors are more common in women than men. About two thirds of all retroperitoneal leiomyosarcomas[40,43,48] and over three fourths of all vena cava leiomyosarcomas occur in women.[94] The significance of this observation is not clear, although growth and proliferation of smooth muscle tissue in women have been noted to coincide with pregnancy as well as estrogenic stimulation (see Chapter 18). Children rarely develop these tumors,[4,34,39] but when they do, the prognosis seems to be similar to that of adults,[2] despite some reports to the contrary.[39]

Reports in the literature as well as our experience at the AFIP indicate that leiomyosarcomas are rarely induced by radiation.[12,32,54,58] Such tumors are largely curiosities, and it is much more common to see fibrosarcomas, osteosarcomas, and malignant fibrous histiocytomas induced by radiation. Leiomyosarcomas may develop as a second malignancy in the setting of bilateral (hereditary) retinoblastoma. In the past some have attributed this to radiation,[8] but we have seen these tumors develop well outside the field of radiation and believe them to be the direct result of deletions in the RB1 locus. A recent study by Stratton et al.[33] indicates that deletions or mutations of the RB1 locus can be identified in a small number of leiomyosarcomas that occur on a sporadic basis.

There is little evidence that leiomyomas undergo malignant transformation with any degree of regularity. Well-differentiated areas resembling leiomyoma are often found within a leiomyosarcoma, but this by no means proves that malignant transformation occurred. In fact, the predilection of leiomyosarcomas for deep soft tissue as opposed to the superficial location of leiomyomas provides some evidence to the contrary. Leiomyosarcomas have also been associated with the production of beta-human chorionic gonadotropin.[15] Experimentally the tumors may be induced in rabbits by intramuscular deposition of nickel subsulphide.[11] One alleged leiomyosarcoma occurred on the diaphragmatic surface of an asbestos worker, although the illustrations in this case cast some doubt on the diagnosis.[5]

Although all leiomyosarcomas of soft tissue are histologically similar, it is useful to divide them into three geographic groups because of certain clinical and biological differences. The location of leiomyosarcoma is important in determining the prognosis. *Leiomyosarcomas of deep soft tissue,* particularly the retroperitoneum, are the most common group and serve as the prototype, since they illustrate best the range of histological changes common to these tumors, the problems inherent in histological evaluation, and occasionally the inability to predict biological behavior from the histological appearance alone. *Leiomyosarcomas of cutaneous and subcutaneous tissue* are a second group, usually having a good prognosis because of their superficial location. They can be likened to atypical fibroxanthoma and superficial forms of malignant fibrous histiocytoma (Chapter 15), which have a highly atypical appearance but a favorable clinical course because of their limited clinical stage. The last group is *leiomyosarcomas of vascular origin,* which are relatively rare. These tumors usually arise in association with medium-sized or large veins.

LEIOMYOSARCOMAS OF DEEP SOFT TISSUE

Leiomyosarcomas of deep soft tissue arise principally in the retroperitoneal space and abdominal cavity. According to Golden and Stout[40] and the Soft Tissue Task Force,[28] about half of all soft tissue leiomyosarcomas occur in the retroperitoneum, making it the single most common soft tissue site. Leiomyosarcomas also occur in intraabdominal locations such as the omentum and mesentery[45,51] and infrequently in deep soft tissue sites unrelated to vessels. Smooth muscle tumors presenting as pedunculated masses attached to the serosal surfaces of the viscera, particularly the stomach, are traditionally considered gastrointestinal tract lesions and are not included in the present discussion.

Clinical findings

About two thirds of retroperitoneal leiomyosarcomas occur in women.[48] The median age at the time of presentation is 60 years,[48] a finding that is roughly comparable to other retroperitoneal sarcomas such as liposarcomas and malignant fibrous histiocytoma. This contrasts with the younger age of patients with gastrointestinal leiomyosarcomas, which probably become symptomatic at an earlier

stage. The presenting signs and symptoms are relatively nonspecific and include an abdominal mass or swelling, pain, weight loss, nausea, or vomiting. By means of CT scan and angiography the lesions can be localized to the retroperitoneal space, although they cannot be distinguished from other retroperitoneal sarcomas.[41] They appear hypovascular or moderately vascular and derive their main arterial supply from the lumbar arteries, with ancillary supply from vessels such as the celiac, superior mesenteric, inferior mesenteric, and renal arteries. Displacement and distortion of normal vessels are common findings, and in some cases neovascularity may also be observed.[41] The use

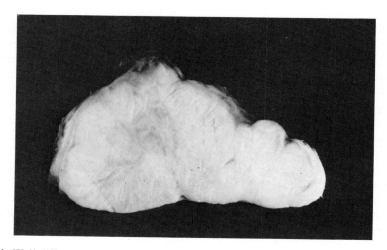

FIG. 19-1. Well-differentiated leiomyosarcoma displaying a whorled appearance similar to a leiomyoma on cut section.

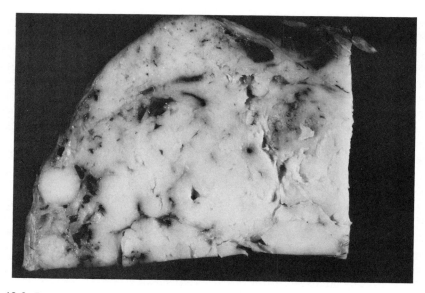

FIG. 19-2. Poorly differentiated leiomyosarcoma characterized by fleshy white tissue with hemorrhage and necrosis.

of indium-111-antimyosin, which is taken up by neoplastic muscle cells, has been suggested as a means of identifying these tumors preoperatively.[4] At surgery the masses are usually quite large and often unresectable. In our experience with 36 leiomyosarcomas of the retroperitoneum, the mean size was about 16 cm, with a range of 7.5 to 35 cm and an average weight of approximately 1600 g.[48] They commonly involve other structures such as the kidney, pancreas, and vertebral column by direct extension. Some tumors have a white-gray whorled appearance resembling a leiomyoma on cut sections (Fig. 19-1). More often the tumors are fleshy white-gray masses with foci of hemorrhage and necrosis and are therefore indistinguishable from other sarcomas (Fig. 19-2). Cysts may be present and occasionally are so striking that these tumors may be mistaken on gross inspection for cystic neurilemomas.

Compared with retroperitoneal lesions, tumors arising from the deep soft tissues of the extremities are far less common and seem to affect the sexes equally. Only 27 cases were identified by Gustafson et al.[10] in a 22-year review of a Swedish population in Lund. These tumors present as an enlarging mass, usually in the lower extremity. Although on gross inspection they resemble those in the retroperitoneum, they are usually considerably smaller (8 cm) when diagnosed initially.

Microscopic findings

As a group retroperitoneal and deep soft tissue leiomyosarcomas probably display the greatest variety of patterns of any soft tissue leiomyosarcomas. The typical cell of the leiomyosarcoma is elongated and has an abundant cytoplasm that varies tinctorially from pink to deep red in sections stained with hematoxylin-eosin stain. The nucleus is usually centrally located and blunt ended or "cigar shaped" (Fig. 19-3, A). In some smooth muscle cells a vacuole may be seen at one end of the nucleus, causing a slight indentation so that the nucleus assumes a concave rather than a convex contour (Figs. 19-3, A, 19-4, and 19-5). In less well-differentiated tumors the nucleus is larger and more hyperchromatic and often loses its central location (Figs. 19-3, B, and 19-6). Multinucleated giant cells are common. Likewise, depending on the degree of differentiation, the appearance of the cytoplasm varies. Differentiated cells have numerous well-oriented myofibrils that are demonstrable as deep red, longitudinally placed parallel lines running the length of the cell on staining with the Masson trichrome stain (Fig. 19-7). With phosphotungstic acid-hematoxylin (PTAH) staining the striations are purple. In poorly differentiated cells the longitudinal striations are less numerous, poorly oriented, and therefore more difficult to identify. In some tumors the cytoplasm may have a "clotted" appearance as a result of clumping of the myofilamentous material (Fig. 19-8). When this phenomenon occurs it may be quite difficult to identify linear striations. Glycogen can usually be demonstrated (PAS) within the cytoplasm of leiomyosarcomas (Fig. 19-9, A), and in better differentiated tumors a delicate reticulin network is present between cells (Fig. 19-9, B).

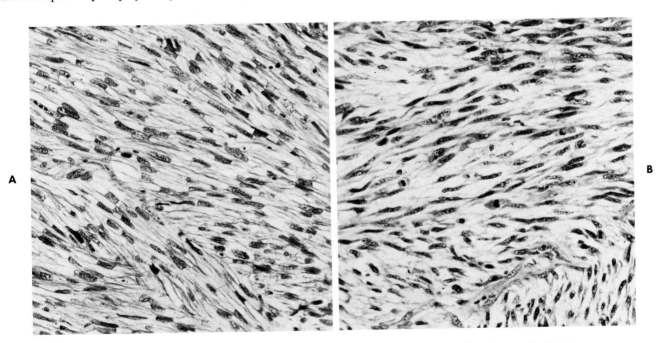

FIG. 19-3. A, Cytological features of well-differentiated leiomyosarcoma showing regular blunt-ended nuclei; occasional cells have perinuclear vacuoles. (×250.) **B,** Less well-differentiated leiomyosarcoma showing more pleomorphic nuclei and darkly staining cytoplasm. (×250.)

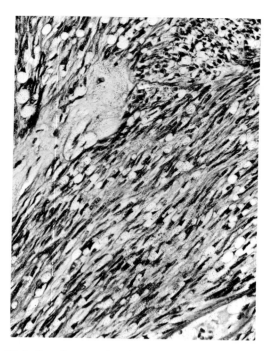

FIG. 19-4. Prominent perinuclear vacuolization within a leiomyosarcoma. Nuclei may become indented by vacuoles. (×250.)

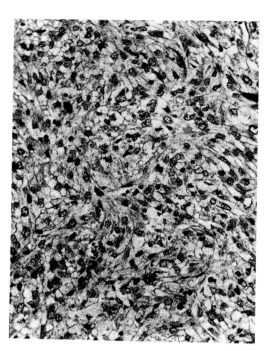

FIG. 19-5. Leiomyosarcoma composed of short fascicles of cells with perinuclear vacuoles. Tumors with this appearance are occasionally mistaken for clear cell carcinoma of kidney with spindling. (×180.)

As a rule, most retroperitoneal and soft tissue leiomyosarcomas are moderately differentiated tumors, often displaying sharply marginated borders (Fig. 19-10). They are composed of slender or slightly plump cells that are arranged in fascicles of varying sizes. In well-differentiated areas the fascicles intersect at right angles so that it is possible to see transverse and longitudinal sections side by side, similar to the pattern of a uterine myoma (Fig. 19-11). In most areas, however, the pattern is never that orderly, and it more closely resembles the intertwining fascicular growth of a fibrosarcoma (Fig. 19-12). In occasional leiomyosarcomas the nuclei may align themselves so as to create palisades similar to a neurilemoma (Fig. 19-13). These tumors can pose considerable problems in differential diagnosis. The staining characteristics of the cells, including the presence of cytoplasmic glycogen and linear striations and the absence of S-100 protein, may ultimately be the only means of distinguishing well-differentiated leiomyosarcomas with palisading from neurilemomas. Hyalinization is a relatively common, but usually focal, feature of many leiomyosarcomas (Fig. 19-14). The number of mitotic figures varies greatly, but over 80% of retroperitoneal leiomyosarcomas average 5 or more mitoses per 10 high-power fields (HPF)[48] (see criteria of malignancy, below). A small number of retroperitoneal leiomyosarcomas are anaplastic tumors, superficially resembling malignant fi-

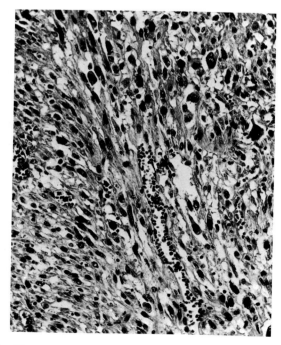

FIG. 19-6. Poorly differentiated leiomyosarcoma showing ill-defined fascicles made up of rather pleomorphic cells. (×180.)

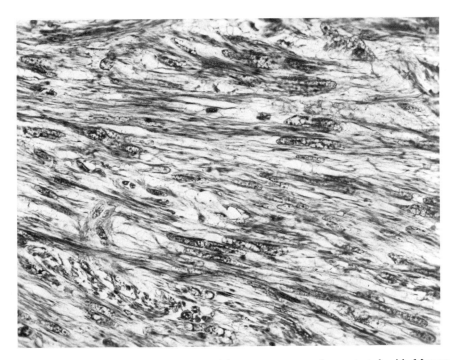

FIG. 19-7. Longitudinal striations within a leiomyosarcoma as demonstrated with Masson trichrome stain. (×400.)

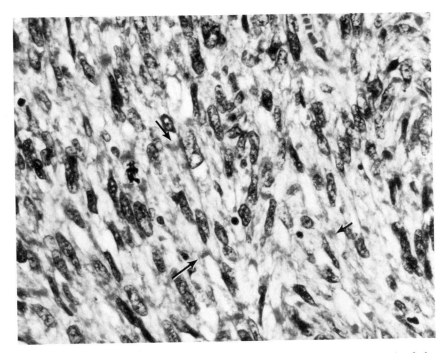

FIG. 19-8. Leiomyosarcoma showing "clotted" appearance of cytoplasm as a result of clumping of myofibrils *(arrows)*. (×400.)

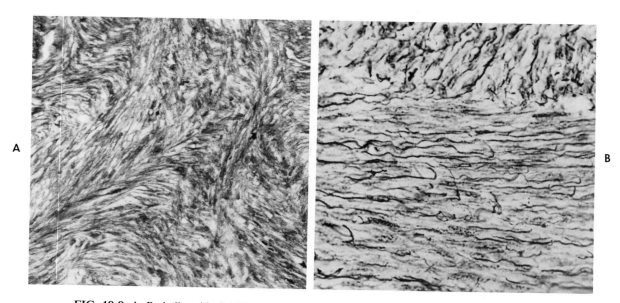

FIG. 19-9. A, Periodic acid–Schiff stain showing glycogen deposits throughout cytoplasm of leiomyosarcoma. (×160.) **B,** Reticulin preparation illustrating fine interstitial fibers in leiomyosarcoma. (×250.)

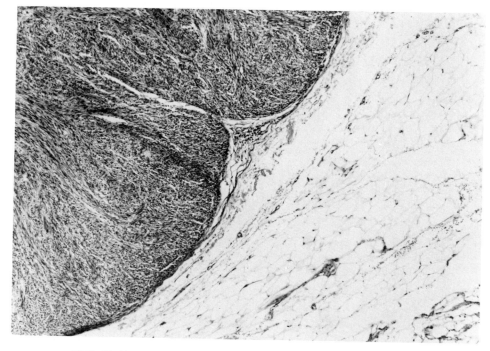

FIG. 19-10. Sharply marginated border of a leiomyosarcoma. (×100.)

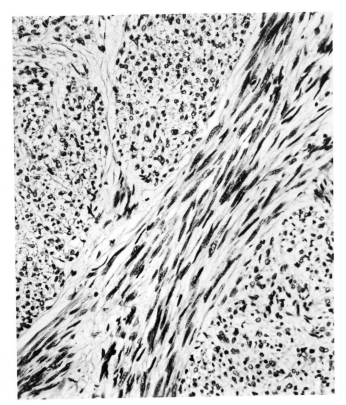

FIG. 19-11. Relatively well-differentiated leiomyosarcoma depicting fascicles of cells intersecting each other at right angles. (×250.)

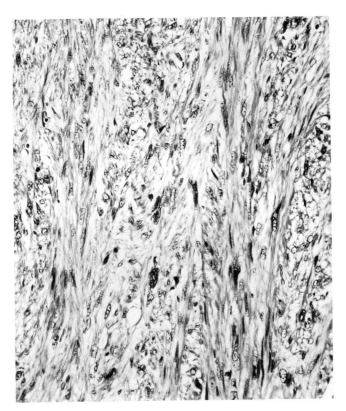

FIG. 19-12. Moderately well-differentiated leiomyosarcoma with less orderly fascicular pattern than is seen in Fig. 19-11 and more pleomorphism of cells. (×250.)

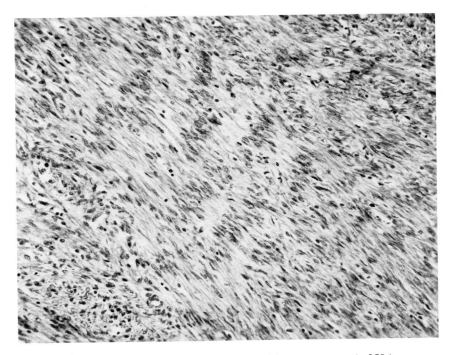

FIG. 19-13. Nuclear palisading within a leiomyosarcoma. (×250.)

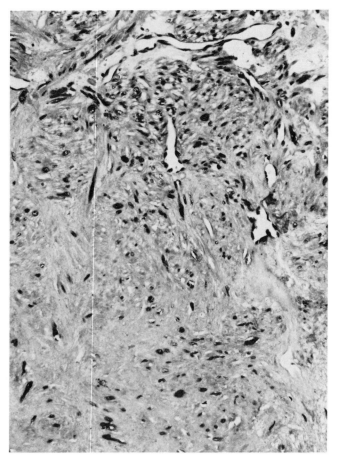

FIG. 19-14. Leiomyosarcoma showing extensive hyalinization. (×160.)

brous histiocytoma (Figs. 19-15 to 19-17). They contain numerous pleomorphic giant cells with deeply eosinophilic cytoplasm intimately admixed with a complement of more uniform-appearing spindled and rounded cells (Fig. 19-17). In contrast to malignant fibrous histiocytoma, these tumors have less interstitial collagen, few inflammatory cells, and at least some cytoplasmic glycogen. In addition, it is usually possible to document myogenic differentiation within the less pleomorphic cells. Necrosis, hemorrhage, and mitotic figures are frequent in these pleomorphic tumors. Osteoclastic giant cells are an infrequent feature of leiomyosarcomas.[37] Sarcomas with combined features of liposarcoma and leiomyosarcoma have been reported recently.[49]

Epithelioid leiomyosarcoma

There are several distinctly uncommon features in leiomyosarcomas. "Epithelioid changes" may occur in smooth muscle tumors. The cells become rounded, and there is often a concomitant "vacuolar" or "clear cell" change in the cytoplasm. This feature may be seen focally in otherwise

typical smooth muscle tumors. Tumors composed predominantly or exclusively of epithelioid smooth muscle cells are also termed *leiomyoblastoma* and are discussed in detail in Chapter 20.

Myxoid leiomyosarcoma

Myxoid change may occur within leiomyosarcomas. It is occasionally so extensive that the tumors appear grossly gelatinous. Although these so-called myxoid leiomyosarcomas have been reported most commonly in the uterus,[45,47] they do develop in conventional soft tissue locations as well. The spindled muscle cells are separated by pools of hyaluronic acid, and in cross-section the fascicles may resemble the cords of tumor seen in a myxoid chondrosarcoma (Figs. 19-18 and 19-19). Because these tumors are quite hypocellular relative to conventional leiomyosarcomas, mitotic rates estimated by counting high-power fields are usually deceptively low, giving the false impression of benignancy. In the experience of King et al.[45] tumors averaging between 0 and 2 mitoses/10 HPF have proved to be aggressive. Four of their six patients died of disease, one was alive with disease, and one died of other causes but was known to have residual tumor at death. Thus these tumors must be considered fully malignant. It is quite possible that spillage of the gelatinous matrix at the time of surgery contributes to the common phenomenon of local recurrence.

Granular cell leiomyosarcoma

Rarely leiomyosarcomas contain cells with granular eosinophilic cytoplasm.[21] This change corresponds to the presence of numerous granules that stain positively for PAS and are resistant to diastase and ultrastructurally are similar to the phagolysosomes seen in granular cell tumor.

Criteria of malignancy

Determining suitable criteria of malignancy in smooth muscle tumors is a difficult problem because these tumors represent a biological continuum in which one is forced to draw certain arbitrary lines in designating some "benign" and others "malignant." Although a number of features such as size, cellularity, atypia, and necrosis correlate to some extent with malignancy, none seems to be as accurate or as reproducible in predicting metastasis as mitotic activity.[46,48] Consequently it is this feature that we rely on most heavily in evaluating these tumors. The importance of a representative mitotic rate obviously implies that smooth muscle tumors of soft tissue be carefully sampled as has been recommended for uterine lesions. Actual levels of mitotic activity that seem to be suitable in evaluating uterine tumors are not valid for soft tissue tumors, as they would result in a significant level of underdiagnosis. For instance, uterine lesions having between 5 and 9 mitoses/10 HPF are considered borderline lesions,[94] but in soft tissue this level

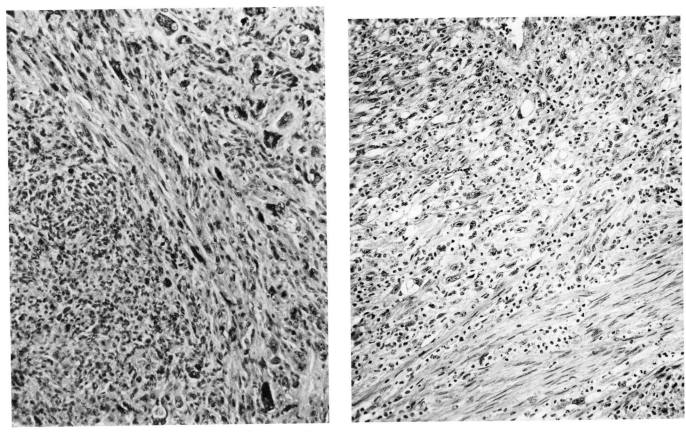

FIG. 19-15. Leiomyosarcoma with pleomorphic areas that resemble a malignant fibrous histiocytoma *(top right)*. (×160.)

FIG. 19-16. Leiomyosarcoma with pleomorphic areas resembling inflammatory form of malignant fibrous histiocytoma. (×160.)

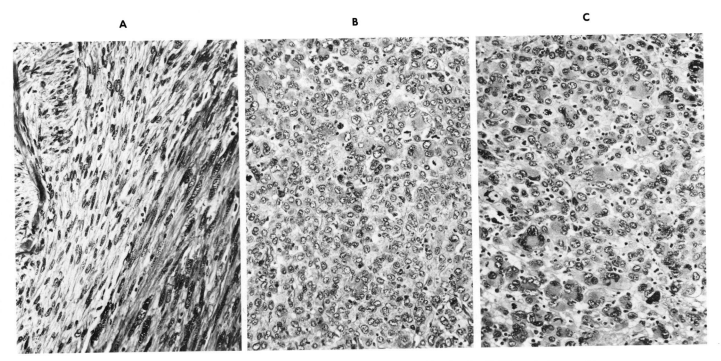

FIG. 19-17. Leiomyosarcoma containing well-differentiated **(A)**, round cell **(B)**, and pleomorphic areas **(C)**. (**A** to **C**, ×160.)

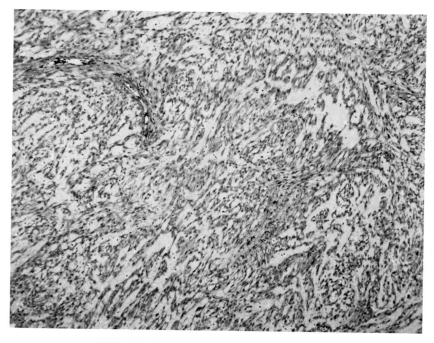

FIG. 19-18. Myxoid leiomyosarcoma. (×100.)

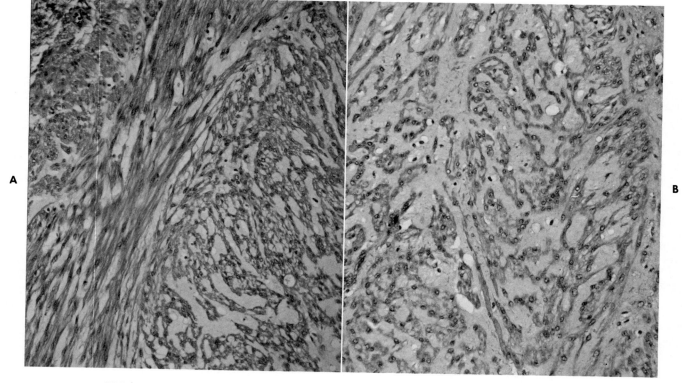

FIG. 19-19. A, Myxoid leiomyosarcoma showing separation of spindled cells. **B,** In cross-section myxoid leiomyosarcomas may have a cordlike pattern reminiscent of myxoid chondrosarcomas. (**A** and **B,** ×250.)

of mitotic activity almost always signifies a tumor that is capable of metastasis.[48] Retroperitoneal smooth muscle tumors having 5 mitoses/10 HPF should be considered malignant, since most patients with tumors of this type will succumb to the disease in our experience. Tumors having between 1 and 4 mitoses/10 HPF are best considered potentially malignant, especially if they are large and have areas of necrosis and significant nuclear atypia. Unfortunately, even when these stringent criteria are used, it is never possible to be absolutely certain about the benignity of large smooth muscle tumors of soft tissue, even if their histological features lead one to conclude they are benign. In our experience histologically benign smooth muscle tumors of the retroperitoneum have metastasized after long latent periods of 30 to 40 years, leading us to conclude that the vast majority of retroperitoneal smooth muscle tumors are potentially malignant. It is essential, however, to be certain of the precise location in evaluating smooth muscle tumors presumed to be of retroperitoneal origin, since mitotically active leiomyomas that have become detached from the uterus or parametria may be confused with a well-

differentiated leiomyosarcoma (see Chapter 18). Moreover, as recently emphasized by Wolff et al.,[38] many lesions formerly regarded as "leiomyomas" or "fibroleiomyomatous hamartomas" of the lung are in actuality metastases from extremely well-differentiated leiomyosarcomas of soft tissue or uterine origin in which mitotic rates were less than 1/10 HPF.

Ultrastructural and immunohistochemical findings

Leiomyosarcomas are characterized by many of the same features as normal smooth muscle cells, but in general they are less developed. Differentiated leiomyosarcomas have deeply clefted nuclei and numerous well-oriented, thin (6 to 8 nm) myofilaments and dense bodies that occupy a large portion of the cell (Fig. 19-20). Pinocytotic vesicles and intercellular connections are conspicuous, and basal lamina invests the entire cell membrane. The presence of these features is diagnostic of smooth muscle cell, even without the benefit of the light microscopic findings. On the other hand, poorly differentiated tumors show a loss of myofilaments as rough endoplasmic reticulum and free ribosomes

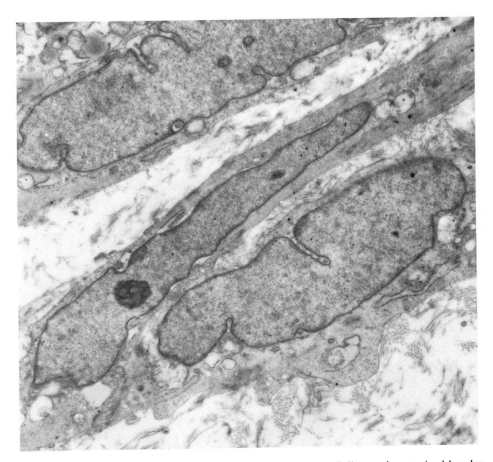

FIG. 19-20. Electron micrograph of metastatic leiomyosarcoma. Cells are characterized by elongated shape, deeply grooved nuclei, and numerous thin filaments with dense bodies.

assume greater prominence.[7] Pinocytotic vesicles and intercellular attachments are sparse, and basal lamina may be incomplete or lacking altogether. In these tumors all of these features must be evaluated in toto and interpreted in conjunction with the light microscopic findings for diagnostic purposes. The importance of the light microscopic findings should not be minimized in these situations because some leiomyosarcomas may assume "a diagnostic growth pattern at the light microscopic level prior to or possibly without developing the specific organelles of smooth muscle cells."[18] On the other hand, it should be emphasized that the mere presence of thin myofilaments with dense bodies does not identify a smooth muscle cell. Thin myofilaments are a nonspecific finding and can be seen in a variety of tumors where they typically occur beneath the cytoplasmic membrane.

Localization of muscle antigens by means of immunohistochemistry has become an increasingly popular adjunctive procedure in the diagnosis of these neoplasms. Over the last several years issues have been raised concerning the specificity and sensitivity of various muscle antigens and their related antibodies in diagnosis. The appearance of commercially available antibodies that perform well on formalin-fixed tissues has, to a large extent, ameliorated the situation, yet it is imperative that the pathologist be aware of the distribution of various muscle antigens within normal nonmuscle tissues so as to avoid serious errors in diagnosis. Muscle specific actin (HHF35)[36] can be detected within most leiomyosarcomas.[1,25,34,65] Desmin is more variable, however, and has been documented in half[1] to nearly one hundred percent of tumors,[65] depending on the series. Although there seems to be general agreement that the presence of desmin diffusely throughout a tumor is usually indicative of myoid differentiation, the presence of either actin or desmin focally should not necessarily be equated with myoid lineage, since myofibroblasts in a variety of neoplastic and nonneoplastic conditions also display this phenotype.[29,30] It has also been demonstrated that tumors with definite ultrastructural features of leiomyosarcomas may lack both antigens. Smooth muscle tumors are also one of the mesenchymal lesions in which keratin immunoreactivity has been reported.[3,16,17,23] The immunoreactivity is usually localized to a perinuclear zone and coexists with desmin. This immunoreactivity is due to the presence of keratins 8 and 18,[16] which are present in simple (nonstratified) epithelium and some mesenchymal tissues. Other antigens that have been sporadically identified within leiomyosarcomas include S-100 protein, Leu-7, myelin basic protein, epithelial membrane antigen, and cathepsin B.[65]

Differential diagnosis

The differential diagnosis of leiomyosarcomas traditionally includes other sarcomas that are composed of fascicles

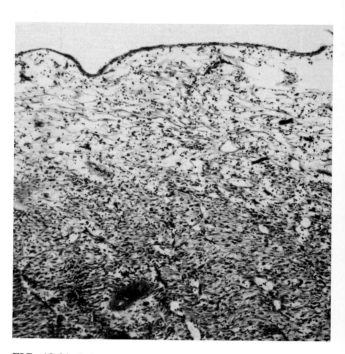

FIG. 19-21. Inflammatory fibromyxoid pseudotumor of bladder showing submucosal myxoid area with deeper cellular area. (×15.)

of moderately differentiated spindle cells, such as fibrosarcoma and malignant schwannoma. Although the low-power appearance of all three can be quite similar, there is usually a greater tendency to see a close juxtaposition of longitudinally and transversely cut fascicles in a leiomyosarcoma. The cytological features play a more important role in differential diagnosis, however. Compared with the cells of leiomyosarcoma, those of a fibrosarcoma tend to be tapered, whereas those of a malignant schwannoma are wavy, buckled, and distinctly asymmetrical. Usually neither malignant schwannomas nor fibrosarcomas contain glycogen, and although both occasionally display fuchsinophilia of the cytoplasm, neither has longitudinal striations. There are, in addition to the above lesions, reactive fibroblastic lesions occurring in the submucosa of various parenchymal organs, which are commonly confused with leiomyosarcomas or even rhabdomyosarcomas. Many of these lesions have been reported in the bladder, where some have been associated with prior instrumentation. We have also encountered them in the vagina, endometrium, larynx, and oral cavity. They have been termed *postoperative spindle cell nodule,*[24] *inflammatory pseudotumor,*[22] and *pseudosarcomatous fibromyxoid tumor.*[26] They are composed of bipolar or stellate fibroblasts, having bizarre nuclei and a light basophilic cytoplasm, set in a myxoid stroma containing inflammatory cells (Figs. 19-21 and 19-22). Mitotic figures may be encountered, although atypical mitotic figures are not seen.

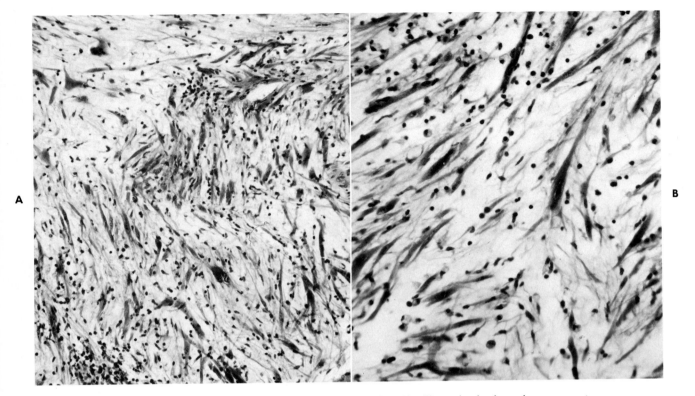

FIG. 19-22. Inflammatory fibromyxoid pseudotumor of bladder illustrating haphazard arrangement of fibroblasts and scattered inflammatory cells (**A**). Cells have bipolar or multipolar shape and prominent nuclei and nucleoli (**B**). (**A**, ×160; **B**, ×250.)

The principal features that we have found helpful in distinguishing these bizarre reactive lesions from leiomyosarcoma are the less-ordered arrangement of the cells with respect to one another, the basophilic hue of the cytoplasm, and the absence of distinct linear striations. In the limited number of cases we have studied, the cells have been strongly positive for vimentin but negative for desmin.

Behavior and treatment

Retroperitoneal leiomyosarcomas are a highly aggressive group of tumors that are often so large that total resection is impossible. Consequently, they may cause death not only by distant metastasis but also by local extension. The survival figures differ in various series and are obviously influenced by the criteria of malignancy, proportion of high-grade versus low-grade tumors, and length of the follow-up period. Kay and McNeill[44] reported a survival rate of nil; Wile et al.,[50] 6%; Ranchod and Kempson,[46] 16% (with a 2-year follow-up period); and Shmookler and Lauer reported 29% (from 5-year actuarial data).[48] In our experience with 30 cases with follow-up data, 17 developed distant metastasis, with the liver and the lung being the two most common sites.[48] Other sites include the skin, soft tissue, and bone. The behavior of leiomyosarcomas in deep soft tissues of the extremities is far better than those of the retroperitoneum. Gustafson et al.[10] report a 64% 5-year survival rate. Independent risk factors for tumor-related deaths included age over 60 years and intratumoral vascular invasion. Although not statistically significant, DNA aneuploidy and tumor necrosis were also associated with a poor prognosis.

CUTANEOUS AND SUBCUTANEOUS LEIOMYOSARCOMAS

Superficial leiomyosarcomas account for 2% to 3% of all superficial soft tissue sarcomas.[64] They occur at almost any age but are most common between the fifth and seventh decades. Although Stout and Hill[64] originally commented on the predilection of the tumors for women, recent reports indicate the disease is far more common in men by a ratio of 2:1 or 3:1.[54] Like their benign counterparts, they usually occur on the extremities and show a predilection for the hair-bearing extensor surfaces.[54] Unlike subcutaneous leiomyomas, most are solitary lesions, and the presence of multiple superficial leiomyosarcomas should always suggest the possibility of metastasis from another soft tissue site such as the retroperitoneum.[42] In a few cases the tumor has developed at the site of previous irradiation.[54,58] Superficial leiomyosarcomas should be divided into two groups: those which are predominantly or exclusively intradermal (cutaneous) and those which involve the subcutis. Cutaneous tumors are usually quite small, averaging less than 2 cm when first detected. They often produce surface changes in the overlying epidermis such as discoloration, umbilication, and ulceration. Subcutaneous tumors, on the other hand, grow faster, achieve a larger size by the time of biopsy, and produce few changes in the skin aside from elevation. Pain is usually a prominent symptom in both types. Because of the rarity of these lesions, they are seldom correctly diagnosed preoperatively.

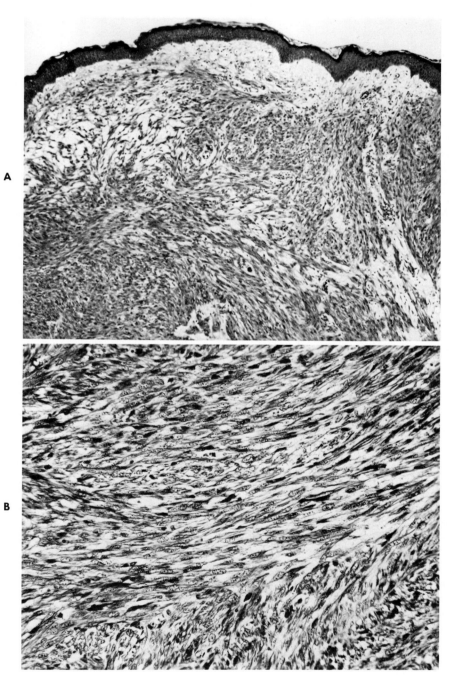

FIG. 19-23. Superficial leiomyosarcoma arising from dermis. (**A,** ×60; **B,** ×160.)

Gross and microscopic findings

Grossly, these leiomyosarcomas usually have a gray-white whorled appearance and a varying degree of circumscription. Those in the dermis appear ill-defined by virtue of the intricate blending of tumor fascicles with the surrounding collagen and pilar arrector muscle. Those in the subcutis, in contrast, appear circumscribed owing to the fact that they compress the surrounding tissue, creating a pseudocapsule. Most superficial leiomyosarcomas resemble retroperitoneal leiomyosarcomas in basic organization (Fig. 19-23). Most are moderately well-differentiated tumors, differing principally by the lack of regressive or degenerative changes. Hemorrhage, necrosis, hyalinization, and myxoid change are rarely encountered, and this is probably a reflection of the smaller size of these lesions. Giant cells may be present, but, as in retroperitoneal tumors, it is rather uncommon to encounter a tumor that has a predominantly pleomorphic appearance. Mitotic figures, including atypical forms, are easily identified within these tumors. In the largest series reported by Fields and Helwig,[54] 80% of these tumors had more than 2 mitoses/10 HPF. We have generally employed the same criteria of histological malignancy for these tumors as has been proposed earlier for retroperitoneal tumors, recognizing that the better course of these tumors is directly attributable to the superficial location and small size, rather than to intrinsic histological differences.

Behavior and treatment

The behavior of this tumor is quite good and is analogous to the favorable prognosis in other forms of sarcomas that are restricted to the superficial soft tissue (see Chapter 15). Although recurrences develop in almost half of the patients,[54] metastases are infrequent and seem to correlate well with the depth of the original tumor. In the experience of Fields and Helwig,[54] tumors confined to the dermis did not metastasize, whereas those involving the subcutis metastasized in one third of the cases. This same trend was noted by Dahl and Angervall,[53] who observed metastasis in about 10% of cutaneous lesions and 40% of subcutaneous lesions. The high rate of metastasis (50%) noted in the early report of Stout and Hill[64] reflects the fact that most of their cases were subcutaneous lesions and some even penetrated deep soft tissue, a phenomenon that substantially alters the outcome for the worse. Metastatic spread occurs hematogenously to the lung, although regional lymph nodes were noted in about 25% of Stout and Hill's cases[64] and have been noted in sporadic case reports.[63]

Because many of these lesions are potentially curable, every effort should be made to eradicate the tumor initially with wide excision. Lesions allowed to recur run an increased risk of eventual metastasis because there is a distinct tendency for recurrent lesions to be larger and to involve deeper structures.[54] Radiotherapy has been employed, but it has not been particularly efficacious.[62]

LEIOMYOSARCOMAS OF VASCULAR ORIGIN

Leiomyosarcomas of vascular origin comprise a seemingly rare group of tumors as illustrated by the fact that only a few hundred cases have been reported in the literature since the initial report by Perl in 1871, and only isolated instances are recorded in several large autopsy series. Hallock et al.[82] noted one case in 34,000 autopsies from the University of Minnesota; Abell[68] reported 2 out of 14,000 autopsies at the University of Pennsylvania; and Dorfman and Fisher[78] found none out of 30,000 autopsies at the Johns Hopkins Hospital. Yet it should be emphasized that several features of this disease probably significantly affect its detection, diagnosis, and incidence. Lesions arising from major vessels such as the vena cava are most likely to produce symptoms leading to their detection. Conversely, tumors arising from small vessels, vessels subserved by ancillary tributaries, or vessels in deep locations probably go unrecognized in a significant percentage of cases. It is difficult, therefore, to be certain what percentage of leiomyosarcomas of the retroperitoneum or other deep soft tissue sites may actually be of vascular origin. Hashimoto et al.[42] recently documented that at least one quarter of leiomyosarcomas of peripheral soft tissue in their experience arose from or involved a vessel. Thus the recorded experience with vascular leiomyosarcomas is a rather biased one, which probably underestimates the true incidence and possibly also conveys a false impression concerning clinical behavior.

Clinical findings

The frequency distribution of vascular leiomyosarcomas parallels in a crudely inverse fashion the pressure within the vascular bed. Leiomyosarcomas are most common in large veins such as the vena cava, far less common in the pulmonary artery, and exceedingly rare in systemic arteries. In the extensive review published by Kevorkian and Cento[94] of cases reported up to the early 1970s, 33 cases arose in the inferior vena cava, whereas 35 collectively affected other medium-sized or large veins. Ten occurred in the pulmonary artery alone, and eight arose in systemic arteries. One report has indicated the unique occurrence of a leiomyosarcoma in a surgically created arteriovenous fistula.[113] The symptoms related to these tumors are diverse and are determined by the location of the tumor, rate of growth, and degree of collateral blood flow or drainage in an affected part.

Inferior vena cava leiomyosarcoma

These tumors occur in mid- or late-adult life with an average patient age of about 50 years. Between 80% and 90% of patients are women. The location of the tumor within the vessel is significant because it determines the type of symptoms and surgical resectability. Most tumors arise in the upper third or suprahepatic region.[73] Affected patients develop the Budd-Chiari syndrome, with hepatomegaly, jaundice, and massive ascites. Nausea, vomiting, and lower extremity edema may also be present. These tumors are surgically unresectable. Tumors of the midsegment involve the region between the renal veins and hepatic veins, and the symptoms are those of right upper quadrant pain and tenderness, frequently mimicking biliary tract disease. Extension into the hepatic veins may cause some of the symptoms of the Budd-Chiari syndrome, whereas extension into the renal veins will result in varying degrees of renal dysfunction, from mild elevation of the blood urea nitrogen to nephrotic syndrome. Some of these lesions are surgically resectable. Lesions arising below the renal veins cause lower leg edema, but unless they have spread extensively beyond the confines of the vessel, they are often amenable to surgical excision. In a few cases of vena cava leiomyosarcomas, abnormalities of red blood cell morphology and a consumption coagulopathy have been observed.[111] Although previously an antemortem diagnosis of these lesions was difficult, selective arteriography and vena cavography can be used to define the presence and extent of the mass.[73] Metastases develop in about half of cases to sites such as the lung, kidney, pleura, chest wall, liver, and bone.[74]

Leiomyosarcomas of other veins

Unlike vena cava lesions, those in other veins affect the sexes equally and most often arise in the veins of the lower extremity, including the saphenous, iliac, and femoral veins. They usually present as mass lesions of variable duration that occasionally produce lower leg edema. Pressure on nerves coursing close to the affected vessel may produce additional symptoms of numbness. Angiographically the lesions are highly vascular and create compression of the accompanying artery. The compression appears to be the result of entrapment of the artery that resides within the same preformed fibrous sheath (conjunctiva vasorum) as the vein. Since incisional biopsy of intravascular sarcomas can give rise to considerable seeding of tumor by hemorrhage, it has been suggested that thorough radiographic evaluation be followed by needle biopsy in selected cases.[71] The behavior of this group of leiomyosarcomas has been a controversial topic.[71,95] Although one series suggested that small intravascular leiomyosarcomas might have a relatively good prognosis,[95] all six cases reported by Berlin et al.[71] developed metastases, even those with relatively low mitotic rates. However, all but one of the tumors exceeded 4 cm in diameter.

Pulmonary artery leiomyosarcoma

Pulmonary artery leiomyosarcomas are the most common form of arterial leiomyosarcoma. They occur in adults and display no predilection for either sex. Their symptoms are referable to decreased pulmonary outflow, including chest pain, dyspnea, palpitations, dizziness, syncopal attacks,

and eventual right heart failure. Until recently the diagnosis was inevitably made at autopsy. Most of these tumors arise at the base of the heart and grow distally into the left and right main pulmonary arteries.

Gross and microscopic findings

In almost all reported cases, vascular leiomyosarcomas are described as polypoid or nodular masses that are firmly attached to the vessel at some point and have spread for a variable extent along its surface. The rare cases describing extensive spread along the vena cava into the right heart, however, may be cases of intravenous leiomyomatosis that were originally misdiagnosed.[89] (See Chapter 18.) In the case of thin-walled veins, extension to the adventitial surfaces and adjacent structures is a relatively early event, whereas in arteries the integrity of the internal elastic lamina is often preserved so that spread outside the vessel does not occur. Histologically the tumors are basically similar to those in the retroperitoneum, although they usually do not show as prominent a degree of hemorrhage or necrosis (Fig. 19-24). Mitoses, in our experience, are rather easy to identify in these tumors, and the histological criteria of malignancy previously discussed are equally applicable to these lesions. In fact, in our experience true leiomyomas arising from vessels are extremely rare, and this diagnosis should be made with extreme caution and only after the lesion has been extensively sampled.

Behavior and treatment

The morbidity and mortality associated with these tumors are primarily a result of direct extension of these tumors along vessels, with compromise of the circulation. Only about half of the patients will actually have metastases documented at the time of surgery or autopsy, and these occur mainly in the liver or lung and less often in regional lymph nodes or intraabdominal organs. Unfortunately, owing to the fact that only about half of the cases have been diagnosed antemortem in the past, there is little information concerning the results of therapy. It might be anticipated that more sophisticated angiographic techniques leading to earlier diagnosis and therapy would improve survival rates, which thus far have been poor. In 1973, Stuart and Baker,[106] analyzing 10 cases occurring in the vena cava that were treated surgically, noted that of the 5 patients followed up longer than 1 year, all died. In a more recent series by Burke and Virmani,[74] only 7 of 13 inferior vena cava sarcomas developed metastases. One of the greatest problems in the treatment of this disease is that the particular location may make surgical resection impossible. This is true in suprahepatic lesions where ligation of the cava and partial hepatectomy have never been accomplished. Middle caval lesions may be resected with difficulty but require removal of one kidney and pelvic transplantation of the other if radiation is contemplated.

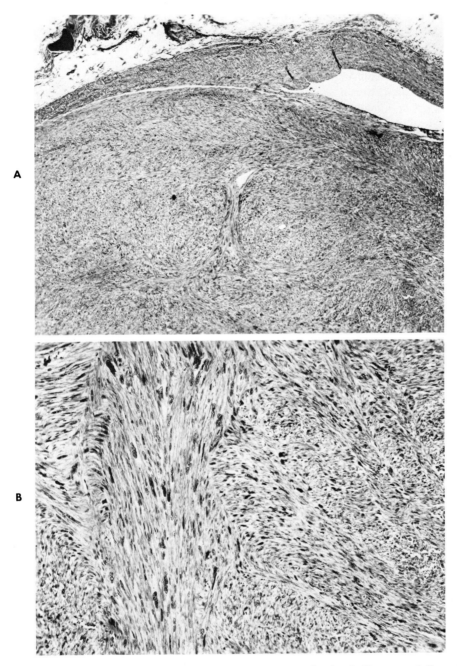

FIG. 19-24. Leiomyosarcoma arising from the media of a small vein. **A,** Tumor partially occludes lumen and grows outward as well. (×40.) **B,** Most vascular leiomyosarcomas are moderately well-differentiated tumors similar to retroperitoneal tumors. (×100.)

MISCELLANEOUS SARCOMAS OF VASCULAR ORIGIN

Nonmyogenic sarcomas arising from vessels are a veritable potpourri of lesions that are difficult to classify.* In contrast to the foregoing group, most of these peculiar hybrid lesions occur more often in the arterial system, particularly the pulmonary artery, where they tend to present in middle age with a constellation of symptoms associated with right ventricular outflow obstruction or pulmonary emboli.[74] Most arising in this location probably arise from the base of the heart, although it is difficult to exclude origin from the valve or even the heart itself. Aortic sarcomas tend to develop in older patients and involve the lower portion of the vessel. They are associated with a myriad of symptoms related to systemic embolization.[74] Arterial sarcomas grow in an intraluminal fashion similar to leiomyosarcomas, but there is a tendency for such lesions to creep along the vessel wall, splitting apart the layers of intima and media in their paths. This form of spreading has been termed *intimal sarcomatosis* by Hedinger.[85] Histologically, a variety of terms have been applied to these tumors, including *pleomorphic sarcoma, intimal sarcoma,*[69,85,99] *undifferen-tiated sarcoma,*[103] *fusocellular sarcoma, malignant mesenchymoma,*[81] *chondrosarcoma,*[87] and *osteosarcoma.*[97,99] The terms serve to emphasize the fact that these tumors are, in general, highly pleomorphic tumors composed of haphazardly arranged giant cells and spindle cells.

The largest institutional review of arterial sarcomas published recently from the Armed Forces Institute of Pathology analyzed 11 and 16 cases from the aorta and pulmonary artery, respectively.[74] Histologically the sarcomas in both locations were for the most part pleomorphic, intimal-based lesions. Of the 17 cases reported, three had the pattern of angiosarcoma and three osteosarcoma, whereas the remainder were pleomorphic sarcomas that were difficult to classify. Other reports have documented the presence of cartilage or skeletal muscle differentiation in these tumors.[81,98]

The fact that these tumors occur in a different set of vessels, show a strikingly different histological appearance, and often remain confined to the superficial portions of the vessel suggests the possibility that these tumors may represent *intimal sarcomas,* in contrast to the previous group, which are more properly considered sarcomas of medial or adventitial origin. Because of their location, diagnosis is rarely made antemortem, and death from local tumor extension, particularly to the lungs, is the rule.

*References 69, 81, 87, 97, 99, 103.

REFERENCES
General

1. Azumi N, Ben-Ezra J, Battifora H: Immunophenotypic diagnosis of leiomyosarcomas and rhabdomyosarcomas with monoclonal antibodies to muscle-specific actin and desmin in formalin-fixed tissue. *Mod Pathol* 1:469, 1988.
2. Botting AJ, Soule EH, Brown AL: Smooth muscle tumors in children. *Cancer* 18:711, 1965.
3. Brown DC, Theaker JM, Banks PM, et al: Cytokeratin expression in smooth muscle and smooth muscle tumours. *Histopathology* 11:477, 1987.
4. Cox PH, Verweij J, Pillay M, et al: Indium 111 antimyosin for the detection of leiomyosarcoma and rhabdomyosarcoma. *Eur J Nucl Med* 14:50, 1988.
5. Dionne GP, Beland JE, Wang N-S: Primary leiomyosarcoma of the diaphragm of an asbestos worker. *Arch Pathol Lab Med* 100:398, 1976.
6. Evans DJ, Lampert IA, Jacobs M: Intermediate filaments in smooth muscle tumors. *J Clin Pathol* 36:57, 1983.
7. Ferenczy A, Richart RM, Okagaki T: A comparative ultrastructural study of leiomyosarcoma, cellular leiomyoma, and leiomyoma of the uterus. *Cancer* 28:1004, 1971.
8. Font RL, Jurco S, Brechner RJ: Postradiation leiomyosarcoma of the orbit complicating bilateral retinoblastoma. *Arch Ophthalmol* 101:1557, 1983.
9. Gabbiani G, Csank-Brassert J, Schneeberger JC, et al: Contractile proteins in human cancer cells. *Am J Pathol* 83:457, 1976.
10. Gustafson P, Willen H, Baldetorp B, et al: Soft tissue leiomyosarcoma: a population-based epidemiologic and prognostic study of 48 patients, including cellular DNA content. *Cancer* 70:114, 1992.
11. Hildebrand HF, Biserte G: Nickel subsulphide-induced leiomyosarcoma in rabbit white skeletal muscle. *Cancer* 43:1358, 1979.
12. Hutton KA, Swift RI, Urban M, et al: Leiomyosarcoma of the chest wall following treatment of Hodgkin's disease. *Eur J Surg Oncol* 18:388, 1992.
13. Lack EE: Leiomyosarcomas in childhood: a clinical and pathologic study of 10 cases. *Pediatr Pathol* 6:181, 1986.
14. Laskin WB, Silverman TA, Enzinger FM: Postradiation soft tissue sarcomas: an analysis of 53 cases. *Cancer* 62:2330, 1988.
15. Meredith RF, Wagman LD, Piper JA, et al: Beta-chain human chorionic gonadotropin-producing leiomyosarcoma of the small intestine. *Cancer* 58:131, 1986.
16. Miettinen M: Immunoreactivity for cytokeratin and epithelial membrane antigen in leiomyosarcomas. *Arch Pathol Lab Med* 112:637, 1988.
17. Miettinen M: Keratin subsets in spindle cell sarcomas: keratins are widespread but synovial sarcoma contains a distinctive keratin polypeptide pattern and desmoplakins. *Am J Pathol* 138:505, 1991.
18. Morales AR, Fine G, Pardo V, et al: The ultrastructure of smooth muscle tumors with a consideration of the possible relationship of glomangioma, hemangiopericytomas, and cardiac myxomas. *Pathol Annu* 10:65, 1975.
19. Mukai K, Schollmeyer JV, Rosai J: Immunohistochemical localization of actin. *Am J Surg Pathol* 5:91, 1981.
20. Nadji N, Morales AR: *Immunoperoxidase techniques: a practical approach to tumor diagnosis,* Chicago, 1986, American Society of Clinical Pathologists Press.
21. Nistal M, Raniagua R, Picazo ML, et al: Granular changes in vascular leiomyosarcoma. *Virchows Arch (Pathol Anat)* 386:239, 1980.
22. Nochomovitz LE, Orenstein JM: Inflammatory pseudotumor of the urinary bladder: possible relationship to nodular fasciitis: two case reports, cytologic observations, and ultrastructural observations. *Am J Surg Pathol* 9:366, 1985.

23. Norton AJ, Thomas JA, Isaacson PG: Cytokeratin-specific mono-clonal antibodies are reactive with tumours of smooth muscle deri-vation: an immunohistochemical and biochemical study using anti-bodies to intermediate filament cytoskeletal proteins. *Histopathology* 11:487, 1987.

24. Proppe KH, Scully RE, Rosai J: Postoperative spindle cell nodules of genitourinary tract resembling sarcomas: a report of eight cases. *Am J Surg Pathol* 8:101, 1984.

25. Rangdaeng S, Truong LD: Comparative immunohistochemical stain-ing for desmin and muscle-specific actin: a study of 576 cases. *Am J Clin Pathol* 96:32, 1991.

26. Ro JY, Ayala AG, Ordonez NG, et al: Pseudosarcomatous fibro-myxoid tumor of the urinary bladder. *Am J Clin Pathol* 86:583, 1986.

27. Robinson E, Neugut AI, Wylie P: Clinical aspects of postirradiation sarcomas. *J Natl Cancer Inst* 80:233, 1988.

28. Russell WO, Cohen J, Enzinger FM, et al: A clinical and patholog-ical staging system for soft tissue sarcomas. *Cancer* 40:1562, 1977.

29. Schuerch W, Skalli O, Seemayer TA, et al: Intermediate filament proteins and actin isoforms as markers for soft tissue tumor differ-entiation and origin. I. Smooth muscle tumors. *Am J Pathol* 128:91, 1987.

30. Skalli O, Schuerch W, Seemayer T, et al: Myofibroblasts from di-verse pathologic settings are heterogeneous in their content of actin isoforms and intermediate filament proteins. *Lab Invest* 60:275, 1989.

31. Stallard D, Sundaram M, Johnson FE, et al: Case report 747: leio-myosarcoma of great saphenous vein. *Skeletal Radiol* 21:399, 1992.

32. Stevens GN, Tattersall MH, Stalley P: Leiomyosarcoma following therapeutic irradiation for ankylosing spondylitis. *Br J Radiol* 63:730, 1990.

33. Stratton MR, Williams S, Fisher C, et al: Structural alterations of the RB1 gene in human soft tissue tumours. *Br J Cancer* 60:202, 1989.

34. Swanson PE, Wick MR, Dehner LP: Leiomyosarcoma of somatic soft tissues in childhood: an immunohistochemical analysis of six cases with ultrastructural correlation. *Hum Pathol* 22:569, 1991.

35. Torosian MH, Friedrich C, Godbold J, et al: Soft-tissue sarcoma: initial characteristics and prognostic factors in patients with and with-out metastatic disease. *Semin Surg Oncol* 4:13, 1988.

36. Tsukada T, Tippens D, Mar H, et al: HHF35, a muscle-actin-specific monoclonal antibody. I. Immunocytochemical and biochemical char-acterization. *Am J Pathol* 126:51, 1987.

37. Wilkinson N, Fitzmaurice RJ, Turner PG, et al: Leiomyosarcoma with osteoclast-like giant cells. *Histopathology* 20:446, 1992.

38. Wolff M, Silva F, Kaye G: Pulmonary metastases (with admixed epithelial elements) from smooth muscle neoplasms: report of nine cases, including three males. *Am J Surg Pathol* 3:325, 1979.

39. Yannopoulos K, Stout AP: Smooth muscle tumors in children. *Cancer* 15:958, 1962.

Leiomyosarcomas of retroperitoneum and deep soft tissues

40. Golden T, Stout AP: Smooth muscle tumors of the gastrointestinal tract and retroperitoneal tissues. *Surg Gynecol Obstet* 73:784, 1941.

41. Granmayeh M, Jonsson K, McFarland W, et al: Angiography of ab-dominal leiomyosarcoma. *Am J Roentgenol* 130:725, 1978.

42. Hashimoto H, Daimaru Y, Tsuneyoshi M, et al: Leiomyosarcoma of the external soft tissues. *Cancer* 57:2077, 1986.

43. Hashimoto H, Tsuneyoshi M, Enjoji M: Malignant smooth muscle tumors of the retroperitoneum and mesentery: a clinicopathologic analysis of 44 cases. *J Surg Oncol* 28:177, 1985.

44. Kay S, McNeill DD: Leiomyosarcoma of the retroperitoneum. *Surg Gynecol Obstet* 129:285, 1969.

45. King ME, Dickersin GR, Scully RE: Myxoid leiomyosarcoma of the uterus: a report of six cases. *Am J Surg Pathol* 6:589, 1982.

46. Ranchod M, Kempson RL: Smooth muscle tumors of the gastroin-testinal tract and retroperitoneum. *Cancer* 39:255, 1977.

47. Salm R, Evans DJ: Myxoid leiomyosarcoma. *Histopathology* 9:159, 1985.

48. Shmookler BM, Lauer DH: Retroperitoneal leiomyosarcoma: a clin-icopathologic analysis of 36 cases. *Am J Surg Pathol* 7:269, 1983.

49. Suster S, Wong TY, Moran CA: Sarcomas with combined features of liposarcoma and leiomyosarcoma: study of two cases of an un-usual soft-tissue tumor showing dual lineage differentiation. *Am J Surg Pathol* 17:905, 1993.

50. Wile AG, Evans HL, Romsdahl MM: Leiomyosarcoma of soft tis-sue: a clinicopathologic study. *Cancer* 48:1022, 1981.

51. Yannopoulos K, Stout AP: Primary solid tumor of the mesentery. *Cancer* 16:914, 1963.

Cutaneous and subcutaneous leiomyosarcomas

52. Chaves E, Sa HH, Gadelha N, et al: Leiomyosarcoma in the skin. *Acta Dermatol Venereol* 52:288, 1972.

53. Dahl I, Angervall L: Cutaneous and subcutaneous leiomyosarcoma: a clinicopathologic study of 47 patients. *Pathologia Europaea* 9:307, 1974.

54. Fields JP, Helwig EB: Leiomyosarcoma of the skin and subcutane-ous tissue. *Cancer* 47:156, 1981.

55. Haim S, Gellei B: Leiomyosarcoma of the skin: report of two cases. *Dermatologica* 140:30, 1970.

56. Headington JT, Beals TF, Niederhuber JE: Primary leiomyosarcoma of skin: a report and critical appraisal. *J Cutan Pathol* 4:308, 1977.

57. Heieck JJ, Organ CH Jr: Leiomyosarcoma of the scalp in a new-born. *Arch Dermatol* 102:213, 1970.

58. Hietanen A, Sakai Y: Leiomyosarcoma in an old irradiated lupus lesion. *Acta Dermatol Venereol* 40:167, 1960.

59. Jain SP: Leiomyosarcoma in the skin: a case report. *Indian J Surg* 31:638, 1969.

60. Orellana-Diaz O, Hernandez-Perez E: Leiomyoma cutis and leio-myosarcoma: a 10-year study and a short review. *J Dermatol Surg Oncol* 9:283, 1983.

61. Pense AK, Saxena O: Superficial leiomyosarcoma: report of a case. *Indian J Pathol Bacteriol* 12:120, 1969.

62. Phelan JT, Sherer W, Mesa P: Malignant smooth muscle tumors (leiomyosarcomas) of soft tissue origin. *N Engl J Med* 266:1027, 1962.

63. Rising JA, Booth E: Primary leiomyosarcoma of the skin with lym-phatic spread. *Arch Pathol* 81:94, 1966.

64. Stout AP, Hill WT: Leiomyosarcoma of the superficial soft tissue. *Cancer* 11:844, 1964.

65. Swanson PE, Stanley MW, Scheithauer BW, et al: Primary cutane-ous leiomyosarcoma: a histologic and immunohistochemical study of 9 cases with ultrastructural correlations. *J Cutan Pathol* 15:129, 1988.

66. Tappeiner J, Wodniansky P: Solitaeres Leiomyom-Leiomyosarkom. *Hautarzt* 12:160, 1961.

67. Wang P, Hornstein OP, Schricker KTH: Kutanes Leiomyosarkom und osteomedullaeres Plasmozytom mit Nachweis von IgA kappa-Paraprotein in Serum und Hauttumor. *Hautarzt* 27:441, 1976.

Vascular leiomyosarcomas and related lesions

68. Abell MR: Leiomyosarcoma of inferior vena cava: review of litera-ture and report of two cases. *Am J Clin Pathol* 28:272, 1957.

69. Altman NH, Shelley WM: Primary intimal sarcoma of the pulmo-nary artery. *Johns Hopkins Med J* 133:214, 1973.

70. Aufrecht E: Ein Myom der Vena Saphena. *Virchows Arch (Pathol Anat)* 44:133, 1868.

71. Berlin O, Stener B, Kindblom L, et al: Leiomyosarcomas of venous origin in the extremities: a correlated clinical, roentgenologic, and

morphologic study with diagnostic and surgical implications. *Cancer* 54:2147, 1984.

72. Birkenstock WE, Lipper S: Leiomyosarcoma of the right common iliac artery: a case report. *Br J Surg* 63:81, 1976.

73. Brewster DC, Athanasoulin CA, Darling RC: Leiomyosarcoma of the inferior vena cava: diagnosis and surgical management. *Arch Surg* 111:1081, 1976.

74. Burke AP, Virmani R: Sarcomas of the great vessels: a clinicopathologic study. *Cancer* 71:1761, 1993.

75. Cardell BS, McGill DAF, Williams R: Leiomyosarcoma of inferior vena cava producing Budd-Chiari syndrome. *J Pathol* 104:283, 1971.

76. Demers ML, Curley SA, Romsdahl MM: Inferior vena cava leiomyosarcoma. *J Surg Oncol* 51:89, 1992.

77. Deutsch V, Fraenkel O, Frand V, et al: Leiomyosarcoma of the inferior vena cava presenting into the right atrium. *Br Heart J* 30:571, 1968.

78. Dorfman HD, Fisher ER: Leiomyosarcoma of the greater saphenous vein. *Am J Clin Pathol* 39:73, 1963.

79. Griffin AS, Sterchi JM: Primary leiomyosarcoma of the inferior vena cava: a case report and review of the literature. *J Surg Oncol* 34:53, 1987.

80. Haber IM, Truong L: Immunohistochemical demonstration of the endothelial nature of aortic intimal sarcoma. *Am J Surg Pathol* 12:798, 1988.

81. Hagstrom L: Malignant mesenchymoma in pulmonary artery and right ventricle. *Acta Pathol Microbiol Scand* 51:87, 1961.

82. Hallock P, Watson CJ, Berman L: Primary tumor of inferior vena cava with clinical features suggestive of Chari's disease. *Arch Intern Med* 66:50, 1940.

83. Hayata T, Sato I: Primary leiomyosarcoma arising in the trunk of pulmonary artery: a case report and review of the literature. *Acta Pathol Jpn* 27:137, 1977.

84. Hayes FL, Farha SJ, Brown RL: Primary leiomyosarcoma of the pulmonary artery. *Am J Cardiol* 34:615, 1974.

85. Hedinger E: Ueber Intima Sarkomatose von Venen und Arterien in sarkomatoesen Strumen. *Virchows Arch (Pathol Anat)* 164:199, 1901.

86. Henrichs KJ, Wenisch HJC, Hofmann W, et al: Leiomyosarcoma of the pulmonary artery. *Virchows Arch (Pathol Anat)* 383:207, 1979.

87. Hohbach C, Mall W: Chondrosarcoma of the pulmonary artery. *Beitr Pathol* 160:298, 1977.

88. Johansen JK, Nielsen R: Leiomyosarcoma of the inferior vena cava: report of a case. *Acta Chir Scand* 137:181, 1971.

89. Jonasson D, Pritchard J, Long L: Intraluminal leiomyosarcoma of the inferior vena cava. *Cancer* 19:1311, 1966.

90. Jurayj MN, Midell AJ, Bederman S, et al: Primary leiomyosarcoma of the inferior vena cava: report of a case and review of the literature. *Cancer* 26:1349, 1970.

91. Justiniani FR, Cohen GH, Roen SA, et al: Budd-Chiari syndrome due to leiomyosarcoma of the inferior vena cava. *Am J Dig Dis* 18:337, 1973.

92. Kapsinow R, Brierre JT: Leiomyosarcoma of the inferior vena cava. *J La State Med Soc* 126:400, 1974.

93. Karmody AM, Zaman SN, Sarfeh JI: Leiomyoma of external iliac vein. *N Y State J Med* 77:2279, 1977.

94. Kevorkian J, Cento JP: Leiomyosarcoma of large arteries and veins. *Surgery* 73:39, 1973.

95. Leu HJ, Makek M: Intramural venous leiomyosarcomas. *Cancer* 57:1395, 1986.

96. Light HG, Peskin GW, Ravdin IS: Primary tumors of the venous system. *Cancer* 13:818, 1960.

97. McConnel TH: Bony and cartilaginous tumor of the heart and great vessels. *Cancer* 25:611, 1970.

98. McGlennen RC, Manivel JC, Stanley SJ, et al: Pulmonary artery trunk sarcoma: a clinicopathological, ultrastructural, and immunohistochemical study of four cases. *Mod Pathol* 2:486, 1989.

99. Murphy MSN, Meckstroth GV, Merkel BH, et al: Primary intimal sarcoma of pulmonary valve and trunk with osteogenic sarcomatous elements. *Arch Pathol Lab Med* 100:649, 1976.

100. Nonomura A, Kurumaya H, Kono J, et al: Primary pulmonary artery sarcomas: report of two autopsy cases studied by immunohistochemistry and electron microscopy, and review of 110 cases reported in the literature. *Acta Pathol Jpn* 38:883, 1988.

101. Radhakrishanan J, Alrenga DP, Ghosh BC: Isolated hepatic metastasis from renal vein leiomyosarcoma. *Arch Pathol Lab Med* 102:606, 1978.

102. Salaquarda F: Leiomyoma of the inferior vena cava. *Zentralbl Allg Pathol* 105:405, 1964.

103. Shmookler BM, Marsh HB, Roberts WC: Primary sarcoma of the pulmonary trunk and of left main pulmonary artery: a rare cause of obstruction to right ventricular outflow. *Am J Med* 63:263, 1977.

104. Smout MS, Fisher JH: Leiomyosarcoma of the saphenous vein. *Can Med Assoc J* 83:1066, 1960.

105. Stringer BD: Leiomyosarcoma of artery and vein. *Am J Surg* 134:90, 1977.

106. Stuart FP, Baker WH: Palliative surgery for leiomyosarcoma of the inferior vena cava. *Ann Surg* 177:237, 1973.

107. Taheri SA, Conner GW: Leiomyosarcoma of iliac veins. *Surgery* 94:516, 1983.

108. Thijs LG, Kroon TAJ, Van Leevwen TM: Leiomyosarcoma of the pulmonary trunk associated with pericardial effusion. *Thorax* 29:490, 1974.

109. Thomas MA, Fine G: Leiomyosarcoma of the veins: report of two cases and review of literature. *Cancer* 13:96, 1960.

110. Varela-Duran J, Oliva H, Rosai J: Vascular leiomyosarcoma: the malignant counterpart of vascular leiomyoma. *Cancer* 44:1684, 1979.

111. Wackers FJT, Vander Schoot JB, Hampe JF: Sarcoma of the pulmonary trunk associated with hemorrhagic tendency: a case report and review of the literature. *Cancer* 23:339, 1969.

112. Wang NS, Seemayer TA, Ahmed MN, et al: Pulmonary leiomyosarcoma associated with an arteriovenous fistula. *Arch Pathol* 98:100, 1974.

113. Weinreb W, Steinfeld A, Rodil J, et al: Leiomyosarcoma arising in an arteriovenous fistula. *Cancer* 52:390, 1983.

114. Wilder JR, Lotfi MW: Leiomyoma of the saphenous vein. *Postgrad Med* 50:154, 1971.

115. Wray RC, Dawkins H: Primary smooth muscle tumours of the inferior vena cava. *Ann Surg* 174:1009, 1971.

116. Wright EP, Virmani R, Glick AD, et al: Aortic intimal sarcoma with embolic metastasis. *Am J Surg Pathol* 9:890, 1985.

CHAPTER 20

EPITHELIOID SMOOTH MUSCLE TUMORS

In 1960 Martin et al.[32] described six cases of an unusual round cell myogenic tumor of the stomach. Two years later Stout[45] added his experience with 69 similar cases, two of which were malignant. He emphasized the high rate of misdiagnosis because of the unusual morphological alteration of the smooth muscle cell and suggested the term "leiomyoblastoma" (bizarre leiomyoma) because it did not expressly connote benignancy or malignancy. He furthermore believed that identification of potentially malignant leiomyoblastomas was difficult and not always possible. In time the term "leiomyoblastoma" came to imply a biologically indeterminate group of smooth muscle tumors characterized by a peculiar polygonal or "epithelioid" cell, often with clear cytoplasm. Use of this term has waned with the belief that these tumors should be evaluated like conventional smooth muscle tumors and provisionally separated into benign and malignant forms. Most recently the principal controversy has centered on the issue of differentiation. These tumors rarely show clear-cut features of muscle differentiation ultrastructurally and do not have the same immunophenotypic profile as ordinary leiomyomas and many leiomyosarcomas. For this reason the term "gastrointestinal stromal tumor" has become increasingly popular for a variety of mesenchymal tumors of the gastrointestinal tract, including epithelioid smooth muscle tumors, traditional leiomyosarcomas, spindle cell tumors with possible neural differentiation, and even tumors that may show autonomic differentiation (plexosarcoma).* This term serves a convenient and appropriate taxonomic function for gastrointestinal pathologists, but it is inherently contradictory for soft tissue neoplasms. Thus, the authors, along with the World Health Organization Committee for the Classification of Soft Tissue Tumors, have continued to use the term "epithelioid smooth muscle tumor," recognizing that these lesions at best only partially resemble smooth muscle tumors. Since epithelioid smooth muscle tumors occur principally in the gastrointestinal tract (particularly the stomach), the collective experience relating to the soft tissue counterpart

is virtually anecdotal. For want of better data, the data derived from gastrointestinal lesions must be accepted and then applied to soft tissue neoplasms, with the understanding that in time, refinements in these concepts may become necessary.

CLINICAL FINDINGS

Epithelioid smooth muscle tumors may be found in a number of sites, but they show a striking predilection to occur within the abdominal cavity, gastrointestinal tract, and uterus. Of the 155 leiomyoblastomas reviewed by Pizzimbono et al.,[40] 146 occurred in the stomach, three in the small intestine, four in the omentum and mesentery, two in the uterus, and one in the retroperitoneum. Rare cases have been reported in the neck and vulva[41] and recently in the skin.[46] In our experience it is highly unusual to encounter a pure epithelioid smooth muscle tumor in the soft tissues of the extremity, although occasionally focal epithelioid changes may occur within an otherwise typical smooth muscle tumor. Because gastric epithelioid smooth muscle tumors are so common relative to those in other sites, these tumors are considered in this chapter along with the rare soft tissue counterpart.

Epithelioid smooth muscle tumors of gastric origin

These tumors occur principally during mid- or late-adult life, and only rare cases have been recorded in patients younger than age 20 years.[12,45] Males are more often affected than females.[2] According to Appelman and Helwig,[3] about four fifths of epithelioid smooth muscle tumors of the stomach are histologically and biologically benign and would be classified as epithelioid leiomyomas, whereas the remainder are leiomyosarcomas. Certain topographical differences have been noted between the benign and malignant forms. Epithelioid leiomyosarcomas tend to be more common in the proximal portion of the stomach (cardia, fundus) and the posterior wall, whereas epithelioid leiomyomas are more common on the anterior wall.[3] Regardless of the degree of malignancy, the majority present with signs or symptoms of upper gastrointestinal tract hemorrhage

---

*References 30, 33, 34, 37, 39, 43, 48, 50, 51, 54.

manifested by hematemesis, melena, or blood loss anemia. Unusual signs include bilateral leg edema from venous obstruction, microangiopathic hemolytic anemia,[40] and acute intraabdominal hemorrhage.[24] These tumors arise from the muscularis propria and may grow in an endophytic or exophytic fashion. They can extend into the gastrocolic ligament and greater omentum, sometimes retaining only a tenuous relationship with the stomach by means of a narrow stalk. A few tumors may grow in both directions, assuming a dumbbell or hourglass shape. In most cases roentgenographic studies document the presence of a filling defect in the stomach, occasionally with overlying ulceration. CT scans detect lesions as small as 1 cm, particularly if there is clinical suspicion of a gastric lesion and care is taken to obtain a number of different views.

In contrast to the usual form of the disease just described, gastric epithelioid leiomyosarcomas may occur in association with functioning extraadrenal or adrenal paragangliomas and pulmonary chondromas.[6,7] This unusual triad, first recognized by Carney (Carney's triad), occurs predominantly, but not exclusively, in young females. The average age is about 16 years. Usually the disease is heralded by signs or symptoms related to the gastric tumor, followed at some time later by signs or symptoms of paraganglioma or pulmonary chondroma. However, only about one quarter of patients studied to date have manifested the full triad,[7] the remainder having developed only two of the three tumors. The gastric tumors usually involve the body and antrum, may be multiple, and typically result in a multibosselated deformity of the antrum, especially apparent on the serosal surface. The gross appearance of these leiomyosarcomas contrasts rather strikingly with the conventional form of gastric epithelioid leiomyosarcoma. The paragangliomas are most often located in the mediastinum. The chondromas are often multiple and appear to be pure chondroid tumors, lacking an epithelial component as is seen in chondroid hamartomas. They may or may not be calcified. There is no evidence that this unusual complex is inherited. Chromosome studies and studies of cellular immunity have likewise been noncontributory. Yet it is indisputable that the early age of onset, the predilection for women, the multiplicity of tumors, and, above all, the association of three tumors that otherwise are very rare, are indicative of a distinctive entity. Because of the life-threatening consequences of this complex, Carney has recommended that patients who manifest any of these three tumors at an early age (less than 35 years) be followed up periodically for evidence of the other two. It is also important to recognize that despite the fact that the gastric tumors have been classified as "leiomyosarcomas," long survival times have been noted even in the face of nodal or hepatic metastasis, a phenomenon seldom noted in conventional epithelioid leiomyosarcomas. Persson et al.[38] recently documented four cases of young individuals with metastatic epithelioid leiomyosarcoma, with survival rates ranging from 17 to 48, years who had been treated only surgically, one of whom had Carney's complex. It is important to be aware of the fact that indolent forms of gastric epithelioid leiomyosarcoma occur in young persons.

Epithelioid smooth muscle tumors of soft tissue

These tumors arise principally from omentum and mesentery and less often retroperitoneum, where they are usually large white-gray masses with areas of hemorrhage or cyst formation (Fig. 20-1). In our experience the majority of these lesions are malignant, and the symptoms produced

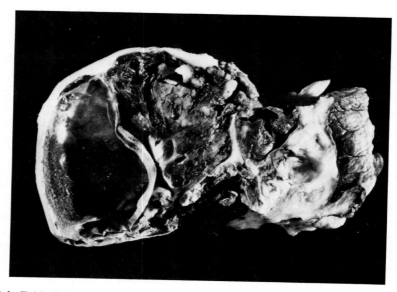

FIG. 20-1. Epithelioid leiomyoma of omentum (benign leiomyoblastoma) showing hemorrhage and extensive cystic change.

are quite similar to those of intraabdominal and retroperitoneal leiomyosarcomas and include the presence of a mass, weight loss, fever, nausea, and vomiting.

MICROSCOPIC FINDINGS
Epithelioid leiomyoma (benign leiomyoblastoma)

Epithelioid leiomyomas of both soft tissue and stomach are essentially identical and are composed of nodules of short spindled and rounded cells that grow in sheets rather than fascicles. The nodules vary in cellularity and proportion of spindled and rounded cells, so that with low-power views, the tumor often has a variegated appearance. The predominant cell of epithelioid leiomyoma has a short spindled or fusiform shape and an amphophilic or slightly eosinophilic cytoplasm, often with a fine fibrillary quality (Fig. 20-2, A). The nucleus is round or oval and centrally located. It is usually not possible to demonstrate distinct myofibrils within the cells by light microscopy, and at best only delicate fuchsinophilic wisps are evident within the cytoplasm. These fusiform cells usually blend gradually with cells having pathognomonic epithelioid features (Figs. 20-2, B, 20-3, and 20-5). They are notable for their round shape, abundant amphophilic or clear cytoplasm, and centrally placed nucleus (Fig. 20-2, B). There is occasionally a vacuolar change in the cytoplasm. In some cases a distinct vacuole may displace the nucleus to one side, creating a signet-ring cell (see Figs. 20-6 and 20-7). Tumors composed of a predominance of signet-ring cells may be mistaken for liposarcomas or mucinous carcinomas by those unfamiliar with their appearance. As emphasized originally by Stout, the vacuoles of these signet-ring cells, however, do not stain for fat, mucosubstances, or glycogens and, therefore, can be readily distinguished from those of liposarcoma or carcinoma. In fact, these vacuoles seem to represent an artifact of formalin fixation because they are not present in frozen sections or in material fixed for electron microscopy. In addition to the spindled and epithelioid cells, multinucleated giant cells are sometimes present, and occasionally their nuclei may appear slightly hyperchromatic.hange are sometimes present. These tumors are distinguished from epithelioid leiomyosarcomas principally on the basis of mitotic figures, size, and cellularity (see Criteria of Malignancy below).

Epithelioid leiomyosarcoma (malignant leiomyoblastoma)

Most epithelioid leiomyosarcomas are similar to their benign counterparts and are composed of an admixture of fusiform and epithelioid cells (Figs. 20-4 to 20-9), although there is a tendency for the epithelioid cells to predominate.

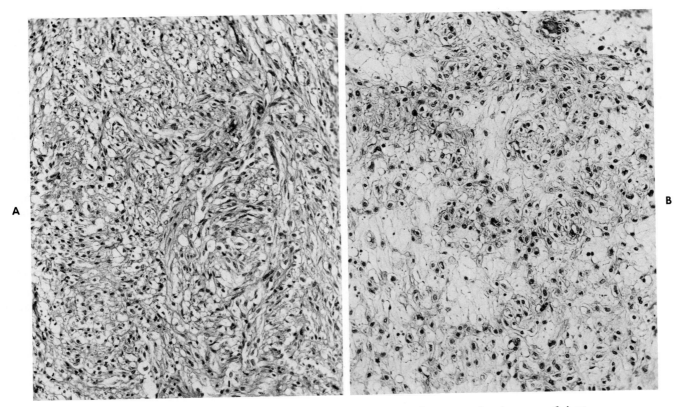

A   **B**

FIG. 20-2. Epithelioid leiomyoma (benign leiomyoblastoma) of omentum showing areas of short spindled cells **(A),** which are found in association with areas containing classic rounded cells with clear cytoplasm **(B).** (**A,** ×125; **B,** ×165.)

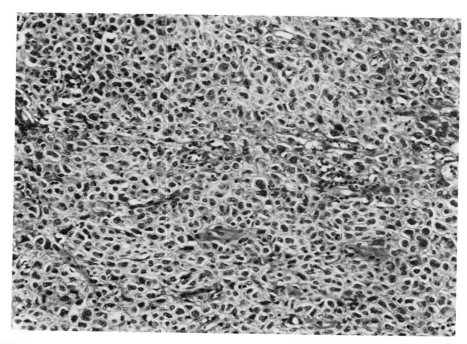

FIG. 20-3. Epithelioid leiomyoma of omentum composed exclusively of rounded cells with little or no clear cell change of the cytoplasm. (×160.)

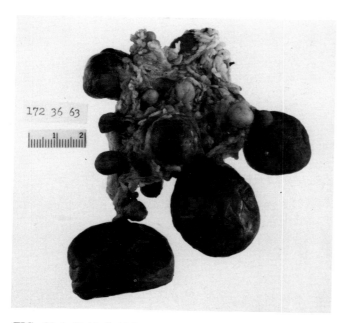

FIG. 20-4. Epithelioid leiomyosarcoma of omentum presenting as multiple nodules, suggestive of metastatic carcinoma or even mesothelioma.

In malignant forms the cells are less mature, as evidenced by the less abundant cytoplasm and greater degree of pleomorphism and mitotic activity. The tumors are frequently punctuated with microscopic cysts (Fig. 20-10). A small number of epithelioid leiomyosarcomas are qualitatively

different and bear a vague similarity to a glomus tumor in that they are composed principally of small rounded cells with scant cytoplasm (Fig. 20-11, *B*). The cells may be arranged in sheets, in small whorls around blood vessels, in a pseudoalveolar pattern, or in a pattern resembling a hemangiopericytoma (Fig. 20-11, *C*). The latter forms of epithelioid leiomyosarcoma are sometimes very difficult to recognize out of context; consequently, one must rely heavily on identification of areas resembling conventional smooth muscle tumor (Fig. 20-11, *A*). Usually the metastases from epithelioid leiomyosarcomas resemble the parent growth, although the mitotic rates may be quite different. Occasionally, isolated metastases in liver or lymph nodes may be difficult to diagnose because of their similarity to metastatic carcinoma or carcinoid tumor (Fig. 20-12). This situation most frequently arises in patients who have had gastrointestinal leiomyosarcomas resected previously and who present years later with metastatic disease. Obviously there is no substitute for review of the original material coupled with the appropriate special staining procedures for mucin and neurosecretory granules.

ULTRASTRUCTURAL AND IMMUNOHISTOCHEMICAL FINDINGS

A number of ultrastructural studies of epithelioid smooth muscle tumors have appeared, although it is not always clear whether these tumors were considered benign or malignant. The tumors have varied: some showed all the characteristics of smooth muscle cells[21,26,42] (thin myofila-

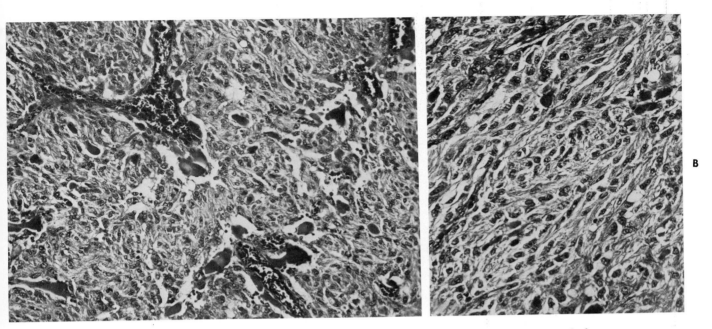

FIG. 20-5. Epithelioid leiomyosarcoma (malignant leiomyoblastoma) showing areas composed of short spindles of fusiform cells (**A**) that have a fine fibrillary quality to the cytoplasm (**B**). (**A**, ×160; **B**, ×250.)

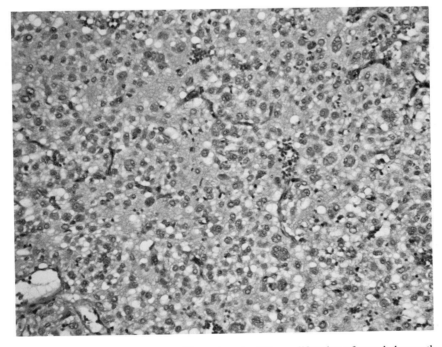

FIG. 20-6. Epithelioid leiomyosarcoma illustrating sheetlike proliferation of rounded smooth muscle cells. (×200.)

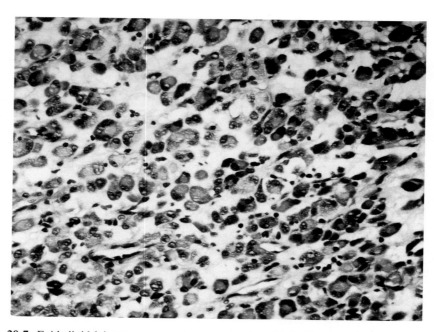

FIG. 20-7. Epithelioid leiomyosarcoma depicting classic epithelioid cells with extreme vacuolar change of the cytoplasm. These so-called signet-ring cells often cause confusion with carcinoma or liposarcoma.

ments, cytoplasmic and subplasmalemmal dense bodies, pinocytotic vesicles, basal lamina, and intercellular junctions), while others have few of these features.[52] Although sampling may account for some of the differences in the published reports, it is unlikely that it accounts for all of them. In general, myofilaments seem to be less well represented in these tumors compared with conventional smooth muscle tumors (Fig. 20-13), an observation that correlates with our inability to demonstrate linear striations in most of these tumors by light microscopy. When present, myofilaments are sparsely distributed at the periphery of the cytoplasm. The clear or vacuolated cytoplasm, which is so characteristic of these tumors by light microscopy, is usually absent by electron microscopy,[9,21,42] although it seems to correspond topographically to cells with a low cytoplasmic density, due in part to greater dispersion of organelles.[11] Thus most investigators have considered the vacuole per se an unusual but consistent artifact of formalin fixation.

The prevalence of muscle antigens within these tumors has been a vexing and frustrating question, and it is nearly impossible to precisely compare data published in the literature for a number of reasons. First, the experience cited in the literature is based almost exclusively on gastrointestinal stromal tumors in which little attempt is made to subclassify the lesions into epithelioid versus nonepithelioid types or to specify a precise location that may have a bearing on both histological appearance and immunophenotype.

Second, the sensitivity of various antibodies, type of fixation, and preparation of tissue (fixed versus frozen) have varied greatly from study to study.* Even so, there seems to be a general acknowledgement that epithelioid smooth muscle tumors do not express muscle antigens to the extent that conventional smooth muscle tumors do, although all express vimentin. In the experience cited by Ma et al.[31] about half of 19 epithelioid smooth muscle tumors from all gastrointestinal sites expressed smooth muscle or muscle-specific actin, whereas none expressed desmin. Neural markers (neurofilament protein, glial fibrillary acidic protein, and S-100 protein) were also negative. However, in other studies a variable percentage of tumors have expressed S-100 protein[37,39,48] as well as other neural markers such as neuron-specific enolase and protein gene product.[48] The unexpected presence of neural markers within these lesions has led authors to suggest that some of these tumors may show either neural or bidirectional differentiation.[48] Still others have observed that S-100 protein is more apt to be present in small bowel lesions and have proposed the intriguing idea that the histological appearance of gastrointestinal stromal tumors is site related.[39] There do not appear to be significant differences in immunophenotype between benign and malignant lesions. The authors and others have recently observed CD34 in a significant number

*References 34, 37, 39, 43, 48, 50, 51, 54.

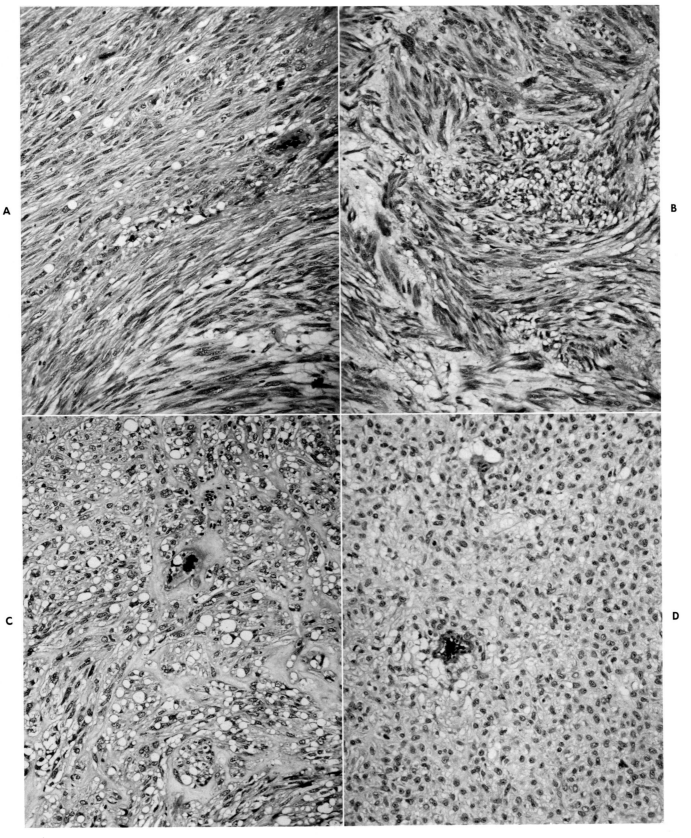

FIG. 20-8. Epithelioid leiomyosarcoma showing a variety of patterns, all within the same tumor. **A** and **B** have features of conventional leiomyosarcoma, whereas **C** and **D** display epithelioid features. Cytoplasmic vacuolization is especially prominent in **C**. (**A** to **D**, ×160.)

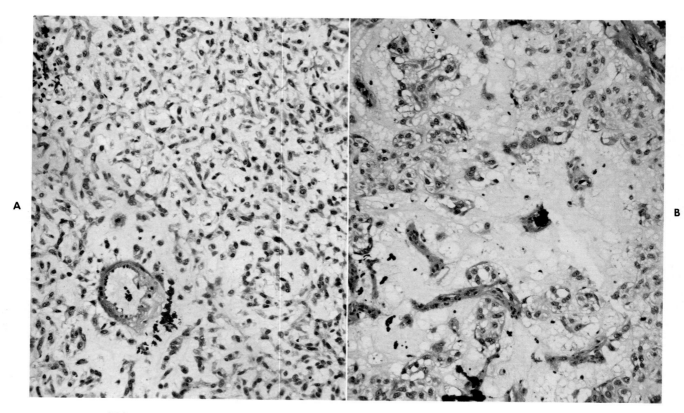

FIG. 20-9. Epithelioid leiomyosarcoma showing myxoid change of stroma. In **A**, cells have a rounded to slightly spindled shape, whereas in **B**, they are uniformly rounded. (**A** and **B**, ×160.)

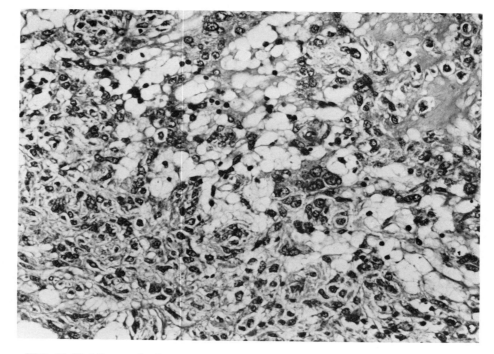

FIG. 20-10. Microcystic change occurring within an epithelioid leiomyosarcoma. (×250.)

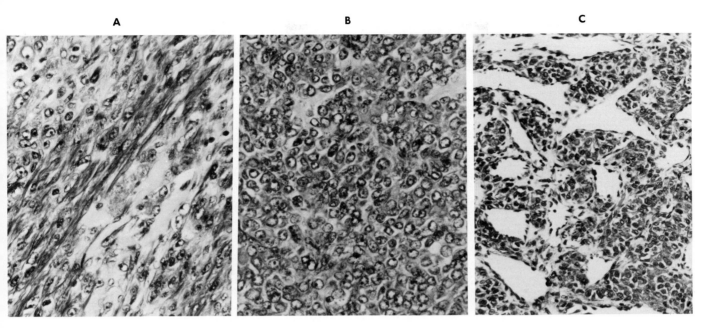

FIG. 20-11. Poorly differentiated epithelioid leiomyosarcoma. Tumor consists predominantly of sheets of small rounded cells **(B)**, which are focally arranged in a pericytoma pattern **(C)**. Tumor could be identified by virtue of areas **(A)** resembling conventional leiomyosarcoma. **(A** to **C,** ×250.)

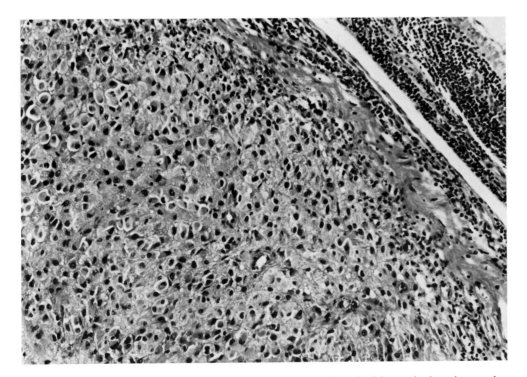

FIG. 20-12. Epithelioid leiomyosarcoma metastatic to a lymph node. Metastatic deposits may be mistaken for carcinoma. (×160.)

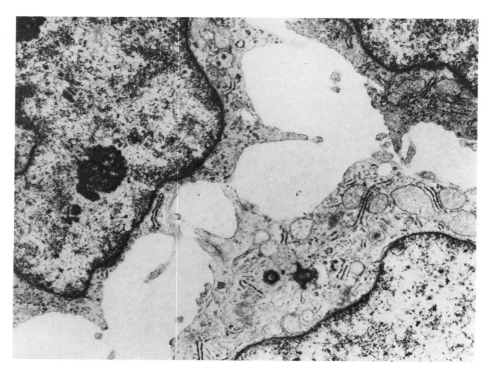

FIG. 20-13. Electron microscopic view of gastric leiomyoblastoma. Cells have cytoplasm of relatively low electron density, and in this case they were devoid of myofilaments. Vacuolar cytoplasmic change seen in light microscopic material is usually not seen in material preserved for electron microscopy. (Courtesy Dr. Jerome B. Taxy, Baltimore, Maryland.)

of epithelioid smooth muscle tumors, although the diagnostic utility of this antigen and its relationship to various histological parameters are yet to be determined.

The bewildering array of immunohistochemical findings does not serve to identify the lineage of this tumor but does leave one with the unmistakable belief that these lesions are different from the common leiomyomas and leiomyosarcomas encountered in the uterus or soft tissue. It has been argued that the presence of actins in these tumors indicates smooth muscle differentiation but possibly of a rather primitive degree.

CRITERIA OF MALIGNANCY
Size and mitotic activity

In the absence of data based on epithelioid smooth muscle tumors of soft tissue, the data derived from gastrointestinal lesions are used. Mitotic activity and size are the two most important, albeit interdependent, parameters of outcome. In the studies of Appelman and Helwig[3] and Byard et al.,[5] there was a strong correlation between mitotic activity and metastatic rate (Table 20-1). Tumors having less than one mitotic figure per 50 HPF had a metastatic rate of 2% compared with those having more than 10 mitoses per 50HPF, which metastasized in all instances. Ueyama et

Table 20-1. Relationship between mitotic rate and metastatic rate in gastric stromal tumors with epithelioid features

Author	No. mitoses	Metastasis (%)
Appelman	0 per 50 HPF	2
	1 to 5 per 50 HPF	13
	>10 per 50 HPF	100
Byard	<10 per 10 HPF	5
	>10 per 10 HPF	100

al.,[51] using the criteria of more than five mitoses per 50 HPF, identified 32 sarcomas from a pool of 120 gastrointestinal stromal tumors. Of patients in this group who were followed up, nearly half succumbed to their disease, while none of the patients with benign lesions succumbed. This study would suggest that a finding of five mitoses per 50 HPF identifies lesions with a high risk of metastasis, but it does not ensure that lesions with fewer mitoses cannot metastasize. Consequently, we have often made the diagnosis of malignancy when the levels of mitotic activity were somewhat less but the lesion was large (greater than 6 cm).

In the extreme case we believe that the diagnosis of low-grade sarcoma should also be entertained in mitotically inactive lesions that are extremely large and locally invasive, since such lesions in our experience can produce metastasis. Once a diagnosis of malignancy is made by histological criteria, evaluation of size can yield additional information about metastatic risk.

It is clear from the foregoing discussion that there will be situations in which the level of malignancy is indeterminate. These could include an extremely small (1 to 2 cm) histologically malignant lesion perhaps discovered incidentally. We believe it justifiable to designate such lesions as tumors of borderline or indeterminate malignancy. Hopefully, this approach guarantees good follow-up for the patient.

DNA ploidy and proliferation studies

A number of studies have investigated the relationship between DNA ploidy and malignancy.[15,16] In general there is a positive correlation between aneuploidy and malignancy as determined by histological criteria. However, considerable overlapping exists, such that DNA ploidy analysis is not useful in the individual case.[16] Evaluation of proliferation cell nuclear antigen correlates well with malignancy.[19,54] Sarcomas have more stainable antigen than benign tumors and, in some studies levels of this antigen, correlate well with survival rates.[19]

BEHAVIOR AND TREATMENT

Most data regarding the behavior and treatment of epithelioid smooth muscle tumors are derived from experience with gastrointestinal tract lesions. Pizzimbono et al.,[40] in reviewing the collective experience from the literature, which showed that over 90% of these tumors were gastric tumors, concluded that about 17% ultimately metastasized. About three fourths of metastasizing lesions had documented metastasis at the time of the initial surgery, while the remainder developed metastases subsequent to surgery. Metastases occur most commonly in the liver and peritoneal surfaces. In a large follow-up study in Japan, the 10-year survival rate for malignant gastrointestinal stromal tumors from all sites was 48%.[51] However, the 10-year survival rate for gastric tumors was significantly better (74%) than that of intestinal lesions (17%).

The extent of surgical excision of gastric lesions does not affect survival rates. Total or subtotal gastrectomy offered no better chance for survival than segmental resections, provided the tumor was completely excised.[3] Unfortunately there are no collective data relative to the behavior of epithelioid smooth muscle tumors of soft tissue. It has been our impression that the majority of these lesions in soft tissue are malignant and, therefore, capable of metastasis. The few reported cases in the literature have behaved in an aggressive fashion. One case that involved the transverse mesocolon and possessed two or three mitoses per 50 HPF metastasized within 5 years,[11] while another case reported by Wellman,[53] which was in the retroperitoneum and had 12 mitoses per 50 HPF, was widely metastatic to the peritoneal surfaces at the time of surgery. Suster[46] recently reported five epithelioid leiomyosarcomas of the skin and subcutis, one of which killed the patient. Clearly, tumors judged histologically malignant should be widely excised and treated in the same manner as leiomyosarcomas of comparable grade. Those considered histologically benign or of indeterminate malignancy should nonetheless be completely excised and the patient carefully followed up for evidence of recurrence.

REFERENCES

1. Abramson DJ: Gastric leiomyoblastoma. *Ann Surg* 178:625, 1973.
2. Appelman HD: Smooth muscle tumors of the gastrointestinal tract: what we know that Stout didn't know. *Am J Surg Pathol* 10(suppl):83, 1986.
3. Appelman HD, Helwig EB: Gastric epithelioid leiomyoma and leiomyosarcoma (leiomyoblastoma). *Cancer* 38:708, 1976.
4. Bose B, Candy J: Gastric leiomyoblastoma. *Gut* 11:875, 1970.
5. Byard RW, Barr JR, Naidoo SP, et al: Gastric stromal tumors with epithelioid features: clinicopathological features of 22 cases. *Surg Pathol* 3:281, 1990.
6. Carney JA: The triad of gastric epithelioid leiomyosarcoma, functioning extraadrenal paraganglioma, and pulmonary chondroma. *Cancer* 43:374, 1979.
7. Carney JA: The triad of gastric epithelioid leiomyosarcoma, pulmonary chondroma, and functioning extraadrenal paraganglioma: a five year review. *Medicine (Baltimore)* 62:159, 1983.
8. Chang V, Aikawa M, Druet R: Uterine leiomyoblastoma: ultrastructural and cytological studies. *Cancer* 39:1563, 1977.
9. Cooper PN, Hardy GJ, Dixon MF: A flow cytometric, clinical, and histological study of stromal neoplasms of the gastrointestinal tract. *Am J Surg Pathol* 16:163, 1992.
10. Cornog JL: Gastric leiomyoblastoma: a clinical and ultrastructural study. *Cancer* 34:711, 1974.
11. Cornog JL: The ultrastructure of leiomyoblastoma. *Arch Pathol* 87:404, 1969.
12. DeCastro FJ, Olsen WR, Littler ER: Gastric leiomyoblastoma in an adolescent. *Am J Surg* 123:614, 1972.
13. Eimoto T, Miyake M, Sasaki T: Vascular leiomyoblastoma of the stomach. *Acta Pathol Jpn* 29:277, 1979.
14. El-Naggar AK, McLemore D, Garnsey L, et al: Gastrointestinal stromal tumors: DNA flow-cytometric study of 58 patients with at least five years of follow-up. *Mod Pathol* 2:511, 1988.
15. Evans HL: Smooth muscle tumors of the gastrointestinal tract: a study of 56 cases followed for a minimum of 10 years. *Cancer* 56:2242, 1985.
16. Flint A, Appelman HD, Beckwith AL: DNA analysis of gastric stromal neoplasm: correlation with pathologic features. *Surg Pathol* 2:117, 1989.
17. Franquemont DW, Frierson HF: Muscle differentiation and clinicopathologic features of gastrointestinal stromal tumors. *Am J Surg Pathol* 16:947, 1992.

18. Frimodt-Moller PC, Klunder KB, Svanholm H: Benign and malignant epithelioid leiomyoma (leiomyoblastoma of the stomach). *Acta Chir Scand* 145:257, 1979.

19. Goldblum JR, Mandell SH, Appelman HD, et al: Proliferating cell nuclear antigen and p53 antigen expression in gastrointestinal stromal tumors. *Am J Clin Pathol* 98:351, 1992.

20. Gupta RK, Chandler JP: Leiomyoblastoma of the stomach. *Ann Surg* 161:562, 1965.

21. Hajdu SI, Erlandson RA, Paglia MA: Light and electron microscopic studies of a gastric leiomyoblastoma. *Arch Pathol* 93:36, 1972.

22. Hjermstad BM, Sobin LH, Helwig EB: Stromal tumors of the gastrointestinal tract: myogenic or neurogenic. *Am J Surg Pathol* 11:383, 1987.

23. Kay S, Still WJS: A comparative electron microscopic study of a leiomyosarcoma and bizarre leiomyoma (leiomyoblastoma) of the stomach. *Am J Clin Pathol* 52:403, 1969.

24. Kelsey JR Jr: Leiomyoblastoma of the stomach presenting as acute intraperitoneal hemorrhage. *Gastroenterology* 51:539, 1966.

25. Kiyabu MT, Bishop PC, Parker JW, et al: Smooth muscle tumors of the gastrointestinal tract: flow cytometric quantitation of DNA and nuclear antigen content and correlation with histologic grade. *Am J Surg Pathol* 12:954, 1988.

26. Knapp RH, Wick MR, Goellner JR: Leiomyoblastomas and their relationship to other smooth-muscle tumors of the gastrointestinal tract. *Am J Surg Pathol* 8:449, 1984.

27. Kurman RJ, Norris HJ: Mesenchymal tumors of the uterus. VI. Epithelioid smooth muscle tumors including leiomyoblastoma and clear-cell leiomyoma. *Cancer* 37:1853, 1976.

28. Langley JR: Gastric and extragastric leiomyoblastoma: report of six new cases with a review of the literature. *Am Surg* 42:369, 1976.

29. Lavin P, Hajdu SI, Foote FW: Gastric and extragastric leiomyoblastomas. *Cancer* 29:305, 1972.

30. Lewin K, Appelman HD: Tumors of the stomach. In: *Atlas of tumor pathology*, Armed Forces Institute of Pathology, Washington, D.C. (in press).

31. Ma CK, Amin MB, Kintanar E, et al: Immunohistochemical characterization of gastrointestinal stromal tumors: a study of 82 cases compared with 11 cases of leiomyomas. *Mod Pathol* 6:139, 1993.

32. Martin JF, Bazin P, Feroldi J, et al: Tumeurs myoides intra-murales de l'estomac: considerations microscopiques à propos de 6 cas. *Ann Anat Pathol (Paris)* 5:484, 1960.

33. Mazur MT, Clark HB: Gastric stromal tumors: reappraisal of histogenesis. *Am J Surg Pathol* 7:507, 1983.

34. Miettinen M: Gastrointestinal stromal tumors: an immunohistochemical study of cellular differentiation. *Am J Clin Pathol* 89:601, 1988.

35. Min K-W: Small intestinal stromal tumors with skeinoid fibers: clinicopathological, immunohistochemical, and ultrastructural investigations. *Am J Surg Pathol* 16:145, 1992.

36. Morales AR, Fine G, Pardo V, et al: The ultrastructure of smooth muscle tumors with a consideration of the possible relationship of glomangioma, hemangiopericytomas, and cardiac myxomas. *Pathol Annu* 10:65, 1975.

37. Newman PL, Wadden C, Fletcher CDM: Gastrointestinal stromal tumors: correlation of immunophenotype with clinicopathologic features. *J Pathol* 164:107, 1991.

38. Persson S, Kindblom LG, Angervall L, et al: Metastasizing gastric epithelioid leiomyosarcomas (leiomyoblastomas) in young individuals with long-term survival. *Cancer* 70:721, 1992.

39. Pike AM, Lloyd RV, Appelman HD: Cell markers in gastrointestinal stromal tumors. *Hum Pathol* 19:830, 1988.

40. Pizzimbono CA, Higa E, Wise L: Leiomyoblastoma of the lesser sac: case report and review of the literature. *Am Surg* 39:692, 1973.

41. Rachman R, Meranze DR, Zibelman CS, et al: Malignant leiomyoblastoma. *Am J Clin Pathol* 49:556, 1968.

42. Salazar H, Totten RS: Leiomyoblastoma of the stomach: an ultrastructural study. *Cancer* 25:176, 1970.

43. Saul SH, Rast ML, Brooks JJ: The immunohistochemistry of gastrointestinal stromal tumors: evidence supporting origin from smooth muscle. *Am J Surg Pathol* 11:464, 1987.

44. Smithwick W, Biesecker JL, Leand PM: Leiomyoblastoma: behavior and prognosis. *Cancer* 24:996, 1969.

45. Stout AP: Bizarre smooth muscle tumors of the stomach. *Cancer* 15:400, 1962.

46. Suster S: Epithelioid leiomyosarcoma of the skin and subcutaneous tissue: clinicopathologic, immunohistochemical, and ultrastructural study of five cases. *Am J Surg Pathol* 18:232, 1994.

47. Tallqvist G, Salmela H, Lindstrom BL: Leiomyoblastoma of the stomach. *Acta Pathol Microbiol Scand* 71:194, 1967.

48. Thompson EM, Evans DJ: The significance of PGP 9.5 in tumours: an immunohistochemical study of gastrointestinal stromal tumours. *Histopathology* 17:175, 1990.

49. Tisell LE, Angervall L, Dahl I, et al: Recurrent and metastasizing gastric leiomyoblastoma (epithelioid leiomyosarcoma) associated with multiple pulmonary chondrohamartomas: long survival of a patient treated with repeated operations. *Cancer* 41:259, 1978.

50. Tsutsumi Y, Kubo H: Immunohistochemistry of desmin and vimentin in smooth muscle tumors of the digestive tract. *Acta Pathol Jpn* 38:455, 1988.

51. Ueyama T, Guo K-J, Hashimoto H, et al: A clinicopathologic and immunohistochemical study of gastrointestinal stromal tumors. *Cancer* 69:947, 1992.

52. Weiss RA, Mackay B: Malignant smooth muscle tumors of the gastrointestinal tract. *Ultrastruct Pathol* 2:231, 1981.

53. Wellman K: Bizarre leiomyoblastoma of the retroperitoneum: report of a case. *J Pathol Bacteriol* 94:447, 1967.

54. Yu CC-W, Fletcher CDM, Newman PL, et al: A comparison of proliferating cell nuclear antigen (PCNA) immunostaining, nucleolar organizer region (AgNOR) staining, and histological grading in gastrointestinal stromal tumors. *J Pathol* 166:147, 1992.

CHAPTER 21

RHABDOMYOMA

STRIATED MUSCLE TISSUE: DEVELOPMENT AND STRUCTURE

Skeletal muscle is primarily formed within myotomes, which are arranged in segmental pairs along the spine and make their first appearance in the cephalic region during the third week of intrauterine life. In the region of the anterior head and neck, skeletal muscle may also develop from mesenchyme that is derived from the neural crest (mesectoderm).

At the earliest stage of muscle development, primitive mesenchymal cells differentiate along two lines: (1) fibroblasts, loosely arranged spindle-shaped cells having the capacity to form collagen, and (2) myoblasts, round or oval cells with single centrally positioned nuclei and granular eosinophilic cytoplasm. Over the next few weeks the individual myoblasts assume a more elongated bipolar shape with slender symmetrically arranged processes and nonstriated longitudinal myofibrils that are laid down first in the peripheral portion of the cytoplasm; this is followed by successive alignment and fusion of the individual myoblasts into myotubes with multiple centrally placed nuclei (myotubular stage) (Figs. 21-1 and 21-2). During the seventh to tenth weeks of intrauterine development, as differentiation progresses, the myofibrils become thicker and more numerous by longitudinal division and develop increasingly distinct cross-striations. Finally, during the eleventh to fifteenth weeks the nucleus is moved from its initial central position toward the periphery of the muscle fiber. Muscles derived from the cervical and thoracic myotomes mature earlier than those arising more distally.

Ultrastructurally the individual myofibrils are composed of two types of myofilaments: thin (actin) filaments measuring 50 to 70 nm in diameter and thick (myosin) filaments measuring 140 to 160 nm in diameter. The thin filaments are laid down first in a random fashion, but later they become rearranged and form parallel bundles together with thick filaments and polyribosomes. In cross-sections the thin filaments surround the thick filaments in distinct, evenly spaced hexagonal patterns.

Mature striated muscle consists of parallel arrays of closely packed myofibrils embedded within sarcoplasm and enveloped by a thin sarcolemmal sheath. Each of the myofibrils shows distinct cross-banding, light and dark bands caused by the periodic arrangement and interdigitation of the thin and thick myofilaments. In this arrangement, I (isotropic) bands, A (anisotropic) bands, and H bands can be distinguished. The I band consists solely of thin (actin) filaments and is divided in its center by the Z line or disc, which is thought to serve as an attachment site for the sarcomeres, the repeating individual units of the muscle fiber. The adjacent A band is a zone of overlapping thin and thick (actin and myosin) filaments; it is separated by the H band, which consists only of thick myofilaments. The width of the individual bands and sarcomeres varies and depends on the state of muscle contraction (Fig. 21-3).

Closely associated with the parallel arrays of myofilaments and the surrounding sarcoplasm are mitochondria, a canalicular network of endoplasmic reticulum, a small Golgi complex, ribosomes, and glycogen and lipid granules. These organelles are confined by a sarcolemmal membrane that measures approximately 70 nm in thickness and is covered by a basal lamina. The sarcolemmal nuclei measure 6 to 12 μm in greatest diameter and contain one or two small nucleoli; they are located at the periphery of the myofibrils beneath the sarcolemmal membrane. Satellite cells—reserve cells and possible precursors of myoblasts that play a role in the regeneration of striated muscle tissue—are situated in the endomysium between the sarcolemmal membrane and basal lamina.

CLASSIFICATION OF RHABDOMYOMA

Although, as a general rule, benign soft tissue neoplasms outnumber malignant neoplasms by a sizable margin, this does not hold true for the neoplasms of striated muscle tissue. In this particular group of neoplasms, rhabdomyomas (the benign tumors of striated muscle tissue) are considerably less common than rhabdomyosarcomas; according to our data, they amount to no more than 2% of all striated muscle tumors.

Among rhabdomyomas four clinically and morphologi-

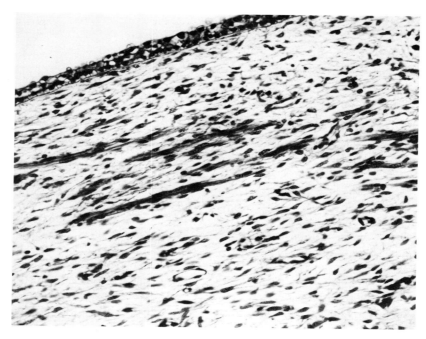

FIG. 21-1. Developing striated muscle in the soft tissue of a 9-week-old fetus. Note the close resemblance to botryoid-type embryonal rhabdomyosarcoma (Fig. 22-23). (×250.)

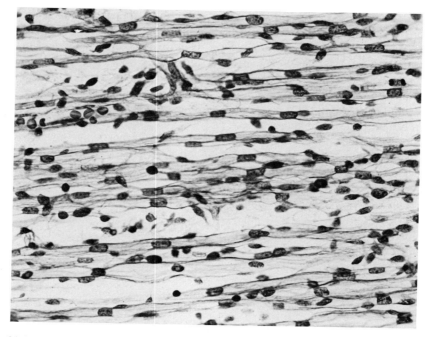

FIG. 21-2. Myotube stage in the development of striated muscle bearing a close resemblance to both fetal rhabdomyoma (Fig. 21-13) and the "tubular" type of embryonal rhabdomyosarcoma (Fig. 22-14). (×395.)

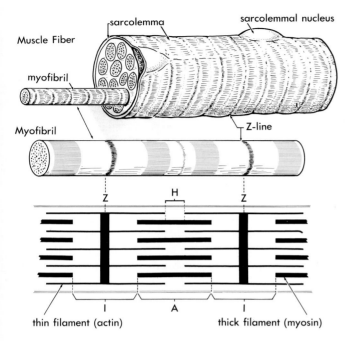

Muscle Fiber

sarcolemma

sarcolemmal nucleus

myofibril

Myofibril

Z-line

Z   H   Z

thin filament (actin)   thick filament (myosin)

I   A   I

FIG. 21-3. Schematic drawing of muscle fiber, myofibril, and sliding actin and myosin filaments during rest phase of muscle contraction.

cally different types can be distinguished: (1) the *adult type,* a slowly growing lesion that is nearly always found in the head and neck area of older persons; (2) the *fetal type,* a rare process that also affects mainly the head and neck region but occurs in both children and adults; (3) the *genital type,* a tumorlike polypoid mass that has been described so far only in the vagina and vulva of middle-aged women; and (4) the *rhabdomyomatous mesenchymal hamartoma,* a peculiar striated muscle proliferation that occurs chiefly in the periorbital and perioral region of infants and young children.

Rhabdomyoma of the heart is a well-established hamartomatous process that is frequently encountered in association with tuberous sclerosis of the brain, sebaceous adenomas, and various other hamartomatous lesions of the kidney and other organs. Cardiac rhabdomyoma occurs chiefly but not exclusively in patients of the pediatric age-group and usually manifests as a multifocal or rarely diffuse process involving the myocardium of both ventricles and the interventricular septum.[10] Clinically the lesion may be asymptomatic or may cause cardiac arrhythmia, tachycardia, or even sudden cardiac death. Spontaneous regression of the tumor has been observed in some cases.[3] To our knowledge, the concurrence of cardiac and extracardiac rhabdomyoma in the same patient has not been observed. Nor has extracardiac rhabdomyoma been found in association with manifestations of the tuberous sclerosis complex.

The terms *rhabdomyoblastoma* has been used as synonym for well-differentiated rhabdomyosarcoma or as a descriptive term in reports of granular cell tumor *(granular cell myoblastoma),* a condition that is of Schwann cell rather than muscle origin (see Chapter 31).

ADULT RHABDOMYOMA

The adult type of rhabdomyoma, like the other two types, is a rare but morphologically characteristic lesion; only about 90 cases have been reported in the literature, including several cases with multifocal lesions in the same general area. The terms *extracardiac rhabdomyoma*[2,3] and *rhabdomyoma purum*[14,31] have also been employed in the literature to describe this tumor. As previously pointed out, there is no etiological relationship between adult rhabdomyoma and *granular cell myoblastoma (Abrikossoff's tumor*[1]*).*

Clinical findings

The process usually presents as a solitary round or polypoid mass in the neck region that causes neither tenderness nor pain but may compress or displace the tongue or may protrude into and partially obstruct the pharynx or larynx. As a consequence, it may cause hoarseness or progressive difficulties in breathing or swallowing. It has also been reported as an incidental finding at autopsy or during radical neck dissection for an unrelated cause. It is a slowly growing process, and several of the reported cases have been known to be present for many years. Parsons and Puro,[34] for instance, reported a 74-year-old patient who had rhabdomyoma of the sternohyoid muscle for no fewer than 55 years.

Most cases occur in adults older than 40 years (median age 60 years), and so far only one typical example has been described in a child.[38] Men are involved more commonly than women, but apparently there is no predilection for any particular race. The principal site of the tumor is the neck, where it seems to arise from the branchial musculature of the third and fourth branchial arches. The tumor is found most frequently in the region of the larynx,[6,7,14,26] pharynx,[4,18,32,40] and the floor of the mouth or base of the tongue.[25,33,44] It may also involve the soft palate and the uvula,[9,12,21] usually as an extension of a pharyngeal rhabdomyoma. Isolated examples have been encountered in the somatic muscles of the lateral neck (sternocleidomastoid[35] and sternohyoid[34]), the lower lip and cheek,[39] and the orbit.[34] One unusually large example, which was found incidentally at autopsy, extended from the supraclavicular region into the upper mediastinum.[30] Another, a rhabdomyoma of typical histological appearance, occurred in the wall of the stomach of a 47-year-old woman.[41] It is remarkable that there is no record of an adult rhabdomyoma arising in the muscles of the limbs.

The majority of adult rhabdomyomas are solitary, but about 20% are multifocal, mostly involving the general area of the neck.* For example, the patient reported by Parsons and Puro[34] and Goldman,[19] who had an adult rhabdomyoma of the left neck, developed a second tumor of similar appearance in the left vocal cord, which was found at autopsy. Walker and Laszewski[42] reported a rhabdomyoma of the tongue that recurred after 21 years on both sides of the neck; it was diagnosed by fine-needle aspiration biopsy.

---

*References 2, 5, 8, 15, 17, 20, 24, 36.

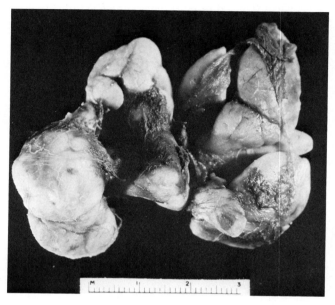

FIG. 21-4. Adult rhabdomyoma. A multilobulated tan-brown tumor removed from the floor of the mouth of an 81-year-old woman.

Pathological findings

As a rule, the tumor is well defined, rounded, or coarsely lobulated and ranges from 0.5 to 10 cm in greatest diameter with a median size of 3 cm (Fig. 21-4). On cut section it has a finely granular, gray-yellow to red-brown color (Fig. 21-5).

Microscopically it is composed of tightly packed, large, round or polygonal cells, 15 to 150 μm in diameter and separated from one another by thin fibrous septa and narrow vascular channels. The cells have deeply acidophilic, finely granular cytoplasm, one or rarely two peripherally placed vesicular nuclei, and one or more small nucleoli (Fig. 21-6). Many of the cells are vacuolated as the result of removal of intracellular glycogen during processing; some of the vacuolated cells, in fact, contain merely a small central acidophilic cytoplasmic mass connected by thin strands of cytoplasm to a condensed rim of cytoplasm at the periphery (spider cells), but these cells are much more conspicuous in cardiac than extracardiac rhabdomyomas (Fig. 21-7). Mitotic figures are nearly always absent.[13,21,24]

Cross-striations can be discerned in most cases, but sometimes they are detected only after a prolonged search (Fig. 21-8, A); additional features present in many cases are intracytoplasmic rodlike or "jackstraw"-like crystalline structures, first described by Moran and Enterline[32] in 1964 (Fig. 21-8, B). Both cross-striations and crystalline structures are identified much more readily with the phosphotungstic acid–hematoxylin (PTAH) stain than with the hematoxylin-eosin preparation; moreover, many cells contain intracellular lipid demonstrable with the oil red O preparation. The cells also stain positively for immunoreactive myoglobin, desmin, and alpha-smooth muscle and less commonly for vimentin, S-100 protein, and Leu-7[8,22,24] (Fig. 21-9).

Gibas and Miettinen,[18] in a cytogenetic study of a recur-

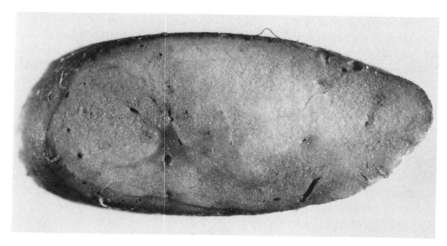

FIG. 21-5. Adult rhabdomyoma in cross-section showing a well-vascularized, finely granular surface.

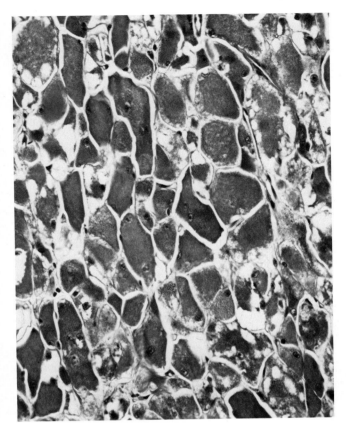

FIG. 21-6. Adult rhabdomyoma composed of variously sized, deeply eosinophilic polygonal cells with small, peripherally placed nuclei and occasional intracellular vacuoles. (×250.)

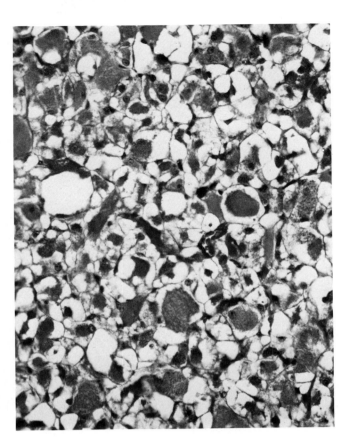

FIG. 21-7. Adult rhabdomyoma. Another portion of tumor shown in Fig. 21-6 having a more pronounced vacuolated appearance, probably secondary to removal of intracellular glycogen by the fixative. (×250.)

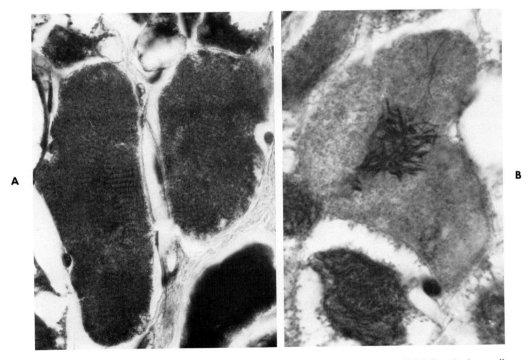

FIG. 21-8. Adult rhabdomyoma. **A,** Cell with cross-striations. (PTAH; ×630.) **B,** "Jackstraw"-like crystalline intracellular structures, probably representing Z-band material. (×1000.)

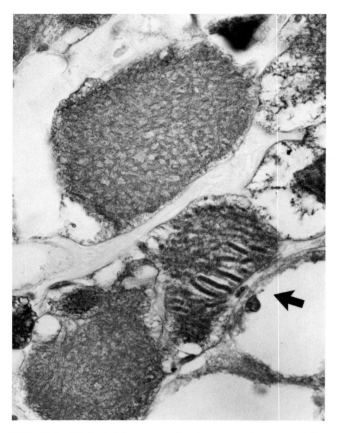

FIG. 21-9. Adult rhabdomyoma showing strong immunostaining for myoglobin. Note cross-banding at arrow. (×400.)

rent parapharyngeal rhabdomyoma in a 64-year-old man, found reciprocal translocation of chromosomes 15 and 17 and minor clone abnormality in the long arm of chromosome 10. They concluded that this finding lends support to the notion that the adult rhabdomyoma is a true neoplasm rather than a hamartoma.

Ultrastructural findings

There is good agreement among most observers as to the ultrastructure of adult rhabdomyoma.[9,21,29,37] The cytoplasm contains, in addition to a variable number of mitochondria with linear cristae and deposits of glycogen, thin and thick myofilaments showing different degrees of differentiation and measuring 50 to 70 nm and 135 to 150 nm in diameter, respectively. Distinct Z lines are readily discernible within the I band, but sometimes A, H, M, and N bands are also apparent (Figs. 21-10 and 21-11). Cornog and Gonatas[11] identified the crystalline intracytoplasmic inclusions as hypertrophied Z bands and pointed out their close resemblance to structures found in nemaline myopathy. There are also "triads," trigonal arrays of actin and my-

osin filaments that can be seen in cross-section[43] and parallel rows of electron-dense particles within the mitochondria.[28,36,44] The individual cells are surrounded by a thin basal lamina with focal infoldings of the plasma membrane in some of the cells.[9] Kay et al.[25] compared the ultrastructure of cardiac rhabdomyoma and adult rhabdomyoma and noted better organization and more prominent Z lines in cardiac rhabdomyoma.

Differential diagnosis

Problems in diagnosis are unlikely for anyone familiar with the characteristic picture of the tumor. Yet in the earlier literature, granular cell tumor (granular cell myoblastoma)[1] and adult rhabdomyoma were often confused, although the cells of granular cell tumor tend to be less well defined and lack the characteristic vacuolation caused by intracellular glycogen; they are also devoid of cross-striations and usually are associated with more collagen. Moreover, the cells of granular cell tumors contain numerous lysosomes and abundant intracellular acid phosphatase.[6] S-100 protein expression is more pronounced in granular cell tumors than in rhabdomyoma.

Hibernoma also enters into differential diagnosis because of the frequent intracytoplasmic vacuoles and the presence of intracellular lipid. This tumor, however, is composed of small deeply eosinophilic granular cells that frequently contain distinct and variably sized lipid droplets in the cytoplasm. *Reticulohistiocytoma,* another lesion that must be included in differential diagnosis, usually consists of an intimate mixture of deeply acidophilic histiocytes and fibroblasts intermingled with xanthoma cells, multinucleated giant cells, and chronic inflammatory elements. Typically, none of these cells contains glycogen. Glycogen is also absent in the epithelioid type of fibrous histiocytoma. Crystal-storing histiocytosis associated with lymphoplasmacytic neoplasms may also simulate adult rhabdomyoma, but in this lesion the crystal-storing cells stain positively for immunoglobulin and CD68 (KP1) but are negative for skeletal muscle markers and S-100 protein.[23]

Rhabdomyoma of the heart bears a close resemblance to adult rhabdomyoma, but its cells show a greater degree of vacuolation and a greater number of giant cells. Cardiac rhabdomyoma is a well-established hamartomatous process that is frequently encountered in association with tuberous sclerosis of the brain, sebaceous adenomas, and various other hamartomatous lesions of the kidney and other organs.

Rhabdomyosarcoma is always less well defined and characteristically is composed of poorly differentiated and pleomorphic round or spindle-shaped cells associated with varying numbers of rhabdomyoblasts. Mitotic figures are common in rhabdomyosarcoma but are absent or very rare in adult rhabdomyoma. *Oncocytoma* and *paraganglioma* must also be included in differential diagnosis.

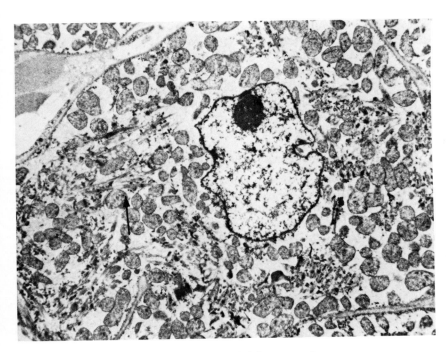

FIG. 21-10. Electron micrograph of adult rhabdomyoma showing association of mitochondria and short bundles of thin and thick myofilaments *(arrow)*. (From Bagby RA, Packer JT, Iglesias RG: *Arch Otolaryngol* 102:101, 1976. Copyright 1976, American Medical Association.)

Prognosis and therapy

The tumor is readily amenable to therapy but may recur locally if incompletely excised. In one series of 19 cases with follow-up information the tumor recurred in eight (42%) of the cases.[24] Examples of multiple and late recurrences have also been described.[24,50] Andersen and Elling[4] reported three recurrences within 35 years. Spontaneous regression, as in some cases of cardiac rhabdomyoma, has not been observed.

FETAL RHABDOMYOMA

Fetal rhabdomyoma is even rarer in our experience than adult-type rhabdomyoma, and only a small number of cases have been recorded in the medical literature. Awareness of the existence of this tumor, however, is of considerable importance because of its close similarity to rhabdomyosarcoma; in fact, failure to recognize this lesion as a benign process may lead to excessive and unnecessary therapy. Diagnosis of this tumor may be difficult, since it is marked by a variable histological pattern that ranges from immature, predominantly myxoid tumors to tumors showing a high degree of cellular differentiation and hardly any myxoid matrix. The former have been described as the *myxoid*[50] or *classic*[53] *type of fetal rhabdomyoma,*[50] the latter

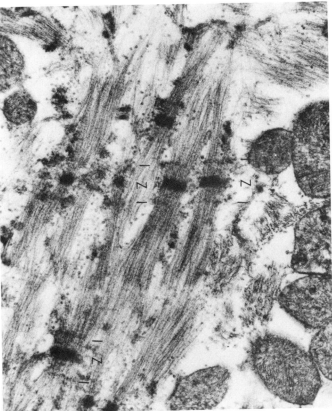

FIG. 21-11. Electron micrograph of adult rhabdomyoma. Bundles of actin and myosin filaments with clearly discernible Z lines flanked by distinct I bands. (From Bagby RA, Packer JT, Iglesias RG: *Arch Otolaryngol* 102:101, 1976. Copyright 1976, American Medical Association.)

variously as the *intermediate,*[53] *cellular,*[50] or *juvenile type*[47] *of fetal rhabdomyoma*. Intermediate forms between these two types are not uncommon. There is also a third and still ill-defined morphological variant of this tumor that is marked by prominent neural involvement akin to neuromuscular hamartoma. Fetal rhabdomyoma is also a rare manifestation of the *nevoid basal cell carcinoma syndrome*.[48,51]

Clinical features

The age incidence varies slightly according to the prevailing histological type. Tumors of the predominantly *myxoid type* mainly affect boys during the first year of life and are rare in older patients. In the series of Kapadia et al.[53] for instance, 6 of the 8 patients with this type of tumor were infants younger than 1 year of age. The favorite sites of the myxoid type are the subcutaneous tissue and the submucosa of the head and neck, especially the pre- and postauricular regions.[49,53,56] The *intermediate type* affects adults more often than children. It almost exclusively occurs in the region of the head and neck, including the orbit, tongue, nasopharynx, and soft palate.[45,46,52,53] In both types, males outnumber females by a ratio of approximately 3:1.

There are only a few reports in the literature of fetal rhabdomyomas associated with multiple basal cell carcinomas and various osseous anomalies.[48,51,54] In one case, described by Dahl et al.,[48] two fetal rhabdomyomas in the left thigh and the chest wall were associated with multiple basal cell carcinomas and anomalies of the eye and rib (bifurcated rib). In another case reported by DiSanto et al.,[51] a very large fetal rhabdomyoma, extending from the mediastinum to the retroperitoneum, was removed from a 6-year-old girl who had multiple osseous anomalies and a family history of nevoid basal cell carcinoma.

Pathological findings

On gross examination the tumors are well to moderately well circumscribed and average 2 to 6 cm in greatest diameter. Mucosal lesions tend to be polypoid or pedunculated. On section they are gray-white to pink, often with a mucoid, glistening surface. Unlike rhabdomyosarcoma, fetal rhabdomyoma is primarily a superficial tumor and is found more often in the subcutis or submucosa than in muscle. Most are solitary, but multicentric fetal rhabdomyomas have been reported in association with the nevoid basal cell carcinoma syndrome.[48,54]

Under the microscope two closely related types can be distinguished. The *myxoid type* is chiefly composed of primitive oval or spindle-shaped cells with indistinct cytoplasm, interspersed muscle fibers, and a richly myxoid matrix (Figs. 21-12 to 21-14). The slender, eosinophilic muscle fibers vary little in size and shape and bear a close resemblance to those found in the myotubular stage of mus-

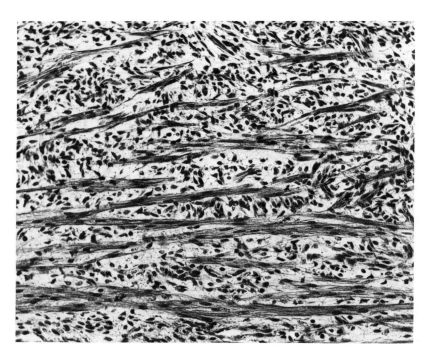

FIG. 21-12. Fetal rhabdomyoma, myxoid type, removed from the postauricular region of a 2-month-old girl. The lesion is composed of an intimate mixture of primitive, round and spindle-shaped mesenchymal cells and differentiated myofibrils within a richly myxoid background. (×450.)

cle development. They may be difficult to discern with hematoxylin-eosin staining and are best seen with phosphotungstic acid–hematoxylin staining or the Masson trichrome stain. Cross-striations are rare in the majority of cases. Sometimes, focal proliferation of abundant muscle fibers makes it difficult to draw a sharp line between tumor and normal muscle tissue (Fig. 21-15).

The *intermediate type* is characterized by the presence

of numerous differentiated muscle fibers, less conspicuous or absent spindle-shaped mesenchymal cells, and little or no myxoid stroma. The predominant cells are broad, strap-shaped muscle cells with abundant eosinophilic cytoplasm, centrally located vesicular nuclei, and frequent cross-striations; many of the cells contain glycogen and are often vacuolated (Figs. 21-16 and 21-17). Like adult rhabdomyomas, the muscle cells stain positively for myoglobin,

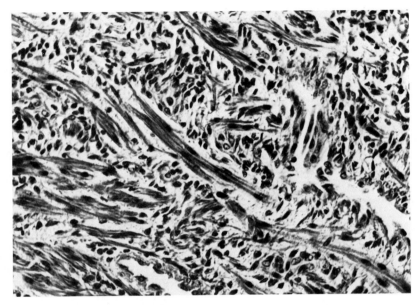

FIG. 21-13. Fetal rhabdomyoma, myxoid type. Unlike embryonal rhabdomyosarcoma, the muscle cells vary little in shape and size, and there is no mitotic activity. Cells with cross-striations were rare in this tumor. (Trichrome; ×550.)

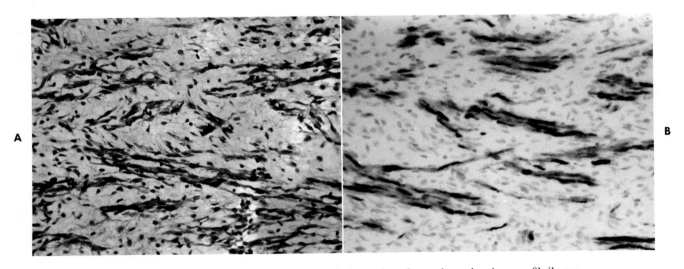

FIG. 21-14. Fetal rhabdomyoma of the postauricular region of a newborn showing myofibrils separated by a prominent myxoid matrix and scattered small mesenchymal cells **(A)** (×160) and positive staining of the myofibrils for immunoreactive desmin **(B)**. (×260.)

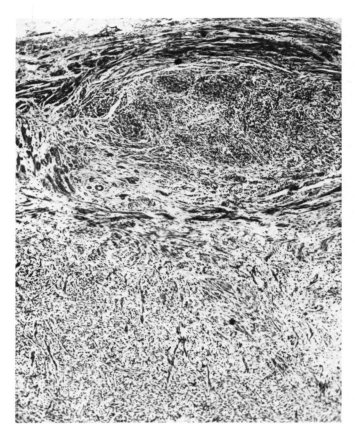

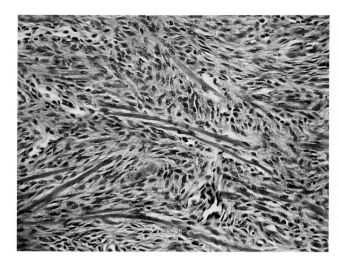

FIG. 21-16. Fetal rhabdomyoma, intermediate (cellular) type. Prominent spindle cell pattern with interspersed differentiated eosinophilic myofibrils containing cross-striations. (×450.)

FIG. 21-15. Fetal rhabdomyoma. The better differentiation of the muscle tissue at the periphery helps in the distinction from embryonal rhabdomyosarcoma. (Masson trichrome stain; ×35.)

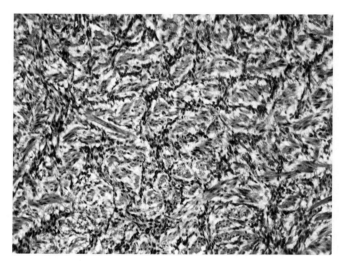

FIG. 21-17. Fetal rhabdomyoma, intermediate (cellular) type consisting of intersecting bundles of differentiated myofibrils separated by strands of small undifferentiated spindle cells. (×260.)

desmin, and muscle-specific actin.[53] In some cases there is mild cellular pleomorphism, but marked cellular atypia is not a feature of the disease, as it is in embryonal rhabdomyosarcoma. Transitional forms between the myxoid and intermediate types are not rare.[58] In fact, age and duration may play a role in the maturation of some tumors, as suggested by the older age of the average patient with the intermediate (cellular) type and the reported long duration of some cases. Mitotic figures are rare or absent in most cases. No mitotic figures were found in 19 of 24 fetal rhabdomyomas described by Kapadia et al.[53]

In addition to the myxoid and intermediate types there are also sporadic fetal rhabdomyoma-like tumors that are intimately associated with peripheral nerves reminiscent of neuromuscular hamartoma (benign Triton tumor). In the past we have seen two such cases in the head and neck region, and Zwick et al.[59] described such a tumor that seemed to arise in the mandibular division of the trigeminal nerve.

Ultrastructurally the differentiated muscle cells consist of organized bundles of thick (myosin) and thin (actin) myo-

filaments with the characteristic banding in some of the more differentiated muscle cells (Fig. 21-18). Rodlike cytoplasmic inclusions or hypertrophied Z-band materials have been described but seem to be much less common than in adult rhabdomyoma.[45,47,58] The differentiated cells also contain considerable amounts of intracellular glycogen and a small number of mitochondria. The intervening small spindle cells are devoid of any specific cellular differentiation.

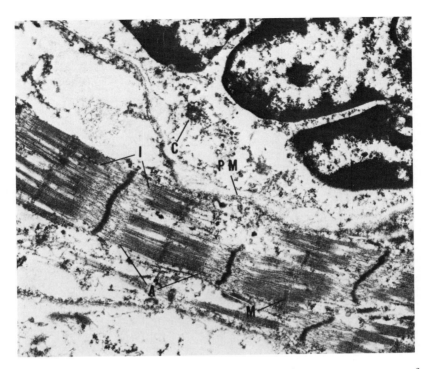

FIG. 21-18. Electron micrograph of fetal rhabdomyoma showing mature appearance of muscle fiber with isotropic *(I)* and anisotropic *(A)* segments and intervening Z and M lines. *C,* Centriole; *PM,* plasma membrane. (×18,700.)

Differential diagnosis

Distinction from *embryonal and spindle cell rhabdomyosarcomas* is the principal problem in diagnosis; unlike rhabdomyosarcoma, fetal rhabdomyoma tends to be fairly well circumscribed and is superficially located. Mitotic figures are rare, and the tumor lacks a significant degree of cellular pleomorphism and areas of necrosis. As has already been pointed out, considerable cellularity, a mild degree of cellular pleomorphism, and occasional mitotic figures do not rule out this diagnosis.[53]

Caution in the differential diagnosis must also be exercised because of the possible malignant transformation of fetal rhabdomyoma. We have encountered one case in which the initial lesion, biopsied at 3 weeks of age, seemed to be characteristic of fetal rhabdomyoma, whereas the recurrent tumor, excised at 23 months, showed a much greater degree of cellularity and mitotic activity and was indistinguishable from embryonal rhabdomyosarcoma. Another possible case of "cellular fetal rhabdomyoma with malignant transformation" was reported by Kodet et al.[55] in the tongue of an 18-month-old infant.

Infantile (desmoid-type) fibromatosis may bear a close resemblance to fetal rhabdomyoma, especially if the tumor diffusely infiltrates muscle tissue and contains numerous residual muscle fibers that have been entrapped by the proliferating fibroblasts. Fetal rhabdomyoma, however, is better circumscribed than fibromatoses, is situated in the subcutis rather than in muscle tissue, and lacks the fasciculated spindle cell pattern. In addition, interspersed fat cells, a frequent feature of diffuse infantile fibromatosis, are absent in fetal rhabdomyoma. Other lesions that must be considered in differential diagnosis are fibrosarcoma and leiomyosarcoma.

Prognosis and therapy

Fetal rhabdomyoma is a benign condition that is readily curable by local excision. It is a slowly growing process, and several examples are known to have been present for years with little change in size or histological picture except for interstitial fibrosis. The exact pathogenesis of fetal rhabdomyoma is still obscure; it may be a hamartomatous growth, as suggested by association of the tumor with the nevoid basal cell carcinoma syndrome, or it may be a true neoplasm. There is, however, no valid support for the contention that fetal rhabdomyoma is an early stage in the development of adult rhabdomyoma.

GENITAL RHABDOMYOMA

Although this condition bears some resemblance to both adult and fetal rhabdomyoma, it is sufficiently different in

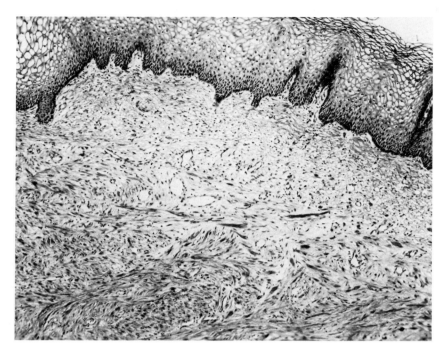

FIG. 21-19. Genital (vaginal) rhabdomyoma. Submucosal proliferation of striated muscle cells separated by varying amounts of myxoid material and collagen. (×60.)

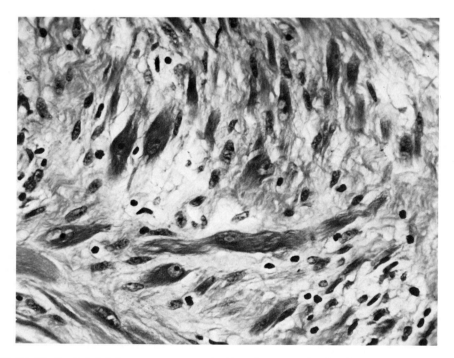

FIG. 21-20. Genital rhabdomyoma composed of loosely arranged striated muscle cells and fibroblasts. (×400.)

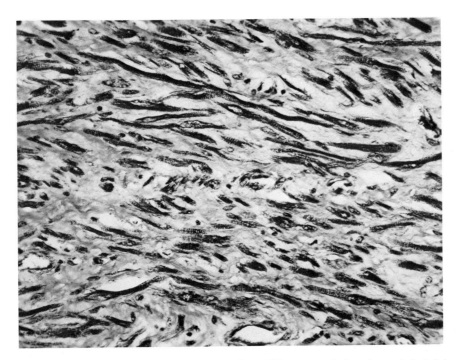

FIG. 21-21. Striated muscle fibers with clearly discernible cross-striations in genital rhabdomyoma. (PTAH; ×250.)

its clinical and microscopic manifestations to qualify as a separate entity. So far only a small number of cases have been described,[60-62,64,69] including some that were reported as fetal rhabdomyoma.[50] All arose as a slowly growing "polypoid" mass or "cyst" in the vagina or vulva of young or middle-aged women. Most were asymptomatic and were found on routine physical examination; some caused dyspareunia, others were first noted because of mucosal erosion and hemorrhage. A similar lesion in the prostate of a 19-year-old man has also been described.[73]

Microscopically, the excised tumor usually forms a polypoid or cauliflower-like mass covered by epithelium and rarely measuring more than 3 cm in greatest diameter. Under the microscope it consists of scattered, more or less mature muscle fibers showing distinct cross-striations and a matrix containing varying amounts of collagen and mucoid material (Figs. 21-19 to 21-21). As in other rhabdomyomas the cells are immunoreactive with desmin, myoglobin, actin, and myosin antibodies.[66] Electron microscopic examination of the lesion reveals a large nucleus with a prominent dense nucleolus and arrays of thick and thin myofilaments with Z lines and A and I bands, together with intracytoplasmic bodies and basal lamina. There are also attachment plaques or peripheral couplings.[61,64]

The lesion pursues a benign course and is adequately treated by local excision. As with other types of rhabdomyoma, it is still undecided whether the lesion is a hamartomatous growth or a neoplasm. Genital rhabdomyoma must be

distinguished from benign vaginal polyps; the latter lack striated muscle cells and are marked by cellular atypia.

RHABDOMYOMATOUS MESENCHYMAL HAMARTOMA OF SKIN

This process consists of multiple or solitary, small dome-shaped papules or polypoid pedunculated lesions that occur principally in the face and neck of newborns and infants with a predilection for the periorbital or periauricular regions. They range in size from a few millimeters to 1 or 2 centimeters. Microscopically the lesions are located in the subcutis and are composed of poorly oriented or perpendicular bundles of well-differentiated skeletal muscle, interspersed with islands of fat, fibrous tissue, and occasionally proliferated nerves.[67,69,71,72,75] Sahn et al.[74] report one case in which contraction of the muscle caused "spontaneous and independent movement of the projections during feeding." Associated congenital abnormalities have also been observed.[70,74] Rhabdomyomatous mesenchymal hamartoma must be distinguished from the rare and much less well-differentiated cutaneous embryonal rhabdomyosarcoma.[68]

MISCELLANEOUS LESIONS MIMICKING BENIGN STRIATED MUSCLE TUMORS

Various benign lesions of striated muscle may be confused with benign rhabdomyoma; Durm[76] described supernumerary muscles in the popliteal fossa and ankle region of young adults that presented as tumorlike masses and were identified as accessory hamstring and soleus muscles. Similar accessory muscles may occur in the hand, fingers, and other portions of the body. Some may be bilateral. Likewise, unilateral or bilateral hypertrophy of the masseter muscle may be mistaken for a muscle tumor.[78] We have no experience with this lesion, but according to Waldhart and Lynch,[79] this condition occurs chiefly in young adults and is often accompanied by bony overgrowth or a spur at the angle of the mandible. Benign skeletal muscle differentiation has also been observed in the uterus and in a uterine leiomyoma.[77] Another benign muscular lesion, the neuromuscular hamartoma or benign Triton tumor, is described in Chapter 31.

REFERENCES
Adult rhabdomyoma

1. Abrikossoff A: Über Myome, ausgehend von der quergestreiften willkürlichen Muskulatur. *Virchows Arch (Pathol Anat)* 260:215, 1926.
2. Albrechtsen R, Ebbesen F, Van Pedersen SV: Extracardiac rhabdomyoma: light and electron microscopic studies of two cases in the mandibular area with review of previous reports. *Acta Otolaryngol* 78:458, 1974.
3. Alkalay AL, Ferry DA, Lin B, et al: Spontaneous regression of cardiac rhabdomyoma in tuberous sclerosis. *Clin Pediatr* 26:532, 1987.
4. Andersen CB, Elling F: Adult rhabdomyoma of the oropharynx recurring three times within thirty-five years. *Acta Pathol Microbiol Immunol Scand* 94A:281, 1986.
5. Assor D, Thomas JR: Multifocal rhabdomyoma: report of a case. *Arch Otolaryngol* 90:489, 1969.
6. Bagby RA, Packer JT, Iglesias RG: Rhabdomyoma of the larynx. *Arch Otolaryngol* 102:101, 1976.
7. Battifora HA, Eisenstein R, Schild JA: Rhabdomyoma of larynx: ultrastructural study and comparison with granular cell tumors (myoblastomas). *Cancer* 23:183, 1969.
8. Blaauwgeers JL, Troost D, Dingemans KP, et al: Multifocal rhabdomyoma of the neck: report of a case studied by fine-needle aspiration, light and electron microscopy, histochemistry and immunohistochemistry. *Am J Surg Pathol* 13:791, 1989.
9. Bock D, Bock P: Rhabdomyoma of the soft palate: fine structural details of a highly differentiated muscle tumor. *Histol Histopathol* 2:285, 1987.
10. Burke AP, Virmani R: Cardiac rhabdomyoma: a clinicopathologic study. *Mod Pathol* 4:70, 1991.
11. Cornog JL Jr, Gonatas NK: Ultrastructure of rhabdomyoma. *J Ultrastruct Res* 20:433, 1967.
12. Czernobilsky B, Cornog JL, Enterline HT: Rhabdomyoma: report of a case with ultrastructural and histochemical studies. *Am J Clin Pathol* 49:782, 1968.
13. Enzinger FM: Adult rhabdomyoma: letter to the case. *Pathol Res Pract* 183:512, 1988.
14. Ferlito A, Frugoni P: Rhabdomyoma purum of the larynx. *J Laryngol Otol* 89:1131, 1975.
15. Fortson JK, Prunes FS, Lang AG: Adult multifocal extracardiac rhabdomyoma. *J Natl Med Assoc* 85:147, 1993.
16. Fu Y, Perzin K: Nonepithelial tumors of the nasal cavity, paranasal sinuses, and nasopharynx: a clinicopathologic study. V. Skeletal muscle tumors: rhabdomyoma and rhabdomyosarcoma. *Cancer* 37:364, 1976.
17. Gardner DG, Corio RL: Multifocal adult rhabdomyoma. *Oral Surg Oral Med Oral Pathol* 56:76, 1983.
18. Gibas Z, Miettinen M: Recurrent parapharyngeal rhabdomyoma: evidence of neoplastic nature of the tumor from cytogenetic study. *Am J Surg Pathol* 16:721, 1992.
19. Goldman L: Multicentric benign rhabdomyoma of skeletal muscle. *Cancer* 16:1609, 1963.
20. Golz R: Multifocal adult rhabdomyoma: case report and literature review. *Pathol Res Pract* 183:512, 1988.
21. Heiden CL, Steuer G, Marguart KH: Ein Rhabdomyoma des weichen Gaumens. *Laryngol Rhinol Otol (Stuttg)* 57:796, 1978.
22. Helliwell TR, Sissons MC, Stoney PJ, et al: Immunochemistry and electron microscopy of head and neck rhabdomyoma. *J Clin Pathol* 41:1058, 1988.
23. Kapadia SB, Enzinger FM, Heffner DK, et al: Crystal-storing histiocytosis associated with lymphoplasmacytic neoplasms: report of three cases mimicking adult rhabdomyoma. *Am J Surg Pathol* 17:461, 1993.
24. Kapadia SB, Meis JM, Frisman DM, et al: Adult rhabdomyoma of the head and neck: a clinicopathologic and immunophenotypic study. *Hum Pathol* 24:608, 1993.
25. Kay S, Gerszten E, Dennison S: Light and electron microscopic study of a rhabdomyoma arising in the floor of the mouth. *Cancer* 23:708, 1969.
26. Kirkengaard L, Winther LK: Rhabdomyoma of the hypopharynx and larynx: report of two cases and a review of the literature. *J Laryngol Otol* 90:1041, 1976.
27. Knowles DM II, Jakobiec FA: Rhabdomyoma of the orbit. *Am J Ophthalmol* 80:1011, 1975.
28. Konrad EA, Meister P, Hübner G: Extracardiac rhabdomyoma: report of different types with light microscopic and ultrastructural studies. *Cancer* 49:898, 1982.
29. Lehtonen E, Asikainen U, Badley RA: Rhabdomyoma: ultrastructural features and distribution of desmin, muscle type, of intermediate filament protein. *Acta Pathol Microbiol Immunol Scand* 90A:125, 1982.
30. Miller R, Kurtz SM, Powers JM: Mediastinal rhabdomyoma. *Cancer* 42:1983, 1978.
31. Misch KA: Rhabdomyoma purum: a benign rhabdomyoma of tongue. *J Pathol Bacteriol* 75:105, 1958.
32. Moran JJ, Enterline HT: Benign rhabdomyoma of the pharynx: a case report, review of the literature, and comparison with cardiac rhabdomyoma. *Am J Clin Pathol* 42:174, 1964.
33. Oloffson J: Extracardiac rhabdomyoma. *Acta Otolaryngol* 74:139, 1972.
34. Parsons HG, Puro HE: Rhabdomyoma of skeletal muscle: report of a case. *Am J Surg* 89:1187, 1955.
35. Ross CF: Rhabdomyoma of sternomastoid. *J Pathol Bacteriol* 95:556, 1968.
36. Scrivner D, Meyer JS: Multifocal recurrent adult rhabdomyoma. *Cancer* 46:790, 1980.
37. Silverman JF, Kay S, Chang CH: Ultrastructural comparison between skeletal muscle and cardiac rhabdomyomas. *Cancer* 42:189, 1978.
38. Solomon MP, Tolete-Velcek F: Lingual rhabdomyoma (adult variant) in a child. *J Pediatr Surg* 14:91, 1979.
39. Tandler B, Rossi EP, Stein M, et al: Rhabdomyoma of the lip: light and electron microscopical observations. *Arch Pathol* 89:118, 1970.
40. Tanner NS, Carter RL, Clifford P: Pharyngeal rhabdomyoma: an unusual presentation. *J Laryngol Otol* 92:1029, 1978.

41. Tuazon R: Rhabdomyoma of the stomach. *Am J Clin Pathol* 52:37, 1969.

42. Walker WP, Laszewski MJ: Recurrent adult rhabdomyoma diagnosed by fine-needle aspiration cytology: report of a case and review of the literature. *Diagn Cytopathol* 6:354, 1990.

43. Warner TF, Goell W, Sundharades M, et al: Adult rhabdomyoma: ultrastructure and immunocytochemistry. *Arch Pathol Lab Med* 105:608, 1981.

44. Wyatt RB, Schochet SS Jr, McCormick WF: Rhabdomyoma: light and electron microscopic study of a case with intranuclear inclusions. *Arch Otolaryngol* 92:32, 1970.

Fetal rhabdomyoma

45. Bozic C: Fetal rhabdomyoma of the parotid gland in an infant: histological, immunohistochemical, and ultrastructural features. *Pediatr Pathol* 6:139, 1986.

46. Corio RL, Lewis DM: Intraoral rhabdomyomas. *Oral Surg Oral Med Oral Pathol* 48:525, 1979.

47. Crotty PL, Nakleh RE, Dehner LP: Juvenile rhabdomyoma: an intermediate form of skeletal muscle tumor in children. *Arch Pathol Lab Med* 117:43, 1993.

48. Dahl I, Angervall L, Save-Soderbergh J: Foetal rhabdomyoma. *Acta Pathol Microbiol Scand* 84:107, 1976.

49. Dehner LP, Enzinger FM, Font RL: Fetal rhabdomyoma: an analysis of nine cases. *Cancer* 30:160, 1972.

50. Di Sant Agnese PA, Knowles DM: Extracardiac rhabdomyoma: a clinicopathologic study and review of the literature. *Cancer* 46:780, 1980.

51. DiSanto S, Abt AB, Boal DK, et al: Fetal rhabdomyoma and nevoid basal cell carcinoma syndrome. *Pediatr Pathol* 12:441, 1992.

52. Gardner DG, Corio RL: Fetal rhabdomyoma of the tongue, with a discussion of the two histologic variants of this tumor. *Oral Surg Oral Med Oral Pathol* 56:293, 1983.

53. Kapadia SB, Meis JM, Frisman DM, et al: Fetal rhabdomyoma of the head and neck: a clinicopathologic and immunophenotypic study of 24 cases. *Hum Pathol* 24:754, 1993.

54. Klijanienko J, Caillaud JM, Micheau C, et al: Naevomatose basocellulaire associée à un rhabdomyome foetal multifocal: Une observation. *Presse Méd* 17:2247, 1988.

55. Kodet R, Fajstavr J, Kabelka Z, et al: Is fetal cellular rhabdomyoma an entity or a differentiated rhabdomyosarcoma? A study of patients with rhabdomyoma of the tongue and sarcoma of the tongue enrolled in the intergroup rhabdomyosarcoma studies I, II, and III. *Cancer* 67:2907, 1991.

56. Simha M, Doctor V, Dalal S, et al: Postauricular fetal rhabdomyoma: light and electron microscopic study. *Hum Pathol* 13:673, 1982.

57. Walter P, Guerbaoui M: Rhabdomyoma foetal: Etude histologique et ultrastructurale d'une nouvelle observation. *Virchows Arch (Pathol Anat)* 371:59, 1976.

58. Whitten RO, Benjamin DR: Rhabdomyoma of the retroperitoneum: a report of a tumor with both adult and fetal characteristics: a study by light and electron microscopy, histochemistry, and immunochemistry. *Cancer* 59:818, 1987.

59. Zwick DL, Livingston K, Clapp L, et al: Intracranial trigeminal nerve rhabdomyoma/choristoma in a child: a case report and discussion of possible histogenesis. *Hum Pathol* 20:390, 1989.

Genital rhabdomyoma

60. Ceremsak RJ: Benign rhabdomyoma of the vagina. *Am J Clin Pathol* 52:604, 1969.

61. Chabrel CM, Beilby JOW: Vaginal rhabdomyoma. *Histopathology* 4:645, 1980.

62. Gad A, Eusebi V: Rhabdomyoma of the vagina. *J Pathol* 115:179, 1975.

63. Gee DC, Finckh ES: Benign vaginal rhabdomyoma. *Pathology* 9:263, 1977.

64. Gold JH, Bossen EH: Benign vaginal rhabdomyoma: a light and electron microscopic study. *Cancer* 37:2283, 1976.

65. Leone PG, Taylor HB: Ultrastructure of a benign polypoid rhabdomyoma of the vagina. *Cancer* 31:1414, 1973.

66. Vilela DS, Pizarro AG, Suarez MR: Vaginal rhadomyoma and adenosis. *Histopathology* 16:393, 1990.

Rhabdomyomatous mesenchymal hamartoma of skin

67. Ashfaq R, Timmons CF: Rhabdomyomatous mesenchymal hamartoma of skin. *Pediatr Pathol* 12:731, 1992.

68. Chang Y, Dehner LP, Egbert B: Primary cutaneous rhabdomyosarcoma. *Am J Surg Pathol* 14:977, 1990.

69. Hayes M, van der Westhuizen N: Congenital rhabdomyomatous mesenchymal hamartoma (letter). *Am J Dermatopathol* 14:64, 1992.

70. Hendrick SJ, Sanchez RL, Blackwell SJ, et al: Striated muscle hamartoma: description of two cases. *Pediatr Dermatol* 3:153, 1986.

71. Mills AE: Rhabdomyomatous mesenchymal hamartoma of skin. *Am J Dermatopathol* 11:58, 1989.

72. Mills E: Congenital rhabdomyomatous mesenchymal hamartoma (letter). *Am J Dermatopathol* 13:429, 1991.

73. Morra MN, Manson AJ, Gavrell GJ: Rhabdomyoma of prostate. *Urology* 39:271, 1992.

74. Sahn EE, Garen PD, Pai GS, et al: Multiple rhabdomyomatous mesenchymal hamartomas of skin. *Am J Dermatopathol* 12:485, 1990.

75. White G: Congenital rhabdomyomatous mesenchymal hamartoma (letter). *Am J Dermatopathol* 12:539, 1990.

Miscellaneous lesions mimicking benign striated muscle tumors

76. Durm AW: Anomalous muscle simulating soft tissue tumors on the lower extremities. *J Bone Joint Surg* 47A:1397, 1965.

77. Martin-Reay DG, Christ ML, LaPata RE: Uterine leiomyoma with skeletal muscle differentiation: report of a case. *Am J Clin Pathol* 96:344, 1991.

78. Wade MW, Roy EW: Idiopathic masseter muscle hypertrophy. *J Oral Surg* 29:196, 1971.

79. Waldhart E, Lynch JB: Benign hypertrophy of the masseter muscles and mandibular angles. *Arch Surg* 102:115, 1971.

CHAPTER 22

RHABDOMYOSARCOMA

The concept of what constitutes rhabdomyosarcoma has been the subject of considerable change over the years. Sporadic cases of this tumor have been described since the early nineteenth century, but most were treated as curiosities or as striking examples of the close resemblance between sarcoma and developing normal tissue, and there were often lengthy debates as to their histogenesis.[125,130,178,221] In fact, in some of the earlier studies, Wilms' tumor and malignant mixed mesodermal tumors of the urogenital tract were included among the rhabdomyosarcomas.

Much later, in the 1930s and 1940s, the diagnosis of adult or pleomorphic rhabdomyosarcoma gained in popularity, and most of the rhabdomyosarcomas reported during this period were of this type.[70,152,201] These tumors occurred mainly in the muscles of the lower extremity and affected patients between 50 and 70 years of age. They displayed a striking degree of cellular pleomorphism, but cells with cross-striations were absent in most instances. It was soon realized that most of these tumors were in fact other types of pleomorphic sarcomas, especially malignant fibrous histiocytomas.

During this period it also became evident that many childhood sarcomas formerly diagnosed merely as "round or spindle cell sarcomas" were rhabdomyosarcomas of the embryonal or alveolar type. Knowledge of these tumors was fostered by the introduction of newer and much more effective modes of therapy: Before 1960 childhood rhabdomyosarcoma was known as an almost uniformly fatal neoplasm that recurred and metastasized in a high percentage of cases. During the last 3 decades, however, it has been shown that this tumor responds well to multidisciplinary therapy—encompassing biopsy or conservative surgery, multiagent chemotherapy, and radiotherapy—and that the majority of children treated by these modalities remain free of recurrent and metastatic disease. The many publications of the Intergroup Rhabdomyosarcoma Studies have greatly contributed to our understanding of childhood rhabdomyosarcomas and especially the effect of the various treatment modalities on the survival of patients with this tumor.*

INCIDENCE

Rhabdomyosarcoma is not only the most common soft tissue sarcoma of children under 15 years of age but also one of the most common soft tissue sarcomas of adolescents and young adults. It is definitely rare in persons older than 45 years. There were 234 rhabdomyosarcomas (19%) among 1215 sarcomas reviewed and staged by the Task Force of Soft Tissue Tumors,[180] and there were 379 rhabdomyosarcomas (19%) among 2000 malignant soft tissue tumors collected at the Mayo Clinic.[127] Enjoji and Hashimoto[51] reported 89 rhabdomyosarcomas (11.8%) among 752 malignant soft tissue tumors.

HISTOLOGICAL CLASSIFICATION

Rhabdomyosarcomas vary widely in histological appearance, depending on the degree of cellular differentiation, extent of cellularity, and growth pattern. Most of these tumors can be classified as one of four histological categories: embryonal, botryoid, alveolar, or pleomorphic rhabdomyosarcoma. This classification was first suggested by Horn and Enterline in 1958[89] and adopted by the World Health Organization Classification of Soft Tissue Tumors in 1969.[53] There is considerable overlapping among the various categories, and sometimes it is difficult to decide in which category the tumor should be placed. There also are rare and unusual examples of this tumor for which an exact diagnosis as to histological category is difficult, even if the tumor can be clearly identified as rhabdomyosarcoma. More recently spindle cell rhabdomyosarcoma has been added as another subtype of the embryonal form.[20]

Embryonal rhabdomyosarcoma, the first and most common of the four categories, accounts for 50% to 60% of all rhabdomyosarcomas. It affects mainly but not exclusively

*References 27, 67, 87, 128, 129, 145.

children between birth and 15 years of age and occurs predominantly in the region of the head and neck, including the orbit, the genitourinary tract, and the retroperitoneum, but it may also be encountered in the extremities. Microscopically it bears a close resemblance to various stages in the development of normal muscle tissue and ranges in its morphological spectrum from poorly differentiated monomorphic round cell tumors with hardly any rhabdomyoblastic differentiation to extremely well-differentiated neoplasms consisting almost entirely of rhabdomyoblasts with cross-striations. There are also pleomorphic variants, and it is sometimes quite difficult to draw a sharp line between the childhood and adult forms of pleomorphic rhabdomyosarcoma. *Spindle cell rhabdomyosarcoma* is a subtype of embryonal rhabdomyosarcoma marked by its favorable clinical behavior.

Botryoid embryonal rhabdomyosarcoma is essentially a variant of the embryonal type. It accounts for no more than 5% to 10% of all rhabdomyosarcomas and is characterized by a polypoid grapelike growth pattern, a paucity of cells, and an abundance of richly mucoid, myxoma-like stroma. Its distinctive microscopic appearance is the result of unrestricted growth rather than an intrinsic feature of the tumor. It may be encountered in portions of any embryonal rhabdomyosarcoma, but it is most frequently seen in tumors taking origin in mucosa-lined hollow visceral organs such as the vagina and urinary bladder.[2,11,89]

Alveolar rhabdomyosarcoma is the second most common type of rhabdomyosarcoma. It was first described by Riopelle and Thériault[174] in 1956 and later by Enterline and Horn[52] and others.[54,154] It accounts for approximately 20%

of all rhabdomyosarcomas, and afflicts most often persons between 10 and 25 years of age; it has an anatomical distribution similar to that of embryonal rhabdomyosarcoma except for a much greater incidence in the upper and lower extremities. The collective terms *embryonal alveolar rhabdomyosarcoma*[195] and *juvenile rhabdomyosarcoma*[202] have been employed to stress the close clinical and morphological relationship between the embryonal and alveolar types.

Pleomorphic rhabdomyosarcoma, a tumor that is sometimes described as the "classical" type of rhabdomyosarcoma, probably accounts for less than 5% of all rhabdomyosarcomas. It may affect patients of any age but has its peak incidence in patients older than 40 years. It is primarily a tumor of the large muscles of the extremities, particularly the muscles of the thigh. Diagnosis is difficult not only because of the consistent absence of typical rhabdomyoblasts with cross-striations but also because of the close resemblance of this tumor to malignant fibrous histiocytoma and other pleomorphic sarcomas.[38,66,117]

Overlapping among the various types of rhabdomyosarcoma is common, and mixed forms such as embryonal rhabdomyosarcoma with focal alveolar or pleomorphic features are not rare. For staging and prognostic purposes, mixed forms with embryonal and alveolar features are best classified as rhabdomyosarcomas of the alveolar type.

CLINICAL FINDINGS
Age and sex incidence

Despite the striking diversity in location, clinical presentation, and histological picture, rhabdomyosarcoma has a fairly uniform age incidence; it occurs predominantly in in-

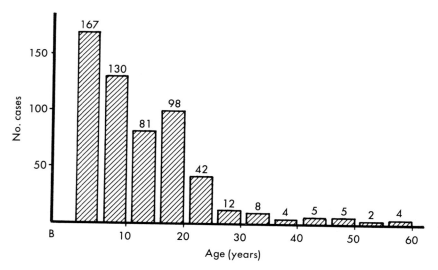

FIG 22-1. Age distribution of 558 cases of rhabdomyosarcoma reviewed at the AFIP during a 10-year period. More than half of the cases occurred during the first 10 years of life; most of these were of the embryonal type. The second peak lies between 15 and 20 years of age; it is a result of the preponderance of alveolar rhabdomyosarcoma in this age-group.

fants and children and somewhat less frequently in adolescents and young adults. In the series of Ragab et al.[160] of 1561 patients with rhabdomyosarcomas, 5% were younger than 1 year of age. About 2% of tumors are present at birth. Rhabdomyosarcomas are rare in patients older than 40 years[132,136,189] (Fig. 22-1).

The median age of 440 patients with embryonal rhabdomyosarcomas, diagnosed at the AFIP during a 10-year period, was 8 years; the median age of 118 patients with alveolar rhabdomyosarcomas seen during the same period was 16 years. The median age varies somewhat according to the histological type: embryonal rhabdomyosarcomas, including those of the botryoid type, are found mostly in infants and children; alveolar rhabdomyosarcomas are observed mainly in adolescents and young adults; pleomorphic rhabdomyosarcomas occur mostly in older persons, with a reported range in median age from 50 to 56 years.[66,89,117] There is also some correlation between tumor location and age; for example, rhabdomyosarcomas of the urinary bladder, prostate, vagina, and middle ear tend to occur in a younger age-group (median age, 4 years) than those in the paratesticular region (median age, 14 years) or the extremities (median age, 14 years).

Males are affected more commonly than females by a ratio of approximately 1.3:1, but the male preponderance is less pronounced among cases occurring in adolescents and young adults as well as in patients with rhabdomyosarcomas of the alveolar type. Blacks are less commonly involved than whites, but this may be a sampling error, and further data in this regard are needed.[220]

Localization and clinical complaints

Although rhabdomyosarcomas may arise anywhere in the body, they occur predominantly in three regions: the head and neck, the genitourinary tract and retroperitoneum, and the upper and lower extremities. Tumors in the head and neck region and the genitourinary tract and retroperitoneum outnumber those in the extremities by a sizable margin. Table 22-1 shows the anatomical distribution of rhabdomyosarcomas reviewed and diagnosed at the AFIP during a 10-year period.

Rhabdomyosarcoma of the head and neck

This is the principal location of rhabdomyosarcoma; 246 (44%) of 558 cases occurred in this general region. The orbit, nasal cavity, and nasopharynx were the leading sites, followed in frequency by the ear and ear canal, paranasal sinuses, soft tissues of the face (cheek) and neck, and the oral cavity, including the tongue, lip, and palate. In the series of Dito and Batsakis,[43] 54 (31.8%) of the 170 cases occurred in the orbit and 49 (28.8%) in the nasopharynx and the nasal and oral cavities. In another series of 202 head and neck rhabdomyosarcomas, 26% affected the orbit and eye and 46% parameningeal sites.[205] Numerous additional reviews of rhabdomyosarcomas in the head and neck region have been published.[47,127,200] As a rule, the tumors in this general region grow rapidly, often in an infiltrative and destructive manner, particularly if the initial treatment is inadequate or delayed. Many invade bone. Detailed x-ray examination, including CT scan or MRI, is indicated in these cases in order to obtain a clear picture of the size and spatial relationship of the tumor and the extent of bone destruction.[32] Nonorbital rhabdomyosarcomas of this region are often referred to collectively as *parameningeal rhabdomyosarcomas* because of their potential intracranial extension and seeding, and, hence, their less favorable course.[15,169]

Rhabdomyosarcoma of the orbit

This is the second most common site of rhabdomyosarcoma in our cases (Table 22-1). As a rule, the neoplasm manifests as a rapidly enlarging painless mass in the upper and inner quadrant of the orbit and causes protrusion and displacement of the globe, usually in a downward or temporal direction, blurred vision, and diplopia; in general, there is little change in visual acuity. Extension into the eyelids is a common occurrence and is associated with marked edema of the lids and conjunctivae, ptosis, and sometimes conjunctival ulceration. In this location, the polypoid subconjunctival growth often displays the characteristics of a botryoid-type embryonal rhabdomyosarcoma. The expanding orbital tumor may also erode into the paranasal sinuses and the base of the skull, where it may spread along the meningeal membranes.

Several examples of orbital rhabdomyosarcomas have

Table 22-1. Anatomical distribution of rhabdomyosarcoma (AFIP, 558 cases)

Anatomical location	Number	Percent
Head and neck		
Orbit, eyelid, skull	109	19.5
Nasal cavity, nasopharynx, palate, mouth, pharynx	73	13.1
Sinuses, cheek, neck	47	8.4
Ear, mastoid	17	3.1
Trunk		
Paratesticular region	114	20.4
Retroperitoneum, pelvis	46	8.2
Chest wall, back, flank, abdominal wall	41	7.3
Urinary bladder, prostate	25	4.5
Vagina, vulva	5	0.9
Extremities		
Upper extremity	41	7.4
Lower extremity	40	7.2
TOTAL	558	100.0

been reported in the earlier literature,[130,221] but Calhoun and Reese[18] were the first to draw attention to the relatively high incidence of this tumor in this location. Similar but larger series of cases were reported by Porterfield and Zimmerman[156] and others.[87,96]

Rhabdomyosarcoma of the nasal cavity and nasopharyngeal region

Rhabdomyosarcomas in this region are often slow to be recognized and may be confused initially with enlarged adenoids, juvenile nasopharyngeal angiofibroma, or a protracted infection that has failed to respond to conventional therapy. The symptoms vary considerably: the enlarging growth may cause increasing difficulties in breathing or swallowing, hoarseness, or alteration of voice. It may fill the nasal cavity and may protrude from one or both nostrils as a gelatinous and not infrequently hemorrhagic polypoid mass. Occasionally it invades the soft or hard palate, the sphenoid or maxillary sinus, and the base of the skull or the floor of the orbit. Rarely, large bulky lesions present as subcutaneous masses in the infraauricular region or the cheek.[19,42,65,102,218] Less commonly the tumor is encountered in the paranasal sinuses,[123] soft palate,[126] oral cavity,[147] tongue,[116] epiglottis, and larynx.[42,176] Table 22-1 shows that 13% of rhabdomyosarcomas in the AFIP series occurred in this general area.

Rhabdomyosarcoma of the middle ear, ear canal, and mastoid

Clinically, patients with this tumor—usually children between ages 2 and 8 years—present with a history of loss of hearing, otalgia, and hemorrhagic or purulent discharge from the ear canal; not surprisingly, many cases are misdiagnosed initially as otitis media. There may also be clouding or opacity of the mastoid cells or sinuses, suggesting mastoiditis or sinusitis. Physical examination usually reveals a gray to purple, fleshy, friable polypoid mass within the ear canal that has penetrated the tympanum and has infiltrated the surrounding soft tissue, causing diffuse swelling in the periauricular region. Paralysis of the facial or other cranial nerves may accompany these symptoms.[6,28,40,94] In one of our cases the tumor extended into the temple and nasopharynx, and in another there was invasion of the cranial cavity. Radiological examination, preferably with tomograms and CT scans, may demonstrate destruction of the petrous portion of the temporal bone, the bony labyrinth, the osseous wall of the auditory canal, and portions of the sphenoid bone.[158,219]

Rhabdomyosarcoma of the genitourinary tract and retroperitoneum

The overall incidence of this group in our cases is slightly lower than that of head and neck rhabdomyosarcomas; among a total of 558 cases observed in a 10-year period,

190 (34%) were situated in this general area. The principal locations were the paratesticular region (114 cases), retroperitoneum (46 cases), prostate (15 cases), urinary bladder (10 cases), and the region of the common bile duct (8 cases) (see Table 22-1). As with most rhabdomyosarcomas of the head and neck region, nearly all (95%) were of the embryonal type and only 5% were of the alveolar type.

In many instances, particularly those in which the tumor reaches a large size, exact determination of the site of origin is difficult, and distinction between tumors arising from specific organs such as the urinary bladder and prostate and those arising from the surrounding retroperitoneum or pelvis is not always possible. In general, effective therapy of rhabdomyosarcomas in the retroperitoneum and pelvic region is more difficult than that of paratesticular rhabdomyosarcomas.[60,92]

Rhabdomyosarcoma of the paratesticular region

The paratesticular region is the most common single site of rhabdomyosarcoma in the AFIP cases. This is predominantly a tumor of adolescents, and half of our cases occurred in patients between 7 and 18 years of age, with a median age of 15 years. Generally tumors at this site manifest as unilateral, firm, painless masses that have been present for a few weeks or months and are usually located at the upper pole of the testis. They may also involve the spermatic cord and the epididymis but usually are separate from the testis proper. There is a high incidence of retroperitoneal or paraaortic lymph node involvement[124,165] a feature that is easily overlooked and must be considered when planning therapy. Clinically the condition must be distinguished from hernia, hydrocele, spermatocele, and adenomatoid tumor. Microscopically, it must be separated from malignant teratoma with a prominent rhabdomyoblastic component. Since Rokitansky's first description in 1849,[178] numerous examples of this tumor have been reported in the literature,[14,110,167] including many involving the spermatic cord and the epididymis.[216]

Rhabdomyosarcoma of the urinary bladder and prostate

This is not only the most common bladder tumor in children under 10 years of age, but is also the most common location of rhabdomyosarcoma occurring during infancy. It originates mainly in the submucosa of the posterior bladder wall, with particular preference for the regions of the bladder neck and trigone; characteristically it grows into the lumen of the urinary bladder as a grapelike, richly mucoid, multinodular or polypoid mass with a broad base that causes not infrequently obstruction of the internal urethral orifice and prostatic urethra. This in turn results in incontinence and difficulties of urination and, when the mucosa becomes necrotic or ulcerated, in gross hematuria. Retention of urine ultimately leads to hydroureter and hydronephrosis. The tumor may also spread diffusely along the submucosa or may penetrate the bladder wall and invade the perivesical region, displacing the rectum and sigmoid. Excretory cystograms usually reveal a vesical filling defect. Prostatic tumors may cause bilateral ureteral obstruction and renal failure. Rhabdomyosarcomas of the urinary bladder and prostate, as well as those of the vagina and anus, ordinarily exhibit the microscopic picture of a botryoid rhabdomyosarcoma.

Since Mostofi and Morse[140] reported, in 1952, 10 examples of this tumor in children between 5 weeks and 9 years of age, numerous additional examples have been recorded in the urinary bladder[99,166,209] (including one in a patient with bilharziasis[155]) and the prostate.[17,99,164] Joshtri et al.[97] described a case occurring in an adult. Semerdjian et al.[190] reported a tumor of characteristic appearance in a 4-year-old boy who had multiple anomalies and had an exstrophied bladder that was repaired shortly after birth. There are also early examples of this tumor in the AFIP cases that were initially misinterpreted as "myxoma" or "polyposis of the bladder in children."

Rhabdomyosarcoma of the common bile duct

This rare tumor arises from the submucosa of the common bile duct and may extend into the porta hepatis or the ampulla of Vater. It grows insidiously and forms a mass in the porta hepatis with or without abdominal distention. It frequently causes weight loss, intermittent jaundice with fever, hepatomegaly, constipation, nausea, and vomiting accompanied by elevation of bilirubin and alkaline phosphatase. Not surprisingly, some of the cases have been initially misdiagnosed as infectious hepatitis. Most are rhabdomyosarcomas of the botryoid type, with typical myxoid grapelike gross and microscopic appearances.[33,93,122,144,182]

Additional examples of rhabdomyosarcoma in the trunk region have been described in the retroperitoneum,[92,171] pelvis,[64,79,92] uterus,[75,82] cervix, vagina,[25,34,44,114] labium, and vulva,[25,206] and in the perineum and perianal region.[162,193,199]

Rhabdomyosarcoma of the limbs

Rhabdomyosarcomas of the extremities are considerably less common than those in the head and neck region and the genitourinary tract. As shown in Table 22-1, only 14.6% of cases occurred in this location, with a similar incidence in the upper and lower extremities. The incidence of these tumors was much higher, however, in the Intergroup Rhabdomyosarcoma Studies I and II, with 18% of childhood rhabdomyosarcomas occurring in the lower extremity and 12% in the upper extremity.[80] In our material the forearms, hands, or feet were more often involved than other portions of the extremities, and alveolar rhabdomyosarcomas outnumbered embryonal rhabdomyosarcomas by a ratio of 4:3. There were only a few examples of pleomorphic rhabdomyosarcomas in this location, mostly affecting adults.

Most of the neoplasms in the limbs present as slowly or, more often, rapidly enlarging masses that usually are deep

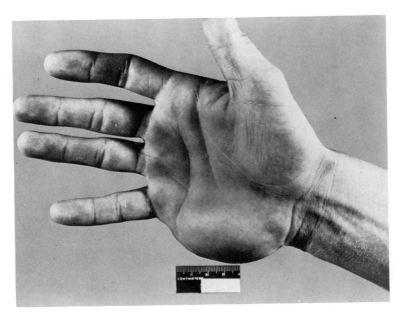

FIG. 22-2. Alveolar rhabdomyosarcoma of the hypothenar eminence of the right hand in a 20-year-old man.

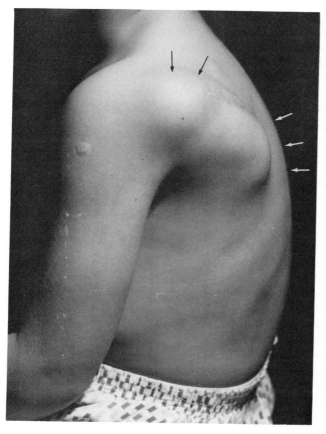

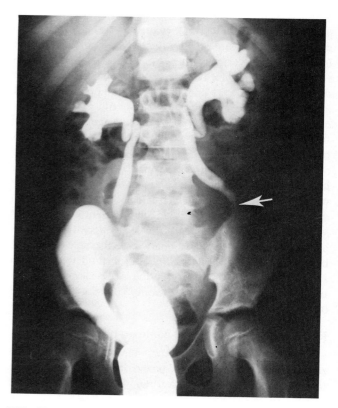

FIG. 22-3. Embrymal rhabdomyosarcoma *(arrows)* involving the scapular musculature of a 6-year-old boy.

FIG. 22-4. Roentgenogram of an embryonal rhabdomyosarcoma of the pelvic retroperitoneum in a 9-year-old boy. Intravenous pyelogram (IVP) showing deviation and compression of both ureters with bilateral hydroureter and hydronephrosis *(arrow)*.

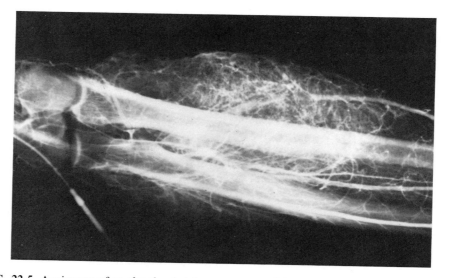

FIG. 22-5. Angiogram of an alveolar rhabdomyosarcoma of the left forearm in a 15-year-old boy showing displacement and narrowing of radial artery, neovascularity, and extravasated contrast material.

seated and are intimately associated with striated muscle tissue. As a rule, they are neither painful nor tender, despite evidence of rapid growth during the preoperative period (Fig. 22-2). Larger examples may cause pain or other neurological disturbances as a result of pressure exerted by the tumor on peripheral nerves. Erosion of bone is rare and is associated mainly with rhabdomyosarcomas of the hands and feet. Similar deep-seated rhabdomyosarcomas occur in the muscles of the chest and abdominal wall and the neck region (Fig. 22-3).

Soule et al.[198] reported that 61 (27%) of 229 rhabdomyosarcomas occurred in the limb and limb girdles; 40 were of the "solid" type and 21 of the alveolar type. LaQuaglia et al.[110] and others[29,69,85,172] reviewed their experience with childhood rhabdomyosarcoma in the extremities, including detailed accounts of the various therapeutic aspects of the disease when it occurs in this location. Radiographs and angiographs show no specific features that would permit a reliable diagnosis as to the type of tumor (Figs. 22-4 and 22-5).

GROSS FINDINGS

Macroscopically there is little that is characteristic of this tumor, and, as in other types of rapidly growing sarcomas, the gross appearance reflects the degree of cellularity, the relative amounts of collagenous or myxoid stroma, and the presence and extent of secondary changes such as hemorrhage, necrosis, and ulceration. In general, tumors growing into body cavities, like those in the nasopharynx and the urinary bladder, are fairly well circumscribed, multinodular, or distinctly polypoid with a glistening, gelatinous, gray-white surface that often shows on cross-section patchy areas of hemorrhage or cyst formation. Deep-seated tumors involving or arising in the musculature, like most rhabdomyosarcomas in the extremities, are usually less well defined and nearly always infiltrate the surrounding tissues. They are more firm and rubbery and have a mottled gray-white to pink-tan, smooth or finely granular, often bulging surface. They rarely reach a large size and average 3 or 4 cm in greatest diameter. There are often areas of focal necrosis and cystic degeneration (Figs. 22-6 and 22-7).

MICROSCOPIC FINDINGS
Embryonal rhabdomyosarcoma

The embryonal type is found in about 3 out of 4 rhabdomyosarcomas; it mostly affects children younger than 10 years of age, but it also occurs in adolescents and young adults; it is rare in patients older than 40 years. Embryonal rhabdomyosarcoma bears a close resemblance to various stages in the embryogenesis of normal skeletal muscle, but its pattern is much more variable and ranges from poorly differentiated tumors that are very difficult to diagnose without immunohistochemical or electron microscopic examination to well-differentiated neoplasms that resemble the appearance of fetal muscle. Features common to most are (1) varying degrees of cellularity with alternating densely packed, hypercellular areas and loosely textured myxoid areas; (2) a mixture of poorly oriented, small, undifferentiated, hyperchromatic round or spindle-shaped cells and a varying number of differentiated cells with eosinophilic cytoplasm characteristic of rhabdomyoblasts; and (3) a matrix containing little collagen and varying amounts

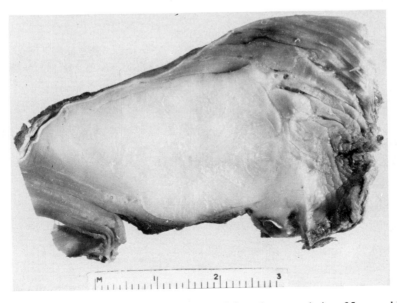

FIG. 22-6. Cross-section of rhabdomyosarcoma of the soleus muscle in a 35-year-old man.

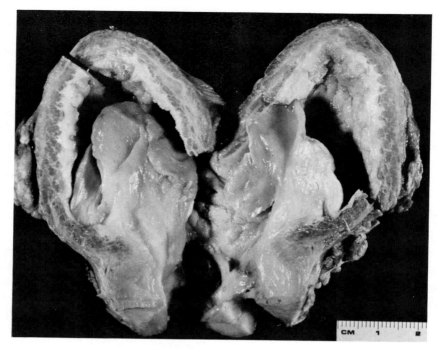

FIG. 22-7. Botryoid-type embryonal rhabdomyosarcoma of the urinary bladder in a 3-year-old child. Note the polypoid and myxoid appearance of the tumor.

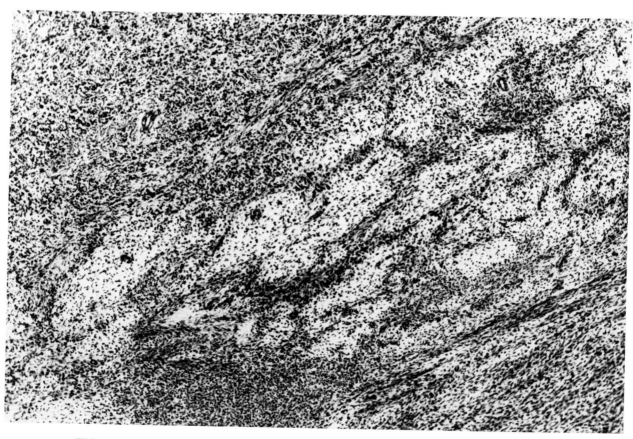

FIG. 22-8. Embryonal rhabdomyosarcoma showing alternating cellular and myxoid areas, a characteristic feature of this tumor. (×100.)

of myxoid material. Cross-striations are discernible in 50% to 60% of cases (Fig. 22-8). Schmidt et al.[183] distinguished primitive (less than 10% rhabdomyoblasts), intermediate (10% to 50% rhabdomyoblasts), and well-differentiated (greater than 50% rhabdomyoblasts) forms of embryonal rhabdomyosarcoma.

The least well differentiated examples of this tumor correspond in appearance to developing muscle at the fifth to eighth weeks of gestation. They consist for the most part of small round or spindle-shaped cells with darkly staining hyperchromatic nuclei and indistinct cytoplasm. The nuclei vary slightly in size and shape—more so than those of the solid form of alveolar rhabdomyosarcoma—have one or two small nucleoli, and usually show a high rate of mitotic activity. Differentiated rhabdomyoblasts are either absent entirely or are confined to a few small areas, making it mandatory to examine multiple sections from different portions of the tumor and requiring adjunctive diagnostic procedures for confirmation of diagnosis in most cases (Figs. 22-9 and 22-10, A and B).

Better differentiated examples of the round cell and spindle type possess, in addition to the primitive or undifferentiated cellular areas, larger round or oval, eosinophilic cells characteristic of rhabdomyoblasts; the cytoplasm of these cells contains granular material or deeply eosinophilic masses of stringy or fibrillary material concentrically arranged near or around the nucleus. Cross-striations are rare in the rounded cells, and if present are usually confined to narrow bundles of concentrically arranged myofibrils at the circumference of the rhabdomyoblast. Degenerated rhabdomyoblasts with a glassy or hyalinized deeply eosinophilic cytoplasm and pyknotic nuclei but without cross-striations are a frequent feature of this tumor (Fig. 22-10, C and D).

Cross-striations are more readily discernible in embryonal rhabdomyosarcomas having a more prominent spindle cell component, tumors that might be regarded as the morphological equivalent of normal muscle at the ninth to fifteenth weeks of intrauterine development; these neoplasms are mainly composed of a mixture of undifferentiated cells and differentiated fusiform or elongated cells that are readily identifiable as rhabdomyoblasts under the light microscope. The rhabdomyoblasts range from slender spindle-shaped cells with a small number of peripherally placed

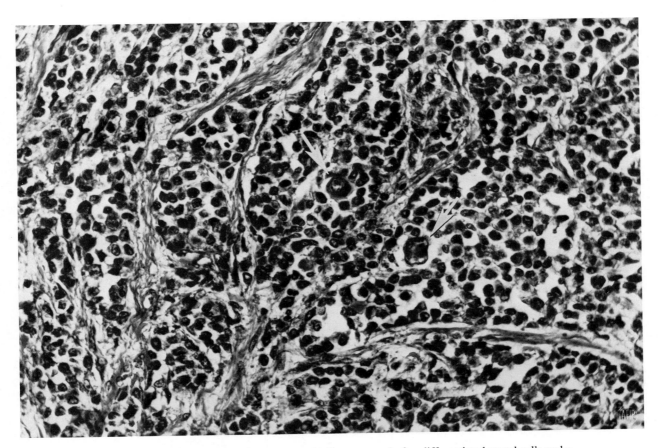

FIG. 22-9. Embryonal rhabdomyosarcoma chiefly composed of undifferentiated round cells and a few scattered rhabdomyoblasts *(white arrows)*. (×250.)

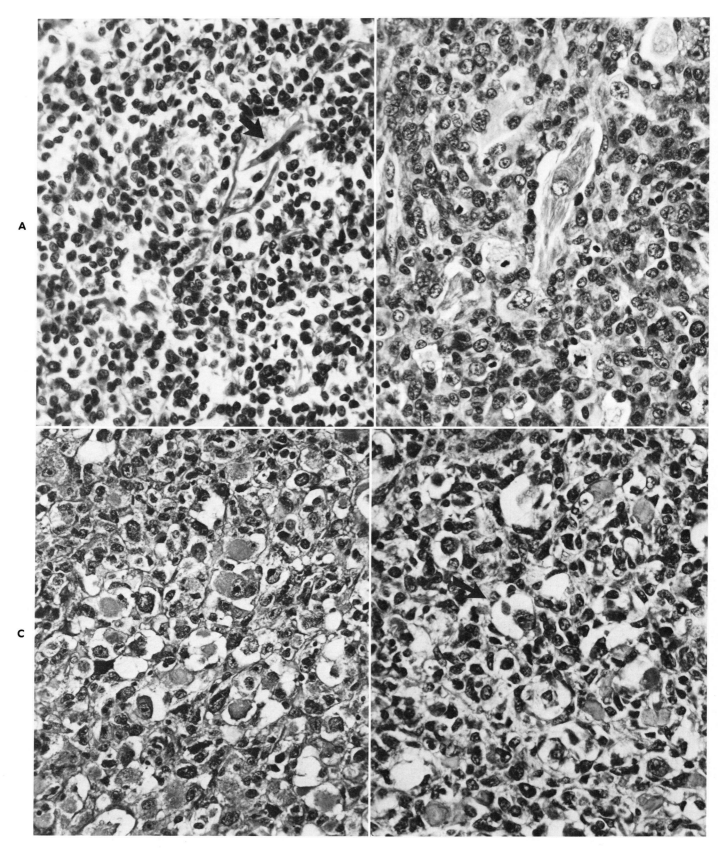

FIG. 22-10. Embryonal rhabdomyosarcoma showing varying degrees of cellular differentiation, (**A** to **D**) including elongated and rounded rhabdomyoblasts with vacuolization caused by deposits of intracellular glycogen (**C** and **D**). (**A** to **C**, ×250; **D**, ×400.)

myofibrils to larger eosinophilic cells having a strap, ribbon, tadpole, or racquet shape, with one or two centrally positioned nuclei and prominent nucleoli and with or without cross-striations. Cross-striations in neoplastic cells differ from those in residual or entrapped muscle cells by their more irregular distribution and the fact that they often traverse only part of the tumor cell. Intracellular granules may be confused with cross-striations, but their granular nature is readily apparent by careful examination of the cell under oil immersion. Sometimes the strap-shaped cells are sharply angulated and form a diagnostically useful "zigzag" or "broken straw" pattern. Most of these tumors show only a moderate degree of cellular pleomorphism (Figs. 22-11 to 22-16).

Embryonal rhabdomyosarcomas with a prominent degree of cellular pleomorphism are rare and are difficult to distinguish from adult pleomorphic rhabdomyosarcomas, except for the more frequent occurrence of cross-striations in childhood tumors. According to Kodet et al.,[107] the cellular pleomorphism adversely affects the outcome only if it is diffuse and involves the entire neoplasm.

There are also extremely well-differentiated embryonal rhabdomyosarcomas that consist almost entirely of well-differentiated rounded, spindle-shaped, or polygonal rhabdomyoblasts with abundant eosinophilic cytoplasm and frequent cross-striations (Figs. 22-17 to 22-19). Some of these differentiated tumors are found in recurrent or metastatic neoplasms after prolonged therapy, possibly due to the "selective destruction of undifferentiated tumor cells."[137]

Glycogen is demonstrable in most cases of rhabdomyosarcoma regardless of type; when it is removed during fixation, multivacuolated cells or "spider cells" result; these are large multivacuolated rhabdomyoblasts with narrow strands of cytoplasm connecting the center of the cell with its periphery.[125] The centrally located nuclei and the irregular shape of the cytoplasmic vacuoles help to distinguish these cells from the more rounded lipid-filled vacuoles of lipoblasts (Figs. 22-10, *C* and *D,* and 22-18, *C*). In contrast to alveolar rhabdomyosarcoma, multinucleated giant cells are rare in the embryonal type.

Occasionally, embryonal rhabdomyosarcoma may display, in addition to its rhabdomyoblastic component, foci of immature cartilaginous or osseous tissue, or both. These tumors may occur at any age and any location, but seem to be more common in the genitourinary tract and the retroperitoneum. Daya and Scully[34] observed cartilaginous differentiation in 45% of rhabdomyosarcomas of the uterine cervix.

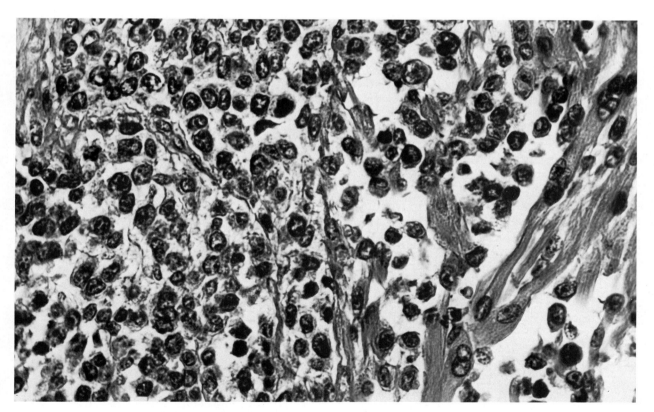

FIG. 22-11. Embryonal rhabdomyosarcoma consisting of poorly differentiated cells and a few differentiated straplike rhabdomyoblasts. (×350.)

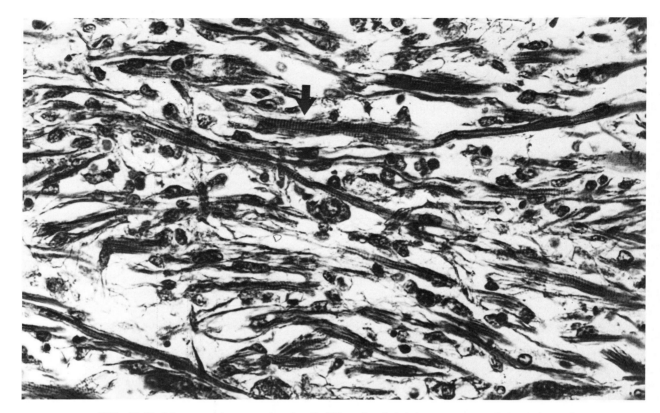

FIG. 22-12. Masson trichrome stain of well-differentiated rhabdomyosarcoma of the embryonal type with distinct cross-striations in most of the tumor cells *(arrow)*. (×395.)

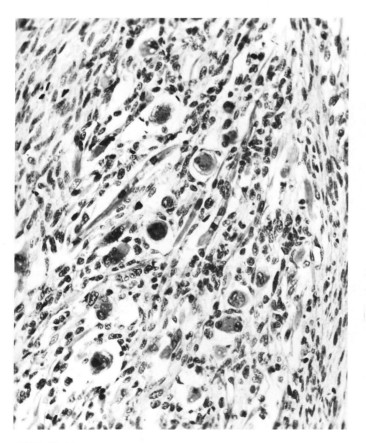

FIG. 22-13. Embryonal rhabdomyosarcoma with loosely arranged rounded and elongated rhabdomyoblasts as well as undifferentiated tumor cells. (×225.)

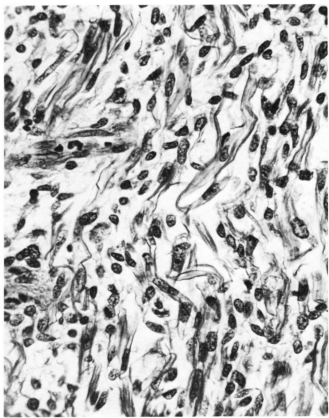

FIG. 22-14. Embryonal rhabdomyosarcoma resembling the tubular stage of fetal muscle. (×395.)

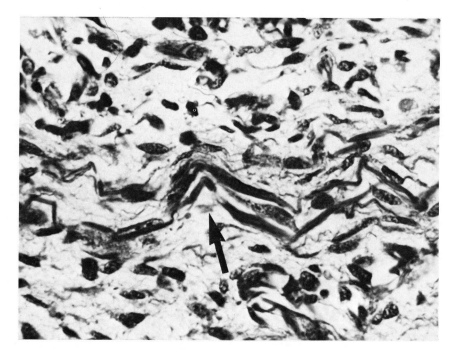

FIG. 22-15. Embryonal rhabdomyosarcoma with elongated rhabdomyoblasts showing a distinct angulation of the muscle fibers *(arrow),* a feature that may aid in diagnosis ("broken straw" sign). (×615.)

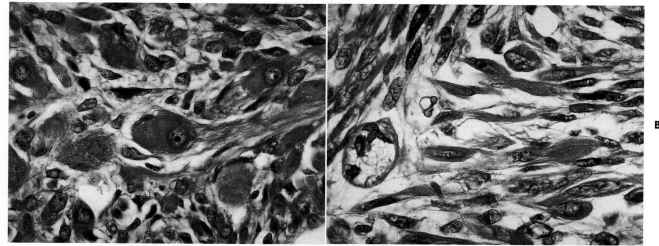

FIG. 22-16. Typical round, ribbon-shaped, and strap-shaped rhabdomyoblasts in embryonal rhabdomyosarcoma. The tumor occurred in the retroperitoneum of a 5-year-old boy. (**A** and **B,** ×630.)

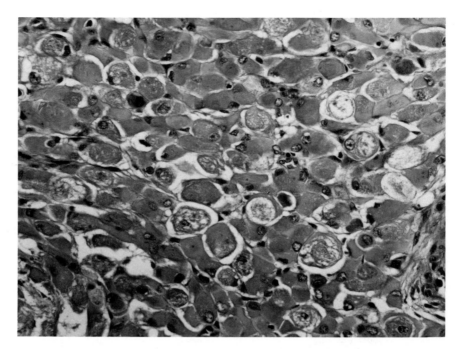

FIG. 22-17. Embryonal rhabdomyosarcoma consisting almost entirely of differentiated rhabdomyoblasts, a feature occasionally encountered in recurrent tumors following inadequate therapy. (×450.)

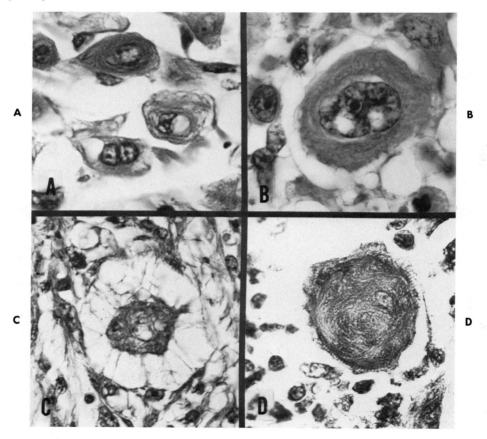

FIG. 22-18. Rhabdomyoblasts showing filamentous stringy material surrounding the nucleus and occasional juxtanuclear vacuoles **(A)**, perinuclear bundles of myofilaments **(B)**, vacuolated cytoplasm secondary to removal of glycogen ("spiderweb" cell) **(C)**, and radiating cross-striations at the periphery **(D)**. (**A**, ×660; **B**, ×1000; **C**, ×485; **D**, ×1000.)

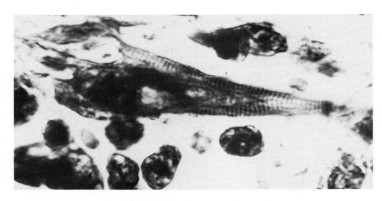

FIG. 22-19. Rhabdomyoblast with distinct cross-striations in its cytoplasm. (×1100.)

Spindle cell rhabdomyosarcoma

Spindle cell rhabdomyosarcoma is a subtype of embryonal rhabdomyosarcoma. Distinction from embryonal rhabdomyosarcoma is warranted because of its more favorable clinical course. The tumor simulates fibrosarcoma or leiomyosarcoma (leiomyomatous rhabdomyosarcoma) by the parallel orientation of uniform spindle cells with eosinophilic fibrillary cytoplasm and elongated hyperchromatic nuclei separated by abundant, partly hyalinized stromal collagen. In addition to the characteristic fasciculated arrangement of the tumor cells there may also be a focal storiform growth pattern. Immunostaining is similar to that of embryonal rhabdomyosarcoma. Clinically this subtype is most often encountered in tumors of the paratesticular region and the head and neck but may also be present at other sites such as the extremities[20,49,113] (Fig. 22-20). A peculiar and probably related desmoplastic and pleomorphic spindle cell sarcoma that displayed the morphological and immunohistochemical features of both spindle cell rhabdomyosarcoma and infantile fibrosarcoma was described by Lundgren et al.[120] as *infantile rhabdomyofibrosarcoma*.

Botryoid-type rhabdomyosarcoma

This term, which is derived from the Greek word for grapes, describes a variant of embryonal rhabdomyosarcoma characterized grossly by its polypoid (grapelike) growth and microscopically by its relative sparsity of cells and abundance of mucoid stroma, often resulting in a myxoma-like picture (Figs. 22-21 to 22-23). The tumor usually arises in the submucosa and is covered by epithelium that may be hyperplastic or may undergo squamous changes, sometimes mimicking carcinoma. Commonly there is a submucosal zone of increased cellularity that has been described as a "cambium layer" in analogy to the zone of maximum growth in a tree (Fig. 22-24). In most cases careful search will disclose scattered spindle-shaped or rounded eosinophilic rhabdomyoblasts in either the cellular

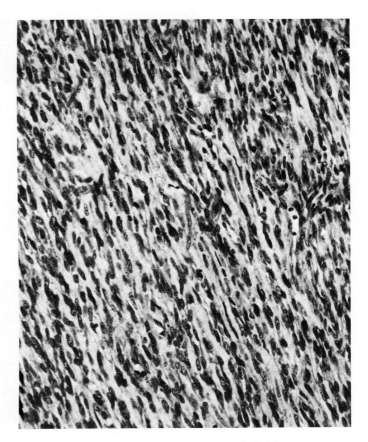

FIG. 22-20. Spindle cell type of embryonal rhabdomyosarcoma with distinct cross-striations in several portions of the neoplasm. The tumor was removed from the abdominal musculature of a 12-year-old boy. (×250.)

or underlying myxoid areas (Figs. 22-25 to 22-27). Sometimes only a few portions of the tumor show the typical botryoid pattern, and most of the tumor is indistinguishable from more cellular forms of embryonal rhabdomyosarcoma (Fig. 22-28).

The majority of botryoid rhabdomyosarcomas are found in mucosa-lined hollow organs such as the nasal cavity, na-

sopharynx, bile duct, urinary bladder, and vagina; tumors of this type may also be encountered in areas where the expanding neoplasm reaches the body surface as in some rhabdomyosarcomas of the eyelid or the anal region. Obviously, its unrestricted growth in body cavities or on body surfaces accounts for its characteristic edematous and grapelike appearance.

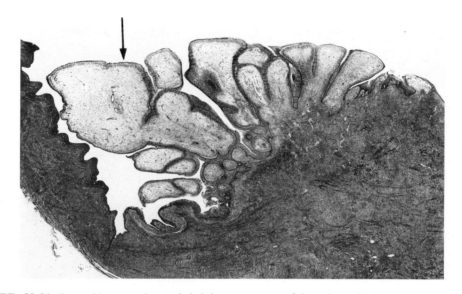

FIG. 22-21. Botryoid-type embryonal rhabdomyosarcoma of the urinary bladder. Note polypoid and myxoid appearance of the tumor and submucosal hypercellular "cambium" layer *(arrow)*. (×10.)

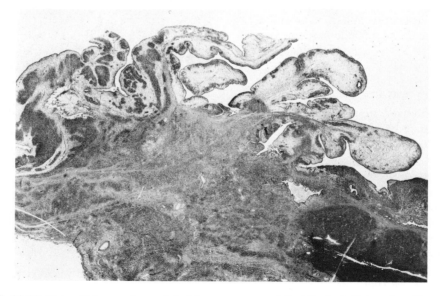

FIG. 22-22. Botryoid-type embryonal rhabdomyosarcoma of the bile duct. Note polypoid growth and alternating myxoid and cellular areas. (×5.)

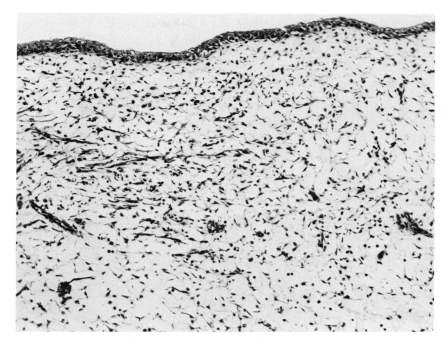

FIG. 22-23. Botryoid-type embryonal rhabdomyosarcoma consisting chiefly of haphazardly arranged primitive mesenchymal cells and occasional strap-shaped rhabdomyoblasts with eosinophilic cytoplasm. (×100.)

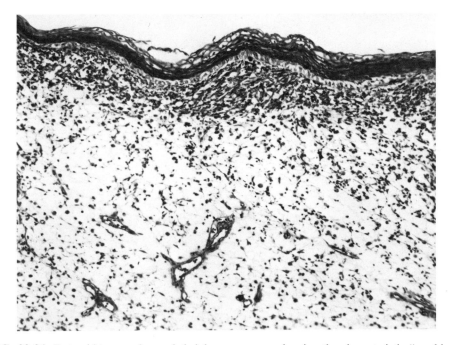

FIG. 22-24. Botryoid-type embryonal rhabdomyosarcoma showing the characteristic "cambium" layer, a submucosal zone of markedly increased cellularity. (×100.)

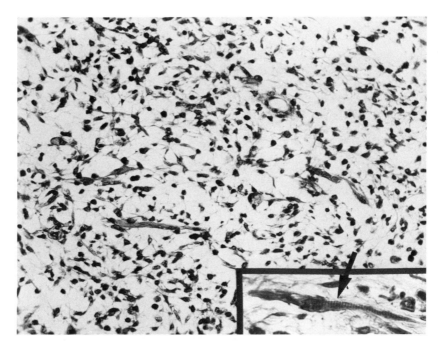

FIG. 22-25. Botryoid-type embryonal rhabdomyosarcoma. Inset shows elongated rhabdomyoblast with cross-striations *(arrow)*. (×210.)

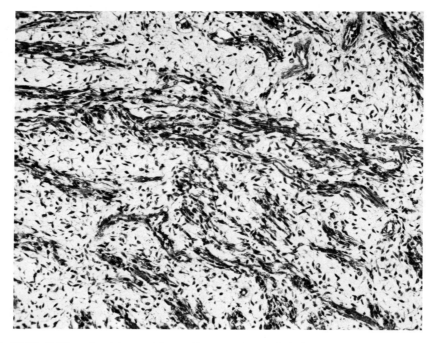

FIG. 22-26. Differentiated form of botryoid-type embryonal rhabdomyosarcoma with numerous strap-shaped and ribbon-shaped rhabdomyoblasts. (×130.)

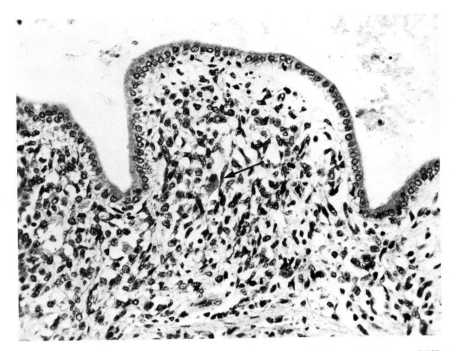

FIG. 22-27. Embryonal rhabdomyosarcoma of the biliary tract with botryoid features. Differentiated rhabdomyoblasts at arrow. (×195.)

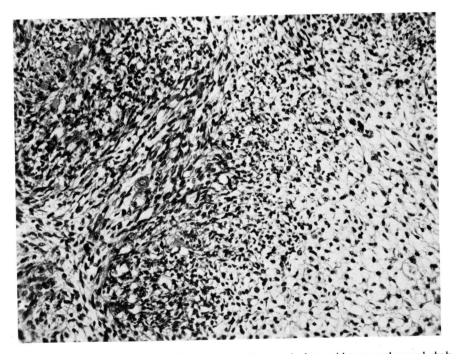

FIG. 22-28. Transition between cellular and myxoid areas in botryoid-type embryonal rhabdomyosarcoma. (×160.)

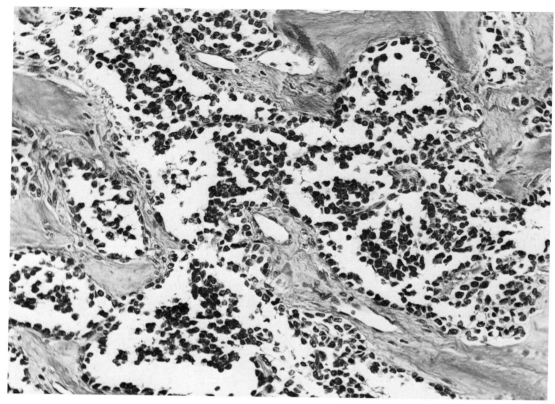

FIG. 22-29. Alveolar rhabdomyosarcoma. Note variously sized loosely textured aggregates of tumor cells separated by irregularly shaped fibrous trabeculae. (×210.)

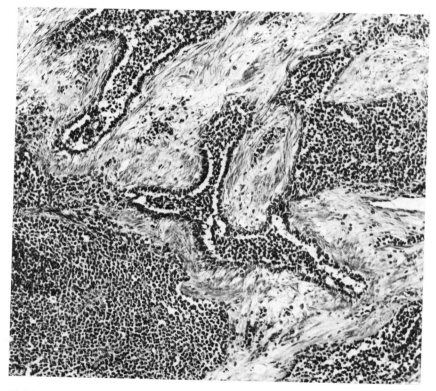

FIG. 22-30. Alveolar rhabdomyosarcoma showing mixture of solid and alveolar areas in the same tumor. (×100.)

Alveolar rhabdomyosarcoma

The alveolar type of rhabdomyosarcoma is composed largely of ill-defined aggregates of poorly differentiated round or oval tumor cells that frequently show central loss of cellular cohesion and formation of irregular "alveolar" spaces. The individual cellular aggregates are separated and surrounded by frameworks of dense, frequently hyalinized fibrous septa that surround dilated vascular channels. Characteristically the cells at the periphery of the alveolar spaces are well preserved and adhere in a single layer to the fibrous septa, in a manner somewhat reminiscent of an adenocarcinoma or papillary carcinoma (Figs. 22-29 and 22-30). The cells in the center of the alveolar spaces tend to be more loosely arranged or "freely floating"; they are often poorly preserved and show evidence of degeneration and necrosis. In rare instances, viable cells are virtually absent, and the tumor consists merely of a coarse sievelike or honeycomb-like meshwork of thick fibrous trabeculae surrounding small loosely textured groups of severely degenerated cells with pyknotic nuclei and necrotic cellular debris[54] (see Fig. 22-38).

There are also "solid" forms of this tumor that lack an alveolar pattern entirely and are composed of densely packed groups or masses of tumor cells resembling the round cell areas of embryonal rhabdomyosarcoma but showing a more uniform cellular picture with little or no fibrosis. These solidly cellular areas are more commonly encountered at the periphery of the tumor and probably represent the most active and most cellular stage of growth. It is important not to confuse the solid form of alveolar rhabdomyosarcoma with the undifferentiated form of embryonal rhabdomyosarcoma, since the former carries a less favorable prognosis. Distinction may be difficult, but in most cases examination of the solid tumors will show, in addition to the uniform cellular pattern, incipient alveolar features (Figs. 22-30 to 22-33). Cytogenetic studies will also help in differential diagnosis.[54,213] There are also rare cases in which the cells have abundant pale-staining, glycogen-containing cytoplasm and vaguely resemble clear cell carcinoma or clear cell malignant melanoma *(clear cell rhabdomyosarcoma)* (Fig. 22-34). Multivacuolated or "spider" cells are rare.

The individual cells in both alveolar and solid portions of the tumor range from 10 to 15 μm in diameter and tend

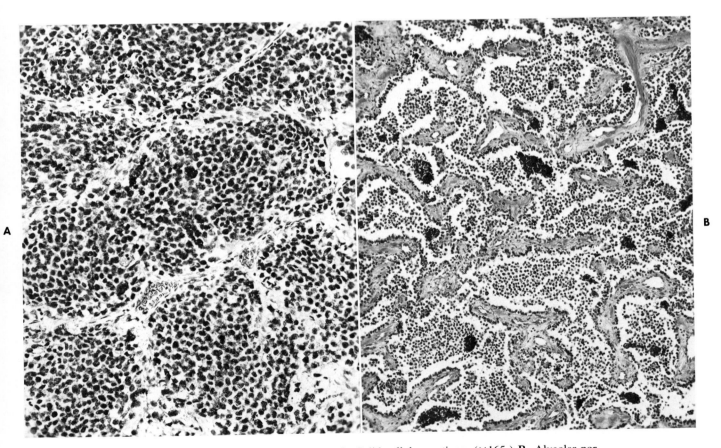

FIG. 22-31. Alveolar rhabdomyosarcoma. **A,** Solid cellular portions. (×165.) **B,** Alveolar portion. (×80.)

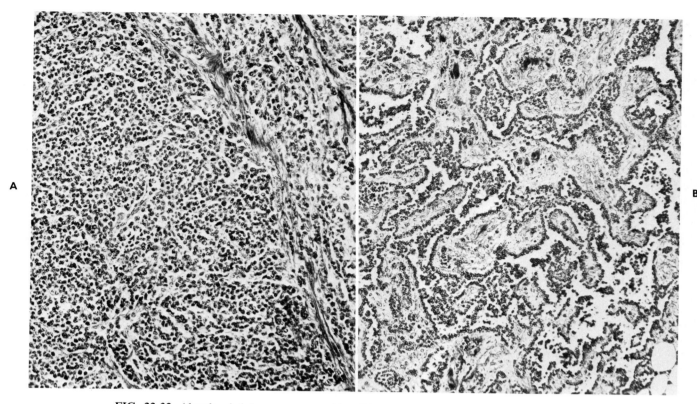

A

B

FIG. 22-32. Alveolar rhabdomyosarcoma with solid round cell areas (A) and alveolar areas (B). In general, the solid areas are more common in the peripheral portion of the tumor. (A, ×110; B, ×120.)

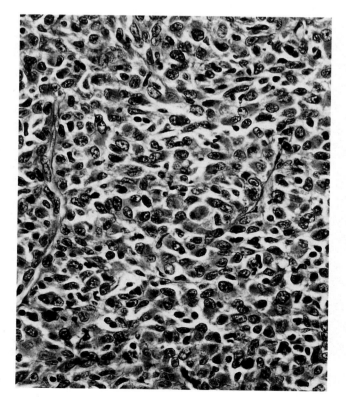

FIG. 22-33. "Solid" type of rhabdomyosarcoma. This tumor did not show a focal alveolar pattern but stained strongly for vimentin, muscle-specific actin, and desmin. (×350.)

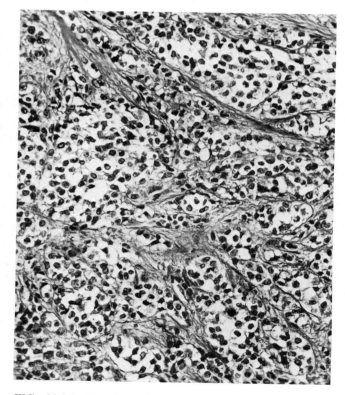

FIG. 22-34. Alveolar rhabdomyosarcoma consisting predominantly of nests of rounded rhabdomyoblasts with abundant pale-staining (glycogen-containing) cytoplasm, a "clear cell" variant of this tumor. (×180.)

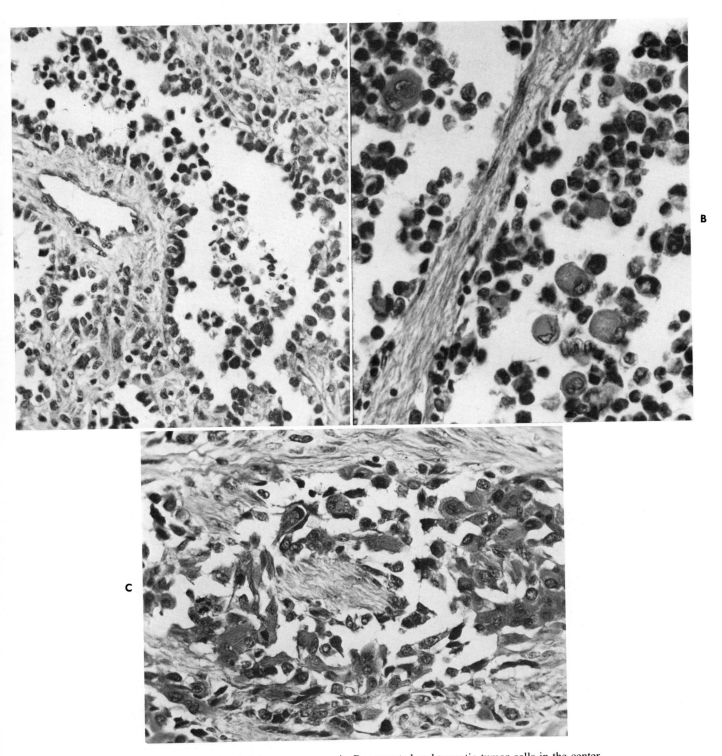

FIG. 22-35. Alveolar rhabdomyosarcoma. **A,** Degenerated and necrotic tumor cells in the center of the alveolar spaces and a single layer of viable tumor cells attached to the intervening fibrous septa. (×350.) **B,** Mixture of "floating" rhabdomyoblasts and degenerated tumor cells with pyknotic nuclei. (×450.) **C,** Differentiated deeply eosinophilic rhabdomyoblasts. (×450.) Rhabdomyoblasts with cross-striations are much less common in the alveolar type than in the embryonal type of rhabdomyosarcoma.

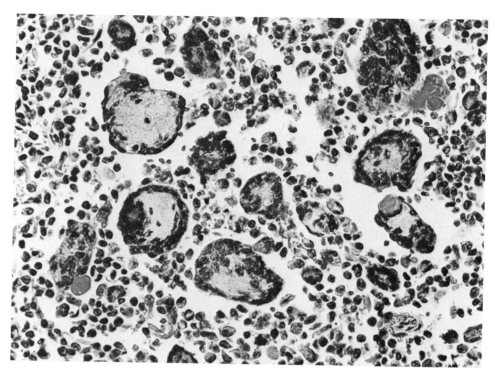

FIG. 22-36. Multinucleated giant cells with peripherally placed "wreathlike" nuclei, a characteristic and diagnostically useful feature of many alveolar rhabdomyosarcomas. (×650.)

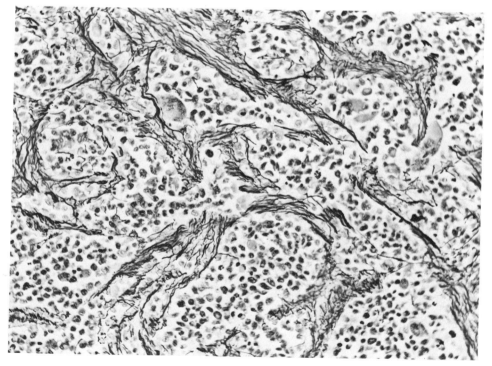

FIG. 22-37. Alveolar rhabdomyosarcoma. Collagen is confined to intervening fibrous septa. (Reticulin preparation; ×210.)

to have round or oval hyperchromatic nuclei with scanty amounts of indistinct cytoplasm. Bulbous or club-shaped cells, sometimes with deeply eosinophilic cytoplasm, are often seen protruding from the fibrous walls into the lumen of the alveolar spaces. Mitotic figures are common and range from 5 to 30/10 HPF.

Neoplastic rhabdomyoblasts with pronounced stringy or granular eosinophilic cytoplasm are less common in alveolar than in embryonal rhabdomyosarcoma and are present in no more than about 30% of cases. Most of the rhabdomyoblasts within the alveolar spaces have rounded or oval configurations (Fig. 22-35, *A, B,* and *C*); but those located in or attached to the fibrous septa tend to be strap shaped or spindle shaped. If cross-striations are present, they are almost exclusively found in the spindle-shaped cells.

In contrast to embryonal rhabdomyosarcoma, multinucleated giant cells are a prominent and diagnostically important feature of alveolar rhabdomyosarcoma. Usually the giant cells possess multiple, peripherally placed nuclei within a pale-staining or weakly eosinophilic cytoplasm (Fig. 22-36). We have never been able to detect cross-striations in these cells, and according to ultrastructural studies by Churg and Ringus,[23] they do not contain myofilaments. Yet

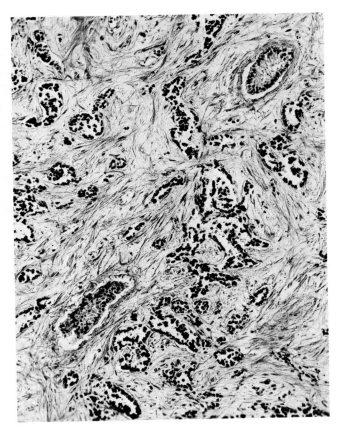

FIG. 22-38. Metastatic alveolar rhabdomyosarcoma showing marked desmoplasia. (×100.)

transitional forms between rhabdomyoblasts and giant cells suggest that the latter are formed by cellular fusion. Collagen formation is usually confined to the intervening septa (Fig. 22-37), but occasionally large portions of the tumor are obliterated by extensive fibroplasia (Fig. 22-38). As has already been mentioned, mixed types with embryonal and alveolar features should be classified as alveolar rhabdomyosarcomas.

Most examples of alveolar rhabdomyosarcoma seem to originate in muscle tissue, and entrapment of normal muscle fibers is common. These fibers are apt to be mistaken for neoplastic rhabdomyoblasts with cross-striations, a feature that sometimes results in the correct diagnosis for the wrong reason.

Metastatic alveolar rhabdomyosarcomas in lymph nodes, the lung, and other viscera also display a distinct alveolar pattern, making it unlikely that this pattern is merely the result of infiltrative growth along the fibrous framework of the involved musculature (Fig. 22-39). There are also cases of diffuse bone marrow metastasis that have been mistaken for leukemia.

Pleomorphic rhabdomyosarcoma

Although numerous examples of pleomorphic rhabdomyosarcoma have been described in the earlier literature,[70,117,201] most of these tumors were probably malignant fibrous histiocytomas or other pleomorphic soft tissue sarcomas. Even today clear distinction of this tumor from other forms of pleomorphic sarcoma remains a difficult problem, and in the absence of cells with cross-striations, immunostaining for desmin and myoglobin or ultrastructural studies, or both, are essential for diagnosis.

Pleomorphic rhabdomyosarcoma can be distinguished from embryonal and alveolar rhabdomyosarcoma by the association of loosely arranged, haphazardly oriented, large, round or pleomorphic cells with hyperchromatic nuclei and deeply eosinophilic cytoplasm (Figs. 22-40 to 22-42). As in embryonal rhabdomyosarcoma, there are racquet-shaped and tadpole-shaped rhabdomyoblasts, but these are generally of larger size and more irregular in outline. Cells with cross-striations are commonly found in embryonal rhabdomyosarcomas with focal pleomorphic features but are virtually nonexistent in adult pleomorphic rhabdomyosarcomas.[38,118,136] For instance, Gaffney et al.[66] failed to find cross-striations in 11 cases of pleomorphic rhabdomyosarcoma even though 10 of the tumors stained positively for desmin and myoglobin and two showed the typical ultrastructural features of rhabdomyosarcoma. In addition to desmin and myoglobin, immunostaining for muscle-specific actin with HHF35 will help to rule out other types of pleomorphic sarcoma, especially malignant fibrous histiocytoma. Rarely, desmin positive cells are found in malignant fibrous histiocytoma, but the large eosinophilic giant cells of this tumor often have a finely vacuolated

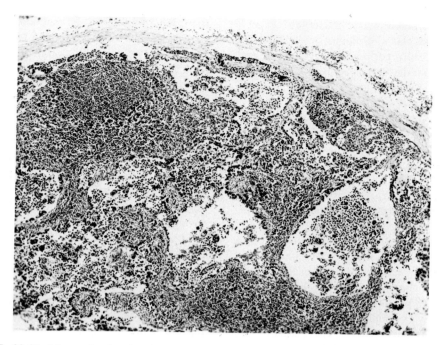

FIG. 22-39. Metastatic alveolar rhabdomyosarcoma. The alveolar pattern is present in the primary tumor as well as in the metastases. (×210.)

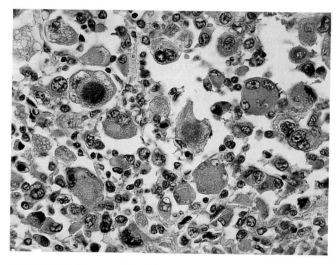

FIG. 22-40. Pleomorphic rhabdomyosarcoma of the retroperitoneum in a 67-year-old woman. The tumor stained positively for muscle-specific actin and desmin. (Masson trichrome stain; ×350.)

cytoplasm (unlike the coarsely vacuolated "spider-web" cells of rhabdomyosarcoma) and are associated with occasional xanthoma cells and a prominent inflammatory component. Moreover, the cells of malignant fibrous histiocytoma contain no or much less glycogen than

pleomorphic rhabdomyosarcomas. Embryonal rhabdomyosarcomas with focal pleomorphic features should be classified as embryonal rhabdomyosarcomas.

SPECIAL DIAGNOSTIC PROCEDURES
Special stains

Although many rhabdomyosarcomas can be positively diagnosed with hematoxylin-eosin stained sections on the basis of their histological features or patterns, many poorly differentiated sarcomas masquerade as rhabdomyosarcomas, and ancillary diagnostic procedures are often essential for an objective and reliable diagnosis. During the past decade conventional special stains, such as the PAS preparation or the Masson trichrome stain, have become much less important for diagnosis and have been largely replaced by immunohistochemical procedures or electron microscopic study of the tumor, or both. Despite the greatly diminished role of conventional stains, Masson trichrome stain, PTAH, and iron-hematoxylin stain complement the morphological findings and facilitate the scanning of multiple sections for the presence of differentiated cells (rhabdomyoblasts) among poorly differentiated cellular elements. These stains, however, lack specificity and stain both myofibrils and other cellular and extracellular structures. Other stains, such as the PAS preparation with and without diastase, are useful in the differential diagnosis of small cell tumors, since most rhabdomyosarcomas contain

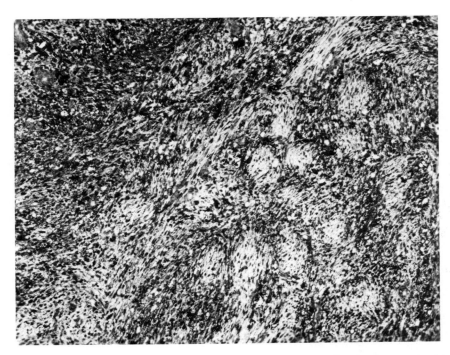

FIG. 22-41. PAS preparation of embryonal rhabdomyosarcoma revealing large amounts of irregularly distributed glycogen. (×100.)

considerable amounts of intracellular PAS-positive glycogen; in many tumors the glycogen is rather irregularly distributed and as a rule is much more conspicuous in well-differentiated than poorly differentiated tumor cells (Fig. 22-41). Extracellular mucinous material stains positively with colloidal iron and alcian blue and is removed by prior treatment of the sections with hyaluronidase. Reticulin preparations usually reveal little interstitial collagen, but fibrosis may be marked in tumors of the alveolar type (Figs. 22-37 and 22-38).

Immunohistochemical procedures

Many immunohistochemical markers have been applied to the diagnosis of rhabdomyosarcoma, but their diagnostic value, sensitivity, and specificity vary substantially, and not all of the reported markers are available commercially. Of the various markers, antibodies against desmin (for the muscle type of intermediate filaments),[3-5,8,133] muscle-specific actin (HHF35),[8,36,142,170,177] and myoglobin[26,57,104,141] seem to be most useful for diagnostic purposes. These markers can be used with frozen and alcohol-fixed material as well as with formalin-fixed tissue, even after years in paraffin (Figs. 22-42 and 22-43).

In general, the intensity of the immunostaining for myoglobin, desmin, and muscle-specific actin is proportional to the degree of rhabdomyoblastic differentiation. Thus immunostaining is most intense in well-differentiated tumors that contain morphologically recognizable round or strap-shaped rhabdomyoblasts and is least prominent in primitive or poorly differentiated rhabdomyosarcomas, the problem cases that cause most of the difficulties in diagnosis. In many cases, "committed" primitive or undifferentiated small cells that are morphologically not recognizable as rhabdomyoblasts stain positively for muscle-specific actin and desmin but usually do not stain for myoglobin. According to Erlandson,[56] poorly differentiated rhabdomyoblasts may be recognized with HHF35 before becoming immunoreactive for desmin. Immunoreactivity for muscle-specific actin, desmin, and myoglobin is also shared by rhabdomyosarcomas of the alveolar and pleomorphic types. Use of desmin and HHF35 does not help to distinguish rhabdomyosarcomas from leiomyosarcomas.[170]

Other somewhat less sensitive markers that have been used in the diagnosis of rhabdomyosarcoma include antibodies for fast, slow, and fetal myosin,[35,58,59] creatine kinase (isoenzymes MM and BB),[37,98,212] beta-enolase,[179] Z-protein,[143] titin,[149] and vimentin.[3,106,138,188] Vimentin is coexpressed in virtually all rhabdomyosarcomas but is more prominent in undifferentiated than well-differentiated tumors. Very primitive rhabdomyosarcomas may stain negatively for vimentin, however.[138] Since vimentin is present in a variety of sarcomas and carcinomas, its diagnostic utility is minimal. Cytokeratin and S-100 protein have also

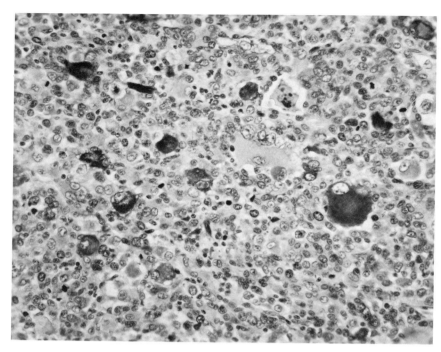

FIG. 22-42. Pleomorphic rhabdomyosarcoma stained with positive immunostaining for myoglobin. (×350.)

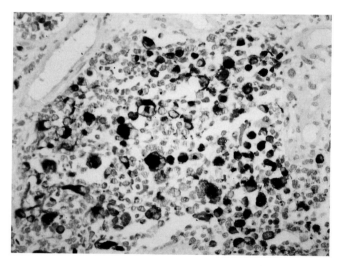

FIG. 22-43. Embryonal rhabdomyosarcoma with positive immunostaining for desmin. (×250.)

been demonstrated in occasional undifferentiated tumor cells and rhabdomyoblasts, respectively.[24,134] Of course, many malignant Triton tumors (malignant peripheral nerve sheath tumors with rhabdomyoblastic differentiation) contain, in addition to rhabdomyoblasts, nerve sheath elements that stain positively for S-100 protein.

More recently, immunohistochemical expression of myo-

genic regulatory protein (MyoD1), a muscle regulatory gene that is present during normal skeletal muscle myogenesis, was used in the identification of rhabdomyosarcoma and other tumors showing myogenic differentiation; this protein has also been demonstrated in tumors other than rhabdomyosarcoma.[41]

Caution in interpretation is advisable with all staining techniques because entrapped normal or degenerated muscle fibers may give a false-positive reaction. One must also be aware, as Eusebi et al.[57] have pointed out, that there may be diffusion and passive uptake of myoglobin by nonmuscular tumor cells and that myoglobin may be demonstrable in carcinoma cells that have invaded striated muscle. Confusion may also be caused by interspersed reactive or neoplastic myofibroblasts staining positively for both desmin and muscle-specific actin.[170]

Ultrastructural findings

The ultrastructure of rhabdomyosarcoma bears a striking resemblance to that of embryonal muscle tissue in varying stages of development, but there is a much wider spectrum in the appearance of the tumor cells. The tumor cells range from primitive undifferentiated cells with few organelles to highly differentiated cells with abundant but often incomplete sarcomeres. In the least well-differentiated cells the cytoplasm may contain only scattered or parallel bundles of thin (actin) myofilaments, measuring 6 to 8 nm in diam-

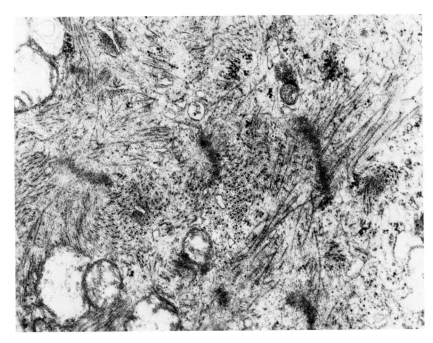

FIG. 22-44. Ultrastructure of embryonal rhabdomyosarcoma showing typical mixture of thick (myosin) and thin (actin) fibrils in longitudinal and cross-section with distinct Z banding in several places.

eter; this is a nonspecific finding that does not permit a reliable diagnosis of rhabdomyosarcoma; better differentiated cells are characterized by distinct bundles of thick (myosin) filaments, ranging from 12 to 15 nm in diameter, with attached ribosomes having an Indian file arrangement (ribosome and myosin complex), a feature that is characteristic of rhabdomyoblastic differentiation. Further cellular maturation is marked by alternating thin (actin) and thick (myosin) filaments in a parallel arrangement, with a characteristic hexagonal pattern seen on cross-sections and rodlike structures or discs composed of Z-band material. In many tumors, there are also well-differentiated rhabdomyoblasts with distinct sarcomeres, including the characteristic A and I banding and clearly discernible Z lines* (Fig. 22-44). Entrapped degenerated muscle fibers can be recognized ultrastructurally by the presence of autolysosomes.[187]

In addition to the myofilaments, the cytoplasm of the rhabdomyoblasts contains a prominent Golgi apparatus and a varying number of mitochondria and glycogen particles. There are also small lysosomes, droplets of lipid, occasional pinocytotic vesicles, and complete or incomplete basal lamina. The multinucleate giant cells, characteristic of the alveolar type, have neither myofilaments nor basal laminae.[23] Gaffney et al.,[66] examining six cases of pleo-

morphic rhabdomyosarcoma, found the typical ultrastructural features of this tumor in only two cases. The remaining four cases showed merely collections of nonspecific filamentous material. The latter feature was also emphasized in another electron microscopic study of pleomorphic rhabdomyosarcoma.[90]

Cytogenetic findings

The most common chromosomal abnormality, characteristic of the alveolar type, is the translocation between chromosomes 2 and 13 t(2;13)(q37;q14), but other changes, including translocations, structural abnormalities, and nonrandom chromosome alterations, have also been described in other histological types of rhabdomyosarcoma.[31,48,50,211] Shapiro et al.[191] and others[13,215] studied the chromosomal sublocalization of the t(2;13) translocation breakpoint in alveolar rhabdomyosarcoma. Olegard et al.[148] described an embryonal rhabdomyosarcoma with 100 chromosomes but no structural aberrations (see Chapter 5).

DIFFERENTIAL DIAGNOSIS

Poorly differentiated round and spindle cell sarcomas, especially when occurring in children or young adults, constitute the most common problem in differential diagnosis. Included in this group are neuroblastoma, neuroepithelioma, Ewing's sarcoma, poorly differentiated angiosarcoma, synovial sarcoma, malignant melanoma, melanotic

---

*References 56, 90, 101, 102, 131, 139, 151.

neuroectodermal tumor of infancy, granulocytic sarcoma, and malignant lymphoma. Small cell carcinoma must also be considered when the tumor occurs in a patient older than 45 years. Differential diagnosis requires not only careful evaluation of the clinical data, the age of the patient, and the location of the lesion, but also painstaking examination of multiple sections for specific features such as rhabdomyoblasts, rosettes, biphasic cellular or vascular differentiation, and intracellular pigment as well as immunohistochemical assessment of the tumor with multiple markers. Special stains may also help in differential diagnosis: intracellular glycogen, for example, which stains positively for PAS and can be removed by diastase, is demonstrable in most rhabdomyosarcomas, Ewing's sarcomas, and malignant melanomas, but is absent in most primitive neuroectodermal tumors, synovial sarcomas, and malignant lymphomas. Other stains useful in differential diagnosis are the Leder stain for naphthol AS-D chloracetate esterase and Fontana's stain or Warthin-Starry preparation for melanin.

Malignant rhabdoid tumor is another rare neoplasm that bears a close resemblance to rhabdomyosarcoma. It occurs not only in the kidney, where it was first described as a variant of Wilms' tumor, but is also found in the soft tissues, although it apparently does not have any predilection for a particular site. The tumor is readily separated from rhabdomyosarcoma on the basis of immunohistochemical studies: the large acidophilic round or polygonal cells of this tumor do not accept immunostains for desmin or myoglobin, but stain positively for keratin (see Chapter 38).[108,197,214]

Alveolar soft part sarcoma is composed of large polygonal cells with vesicular nuclei separated by thin-walled vascular channels. Typically the cells contain intracellular PAS-positive crystalline material that is not removed by diastase digestion (see Chapter 38).

Problems in diagnosis may also be caused by benign reactive and neoplastic lesions, such as polypoid cystitis, polyps and pseudosarcomas of the vagina and vulva with atypical stromal cells,[146,150] pseudosarcoma of the vagina during pregnancy, infectious granuloma, proliferative myositis, granular cell tumor, and fetal rhabdomyoma. Conversely, we have also encountered sparsely cellular botryoid-type rhabdomyosarcomas that were initially misinterpreted as *myxomas*. In these cases consideration of age and location will usually provide the correct diagnosis, since myxomas are virtually nonexistent in children and almost never occur in visceral organs. For the differential diagnosis from *fetal rhabdomyoma* see Chapter 21.

Tumors with heterologous rhabdomyoblastic components

Focal rhabdomyoblastic differentiation occurs in a variety of malignant neoplasms; rhabdomyoblasts are a more or less prominent component of malignant mixed mesoder-

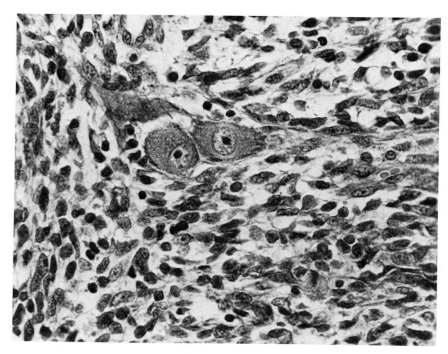

FIG. 22-45. Malignant ectomesenchymoma of the scrotum in a 20-year-old man showing mature ganglion cells with a rhabdomyosarcoma-like tumor. Cells with cross-striations were present in another portion of this neoplasm. (×440.)

mal tumors of the uterus, cervix, or ovary, carcinosarcomas of the breast and stomach, pulmonary blastomas, nephroblastomas, and mixed-type hepatoblastomas; in fact, in rare examples of these neoplasms, as in some Wilms' tumors, the rhabdomyoblastic component may dominate the microscopic picture. Rhabdomyoblastic differentiation is also encountered in malignant or immature teratomas but rarely as a major element. In most of these tumors, the rhabdomyoblastic component is accompanied by malignant epithelial and other mesenchymal elements such as cartilage and bone. Metaplastic cartilage may also be present in otherwise typical rhabdomyosarcomas.

Rhabdomyoblastic differentiation is also a feature of various neuroectodermal neoplasms, notably malignant schwannoma (malignant Triton tumor and malignant glandular Triton tumor), ganglioneuroma (ectomesenchymoma), and medulloepithelioma. Malignant Triton tumors chiefly occur in patients older than 30 years who have manifestations of neurofibromatosis.[30] Malignant ectomesenchymoma is primarily a tumor of children and is not known to be associated with neurofibromatosis; it consists of a mix-

ture of rhabdomyoblastic elements, mature ganglion cells, and neuroma-like structures (Fig. 22-45).[103] We have observed one case in which the initial tumor showed the features of an embryonal rhabdomyosarcoma, and the recurrent tumor was indistinguishable from a ganglioneuroma save for a few peripherally located groups of rhabdomyoblasts (Fig. 22-46, A and B). We have also reviewed a case of concurrent rhabdomyosarcoma of the retroperitoneum and pheochromocytoma in a 46-year-old woman.

Malignant mesenchymoma with a distinct rhabdomyoblastic component does occur, but it is very rare in our experience, particularly if rhabdomyosarcomas with cartilaginous or osseous metaplasia are excluded and diagnosed as rhabdomyosarcomas rather than malignant mesenchymomas. We have seen a few cases, however, in which rhabdomyosarcomatous areas were associated with areas indistinguishable from liposarcoma or osteosarcoma. Rhabdomyoblastic differentiation also occurs in dedifferentiated chondrosarcomas and in polypoid sarcomas of the pulmonary trunk, both tumors that may be considered as variants of malignant mesenchymoma. The various heterologous

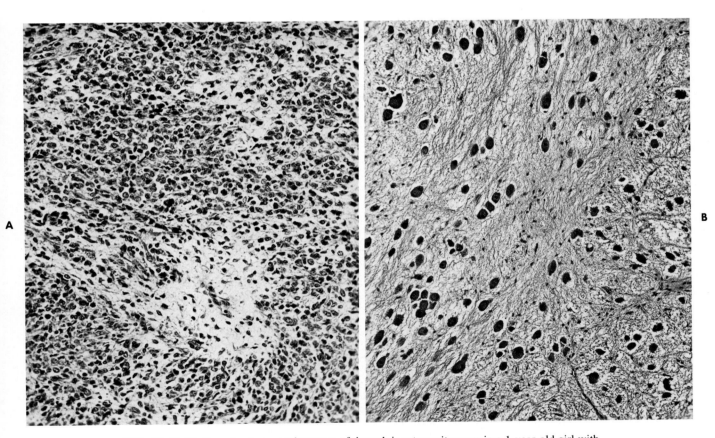

FIG. 22-46. Malignant ectomesenchymoma of the pelvic retroperitoneum in a 1-year-old girl with rhabdomyosarcomatous features in the initial specimen (**A**) and ganglioneuroma-like picture in the material obtained at autopsy (**B**). Rhabdomyoblasts with cross-striations and typical ganglion cells were present in the surgical material and occasional rhabdomyoblasts in the ganglioneuroma-like tumor obtained at autopsy. (**A,** ×195; **B,** ×100.)

Tumors with heterologous rhabdomyoblastic components

Malignant peripheral nerve sheath tumor (malignant Triton tumor)
Ectomesenchymoma
Medulloepithelioma
Medulloblastoma
Congenital pigmented nevus (giant nevus)
Dedifferentiated chondrosarcoma and osteosarcoma
Malignant mesenchymoma
Carcinosarcoma, especially of breast, stomach, and urinary bladder
Pulmonary blastoma
Hepatoblastoma
Wilms' tumor (mesonephroma)
Malignant mixed müllerian tumor of the uterus, cervix, ovary, or retroperitoneum
Germ cell tumors (seminoma, teratoma)
Sertoli-Leydig cell tumor
Thymoma

Clinical staging of patients with rhabdomyosarcoma (Intergroup Rhabdomyosarcoma Studies classification)*

Group I
Localized disease, completely resected (regional nodes not involved)
Confined to muscle or organ of origin
Contiguous involvement with infiltration outside the muscle or organ of origin, as through fascial planes

Group II
Grossly resected tumor with microscopic residual disease
No evidence of gross residual tumor; no evidence of regional node involvement
Regional disease, completely resected (regional nodes involved or extension of tumor into an adjacent organ, or both); all tumor completely resected with no microscopic residual tumor
Regional disease with involved nodes, grossly resected, but with evidence of microscopic residual disease

Group III
Incomplete resection or biopsy with gross residual disease

Group IV
Distant metastatic disease present at onset (lung, liver, bones, bone marrow, brain, and distant muscle and nodes)

*From Maurer HM, et al: *Cancer* 61:209, 1988.

neoplasms with focal rhabdomyoblastic differentiation are listed in the box above (see also Chapter 38).

PROGNOSIS AND THERAPY

During the past 30 or 40 years the prognosis of rhabdomyosarcoma has improved dramatically: prior to 1960 the prognosis was extremely poor, and there were few survivors even after radical, often destructive and disfiguring surgical therapy. In a 1963 follow-up study[53] based on 147 cases from the files of the AFIP, 90% of the patients died of the disease within a period of 5 years. In another AFIP study,[54] which was devoted exclusively to alveolar rhabdomyosarcomas, the 5-year mortality rate was 98%. Others reported similar discouraging data: in 1965, Masson and Soule[127] reported a 5-year death rate of 88%, and in 1962, Dito and Batsakis[43] reported a 5-year death rate of 94%, based on 170 rhabdomyosarcomas of the head and neck, with an average survival time of 16 months.

Since the early 1960s there has been a remarkable improvement in the survival rates of patients with rhabdomyosarcoma because of a multidisciplinary therapeutic approach that consisted of biopsy or surgical removal of the neoplasm and multiagent chemotherapy with or without radiotherapy. As a rule, treatment is carried out after biopsy or resection and careful, comprehensive assessment of tumor stage or tumor group with x-ray, CT scan, MRI, and, if necessary, angiograms. Recommendations for therapy chiefly depend on the stage or clinical group of the disease and the site of the tumor following accurate microscopic diagnosis. Since rhabdomyosarcomas tend to metastasize to the bone marrow, bone marrow aspiration should be part of the staging process.

The Intergroup Rhabdomyosarcoma Study II, confined to patients younger than 21 years with a confirmed diagnosis of rhabdomyosarcoma, distinguishes four groups (see the box above). Standard therapy for group I and II tumors is a regimen of three chemotherapeutic agents, chiefly vincristine (V), dactinomycin (A), and cyclophosphamide (C). The basic therapy for group I tumors is VA. For group II tumors, intensive VA or repetitive-pulse VAC and radiotherapy and for group III and IV tumors, repetitive-pulse VAC with or without adriamycin is used, with radiotherapy to the sites of the primary tumor and the metastasis.[128,129] The dosage of radiation given for residual gross disease usually ranges from 3000 to 5500 rad over a 6-week period.

Specific locations require specific modes of therapy: in

rhabdomyosarcomas of the orbit, for instance, complete control is accomplished with biopsy, systemic chemotherapy, and radiation alone.[87,129] Excellent results are also achieved in rhabdomyosarcomas of the paratesticular region with radical orchiectomy with clear margins, radical retroperitoneal lymph node resection, and chemotherapy.[110,167] Tumors in the parameningeal and paraspinal regions require extended radiation and intrathecal chemotherapy to reduce local failure and spread of the disease.[45,169,205] Preoperative radiotherapy or chemotherapy in rhabdomyosarcomas of the urinary bladder and prostate usually allows less extensive surgical therapy and better functional preservation.[166] Total excision of the tumor is part of the recommended therapy in rhabdomyosarcomas occurring in the trunk and extremities.[69,80]

According to the Intergroup Rhabdomyosarcoma Study II,[129] prognosis is excellent for group I and II tumors, with 5-year survival rates of 85% and 88%, respectively (excluding alveolar rhabdomyosarcomas of the extremities); survival rates are less favorable with group III tumors (66% 5-year survival rate) (excluding some pelvic tumors) and poor with group IV tumors (26% 5-year survival rate). The overall 5-year survival rate for IRS II tumors in 999 patients, including alveolar rhabdomyosarcomas of the extremities and pelvic tumors, is 63%, an 8% increase over IRS group I tumors. Patients with local recurrence or distant metastatic disease at the time of diagnosis or during therapy rarely survive.[45,163] As with other types of sarcomas, the adequacy of early therapy decides the outcome of the disease. Other large studies, based in part on a TNM staging system, report similar or slightly less favorable results.[62,74,84,175]

Additional factors that may influence the clinical course of the disease and necessitate more intensive therapy include the anatomical site and histological type of the tumor. In general, rhabdomyosarcomas in parameningeal sites of the head and neck and paraspinal region, bladder and prostate, biliary tract, retroperitoneum, perineum, and extremities carry a less favorable prognosis than those in the orbit and the genitourinary region, including the prostate but not the bladder. Orbital tumors studied in the Intergroup Rhabdomyosarcoma Study II had a 92% 5-year survival rate.[10,27,69,129,163] Late detection and large size of the tumor, difficulties encountered in surgical removal or extension into the meninges, with or without spinal fluid spread, and an increased rate of lymph node metastasis are mostly responsible for the prognostic differences related to the various anatomical sites. The patients' age may also influence the survival rate: the clinical course tends to be more favorable in children than in adolescents and adults.

There is also a definite link between prognosis and histological type. Patients with alveolar or pleomorphic rhabdomyosarcoma have a less favorable prognosis than those with rhabdomyosarcoma of the embryonal and especially

---

Favorable and unfavorable factors in rhabdomyosarcoma

I. Prognostically favorable factors

Infants and children
Orbital or genitourinary (nonbladder) location
Small size (<5 cm)
Botryoid or spindle cell type
Localized noninvasive tumor without regional lymph node involvement or distant metastasis
Complete initial resection

II. Prognostically unfavorable factors

Adults
Location in head and neck (nonorbital), paraspinal region, abdomen, biliary tract, retroperitoneum, perineum, or extremities
Large size (>5 cm)
Alveolar or pleomorphic type
Local tumor invasion, especially parameningeal or paraspinal region, sinuses, or skeleton
Local recurrence
Local recurrence during therapy
Regional lymph node involvement or distant metastasis
Incomplete initial excision or unresectability

---

the botryoid or spindle cell type.[20,54,67,74,194] Ruymann et al.,[182] reporting on a series of 103 biliary tract rhabdomyosarcomas, found that 30 were of the alveolar type; 15 of the 30 were group IV tumors, indicating a high proportion of early and distant metastasis. Hays et al.[81] reported that in group I or II tumors the death rate of the alveolar type was 44% and of the embryonal type 13.5%. The higher frequency of alveolar rhabdomyosarcoma in the extremities also explains the less favorable clinical course of tumors arising at this site. There is, however, no agreement as to the predictive value of the degree of cellular differentiation. Some doubt that cellular differentiation improves the response to chemotherapy and the prognosis;[217] Others report that patients with primitive (undifferentiated) or pleomorphic types of rhabdomyosarcomas have a less favorable clinical course than those with the well-differentiated types.[74] The mitotic rate is of little value in predicting therapeutic response and outcome of the disease, since it is elevated in most rhabdomyosarcomas.[10,76,183] (See box above.)

Flow cytometric DNA analysis is of doubtful value in predicting the clinical course. In the study by Shapiro et al.[191] one third of unresectable tumors had diploid tumor cell lines and none of the patients with diploid tumors survived. Others reported similar results.[22,109] Boyle et al.[17]

and Molenaar et al.,[135] on the other hand, observed aneuploidy in all of their cases. Some reviewers suggested that aneuploid tumors showed a better response to chemotherapy.

Long-term complications resulting from therapy depend on the location of the primary tumor. On occasion treatment may cause cataracts, xerophthalmia and craniofacial deformities, enteritis, acute or chronic diarrhea, intestinal obstruction, cystitis, hematuria, neutropenia, excessive weight loss, and other complications.[163,169] Radiation therapy may affect growth and induce secondary tumors. There are also cases in which sarcoma of bone or leukemia developed following successful treatment of rhabdomyosarcoma.[84,86,100] Occasionally diffuse bone marrow involvement of an undifferentiated rhabdomyosarcoma may lead to a mistaken diagnosis of leukemia.[21,61]

Recurrence

Inadequately treated tumors grow in an infiltrative, destructive manner and recur in a high percentage of cases. Recurrence may herald metastasis, but by no means do all cases that recur metastasize. Bone does not constitute an effective barrier to growth of the tumor, and bone invasion is a frequent finding, particularly with rhabdomyosarcomas of the head and neck region and the hands and feet. In the head and neck the tumors tend to erode and destroy the bony walls of the orbit and sinuses, the temporal or mastoid bone, and the base of the skull; they may prove fatal because of extensive meningeal spread (parameningeal rhabdomyosarcomas) and spinal cord "drop metastases."[68,161,169] Tefft et al.[207] reported that 20 of 57 cases located at parameningeal sites (nasopharynx, middle ear, paranasal sinuses) developed extension (or metastasis) to the meninges or subarachnoidal fluid. Meningeal spread may also occur with rhabdomyosarcomas at other sites.

Metastasis

Metastases develop during the course of the disease or, in about 20% of cases, are present at diagnosis.[112] Major sites of metastases are the lung, lymph nodes, and bone marrow, followed by the heart, brain, meninges, pancreas, liver, and kidney. The lungs are involved in at least two thirds of cases with metastasis.[168] The incidence of lymph node metastasis largely depends on the location of the tumor. It is greater with rhabdomyosarcomas of the prostate, paratesticular region, and extremities than with those of the orbit and head and neck.[112] In fact, exploration and biopsy of ipsilateral retroperitoneal lymph nodes is recommended in the assessment of paratesticular rhabdomyosarcomas.[167] Pratt et al.[159] reported a high incidence of metastasis to the heart: in their series of 23 fatal cases, 17 metastasized to the lung and eight to both the bone marrow and the heart. There are also rare reports of multiple skin metastases as the primary manifestation of the disease.[77]

Microscopically the recurrent and metastatic lesions may be less well differentiated than the primary growth, but unlike most other types of sarcoma, some recurrent or metastatic lesions, for unknown reasons, show a higher degree of differentiation (Fig. 22-18). We have observed three cases where positive diagnosis of rhabdomyosarcoma was possible only after rhabdomyoblasts with cross-striations were found in the pulmonary metastases. Molenaar et al.[137] reported similar cytological "differentiation" in childhood rhabdomyosarcomas following polychemotherapy and suggested that this may be due to "selective destruction of undifferentiated tumor cells." This phenomenon was also demonstrated in vitro by Lollini et al.[119]

DISCUSSION

Although rhabdomyosarcomas are frequently described as tumors of muscle origin, most of these tumors probably arise from stores of primitive or undifferentiated mesenchyme having the capacity for rhabdomyoblastic differentiation or perhaps from embryonal muscle tissue that has been displaced during the early stages of tissue development.

Origin from undifferentiated mesenchymal tissue is supported by the presence of morphologically typical examples of rhabdomyosarcoma in areas in which normally striated muscle tissue is absent, as in the regions of the common bile duct and the urinary bladder, or in areas in which striated muscle is scanty, as in the nasal cavity, middle ear, and vagina. It is further supported by the occurrence of characteristic rhabdomyosarcomatous elements in carcinosarcomas and other heterologous tumors of the lung, kidney, breast, liver, and uterus as well as in a small percentage of malignant teratomas. The plasticity of mesenchyme in infants may account for the age prevalence of rhabdomyosarcomas. There is little support for origin from metaplastic smooth muscle tissue, however. Molenaar et al.,[136] attempting to explain the relative rarity of rhabdomyosarcomas in adults, speculated that childhood rhabdomyosarcomas and adult malignant fibrous histiocytomas may arise from a common type of primitive mesenchymal cell and that malignant fibrous histiocytoma may represent the adult counterpart of rhabdomyosarcoma. Yet if this were the case one would expect to find a greater number of intermediate forms between these two tumors.

Rhabdomyosarcomas that grow within the muscles of the extremities or other regions of the body may arise from dedifferentiated muscle cells, but this, too, is rather unlikely, since normal muscle tissue does not respond to injury by mitotic proliferation and therefore may not be capable of neoplastic transformation. It is conceivable that in addition to primitive mesenchyme, satellite or reserve cells—undifferentiated rhabdomyoblast-like cells or satellite cells that are retained within normal muscle tissue—may play a role in the histogenesis of some of these tumors.

Little is known about the underlying cause of the rhabdomyoblastic proliferations and the stimulus that may induce such growths. Genetic factors are implicated by the rare occurrence of the disease in siblings,[91] the occasional presence of the tumor at birth, and the association of the disease with other neoplasms in the same patient. Rhabdomyosarcoma has been described in conjunction with a rhabdomyosarcomatous tumor of the kidney,[105] congenital retinoblastoma,[96,114] neurofibromatosis,[30] familial polyposis,[7] multiple lentigines syndrome,[83] and a variety of congenital anomalies.[181] One of our patients, a 41-year-old man with rhabdomyosarcoma of the lower leg, had suffered from familial muscular dystrophy of the scapulohumeral type and bilateral cataracts since the age of 18 years. Li and Fraumeni[115] found among 418 reported cases of rhabdomyosarcoma five families in which a second child (three siblings and two cousins) had a soft tissue sarcoma, and in which the parents, grandparents, and other relatives of these children had a high incidence of carcinoma. Genetic fac-

tors, of course, are also implicated by the described cytogenetic anomalies, especially in cases of alveolar rhabdomyosarcoma.[31,48,50,211]

One can only speculate as to whether extrinsic factors play a role in the pathogenesis of the disease. In our material and in the literature there are several cases in which the patient gave a history of trauma to the area in which the tumor later developed.[52,89,190] Over the past years we have encountered cases at sites of injury by a machine gun bullet, extraction of a molar, femoral fracture following a fall, traumatic scrotal hematoma, and injury caused by a fall on the spine. Cureton and Griffiths[29] described a rhabdomyosarcoma developing in the adductor pollicis of a 33-year-old man 9 years after a crush injury of the hand. Perhaps occasionally trauma serves as a trigger mechanism, but certainly the number of these cases is very small and does not exceed the number of such cases found in association with other types of malignant soft tissue tumors.

REFERENCES

1. Agamanolis DP, Dasu S, Krill CE: Tumors of skeletal muscle. *Hum Pathol* 17:778, 1986.
2. Albores-Saavedra J, Butler JJ, Martin RG: Rhabdomyosarcoma: clinicopathological considerations and report of 85 cases. In *Tumors of bone and soft tissue*, Chicago, 1965, Year Book Medical Publishers.
3. Altmannsberger M, Dirk T, Osborn M, et al: Immunohistochemistry of cytoskeletal filaments in the diagnosis of soft tissue tumors. *Semin Diagn Pathol* 3:306, 1986.
4. Altmannsberger M, Osborn M, Treuner J, et al: Diagnosis of human childhood rhabdomyosarcoma by antibodies to desmin, the structural protein of muscle specific intermediate filaments. *Virchows Arch (Cell Pathol)* 39:203, 1982.
5. Altmannsberger M, Weber K, Droste R, et al: Desmin is a specific marker for rhabdomyosarcomas of human and rat origin. *Am J Pathol* 118:85, 1985.
6. Angervall L, Dahl I, Ekedahl C: Embryonal rhabdomyosarcoma in the external ear. *Acta Otolaryngol* 73:513, 1972.
7. Armstrong SJ, Duncan AW, Mott MG: Rhabdomyosarcoma with familial adenomatous polyposis. *Pediatr Radiol* 21:445, 1991.
8. Azumi N, Ben-Ezra J, Battifora H: Immunophenotypic diagnosis of leiomyosarcomas and rhabdomyosarcomas with monoclonal antibodies to muscle-specific actin and desmin in formalin fixed tissue. *Mod Pathol* 1:469, 1988.
9. Bacon HE, Herabat T: Pararectal rhabdomyosarcoma. *Dis Colon Rectum* 17:365, 1974.
10. Bale PM, Parsons RE, Stevens MM: Diagnosis and behavior of juvenile rhabdomyosarcoma. *Hum Pathol* 14:596, 1983.
11. Bale PM, Reye RD: Rhabdomyosarcoma in childhood. *Pathology* 7:101, 1975.
12. Barnes L, Pietruszka M: Rhabdomyosarcoma arising within a cystosarcoma phyllodes: case report and review of the literature. *Am J Surg Pathol* 2:423, 1978.
13. Barr FG, Holick J, Nycum L, et al: Localization of the t(2;13) breakpoint of alveolar rhabdomyosarcoma on a physical map of chromosome 2. *Genomics* 13:1150, 1992.
14. Batsakis JG: Urogenital rhabdomyosarcoma: histogenesis and classification. *J Urol* 90:180, 1963.
15. Berry MP, Jenkin RDT: Parameningial rhabdomyosarcoma in the young. *Cancer* 48:281, 1981.
16. Böcker W: Ultrastrukturelle Untersuchungen zur Differenzierung von Rhabdomyoblasten in gemischten Schleimhautsarkomen des Uterus. *Zentralbl Allg Pathol* 119:318, 1975.
17. Boyle ET Jr, Reiman HM, Kramer SA, et al: Embryonal rhabdomyosarcoma of bladder and prostate: nuclear DNA patterns studied by flow cytometry. *J Urol* 140:1119, 1988.
18. Calhoun EFP Jr, Reese AR: Rhabdomyosarcoma of the orbit. *Arch Ophthalmol* 27:558, 1942.
19. Canalis RF, Jenkens HA, Hemenway WG: Nasopharyngeal rhabdomyosarcoma: a clinical perspective. *Arch Otolaryngol* 104:122, 1978.
20. Cavazzana AO, Schmidt D, Ninfo V, et al: Spindle cell rhabdomyosarcoma: a prognostically favorable variant of rhabdomyosarcoma. *Am J Surg Pathol* 16:229, 1992.
21. Cho KR, Olson JL, Epstein JI: Primitive rhabdomyosarcoma presenting with diffuse bone marrow involvement: an immunohistochemical and ultrastructural study. *Mod Pathol* 1:23, 1988.
22. Chou P, Shen-Schwarz S, Crawford S, et al: DNA analysis of genitourinary rhabdomyosarcoma in children. *Surg Pathol* 4:145, 1991.
23. Churg A, Ringus J: Ultrastructural observations on the histogenesis of alveolar rhabdomyosarcoma. *Cancer* 41:1355, 1978.
24. Coindre JM, de Mascarel A, Trojani M, et al: Immunohistochemical study of rhabdomyosarcoma: unexpected staining with S-100 protein and cytokeratin. *J Pathol* 155:127, 1988.
25. Copeland LJ, Sneige N, Stringer A, et al: Alveolar rhabdomyosarcoma of the female genitalia. *Cancer* 56:849, 1985.
26. Corson JM, Pinkus GS: Intracellular myoglobin: a specific marker for skeletal muscle differentiation in soft tissue sarcomas—an immunoperoxidase study. *Am J Pathol* 103:384, 1981.
27. Crist WM, Garnsey L, Beltangady MS, et al: Prognosis in children with rhabdomyosarcoma: a report of the Intergroup Rhabdomyosarcoma Studies I and II. *J Clin Oncol* 8:443, 1990.
28. Cunningham MD, Kung FH: Combined therapy for middle ear rhabdomyosarcoma. *Am J Dis Child* 124:401, 1972.
29. Cureton RJ, Griffiths JD: Rhabdomyosarcoma of the hand following severe trauma. *Br J Surg* 44:509, 1956-1957.
30. Daimaru Y, Hashimoto H, Enjoji M: Malignant "Triton" tumors: a

clinicopathologic and immunohistochemical study of nine cases. *Hum Pathol* 15:768, 1984.

31. Dal Cin P, Brock P, Aly MS, et al: A variant (2;13) translocation in rhabdomyosarcoma. *Cancer Genet Cytogenet* 55:191, 1991.

32. Danziger J, Handel SF, Jing BS, et al: Computerized tomography in rhabdomyosarcoma of the head and neck. *Cancer* 44:463, 1979.

33. Davis GL, Kissane JM, Ishak KG: Embryonal rhabdomyosarcoma (sarcoma botryoides) of the biliary tree. *Cancer* 24:333, 1969.

34. Daya DA, Scully RE: Sarcoma botryoides of the uterine cervix in young women: a clinicopathologic study of 13 cases. *Gynecol Oncol* 229:290, 1988.

35. deJong AS, van Vark M, Albus-Lutter CE, et al: Myosin and myoglobin as tumor markers in the diagnosis of rhabdomyosarcoma: a comparative study. *Am J Surg Pathol* 8:521, 1984.

36. deJong AS, van Kessel-van Vark M, Albus-Lutter CE et al: Skeletal muscle actin as tumor marker in the diagnosis of rhabdomyosarcoma in childhood. *Am J Surg Pathol* 9:467, 1985.

37. deJong AS, van Kessel-van Vark M, Albus-Lutter CE, et al: Creatin kinase subunits M and B as markers in the diagnosis of poorly differentiated rhabdomyosarcomas in children. *Hum Pathol* 16:924, 1985.

38. deJong AS, van Kessel-van Vark M, Albus-Lutter CE: Pleomorphic rhabdomyosarcoma in adults: immunohistochemistry as a tool for its diagnosis. *Hum Pathol* 18:298, 1987.

39. Denk H, Krepler R, Artlieb U, et al: Proteins of intermediate filaments: an immunohistochemical and biochemical approach to the classification of soft tissue tumors. *Am J Pathol* 110:193, 1983.

40. Deutsch M, Felder H: Rhabdomyosarcoma of the ear-mastoid. *Laryngoscope* 84:586, 1974.

41. Dias P, Parham DM, Shapiro DN, et al: Myogenic regulatory protein (MyoD1) expression in childhood solid tumors: diagnostic utility in rhabdomyosarcoma. *Am J Pathol* 137:1283, 1990.

42. Dito WR, Batsakis JG: Intraoral, pharyngeal, and nasopharyngeal rhabdomyosarcoma. *Arch Otolaryngol* 77:123, 1963.

43. Dito WR, Batsakis JG: Rhabdomyosarcoma of the head and neck: appraisal of biologic behavior in 170 cases. *Arch Surg* 84:582, 1962.

44. Doederlein G: Traubenfoermige Scheidensarkome des Kindes und die Moeglichkeit ihrer Heilung. *Zieglers Beitr* 103:226, 1939.

45. Donaldson SS: The value of adjuvant chemotherapy in the management of sarcomas in children. *Cancer* 55:2184, 1985.

46. Donaldson SS, Belli JA: A rational clinical staging system for childhood rhabdomyosarcoma. *J Clin Oncol* 2:135, 1984.

47. Donaldson SS, Castro JR, Wilbur JR, et al: Rhabdomyosarcoma of head and neck in children: combination treatment by surgery, irradiation, and chemotherapy. *Cancer* 31:26, 1973.

48. Douglass EC, Shapiro DN, Valentine M, et al: Alveolar rhabdomyosarcoma with the t(2;13): cytogenetic findings and clinicopathologic correlations. *Med Pediatr Oncol* 21:83, 1993.

49. Edel G, Wuisman P, Erlemann R: Spindle cell (leiomyomatous) rhabdomyosarcoma, a rare variant of embryonal rhabdomyosarcoma. *Pathol Res Pract* 189:102, 1993.

50. Engel R, Ritterbach J, Schwabe D, et al: Chromosome translocation (2;13) (q37;q14) in a disseminated alveolar rhabdomyosarcoma. *Eur J Pediatr* 148:69, 1988.

51. Enjoji M, Hashimoto H: Diagnosis of soft tissue sarcomas. *Pathol Res Pract* 178:215, 1984.

52. Enterline HT, Horn RC: Alveolar rhabdomyosarcoma: a distinctive tumor type. *Am J Clin Pathol* 29:356, 1958.

53. Enzinger FM, Lattes R, Torloni H: Histological typing of soft tissue tumours. In *International histological classification of tumors*, No. 3, Geneva, 1969, World Health Organization.

54. Enzinger FM, Shiraki M: Alveolar rhabdomyosarcoma: an analysis of 110 cases. *Cancer* 24:18, 1969.

55. Erlandson RA: Cytoskeletal proteins, including myofilaments in human tumors. *Ultrastruct Pathol* 13:155, 1989.

56. Erlandson RA: The ultrastructural distinction between rhabdomyosarcoma and other undifferentiated sarcomas. *Ultrastruct Pathol* 11:83, 1987.

57. Eusebi V, Bondi A, Rosai J: Immunohistochemical localization of myoglobin in nonmuscular cells. *Am J Surg Pathol* 8:51, 1984.

58. Eusebi V, Cecarelli C, Gorca L, et al: Immunocytochemistry of rhabdomyosarcoma: the use of four different markers. *Am J Surg Pathol* 10:293, 1986.

59. Eusebi V, Rilke F, Ceccarelli C, et al: Fetal heavy chain skeletal myosin: an oncofetal antigen expressed by rhabdomyosarcoma. *Am J Surg Pathol* 10:680, 1986.

60. Exelby PR, Ghavimi F, Jereb B: Genitourinary rhabdomyosarcoma in children. *J Pediatr Surg* 13:746, 1978.

61. Fitzmaurice RJ, Johnson PR, Yin JA, et al: Rhabdomyosarcoma presenting as "acute leukaemia." *Histopathology* 18:173, 1991.

62. Flamant F, Hill C: The improvement in survival associated with combined chemotherapy in childhood rhabdomyosarcoma: a historical comparison of 345 patients in the same center. *Cancer* 53:2417, 1984.

63. Flamant F, Rodary C, Voute PA, et al: Primary chemotherapy in the treatment of rhabdomyosarcoma in children: trial of international society of pediatric oncology (SIOP) preliminary results. *Radiother Oncol* 3:227, 1985.

64. Fleming ID, Etcubanas E, Patterson R, et al: The role of surgical resection combined with chemotherapy and radiation in the management of pelvic rhabdomyosarcoma. *Ann Surg* 199:509, 1984.

65. Fu YS, Perzin KH: Nonepithelial tumors of the nasal cavity, paranasal sinuses, and nasopharynx: a clinicopathological study. V. Skeletal muscle tumors (rhabdomyoma and rhabdomyosarcoma). *Cancer* 37:364, 1976.

66. Gaffney EF, Dervan PA, Fletcher CD: Pleomorphic rhabdomyosarcoma in adulthood: analysis of 11 cases with definition of diagnostic criteria. *Am J Surg Pathol* 17:601, 1993.

67. Gaiger AM, Soule EH, Hewton WA Jr, et al: Pathology of rhabdomyosarcoma: experience of the Intergroup Rhabdomyosarcoma Study, 1972-1978. *Natl Cancer Inst Monogr* 56:19, 1981.

68. Gerson JM, Jaffe, N, Donaldson M, et al: Meningeal seeding from rhabdomyosarcoma of the head and neck with base of the skull invasion: recognition of the clinical evolution and suggestions for management. *Med Pediatr Oncol* 5:137, 1978.

69. Ghavimi F, Mandell LR, Heller G, et al: Prognosis in childhood rhabdomyosarcoma of the extremity. *Cancer* 64:2233, 1989.

70. Glasunow M: Ueber unreife, begrenzt und destruierend wachsende Rhabdomyoblastome. *Frankfurt Ztschft f Path* 45:328, 1933.

71. Gonzalez-Crussi F, Black-Schaffer S: Rhabdomyosarcoma of infancy and childhood: problems of morphologic classification. *Am J Surg Pathol* 3:157, 1979.

72. Gonzalez-Crussi F, Goldschmidt RA, Hsueh W, et al: Infantile sarcoma with intracytoplasmic filamentous inclusions. *Cancer* 49:2365, 1982.

73. Gulati SM, Sharma RC, Iyengar B, et al: Rhabdomyosarcoma of the spermatic cord. *Indian J Cancer* 15:81, 1978.

74. Harms D, Schmidt D, Treuner J: Soft tissue sarcomas in childhood: a study of 262 cases including 169 cases of rhabdomyosarcoma. *Z Kinderchir* 40:140, 1985.

75. Hart W, Craig JR: Rhabdomyosarcomas of the uterus. *Am J Clin Pathol* 70:217, 1978.

76. Hawkins HK, Cancho-Velasquez JV: Rhabdomyosarcoma in children: correlation of form and prognosis in one institution's experience. *Am J Surg Pathol* 11:531, 1987.

77. Hayashi K, Ohtsuki Y, Takahashi K, et al: Congenital alveolar rhabdomyosarcoma with multiple skin metastases: report of a case. *Acta Pathol Jpn* 38:241, 1988.

78. Hays DM: New approach to the surgical management of rhabdomyosarcoma in childhood. *Chir Pediatr* 31:197, 1990.

79. Hays DM: Pelvic rhabdomyosarcomas in childhood: diagnosis and concepts of management reviewed. *Cancer* 45:1810, 1980.

80. Hays DM: Rhabdomyosarcoma. *Clin Orthop* 289:36, 1993.

81. Hays DM, Newton W Jr, Soule EH, et al: Mortality among children with rhabdomyosarcomas of alveolar histologic subtype. *J Pediatr Surg* 18:412, 1983.

82. Hays DM, Shimada H, Raney RB Jr, et al: Clinical staging and treatment results in rhabdomyosarcoma of the female genital tract among children and adolescents. *Cancer* 61:1893, 1988.

83. Heney D, Lockwood L, Alliabone EB, et al: Nasopharyngeal rhabdomyosarcoma and multiple lentigines syndrome: a case report. *Med Pediatr Oncol* 20:227, 1992.

84. Hensley MF, Cangir A, Culbert SJ: Acute granulocytic leukemia following successful treatment of rhabdomyosarcoma. *Am J Dis Child* 131:1417, 1977.

85. Heyn R, Beltangady M, Hays D, et al: Results of intensive therapy in children with localized alveolar extremity rhabdomyosarcoma: a report from the Intergroup Rhabdomyosarcoma Study. *J Clin Oncol* 7:200, 1989.

86. Heyn R, Haeberlen V, Newton WA, et al: Second malignant neoplasm in children treated for rhabdomyosarcoma: Intergroup Rhabdomyosarcoma Study Committee. *J Clin Oncol* 11:262, 1993.

87. Heyn R, Ragab A, Raney RB, et al: Late effects of therapy in orbital rhabdomyosarcoma in children: a report from the Intergroup Rhabdomyosarcoma Study. *Cancer* 57:1738, 1986.

88. Himmell S, Siegel H: Congenital embryonal orbital rhabdomyosarcoma in a newborn. *Arch Ophthalmol* 77:662, 1967.

89. Horn RC, Enterline HT: Rhabdomyosarcoma: a clinicopathological study of 39 cases. *Cancer* 11:181, 1958.

90. Horvat BL, Caines M, Fisher ER: The ultrastructure of rhabdomyosarcoma. *Am J Clin Pathol* 53:555, 1970.

91. Howard GM, Casten VG: Rhabdomyosarcoma of the orbit in brothers. *Arch Ophthalmol* 70:319, 1963.

92. Huang CJ: Rhabdomyosarcoma involving the genitourinary organs, retroperitoneum, and pelvis. *J Pediatr Surg* 21:101, 1986.

93. Isaacson C: Embryonal rhabdomyosarcoma of the ampulla of Vater. *Cancer* 41:365, 1978.

94. Jaffe BF, Fox JE, Batsakis JG: Rhabdomyosarcoma of the middle ear and mastoid. *Cancer* 27:29, 1971.

95. Jaffe N, Filler RM, Farber S, et al: Rhabdomyosarcoma in children. improved outlook with a multidisciplinary approach. *Am J Surg* 125:482, 1973.

96. Jones IS, Reese AB, Krout J: Orbital rhabdomyosarcoma: an analysis of 62 cases. *Trans Am Ophthalmol Soc* 63:223, 1965.

97. Joshtri DP, Wessely Z, Seery WH, et al: Rhabdomyosarcoma of the bladder in an adult: case report and review of the literature. *J Urol* 96:214, 1966.

98. Kahn HJ, Yeger H, Kassim O, et al: Immunohistochemical and electron microscopic assessment of childhood rhabdomyosarcoma: increased frequency of diagnosis over routine histologic methods. *Cancer* 51:1897, 1983.

99. Kamat MR, Kulkarni JN, Tongaonkar HB, et al: Rhabdomyosarcoma of the bladder and prostate in children. *J Surg Oncol* 48:180, 1991.

100. Kaplinsky C, Frisch A, Cohen IJ, et al: T-cell acute lymphoblastic leukemia following therapy of rhabdomyosarcoma. *Med Pediatr Oncol* 20:229, 1992.

101. Kastendieck H, Bocker W, Husselmann H: Zur Ultrastruktur und formalen Pathogenese des embryonalen Rhabdomyosarkoms. *Z Krebsforsch* 86:55, 1976.

102. Katenkamp D, Stiller D, Kuttner K, et al: Untersuchungen zur submikroskopischen Zytologie botyroider (Rhabdomyo-) Sarkome des Nasenrachens. *Zentralbl Allg Pathol* 123:508, 1979.

103. Kawamoto EH, Weidner N, Agostini RM Jr, et al: Malignant ectomesenchymoma of soft tissue: report of two cases and review of the literature. *Cancer* 59:1791, 1987.

104. Kindblom L-G, Seidal T, Karlsson K: Immunohistochemical localization of myoglobin in human muscle tissue and embryonal and alveolar rhabdomyosarcoma. *Acta Pathol Microbiol Immunol Scand* 90A:167, 1982.

105. Kirk RC, Zimmerman LE: Rhabdomyosarcoma of the orbit in a survivor of rhabdomyosarcoma of the kidney. *Arch Ophthalmol* 81:559, 1969.

106. Kodet R: Rhabdomyosarcoma in childhood: an immunohistochemical analysis with myoglobin, desmin, and vimentin. *Pathol Res Pract* 185:207, 1989.

107. Kodet R, Newton WA Jr, Hamoudi AB, et al: Childhood rhabdomyosarcoma with anaplastic (pleomorphic) features: a report of the Intergroup Rhabdomyosarcoma Study. *Am J Surg Pathol* 17:443, 1993.

108. Kodet R, Newton WA Jr, Sachs N, et al: Rhabdoid tumors of soft tissues: a clinicopathologic study of 26 cases enrolled on the Intergroup Rhabdomyosarcoma Study. *Hum Pathol* 22:674, 1991.

109. Kowal-Vern A, Gonzalez-Crussi F, Turner J, et al: Flow and image cytometric DNA analysis in rhabdomyosarcoma. *Cancer Res* 50:6023, 1990.

110. LaQuaglia MP, Ghavimi F, Heller G, et al: Mortality in pediatric paratesticular rhabdomyosarcoma: a multivariate analysis. *J Urol* 142:473, 1989.

111. LaQuaglia MP, Ghavimi F, Penenberg D, et al: Factors predictive of mortality in pediatric extremity rhabdomyosarcoma. *J Pediatr Surg* 25:238, 1990.

112. Lawrence W, Gehan EA, Hays DM, et al: Prognostic significance of staging factors of the UICC staging system in childhood rhabdomyosarcoma: a report from the Intergroup Rhabdomyosarcoma Study (IRS-II). *J Clin Oncol* 5:46, 1987.

113. Leuschner I, Newton WA Jr, Schmidt D, et al: Spindle cell variants of embryonal rhabdomyosarcoma in the paratesticular region: a report of the Intergroup Rhabdomyosarcoma Study. *Am J Surg Pathol* 17:221, 1993.

114. Levene M: Congenital retinoblastoma and sarcoma botryoides of the vagina: report of a case. *Cancer* 13:532, 1960.

115. Li FP, Fraumeni JF Jr: Rhabdomyosarcoma in children: epidemiologic study and identification of a familial cancer syndrome. *J Natl Cancer Inst* 43:1365, 1969.

116. Liebert PS, Stool SE: Rhabdomyosarcoma of the tongue in an infant. *Ann Surg* 178:621, 1973.

117. Linscheid RL, Soule EH, Henderson ED: Pleomorphic rhabdomyosarcomata of the extremities and limb girdles. A clinicopathological study. *J Bone Joint Surg* 47A:715, 1965.

118. Lloyd RV, Hajdu SI, Knapper WH: Embryonal rhabdomyosarcoma in adults. *Cancer* 51:557, 1983.

119. Lollini PL, De Giovanni C, Del Re B, et al: Myogenic differentiation of human rhabdomyosarcoma cells induced in vitro by antineoplastic drugs. *Cancer Res* 49:3631, 1989.

120. Lundgren L, Angervall L, Stenman G, et al: Infantile rhabdomyofibrosarcoma: a high grade sarcoma distinguishable from infantile fibrosarcoma and rhabdomyosarcoma. *Hum Pathol* 24:785, 1993.

121. Mahour GH, Soule EH, Mills SD, et al: Rhabdomyosarcoma in infants and children: a clinicopathological study of 75 cases. *J Pediatr Surg* 2:402, 1967.

122. Majmudar B, Kumar VS: Embryonal rhabdomyosarcoma (sarcoma botryoides) of the common bile duct. *Hum Pathol* 7:705, 1976.

123. Makishima K, Iwasaki H, Horie A: Alveolar rhabdomyosarcoma of the ethmoid sinus. *Laryngoscope* 85:400, 1975.

124. Malek RS, Kelalis PP: Paratesticular rhabdomyosarcoma in childhood. *J Urol* 118:450, 1977.

125. Marchand F: Ueber eine Geschwulst aus quergestreiften Muskelfasern mit ungewöhnlichem Gehalte an Glykogen nebst Bemerkungen ueber das Glycogen in einigen fötalen Geweben. *Virchows Arch (Pathol Anat)* 100:42, 1885.

126. Martin GE, Alexander WA: Case of rhabdomyosarcoma of soft palate. *J Laryngol* 39:312, 1924.

127. Masson JK, Soule EH: Embryonal rhabdomyosarcoma of the head and neck: report of 88 cases. *Am J Surg* 110:585, 1965.

128. Maurer HM, Beltangady M, Gehan EA, et al: The Intergroup Rhabdomyosarcoma Study I: a final report. *Cancer* 61:209, 1988.

129. Maurer HM, Gehan EA, Beltangady M, et al: The Intergroup Rhabdomyosarcoma Study II. *Cancer* 71:1904, 1993.

130. Mayer L: Quergestreifte Muskelfasern inmitten einer Augenhöhlengeschwulst. *Virchows Arch (Pathol Anat)* 37:417, 1866.

131. Mierau GW, Favara BE: Rhabdomyosarcoma in children: ultrastructural study of 31 cases. *Cancer* 46:2035, 1980.

132. Miettinen M: Rhabdomyosarcoma in patients older than 40 years of age. *Cancer* 62:2060, 1988.

133. Miettinen M, Lehto V-P, Badley RA, et al: Alveolar rhabdomyosarcoma: demonstration of the muscle type of intermediate filament protein, desmin, as a diagnostic aid. *Am J Pathol* 108:246, 1982.

134. Miettinen M, Rapola J: Immunohistochemical spectrum of rhabdomyosarcoma and rhabdomyosarcoma-like tumors: expression of cytokeratin and the 68-kd neurofilament protein. *Am J Surg Pathol* 13:120, 1989.

135. Molenaar WM, Dam-Meiring A, Kamps WA, et al: DNA-aneuploidy in rhabdomyosarcomas compared with other sarcomas of childhood and adolescence. *Hum Pathol* 19:573, 1988.

136. Molenaar WM, Oosterhuis AM, Ramaekers FCS: The rarity of rhabdomyosarcomas in the adult: a morphologic and immunohistochemical study. *Pathol Res Pract* 180:400, 1985.

137. Molenaar WM, Oosterhuis JW, Kamps WA: Cytological "differentiation" in childhood rhabdomyosarcoma following polychemotherapy. *Hum Pathol* 15:973, 1984.

138. Molenaar WM, Oosterhuis JW, Oosterhuis AM, et al: Mesenchymal and muscle-specific intermediate filaments (vimentin and desmin) in relation to differentiation in childhood rhabdomyosarcoma. *Hum Pathol* 16:838, 1985.

139. Morales AR, Fine G, Horn RC Jr: Rhabdomyosarcoma: an ultrastructural appraisal. *Pathol Annu* 7:81, 1972.

140. Mostofi FK, Morse WH: Polypoid rhabdomyosarcoma (sarcoma botryoides) of bladder in children. *J Urol* 67:681, 1952.

141. Mukai K, Rosai J, Hallaway BE: Localization of myoglobin in normal and neoplastic human skeletal muscle cells using an immunoperoxidase method. *Am J Surg Pathol* 3:373, 1979.

142. Mukai K, Schollmeyer J, Rosai J: Immunohistochemical localization of actin: applications in surgical pathology. *Am J Surg Pathol* 5:91, 1981.

143. Mukai M, Iri H, Torikata C, et al: Immunoperoxidase demonstration of a new muscle protein (Z-protein) in myogenic tumors as a diagnostic aid. *Am J Pathol* 114:164, 1984.

144. Nagaraj HS, Kmetz DR, Leitner C: Rhabdomyosarcoma of the bile ducts. *J Pediatr Surg* 12:1071, 1977.

145. Newton WA Jr, Soule EH, Hamoudi AB, et al: Histopathology of childhood sarcomas, Intergroup Rhabdomyosarcoma Studies I and II: clinicopathologic correlation. *J Clin Oncol* 6:67, 1988.

146. Norris HJ, Taylor HB: Polyps of the vagina: a benign lesion resembling sarcoma botryoides. *Cancer* 19:227, 1966.

147. O'Day RA, Soule EH, Gores RJ: Embryonal rhabdomyosarcoma of the oral soft tissues. *Oral Surg Oral Med Oral Pathol* 20:85, 1965.

148. Olegard C, Mandahl N, Heim S, et al: Embryonal rhabdomyosarcoma with 100 chromosomes but no structural aberrations. *Cancer Genet Cytogenet* 60:198, 1992.

149. Osborn M, Hill C, Altmannsberger M, et al: Monoclonal antibodies to titin in conjunction with antibodies to desmin separate rhabdomyosarcomas from other tumor types. *Lab Invest* 55:101, 1986.

150. Östör AG, Fortune DW, Riley CB: Fibroepithelial polyps with atypical stromal cells (pseudosarcoma botryoides) of vulva and vagina: a report of 13 cases. *Int J Gynecol Pathol* 7:351, 1988.

151. Overbeck L. Elektronenmikroskopische Untersuchungen des embryonalen Rhabdomyosarkoms. *Frankf Ztschrft f Pathol* 77:49, 1967.

152. Pack GT, Eberhart WF: Rhabdomyosarcoma of skeletal muscle: report of 100 cases. *Surgery* 32:1023, 1952.

153. Parham DM, Webber B, Holt H, et al: Immunohistochemical study of childhood rhabdomyosarcomas and related neoplasms: results of an Intergroup Rhabdomyosarcoma Study project. *Cancer* 67:3072, 1991.

154. Patton RB, Horn RC Jr: Rhabdomyosarcoma: clinical and pathological features and comparison with human fetal and embryonal skeletal muscle. *Surgery* 52:572, 1962.

155. Pieterse HF: Sarcoma botryoides and vesical bilharziasis. *S Afr Med J* 47:2148, 1973.

156. Porterfield JF, Zimmerman LE: Rhabdomyosarcoma of the orbit: a clinicopathologic study of 55 cases. *Virchows Arch (Pathol Anat)* 335:329, 1962.

157. Potenza AD, Winslow DJ: Rhabdomyosarcoma of the hand. *J Bone Joint Surg* 43A:700, 1961.

158. Potter GD: Embryonal rhabdomyosarcoma of the middle ear in children. *Cancer* 19:221, 1966.

159. Pratt CB, Hustu HO, Kumar APM, et al: Treatment of childhood rhabdomyosarcoma at St. Jude Children's Research Hospital 1962-1978. *Natl Cancer Inst Monogr* 56:93, 1981.

160. Ragab AH, Heyn R, Tefft M, et al: Infants younger than 1 year of age with rhabdomyosarcoma. *Cancer* 58:2606, 1986.

161. Raney RB: Spinal cord "drop metastases" from head and neck rhabdomyosarcoma: proceedings of the tumor board of the Children's Hospital of Philadelphia. *Med Pediatr Oncol* 4:3, 1978.

162. Raney RB Jr, Crist W, Hays D, et al: Soft tissue sarcoma of the perineal region in childhood: a report from the Intergroup Rhabdomyosarcoma Studies I and II, 1972 through 1984. *Cancer* 65:2787, 1990.

163. Raney RB Jr, Crist WM, Maurer HM, et al: Prognosis of children with soft tissue sarcoma who relapse after achieving a complete response: a report from the Intergroup Rhabdomyosarcoma Study I. *Cancer* 52:44, 1983.

164. Raney RB Jr, Gehan EA, Hays DM, et al: Primary chemotherapy with and without radiation therapy and/or surgery for children with localized sarcoma of the bladder, prostate, vagina, uterus, and cervix: a comparison of the results in Intergroup Rhabdomyosarcoma Studies I and II. *Cancer* 66:2072, 1990.

165. Raney RB Jr, Hays DM, Lawrence W Jr, et al: Paratesticular rhabdomyosarcoma in childhood. *Cancer* 42:729, 1978.

166. Raney RB Jr, Heyn R, Hays DM, et al: Sequelae of treatment in 109 patients followed for 5 to 15 years after diagnosis of sarcoma of the bladder and prostate: a report of the Intergroup Rhabdomyosarcoma Study Committee. *Cancer* 71:2387, 1993.

167. Raney RB Jr, Tefft M, Lawrence W, et al: Paratesticular sarcoma in childhood and adolescence. *Cancer* 60:2337, 1987.

168. Raney RB Jr, Tefft M, Maurer HM, et al: Disease pattern and survival rate in children with metastatic soft-tissue sarcoma: a report from the Intergroup Rhabdomyosarcoma Study (IRS) I. *Cancer* 62:1257, 1988.

169. Raney RB Jr, Tefft M, Newton WA, et al: Improved prognosis with intensive treatment of children with cranial soft tissue sarcomas arising in nonorbital parameningeal sites. *Cancer* 59:147, 1987.

170. Rangdaeng S, Truong LD: Comparative immunohistochemical staining for desmin and muscle specific actin: a study of 576 cases. *Am J Clin Pathol* 96:32, 1991.

171. Ransom JL, Pratt CB, Hustu HO, et al: Retroperitoneal rhabdomyosarcoma in children: results of multimodality therapy. *Cancer* 45:845, 1980.

172. Ransom JL, Pratt CB, Shanks E: Childhood rhabdomyosarcoma of the extremity: results of combined modality therapy. *Cancer* 40:2810, 1977.

173. Reboul-Marty J, Quintana E, Mosseri V, et al: Prognostic factors of alveolar rhabdomyosarcoma in childhood: an International Society of Pediatric Oncology Study. *Cancer* 68:493, 1991.

174. Riopelle JL, Thériault JP: Sur une forme méconnue de sarcome des

parties molles: Le rhabdomyosarcome alvéolaire. *Ann Anat Pathol (Paris)* 1:88, 1956.

175. Rodary C, Flamant F, Donaldson SS: An attempt to use a common staging system in rhabdomyosarcoma: a report of an international workshop initiated by the International Society of Pediatric Oncology (SIOP). *Med Pediatr Oncol* 17:210, 1989.

176. Rodriguez LA, Ziskind J: Rhabdomyosarcoma of larynx. *Laryngoscope* 80:1733, 1970.

177. Roholl PJM, Elbers HR, Prinsen I, et al: Distribution of actin isoforms in sarcomas: an immunohistochemical study. *Hum Pathol* 21:1269, 1990.

178. Rokitansky K: Ein aus quergestreiften Muskelfasern constituirtes Aftergebilde. *Z Wiener Aerzte*, 1849.

179. Royds JA, Variend S, Timperley WR, et al: An investigation of beta enolase as a histologic marker of rhabdomyosarcoma. *J Clin Pathol* 37:905, 1984.

180. Russell WO, Cohen HJ, Enzinger FM, et al: A clinical and pathological staging system for soft tissue sarcomas. *Cancer* 40:1562, 1977.

181. Ruymann FB, Maddux HR, Ragab A, et al: Congenital anomalies associated with rhabdomyosarcoma: an autopsy study of 115 cases: a report from the Intergroup Rhabdomyosarcoma Study Group. *Med Pediatr Oncol* 16:33, 1988.

182. Ruymann FB, Raney B, Crist WM, et al: Rhabdomyosarcoma of the biliary tree in childhood: a report from the Intergroup Rhabdomyosarcoma Study. *Cancer* 56:575, 1985.

183. Schmidt D, Reimann O, Treuner J, et al: Cellular differentiation and prognosis in embryonal rhabdomyosarcoma: a report from the Cooperative Soft Tissue Sarcoma Study 1981 (CWS 81). *Virchows Arch (Pathol Anat)* 409:183, 1986.

184. Schmidt RA, Cone R, Haas JE, et al: Diagnosis of rhabdomyosarcomas with HHF35, a monoclonal antibody directed against muscle actins. *Am J Pathol* 131:19, 1988.

185. Scupham R, Gilbert EF, Wilde J, et al: Immunohistochemical studies of rhabdomyosarcoma. *Arch Pathol Lab Med* 110:818, 1986.

186. Seidal T: Rhabdomyosarcoma: Definition and diagnosis, thesis. Gothenburg University, Gothenburg, Sweden, 1988, Department Pathology II.

187. Seidal T, Kindblom LG: The ultrastructure of alveolar and embryonal rhabdomyosarcoma: a correlative and electron microscopic study of 17 cases. *Acta Pathol Microbiol Immunol Scand* 92A:231, 1984.

188. Seidal T, Kindblom LG, Angervall L: Myoglobin, desmin, and vimentin in ultrastructurally proven rhabdomyomas and rhabdomyosarcomas: an immunohistochemical study utilizing a series of monoclonal and polyclonal antibodies. *Appl Pathol* 5:201, 1987.

189. Seidal T, Kindblom LG, Angervall L: Rhabdomyosarcoma in middle-aged and elderly individuals. *APMIS* 97:236, 1989.

190. Semerdjian HS, Texter JH, Yawn DH: Rhabdomyosarcoma occurring in repaired exstrophied bladder: a case report. *J Urol* 108:354, 1972.

191. Shapiro DN, Parham DM, Douglass EC, et al: Relationship of tumor cell ploidy to histologic subtype and treatment outcome in children and adolescents with unresectable rhabdomyosarcoma. *J Clin Oncol* 9:159, 1991.

192. Shapiro DN, Valentine MB, Sublett JE, et al: Chromosomal sublocalization of the 2;13 translocation breakpoint in alveolar rhabdomyosarcoma. *Genes Chromosom Cancer* 4:241, 1992.

193. Sharp WC Jr, Helwig EB: Sarcoma botryoides (embryonal rhabdomyosarcoma) of the anus. *J Dis Child* 97:845, 1959.

194. Shimada H, Newton WA, Soule EH, et al: Pathology of fatal rhabdomyosarcoma: report of Intergroup Rhabdomyosarcoma Study (IRS-I and IRS-III). *Cancer* 59:459, 1987.

195. Shuman R: Mesenchymal tumors. In Anderson WAD: *Pathology*, ed 4, St. Louis, 1961, CV Mosby.

196. Smith MT, Armbrustmacher VM, Violett TW: Diffuse meningeal rhabdomyosarcoma. *Cancer* 47:2081, 1981.

197. Sotello-Avila C, Gonzales-Crussi F, de Mello D, et al: Renal and extrarenal rhabdoid tumors in children: a clinicopathologic study of 14 patients. *Semin Diagn Pathol* 3:151, 1986.

198. Soule EH, Geitz M, Henderson ED: Embryonal rhabdomyosarcomas of the limbs and limb-girdles: a clinicopathologic study of 61 cases. *Cancer* 23:1336, 1969.

199. Srouji MN, Donaldson MH, Chatten J, et al: Perianal rhabdomyosarcoma in childhood. *Cancer* 38:1008, 1976.

200. Stobbe GD, Dargeon HW: Embryonal rhabdomyosarcoma of head and neck in children and adolescents. *Cancer* 3:826, 1950.

201. Stout AP: Rhabdomyosarcoma of the skeletal muscles. *Ann Surg* 123:447, 1946.

202. Stout AP, Lattes R: Tumors of the soft tissues. In *Atlas of tumor pathology*, 1966, Armed Forces Institute of Pathology, second series, fascicle 1, Washington, DC.

203. Suit HD, Russell WO, Martin RG: Management of patients with sarcoma of soft tissue in an extremity. *Cancer* 31:1247, 1973.

204. Sulser H: Das Rhabdomyosarkom: Alters- und Geschlechtsverteilung, Lokalisation, pathologische Anatomie und Prognose. *Virchows Arch (Pathol Anat)* 379:35, 1978.

205. Sutow WW, Lindberg RD, Gehan EA, et al: Three-year relapse-free survival rates in childhood rhabdomyosarcoma of the head and neck: report from the Intergroup Rhabdomyosarcoma Study. *Cancer* 49:2217, 1982.

206. Talerman A: Sarcoma botryoides presenting as a polyp on the labium majus. *Cancer* 32:994, 1973.

207. Tefft M, Fernandez C, Donaldson M, et al: Incidence of meningeal involvement by rhabdomyosarcoma of the head and neck in children: a report of the Intergroup Rhabdomyosarcoma Study (IRS). *Cancer* 42:253, 1978.

208. Tefft M, Fernandez CH, Moon TE: Rhabdomyosarcoma: response with chemotherapy prior to radiation in patients with gross residual disease. *Cancer* 39:665, 1977.

209. Timmons JW Jr, Burgert EO Jr, Soule EH, et al: Embryonal rhabdomyosarcoma of the bladder and prostate in childhood. *J Urol* 113:694, 1975.

210. Toker C: Embryonal rhabdomyosarcoma, an ultrastructural study. *Cancer* 21:1164, 1968.

211. Trent J, Casper J, Meltzer P, et al: Nonrandom chromosome alterations in rhabdomyosarcoma. *Cancer Genet Cytogenet* 16:189, 1985.

212. Tsokos M, Howard R, Costa J: Immunohistochemical study of alveolar and embryonal rhabdomyosarcoma. *Lab Invest* 48:148, 1983.

213. Tsokos M, Webber BL, Parham DM, et al: Rhabdomyosarcoma: a new classification scheme related to prognosis. *Arch Pathol Lab Med* 116:847, 1992.

214. Tsuneyoshi M, Daimaru Y, Hashimoto H, et al: Malignant soft tissue neoplasms with the histologic features of renal rhabdoid tumors: an ultrastructural and immunohistochemical study. *Hum Pathol* 16:1235, 1985.

215. Valentine M, Douglass EC, Look AT: Closely linked loci on the long arm of chromosome 13 flank a specific 2;13 translocation breakpoint in childhood rhabdomyosarcoma. *Cytogenet Cell Genet* 52:128, 1989.

216. Walker WF, McCameron HD: Rhabdomyosarcoma of the epididymis. *Br J Surg* 49:319, 1961-1962.

217. Weichert KA, Bove KC, Aron BS, et al: Rhabdomyosarcoma in children: a clinicopathologic study of 35 patients. *Am J Clin Pathol* 66:692, 1976.

218. White A, Verma PL, Bullimore J: Rhabdomyosarcoma of the nasopharynx. *J Laryngol* 88:271, 1974.

219. Wiatrak BJ, Pensak ML: Rhabdomyosarcoma of the ear and temporal bone. *Laryngoscope* 99:1188, 1989.

220. Young JL, Miller RW: Incidence of malignant tumors in U.S. children. *J Pediatr* 86:254, 1975.

221. Zenker K: Ein Fall von Rhabdomyosarcom der Orbita. *Virchows Arch (Pathol Anat)* 120:536, 1890.

CHAPTER 23

BENIGN TUMORS AND TUMORLIKE LESIONS OF BLOOD VESSELS

Hemangiomas are benign neoplasms that closely resemble normal vessels. So faithfully is this facsimile produced that it is difficult to distinguish clearly among neoplasm, hamartoma, and vessel malformation. Although most diagnostic problems center on this issue, there are no completely reliable guidelines for making this distinction. Stout[9] implied this distinction could be made histologically when he stated that a vascular tumor, in contrast to a hamartoma, contained a greater complement of endothelial cells than was necessary to line its lumina. By this definition certain locally aggressive but well-differentiated vascular lesions (e.g., angiomatosis) would be considered hamartomas, whereas reactive lesions with a surfeit of endothelial cells (e.g., papillary endothelial hyperplasia) would be considered neoplastic. Others have suggested that classification can be made on the basis of the clinical presentation, contending that those present at birth or those appearing during early childhood are congenital and are, therefore, tissue malformations rather than true tumors.[158] However, it is likely that some congenital lesions may not become clinically apparent until adult life, depending on their location and rate of growth. In view of these limitations, we have made no attempt to rigorously separate hamartomas and malformations from benign neoplasms and have for purposes of discussion considered most benign vascular lesions encountered by the surgical pathologist as hemangiomas. Thus we have defined *hemangioma* in the broadest sense of the word as a benign but nonreactive process in which there is an increased number of normal or abnormal-appearing vessels. It will be obvious to most, however, that lesions such as the arteriovenous hemangioma could just as appropriately be considered malformations.

Hemangiomas may be of two general types: those which are more or less localized to one area and those which involve large segments of the body such as an entire extremity. The latter type, known as *angiomatosis*, deserves specific mention because of the inherent problems it poses in diagnosis and therapy. Localized hemangiomas, however, are far more common and account for most of the vascular tumors encountered in daily practice. They have been classified in the literature according to clinical, radiographic, and pathological criteria, although no one system is entirely satisfactory. Of necessity the classification of hemangiomas in this chapter is based primarily on pathological changes; we have indicated the clinical and radiological features when appropriate. Moreover, certain conditions such as granuloma pyogenicum and angiolymphoid hyperplasia (epithelioid hemangioma), which in the past have been variably classified as reactions and tumors, are considered benign neoplasms.

NORMAL STRUCTURE AND FUNCTION

The vasculature is divided into arterial and venous components joined by a network of capillaries. The arteries represent a system of dichotomously branching conduits that serve to regulate pressure and deliver blood to the capillary bed, while the thin-walled veins return blood to the heart under lower pressures. The capillaries along with the terminal venules are the principal sites of gas exchange. Larger venules (postcapillary venules) are sensitive to vasoactive amines; hence, they represent the most permeable portions of the vascular tree. During the inflammatory response there is morphological evidence that the venous endothelium[22,23] actively contracts to form intercellular spaces that allow the egress of cells and fluid.

In addition to its traditional role as a lining and barrier cell of the vascular system, the endothelium engages in a variety of synthetic functions and is finely tuned to respond to a number of chemicals, properties discovered as a result of the ability to culture endothelial cells in vitro.[24] Its functions and phenotype are dependent on the tissue, local microenvironment, and activation by cytokines. For example, the surface expression of major histocompatibility antigens can be induced on endothelial cells by cytokines. Basic properties of endothelial metabolism include its ability to transport macromolecules through its system of pinocytotic vesicles, its receptor-mediated uptake of low-density lipoproteins, and its uptake of sugars and amino acids. It also synthesizes and maintains the integrity of its basement membrane of collagen, fibronectin, and laminin. Endothelium possesses both procoagulant and anticoagulant properties. It synthesizes factor VIII–associated antigen (von Willebrand factor), one of the two components of the factor VIII complex,[19] factor V, and plasminogen activator. Thrombomodulin, a surface endothelial protein, indirectly promotes the proteolysis of factors V and VIII. When appropriately stimulated, endothelial cells produce prostacyclin, a potent inhibitor of platelet aggregation and a vasodilator. By virtue of its interactions with various mediators, the endothelium, particularly of the microcirculation, is an important regulator of vascular tone and permeability. Angiotensin-converting enzyme and endothelin, a potent vasoconstrictor, are manufactured by endothelium. Finally, endothelium participates in the overall functioning of the immune system and through its cellular adhesive properties determines the ability of circulating cells to leave the vascular compartment in response to various stimuli. Lymphocytes possess "homing receptors," which are "recognized" by specific molecules (addressins) on the endothelial cell membranes. In response to inflammatory mediators such as interleukin 1, the endothelium acquires adhesive surface proteins. The endothelial leukocyte adhesion molecule 1 permits interleukin 1-stimulated adhesion of neutrophils to endothelium. The intracellular adhesion molecule 1 facilitates adhesion of lymphocytes, neutrophils, and monocytes.

The vascular system develops during the third week of fetal life from mesodermal cells of the "blood islands." Although initially located in the region of the yolk sac, these cells eventually populate the mesenchyme throughout the fetus; the peripheral cells of the islands give rise to endothelial tubes, and the central cells give rise to the hematopoietic elements.[31] As the endothelial tubes develop, they freely anastomose with each other, forming a network that roughly follows the predetermined path of major vessels. The tubes acquire an investiture of pericytes from the surrounding mesenchyme, and in time these primitive vascular cells differentiate into the specific structures of the media and adventitia. The process of new microvessel formation (angiogenesis) is governed by the interaction of agonists and antagonists. Substances that promote angiogenesis include fibroblast growth factor, epidermal growth factor, and alpha-tumor necrosis factor, whereas hydrocortisone, protamine, gamma-interferon, beta-tumor necrosis factor, and beta-transforming growth factor retard angiogenesis. The production of angiogenic factors by normal tissues is tightly controlled, whereas tumors may produce these substances in large amounts and thus have served as a rich source for their isolation and characterization.

At the time of birth the portions of the vascular tree are fully developed as a result of selective growth and regression of the primitive vessels. The arteries in general are thick-walled structures possessing in most instances several layers of smooth muscle cells and varying amounts of elastic tissue. The largest arteries such as the aorta (elastic arteries) have a media that is extensively laced with elastic fibers, whereas the smallest arterioles possess only an internal elastic lamina that divides the intima from the media.

The capillaries represent the smallest vessels, but it is often difficult to determine morphologically the exact point of transition between the smallest vein (or artery) and the capillary. Indeed, the current definition of *capillary* as a vessel, the diameter of which approximates that of the normal erythrocyte (8 μm) is based not only on morphological but also physiological observations.[21] The vessels are composed of a single flattened endothelial cell surrounded by basal lamina and occasional pericytes. The basal lamina is not appreciated by light microscopy but can be inferred by the PAS-positive staining material beneath the endothelium. Although this basic pattern pertains to all capillaries, electron microscopy has demonstrated various alterations from organ to organ. For instance, continuous capillaries consisting of a continuous layer of endothelium and basal lamina are typical of capillaries in skeletal and smooth muscle. Fenestrated capillaries, possessing small pores closed by flaps or diaphragms, are found in endocrine organs, the renal glomerulus, and other sites where rapid exchange of solute material occurs.

Veins parallel the arterial system but are more numerous and appear as partially collapsed structures in tissue sections as a result of their inelasticity. In large and medium-sized veins most of the wall is composed of adventitia made up of muscle fibers and elastic tissue arranged in a less orderly fashion than in the arteries. Small veins possess no elastic tissue and have only a small investiture of smooth muscle. The smallest veins are difficult to distinguish from small arteries, and the distinction at times is best made by the topographical relationship to the capillary.

ULTRASTRUCTURE OF VASCULAR MEMBRANE

The endothelial cell has an elongated shape and measures 25 to 50 μm in length. It is covered on its luminal aspect by a fine coat of carbohydrate-rich material. This nearly imperceptible covering was at one time thought to be the morphological correlate for the nonthrombogenic property of the endothelium, although current evidence suggests that this probably is not true.[28] Beneath the fine cell coat the luminal surface is thrown into small folds or projections. Small micropinocytotic vesicles (60 to 70 nm) dot both the luminal and antiluminal surfaces of the cell and are believed important in the transport of fluid across the cell.[28] The cytoplasm usually contains a small amount of smooth and rough endoplasmic reticulum, free ribosomes, and mitochondria. A variety of filaments are present in endothelium, including thin (actin), intermediate (vimentin), and thick (myosin) filaments. Rod-shaped bodies (Weibel-Palade bodies) measuring 0.1 to 0.3 μm in length and containing an internal structure of parallel tubules are a relatively specific feature of the endothelial cell. They vary in number depending on the type of vessel, and on rare occasions they may also be found in pericytes. Factor VIII–associated antigen has been localized by means of immunoelectron microscopy to these organelles. Intercellular attachments are typically quite prominent in the endothelial cell. Arterioles possess elaborate attachments, whereas venules have less prominent ones, a feature that correlates with the observation that the venules represent preferred sites of permeability changes.

Vascular endothelium rests on a thin basal lamina (50 nm) of nonperiodic collagen, which is synthesized at least in part by the endothelial cells. In some areas in the vascular tree, the basal lamina may have a multilayered appearance. External to the endothelium but enveloped within the basal lamina are the pericytes. These mesenchymal cells have few distinguishing features apart from their branched processes, their close contacts with the endothelial cell, and their investiture by basal lamina. These cells are probably derived from fibroblasts of the surrounding connective tissue and in turn may differentiate into smooth muscle cells of the vessel wall.

HEMANGIOMAS

Hemangioma is one of the most common soft tissue tumors (7% of all benign tumors) and is the most common tumor in infancy and childhood.[60] The majority of hemangiomas are superficial lesions that have a predilection for

Table 23-1. Distribution of hemangiomas (570 cases)*

Location	No. cases
Cutaneous or mucosal hemangiomas	370
Oral cavity	80
Face	75
Arm	60
Leg	50
Scalp	46
Vulva and scrotum	5
Other	54
Liver	109
Central nervous system	43
Heart	16
Bone	12
Gastrointestinal tract, kidney, mesentery	10
Muscle	10
TOTAL	570

*Data modified from Geshickter CF, Keasbey LE: *Am J Cancer* 23:568, 1935.

the head and neck region, but they may also occur internally, notably in organs such as the liver (Table 23-1). The common capillary and cavernous hemangiomas of adults are more frequently encountered in women and may fluctuate in size with pregnancy and menarche; this suggests that the endothelial cells of these tumors may be quite responsive to circulating hormones. Although some vascular tumors regress altogether (e.g., juvenile hemangioma), most persist if untreated but possess a limited growth potential. There is no evidence that they undergo malignant transformation with any degree of regularity. Although isolated cases of this phenomenon have been reported, the early concept of "benign metastasizing hemangiomas" has generally been discredited. Such cases represent well-differentiated angiosarcomas that were improperly diagnosed at the onset (see Chapter 25).

Capillary hemangioma

Capillary hemangiomas comprise the largest single group of hemangiomas. They usually appear during the first few years of life (with the notable exception of the senile or cherry angioma) and are located in the skin or subcutaneous tissue. Typically elevated and red to purple in color, they are composed of a proliferation of capillary-sized vessels lined by flattened endothelium (Fig. 23-1). Architecturally, virtually all capillary hemangiomas are composed of nodules of small capillary-sized vessels, each of which is subserved by a "feeder" vessel. This lobular or grouped arrangement of vessels is a very helpful feature in distinguishing benign and malignant vascular proliferations.[12] The term *lobular hemangioma* has been employed as a generic designation for a number of hemangiomas characterized by this architectural pattern. They include capillary hemangioma of infancy, pyogenic granuloma, and epithelioid hemangioma. Several clinical variants of capillary hemangiomas are discussed below.

Cellular hemangioma of infancy (strawberry nevus, nevus vasculosus, hypertrophic angioma of infancy, benign hemangioendothelioma of infancy). The cellular hemangioma of infancy is an immature form of capillary hemangioma.[65-69,71,72,76-78] It occurs during infancy at a rate of about 1 in every 200 live births.[77] About one fifth of the cases are multiple. In the early stage they may resemble the common birthmark in that they are flat, red lesions that intensify in color when the infant strains or cries. With time they acquire an elevated protruding appearance that distinguishes them from birthmarks and has earned them the fanciful designation of *strawberry nevus*. Deeply situated lesions will impart little color to the overlying skin and consequently may be misdiagnosed preoperatively. These tumors may be located on any body surface but are most common in the region of the head and neck, particularly the parotid, where they seemingly follow the distribution of cutaneous nerves and arteries.

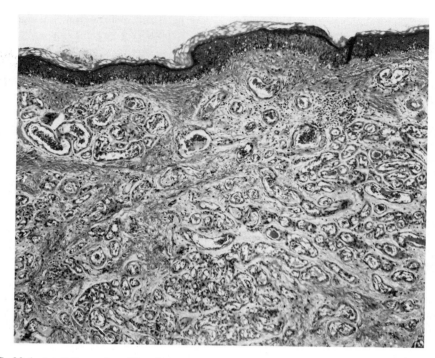

FIG. 23-1. Adult form of capillary hemangioma consisting of small vessels lined by flattened mature endothelium. (×160.)

The evolution of the lesion is quite characteristic. Although described as congenital they actually appear within a few weeks after birth[77] and rapidly enlarge over a period of several months, achieve the largest size in about 6 months, and regress over a period of a few years. Regression is usually accompanied by a fading of the lesion from scarlet to dull red-gray and by a concomitant wrinkling of the once taut skin. It has been estimated that by age 7 years, 75% to 90% have involuted, leaving a small pigmented scar. In those lesions that have ulcerated, the cosmetic defect may be more significant.

The tumors are multinodular masses that are fed by a single normally occurring arteriole.[77] Histologically, the tumor varies with its age. Early lesions are characterized by plump endothelial cells that line vascular spaces with small inconspicuous lumina (Figs. 23-2, A, and 23-3). Mitotic figures may be present in moderate numbers. Mast cells and factor XIII–positive interstitial cells are a consistent feature of these tumors. The former may be important in the production of angiogenic factors that regulate the growth of these tumors.[69] At this early stage of development the vascular nature of the tumor may not be readily apparent unless a reticulin preparation is done that demonstrates connective tissue fibers encircling the myriad of tiny vessels. As the lesions mature and blood flow through the lesion commences, the endothelium becomes flattened and resembles that seen in adult forms of capillary hemangioma (Fig.

23-2, B). Maturation usually begins at the periphery of the tumors but ultimately involves all zones. Regression of the juvenile hemangioma is accompanied by a progressive and diffuse interstitial fibrosis. In unusual cases infarction of the tumor may occur, presumably as a result of thrombosis.

Electron microscopy and immunohistochemistry can be helpful in defining the vascular nature of these tumors.[72,76] Solid nests of endothelium are surrounded by basal lamina and are encircled by a cuff of pericytes (Fig. 23-4). More mature areas, of course, display canalization of the vessels. Weibel-Palade bodies may be present but tend to be scarce in less mature areas. A peculiar crystalline structure has been identified within the endothelium of these tumors.[70,74] Measuring about 0.5 to 2 μm, they have a substructure consisting of parallel lamellar bands with a periodicity of 18 to 30 nm. Their exact significance is unknown, although it is believed that they reflect the immaturity of the endothelium, since similar structures have been noted in human fetal endothelium.

Factor VIII–associated protein can be identified within cellular hemangiomas of infancy but in our experience is often inapparent within the solid or immature-appearing areas and only becomes significant in the well-canalized portions of the tumor (Fig. 23-5).

Treatment of these lesions has to be individualized and depends on factors such as location or rate of growth. When this tumor is in the rapid growth phase, there is often a ten-

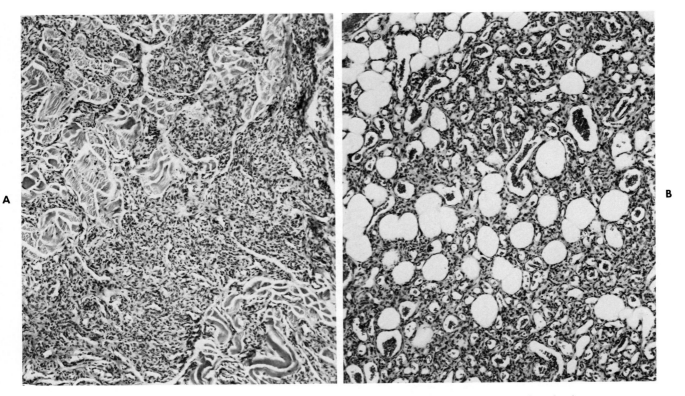

FIG. 23-2. Juvenile form of capillary hemangioma. **A,** Early cellular stage of tumor where luminal differentiation is inconspicuous. (×100.) **B,** Maturation within lesion results in appearance similar to adult form of capillary hemangioma. (×100.)

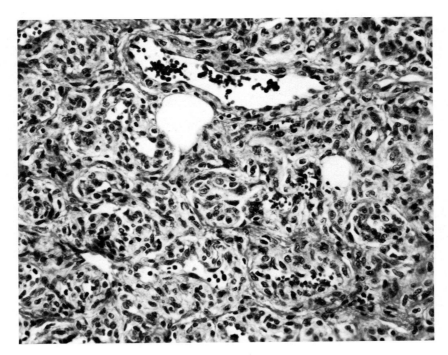

FIG. 23-3. Juvenile hemangioma showing mixture of mature and immature capillary vessels. (×160.)

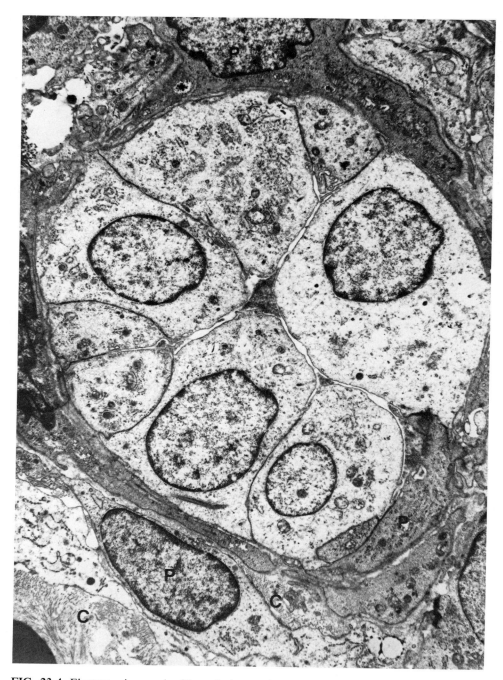

FIG. 23-4. Electron micrograph of juvenile hemangioma. Prominent endothelial cells eclipse lumen. Vessels are surrounded by basal lamina, pericytes *(P),* and collagen *(C).* (From Taxy JB, Battifora H: The electron microscope in the diagnosis of soft tissue tumors. In Trump BF, Jones RT, editors: *Diagnostic electron microscopy,* New York, 1980, John Wiley and Sons.)

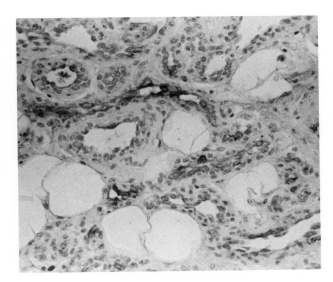

FIG. 23-5. Peroxidase-antiperoxidase stain for factor VIII-associated antigen in a cellular hemangioma of infancy. Note that immature nests of cells do not contain immunoreactive factor VIII-associated antigen, whereas mature endothelium lining canalized vessels does. (×250.)

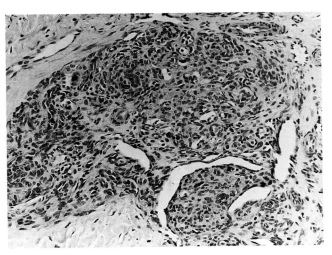

FIG. 23-6. Acquired tufted hemangioma (×100). (Reprinted from Weiss SW, Sobin LH: *WHO classification of soft tissue tumors*, Springer-Verlag, 1994.)

dency to be overzealous in therapy. It has been suggested that these lesions be approached with a policy of "masterful neglect."[44] Small lesions in inconspicuous locations can probably be ignored altogether. Rapidly enlarging lesions that threaten a vital structure (e.g., trachea) or pose cosmetic problems should be treated. Although cryosurgery, injection of sclerosing agents, and irradiation have been employed in the past as initial therapy before resorting to surgery, these methods are becoming obsolete. Systemic steroids are currently used as a means to retard or curtail growth before surgery or to obviate surgery.[44]

Acquired tufted angioma (angioblastoma of Nakagawa). First described by Wilson Jones,[63] this form of hemangioma shares many of the histological features of juvenile hemangioma.[80-83] As implied by its name, it usually occurs in an older group of patients on an acquired basis and is characterized by slowly growing erythematous macules or plaques involving the dermis of the upper portions of the body. Histologically the lesion is made up of nodules of capillary-sized vessels that grow in a "cannonball" fashion throughout the deep dermis. The capillary-sized vessels may be imperfectly canalized so as to give the impression of solid nests of endothelial cells (Fig. 23-6). At the periphery some of the vessels appear flattened or slit-like, as is somewhat reminiscent of Kaposi's sarcoma. Although this tumor is perhaps most similar in its appearance to cellular hemangioma of infancy, it is not arranged in distinct lobules but rather grows in an irregular fashion throughout the dermis. Moreover, with immunohistochemical procedures, most of the solid endothelial nests do not

express factor VIII–associated antigen although other endothelial markers can be identified, suggesting that the cells may represent a more primitive form of endothelial cell. Ultrastructurally endothelial crystalloids similar to those in capillary hemangiomas of infancy have been identified.[81] The usual course of this tumor is that of progressive spread with ultimate stabilization.

Targetoid hemosiderotic hemangioma. Targetoid hemosiderotic hemangioma is a rare vascular tumor that may have areas resembling the patch stage of Kaposi's sarcoma.[84-86] The lesion usually develops as a small violaceous papule with a surrounding ecchymotic halo; this accounts for the descriptive adjective *targetoid* in its name. Most patients are children or young adults. The superficial portion of the tumor consists of dilated ectatic vessels that expand the papillary dermis and lie beneath a hyperkeratotic epidermis. The endothelial cells lining these expanded channels are plump or hobnailed and occasionally form papillary tufts similar to those of Dabska tumor. In the deeper portion of the tumor the vessels are small and attenuated and appear to dissect through the collagen. They are in turn surrounded by collections of inflammatory cells and hemosiderin. It is the deep portions of this tumor that have been likened to the patch stage of Kaposi's sarcoma, progressive lymphangioma, or even well-differentiated angiosarcoma. However, in Kaposi's sarcoma the early vascular proliferation is virtually never surrounded by significant inflammation or hemosiderin as is seen in targetoid hemosiderotic hemangioma.

With the small number of cases and limited follow-up information regarding this tumor it is difficult to make definitive statements as to its proper place in the spectrum of vascular neoplasia. Santa Cruz and Aronberg,[85] who first described the tumor, regard this lesion as benign, based on the eight original cases they described.

Verrucous hemangioma. Verrucous hemangioma is a variant of capillary or cavernous hemangioma that undergoes a reactive hyperkeratosis of the overlying skin and consequently may be confused with a wart or keratosis.[49] The lesions begin during childhood as unilateral lesions in the dermis of the lower extremity. Grossly and histologically, they resemble conventional hemangiomas in their early stage of development. With time the overlying epidermis displays hyperkeratosis, acanthosis, and papillomatosis, features that obscure the vascular nature. These tumors have a propensity to recur locally and to develop satellite lesions if incompletely excised.

Cherry angioma (senile angioma, De Morgan's spots). Cherry angioma is a ruby red papule that measures a few millimeters in diameter and possesses a pale halo zone.[197] It may appear in adolescence but is most common in late adult life. The predilection for the trunk and extremity contrasts with the head and neck location for most childhood hemangiomas. The lesions are located in the superficial corium and consist of dilated thin-walled capillaries, which create an elevation and mild atrophy of the overlying skin.

Cavernous hemangioma

Cavernous hemangiomas are less frequent than capillary hemangiomas but share common age and anatomical distributions. They are most common during childhood and are located in the upper portion of the body. As a result, it has

been suggested that they simply represent massively engorged capillary hemangiomas, a contention supported by the fact that some hemangiomas have a capillary component at the surface and a cavernous component in the deeper portion. However, they differ from capillary hemangiomas

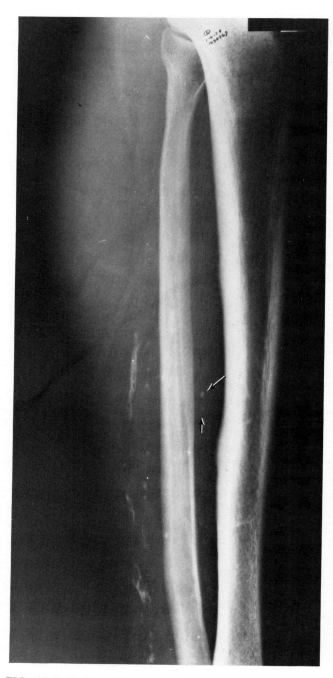

FIG. 23-8. Radiograph of hemangioma having both cavernous and venous features histologically. Note long curvilinear calcifications in addition to phleboliths *(arrows)*. The latter are highly characteristic of cavernous hemangiomas. (Courtesy John Madewell, MD.)

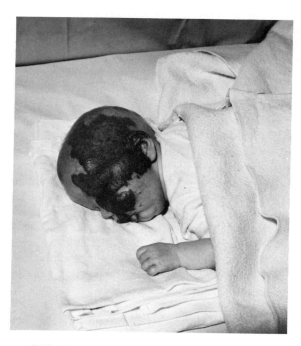

FIG. 23-7. Cavernous hemangioma of the face.

in several important respects. They are usually larger and less circumscribed and more frequently involve deep structures. They show essentially no tendency to regress and may even be locally destructive by virtue of the pressure they exert on neighboring structures. Consequently, the majority of cavernous hemangiomas require surgery, in contrast to their capillary counterparts.

The color and surface appearance of these lesions relate to the location. Superficial lesions are blue puffy masses with an irregular surface caused by the dilatation of the vessels (Fig. 23-7). Deep lesions may impart little or no color to the overlying skin. Radiographically, the large deep lesions appear as localized or diffuse nonhomogeneous water density masses. Tortuous water density channels representing the afferent and efferent blood supplies can occasionally be seen within adjacent fat. Calcification is common and can be of several types (Fig. 23-8). Amorphous or curvilinear calcification is nonspecific, while phlebolith formation is not only more frequent but also a more specific finding. Both are the result of dystrophic calcification within organizing thrombi.[6] Cavernous hemangiomas are composed of large dilated blood-filled vessels lined by flattened endothelium (Fig. 23-9). The vessels may be arranged in a roughly lobular arrangement or in a diffuse haphazard pattern. The walls are occasionally thickened by an adventitial fibrosis, and inflammatory cells may be scattered throughout the stroma. *Sinuosoidal hemangioma* is a vari-

ant of cavernous hemangioma that differs from the latter in several respects.[40] It occurs as a solitary acquired lesion in adults, usually women, and is relatively well demarcated (Fig. 23-10). The thin-walled cavernous vessels ramify with one another to a much greater extent than in a conventional cavernous hemangioma. Papillary infoldings of the endothelium are usually identified, and in two cases reported by Calonje and Fletcher,[40] central infarction of the tumors occurred (Fig. 23-11). Whether these lesions deserve to be considered a distinct entity is not clear, since sinuoidal patterns may be seen within hemangiomas of all types secondary to thrombosis and reorganization.

Several syndromes may be associated with cavernous hemangiomas. Thrombocytopenia purpura complicating giant hemangiomas is known as *Kasabach-Merritt syndrome*.[39,50,52,63] Most of these hemangiomas are large solitary cavernous hemangiomas located on an extremity, although the syndrome has complicated capillary hemangiomas, angiomatosis, or angiosarcomas. Typically the syndrome occurs during infancy, and the onset of purpura is heralded by rapid enlargement of the tumor. The patients develop numerous cutaneous petechiae and ecchymoses, not only in the skin but also in internal organs. Although the pathogenesis is not fully understood, intravascular coagulation and sequestration of platelets within the tumors appears to be one important mechanism.[39] Patients with this syndrome usually require therapy because death from hem-

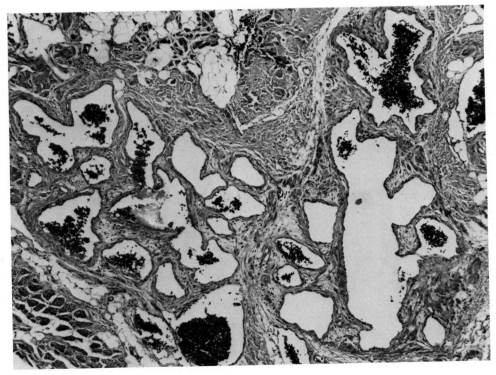

FIG. 23-9. Cavernous hemangioma illustrating large, thin-walled veins. (×25.)

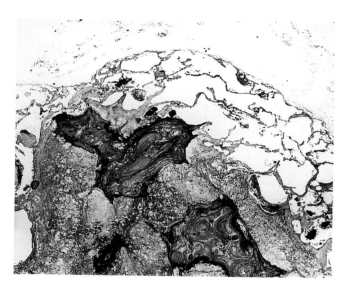

FIG. 23-10. Sinusoidal hemangioma. (×25.) (Case courtesy of Dr. C.D.M. Fletcher.)

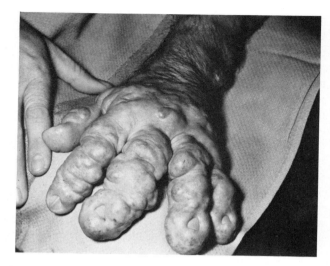

FIG. 23-12. Multiple enchondromas occurring in a patient with Maffucci's syndrome. Patients also develop hemangiomas, usually of the cavernous type.

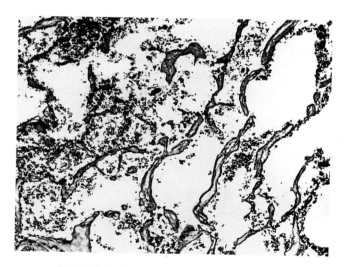

FIG. 23-11. Sinusoidal hemangioma. (×160.)

orrhage and infection approaches 30%, and spontaneous regression of these tumors cannot be anticipated. In most cases surgery is not possible because of the precarious hematological status of the patient and the large size of the tumor. In the past steroids or radiation therapy, or both, were the mainstay of treatment. Several new strategies include the administration of recombinant interferon alfa-2a[45] and pentoxifylline.[42]

A distinctive form of cavernous hemangioma of the skin in association with similar gastrointestinal tract lesions was delineated by Bean in 1958 as *blue rubber bleb nevus syndrome*.[46,197] The term aptly describes the blue cutaneous lesions, which look and feel like rubber nipples. They com-

press easily with pressure, leaving a flaccid wrinkled appearance to the skin, and then regain their shape with cessation of pressure. In addition, most patients have gastrointestinal hemangiomas, usually in the small intestine. These internal lesions commonly bleed so that chronic anemia complicates the course of the disease. Some reported cases have suggested an autosomal dominant mode of inheritance. Because of the diffuse nature of the disease, therapy is aimed at resecting only bleeding lesions from the intestine.

Maffucci's syndrome (dyschondroplasia with vascular hamartomas) is a rare mesodermal dysplasia characterized by multiple hemangiomas and enchondromas (Fig. 23-12). The vascular tumors are usually noted at birth and are of the cavernous type.[197] Other vascular lesions including lymphangiomas and phlebectasias may also be present. Spindle cell hemangioendotheliomas (see Chapter 24) may also occur in Maffucci's syndrome. The cartilaginous tumors typically develop after the vascular lesions and are the result of a defect in endochondral ossification so that there is a marked overgrowth in the cartilage plates. The bones are shortened and have numerous enchondromas and exostoses. Pathological fractures are common, and in about 20% of the patients malignant tumors, usually chondrosarcomas (or rarely angiosarcomas), develop.

Arteriovenous hemangioma

Arteriovenous hemangiomas can be divided into two types: those which occur in deep locations and are associated with varying degrees of arteriovenous shunting and those which occur superficially in the dermis and in which no significant shunting occurs.

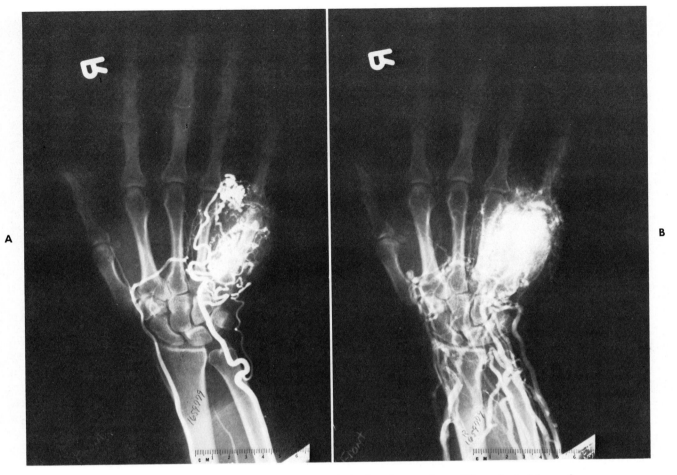

FIG. 23-13. Arteriovenous hemangioma of hand. **A,** Arteriogram shows filling of arterial vessels supplying tumor. **B,** Opacification of tumor in region of fifth metacarpal and filling of draining veins while still in arterial phase. (Courtesy Dr. John Madewell.)

The deep form is the more important type; it usually occurs in young persons and is regarded by some as an arteriovenous malformation.[92,95,197] It can be conceptualized as partial persistence of the fetal capillary bed, causing abnormal connections between the arteries and veins. The lesions may be located in any portion of the body but most commonly affect the head, neck, and lower extremity. Those located close to the skin surface and those associated with large shunts may visibly pulsate or writhe under the influence of the afferent arterial blood flow. This distinctive gross appearance has earned this lesion various names, including *cirsoid aneurysm, racemose hemangioma,* and *arteriovenous aneurysm.* These tumors give rise to a constellation of signs and symptoms indicative of the magnitude of the shunt. Large shunts result in a continuous thrill or bruit over the mass, increased warmth of the skin, marked increase in oxygen saturation of the venous blood, and reflex bradycardia following compression of the fistula

(Branham's sign). When shunting is less significant, the foregoing signs may not be present and the limb will simply display increased girth and enlargement of the veins. Pain may be a prominent symptom as a result of pressure on nerves. In some arteriovenous hemangiomas of bone and soft tissue, hypertrophy of the extremity may be present.[92] Arteriography is indispensable in the diagnosis of these tumors because it demonstrates large tortuous vessels of both the arterial and venous types with early filling of the draining veins[4] (Fig. 23-13). In addition, the lymph vessels may appear hyperplastic on lymphography. Histologically, this form of hemangioma may be quite difficult to diagnose out of context. The diagnosis can sometimes be inferred by the presence of medium-sized or larger arteries and veins in close association with one another (Fig. 23-14, *A*) and by intimal thickening of the veins, suggesting elevated pressure in this portion of the vasculature. Actual continuities or shunts between the arteries and veins, however, are best

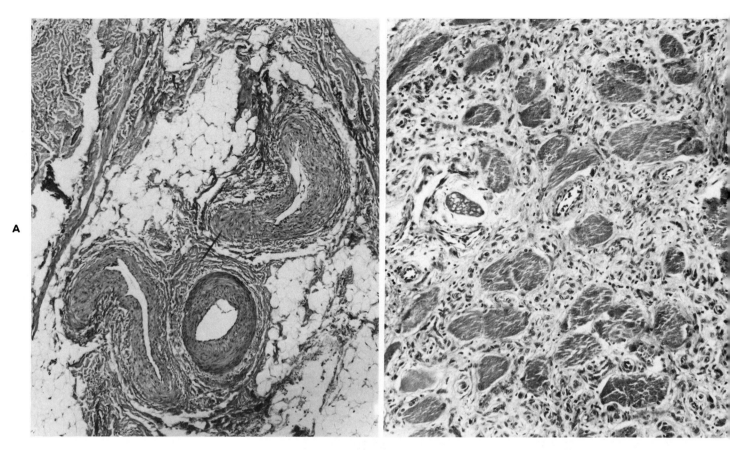

FIG. 23-14. A, Arteriovenous hemangioma illustrating close juxtaposition of arteries and veins in some portions of the tumor. (×100.) **B,** In other areas tumor is indistinguishable from a capillary hemangioma. Same case as Fig. 23-12. (×25.)

documented by serial sections or by corrosion cast evaluation of the vascular network. These studies illustrate numerous fistulae of various sizes, right-angle branch points, and increased tortuosity of vessels.[91] It should be emphasized that these tumors can vary considerably from area to area. In some portions they may simply resemble a capillary or cavernous hemangioma (Fig. 23-14, *B*). Cutaneous manifestations of arteriovenous hemangiomas with fistulae may crudely simulate the appearance of Kaposi's sarcoma (see Chapter 25). These changes have been referred to as *kaposiform angiodermatitis* or *pseudo-Kaposi's sarcoma*.[87,89,93,94] The changes consist of a proliferation of small capillary-sized vessels with thickened walls, in association with fibroblasts and hemosiderin deposits (Figs. 23-15 and 23-16). In our opinion, therefore, the diagnosis of arteriovenous hemangioma of the deep type is best made in conjunction with the radiographic and clinical findings. Treatment of these lesions may prove extremely difficult. Usually the arteriovenous communications within these lesions are small and numerous so that ligation of a few feeding arteries is only partially effective. Cure often requires

a direct surgical excision of the lesion. In extreme cases where the lesions are large and congestive heart failure has ensued, amputation of the affected extremity may offer the only hope for reasonable quality of life.[44]

The second or superficial form of arteriovenous hemangioma occurs uniformly in adults as a small asymptomatic cutaneous nodule in which arteriovenous shunting is absent or clinically insignificant.[90] This unusual lesion was first described by Girard et al,[90] who noted its occurrence during mid-adult life as a solitary blue to red papule localized to the dermis or submucosa of the lips and perioral skin. Others have termed similar lesions *acral arteriovenous tumor*.[88] Histologically, they contain dilated thin-walled veins in the superficial corium or submucosa, while the arteries may be located in these regions or in the deeper areas of the tumor (Figs. 23-17 and 23-18). Although arteriovenous shunts were identified in about one fourth of cases studied, the small size of the vessels involved obviously results in clinically inapparent shunting. Although the etiology of this lesion is unknown, Girard et al.[90] suggest it represents a multicentric hamartoma of the dermal and

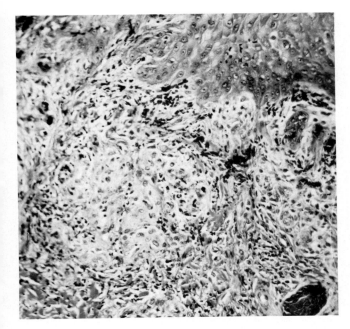

FIG. 23-15. Kaposiform changes in skin overlying arteriovenous fistula. Proliferation of small thick-walled vessel in dermis is seen. (×160.)

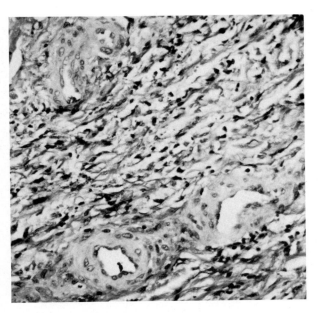

FIG. 23-16. Kaposiform changes in skin overlying arteriovenous fistula. Area is adjacent to that in Fig. 23-15 and shows fibroblasts and hemosiderin deposits adjacent to thick-walled vessels. (×250.)

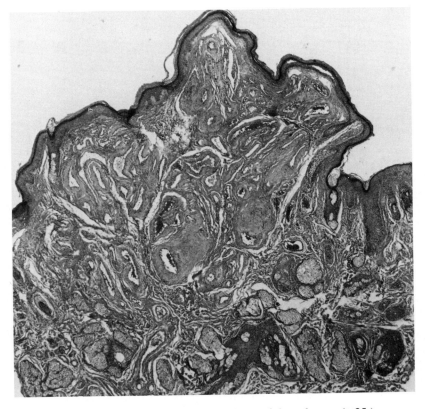

FIG. 23-17. Arteriovenous hemangioma of dermal type. (×25.)

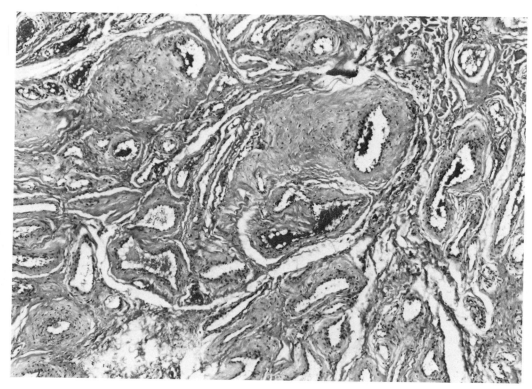

FIG. 23-18. Arteriovenous hemangioma of dermal type depicting thick-walled and thin-walled vessels in close association with one another. (×100.)

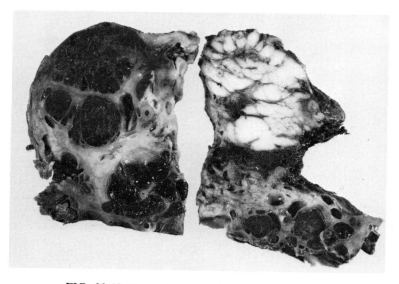

FIG. 23-19. Gross specimen of venous hemangioma.

submucosal plexus of vessels. Although none of the lesions undergo spontaneous regression, they grow slowly, achieve only a small size, and are usually cured by simple excision.

Venous hemangioma

Venous hemangiomas are characteristically tumors that present during adult life and are most common in deep lo-

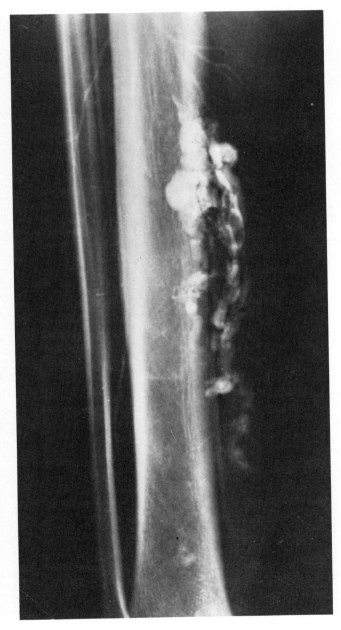

FIG. 23-20. Hemangioma with venous and cavernous features (same case as Fig. 23-8). Venous phase of arteriogram portrays large saccular structures that correspond to tortuous thick-walled muscular veins. (Courtesy Dr. John Madewell.)

cations such as the retroperitoneum, mesentery, and muscles of the extremity where they develop as large masses consisting of congeries of gaping venous vessels (Fig. 23-19). Blood flow is slow within these spaces, and the feeding vessels may be thrombosed. Consequently, these lesions are often not visualized on arteriography but require venography or direct injection to identify their presence and extent[6] (Fig. 23-20). Histologically, they are distinguished from capillary and cavernous hemangiomas by the fact that most of their vessels are thick walled. The muscle within the vessel walls, however, is less well organized than that of normal veins and often blends in a random fashion with the surrounding soft tissue structures (Fig. 23-21). Calcification may also occur within these lesions and represents dystrophic calcification within organizing thrombus material just as it does in cavernous hemangiomas. Some venous hemangiomas may also possess areas that are indistinguishable from a cavernous hemangioma. Recently we have encountered two distinctive venous hemangiomas composed of thick-walled vessels that occurred on the dorsum of the feet in two children with Turner's syndrome.[61] These rather distinctive forms of venous hemangioma may represent one of the various cardiovascular abnormalities associated with this genetic syndrome.

Epithelioid hemangioma (angiolymphoid hyperplasia with eosinophilia, histiocytoid hemangioma)

Epithelioid hemangioma is an unusual but distinctive vascular tumor that was first described by Wells and Whimster[116] as *angiolymphoid hyperplasia with eosinophilia* and subsequently by others as *inflammatory angiomatous nodule, atypical or pseudopyogenic granuloma,*[98,99] and *histiocytoid hemangioma.*[113] The lesions reported in the Japanese literature as *Kimura's disease*[105,120] represent a different entity.

Epithelioid hemangiomas typically occur during early to mid-adult life (age 20 to 40 years) and affect women more often than men. Most are situated superficially in the head and neck, particularly the region around the ear. As a result, they can be detected relatively early as small dull red pruritic plaques. Crusting, excoriation, bleeding, and coalescence of lesions are common secondary features. About half of the patients develop multiple lesions generally occurring in the same area. One unusual case of numerous lesions has been reported in a patient with an inverted ratio of helper to suppressor T cells.[114] Affected patients appear relatively well, although occasionally significant regional lymph node enlargement and eosinophilia of the peripheral blood accompany the lesions. These signs have suggested the possibility of an infectious agent, but to date none has been identified.

Typically these tumors are circumscribed lesions of the subcutis or dermis (Figs. 23-22 to 23-29), but occasionally they involve deep soft tissue and in rare instances involve

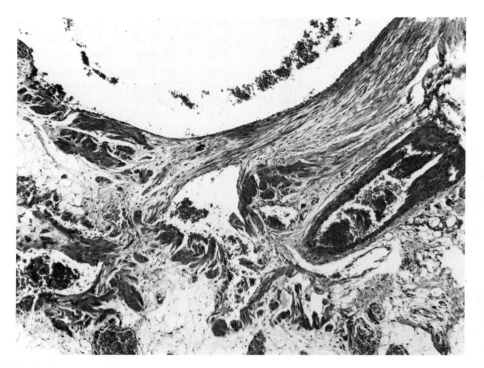

FIG. 23-21. Large thick-walled veins of venous hemangioma. Muscle of vessels blends with surrounding soft tissue. (×60.)

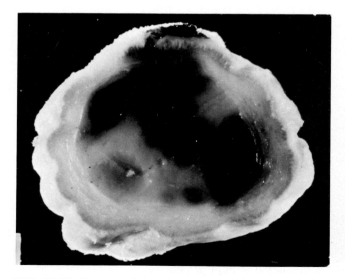

FIG. 23-22. Gross specimen of subcutaneous form of epithelioid hemangioma.

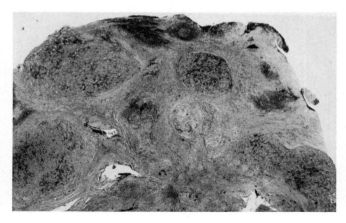

FIG. 23-23. Low-power view of epithelioid hemangioma involving subcutis. Note multinodular growth. (×15.)

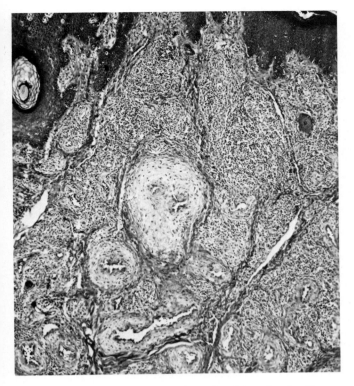

FIG. 23-24. Epithelioid hemangioma involving dermis. Tumor consists of large vessels surrounded by loose myxoid zone. Congeries of smaller capillary-sized vessels surround large vessels. (×60.)

or arise from vessels (Figs. 23-30 and 23-31). Intravascular forms of this tumor not unexpectedly cause diagnostic problems for the pathologist; attention has been focused on this phenomenon by Rosai and Ackerman,[112] who described such lesions as *intravenous atypical vascular proliferation*. Like many other hemangiomas this lesion may have a vague lobular arrangement as a result of the clustering of small capillary-sized vessels around a medium-sized parent vessel (Figs. 23-24 and 23-25). Many of the vessels are lined by distinct epithelioid endothelial cells (Figs. 23-25, 23-26, and 23-28 to 23-30) with scalloped borders that protrude deeply into the lumen in a manner that has been likened to "tombstones" (Fig. 23-28, *B*). In small vessels the endothelium may assume a more conventional appearance (Fig. 23-27). These epithelioid endothelial cells have rounded or lobated nuclei and abundant acidophilic cytoplasm containing occasional vacuoles that represent primitive vascular lumen formation (Fig. 23-28, *A*). Although they possess many of the ultrastructural features of endothelium, including micropinocytotic vesicles, antiluminal basal lamina, and Weibel-Palade bodies, they manifest certain modifications. Adjacent cells are often separated by rather large gaps and interdigitate only along their lateral basal borders by means of tight junctions. Organelles are more abundant in these cells and include increased numbers of mitochondria, smooth and rough endoplasmic reticulum, free ribosomes, and thin cytofilaments. Histochemical reactions demonstrate increased hydrolytic and oxida-

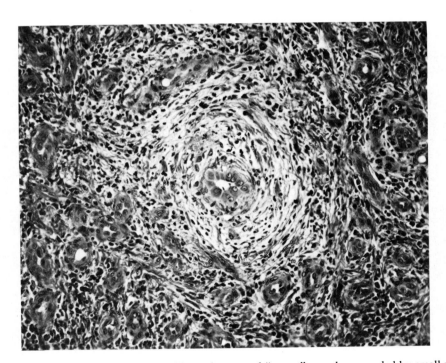

FIG. 23-25. Epithelioid hemangioma illustrating central "parent" vessel surrounded by small vessels and dense inflammation. (×160.)

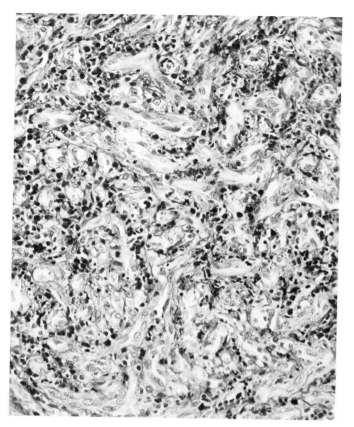

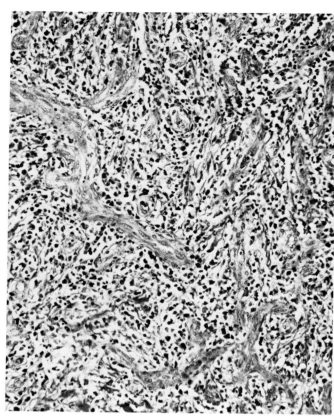

FIG. 23-26. Epithelioid hemangioma. Vessels are lined by pale-staining cuboidal endothelial cells that are admixed with inflammatory elements, predominantly eosinophils. (×250.)

FIG. 23-27. Epithelioid hemangioma in which some areas display more conventional-appearing endothelial cells interspersed with chronic inflammatory cells. (×160.)

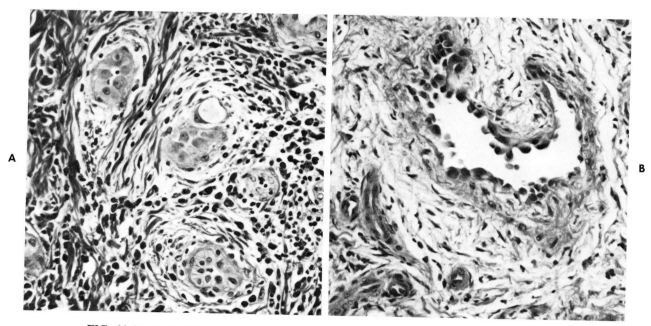

FIG. 23-28. Epithelioid hemangioma. **A,** Occasional vacuolization of endothelial cells. (×250.)
B, "Tombstone"-like arrangement of cells in larger vessels. (×250.)

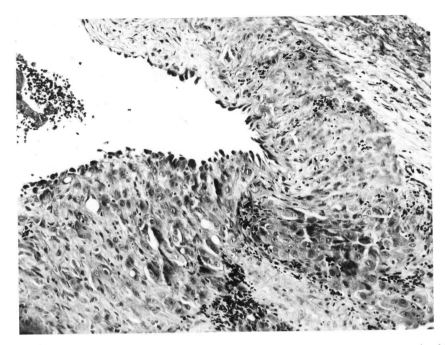

FIG. 23-29. Epithelioid hemangioma involving wall of large vessel. This phenomenon should not be equated with malignancy. (×160.)

tive enzymes and decreased alkaline phosphatase as compared to normal capillary endothelium. A mixture of inflammatory cells surrounds the vessels. Eosinophils are particularly characteristic of these tumors, but lymphocytes, mast cells, and plasma cells are also present (Figs. 23-26 and 23-27). Lymphoid aggregates replete with germinal centers are occasionally present but are believed by some to be a feature of long-standing lesions or a peculiar host response.

Although about one third of these lesions recur, virtually none has produced metastasis. One case reported by Reed and Terazakis[111] evidently gave rise to microscopic metastases in a regional lymph node, but this appears to be a unique event.[109,111] Rare lesions have been noted to regress spontaneously, but usually surgical excision is required. About 80% of reported patients in the literature have responded at least partially to superficial radiotherapy,[106] but cryotherapy and injection of intralesional steroids have not met with success.[109]

Despite their benign nature, considerable controversy still exists as to the basic nature of these lesions, some authors considering them reactive and others neoplastic. In our experience, which reviewed 96 cases of epithelioid hemangioma, we were impressed that over 60% of cases were intimately associated with a large vessel, which showed mural damage or rupture, or both.[101] These observations suggest that at least a significant number of soft tissue epithelioid hemangiomas may be reactive lesions (Figs.

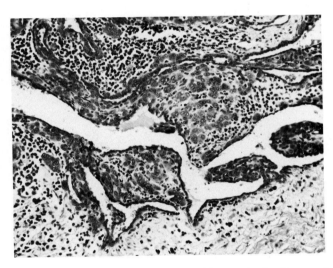

FIG. 23-30. Epithelioid hemangioma with growth of cells around larger vessels. (×160.)

23-32 and 23-33). In this regard a rather impressive case of epithelioid hemangioma was reported to occur in a patient following a popliteal arteriovenous fistula.[108] Others have commented on the high incidence of arteriovenous shunts, particularly in deeply situated forms of epithelioid hemangioma. Although sharing many common histological features and a benign clinical course, the lesions may be pathogenetically heterogeneous.

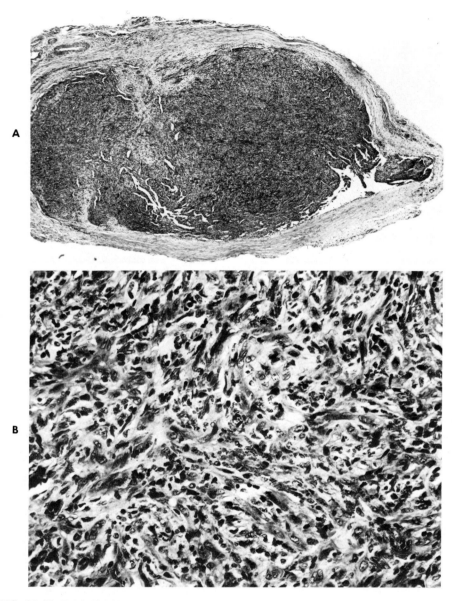

FIG. 23-31. Epithelioid hemangioma arising entirely within a vessel (**A** and **B**) (intravenous atypical vascular proliferation). (**A**, ×25; **B**, ×250.)

There has been considerable speculation concerning the nature and significance of the epithelioid endothelial cell. In our opinion it seems to represent an altered functional state of endothelium, since it may be encountered in benign and malignant vascular tumors as well as in reactive vascular lesions. Rosai et al.,[113] noting the lobated nuclei, the decreased alkaline phosphatase, and the increased acid phosphatase compared with normal endothelium, referred to these cells as *histiocytoid*. The term *histiocytoid hemangioma*,[113] however, has been applied to a heterogeneous group of vascular lesions, including epithelioid hemangioma, hemangioendothelioma of bone, and epithelioid hemangioendothelioma (see Chapter 24), which vary considerably in presentation and behavior. For this reason, we have discouraged the use of *histiocytoid hemangioma* as a strict diagnostic term unless it is modified by some comment as to the level of malignancy of the lesions. It provides, however, an elegant concept for a group of lesions characterized by a peculiar epithelioid (or histiocytoid) endothelial cell.

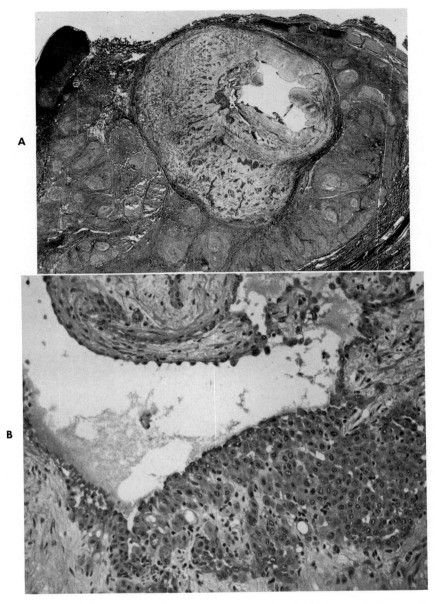

FIG. 23-32. Changes reminiscent of epithelioid hemangioma arising from wall of traumatized vessels. Note prominent lymphocytic infiltrate around lesions (**A**) and solid islands of epithelioid endothelial cells (**B**). (**A,** ×15; **B,** ×160.)

Kimura's disease

First described by Kim in the Chinese literature and later by Kimura et al.[120] in the Japanese literature, this is a chronic inflammatory condition that appears to be endemic in the Asian population and occurs only infrequently in Westerners. Although formerly thought to be identical to epithelioid hemangioma (angiolymphoid hyperplasia), there are many data indicating that these are two entirely unrelated lesions bearing only a few superficial histological similarities.[117,118,121,124]

Kimura's disease presents as lymphadenopathy with or without an associated soft tissue mass. Peripheral eosinophilia is nearly always present. Increased serum IgE, proteinuria, and nephrotic syndrome may also occur as part of the disease.[123,125] Lesions are most frequent in the subcutis of the head and neck area, although lesions have been noted in the groin, extremities, and chest wall. There is a striking male predilection in this disease. The lesions are characterized by dense lymphoid aggregates containing prominent germinal centers (Fig. 23-34). Within the germinal

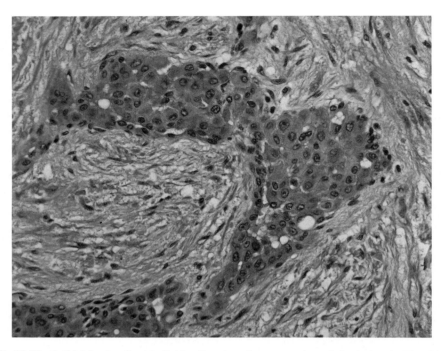

FIG. 23-33. Solid islands of epithelioid cells taken from a portion of the lesion in Fig. 23-32. Islands of endothelial cells can be easily mistaken for squamous carcinoma. (×250.)

center one can occasionally identify nuclear debris, poly-karyocytes, and a delicate eosinophilic matrix. Immunohistochemical procedures reveal that IgE-bearing cells, corresponding to the distribution of dendritic reticulum cells, populate the germinal center. Thin-walled vessels, with the characteristics of postcapillary venules, reside adjacent to the germinal centers, occasionally dipping into the centers. Dense infiltrates of eosinophils adjacent to the lymphoid aggregates occasionally form "eosinophilic abscesses." In the late stages of the disease a dense hyaline fibrosis supervenes. The adherence of the mass to the surrounding structures often triggers alarm on the part of the surgeon regarding the possibility of malignancy. In affected lymph nodes there is an exuberant follicular hyperplasia with preservation of the architecture. The changes within the germinal center are as described above for the soft tissue lesions.

The etiology of this condition is unknown, although the peripheral eosinophilia and elevated serum IgE suggest an immunological reaction to an unknown stimulus. The lesions are benign, although recurrence may develop after surgical excision. There are no instances of malignancy supervening on these peculiar lymphoid proliferations.

Although both Kimura's disease and angiolymphoid hyperplasia have in common a lymphoid infiltrate with eosinophils, there are rather striking differences. The vascular proliferation in Kimura's disease is relatively minor and is eclipsed by the inflammatory component. Moreover, the

vessels in Kimura's disease are not lined by epithelioid endothelium but by more attenuated endothelial cells.

Granulation tissue-type hemangioma (pyogenic granuloma)

The so-called pyogenic granuloma is a polypoid form of capillary hemangioma occurring on the skin and mucosal surfaces. The inflammatory changes that often accompany these tumors may be so pronounced that the lesions bear a striking resemblance to granulation tissue. In fact, most early pathologists considered these lesions to be infectious. Poncet and Dor, credited with the first description, believed these lesions were secondary to infection by Botryomyces organisms, while others implicated pyogenic bacteria, specifically staphylococci. Uncomplicated lesions, however, lack ulceration and inflammation and are quite similar to ordinary capillary hemangiomas except for their distinctive gross appearance and clinical symptoms.

These tumors may occur on either the skin or the mucosal surfaces, although the latter accounts for about 60% of all cases.[136] In the extensive review by Kerr[136] of 289 cases, the following were the most common sites in descending order of frequency: gingiva (64 cases), finger (44 cases), lips (40 cases), face (28 cases), and tongue (20 cases). The sexes are affected approximately equally, and the disease is evenly distributed over all decades. Approximately one third develop following minor trauma. Multi-

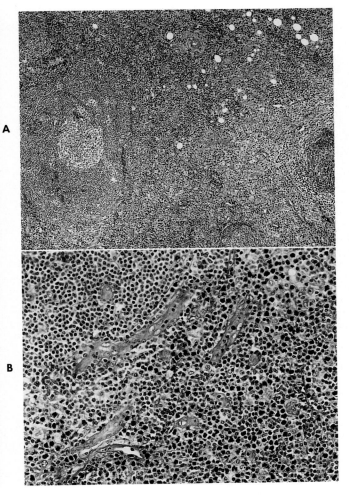

FIG. 23-34. Kimura's disease. (**A** and **B**, ×250.)

ple lesions may develop simultaneously, but this phenomenon almost always occurs in the cutaneous rather than the mucosal form of the disease. Recently there have been a few reports of disseminated (eruptive) forms of pyogenic granuloma,[131,135,146] one following surgical removal of a solitary pyogenic granuloma. Disseminated pyogenic granulomas progress for a limited period of time and ultimately stabilize or regress. The mechanism for these initially alarming presentations is not clear, although some have suggested the release of angiogenic factors by the tumors. In the ordinary case the tumors develop rapidly and achieve their maximal size of several millimeters to a few centimeters within a few weeks or months. The well-established lesion is a polypoid, friable, purple-red mass that bleeds easily and frequently ulcerates. Sessile forms of this tumor also occur, but they tend to be recurrent lesions.

The appearance of these lesions at low magnification should immediately suggest the diagnosis because they are distinctly exophytic growths connected to the skin by stalks of varying diameter (Figs. 23-35 and 23-38, *A*) and occasionally are surrounded by a heaped-up collar of normal tissue. The adjacent epithelium is hyperkeratotic or acanthotic, but the epithelium overlying the lesion itself is flattened, atrophic, or ulcerated (Fig. 23-36). The basic lesion is a lobulated cellular hemangioma[137] set in a fibromyxoid matrix. Each lobule of the hemangioma is made up of a larger vessel, often with a muscular wall and surrounded by congeries of small capillaries. Most lesions, however, are altered by secondary inflammatory changes; as a result they have been likened to granulation tissue. Both acute and chronic inflammatory cells are scattered throughout the lesion but not unexpectedly are most numerous at the surface. Secondary invading microorganisms are occasionally present in the superficial reaches of ulcerated lesions. Stromal edema may widely separate the capillary lumina,

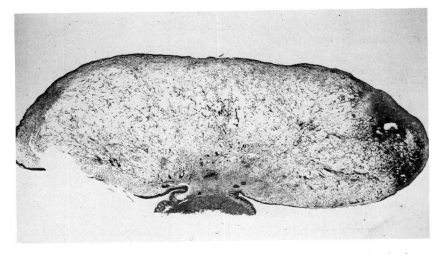

FIG. 23-35. Granulation tissue-type hemangioma (pyogenic granuloma). Lesion is characterized by exophytic growth with attachment to skin or mucosa by means of a narrow stalk. (×15.)

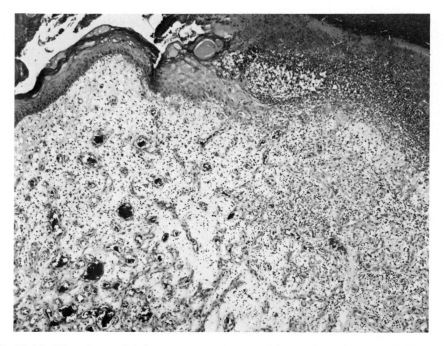

FIG. 23-36. Ulceration and inflammatory exudate overlying surface of pyogenic granuloma. (×60.)

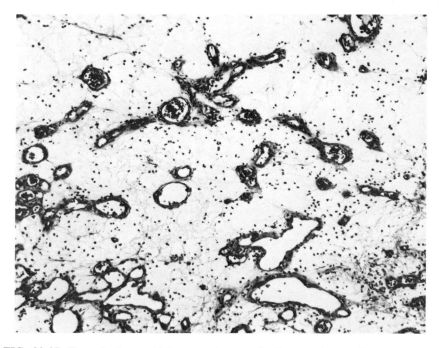

FIG. 23-37. Stromal edema widely separating vessels of pyogenic granuloma. (×100.)

thereby obscuring the lobular arrangement of the tumor (Fig. 23-37). Mitotic activity may be brisk within both the endothelium and stromal fibroblasts when secondary changes such as edema and inflammation are present. In lesions that involute there is evidence suggesting that they develop a progressive stromal and perivascular fibrosis. Rarely the pyogenic granuloma may have areas in which the endothelium has an epithelioid appearance (Fig. 23-38).

The clinical appearance of these lesions is quite characteristic and can serve as a useful diagnostic adjunct to the pathologist in difficult situations where the distinction, for instance, between a well-differentiated angiosarcoma or an angiomatous form of Kaposi's sarcoma must be made. In these situations it is useful to recall that the pyogenic granuloma is a more or less circumscribed lesion, often with a lobular arrangement, in contrast to the rambling poorly confined nature of malignant vascular neoplasms. In particular, the manner in which even well-differentiated angiosarcomas dissect through connective tissue and create irregu-

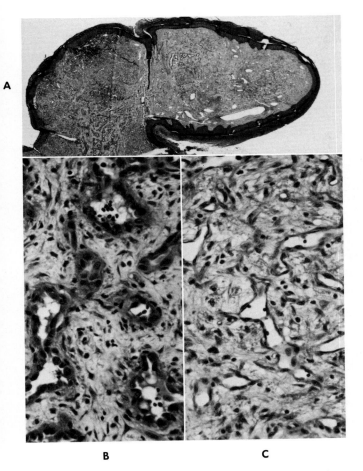

FIG. 23-38. Pyogenic granuloma (**A**) having areas within it characterized by rather normal (**C**) as well as epithelioid (**B**) endothelium. (**A**, ×15; **B** and **C**, ×250.)

lar vascular spaces contrasts sharply with the pyogenic granuloma. Likewise, Kaposi's sarcoma is not well circumscribed and contains, in addition, at least focal cellular zones of spindled cells, which form the traditional slitlike vascular spaces. However, these diagnostic areas are often located in the central or deep areas of the tumor, while the well-differentiated angiomatous component may be seen peripherally or superficially. Thus in certain instances it is evident that a superficial biopsy of a vascular neoplasm may not be an adequate means of excluding malignancy.

Although the pyogenic granuloma is a benign lesion, 16% have been noted to recur in one large series of tumors treated conservatively.[127] However, a significantly lower recurrence rate has been noted in a recent series of 74 cases reported by Mills et al.[139] Recurrence in this disease may present as a solitary nodule or as multiple small satellite nodules around the site of the original lesion.[130,134,141,145,147] The phenomenon of *satellitosis* in this disease has been analyzed by Warner and Wilson-Jones,[145] who found that most of these lesions occurred on the region of the trunk, particularly the scapular area, and the majority had been incompletely excised initially. In contrast to the original tumors, the satellites are usually not pedunculated but rather are sessile and possess an intact surface epithelium. Thus in these respects they may grossly resemble ordinary hemangiomas. Although the rapid development of numerous satellites often causes considerable alarm on the part of the clinician, these lesions usually respond to reexcision and in some instances have even regressed spontaneously.

Granuloma gravidarum. Granuloma gravidarum is a specialized form of pyogenic granuloma that occurs on the gingival surface during pregnancy.[137] It is estimated that gingival changes occur in about 50% of pregnant women but that only about 1% of this group will develop localized tumors.[137] Typically, these lesions develop abruptly during the first trimester and arise from the interdental area of the gum. They are grossly and histologically indistinguishable from the ordinary form of pyogenic granuloma. They regress dramatically following parturition. However, many persist as small mucosal nodules, which are capable of renewed growth at the time of subsequent pregnancies. This unusual tumor has provided some of the most compelling evidence that the pyogenic granuloma lacks the degree of autonomous growth that characterizes most vascular tumors of adulthood. In fact, hormone sensitivity manifested by the granuloma gravidarum has led some to conclude that the lesion should not be regarded as a true neoplasm but rather as an exaggerated hyperplasia resulting from an altered physiological state.

Intravenous pyogenic granuloma. An intravenous counterpart of pyogenic granuloma has been recognized by Cooper et al.[129] This tumor is most common on the neck and upper extremity. It presents as a red-brown intravascular

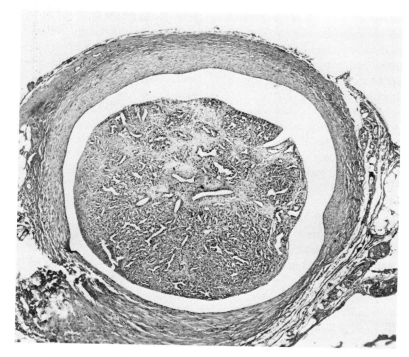

FIG. 23-39. Intravascular form of pyogenic granuloma. (×40.)

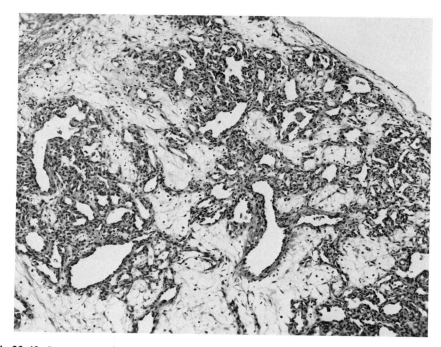

FIG. 23-40. Intravascular form of pyogenic granuloma. In contrast to cutaneous form, there are few secondary changes; lesions consequently show preservation of the lobular arrangements of vessels. (×100.)

polyp that can be easily mistaken for an organizing thrombus (Fig. 23-39). The tumor arises from the vein wall and protrudes deeply into the lumen but remains anchored to the wall by means of a narrow stalk containing the "feeder" vessels. The tumor is covered by a lining of endothelium, and the stroma often contains smooth muscle fibers, presumably remnants of the vein wall. Histologically, they are identical to uncomplicated examples of pyogenic granuloma in that these tumors display no inflammatory or ulcerative change (Fig. 23-40). Like other pyogenic granulomas they are benign and manifest no tendency to spread within the blood stream.

DEEP HEMANGIOMAS OF MISCELLANEOUS SITES

Compared with cutaneous hemangiomas, those involving deep soft tissue structures are quite uncommon (Table 23-1), yet these tumors deserve special mention because it is their unorthodox locations and different clinical presentations that create concern on the part of clinician and pathologist as to the possibility of malignancy.

Intramuscular hemangioma

Skeletal muscle hemangioma is probably the most common form of hemangioma of deep soft tissue, but it is nonetheless rare if one considers the entire spectrum of benign vascular neoplasms. Watson and McCarthy[60] estimated that they account for 0.8% of all benign vascular tumors, a figure that varies depending on the frequency with which incidental hemangiomas are excised at a given institution. The majority of intramuscular hemangiomas occur in young adults, with 80% to 90% manifesting before the age of 30 years.[148] The young age of affected patients and the long duration of symptoms in some cases raise the possibility that many of these tumors may be congenital tumors that slowly give rise to symptoms during late childhood or early adult life. Unlike cutaneous hemangiomas, this form does not show a striking predilection for females and affects the sexes in roughly equal numbers. Although any muscle can be affected, the majority are located in the lower extremity, particularly the muscles of the thigh. In our experience at the AFIP there is some evidence that intramuscular hemangiomas of the capillary type have a greater predilection for the head and neck musculature and in this respect have a distribution similar to the juvenile form of capillary hemangiomas found in infants and young children.[44]

Clinically, these lesions are more likely to pose diagnostic problems than superficial hemangiomas. They present simply as enlarging soft tissue masses with few signs or symptoms to belie their vascular nature. In particular, there is rarely any overlying discoloration of the skin, visible pulsation, or audible bruit. Radiographs and arteriography are far more helpful in suggesting the diagnosis. Plain films may reveal phleboliths in addition to a soft tissue mass, or

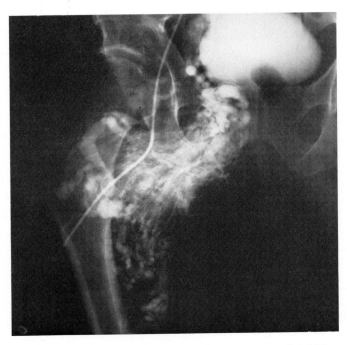

FIG. 23-41. Intramuscular hemangioma involving medial thigh.

arteriography may demonstrate a highly vascular lesion (Fig. 23-41) with early venous runoff. Moreover, the vessels are oriented parallel to one another in a "striated" pattern.[149,150] This pattern is created by the orderly entry and proliferation of vessels between fascicles of muscle and is considered a helpful feature in supporting benignancy. Pain is a frequent but not invariable symptom and is said to be more common in tumors involving long narrow muscles where stretching of the muscle and nerve fibers by the tumor is more intense. Occasionally impairment of function or anatomical deformity occurs. Although a history of trauma is given in about one fifth of cases, there is no indisputable evidence that the lesions are caused by trauma, and it appears more likely that trauma merely aggravates the underlying tumor.

Intramuscular hemangiomas vary greatly in their gross and microscopic appearances, depending on whether they are of the capillary, cavernous, or mixed type, and in many cases it is not possible to sharply classify these types because they are all part of the same histological spectrum.

In general, intramuscular hemangiomas of the capillary type are most common and are most likely to be confused with a malignant tumor. Grossly, they may not appear especially vascular because they vary from tan to yellow or red (Fig. 23-42). They are composed of a myriad of small capillary-sized vessels with plump nuclei that extend between individual muscle fibers (Figs. 23-43 to 23-47). In most areas well-developed lumen formation is apparent, although occasional tumors may have a solidly cellular appearance quite similar to the early stage of the juvenile hemangioma. In occasional cases there may be mitotic activity, intraluminal papillary tufting, and a proliferation of capillary vessels within perineural sheaths (Fig. 23-47). Although seemingly disturbing features, none of these features is indicative of malignancy in these tumors.

On the other hand, the cavernous form of intramuscular hemangioma is easily recognized as a benign vascular tumor (Figs. 23-48 and 23-49). Grossly, they are blue-red masses composed of large vessels lined by bland and mark-

edly attenuated endothelium, which seldom show a significant degree of pleomorphism. However, the presence of adipose tissue within these tumors is common, and at times it may be so conspicuous as to suggest the diagnosis of lipoma. Many of the earlier tumors described as *infiltrating angiolipomas of muscle* or *benign mesenchymoma* may well represent examples of intramuscular hemangiomas possessing a striking fatty overgrowth.

The most important consideration in differential diagnosis of these lesions is the distinction from an angiosarcoma of skeletal muscle. It should be recalled that angiosarcomas of deep soft tissue, specifically skeletal muscle, are quite rare (see Chapter 25); thus a vascular tumor of skeletal muscle is statistically more likely to be benign than malignant. Moreover, intramuscular hemangiomas do not develop the freely anastomosing sinusoidal pattern encountered in most well-differentiated angiosarcomas, nor do they possess nuclear pleomorphism and hyperchromatism. As indicated earlier, some hemangiomas of skeletal muscle contain significant lipomatous components and therefore are occasionally confused with liposarcomas. Although well-differentiated liposarcomas contain a very intricate vascular pattern, they hardly ever show the gaping vessels characteristic of the hemangioma, and they contain, in addition, lipoblasts. Finally, diffuse forms of hemangiomas (angiomatosis) involving skeletal muscle are histologically indistinguishable from the intramuscular hemangiomas. The separation of the two disorders must therefore be based

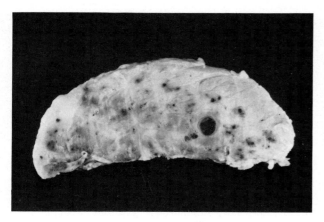

FIG. 23-42. Cut section of intramuscular hemangioma showing replacement of muscle fibers within vessels of various sizes.

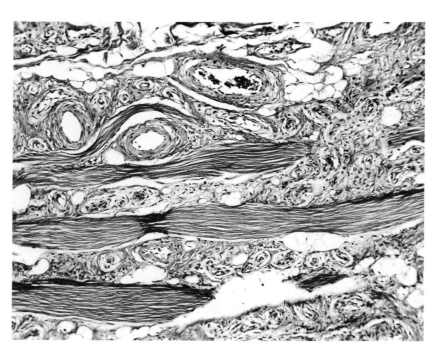

FIG. 23-43. Intramuscular hemangioma illustrating separation of muscle fibers by proliferating vessels. This pseudoinfiltrative pattern is often mistaken for evidence of malignancy. (×115.)

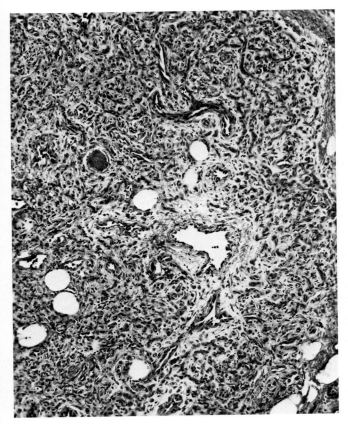

FIG. 23-44. Example of cellular small vessel type of intramuscular hemangioma. (×100.)

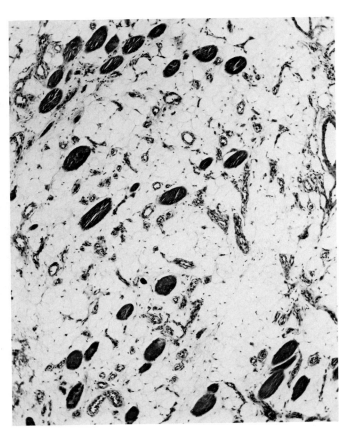

FIG. 23-45. Small vessel type of intramuscular hemangioma showing significant admixture of fat. Such tumors have sometimes been classified as "angiolipomas" of muscle. (×50.)

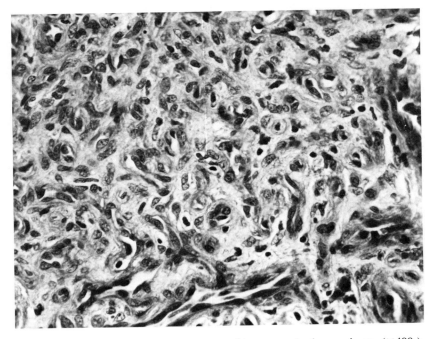

FIG. 23-46. Small vessel (capillary) type of intramuscular hemangioma. (×400.)

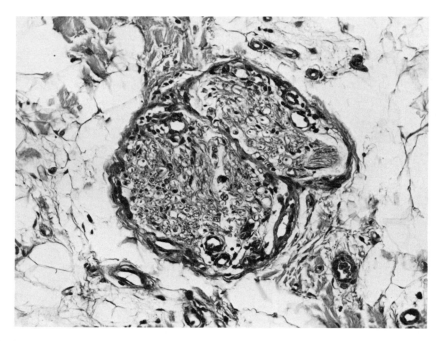

FIG. 23-47. Small capillary vessels involving perineural space in an intramuscular hemangioma. This feature is not indicative of malignancy. (×225.)

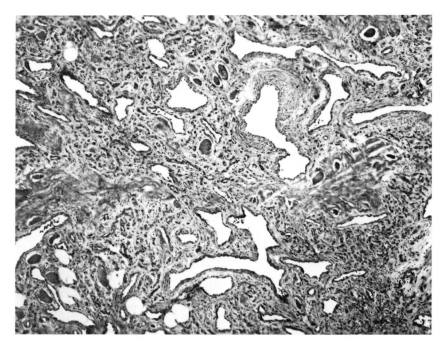

FIG. 23-48. Mixed type of intramuscular hemangioma. Tumor is composed of both small and large vessels. (×60.)

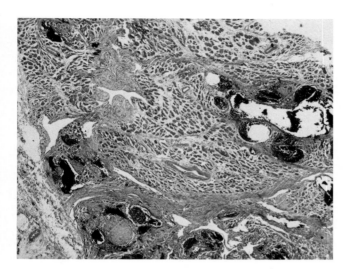

FIG. 23-49. Intramuscular hemangioma of large vessel type. (×25.)

on clinical parameters. In contrast to the intramuscular hemangioma, angiomatosis is usually a congenital or childhood lesion that extensively involves a large body area, including muscle, skin, and bone. Intramuscular hemangiomas are best considered benign tumors possessing a small but definite risk of local recurrence, attributable to the ease and

adequacy of the initial excision. In our experience 18% of patients develop local recurrences, although others have reported recurrences of over 50%.[151] Metastases have not been recorded, however. Treatment is therefore best aimed at complete excision without resorting to radical surgery. Prior embolization of the tumor has been used as a means of facilitating surgical excision.[153]

Synovial hemangioma

Synovial hemangioma is a well-recognized but rare entity. Theoretically it may arise from any synovial-lined surface and therefore may be found along the course of tendons or within a joint space.[167,169,171,172,175] In the former location they present in the same fashion as the common giant cell tumor, namely as painless soft tissue swellings. Origin from synovium in these cases is only assumed because they may also involve superficial structures, and confinement by synovium is often not apparent. Thus the most characteristic form of synovial hemangioma is the intraarticular variety in which the tumor consists of a more or less discrete mass lined by a synovial membrane.[168,170,174] These tumors almost invariably involve the knee joint and classically present as recurrent episodes of pain, swelling, and joint effusion. The symptoms usually begin during childhood and persist several years before the time of diagnosis. In most instances a spongy compressible mass, which decreases in size with elevation, can be palpated over the joint. Plain films of the joint show nonspecific changes in-

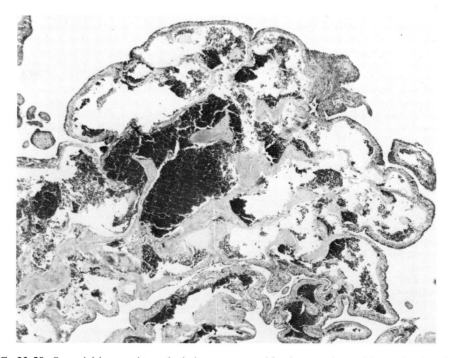

FIG. 23-50. Synovial hemangioma depicting cavernous blood spaces located immediately subjacent to synovial membrane. (×15.)

cluding capsular thickening and vague soft tissue density and rarely erosion of bone or invasion of adjacent muscle. Arteriography is more diagnostic in that the pooling of blood over the mass suggests a vascular tumor. The tumor grows either as a discrete pedunculated lesion or as a diffuse process. Histologically, the tumors are cavernous hemangiomas in which the vessels are separated by an edematous, myxoid, or focally hyalinized matrix occasionally containing inflammatory cells and siderophages (Fig. 23-50). The synovium overlying the tumor is sometimes thrown into villous projections, and its cells contain moderate to marked amounts of hemosiderin pigment (Fig. 23-51). These synovial changes appear to be secondary phenomena but sometimes may be so striking as to raise the possibility of a primary synovitis. Proper evaluation depends on the recognition that the underlying vessels are far too numerous and large for the area in question.

There is no general agreement concerning the pathogenesis of these lesions. It has been suggested by some that those lesions are not neoplasms but represent a reaction to trauma, although such a history is given in only a small number of cases. On the other hand, the young age of most afflicted patients again raises the question as to whether these represent congenital malformations or tumors, especially since occasional patients have been noted to have hemangiomas elsewhere. Treatment of local or pedunculated tumors is relatively easy and consists of simple extirpation.

Diffuse lesions are more difficult to eradicate surgically, and small doses of irradiation have sometimes been advocated.

Hemangioma of peripheral nerve

Hemangiomas arising within the confines of the epineurium are extremely rare tumors, and of the few cases described in the literature several are probably unacceptable because they appear to involve nerve secondarily.[178] Of the acceptable cases[176,177,179,182] there appears to be no characteristic age or anatomical distribution, although most cases occur in patients under the age of 40 years. Pain is a common symptom and may be accompanied by numbness and muscle wasting in the affected region. In one case symptoms of carpal tunnel syndrome were noted as a result of the location of the tumor in the median nerve. Involved nerves have included the trigeminal,[177] ulnar,[177] median,[176,179] posterior tibial,[180] and peroneal nerves.[180] Histologically, the majority of tumors have been cavernous hemangiomas with no features suggesting histological malignancy. Treatment of these benign tumors must be individualized. The benefits of total resection must be balanced against the morbidity of the procedure. Recently complete removal of an intraneural hemangioma was accomplished by intrafascicular dissection using dissecting microscopy.[182] Such an approach offers complete removal with minimal morbidity.

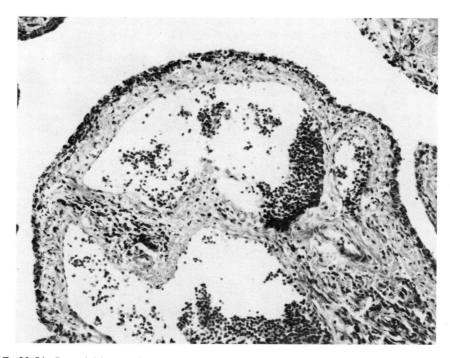

FIG. 23-51. Synovial hemangioma. Pigmentation of synovial cells is a result of presence of hemosiderin. (×60.)

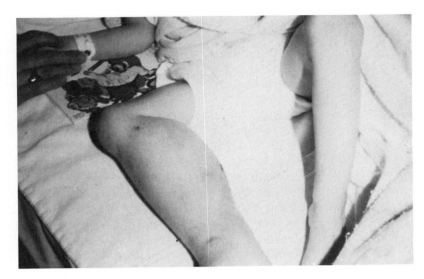

FIG. 23-52. Child with angiomatosis affecting entire lower leg.

ANGIOMATOSIS (DIFFUSE HEMANGIOMA)

Angiomatosis is a rare benign, but clinically extensive, vascular lesion of soft tissue, which almost invariably becomes symptomatic during childhood. These lesions probably begin during early intrauterine life when the limb buds form, grow proportionately with the fetus, and consequently affect large areas of the trunk or extremity (Fig. 23-52). One of us (SWW) has proposed a combined clinicopathological definition for this condition requiring that such lesions be histologically benign and affect a large segment of the body in a contiguous fashion.[193] Involvement may be of two types and consists either of extensive vertical involvment of multiple tissue planes (e.g., subcutis, muscle, and bone) or extensive involvement of tissue of the same type (e.g., multiple muscles). Over half of patients present within the first 2 decades of life, usually with symptoms of diffuse persistent swelling sometimes associated with pain and discoloration. Only rarely is hypertrophy, gigantism, or clinical evidence of arteriovenous shunting present. On CT scan the lesions appear as ill-defined nonhomogenous masses that may resemble sarcoma except for the presence of serpiginous dense areas that correspond to thick-walled, tortuous vessels (Fig. 23-53). Because of the presence of large amounts of fat, these tumors often appear as predominantly fatty tumors (Fig. 23-54). Histologically angiomatosis may assume one of two patterns. The first and more common pattern seen in the vast majority of over 50 cases we have reviewed consisted of a melange of large venous, cavernous, and capillary-sized vessels scattered haphazardly throughout soft tissue (Fig. 23-55). The venous vessels are remarkable for their irregular thick walls, which possess occasional attenuations and herniations of the wall (Figs. 23-56 and 23-57). A rather charac-

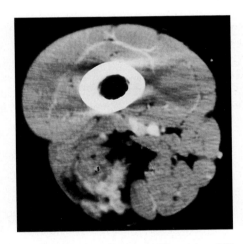

FIG. 23-53. CT scan of angiomatosis illustrating diffuse nonhomogenous regions within muscle. Serpiginous areas *(arrow)* represent tortuous vessels. (Reprinted from *Am J Surg Pathol* 16:764, 1992.)

teristic feature of these veins is the presence of small vessels clustered just adjacent to or within the wall of a large vein (Fig. 23-57). The second pattern, which occurs in a minority of cases, is virtually identical to a capillary hemangioma, except that the nodules of tumor diffusely infiltrate the surrounding soft tissue. The prominent amount of fat present in these lesions has led previous authors to use the term *infiltrating angiolipoma* (Fig. 23-58), suggesting that angiomatosis is probably best regarded as a more generalized mesenchymal proliferation. One unique case, which featured a diffuse proliferation of glomus cells in addition to the vessels, offers some support to the foregoing idea.[193]

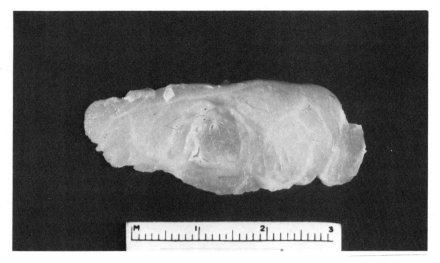

FIG. 23-54. Cut section through a portion of an angiomatosis. Pale appearance of muscle is typical and indicates replacement of fibers by vessels and fat.

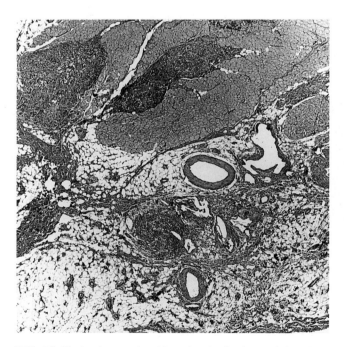

FIG. 23-55. Angiomatosis with variously sized vessels involving muscle and fat. (×60.)

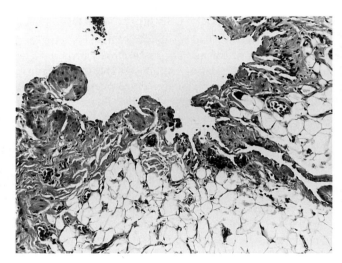

FIG. 23-56. Venous vessel within angiomatosis illustrating irregular wall and herniations. (×250.) (Reprinted from *Am J Surg Pathol* 16:764, 1992.)

In the recent study by Rao and Weiss,[193] nearly 90% of patients experienced recurrences and 40% experienced more than one recurrence within a 5-year period. A somewhat lower recurrence rate was reported by Howat and Campbell.[188] This behavior contrasts with the recurrence rate of intramuscular hemangiomas, which is usually less than 50%. Although there has been speculation that recurrence rates may be higher in younger children affected with this condition, this appears not to be true. Since there is no evidence that such lesions ever progress to frank malignancy, the goal of therapy is to treat the lesions as conservatively as possible, balancing the need for complete surgical extirpation with the morbidity of the procedure.

Diagnosis of these unusual tumors may prove difficult. As indicated in the discussion of intramuscular hemangiomas, the distinction between an angiomatosis and an intramuscular hemangioma is fundamentally made on clinical rather than pathological criteria. However, we believe that

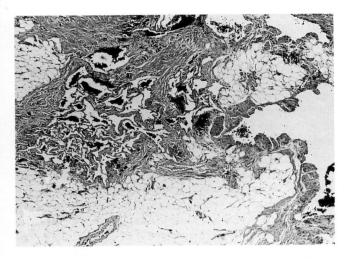

FIG. 23-57. Angiomatosis with small vessels residing adjacent to and within wall of larger vessel. (×60.) (Reprinted from *Am J Surg Pathol* 16:764, 1992.)

the irregular venous channels with clustered small vessels in their walls are quite characteristic of angiomatosis and should certainly in small biopsy specimens prompt a dialogue with the clinician concerning the extent of the lesion.

VASCULAR ECTASIAS

Vascular ectasias are collectively a common group of lesions characterized by localized dilatation of preformed ves-

sels. Although most are cutaneous and share certain common histological features, the clinical presentation and etiology are quite different. Thus in many instances a precise diagnosis depends on a complete knowledge of the clinical history and gross appearance of the lesion in question. Of the many types of vascular ectasias, only the more significant ones are mentioned. The reader is referred to an excellent review of the subject for detailed discussions of the less common forms.[3]

Nevus flammeus (nevus telangiectaticus)

The most common form of ectasia is the nevus flammeus or ordinary birthmark. These lesions are most common on the mid-forehead, eyelids, and nape of the neck.[206,207] It has been estimated that about half of all infants possess a nevus flammeus in the neck; this suggests a possible autosomal dominant mode of inheritance. Typically, the birthmark is a mottled macular lesion ranging in color from light pink to deep purple. Most are dull pink and are referred to as "salmon patches," or facetiously as "the affectionate peck of a stork." Most lesions eventually regress. Those on the forehead and eyelids are quite evanescent and disappear within the first year of life. Lesions on the nape of the neck fade more slowly, and their vestiges may be documented in about 20% of the adult population.

The *port-wine stain (nevus vinosus)* is a specialized form of nevus flammeus. It differs from the latter in several respects; it grows proportionately with the child and demonstrates no tendency to fade. Although it begins as a smooth

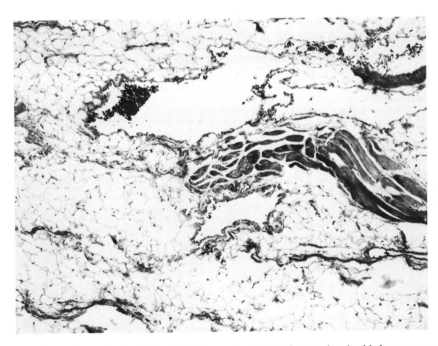

FIG. 23-58. Angiomatosis involving skeletal muscle. Tumor is associated with large amounts of mature fat, sometimes causing confusion with a lipomatosis. (×60.)

red to purple macular lesion on the face or extremity, it often acquires an elevated thickened surface that is more reminiscent of a true hemangioma. Some authors prefer to classify port-wine stain and nevus flammeus as forms of hemangioma.[5] However, histologically only a dilatation of vessels in the mid- and deep dermis is present, and in the early lesion even this change may not be pronounced. Comparison of port-wine stains with normal skin has not indicated any differences in immunostaining for factor VIII–associated protein, basement membrane protein, or fibronectin.[200] There does, however, appear to be a decrease in the number of perivascular nerves, suggesting that lack of neural control of the vascular bed results in their progressive dilatation.[205] Treatment of port-wine stains by laser therapy is under current investigation.[198,199]

Aside from the cosmetic problems it poses, the port-wine stain may indicate the presence of more extensive vascular malformation. Port-wine stains of the face that occur in the distribution of the trigeminal nerve may be associated with ipsilateral vascular malformations of the leptomeninges and occasionally of the retina (Sturge-Weber syndrome, encephalotrigeminal angiomatosis). Seizures, hemiplegia, and mental retardation, which characterize the full-blown syndrome, are the result of cerebral atrophy induced by the meningeal malformation. The Klippel-Trenaunay syndrome includes a port-wine stain associated with varicosities and hypertrophy (gigantism) of an extremity.[202,203] In most instances of this rare condition the lower extremity is affected, and the extensive varicosities and edema appear to be the result of agenesis of the deep venous structures. In a small percent of patients there may be, in addition, a congenital arteriovenous fistula. It has been suggested that this subgroup be separately designated as Parkes-Weber syndrome because the problems in management are different.[202,203] In Parkes-Weber syndrome the major therapeutic thrust must be directed toward reducing or eliminating the arteriovenous fistula in order to prevent supervening congestive heart failure.

Arterial spider

Arterial spiders (nevus araneus) represent another common form of ectasia, but unlike the nevus flammeus they are rarely found at birth. Instead they represent acquired lesions that are associated with altered physiological states (e.g., pregnancy, liver disease, hyperthyroidism); the lesions often regress with restoration of the normal state.[197] Grossly, they are characterized by a small central arteriole or "punctum" from which tiny radial vessels emanate. With application of pressure over the punctum the entire lesion blanches. With release of pressure the lesion reddens in a centrifugal direction. The vascular spider consists of a thick-walled arteriole, which dilates, branches as it approaches the surface epithelium, and eventually anastomoses with small capillaries of the dermis.

Hereditary hemorrhagic telangiectasia (Osler-Weber-Rendu disease)

This disease is characterized by vascular anomalies composed of dilated capillaries and veins of the skin and mucosal membranes.[204] It is inherited as an autosomal dominant disease and commences with the development of numerous small red papules on the skin and mucosa, particularly in the region of the face, lips, oral mucosa, and tongue. Similar lesions may be found in the gastrointestinal, genitourinary, and pulmonary systems. The lesions usually appear in childhood, increase with age, and in the elderly may have an appearance similar to the vascular spider. In contrast to the spider the lesions are prone to bleeding so that the course of the disease is marked by repeated bouts of hemorrhage. Treatment must be supportive because treatment of the ectasias by such modalities as electrocoagulation can result in formation of satellite lesions.

REACTIVE VASCULAR PROLIFERATIONS
Papillary endothelial hyperplasia (vegetant intravascular hemangioendothelioma, intravascular angiomatosis)

Papillary endothelial hyperplasia is an exuberant, usually intravascular, endothelial proliferation that in many respects mimics an angiosarcoma. It was first described by Masson, who designated it vegetant intravascular hemangioendothelioma.[214] He regarded it as a true neoplasm that displays degenerative changes including necrosis and thrombosis as it outgrows its blood supply. Henschen,[211] on the other hand, believed it was a primary endothelial proliferation occurring in response to inflammation and stasis within a vascular bed. His theory rested on the frequency with which this process occurred within vessels of inflamed hemorrhoids, urethral caruncles, and laryngeal polyps. Most evidence to date supports the contention that the lesion is an unusual form of organizing thrombus. Why only some thrombi display this form of organization is not entirely clear.

Although this process may occur in virtually any vessel in the body, only those lesions which present as detectable masses are likely to come to the attention of the surgical pathologist. In our experience such lesions are most commonly located within veins on the head, neck, fingers, and trunk, where they appear as small, firm, superficial (deep dermis or subcutis) masses imparting a red to blue discoloration to the overlying skin (Fig. 23-59).[209] Usually a history of trauma is not elicited. Both appearance and symptoms are nonspecific so that ultimately biopsy is required to establish the identity of the lesion. In addition to its occurrence in a pure form within a dilated vessel, this lesion may be engrafted on a preexisting vascular lesion such as a hemangioma, pyogenic granuloma, or vascular malformation. In these cases the symptoms, appearance, and ultimate prognosis are related to the underlying lesion. In fact, most

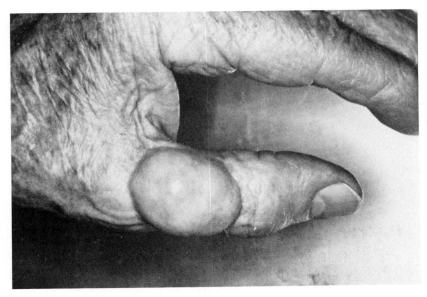

FIG. 23-59. Papillary endothelial hyperplasia presenting as localized nodule on thumb.

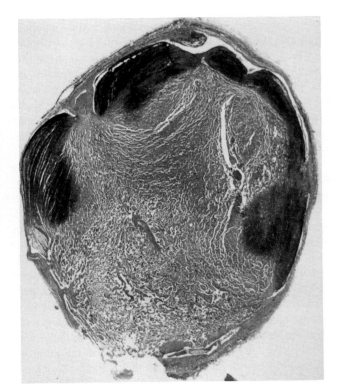

FIG. 23-60. Organizing thrombus within a vessel showing early stages of papillary endothelial hyperplasia at bottom of picture. (×15.)

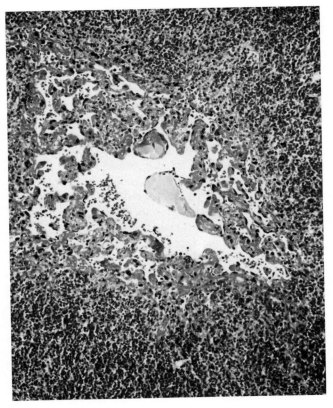

FIG. 23-61. Earliest stage of papillary endothelial hyperplasia. (×160.)

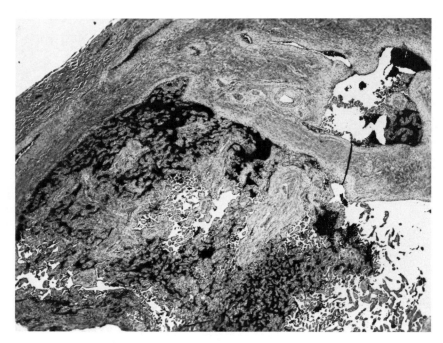

FIG. 23-62. Papillary endothelial hyperplasia occurring within dilated vessel. (×25.)

deeply situated examples of papillary endothelial hyperplasia are those which occur within intramuscular hemangiomas.

In its pure form the lesion is a small (average size, 2 cm), purple-red, multicystic mass containing clotted blood and surrounded by a fibrous pseudocapsule containing residual smooth muscle or elastic tissue of the preexisting vessel wall (Figs. 23-60 to 23-62). In vessels of small caliber that are markedly dilated, little or no muscle is demonstrable within the pseudocapsule. Rarely, rupture of the vessel of origin permits spilling over of the process into surrounding soft tissue, a phenomenon that should not be equated with malignancy. In our experience the vast majority of these lesions are intimately associated with thrombus material, lending support to the idea that they are unusual organizing thrombi. In the early lesion the ingrowth of endothelium along the contours of the thrombus partitions it into coarse papillae with fibrin cores (Figs. 23-61 to 23-64). In the well-established or typical lesion, a myriad of small delicate papillae project into the lumen and closely simulate the tufting growth of the hemangiosarcoma. These papillae are composed of a single layer of endothelium surrounding a collagenized core (Fig. 23-65). The endothelial cells appear plump or swollen but lack significant pleomorphism and mitotic figures (Fig. 23-66). In the late stage, clumping and fusing of the papillae give rise to an anastomosing network of vessels embedded in a loose meshlike stroma of connective tissue.

Ultrastructurally, the cells lining the papillae appear to be differentiated endothelial cells possessing numerous micropinocytotic vesicles at the luminal aspect, tight junctions along the lateral boundaries, and occasional intracytoplasmic Weibel-Palade bodies. Basal lamina invests the antiluminal surface of the cell. In addition, pericytes and undifferentiated cells can be identified on the antiluminal aspects of the endothelial cells.[212] The participation of several cell types is quite similar to the situation encountered in human granulation tissue and is further evidence of the reactive nature of this process.

The most significant aspect of this lesion is the regularity with which it is confused with an angiosarcoma. A helpful point in differential diagnosis is its intravascular location, since angiosarcomas are almost never confined to a vascular lumen. As mentioned earlier, passive extension of this process into soft tissue may occur following vessel rupture. However, even in these cases the intravascular location of most of the lesion, coupled with the reactive changes in the vessel wall suggesting rupture, aid in the proper identification. On very rare occasions papillary endothelial hyperplasia occurs extravascularly as a result of organization of a hematoma,[215] but this diagnosis should be made with caution (Figs. 23-67 and 23-68). Apart from the usual intravascular location, papillary endothelial hyperplasia lacks the frank tissue necrosis, marked pleomorphism, and relatively high mitotic rate that characterize most angiosarcomas.

The prognosis of this lesion is excellent. Essentially all cases are cured by simple excision. Those which do recur

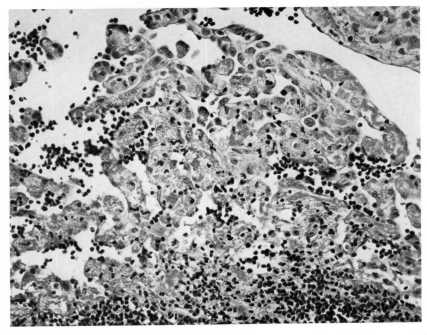

FIG. 23-63. Early stage of papillary endothelial hyperplasia. Thrombus material is present in lower half of picture, while top half shows incipient formation of papillary fronds. (×160.)

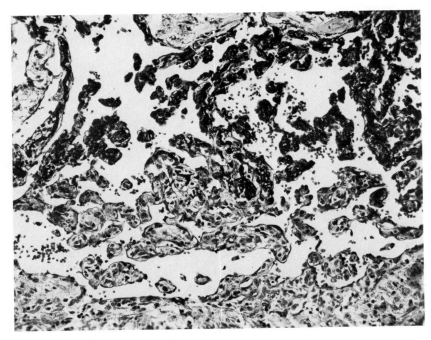

FIG. 23-64. Papillary endothelial hyperplasia with well-developed fronds, some of which still contain fibrin indicated by darkly staining material. (PTAH; ×160.)

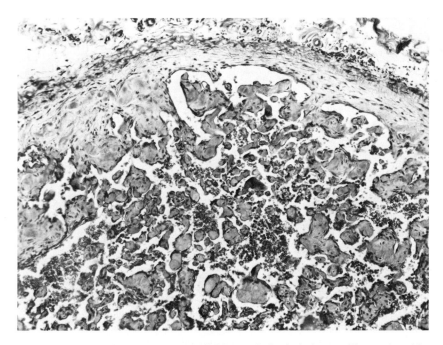

FIG. 23-65. Late stage of papillary endothelial hyperplasia depicting papillary tufts with central hyaline cores. (×100.)

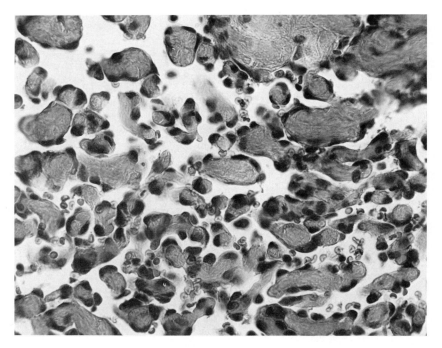

FIG. 23-66. Papillary endothelial hyperplasia. Tufts are lined for the most part by a single layer of endothelial cells devoid of pleomorphism and mitotic activity. (×350.)

are usually those which are superimposed on vascular tumors. The therapy in these cases should be dictated by the nature of the underlying lesions.

Vascular transformation of lymph node (nodal angiomatosis)

First described as *vascular transformation of lymph node*[219] and later as *nodal angiomatosis*,[218] this reactive change of lymph node occurs secondary to lymphatic or venous obstruction, or both, and has been observed particularly in axillary lymph nodes removed at the time of radical mastectomy for breast carcinoma. The change may also occur in lymph nodes removed for a variety of other diagnostic or therapeutic reasons. Typically the change involves the subcapsular space and sinuses in either a segmental or diffuse fashion. In the most readily recognized case the small, ectatic, capillary-sized vessels are well formed (Fig 23-69). Chan et al.[217] have recently emphasized a greater range of changes in this condition than previously appreciated. In extreme examples of vascular transformation the vessels may be closely packed and slightly attenuated so that the resemblance to Kaposi's sarcoma is more than fleeting. Usually, however, there is a maturation of the vessels toward the periphery of the lymph node such that ectatic capillaries are present immediately subjacent to the capsule. Extravasation of erythrocytes occurs, and in exceptional cases hyaline droplets, similar to those in Kaposi's sarcoma, are identified.

There are a number of features that serve to distinguish this lesion from Kaposi's sarcoma. These include the overall preservation of lymph node architecture despite the expansion of the subcapsular and medullary sinuses, the peripheral maturation of the vessels, the lack of vessels arranged in distinct fascicles, and the presence of secondary sclerosis. However, the earliest stages of Kaposi's sarcoma of lymph node, as seen in the patient with acquired immunodeficiency syndrome, may prove exceptionally difficult and at some times impossible to distinguish from vascular transformation of the lymph node.

Glomeruloid hemangioma

Glomeruloid hemangioma is a descriptive term coined by Chan et al.[221] for the reactive vascular proliferations that

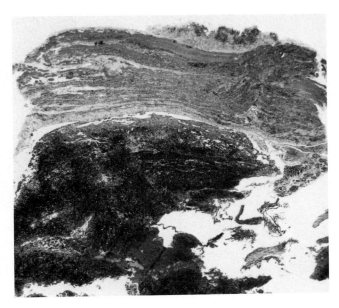

FIG. 23-67. Papillary endothelial hyperplasia occurring within an intramuscular hematoma. (×15.)

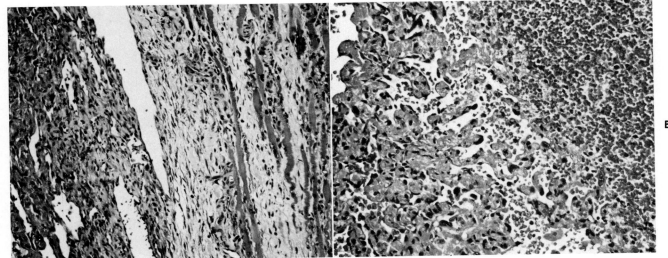

FIG. 23-68. High-power view of Fig. 23-67 illustrating the extravascular location (**A**) of the endothelial proliferation (**B**). (**A** and **B**, ×160.)

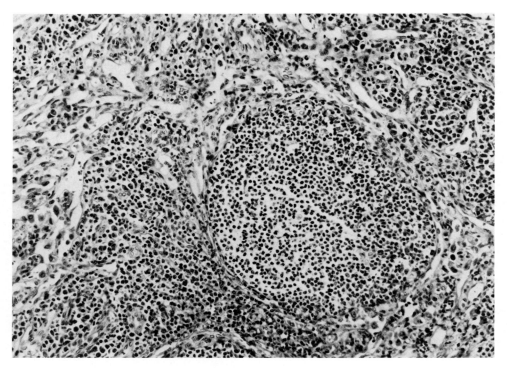

FIG. 23-69. Vascular transformation occurring within a lymph node (nodal angiomatosis). Vessels surround but preserve lymph follicles. Lymph node was removed as part of regional lymph node dissection for carcinoma. (×160.)

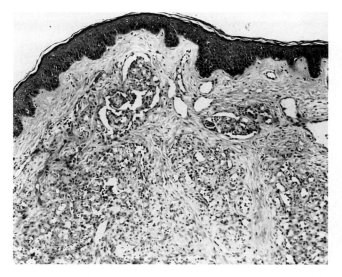

FIG. 23-70. Glomeruloid hemangioma. (×60.) (Case courtesy of C.D.M. Fletcher, M.D.)

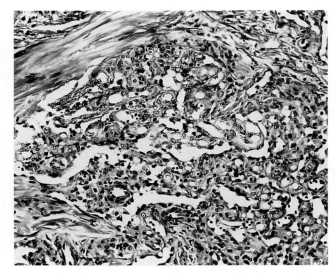

FIG. 23-71. Glomeruloid hemangioma. (×160.) (Case courtesy of C.D.M. Fletcher, M.D.)

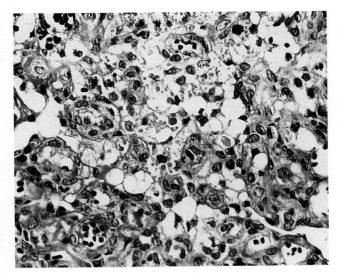

FIG. 23-72. Hyaline droplets of immunoglobulin within glomeruloid hemangioma. (×400.) (Case courtesy of C.D.M. Fletcher, M.D.)

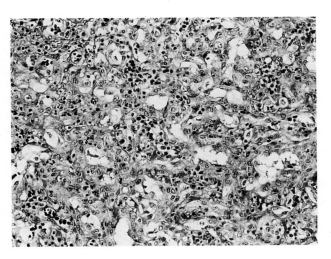

FIG. 23-73. Bacillary angiomatosis showing endothelial cells with clear cytoplasm set amidst an inflammatory background. (×160.)

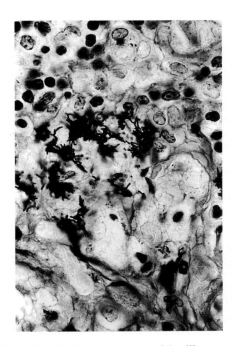

FIG. 23-74. Warthin-Starry staining of bacillary angiomatosis showing numerous clumped rod-shaped organisms. (×400.)

occur in *POEMS syndrome* (Takatsuki syndrome and Crowe-Fukase syndrome).[221-224] This syndrome is characterized by *p*olyneuropathy (peripheral neuropathy, papilledema), *o*rganomegaly (hepatosplenomegaly, lymphadenopathy), *e*ndocrinopathy (amenorrhea, gynecomastia, impotence, adrenal insufficiency, hypothyroidism, glucose intolerance), *M*-protein (plasmacytosis, paraproteinemia, bone lesions), and *s*kin lesions (hyperpigmentation, hypertrichosis, angiomas) and in some instances overlaps with multicentric Castleman's disease.

The vascular lesions develop within the dermis beneath an intact and essentially normal epidermis. In the classic case, glomeruloid nests of capillaries lie within ectatic capillaries creating a "vessel within a vessel" appearance (Figs. 23-70 and 23-71). The intravascular capillaries are lined by normal-appearing endothelium and are filled with erythrocytes. A distinctive feature of the intravascular proliferation are the large round cells filled with eosinophilic globules corresponding to polytypic immunoglobulin (Fig. 23-72). Chan et al.[221] suggest that these cells, which reside principally outside the basal lamina, are closely related to endothelial cells rather than pericytes or smooth muscle cells. Their unusual appearance is probably induced by the presence of cytoplasmic immunoglobulin, which is derived from serum. In some cases of POEMS syndrome the vascular lesions may be indistinguishable from an ordinary capillary hemangioma and in other cases the lesions may show features intermediate between a capillary hemangioma and the classic glomeruloid hemangioma, suggesting that they represent stages of the same process.

Bacillary (epithelioid) angiomatosis

Bacillary (epithelioid) angiomatosis is a pseudoneoplastic vascular proliferation occurring almost exclusively in immunocompromised hosts, which is caused by a recently recognized rikettsia, *Rochalimaea henselae*.[229,230] In the typical case the disease is characterized by numerous red skin lesions, which may resemble Kaposi's sarcoma clinically. In some cases there are also liver, spleen, lymph node, bone, and soft tissue lesions.[225-228,231] A proliferation of capillary-sized vessels lined by plump endothelium with clear cytoplasm typify the skin and soft tissue lesions (Fig. 23-73). Mild atypia and occasional mitotic figures may be present within the endothelial cells. Although the strikingly clear cytoplasm of the endothelial cells bears some similarity to the endothelial changes in epithelioid

hemangioma, there is typically a striking neutrophilic infiltrate within the interstitium along with collections of pink coagulum containing clusters of the organisms that are easily identified on Warthin-Starry staining (Fig. 23-74). On electron microscopy, the organisms appear as bacillary forms with a trilaminar cell wall. In the liver the organisms induce peliotic changes. Large numbers of organisms can be identified around the peliotic zones in the liver.

REFERENCES

General

1. Burgdorf WCH, Mukai K, Rosai J: Immunohistochemical identification of factor VIII–related antigen in endothelial cells of cutaneous lesions of alleged vascular nature. *Am J Clin Pathol* 75:167, 1981.
2. Coffin CM, Dehner LP: Vascular tumors in children and adolescents: a clinicopathologic study of 228 tumors in 222 patients. *Pathol Annu* 1:97, 1993.
3. Esterly NB: Cutaneous hemangiomas, vascular stains, and associated syndromes. *Curr Probl Pediatr* 17:7, 1987.
4. Geshickter CF, Keasbey LE: Tumors of blood vessels. *Am J Cancer* 23:568, 1935.
5. Johnson WC: Pathology of cutaneous vascular tumors. *Int J Dermatol* 15:239, 1976.
6. Madewell JE, Sweet DE: Tumors and tumorlike lesions in or about joints. In Resnick D, Niwayama G, editors: *Diagnosis of bone and joint disorders,* vol 3, Philadelpha, 1981, WB Saunders.
7. Nadji M, Gonzalez MS, Castro A, et al: Factor VIII–related antigen: an endothelial cell marker. *Lab Invest* 42:139A, 1980.
8. Rook A, Wilkinson DS, Ebling FJ, editors: *Textbook of dermatology,* ed 3, vol 1, Oxford, 1979, Blackwell Scientific Publications.
9. Stout AP: Hemangioendothelioma: a tumor of blood vessels featuring vascular endothelial cells. *Ann Surg* 118:445, 1943.
10. Tsang WYW, Chan JKC, Fletcher CDM: Recently characterized vascular tumors of the skin and soft tissues. *Histopathology* 19:489, 1991.
11. Waldo ED, Yuetin JC, Kaye GI: The ultrastructure of vascular tumors: additional observations and a review of the literature. *Pathol Annu* 12:279, 1977.
12. Weiss SW: Vascular tumors: a deductive approach to diagnosis. *Surg Pathol* 2:185, 1989.

Normal structure and function

13. Buonassisi V, Colburn P: Hormone and surface receptors in vascular endothelium. In Altura BM, editor: *Advances in microcirculation,* vol 9, Basel, 1979, S. Karger.
14. Fernando NVP, Movat HZ: The fine structure of the terminal vascular bed. III. Capillaries. *Exp Molec Path* 3:87, 1964.
15. Fojardo LF: The complexity of endothelial cells: a review. *Am J Clin Pathol* 92:241, 1989.
16. Folkman J: How is blood vessel growth regulated in normal and neoplastic tissue? G.H.A. Clowes Memorial Award Lecture. *Cancer Res* 46:467, 1986.
17. Hammersen F: Endothelial contractility—does it exist? In Altura BM, editor: *Advances in microcirculation,* vol 9, Basel, 1979, S. Karger.
18. Haudenschild CC, Cotran RS, Gimbrone MA, et al: Fine structure of vascular endothelium in culture. *J Ultrastruct Res* 50:22, 1975.
19. Hoyer LW: The factor VIII complex: structure and function. *Blood* 58:1, 1981.

20. Jaffe EA, Nachman RL, Becker CG, et al: Culture of human endothelial cells derived from umbilical veins: identification by morphologic and immunologic criteria. *J Clin Invest* 52:2745, 1973.
21. Majno G: Ultrastructure of the vascular membrane. In Hamilton WF, Dow P, editors: *Circulation, handbook of physiology,* vol 3, American Physiology Society, 1965, Washington, DC.
22. Majno G, Palade GE, Schoeff GI: Studies on inflammation. II. The site of action of histamine and serotonin along the vascular tree: a topographic study. *J Biophys Biochem Cytol* 11:607, 1961.
23. Majno G, Shea SM, Leventhal M: Endothelial contraction induced by histamine-type mediators: an electron microscopic study. *J Cell Biol* 42:647, 1969.
24. Messmer K, Hammersen F, editors: *Structure and function of endothelial cells,* Basel, 1983, S. Karger.
25. Rhodin JAG: The ultrastructure of mammalian arterioles and precapillary sphincters. *J Ultrastruct Res* 18:181, 1967.
26. Rhodin JAG: Ultrastructure of mammalian venous capillaries, venules, and small collecting veins. *J Ultrastruct Res* 25:452, 1969.
27. Romanul FCA, Bannister RG: Localized areas of high alkaline phosphatase activity in the terminal arterial tree. *J Cell Biol* 15:73, 1962.
28. Thorgeirsson G, Robertson AL Jr: The vascular endothelium—pathobiologic significance (Review). *Am J Pathol* 93:801, 1978.
29. Toth B, Malick L: Scanning electron microscopic study of the surface characteristics of neoplastic endothelial cells of blood vessels. *J Pathol* 118:59, 1976.
30. Turner RR, Beckstead JH, Warnke RA, et al: Endothelial cell phenotypic diversity. *Am J Clin Pathol* 87:569, 1987.
31. Wagner RC: Endothelial cell embryology and growth. In Altura BM, editor: *Advances in microcirculation,* vol 9, Basel, 1979, S. Karger.
32. Zetter BR: Endothelial heterogeneity: Influence of vessel size, organ localization, and species specificity on the properties of cultured endothelial cells. In Ryan U, editor: *Endothelial cells,* vol 2, Boca Rotan, Florida, 1987, CRC Press.

Hemangiomas (general)

33. Alessi E, Bertani E, Sala F: Acquired tufted angioma. *Am J Dermatopathol* 8:426, 1986.
34. Baker AL, Kahn PC, Binder SC: Gastrointestinal bleeding due to blue rubber bleb nevus syndrome. *Gastroenterology* 61:530, 1971.
35. Behar A, Moran E, Izak G: Acquired hypofibrinogenemia associated with a giant cavernous hemangioma of the liver. *Am J Clin Pathol* 40:78, 1963.
36. Blix S, Aas K: Giant haemangioma, thrombocytopenia, fibrogenopenia, and fibrinolytic activity. *Acta Med Scand* 169:63, 1961.
37. Boley SJ, Morse WE: Hormonally influenced hemangioma. *Arch Surg* 74:482, 1957.
38. Booher RJ: Tumors arising from blood vessels in the hands and feet. *Clin Orthop* 19:71, 1961.
39. Brizel HE, Raccuglia G: Giant hemangioma with thrombocytopenia: radioisotope demonstration of platelet sequestration. *Blood* 26:751, 1965.

40. Calonje E, Fletcher CDM: Sinusoidal hemangioma: a distinctive benign vascular neoplasm within the group of cavernous hemangiomas. *Am J Surg Pathol* 15:1130, 1991.

41. Cohen SR, Wange CI: Steroid treatment of hemangioma of the head and neck in children. *Ann Otol* 81:584, 1972.

42. de Prost Y, Teillac D, Bodemer C, et al: Successful treatment of Kasabach-Merritt syndrome with pentoxifylline. *J Am Acad Dermatol* 25:854, 1991.

43. Edgerton MT: The treatment of hemangiomas with special reference to the role of steroid therapy. *Ann Surg* 163:517, 1976.

44. Edgerton MT, Hiebert JM: Vascular and lymphatic tumors in infancy, childhood, and adulthood: challenge of diagnosis and treatment. *Curr Probl Cancer* 7:1, 1978.

45. Ezekowitz RA, Mulliken JB, Folkman J: Interferon alfa-2a therapy for life-threatening hemangiomas of infancy. *N Engl J Med* 326:1456, 1992.

46. Hagood MF, Gathright JB: Hemangiomatosis of the skin and GI tract. *Dis Colon Rectum* 18:141, 1975.

47. Henley JD, Danielson CFM, Rothenberger SS, et al: Kasabach-Merritt syndrome with profound platelet support. *Am J Clin Pathol* 99:628, 1993.

48. Hoehn JG, Farow CM, Devine KD, et al: Invasive hemangioma of the head and neck. *Am J Surg* 120:495, 1970.

49. Imperial R, Helwig EB: Verrucous hemangioma: a clinicopathologic study of 21 cases. *Arch Dermatol* 96:247, 1967.

50. Inceman S, Tangu Y: Chronic defibrination syndrome due to a giant hemangioma associated with microangiopathic hemolytic anemia. *Am J Med* 46:997, 1969.

51. Johnson KW, Ghormley RK, Dockerty MB: Hemangiomas of the extremities. *Surg Gynecol Obstet* 102:531, 1956.

52. Kasabach HH, Merritt KK: Capillary hemangioma with extensive purpura: report of a case. *Am J Dis Child* 59:1063, 1961.

53. Lasser AE, Stein AF: Steroid treatment of hemangiomas in children. *Arch Dermatol* 108:565, 1973.

54. MacCollum DW, Martin LW: Hemangioma in infancy and childhood: a report based on 6479 cases. *Surg Clin North Am* 36:1647, 1956.

55. Margileth AM, Museles M: Current concepts in diagnosis and management of congenital cutaneous hemangiomas. *Pediatrics* 36:410, 1965.

56. Martin LN, MacCollum DW: Hemangioma in infants and children. *Am J Surg* 101:571, 1961.

57. Nichols GE, Gaffey MJ, Mills SE, et al: Lobular capillary hemangioma: an immunohistochemical study including steroid hormone receptor status. *Am J Clin Pathol* 97:77, 1992.

58. Oughterson AW, Tennant R: Angiomatous tumors of the hands and feet. *Surgery* 5:75, 1939.

59. Pearl CS, Matthews WH: Congenital retroperitoneal hemangioendothelioma with Kasabach-Merritt syndrome. *South Med J* 72:239, 1979.

60. Watson WL, McCarthy WD: Blood and lymph vessel tumors. *Surg Gynecol Obstet* 71:569, 1940.

61. Weiss SW: Pedal hemangioma (venous malformation) occurring in Turner's syndrome: an additional manifestation of the syndrome. *Hum Pathol* 19:1015, 1988.

62. White CW, Sondhein HM, Crouch EC, et al: Treatment of pulmonary hemangiomatosis with recombinant interferon alfa-2a. *N Engl J Med* 320:1197, 1989.

63. Wilson Jones E: Malignant vascular tumors. *Clin Exp Dermatol* 1:287, 1976.

64. Wind MS, Pillari G: Deep soft tissue hemangioma of infancy: Kasabach-Merritt syndrome. *N Y State J Med* 79:373, 1979.

Juvenile hemangioma

65. Bowers RE, Graham EA, Tomlinson KM: Spontaneous cure of strawberry nevi. *Arch Dermatol* 82:667, 1960.

66. Campbell JS: Congenital capillary hemangiomas of the parotid gland: a lesion characteristic of infancy. *N Engl J Med* 254:56, 1956.

67. Goldman RL, Perzik SL: Infantile hemangioma of the parotid gland: a clinicopathological study of 15 cases. *Arch Otolaryngol* 90:605, 1969.

68. Gonzalez-Crussi F, Hull MT, Grosfeld JL, et al: Congenital hemangioendothelioma: immunologic and ultrastructural studies. *Lab Invest* 38:387A, 1978.

69. Gonzalez-Crussi F, Reyes-Mugica M: Cellular hemangiomas (hemangioendotheliomas) in infants: light microscopic, immunohistochemical, and ultrastructural observations. *Am J Surg Pathol* 15:769, 1991.

70. Kumakiri M, Muramoto F, Tsukinaga T, et al: Crystalline lamellae in the endothelial cells of a type of hemangioma characterized by the proliferation of immature endothelial cells and pericytes. *J Am Acad Dermatol* 8:68, 1983.

71. Lister WA: The natural history of strawberry nevi. *Lancet* 1:1429, 1938.

72. McFarland J: A congenital capillary angioma of the parotid gland: considerations of similar cases in the literature. *Arch Pathol* 9:820, 1930.

73. Pasyk KA, Grabb WC, Cherry GW: Cellular hemangioma: light and electron microscopic studies of two cases. *Virchows Arch (Pathol Anat)* 396:103, 1982.

74. Pasyk KA, Grabb WC, Cherry GW: Crystalloid inclusions in endothelial cells of cellular and capillary hemangiomas. *Arch Dermatol* 119:134, 1983.

75. Pasyk KA, Grabb WC, Cherry GW: Ultrastructure of mast cells in growing and involuting stages of hemangiomas. *Hum Pathol* 14:174, 1983.

76. Taxy JB, Gray SR: Cellular angiomas of infancy: an ultrastructural study of two cases. *Cancer* 43:2322, 1979.

77. Walsh TS, Tompkins VN: Some observations on the strawberry nevus of infancy. *Cancer* 9:869, 1956.

78. Wawro NM, Fredrickson RW, Tennant RW: Hemangioma of the parotid gland in the newborn and in infancy. *Cancer* 8:595, 1955.

79. Yasunaga C, Sueshi K, Ohgami H, et al: Heterogeneous expression of endothelial cell markers in infantile hemangioendothelioma: immunohistochemical study of two solitary cases and one multiple one. *Am J Clin Pathol* 91:673, 1989.

Acquired tufted angioma

80. Alessi E, Bertani E, Sala F: Acquired tufted hemangioma. *Am J Dermatopathol* 8:68, 1986.

81. Kumakiri M, Muramoto LF, Tsukinga I, et al: Crystalline lamellae in the endothelial cells of a type of hemangioma characterized by the proliferation of immature endothelial cells and pericytes-angioblastoma (Nakagawa). *J Am Acad Dermatol* 8:68, 1983.

82. Padilla RS, Orkin M, Rosai J: Acquired tufted angioma (progressive capillary hemangioma): a distinctive clinicopathologic entity related to lobular capillary hemangioma. *Am J Dermatopathol* 9:292, 1987.

83. Wilson-Jones E, Orkin M: Tufted angioma (angioblastoma): a benign progressive angioma, not to be confused with Kaposi's sarcoma or low-grade angiosarcoma. *J Am Acad Dermatol* 20:214, 1989.

Targetoid hemosiderotic hemangioma

84. Rapini RP, Golitz LE: Targetoid hemosiderotic hemangioma. *J Cutan Pathol* 17:233, 1990.

85. Santa Cruz DJ, Aronberg J: Targetoid hemosiderotic hemangioma. *J Am Acad Dermatol* 19:550, 1988.

86. Vion B, Frenk E: Targetoid hemosiderotic hemangioma. *Dermatology* 184:300, 1992.

Arteriovenous hemangioma

87. Bluefarb SM, Adams LA: Arteriovenous malformation with angiodermatitis: stasis dermatitis simulating Kaposi's sarcoma. *Arch Dermatol* 96:176, 1967.
88. Connelly MG, Winkelmann RK: Acral arteriovenous tumor: a clinicopathologic review. *Am J Surg Pathol* 9:15, 1985.
89. Earhart RN, Aeling JA, Nuss DD, et al: Pseudo-Kaposi's sarcoma: a patient with arteriovenous malformation and skin lesions simulating Kaposi's sarcoma. *Arch Dermatol* 110:907, 1974.
90. Girard C, Graham JH, Johnson WC: Arteriovenous hemangioma (arteriovenous shunt): a clinicopathological and histochemical study. *J Clin Pathol* 1:73, 1974.
91. Lawton RL, Tidrick RT, Brintall ES: A clinicopathologic study of multiple congenital arteriovenous fistulae of the lower extremities. *Angiology* 8:161, 1957.
92. Reid MR: Abnormal arteriovenous communications acquired and congenital. II. The origin and nature of arteriovenous aneurysms, cirsoid aneurysms, and simple angiomas. *Arch Surg* 10:996, 1925.
93. Rusin LJ, Harrell ER: Arteriovenous fistula: cutaneous manifestations. *Arch Dermatol* 112:1135, 1976.
94. Strutton G, Weedon D: Acro-angiodermatitis: a simulant of Kaposi's sarcoma. *Am J Dermatopathol* 9:85, 1987.
95. Ward CE, Horton BT: Congenital arteriovenous fistulas in children. *J Pediatr* 16:746, 1940.

Epithelioid hemangioma

96. Castro C, Winkelmann RK: Angiolymphoid hyperplasia with eosinophilia in the skin. *Cancer* 34:1969, 1974.
97. Daniels DG, Schrodt R, Fleigelman MT, et al: Ultrastructural study of a case of angiolymphoid hyperplasia with eosinophilia. *Arch Dermatol* 109:870, 1974.
98. Eady RAJ, Cowen T, Wilson-Jones E: Pseudopyogenic granuloma: the histopathogenesis in the light of ultrastructural studies. *Br J Dermatol* 95(suppl):14, 1976.
99. Eady RAJ, Wilson-Jones E: Pseudopyogenic granuloma: enzyme histochemical and ultrastructural study. *Hum Pathol* 8:653, 1977.
100. Fattah A, Fahmy A: Subcutaneous lymphoid hyperplasia with eosinophilia. *Dermatologica* 139:220, 1969.
101. Fetsch JF, Weiss SW: Observations concerning the pathogenesis of epithelioid hemangioma (angiolymphoid hyperplasia). *Mod Pathol* 4:449, 1991.
102. Henry PG, Burnett JW: Angiolymphoid hyperplasia with eosinophilia. *Arch Dermatol* 114:1168, 1978.
103. Kandil E: Dermal angiolymphoid hyperplasia with eosinophilia versus pseudopyogenic granuloma. *Br J Dermatol* 83:405, 1970.
104. Kawada A, Takahashi H, Anzai T: Eosinophilic lymphofolliculosis of the skin (Kimura's disease). *Jpn J Dermatol* 76:61, 1966.
105. Kindblom L-G, Fassina AS: Angiolymphoid hyperplasia with eosinophilia of the skin. *Acta Pathol Microbiol Scand* 89A:271, 1981.
106. Kitabatake T, Kurokawa H, Kurokawa S, et al: Radiotherapy for eosinophilic granuloma of the soft tissue (Kimura's disease). *Strahlentherapie* 144:407, 1972.
107. Mehregan AH, Shapiro L: Angiolymphoid hyperplasia with eosinophilia. *Arch Dermatol* 103:50, 1971.
108. Moesner J, Pallesen R, Sorensen B: Angiolymphoid hyperplasia with eosinophilia (Kimura's disease): a case with dermal lesions in the knee and a popliteal arteriovenous fistula. *Arch Dermatol* 117:650, 1981.
109. Olsen TJ, Helwig EB: Angiolymphoid hyperplasia with eosinophilia: a clinicopathologic study of 116 patients. *J Am Acad Dermatopathol* 12:781, 1985.

110. Peterson WC, Fusaro RM, Goltz RW: Atypical pyogenic granuloma: a case of benign hemangioendotheliosis. *Arch Dermatol* 90:197, 1964.
111. Reed RJ, Terazakis N: Subcutaneous angioblastic lymphoid hyperplasia with eosinophilia (Kimura's disease). *Cancer* 29:489, 1972.
112. Rosai J, Ackerman LR: Intravenous atypical vascular proliferation: a cutaneous lesion simulating a malignant blood vessel tumor. *Arch Dermatol* 109:714, 1974.
113. Rosai J, Gold J, Landy R: The histiocytoid hemangiomas: a unifying concept embracing several previously described entities of skin, soft tissue, large vessels, bone, and heart. *Hum Pathol* 10:707, 1979.
114. Waldo E, Sidhu GS, Stahl R, et al: Histiocytoid hemangioma with features of angiolymphoid hyperplasia and Kaposi's sarcoma: a study by light microscopy, electron microscopy, and immunologic techniques. *Am J Dermatopathol* 5:525, 1983.
115. Wells GC, Summerly R: Subcutaneous lymphoid hyperplasia with eosinophilia. *Proc R Soc Med* 56:728, 1963.
116. Wells GC, Whimster I: Subcutaneous angiolymphoid hyperplasia with eosinophilia. *Br J Dermatol* 81:1, 1969.

Kimura's disease

117. Chan JKC, Hui PK, Ng CS, et al: Epithelioid hemangioma (angiolymphoid hyperplasia with eosinophilia) and Kimura's disease in Chinese. *Histopathology* 15:557, 1989.
118. Googe PB, Harris NL, Mihm MC: Kimura's disease and angiolymphoid hyperplasia with eosinophils: two distinct histopathological entities. *J Cutan Pathol* 14:263, 1987.
119. Hui PK, Chan JKC, Ng CS, et al: Lymphadenopathy of Kimura's disease. *Am J Surg Pathol* 13:177, 1989.
120. Kimura T, Yoshimura S, Ishikawa E: Unusual granulation combined with hyperplastic change of lymphatic tissue. *Trans Soc Pathol Jpn* 37:179, 1948.
121. Kung ITM, Gibson JB, Bannatyne PM: Kimura's disease: a clinicopathological study of 21 cases and its distinction from angiolymphoid hyperplasia with eosinophilia. *Pathology* 16:39, 1984.
122. Kuo TT, Shih L-Y, Chan H-L: Kimura's disease: involvement of regional lymph nodes and distinction from angiolymphoid hyerplasia with eosinophilia. *Am J Surg Pathol* 12:843, 1988.
123. Quinibi WY, Al-Sibai MB, Akhtar M: Mesangioproliferative glomerulonephritis associated with Kimura's disease. *Clin Nephrol* 30:111, 1988.
124. Urabe A, Tsuneyoshi M, Enjoji M: Epithelioid hemangioma versus Kimura's disease: a comparative clinicopathologic study. *Am J Surg Pathol* 11: 758, 1987.
125. Yamada A, Mitsuhashi K, Miyakawa Y, et al: Membranous glomerulonephritis associated with eosinophilic folliculitis of the skin (Kimura's disease): report of a case and review of the literature. *Clin Nephrol* 18:211, 1982.

Granulation tissue-type hemangioma (pyogenic granuloma)

126. Batsakis JG: *Tumors of the head and neck: clinical and pathological considerations.* Vasoformative tumors (Chapter 15). Baltimore, 1979, Williams & Wilkins.
127. Bhaskar SN, Jacoway JR: Pyogenic granuloma: clinical features, incidence, histology, and result of treatment: Report of 242 cases. *J Oral Surg* 24:391, 1966.
128. Choukas NC, Toto PD: Pyogenic granuloma: report of a case. *Oral Surg Oral Med Oral Pathol* 22:194, 1966.
129. Cooper PH, McAllister HA, Helwig EB: Intravenous pyogenic granuloma: a study of 18 cases. *Am J Surg Pathol* 3:221, 1979.
130. Coskey RJ, Mehregan AH: Granuloma pyogenicum with multiple satellite recurrences. *Arch Dermatol* 96:71, 1967.
131. De Kaminsky AR, Otero AC, Kaminsky CA, et al: Multiple disseminated pyogenic granuloma. *Br J Dermatol* 98:461, 1978.

132. Evans CD, Warin RP: Pyogenic granuloma with local recurrences. *Br J Dermatol* 69:106, 1957.

133. Frain-Bell W: Multiple pyogenic granulomata. *Br J Dermatol* 70:428, 1958.

134. Grupper C, Pastel A: Pyogenic granuloma with multiple satellites. *Bull Soc Franc Derm Syph* 76:496, 1969.

135. Juhlin L, Sven-Olaf H, Ponten J, et al: Disseminated granuloma pyogenicum. *Acta Derm Venereol (Stock)* 50:134, 1970.

136. Kerr DA: Granuloma pyogenicum. *Oral Surg Oral Med Oral Pathol* 4:158, 1951.

137. McDonald RH: Granuloma gravidarum. *Am J Obstet Gynecol* 72:1132, 1956.

138. Michelson HE: Granuloma pyogenicum: clinical and histological review of 29 cases. *Arch Dermatol* 12:492, 1925.

139. Mills SE, Cooper PH, Fechner RE: Lobular capillary hemangioma: the underlying lesion of pyogenic granuloma. *Am J Surg Pathol* 4:471, 1980.

140. Montgomery DW, Culver GD: Granuloma pyogenicum. *Arch Dermatol Syph* 26:131, 1932.

141. Nagashima N, Niizuma K: Multiple satellite granuloma telangiectaticum. *Jpn J Dermatol* 82:1, 1972.

142. Rowe L: Granuloma pyogenicum. *AMA Arch Dermatol* 78:341, 1958.

143. Tulevech CB, Cabaud P: Granuloma pyogenicum. *Am J Ophthalmol* 66:957, 1968.

144. Ulbright TM, Santa Cruz DI: Intravenous pyogenic granuloma: a case report with ultrastructural findings. *Cancer* 45:1646, 1980.

145. Warner J, Wilson-Jones E: Pyogenic granuloma recurring with multiple satellites: a report of 11 cases. *Br J Dermatol* 80:218, 1968.

146. Wilson BB, Greer KE, Cooper PH: Eruptive disseminated lobular capillary hemangioma (pyogenic granuloma). *J Am Acad Dermatol* 21:391, 1989.

147. Zaynoun ST, Juljulian HH, Kurban AK: Pyogenic granuloma with multiple satellites. *Arch Dermatol* 9:689, 1974.

Intramuscular hemangioma

148. Allen PW, Enzinger FM: Hemangiomas of skeletal muscle: an analysis of 89 cases. *Cancer* 29:8, 1972.

149. Angervall L, Nielsen JM, Stener B, et al: Concomitant arteriovenous vascular malformation in skeletal muscle. *Cancer* 44:232, 1979.

150. Angervall L, Nilsson L, Stener B, et al: Angiographic, microangiographic, and histologic study of vascular malformation in striated muscle. *Acta Radiol* 7:65, 1968.

151. Beham A, Fletcher CDM: Intramuscular angioma: a clinicopathologic analysis of 74 cases. *Histopathology* 18:53, 1991.

152. Chauhan ND: Skeletal muscle hemangioma. *J Irish Med Assoc* 66:291, 1973.

153. Cohen AJ, Youkey JR, Clagett GP: Intramuscular hemangioma. *JAMA* 249:2680, 1983.

154. Conners JJ, Khan G: Hemangioma of the striated muscle. *South Med J* 70:1423, 1977.

155. Davis JS, Kitlowski EA: Primary intramuscular hemangiomas of striated muscle. *Arch Surg* 20:39, 1930.

156. Fergusson IL: Hemangiomata of skeletal muscle. *Br J Surg* 59:634, 1972.

157. Fulton MN, Sosman MC: Venous angiomas of skeletal muscle. *JAMA* 119:319, 1942.

158. Godanich IF, Capanacci M: Vascular hamartomata and infantile angioectatic osteohyperplasia of the extremities. *J Bone Joint Surg* 44A:815, 1962.

159. Jenkins HR, Delaney PA: Benign angiomatous tumors of skeletal muscles. *Surg Gynecol Obstet* 55:464, 1932.

160. LaSorte AF: Cavernous hemangioma of striated muscle. *Am J Surg* 100:593, 1960.

161. MacDermott EN: Two cases of hemangioma of voluntary muscle: a brief review of the literature. *Br J Surg* 23:252, 1935.

162. Mailer R: Traumatic hemangiomatous tumors of skeletal muscle. *Br J Surg* 23:245, 1935.

163. Scott JES: Hemangiomata in skeletal muscle. *Br J Surg* 44:496, 1957.

164. Shallow TA, Eger SA, Wagner FB: Primary hemangiomatous tumors of skeletal muscle. *Ann Surg* 119:700, 1944.

165. Sutherland AD: Equinus deformity due to hemangioma of calf muscle. *J Bone Joint Surg* 57B:104, 1975.

166. Trias A, Dilenge D: A new approach to the treatment of cavernous hemangioma of skeletal muscle. *J Bone Joint Surg* 54B:770, 1972.

Synovial hemangioma

167. Bate TH: Hemangioma of the tendon sheath. *J Bone Joint Surg* 36A:104, 1954.

168. Bennett GE, Cobey MC: Hemangioma of joints: report of five cases. *Arch Surg* 38:487, 1939.

169. Burman MS, Milgram JE: Hemangioma of tendon and tendon sheath. *Surg Gynecol Obstet* 50:397, 1930.

170. Cobey MC: Hemangioma of joints. *Arch Surg* 46:465, 1943.

171. Harkins HN: Hemangioma of a tendon sheath: report of a case with a study of 24 cases from the literature. *Arch Surg* 34:12, 1937.

172. Lichtenstein L: Tumors of synovial joints, bursae, and tendon sheath. *Cancer* 8:816, 1955.

173. McInerney D, Park WM: Thermographic assessment of synovial hemangioma. *Clin Radiol* 29:469, 1978.

174. Osgood RB: Tuberculosis of the knee joint: angioma of the knee joint. *Surg Clin North Am* 1:665, 1921.

175. Webster GV, Geschickter DF: Benign capillary hemangioma of digital flexor tendon sheath: case report. *Ann Surg* 122:444, 1945.

Hemangioma of peripheral nerve

176. Kojima T, Ide Y, Marumo E, et al: Hemangioma of median nerve causing carpal tunnel syndrome. *Hand* 8:62, 1976.

177. Losli EJ: Intrinsic hemangiomas of the peripheral nerves. *Arch Pathol* 53:226, 1952.

178. Purcell FH, Gurjian ES: Hemangioma of the peripheral nerves. *Ann J Surg* 30:541, 1945.

179. Sato S: Uber das cavernose Angiom des peripherischen Nerven system. *Arch Klin Chir* 100:553, 1913.

180. Sommer R: Uber cavernose Angiome am peripheren Nervensystem. *Dtsch Ztschr Chir* 173:65, 1922.

181. Stewart SF, Bettin ME: The motor significance of hemangioma with report of a case of plexiform telangiectasis of the sciatic nerve and its branches. *Surg Gynecol Obstet* 39:307, 1924.

182. Wood MB: Intraneural hemangioma: report of a case. *Plast Reconstr Surg* 65:74, 1980.

Angiomatosis

183. Bishop BWF: Hemangioma of voluntary muscle. *Br J Surg* 24:190, 1936.

184. DeTakats G: Vascular anomalies of the extremities. *Surg Gynecol Obstet* 55:227, 1932.

185. Doederlein H: An unusually extensive hemangioma of diaphragm and of internal thoracic and abdominal wall as a cause of death in newborn. *Zentralbl Allg Pathol* 71:193, 1938.

186. Gonzalez-Crussi F, Enneking WF, Arean VM: Infiltrating angiolipoma. *J Bone Joint Surg* 48A:1111, 1966.

187. Holden KR, Alexander F: Diffuse neonatal hemangiomatosis. *Pediatrics* 46:411, 1970.

188. Howat AJ, Campbell PE: Angiomatosis: a vascular malformation of infancy and childhood. *Pathology* 19:377, 1987.

189. King DJ: A case resembling hemangiomatosis of the extremities. *J Bone Joint Surg* 28:623, 1946.

190. Kings KLM: Multifocal hemangiomatous malformation: a case report. *Thorax* 30:485, 1975.

191. Koblenzer PJ, Bukowski MJ: Angiomatosis (hamartomatous lymphangiomatosis). *Pediatrics* 28:65, 1961.

192. Lin JJ, Lin F: Two entities in angiolipoma. *Cancer* 34:720, 1974.

193. Rao VK, Weiss SW: Angiomatosis of soft tissue: an analysis of the histologic features and clinical outcome in 51 cases. *Am J Surg Pathol* 16:764, 1992.

194. Stock FE: Diffuse systemic angiomata. *Br J Surg* 41:273, 1953.

Vascular ectasias

195. Alderson MR: Spider naevi: Their incidence in healthy school children. *Arch Dis Child* 38:286, 1963.

196. Barsky SH, Rosen S, Geer DE, et al: The nature and evolution of port wine stains: a computer-assisted study. *J Invest Dermatol* 74:154, 1980.

197. Bean WB: *Vascular spiders and related lesions of the skin.* Springfield, Illinois, 1958, Charles C. Thomas.

198. Buecker JW, Ratz JL, Richfield DF: Histology of port-wine stain treated with carbon dioxide laser. *J Am Acad Dermatol* 10:14, 1984.

199. Finley JL, Arndt KA, Noe J, et al: Argon laser port-wine stain interaction. *Arch Dermatol* 120:613, 1984.

200. Finley JL, Clark RAF, Colvin RB, et al: Immunofluorescent staining with antibodies to factor VIII, fibronectin, and collagenous basement membrane protein in normal skin and port-wine stains. *Arch Dermatol* 118:971, 1982.

201. Finley JL, Noe JM, Arndt KA, et al: Port wine stains: morphologic variations and developmental lesions. *Arch Dermatol* 120:1453, 1984.

202. Letts RM: Orthopedic treatment of hemangiomatous hypertrophy of the lower extremity. *J Bone Joint Surg* 59A:777, 1977.

203. Lindenauer SM: The Klipper-Trenaunay syndrome: varicosity, hypertrophy, and hemangioma with arteriovenous fistula. *Ann Surg* 162:303, 1965.

204. Osler W: On a family form of recurring epistaxis associated with multiple telangiectases of the skin and mucous membranes. *Bull Johns Hopkins Hosp* 12:333, 1901.

205. Smoller B, Rosen S: Port-wine stains: a disease of altered neural modulation of blood vessels. *Arch Dermatol* 122:177, 1986.

206. Tan KL: Nevus flammeus of the nape, glabella, and eyelids. *Clin Pediatr* 11:112, 1972.

207. Wenzl JE, Burgert EO: The spider nevus in infancy and childhood. *Pediatrics* 33:227, 1964.

Papillary endothelial hyperplasia

208. Barr RJ, Graham JH, Sherwin LA: Intravascular papillary endothelial hyperplasia: a benign lesion mimicking angiosarcoma. *Arch Dermatol* 114:723, 1978.

209. Clearkin KP, Enzinger FM: Intravascular papillary endothelial hyperplasia. *Arch Pathol Lab Med* 100:441, 1976.

210. Hashimoto H, Daimaru Y, Enjoji M: Intravascular papillary endothelial hyperplasia: a clinicopathologic study of 91 cases. *Am J Dermatopathol* 5:539, 1983.

211. Henschen F: L'Endovasculite proliferante thrombopoietique dans la lesion vasculaire locale. *Ann Anat Pathol (Paris)* 9:113, 1932.

212. Kreutner A Jr, Smith RM, Trefny FA: Intravascular papillary endothelial hyperplasia: light and electron microscopic observations of a case. *Cancer* 42:2305, 1978.

213. Kuo T, Sayers P, Rosai J: Masson's "vegetant intravascular hemangioendothelioma": a lesion often mistaken for angiosarcoma. *Cancer* 38:1227, 1976.

214. Masson P: Hemangioendotheliome vegetant intravasculaire. *Bull Soc Anat (Paris)* 93:517, 1923.

215. Pins MR, Rosenthal DI, Springfield DS, et al: Florid extravascular papillary endothelial hyperplasia (Masson's pseudoangiosarcoma) presenting as a soft tissue sarcoma. *Arch Pathol Lab Med* 117:259, 1993.

216. Salyer WR, Salyer DC: Intravascular angiomatosis: development and distinction from angiosarcoma. *Cancer* 36:995, 1975.

Vascular transformation of lymph node

217. Chan JKC, Warnke RA, Dorfman R: Vascular transformation of sinuses in lymph nodes: a study of its morphological spectrum and distinction from Kaposi's sarcoma. *Am J Surg Pathol* 15:732, 1991.

218. Fayemi AO, Toker C: Nodal angiomatosis. *Arch Pathol* 99:170, 1975.

219. Haferkamp O, Rosenau W, Lennert K: Vascular transformation of lymph node sinuses due to venous obstruction. *Arch Pathol* 92:81, 1971.

220. Ostrowski ML, Siddiqui T, Barnes RE, et al: Vascular transformation of lymph node sinuses: a process displaying a spectrum of histologic features. *Arch Pathol Lab Med* 114:656, 1990.

Glomeruloid hemangioma

221. Chan JKC, Fletcher CDM, Hicklin GA, et al: Glomeruloid haemangioma: a distinctive cutaneous lesion of multicentric Castleman's disease associated with POEMS syndrome. *Am J Surg Pathol* 14:1036, 1990.

222. Ishikawa AO, Nihei Y, Ishikawa H: The skin changes of POEMS syndrome. *Br J Dermatol* 117:523, 1987.

223. Kanitakis J, Roger H, Soubrier M, et al: Cutaneous angiomas in POEMS syndrome: an ultrastructural and immunohistochemical study. *Arch Dermatol* 124:695, 1988.

224. Zak FG, Solomon A, Fellner MJ: Viscerocutaneous angiomatosis with dysproteinemia phagocytosis: its relationship to Kaposi's sarcoma and lymphoproliferative disorders. *J Pathol* 92:594, 1966.

Bacillary (epithelioid) angiomatosis

225. Baron AL, Steinbach LS, LeBoit PE, et al: Osteolytic lesions and bacillary angiomatosis in HIV infection: radiologic differentiation from AIDS-related Kaposi's sarcoma. *Radiology* 177:77, 1990.

226. Chan JKC, Lewin KJ, Lombard CM, et al: Histopathology of bacillary angiomatosis of lymph node. *Am J Surg Pathol* 15:430, 1991.

227. Cockerell CJ, Bergstresser PR, Myrie-Williams C, et al: Bacillary epithelioid angiomatosis occurring in an immunocompetent individual. *Arch Dermatol* 126:787, 1990.

228. LeBoit PE, Berger TG, Egbert BM, et al: Bacillary angiomatosis: the histopathology and differential diagnosis of a pseudoneoplastic infection in patients with human immunodeficiency virus disease. *Am J Surg Pathol* 13:909, 1989.

229. Reed JA, Brigati DJ, Flynn SD, et al: Immunocytochemical identification of *Rochalimaea henselae* in bacillary (epithelioid) angiomatosis, parenchymal bacillary peliosis, and persistent fever with bacteremia. *Am J Surg Pathol* 16: 650, 1992.

230. Relman DA, Loutit JS, Schmidt TM, et al: The agent of bacillary angiomatosis: an approach to the identification of uncultured pathogens. *N Engl J Med* 323:1573, 1990.

231. Schnella RA, Greco MA: Bacillary angiomatosis presenting as a soft-tissue tumor without skin involvement. *Hum Pathol* 21:567, 1990.

232. Stoler MH, Bonfiglio TA, Steigbigel RT: An atypical subcutaneous infection associated with acquired immune deficiency syndrome. *Am J Clin Pathol* 80:714, 1983.

CHAPTER 24

HEMANGIOENDOTHELIOMA: VASCULAR TUMORS OF INTERMEDIATE MALIGNANCY

The term *hemangioendothelioma* has become an empirically useful designation for those vascular tumors which histologically are intermediate in appearance between a hemangioma and a conventional angiosarcoma. By no means is this a homogeneous group of tumors, since each lesion so designated presents its unique set of histologically unusual or ambiguous features. Some may possess nearly all of the features of a hemangioma but display a greater degree of cellularity and mitotic activity. Others may contain well-formed vascular channels, but they are not arranged in lobules as is the case in most hemangiomas. However, within the spectrum of hemangioendothelioma at least four distinct entities are recognized: (1) epithelioid hemangioendothelioma,[16,17] one of the tumors within the spectrum of "histiocytoid hemangioma"[13]; (2) spindle cell hemangioendothelioma[28]; (3) kaposiform hemangioendothelioma; and (4) malignant endovascular papillary angioendothelioma (Dabska tumor).[35] Not only do these tumors have histological features different from both hemangioma and angiosarcoma, but their biological behavior also warrants their separation from the ordinary hemangioma and angiosarcoma.

EPITHELIOID HEMANGIOENDOTHELIOMA

This epithelioid, angiocentric vascular tumor can occur at almost any age but rarely occurs in childhood[6,16,17]; it affects the sexes about equally. To date no predisposing factors have been identified; in particular, none of the 90 patients that we have studied gave a history of ingestion of oral contraceptives. The tumor develops as a solitary, slightly painful mass in either superficial or deep soft tissue. At least half of cases are closely associated with or arise from a vessel, usually a vein. In some cases occlusion of the vessel accounts for more profound symptoms such as edema or thrombophlebitis. Those tumors

that arise from vessels usually have a variegated, white-red color and superficially resemble organizing thrombi, except that they are firmly attached to the surrounding soft tissue. Those that do not arise from vessels are white-gray and offer little hint of their vascular nature on gross inspection. Calcification is occasionally seen in large deeply situated tumors.

Microscopic features

Lesions that arise from vessels have a characteristic appearance when seen at low power. They expand the vessel, usually preserving its architecture as they extend centrifugally from the lumen to the soft tissue (Fig. 24-1). The lumen is filled with a combination of tumor, necrotic debris, and dense collagen. Unlike the epithelioid hemangi-

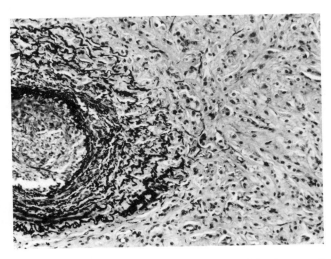

FIG. 24-1. Epithelioid hemangioendothelioma arising from small artery. (Elastic stain; ×160.)

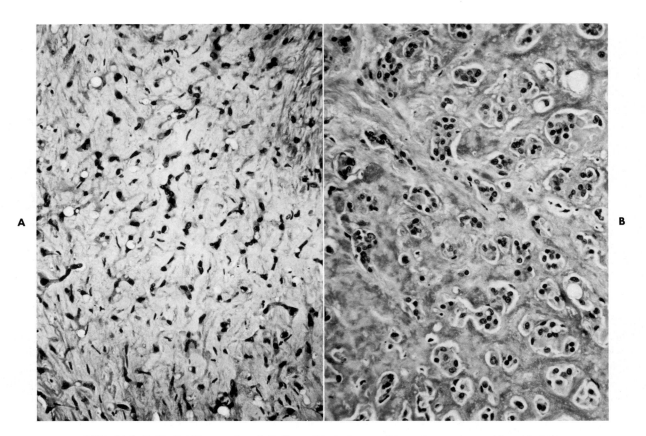

FIG. 24-2. Epithelioid hemangioendothelioma illustrating cordlike pattern and myxoid matrix **(A).** Other areas contain nests of cells and hyalinized stroma **(B).** **(A,** ×160; **B,** ×200.)

oma (see Chapter 23), in which vascular differentiation proceeds through the formation of multicellular, canalized vascular channels, vascular differentiation in these tumors is more primitive and is expressed primarily at the cellular level. The tumors are composed of short strands or solid nests of rounded to slightly spindled endothelial cells (Fig. 24-2). Rarely are large, distinct vascular channels seen, except in the more peripheral portions of the tumor. Instead the tumor cells form small intracellular lumina, which are seen as clear spaces or "vacuoles" that distort or "blister" the cell (Figs. 24-3 to 24-5). Frequently confused with the mucin vacuoles of adenocarcinoma, these miniature lumina occasionally contain erythrocytes. The stroma varies from highly myxoid to hyaline. The myxoid areas are light blue on hematoxylin-eosin staining, and conventional histochemical treatment with aldehyde fuchsin pH 1.0 may reveal sulfated acid mucopolysaccharides. This staining pattern should not be equated with cartilaginous differentiation but simply reflects the tendency of some vascular tumors to produce sulfated acid mucins similar to the ground substance of vessel walls. Although occasional tumors do contain eosinophils and lymphocytes, rarely is this feature as pronounced as it is in the epithelioid hemangioma.

In most cases the tumors appear quite bland and there is virtually no mitotic activity. In about one fourth of cases the tumors contain areas with significant atypia, mitotic activity (greater than 1/10 HPF), focal spindling of the cells, or necrosis. Such features can be correlated with a more aggressive course, as discussed below. When metastases occur in this disease, they usually develop from tumors with these atypical features. Not unexpectedly, metastases also contain these features. In rare instances both primary and metastatic lesions may appear bland cytologically.

Differential diagnosis

The differential diagnosis of this tumor includes metastatic carcinoma (or melanoma) as well as various sarcomas that can assume an epithelioid appearance. In general, carcinomas and melanomas metastatic to soft tissue display far more nuclear atypia and mitotic activity than the epithelioid hemangioendothelioma and are rarely angiocentric. Epithelioid forms of angiosarcoma are composed of solid sheets of very atypical, mitotically active, epithelioid endothelial cells. Necrosis is common, and vascular differentiation is expressed primarily by the formation of irregular sinusoidal vascular channels. Epithelioid sarcoma is per-

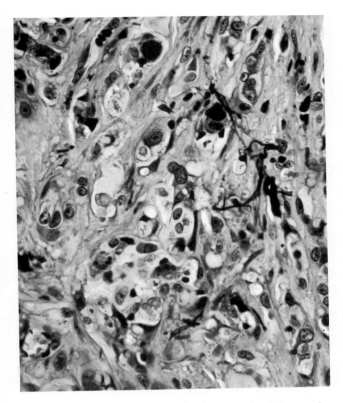

FIG. 24-3. Epithelioid hemangioendothelioma showing vacuoles representing miniature lumina, some containing erythrocytes. (Pentachrome stain; ×400.)

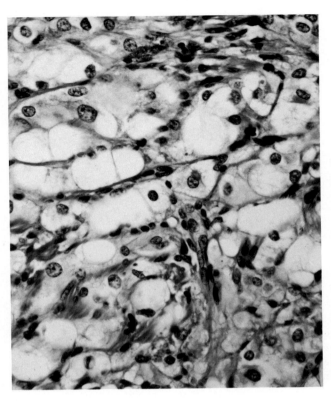

FIG. 24-4. Extreme degree of "vacuolization" within an epithelioid hemangioendothelioma. (×400.)

haps the best mimic of this tumor. Composed of nodules of rounded eosinophilic cells that surround cores of necrotic debris and collagen, epithelioid sarcoma develops primarily as a distal extremity lesion in young individuals. The polygonal cells usually blend and merge with the collagen in a close interplay between cell and stroma. In ambiguous cases, both immunohistochemistry and electron microscopy may provide the most reliable clues of differentiation. With appropriate "cocktails" of monoclonal antibodies directed against a broad spectrum of cytokeratins, immunostaining is positive in virtually all carcinomas and epithelioid sarcomas. Epithelioid hemangioendotheliomas usually do not express cytokeratin, although recent studies of epithelioid vascular tumors have identified cytokeratin in a rare case.[8] With optimal material, factor VIII–associated antigen can be demonstrated within the cytoplasm of most epithelioid hemangioendotheliomas (Fig. 24-6). Accentuation of the staining is often noted around the cytoplasmic minilumina. The cells of epithelioid hemangioendothelioma also bind *Ulex europaeus.* Reticulin staining highlights material around individual cells and groups of cells comprising solid vascular channels (Fig. 24-7). By electron microscopy the cells have characteristics of endothelium, including well-developed basal lamina, pinocytotic vesicles, and occa-

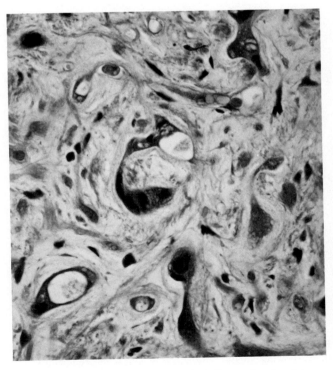

FIG. 24-5. Epithelioid hemangioendothelioma showing intracytoplasmic lumina. (×600.)

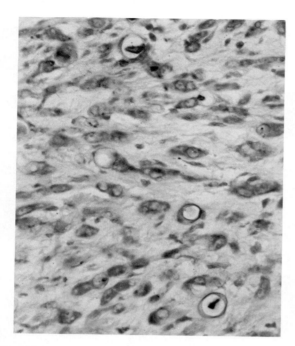

FIG. 24-6. Peroxidase-antiperoxidase stain for factor VIII–associated antigen. Immunoreactivity is present in cytoplasm of most cells and is accentuated around cytoplasmic lumina. (×160.)

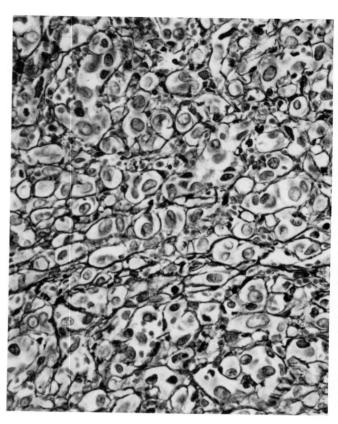

FIG. 24-7. Reticulin staining in epithelioid hemangioendothelioma, showing small nests of cells. (×250.)

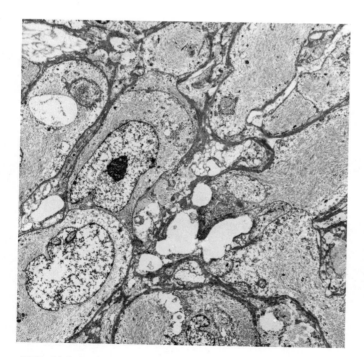

FIG. 24-8. Electron micrograph of epithelioid hemangioendothelioma showing complete investiture of cells with basal lamina, numerous intermediate filaments, and surface-oriented pinocytotic vesicles. (×2200.)

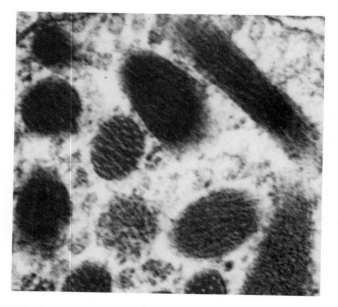

FIG. 24-9. Weibel-Palade body within an epithelioid hemangioendothelioma. In longitudinal section, body has linear substructure; in cross-section, a dot matrix pattern is seen. (×75,200.)

sional Weibel-Palade bodies (Figs. 24-8 and 24-9). They differ from normal endothelium principally by the superabundance of intermediate filaments that crowd the cytoplasm.

Behavior and treatment

Additional follow-up information has confirmed our initial impression that the overall prognosis in this tumor is quite favorable.[17] Of the 46 patients followed up for an average period of 48 months, 6 (13%) developed a local recurrence, and 14 (31%) developed metastasis in regional lymph nodes, lung, liver, and bone (Table 24-1). Fewer than half of the patients who developed metastases died of their disease. This is explained by the fact that half of all metastases are in regional lymph nodes, and excision of these structures may result in cure or at least long-term disease-free survival. Designation of some of these tumors as "malignant" on the basis of the features described earlier has proven merit, since these tumors have a more aggressive course than the ordinary "benign" forms. Histologically, malignant forms have a higher incidence of metastasis and a shorter interval between the time of diagnosis and metastasis. A small percentage of benign-appearing epithelioid hemangioendotheliomas do metastasize and cause death of the patient. Unfortunately, on histological grounds it is neither possible to predict which lesions will metastasize nor which may evolve over a period of time to a malignant lesion. That this evolution does take place has been documented in at least one case in our material. Because of the low-grade nature of these tumors, complete and, ideally, wide local excision without adjuvant radiotherapy or chemotherapy should be the treatment of choice. Histologically malignant forms should be treated similarly to other sarcomas with at least radical local excision. Since the regional lymph nodes represent a common metastatic site, these structures should be evaluated as part of the treatment of this disease.

Epithelioid hemangioendothelioma in other sites

Epithelioid hemangioendotheliomas occur in other sites.[5,7,9-12,16,18] In parenchymal organs there is an even greater tendency for these tumors to be confused with carcinomas. For example, in the lung they were initially believed to be an unusual form of intravascular bronchioloalveolar carcinoma and in the liver a sclerosing form of cholangiocarcinoma. However, their vascular nature has been confirmed in numerous reports.[2-5,7,9] Comparable tumors have also been reported in bone as "angioglomoid tumor"[14] and "myxoid angioblastomatosis."[11,12] We have also seen these tumors arise as primary lesions within lymph nodes[6,17] and even in the brain and meninges.

Although the basic features of the tumor are similar within the various organs, the clinical presentation and disease-related signs and symptoms differ. In the liver and lung the tumor occurs primarily in women and has a striking tendency to present in a multifocal fashion because of extensive growth along small vessels. The death rate from the disease in the lung and liver has been reported as 65% and 35%, respectively, compared with a 13% death rate in soft tissue[15] (Table 24-2). Because of the low-grade nature of these tumors, there has been considerable interest in performing liver transplantation in this disease. In a study by Marino et al.,[10] the projected 5-year survival rate of patients receiving orthotopic liver transplantation was 76%, a figure that compares favorably with patients undergoing the procedure for nonmalignant disease.

Table 24-1. Behavior of epithelioid hemangioendothelioma of soft tissue (46 cases)*†

Recurrence		6 (13%)
Metastasis		14 (31%)
Lung	7	
Lymph node	7	
Died of disease		6 (13%)

*Average follow-up period 48 months.
†From Weiss SW, Ishak KG, Dail DH, et al: *Semin Diagn Pathol* 3:259, 1986.

Table 24-2. Comparison of epithelioid hemangioendothelioma of various organs*

Organ	Age	Sex	Distribution	Angiocentricity	Mortality (%)
Soft tissue	Second to ninth decade	Males = females	Solitary, rarely multifocal cases	Half arise from vessel	13
Bone	First to eighth decade (peak second to third decade)	Slightly more common in males	About half multifocal	?	?
Lung	Median 40 years	More common in females	Most multifocal	Intravascular spread common	65
Liver	Second to ninth decade (average 50 years)	More common in females	Most multifocal	Intravascular spread common	35

*Reprinted from Weiss SW, Ishak KG, Dail DH, et al: *Semin Diagn Pathol* 3:259, 1986.

SPINDLE CELL HEMANGIOENDOTHELIOMA

Described in 1986 as a low-grade angiosarcoma with features of both cavernous hemangioma and Kaposi's sarcoma,[28] spindle cell hemangioendothelioma is an indolent nonmetastasizing lesion that recurs locally and can result in extensive local disease.[24] The tumor occurs in young adults, and the common location is the subcutis or dermis of the distal extremities, particularly the hand. The tumor

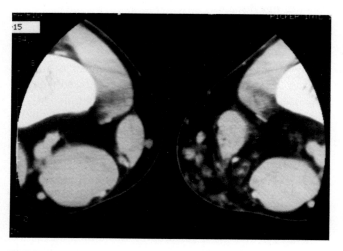

FIG. 24-10. CT scan of thigh of patient with spindle cell hemangioendothelioma. Right side shows numerous subcutaneous soft tissue densities corresponding to tumor. (From *Am J Surg Pathol* 10:521, 1986.)

may be associated with Maffucci's syndrome,[24] Klippel-Trenaunay syndrome,[21] early onset varicosities,[21] and congenital lymphedema,[21,28] and in one case epithelioid hemangioendothelioma.[29] The tumors produce few symptoms apart from the appearance of a mass. Although many cases begin as one nodule, there seems to be a remarkable tendency for lesions to either grow locally or develop multifocally within a generalized area (Fig. 24-10). Grossly the tumors are small, circumscribed reddish nodules that occasionally contain pearly phleboliths that pop out when the tumor is sectioned (Fig. 24-11). When the tumor is viewed at low power one is impressed by the presence of large veins adjacent to the tumor suggesting the presence of a malformation or underlying benign neoplasm, and in about half of cases the lesions may be partially intravascular. Thin-walled vessels that contain organizing thrombi usually suggest an initial diagnosis of cavernous hemangioma (Figs. 24-12 and 24-13). Between the cavernous spaces there is a proliferation of relatively bland-appearing spindled cells (Figs. 24-14 and 24-15). Out of context these areas might suggest Kaposi's sarcoma; however, in contrast to Kaposi's sarcoma, these areas also contain occasional rounded or epithelioid endothelial cells, similar to those of epithelioid hemangioendothelioma (Fig. 24-16). As in the latter tumor, these cells occasionally contain vacuoles or intracytoplasmic lumina (Figs. 24-17 and 24-18). In the extreme case, clusters of vacuolated cells lie within the spindled stroma and are easily mistaken for entrapped fat. Factor VIII–associated antigen can be identified within the endo-

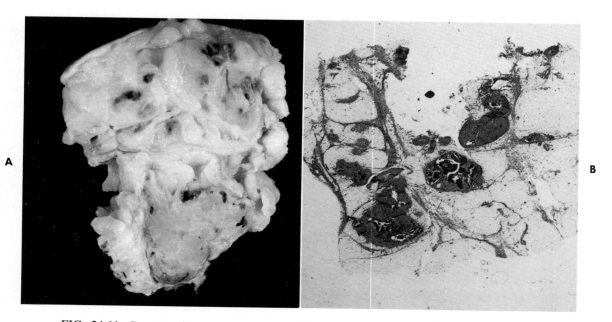

FIG. 24-11. Gross specimen of spindle cell hemangioendothelioma (same case as Fig. 24-10) showing numerous tumor nodules in subcutis **(A)**. Low-power view of tumor illustrating variability in size and degree of cavernous change **(B)**. (×10.) (From *Am J Surg Pathol* 10:521, 1986.)

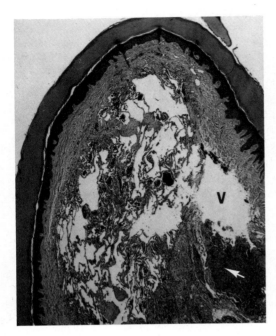

FIG. 24-12. Spindle cell hemangioendothelioma illustrating cavernous spaces *(V)* juxtaposed to solidly cellular spindled areas *(arrow).* (×60.) (From *Am J Surg Pathol* 10:521, 1986.)

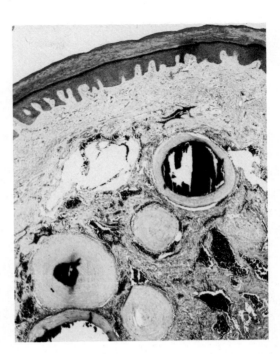

FIG. 24-13. Spindle cell hemangioendothelioma containing numerous phleboliths. (×60.) (From *Am J Surg Pathol* 10:521, 1986.)

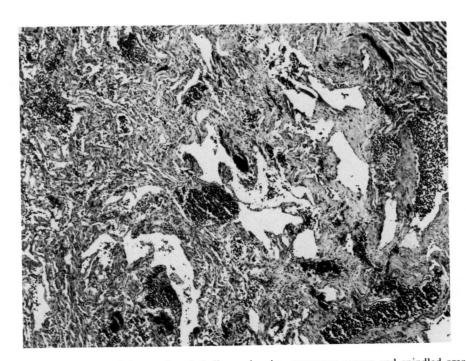

FIG. 24-14. Spindle cell hemangioendothelioma showing cavernous spaces and spindled areas. (×160.) (From *Am J Surg Pathol* 10:521, 1986.)

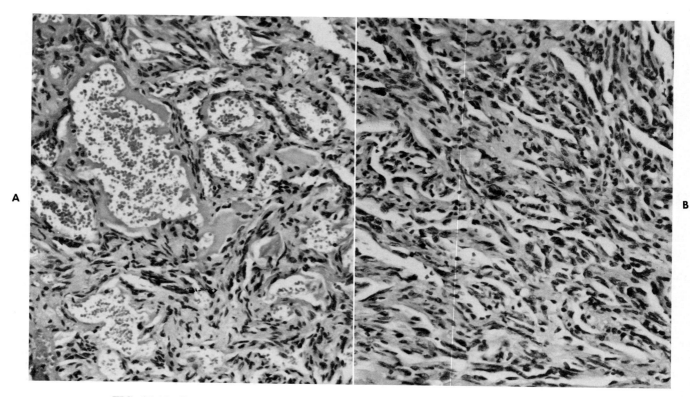

FIG. 24-15. Cavernous spaces (**A**) and spindled areas (**B**) within spindle cell hemangioendothelioma. (**A** and **B**, ×250.) (From *Am J Surg Pathol* 10:521, 1986.)

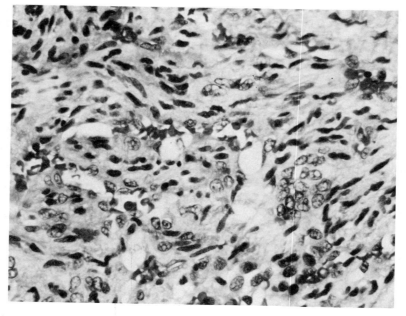

FIG. 24-16. Epithelioid endothelial cells within spindled stroma of spindle cell hemangioendothelioma. (×250.)

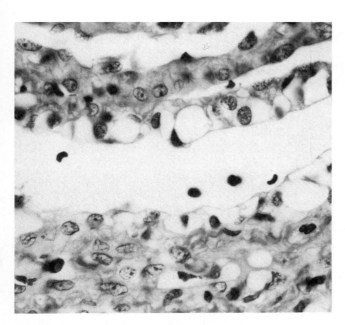

FIG. 24-17. Vacuolization of endothelium within spindle cell hemangioendothelioma. (×630.)

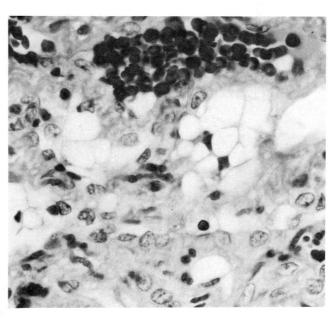

FIG. 24-18. Vacuolated endothelium within stroma of spindle cell hemangioendothelioma. (×630.)

thelium lining the cavernous spaces and within the epithelioid endothelium of the stroma, but is not generally identified within the spindled cells. Electron microscopic findings parallel the immunohistochemical ones in that cells positive for factor VIII–associated antigen have ultrastructural features of endothelium, whereas the spindled cells are less well-differentiated mesenchymal cells resembling fibroblasts.[22]

The recent study by Perkins and Weiss, evaluating approximately 80 cases, indicates that about 60% locally recur.[24] Recurrences develop both within the immediate operative site as well as several centimeters distant to it, suggesting both multifocal as well as true recurrent disease. However, neither regional nor distant metastasis has been documented in this disease. Although our original study reported regional lymph node metastasis in one case,[28] that particular lesion had been both irradiated and progressed to sarcoma, suggesting it was a complication of radiation and not an expression of the natural history of the tumor. Thus, the appropriate therapy is conservative excision for limited disease. Treatment of extensive recurrent disease by surgery may be done depending on the cosmetic needs of the patient and the discomfort associated with the surgery. Certainly the tumor is compatible with normal longevity; one patient in our consultation files was alive and well with this tumor for over 70 years.

The indolent course of this tumor and the lack of metastatic disease has prompted some to suggest that this is not a neoplasm at all, but rather a reactive lesion occurring in response to repeated intravascular thrombosis and recanalization.[21,22] We doubt that this lesion can be explained solely on the basis of thrombosis and recanalization. If so, it should clearly have been recognized in other sites (e.g., hemorrhoids) where thrombosis and recanalization occur with great regularity, and it would not explain rare examples of the tumor that occur in internal sites such as the spleen. We and others[20] believe that the preponderance of evidence suggests that these are either histologically benign neoplasms or malformations in which vascular thrombosis supervenes. This is supported by the intravascular location and the large adjacent vessels that are seen in about half of cases.

KAPOSIFORM HEMANGIOENDOTHELIOMA

The recently described kaposiform hemangioendothelioma is an extremely rare tumor that occurs exclusively during the childhood and teenage years and has features common to both capillary hemangioma and Kaposi's sarcoma.[34] In the past these lesions have been reported anecdotally under a variety of names, including "kaposi-like infantile hemangioendothelioma,"[33] "hemangioma with Kaposi's sarcoma-like features,"[31] and simply "hemangioendothelioma."[32] The lesions occur in either superficial or deep soft tissue, although those in the latter sites, particularly the retroperitoneum, are associated with consumption coagulopathy (Kasabach-Merritt syndrome). A small subset of cases is associated with lymphangiomatosis, which may either antedate the tumor or be discovered contemporaneously.[34]

These gray-white tumor masses are composed of nodules that suggest both capillary hemangioma and Kaposi's sar-

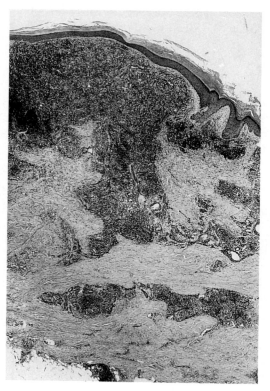

FIG. 24-19. Kaposiform hemangioendothelioma illustrating ill-defined sheets of tumor infiltrating dermis. (×25.)

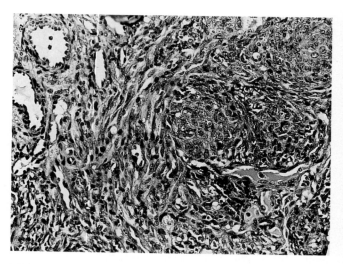

FIG. 24-20. Kaposiform hemangioendothelioma showing spindled zones merging with glomeruloid nests of rounded or epithelioid endothelial cells. Note particulate material within cells in glomeruloid areas. (×160.)

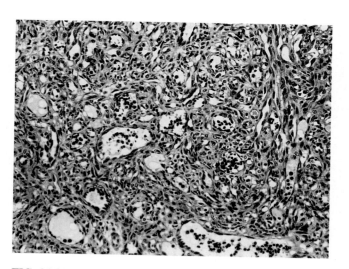

FIG. 24-21. Capillary hemangioma-like areas within a kaposiform hemangioendothelioma. (×240.)

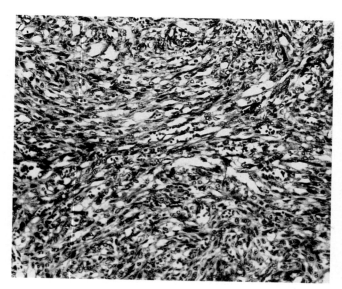

FIG. 24-22. Spindled Kaposi sarcoma-like areas within a kaposiform hemangioendothelioma. (×240.)

coma. The ill-defined nodules contain a mixture of small round capillary-sized vessels that blend with slitlike vessels (Figs. 24-19 to 24-22). Unlike the typical capillary hemangioma, which is made up of distinct lobules of small vessels, this tumor consists of irregular rambling sheets of tumor that infiltrate the soft tissues. Scattered throughout the tumors are glomeruloid nests of rounded or epithelioid endothelial cells with abundant eosinophilic cytoplasm containing fine granules of hemosiderin, hyaline globules, and cytoplasmic vacuoles, similar to those of the epithelioid hemangioendothelioma (Fig. 24-20). Smaller amounts of hemosiderin and hyaline globules are also present in the spindled zones. Red blood cell fragments and microthrombi are also identified between these cells as well as in the spindled endothelium. Atypia is usually minimal within these tumors, as are mitotic figures. In those cases that have developed in the setting of lymphangiomatosis there is usually an abrupt transition between the two lesions (Fig. 24-23).

Immunohistochemically, these tumors bear some, but not all, the markers of vascular endothelium, suggesting that the constituent cells are a less well differentiated or mature form of endothelium. The majority of cells express CD34 but not factor VIII-associated antigen nor do they bind *Ulex europaeus*. Large well-formed "feeder" vessels peripheral to the tumor nodules express conventional vascular endothelial markers. Ultrastructurally the endothelial cells are arranged in cohesive nests with imperfect or partial lumen formation and are invested only partially with basal lamina.

The behavior of this neoplasm is strongly influenced by its site, clinical extent, and the development of any consumption coagulopathy. Tumors located in the retroperitoneum and mediastinum are typically extensive, unresectable lesions associated with Kasabach-Merritt syndrome, which ultimately results in the death of the patient. More limited tumors occurring in the superficial soft tissues are curable with wide local excision. To date none of these tumors has produced distant metastasis, although one case was marked by progressive local metastasis and involvment of regional lymph nodes.[30] Thus the challenge in these cases is not only to eradicate the tumor but also to support patients who have life-threatening hemorrhage from consumption coagulopathy.

As implied, the two most important differential considerations in this disease are capillary (cellular) hemangioma of infancy and Kaposi's sarcoma. Capillary hemangiomas are composed of distinct nodules of small capillary-sized vessels. Although canalization can be imperfect in the early phase of growth, capillary hemangiomas do not display spindling of the cells nor do they contain fragmented red cells and hemosiderin. Kaposi's sarcoma is an exceptionally rare tumor in childhood with the exception of lymphadenopathic forms that have been described in Africa. It is characterized by uniform spindling of the cells and often a striking inflammatory infiltrate peripherally. Although clearly portions of kaposiform hemangioendothelioma may be indistinguishable from Kaposi's sarcoma, the former shows much greater variation from area to area. Recently, transcripts similar to human papillomavirus 16 have been described in Kaposi's sarcoma, occurring both in the setting and outside the setting of acquired immunodeficiency syndrome. In two cases of kaposiform hemangioendothelioma recently studied by us these transcripts were not identified, providing additional evidence for the separate nature of the two diseases.[34]

MALIGNANT ENDOVASCULAR PAPILLARY ANGIOENDOTHELIOMA

This is a rare but distinctive vascular tumor described in 1969 by Dabska.[35] On the basis of her six cases, it appears to be a form of low-grade angiosarcoma occurring in the skin or subcutis of infants and young children, although we have seen rare cases in adults. It may present as either a diffuse subcutaneous swelling or a discrete intradermal tumor that possesses a capacity for deep extension if left untreated. Of the few cases available for review, no particular anatomical site is favored. The tumor is composed of large but well-formed vascular spaces lined by endothelium and partially filled with clear fluid. At low power the tumor may resemble a cavernous lymphangioma (Fig. 24-24), an observation that is reenforced by the finding of lymphocytes within and around the vascular spaces and within the stroma of the tumor. The endothelium lining the spaces var-

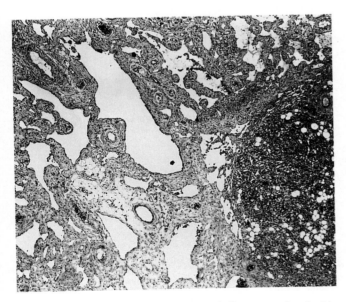

FIG. 24-23. Kaposiform hemangioendothelioma associated with lymphangiomatosis. Lymphangioma is present on left, tumor nodule on right. (×60.)

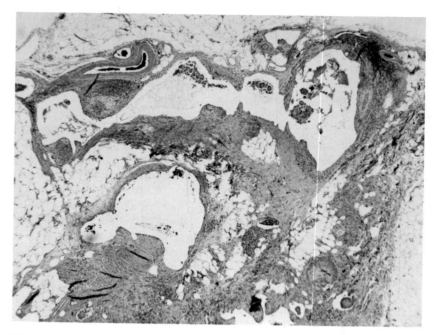

FIG. 24-24. Malignant endovascular papillary angioendothelioma (Dabska tumor). At low power, tumor resembles a cavernous lymphangioma. (×60.)

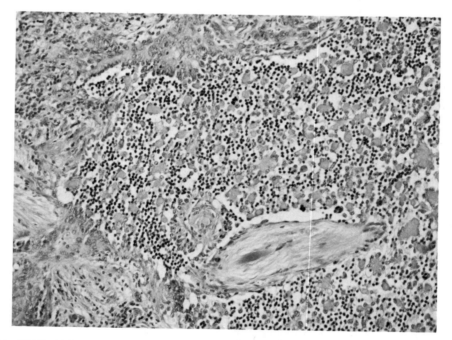

FIG. 24-25. Dabska tumor illustrating tiny neoplastic papillae within the cavernous spaces. (×250.)

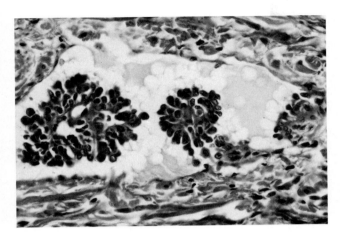

FIG. 24-26. Papillary structures within a Dabska tumor. (×250.)

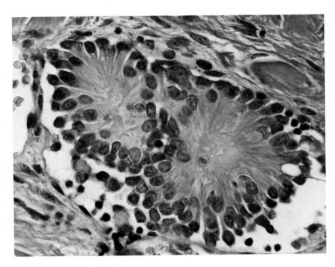

FIG. 24-27. Endovascular papillations of Dabska tumor showing peripheral polarization of endothelial nuclei and central hyaline core. (×630.)

ies from small rounded cells resembling lymphocytes to cuboidal and even columnar cells (Figs. 24-25 to 24-27). The nuclei are often polarized toward the luminal surface of the vessel, thereby heightening the resemblance of the endothelium to epithelium (Fig. 24-27). The distinguishing feature, however, is the manner in which the redundant endothelium creates endovascular papillations with central hyaline cores (Figs. 24-26 and 24-27) composed of accumulated basement membrane material presumably synthesized by the tumor cells.[39] These structures have been compared with renal glomeruli (Fig. 24-26). Intracytoplasmic vacuolization of the endothelium may be observed, a phenomenon seen in other vascular tumors such as Kimura's disease and epithelioid hemangioendothelioma. In some cases there is a close intermingling of endothelial cells with the intravascular lymphocytes, an observation that has led some to suggest that the tumor cells may express some of the properties of the "high" endothelial cell of the postcapillary venule.[37] The cells express factor VIII–associated protein and bind *Ulex europaeus*. They do not express HLA-DR, however.[37] It should be noted that occasionally ordinary angiosarcomas may contain areas where growth of malignant endothelial cells into small vessels may simulate the pattern of malignant endovascular papillary angioendothelioma. However, the latter term should be restricted for low-grade tumors having all of the features mentioned above.

The prognosis of this tumor is good. Despite the presence of regional lymph node metastasis in 2 of 6 patients reported by Dabska, all 6 patients were alive without evidence of disease 4 to 16 years after wide local excision.

REFERENCES
Epithelioid hemangioendothelioma

1. Angervall L, Kindblom L-G, Karlsson K, et al: Atypical hemangioendothelioma of venous origin: a clinicopathologic, angiographic, immunohistochemical, and ultrastructural study of two endothelial tumors within the concept of histiocytoid hemangioma. *Am J Surg Pathol* 9:504, 1985.
2. Bhagavan BS, Dorfman HD, Murthy MSN, et al: Intravascular bronchioloalveolar tumor (IVBAT): a low-grade sclerosing epithelioid angiosarcoma of lung. *Am J Surg Pathol* 6:41, 1982.
3. Corrin B, Manners B, Millard M, et al: Histogenesis of the so-called intravascular bronchiolo-alveolar tumor. *J Pathol* 128:163, 1979.
4. Dail DH, Liebow AA, Gmelich JT, et al: Intravascular, bronchiolar, and alveolar tumor of the lung (IVBAT): an analysis of twenty cases of a peculiar sclerosing endothelial tumor. *Cancer* 51:451, 1983.
5. Dean PJ, Haggitt RC, O'Hara CJ: Malignant epithelioid hemangioendothelioma of the liver in young women: relationship to oral contraceptive use. *Am J Surg Pathol* 9:695, 1985.
6. Ellis GL, Kratochvil FJ: Epithelioid hemangioendothelioma of the head and neck: a clinicopathologic report of twelve cases. *Oral Surg Oral Med Oral Pathol* 61:61, 1986.
7. Fukayama M, Nihei Z, Takizawa T, et al: Malignant epithelioid hemangioendothelioma of the liver spreading through the hepatic veins. *Virchows Arch (Pathol Anat)* 404:275, 1984.
8. Gray MH, Rosenberg AE, Dickersin GR, et al: Cytokeratin expression in epithelioid vascular neoplasms. *Hum Pathol* 21:212, 1990.
9. Ishak KG, Sesterhenn IA, Goodman ZD, et al: Epithelioid hemangioendothelioma of the liver: a clinicopathologic and follow-up study of 32 cases. *Hum Pathol* 15:839, 1984.
10. Marino I, Todo S, Tzakis AG, et al: Treatment of hepatic epithelioid hemangioendothelioma with liver transplantation. *Cancer* 62:2079, 1988.

11. Mirra JM, Kameda N: Myxoid angioblastomatosis of bones: a case report of a rare, multifocal entity with light, ultramicroscopic, and immunopathologic correlation. *Am J Surg Pathol* 9:450, 1985.

12. Reed RJ: Consultation case. *Am J Surg Pathol* 6:159, 1982.

13. Rosai J, Gold J, Landy R: The histiocytoid hemangiomas: a unifying concept embracing several previously described entities of skin, soft tissue, large vessels, bone, and heart. *Hum Pathol* 10:707, 1979.

14. Tang TT, Zuege RC, Babbitt DP, et al: Angioglomoid tumor of bone: a case report. *J Bone Joint Surg* 58A:873, 1976.

15. Tsuneyoshi M, Dorfman HD, Bauer TW: Epithelioid hemangioendothelioma of bone: a clinicopathologic, ultrastructural, and immunohistochemical study. *Am J Surg Pathol* 10:754, 1986.

16. Weiss SW, Enzinger FM: Epithelioid hemangioendothelioma: a vascular tumor often mistaken for a carcinoma. *Cancer* 50:970, 1982.

17. Weiss SW, Ishak KG, Dail DH, et al: Epithelioid hemangioendothelioma and related lesions. *Semin Diagn Pathol* 3:259, 1986.

18. Weldon-Linne CM, Victor TA, Christ ML, et al: Angiogenic nature of the intravascular bronchioloalveolar tumor of the lung. *Arch Pathol Lab Med* 105:174, 1981.

19. Zagzag D, Yang G, Seidman I, et al: Malignant epithelioid hemangioendothelioma arising in an intramuscular lipoma. *Cancer* 71:764, 1993.

Spindle cell hemangioendothelioma

20. Ding J, Hashimoto H, Imayama S, et al: Spindle cell hemangioendothelioma: probably a benign vascular lesion, not a low-grade angiosarcoma. *Virchows Arch (Pathol Anat)* 420:77, 1992.

21. Fletcher CDM, Beham A, Schmid C: Spindle cell hemangioendothelioma: a clinicopathologic study indicative of a nonneoplastic lesion. *Histopathology* 18:291, 1991.

22. Imayama S, Murakamai Y, Hashimoto H, et al: Spindle cell hemangioendothelioma exhibits the ultrastructural features of a reactive vascular proliferation rather than of angiosarcoma. *Am J Clin Pathol* 97:279, 1992.

23. Ono CM, Mitsunaga MM, Lockett LJ: Intragluteal spindle cell hemangioendothelioma: an unusual presentation of a recently described vascular neoplasm. *Clin Orthop* 281:224, 1992.

24. Perkins P, Weiss SW: Spindle cell hemangioendothelioma: a clinicopathologic study of 78 cases. *Mod Pathol* 7:9A, 1994.

25. Scott GA, Rosai J: Spindle cell hemangioendothelioma: report of seven additional cases of a recently described entity vascular neoplasm. *Am J Dermatopathol* 10:281, 1988.

26. Steinbach LS, Omisky SH, Shpall S, et al: MR imaging of spindle cell hemangioendothelioma. *J Comput Assist Tomogr* 15:155, 1991.

27. Terashi H, Itami S, Kurata S, et al: Spindle cell hemangioendothelioma: report of three cases. *J Dermatol* 18:104, 1991.

28. Weiss SW, Enzinger FM: Spindle cell hemangioendothelioma: a low-grade angiosarcoma resembling cavernous hemangioma and Kaposi's sarcoma. *Am J Surg Pathol* 10:521, 1986.

29. Zoltie N, Roberts PF: Spindle cell hemangioendothelioma in association with epithelioid hemangioendothelioma. *Histopathology* 15:544, 1989.

Kaposiform hemangioendothelioma

30. Lai FM, Allen PW, Yuen PM, et al: Locally metastasizing vascular tumor: spindle cell, epithelioid, or unclassified hemangioendothelioma. *Am J Clin Pathol* 96:660, 1991.

31. Niedt GW, Greco MA, Wieczorek R, et al: Hemangioma with Kaposi's sarcoma-like features: report of 2 cases. *Pediatr Pathol* 9:567, 1989.

32. Pearl GS, Matthews WH: Congenital retroperitoneal hemangioendothelioma with Kasabach-Merritt syndrome. *South Med J* 72:239, 1979.

33. Tsang WYW, Chang JKC: Kaposi-like infantile hemangioendothelioma: a distinctive vascular neoplasm of the retroperitoneum. *Am J Surg Pathol* 15:982, 1991.

34. Zukerberg LR, Nickoloff BJ, Weiss SW: Kaposiform hemangioendothelioma of infancy and childhood: an aggressive neoplasm associated with Kasabach-Merritt syndrome and lymphangiomatosis. *Am J Surg Pathol* 17:321, 1993.

Malignant endovascular papillary angioendothelioma

35. Dabska M: Malignant endovascular papillary angioendothelioma of the skin in childhood. *Cancer* 24:503, 1969.

36. Magnin PH, Schroh RG, Barquin MA: Endovascular papillary angioendothelioma in children. *Pediatr Dermatol* 4:332, 1987.

37. Manivel JC, Wick MR, Swanson PE, et al: Endovascular papillary angioendothelioma of childhood: a vascular lesion possibly characterized by "high" endothelial cell differentiation. *Hum Pathol* 17:1240, 1986.

38. Morgan J, Robinson MJ, Rosen LB, et al: Malignant endovascular papillary angioendothelioma (Dabska tumor): a case report and review of the literature. *Am J Dermatopathol* 11:64, 1989.

39. Patterson K, Chandra RS: Malignant endovascular papillary angioendothelioma: a cutaneous borderline tumor. *Arch Pathol Lab Med* 109:671, 1985.

CHAPTER 25

MALIGNANT VASCULAR TUMORS

ANGIOSARCOMA

Angiosarcomas are malignant tumors, the cells of which manifest many of the functional and morphological properties of normal endothelium. They may vary from highly differentiated tumors that resemble hemangiomas to those whose anaplasia makes them difficult to distinguish from carcinomas or melanomas. Consequently, the literature is replete with various terms such as hemangioendothelioma,* lymphangioendothelioma,[91] hemangioblastoma,[143,149,154] lymphangiosarcoma,† and hemangiosarcoma that attest to the wide morphological spectrum and the lack of standardized nomenclature. In this book we use the term *hemangioendothelioma* to refer to tumors that have an appearance intermediate between a benign hemangioma and angiosarcoma and, therefore, might be considered of intermediate or borderline malignancy (Chapter 24). In our experience only a small number of vascular tumors fall into this group. We have employed the all-inclusive term *angiosarcoma* in preference to the terms *hemangiosarcoma* and *lymphangiosarcoma,* which imply similarity of the tumor to cells of capillary or lymphatic endothelium, respectively. We have found the distinction between hemangiosarcomas and lymphangiosarcomas not only difficult but also somewhat arbitrary. By convention, angiosarcomas arising in the setting of lymphedema have been designated lymphangiosarcomas on the presumption that this impressive post hoc phenomenon indicates origin of the tumor from dilated lymphatic vessels. However, it is not established that these tumors uniformly display lymphatic differentiation. In fact, the results of histochemical and electron microscopic studies offer equal support for differentiation of the hemangiomatous type. Although it may be inappropriate at this point to categorically deny the existence of a specific sarcoma of lymphatic endothelium, there seem to be few reliable criteria to make this distinction on histological grounds. With the advent of a variety of monoclonal antibodies, which permit distinction of capillary and lymphatic endothelial cells, more accurate characterization of these tumors may be possible. At this time, however, we believe the less committal term *angiosarcoma* is justified.

Incidence

Angiosarcomas are collectively one of the rarest forms of soft tissue neoplasms. They account for a vanishingly small proportion of all vascular tumors, and they comprise less than 1% of all sarcomas as estimated by a 20-year study at the M.D. Anderson Hospital.[62] Although they may occur in any location in the body, they rarely arise from major vessels and have a decided predilection for skin and superficial soft tissue, a phenomenon that contrasts sharply with the deep location of most soft tissue sarcomas. Analysis of 366 angiosarcomas reviewed at the AFIP during a 10-year period (Table 25-1) shows that one third (121 cases) occurred in the skin, about one fourth (89 cases) in soft tissue, and another one fourth collectively in other sites such as breast, liver, bone, and spleen. The presentation and behavior of these tumors differ depending on location, and a number of reports in the literature document the presentation of various organ-related angiosarcomas.* Hence, angiosarcomas are more properly considered as several closely related tumors rather than as a single entity. We have divided them into five groups:

1. cutaneous angiosarcoma unassociated with lymphedema;
2. cutaneous angiosarcoma associated with lymphedema (lymphangiosarcoma);
3. angiosarcoma of the breast;
4. radiation-induced angiosarcoma; and
5. angiosarcoma of deep soft tissue.

Etiological factors

Chronic lymphedema is the most widely recognized predisposing factor in angiosarcomas of skin and soft tissue,

---

*References 2, 29, 50, 65, 153, 163.
†References 86, 87, 90, 91, 93, 95, 97, 100-108, 111, 113-120, 123-126, 128, 132-136.

*References 8, 18, 20, 24, 45, 58.

yet in our cases only about 10% of tumors are associated with this condition (Table 25-1). Typically lymphedema-associated angiosarcomas occur in women who have undergone radical mastectomy for breast carcinoma and have suffered from chronic severe lymphedema for many years. Chronic lymphedema occurring on a congenital,[101,123,126] idiopathic, traumatic, or infectious basis[98,127,134] also predisposes to angiosarcoma. Several theories have been advanced to explain the association of lymphedema and angiosarcoma. Some have suggested that the growth and proliferation of obstructed lymphatics eventually fail to respond to normal control mechanisms. Others have subscribed to the idea that carcinogens within lymphatic fluid induce the neoplastic change. More recently the concept has been put forth that the lymphedematous extremity represents an "immunologically privileged site"[129] (because of the loss of afferent lymphatic connections) and consequently is unable to perform immunological surveillance of normally occurring mutant cell populations. This notion is supported by the observations that skin grafts survive for long periods when transferred to lymphedematous extremities.[129]

In the past it has been difficult to evaluate the role of radiation in the induction of angiosarcoma, for many patients who had received radiation also had chronic lymphedema. Based on our experience as well as a growing number of reports in the literature, radiation-induced angiosarcomas do occur. Five of the 44 cases reported by Maddox and Evans,[35] 2 of the 44 cases reported by Sordillo et al.,[134] and several other case reports[12,15,70,172] attest to the fact that radiation per se may lead to the development of angiosarcomas. To be considered radiation-induced, these tumors must be biopsy-proven angiosarcomas arising within the radiation field after an interval of several years and must not

be associated with chronic lymphedema. Over half of those cases qualifying as postirradiation angiosarcomas have occurred following radiotherapy for another malignant tumor such as carcinoma of the cervix,[35] ovary,[12] endometrium,[120,172] or breast,[15,167,168,171,174-177] and Hodgkin's disease.[173] Those which follow radiation for genitourinary malignant tumors usually develop on the lower abdominal wall, whereas those following radiation for breast carcinoma usually develop on the chest wall. The lumbar spinal area was the site for those following treatment of Hodgkin's disease.[173] The interval between the radiation and diagnosis has been approximately 12 years.[15,35] Longer intervals, however, have been noted in patients who have received low-dosage radiation for benign conditions such as eczema.[15]

A number of angiosarcomas have developed at the site of defunctionalized arteriovenous fistulas[10,30] or adjacent to foreign material introduced into the body either iatrogenically or accidentally.[5,23,27,30] In an extensive review of the literature provided by Jennings et al.,[27] nine examples of angiosarcoma associated with foreign material were identified. Common to all was a long latent period between the time of introduction of the foreign material and development of the tumor. Although one case occurred within 3 years, the remainder developed more than a decade later. A variety of solid materials were implicated including shrapnel, steel, plastic and dacron graft material,[56] surgical sponges,[5,27] and bone wax.[27] The authors suggest that an exuberant host response in the form of a fibrous tissue capsule around the foreign material may represent an important intermediate step in the development of the sarcoma. Malignant change in a preexisting benign vascular tumor is probably an unusual event. Many cases attesting to this phenomenon probably represent errors in the original diagnosis. In one series of angiosarcomas, however, four occurred in preexisting benign lesions; three arose in port-wine stains, and one arose in an irradiated lymphangioma. Angiosarcomas have also been documented within benign and malignant nerve sheath tumor,[8,11,38] in the setting of neurofibromatosis and as part of a malignant germ cell tumor,[53] and at the site of a herpes zoster lesion.[25] There is one example of angiosarcoma occurring in a patient with xeroderma pigmentosum.[31]

Unfortunately there is little information concerning the possible role of environmental carcinogens in the pathogenesis of soft tissue angiosarcomas. That such factors may exist is suggested by the relatively strong evidence linking various substances to the induction of hepatic angiosarcomas (Kupffer cell sarcomas). About one fourth of hepatic angiosarcomas[19] occur in patients who have received thorium dioxide for cerebral angiography, in vineyard workers exposed to AsO_3-containing insecticides, or in industrial workers exposed to vinyl chloride used in the produc-

Table 25-1. Anatomical distribution of angiosarcomas (AFIP, 1966-1976) (366 cases)

Location	No. cases	Percent
Skin	121	33
Without lymphedema	101	
With lymphedema	20	
Soft tissue	89	24
Breast	30	8
Liver	31	8
Bone	20	6
Spleen	16	4
Heart and great vessels	10	3
Orbit	10	3
Pharynx, oral cavity, and nasal sinuses	13	4
Other	26	7
TOTAL	366	100

tion of synthetic rubber.[3,36,45] A few cases have been recorded in patients receiving long-term androgenic anabolic steroids,[19] and one in a patient receiving estrogen.[24]

Cutaneous angiosarcoma not associated with lymphedema

This is the most common form of angiosarcoma. It primarily affects elderly persons (Tables 25-2 and 25-3) and is usually located on the head and neck, particularly the area of the scalp (Table 25-4) and upper forehead. Since many patients developing angiosarcomas are women with a full head of hair,[72] sun exposure as a tumorigenic agent is questionable. Clinically the appearance of these lesions is variable. Most begin as ill-defined bruiselike areas having an

indurated border and for this reason are apt to be considered benign. In a small number of cases a diagnosis of facial edema is entertained. Large, advanced lesions are elevated, nodular, and occasionally ulcerated (Fig. 25-1). It is difficult to determine the extent of these lesions clinically. This fact, coupled with multifocality noted in about half of

Table 25-2. Age distribution of cutaneous angiosarcomas without lymphedema (AFIP, 1966-1976) (101 cases)

Age (years)	No. cases	Percent
0-11	11	11
11-20	9	9
21-30	6	6
31-40	5	5
41-50	18	18
51-60	10	10
61-70	17	17
>70	22	22
Unspecified	3	2
TOTAL	101	100

Table 25-3. Sex distribution of cutaneous angiosarcomas without lymphedema (AFIP, 1966-1976) (101 cases)

Sex	No. cases	Percent
Male	62	62
Female	31	31
Unknown	8	7
TOTAL	101	100

Table 25-4. Anatomical distribution of cutaneous angiosarcomas without lymphedema (AFIP, 1966-1976) (101 cases)

Location	No. cases	Percent
Head and neck	52	52
Leg	13	13
Trunk	13	13
Arm	8	8
Generalized	2	1
Not specified	13	13
TOTAL	101	100

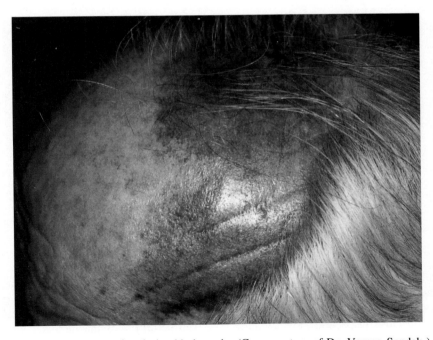

FIG. 25-1. Angiosarcoma of scalp in elderly male. (Case courtesy of Dr. Vernon Sondak.)

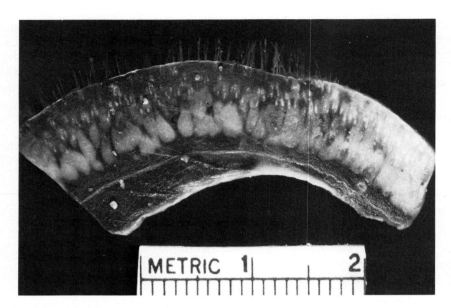

FIG. 25-2. Angiosarcoma of scalp. Hemorrhagic appearance frequently suggests diagnosis of hematoma.

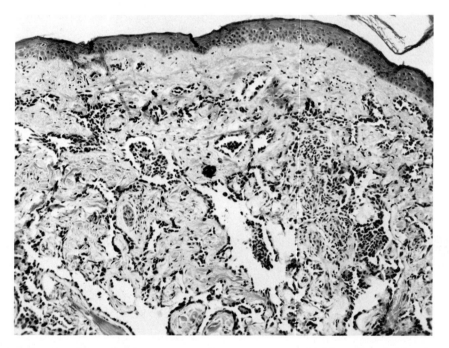

FIG. 25-3. Well-differentiated cutaneous angiosarcoma composed of irregular vascular channels infiltrating dermis. (×100.)

cases, seriously complicates therapy and probably results in suboptimal initial therapy in a large number of cases.

Grossly, the tumors consist of ill-defined hemorrhagic areas (Fig. 25-2), which on close inspection have a microcystic or spongelike quality as a result of the presence of blood-filled spaces. The tumors extensively involve the der-

mis and extend well beyond their apparent gross confines. In poorly differentiated, rapidly growing tumors, deep structures such as subcutis and fascia may also be invaded. The periphery of the tumors contains a fringe of dilated lymphatic vessels surrounded by chronic inflammatory cells and usually small capillaries in which piling up and tufting

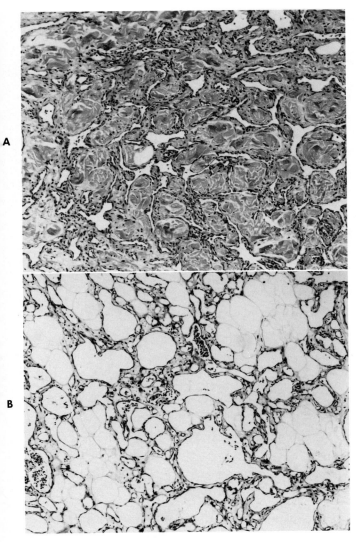

FIG. 25-4. Angiosarcoma dissecting through collagen (**A**) and fat (**B**). (×60.)

of the endothelium suggests incipient malignant change.

Many cutaneous angiosarcomas are well-differentiated to moderately well-differentiated lesions that form distinct vascular channels, albeit of irregular size and shape (Fig. 25-3). Such tumors may at first suggest poorly confined hemangiomas because of the numerous channels and the flattened innocuous appearance of the cells. Yet, in contrast to true hemangiomas, the vascular channels seem to create their own tissue planes, dissecting through the dermal collagen (Fig. 25-4) and fascia or splitting apart groups of subcutaneous fat cells. Moreover, there is a tendency for the channels to communicate with each other, forming an anastomosing network of sinusoids (Figs. 25-4 and 25-5). Although the cells to some extent resemble normal endothelium, they usually have larger, more chromatic nuclei and

often pile up along the lumina, creating the papillations so typical of angiosarcomas (but which may also be seen in reactive vascular proliferation such as papillary endothelial hyperplasia) (Fig. 25-6).

In a small number of cases, cutaneous angiosarcomas may be relatively high-grade tumors that are difficult to distinguish from carcinomas (Figs. 25-7 to 25-9) or high-grade fibrosarcomas (Fig. 25-10). These tumors may have occasional well-differentiated areas, as described earlier, which facilitate diagnosis. Others may be composed exclusively of poorly differentiated areas. The cells in the poorly differentiated tumors may be pleomorphic and usually display prominent mitotic activity. Occasionally a reticulin preparation may be useful in diagnosis as it may clearly outline the vascular lumina, emphasizing that the cells lie on the luminal side of the vessels (Fig. 25-11).

Ultrastructural and histochemical findings. The best-differentiated areas of these tumors possess many of the features of normal endothelium, including a partial investiture of basal lamina along the antiluminal borders (Fig. 25-12), tight junctions between cells, pinocytotic vesicles, and occasional cytofilaments.[78] Weibel-Palade bodies, tubular structures found in normal endothelium, are present in a disappointingly small number of angiosarcomas[34,69,78] and, when present, are few. Poorly differentiated tumors, however, lack many and sometimes all of the foregoing features. However, it has recently been pointed out by Mackay et al.[34] in an ultrastructural study of 47 angiosarcomas, that poorly differentiated areas of angiosarcomas still display topographical features that suggest vascular differentiation. These include a close relationship between tumor cells and erythrocytes such that the latter lie either between or sometimes within the cytoplasm of the former. Ramifying clefts between the cells suggest primitive or abortive vascular (luminal) differentiation. The authors did not note any ultrastructural differences between angiosarcomas arising in lymphedema and those that did not. Alkaline phosphatase, an enzyme found in vascular endothelium, has been identified by some investigators[68] but not by others.[77,79]

Immunohistochemical findings. Whereas confirmation of the diagnosis of angiosarcoma by immunohistochemical methods can be accomplished in some cases,[9,41,42,57,58] use of this modality has been frustrated by the lack of antibodies that are both specific and sensitive for endothelial differentiation. Initial enthusiasm for antibodies directed against factor VIII–associated antigen, the most widely used and relatively sensitive marker for endothelium, was dampened by the finding that less than one fourth of angiosarcomas contained sufficient amounts of the protein to allow demonstration by routine immunohistochemical studies (Fig. 25-13). Because of problems related to diffusion of factor VIII–associated antigen, immunostaining studies for this antigen are difficult to interpret (see Chapter 8). Although nonimmunological binding by *Ulex europaeus,* a

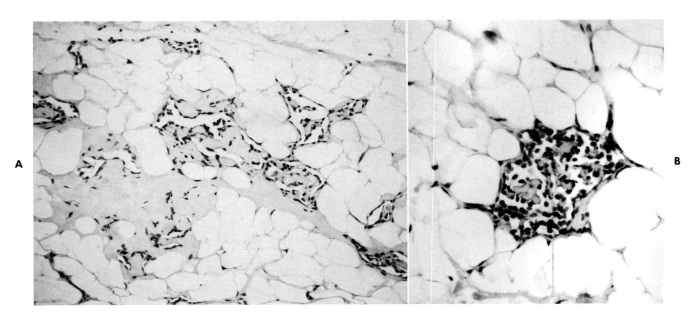

FIG. 25-5. Well-differentiated angiosarcoma diagnosable by virtue of its infiltrative growth (**A**) and papillary ingrowth of endothelium (**B**). (**A**, ×160; **B**, ×250.)

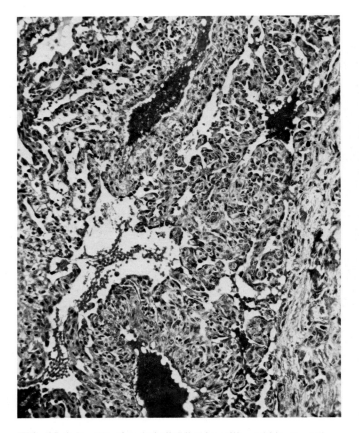

FIG. 25-6. Fronds of endothelial-lined papillae within an angiosarcoma. Although this pattern is quite similar to papillary endothelial hyperplasia (Chapter 23), there is more piling up of cells and more nuclear atypism. (×160.)

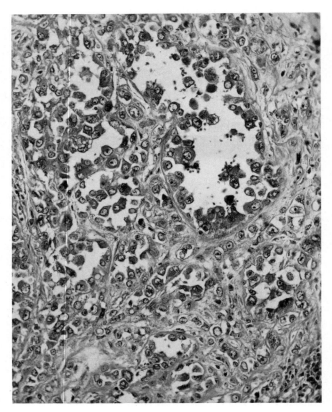

FIG. 25-7. Angiosarcoma showing lumina lined by plump epithelioid endothelial cells. (×160.)

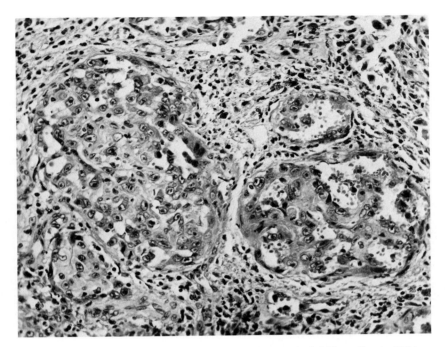

FIG. 25-8. Angiosarcoma composed of rounded epithelial-like cells. (×160.)

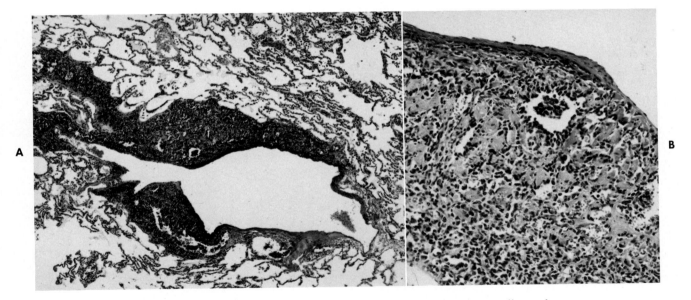

FIG. 25-9. Angiosarcoma metastatic to lung (A). Tumor occasionally shows peculiar tendency to localize around vessels (B). (A, ×100; B, ×160.)

plant lectin, to endothelial cells and their tumors is far more sensitive than factor VIII-AG in identifying angiosarcomas, it is also less specific and has been noted in other soft tissue tumors (e.g., synovial sarcoma, epithelioid sarcoma) as well as some carcinomas. In recent years a number of new antibodies directed against various structural and protein

products of endothelium have been employed. Antibodies to thrombomodulin, an antagonist of factor VIII-AG, decorate most angiosarcomas but also react with various carcinomas and trophoblastic tumors.[61] Likewise, CD34 (human hematopoietic progenitor cell antigen) is expressed by many angiosarcomas[53] and Kaposi's sarcoma but is also

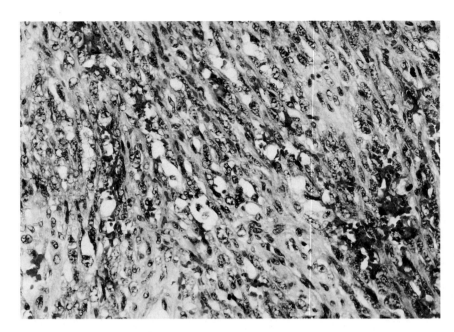

FIG. 25-10. Angiosarcoma with spindled areas resembling a fibrosarcoma. Areas like this also resemble Kaposi's sarcoma except for the fact that they usually appear more pleomorphic. (×250.)

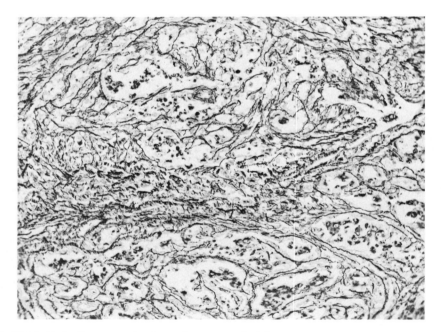

FIG. 25-11. Reticulin preparation in angiosarcoma. Staining accentuates vascular lumina, which may be inapparent in routine staining. (×120.)

seen in a variety of soft tissue tumors including some (e.g., epithelioid sarcoma) that may enter into the differential diagnosis of angiosarcoma.[13,46,56] The most recent acquisition to the immunohistochemical armamentarium is antibodies to CD31 (platelet-endothelial cell adhesion mole-cule), which seems at present to be a highly sensitive and specific antigen for endothelial differentiation. Within the context of soft tissue neoplasia, all benign and malignant vascular tumors express this membrane protein, whereas over 100 soft tissue tumors of nonvascular lineage do not.[17]

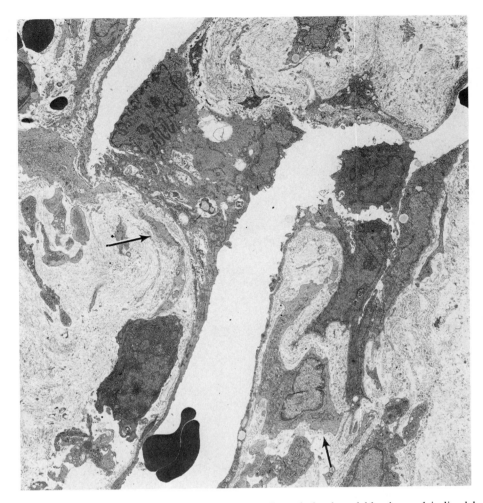

FIG. 25-12. Electron micrograph of angiosarcoma. Irregularly shaped blood vessel is lined by neoplastic endothelial cells possessing segments of basal lamina. Several perithelial cells and their processes are present outside vessel wall *(arrows)*. (Courtesy of Dr. Jerome B. Taxy.)

The most prudent approach to the diagnosis of angiosarcomas, therefore, is to use immunohistochemical studies to rule out other diagnoses that may legitimately enter the differential diagnosis in a given case and to also use a panel of vascular markers that, if positive, could support the diagnosis of angiosarcoma.

Behavior and treatment

The prognosis of cutaneous angiosarcomas is quite poor.[72] This may be explained in part by the delay in seeking medical advice by patients, who were often elderly, as well as by the tendency to underestimate and undertreat the tumors initially. In the largest series, 72 patients reported by Holden et al.,[72] only 12% of patients survived 5 years or longer, with one half dying within 15 months of presentation. A comparably poor outlook was documented by Maddox and Evans[35] in their group of 17 patients, 16 of whom died of complications of the tumor. The most im-

portant factor in determining prognosis seems to be the size of the initial lesions. Tumors less than 5 cm in diameter have a significantly better prognosis than larger lesions.[35] Other factors such as sex, location, and histological grading could not be correlated with prognosis.[72] Death from disease occurs either by local extension of tumor or by metastasis. Usually both recurrences and metastases are noted within 2 years of diagnosis, although in the series of 12 reported by Haustein, the patient died of extensive local disease without metastases.[69]

Sites affected by metastases are most commonly cervical lymph nodes, followed by lung, liver, and spleen. Seven long-term survivors of cutaneous angiosarcomas have been studied by Holden et al.,[72] who noted that they had all received radical radiotherapy, mostly widefield electron beam therapy. Although all had achieved local disease control, two eventually developed late pulmonary metastases (after 10 years).

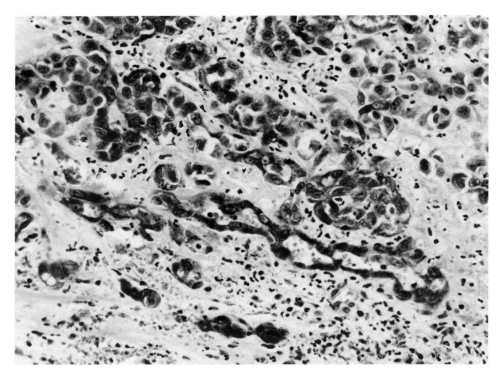

FIG. 25-13. Immunohistochemical localization of factor VIII-AG within an epithelial-appearing angiosarcoma. Antigen was detected within solid clusters of cells as well as those lining lumina. (×250.)

Angiosarcoma associated with lymphedema

In 1948, Stewart and Treves[135] reported six patients who developed vascular sarcomas following radical mastectomy and axillary lymph node dissection for breast carcinoma. Although some of the patients had, in addition, received radiotherapy, the common denominator in each of the cases appeared to be the presence of chronic lymphedema, which usually supervened shortly after the time of mastectomy. Since this original description, approximately 200 cases of vascular sarcomas complicating chronic lymphedema have been recorded. The majority not unexpectedly have occurred in women following mastectomy, although tumors have been documented on the abdominal wall following lymph node dissection for carcinoma of the penis[91] and either the arm or leg affected by congenital,[101] idiopathic, or traumatic lymphedema. Recently reports have noted the association of angiosarcoma in filarial lymphedema as well.[98,133]

The pathogenesis of these unusual tumors is far from understood. It has been suggested that chronic lymphatic obstruction results in an abortive attempt at collateralization that eventually runs awry. However, other explanations obviously must be considered, and localized defects in cellular immunity may play a role, since it has been noted that

homografts transplanted to lymphedematous extremities survive far longer than those transplanted to the normal extremity of the same patient.[129] Moreover, it is possible that radiotherapy plays a secondary role in some cases by enhancing or aggravating the lymphedema.

Clinical findings. About 90% of all angiosarcomas associated with chronic lymphedema occur following mastectomy for breast carcinoma,[139] although the frequency of this complication has been estimated by Shirger[131] as only 0.45% of all women surviving for 5 years following mastectomy. Such patients are women in the seventh decade who have developed a significant degree of lymphedema, usually within a year of mastectomy. The tumors develop within 10 years of the original surgery, although the interval may be as short as 4 years or as long as 27 years. In rare instances the tumor has been reported in postmastectomy patients who have experienced little or no lymphedema. Whether some patients truly have no lymphedema must be questioned because minor degrees of lymphedema in obese patients could go undetected clinically.

When these tumors occur in congenital or idiopathic lymphedema, the affected patients are usually younger, the lymphedema is of longer duration, and any extremity may be affected. Most patients are in the fourth or fifth decade

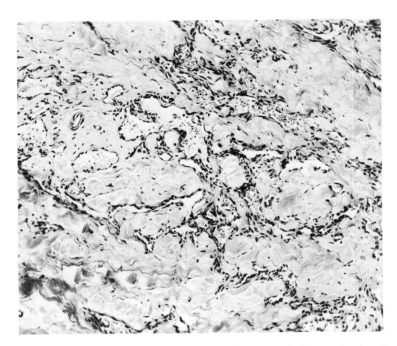

FIG. 25-14. Postmastectomy angiosarcoma (lymphangiosarcoma). Tumor is virtually indistinguishable from cutaneous angiosarcomas arising in patients without lymphedema. (×100.)

and have experienced lymphedema for 19 to 20 years. There is one case of congenital lymphedema and lymphangiosarcoma associated with Maffucci's syndrome.[136]

Regardless of the clinical setting, the onset of cancer is heralded by the development of one or more polymorphic lesions superimposed on the brawny nonpitting edema of the affected extremity. Deeply situated lesions in the subcutis may impart only a mottled purple-red hue to the overlying skin, whereas the superficial lesion can be palpated as distinct nodules that coalesce to form large polypoid growths. Ulceration, accompanied by a serosanguineous discharge, characterizes late lesions. Repeated healing and breakdown give rise to lesions of various stages that spread distally to the hands and feet or proximally to the chest wall or trunk in advanced cases of lymphangiosarcoma.

Microscopic findings. Despite the fact that the term *lymphangiosarcoma* is commonly used, these lesions appear essentially identical to those of the head and neck described in the preceding sections. The hallmark of the lesion is the presence of small capillary-sized vessels composed of obviously malignant cells that infiltrate soft tissue and skin (Fig. 25-14). The lumina may be empty, filled with clear fluid, or engorged with erythrocytes, a finding that has made it difficult to classify these tumors as to blood vessel or lymphatic origin and has led to the suggestion that two lines of differentiation may be present. Lymphocytes are occasionally found around the neoplastic vessels, but because this feature is also seen in other angiosarcomas, it

does not provide sufficient evidence of lymphatic differentiation.

Perhaps the only feature that sets this tumor apart from the conventional angiosarcomas discussed in this chapter and provides some support for lymphatic differentiation is the association of this tumor with areas of so-called lymphangiomatosis.[139] These changes appear to represent premalignant changes of small vessels, presumably lymphatics. The vessels become dilated and appear to form a diffuse ramifying network throughout the soft tissue (Fig. 25-15). They are lined by plump endothelial cells with hyperchromatic nuclei. These areas may merge imperceptibly with areas of frank angiosarcoma or may exist alone in patients who have not yet developed discrete clinical lesions.[120] The question of therapy in this premalignant lesion is problematic. Such patients probably are at risk to develop angiosarcoma and deserve scrupulous follow-up care. However, it seems best to recommend therapy only in those patients who have developed distinct clinical lesions.

Electron microscopic findings. One of the most significant contributions of electron microscopy to the understanding of this disease has been to eradicate any lingering doubt concerning the possibility that these tumors represent carcinomas, specifically late recurrence of the original breast carcinoma.[125,132] Ultrastructurally, the best-differentiated areas of this tumor have features of capillary endothelial cells including numerous pinocytotic vesicles, lateral

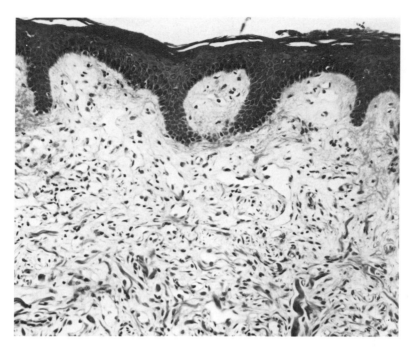

FIG. 25-15. Diffuse proliferation of dermal lymphatic vessels (lymphangiomatosis) containing atypical endothelium. Lesion occurred in a patient a few years following mastectomy for breast carcinoma. Minimal lymphedema was present. Such changes have been considered "premalignant" and may herald onset of frank angiosarcoma (lymphangiosarcoma). (×160).

desmosome-like attachments, and occasionally paranuclear filaments.[101,122] The cells are, furthermore, surrounded by basal lamina outside of which pericytes may be identified. Weibel-Palade bodies have also been identified.[125] There appear to be no differences ultrastructurally between those tumors which arose in lymphedema and those that did not,[34] although in one case reported by Kindblom et al.,[122] the authors also believed that some areas show lymphatic as well as vascular differentiation.

Although electron microscopy can document subtle degrees of endothelial differentiation not appreciated by light microscopy, poorly differentiated tumors understandably contain few ultrastructural features that would permit their recognition. In these areas the cells resemble primitive mesenchymal cells containing abundant rough endoplasmic reticulum, glycogen, few intercellular attachments, and no luminal differentiation.[132]

Cytogenetic findings. Only a few cases of angiosarcoma have been studied cytogenetically. In the one case of Stewart-Treves syndrome reported by Kindblom et al.,[122] 40% of the cells studied had a normal diploid karyotype, whereas the remainder displayed a variety of nonclonal deletions and translocations.

Behavior and treatment. It is difficult to reliably interpret survival data because of the paucity of cases and the fact that early cases have been treated suboptimally by modern standards. Woodward et al.[139] attempted a retrospective analysis of these tumors based on their experience at the Mayo Clinic and that reported in the literature. The mean (actuarial) survival time of patients with lymphangiosarcoma following mastectomy was 19 months, compared with 34 months for those developing the tumor outside this setting. The median survival time of patients with angiosarcoma and lymphedema in the experience of the Memorial Hospital is 31 months.[134] Only 6 of the 40 patients survived 5 years or longer. The salient point in both studies is that long-term survivors have usually been treated by initial radical ablative surgery, either limb disarticulation or hindquarter or forequarter amputation. Patients treated by less radical surgery or by radiation run an unacceptably high risk of local recurrence. It is quite probable that "local recurrence" in this disease is really an expression of extensive multifocal disease, a phenomenon that underscores the need to radically excise the lesions. Metastases to the lung, pleura, and chest wall are very common and account for essentially all of the disease-related deaths.

Angiosarcoma of breast

Angiosarcoma of the breast is a rare tumor, accounting for approximately 1 out of every 1700 to 2000 primary malignant tumors of the breast.[156,157] Despite its highly malignant nature, it may have a deceptively bland appearance, a phenomenon that has led to errors of underdiagnosis attending almost half of the reported cases. Unlike other an-

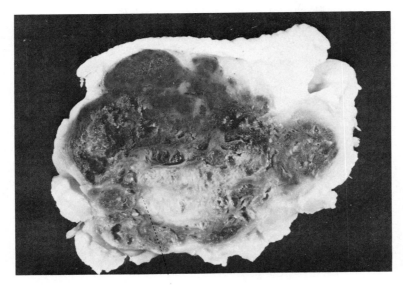

FIG. 25-16. Angiosarcoma of breast. Tumor contains numerous blood-filled cysts.

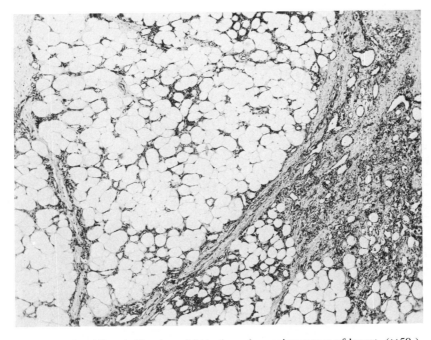

FIG. 25-17. Diffuse infiltration of fatty tissue by angiosarcoma of breast. (×50.)

giosarcomas this type occurs exclusively in women, usually during the third or fourth decade. Only occasional cases have been reported during the postmenopausal period. Several cases have been reported in pregnant women,[149,153,161,162] and at least one case rapidly enlarged with the onset of pregnancy.[156]

These lesions usually develop as rapidly growing masses that cause diffuse enlargement of the breast associated with a blue-red discoloration of the skin. Despite the appreciable size at the time of biopsy, the classic signs of ordinary mammary carcinoma such as skin retraction, nipple discharge, and axillary node enlargement are absent. The tumors are invariably deeply located within the substance of the breast. They usually spread to involve the skin but seldom extend into the pectoral fascia. The tumors are ill-defined, hemorrhagic, spongy masses (Fig. 25-16) sur-

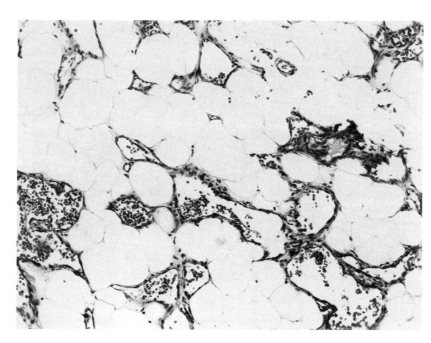

FIG. 25-18. Angiosarcoma of breast illustrating manner in which tumor dissects through fat, isolating groups of cells. (×145.)

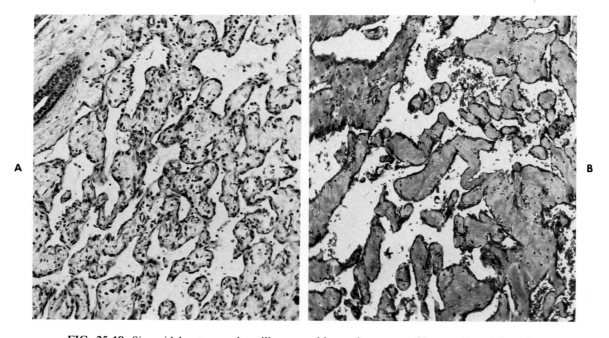

FIG. 25-19. Sinusoidal pattern and papillae created by angiosarcoma of breast. (A and B, ×60.)

rounded by a rim of vascular engorgement. The rim corresponds to a zone of well-differentiated but, nonetheless, neoplastic capillary-sized vessels that can be compared with areas of a hemangioma except that their growth is more permeative. The main tumor mass shows the same changes that characterize other angiosarcomas (Figs. 25-17 to 25-19). Likewise, metastasis may resemble the parent lesion or may show less differentiation. In one unusual case we have reviewed, extramedullary hematopoiesis was present in the metastasis despite its absence in the original tumor.[161]

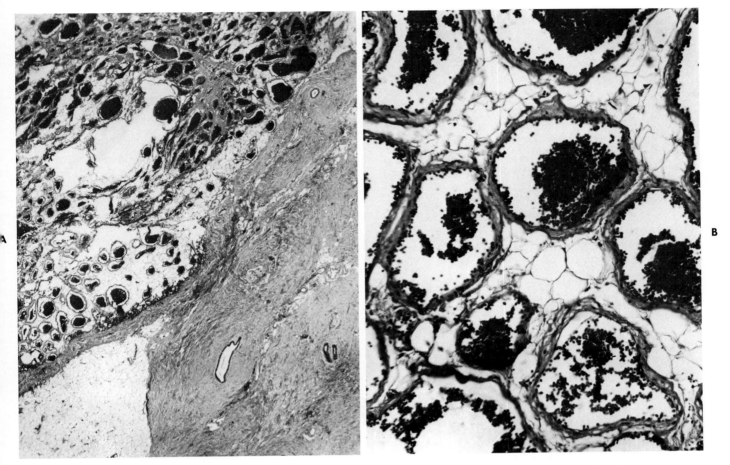

FIG. 25-20. Cavernous hemangioma of breast. **A,** Contrast sharp margins of tumor with those of angiosarcoma. (×25.) **B,** Vessels are well differentiated and have regular lumina. (×250.)

Differential diagnosis of this lesion lies principally in distinguishing it from benign hemangioma or angiolipoma, which on rare occasions involves the breast. In our experience angiosarcomas of the breast are ill-defined lesions almost always containing cellular areas with atypia, mitotic activity, and necrosis. It is the presence of these features that ultimately distinguishes these tumors from hemangiomas. However, because some areas of an angiosarcoma can be well differentiated, it is advisable to totally embed small histologically benign or borderline lesions. Larger lesions presenting the same diagnostic problem should be generously sampled. True hemangiomas or angiolipomas of the breast are usually sharply demarcated from the normal breast tissue (Figs. 25-20 and 25-21). The vessels of the hemangioma are more regular in shape (Fig. 25-20, *B*), while those of the angiolipoma possess the typical microthrombi (Fig. 25-21, *B*).

Behavior and treatment. Angiosarcomas are the most malignant of all breast tumors.[157] Of the approximately 50 cases reported in the literature, about 90% of the patients have died of the disease, usually within 2 years of diagno-sis. Metastasis occurs relatively rapidly after diagnosis and most frequently involves the lungs, skin, and bone. In some instances massive bleeding from metastatic lesions appears to be the immediate cause of death.[152,153,161] However, in a recent study of 40 patients treated at two institutions, the survival rate was much better and could be correlated with the tumor grade. Over three fourths of patients with grade I lesions were alive compared with less than one fifth with grade III lesions.[146]

A similar trend was noted for 15 patients with breast angiosarcoma entered into the Connecticut Tumor Registry.[158] The best chance of survival is offered to those patients who present shortly after onset of symptoms with relatively small lesions and who receive prompt mastectomy.[162] Less radical procedures almost always lead to local recurrence. Axillary lymph node dissections are not essential in the management of this disease, because metastasis to these structures, even in the face of large primary lesions, is quite rare. Adjuvant chemotherapy, particularly with dactinomycin, seems to be effective in some patients.[144]

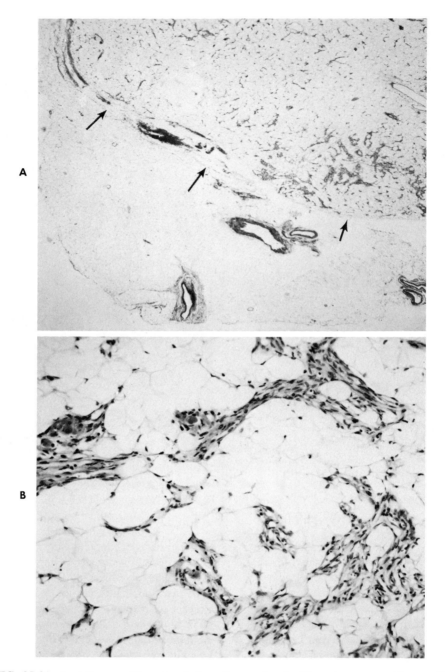

FIG. 25-21. Angiolipoma of breast, a lesion often confused with angiosarcoma of breast. Tumor is **(A)** typically well demarcated from normal breast *(arrows)* and is composed of **(B)** attenuated vascular channels containing microthrombi. (**A,** ×15; **B,** ×160.)

Angiosarcoma of soft tissue

Angiosarcomas arising from and essentially restricted to deep soft tissue comprise a poorly defined group of tumors reported only rarely in the literature. An estimate that one fourth of angiosarcomas are of this type (Table 25-1) most likely is an overestimate of their frequency, since many of these tumors are probably cutaneous angiosarcomas with deep extension. Even allowing for difficulties in ascertaining acceptable cases, it appears that these tumors do not display the relatively homogenous clinical characteristics of other angiosarcomas. Rather these tumors may occur at any age and are evenly distributed throughout all decades (Ta-

Table 25-5. Age distribution of angiosarcomas of soft tissue (AFIP, 1966-1976) (89 cases)

Age (years)	No. cases	Percent
0-10	12	12
11-20	14	16
21-30	16	18
31-40	12	13
41-50	8	10
51-60	11	12
>60	16	19
TOTAL	89	100

Table 25-6. Sex distribution of angiosarcomas of soft tissue (AFIP, 1966-1976) (89 cases)

Sex	No. cases	Percent
Male	58	66
Female	28	32
Unknown	3	2
TOTAL	89	100

Table 25-7. Anatomical distribution of angiosarcomas of soft tissue (AFIP, 1966-1976) (89 cases)

Location	No. cases	Percent
Leg	34	38
Arm	17	19
Trunk	22	25
Head and neck	13	15
Unknown	3	3
TOTAL	89	100

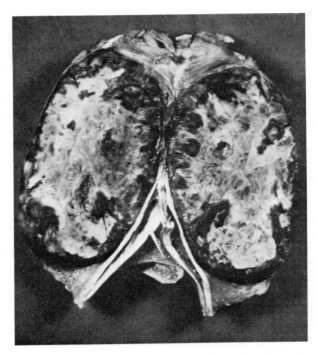

FIG. 25-22. Angiosarcoma of deep soft tissue. Prominent hemorrhage and necrosis characterized the tumor.

bles 25-5 and 25-6). Like the more common soft tissue sarcomas, this form of angiosarcoma has a propensity to occur on the extremities or in the abdominal cavity (Table 25-7), where it presents as a large, markedly hemorrhagic mass (Fig. 25-22). It is not unusual for these tumors to be confused with a chronic hematoma, even following biopsy of tumors, if the biopsy material is limited or nonrepresentative. In the very young the large size of this tumor may result in hematological abnormalities such as thrombocytopenia, high-output cardiac failure from arteriovenous shunting, or even death from massive exsanguination. In histological studies, these tumors show the same range as other angiosarcomas, although they tend to be of a more uniformly high grade. It also appears that deeply situated angiosarcomas have a tendency to display epithelioid change of the endothelium.[164,165] These so-called epithelioid angiosarcomas consist of sheets of highly atypical rounded cells, some of which contain intracytoplasmic lumina. In addition to factor VIII-AG this form of angiosarcoma also commonly coexpresses cytokeratin, and this makes their distinction from carcinoma particularly difficult.

Although angiosarcomas of deep soft tissue should for the most part be considered highly malignant, the paucity of data precludes precise statements concerning the rate of metastasis and optimal mode of therapy. In the experience cited by Fletcher et al.,[164] concerning epithelioid angiosarcoma of deep soft tissue, two thirds of patients (four of six) with sufficient follow-up information developed metastatic disease.

Radiation-induced angiosarcoma

Although not a common postirradiation sarcoma, angiosarcomas have been documented following therapeutic irradiation for tumors of diverse types. In previous decades postirradiation angiosarcomas commonly presented as intraabdominal or abdominal wall masses following radiation for carcinomas of the cervix, ovary, and uterus, with a small number of cases occurring following radiation for various other malignant or benign conditions.[68,70,71] In the last several years, however, the clinical profile seems to be changing. A number of angiosarcomas involving the skin or breast parenchyma in women who have had breast-sparing surgery and radiation for mammary carcinoma often coupled with axillary lymph node dissection have been reported.[166-171,174-176] Most of these patients have not had lymphedema, suggesting that the significant common theme is radiation. Latencies in this group of patients have been relatively short compared with other postirradiation sarcomas and average approximately 5 years with some occurring after 3 years.[171] Nearly all of these tumors have been aggressive high-grade sarcomas. However, cases reported by Moskaluk et al.[169] and Davies et al.[15] involved low-grade or borderline vascular tumors that repeatedly recurred but did not produce metastasis. Thus, it appears that postirradiation sarcomas occurring in the setting of breast-conserving surgery for carcinoma may represent a broader spectrum of lesions than formerly appreciated.

KAPOSI'S SARCOMA

In 1872 Kaposi[249] described five cases of an unusual tumor that principally affected the skin of the lower extremities in a multifocal, often symmetrical fashion. He considered the condition a round cell sarcoma that he termed "idiopathic multiple pigmented sarcoma of the skin." Since his description, there have been dissenting opinions as to whether the lesions are neoplasms or hyperplasia. Those who favor the latter idea have emphasized the waxing and waning course of the disease, instances of regression, and the fact that the tumor does not produce metastatic disease in the manner of conventional sarcomas but rather develops in a multifocal fashion. Although most consider the well-established lesions of Kaposi's sarcoma neoplastic, its course is greatly influenced by the immune status of the individual.

Current evidence suggests that Kaposi's sarcoma is a viral-associated, if not viral-induced, tumor. The geographical distribution of Kaposi's sarcoma in Africa is similar to, although not identical to, that of Burkitt's lymphoma,[260] a tumor associated with a chronic carrier state of Epstein-Barr virus. The variable course of the disease, marked in rare instances by spontaneous regression, is compatible with immunological response to tumor similar to viral-induced tumor in animals.[220,221] The multiplicity of lesions in Kaposi's sarcoma in the absence of a discrete primary tumor indicates multifocal disease compatible with viral infection. Finally, the emergence of Kaposi's sarcoma within certain groups of AIDS patients known to be coinfected with other viruses has reinforced efforts to identify an oncogenic virus for this intriguing tumor.

Identification of a causative agent has not been accomplished, however. It does not appear that HIV can be directly or solely imputed in the pathogenesis of Kaposi's sarcoma for several reasons: (1) Kaposi's sarcoma occurs preferentially within some AIDS risk groups; (2) there is no seroepidemiological association between the chronic form of Kaposi's sarcoma in Africa and HIV infection[186]; and (3) HIV-l sequences have not been identified within Kaposi's sarcoma cells. Although in the past a large body of circumstantial evidence seemed to link cytomegalovirus infections with Kaposi's sarcoma, there have been conflicting data as to whether cytomegalovirus genomic sequences are present in Kaposi's sarcoma cells.[222,243] The issue of a causative agent has been made all the more complicated by the apparent finding of HPV-16–like sequences and HPV-related antigens within this neoplasm[244,279] and by the observation that the HIV-1 tat gene, when introduced into the germ line of mice, can induce lesions quite similar to those of Kaposi's sarcoma.[210,316] Epidemiological studies attempting to identify other agents, common exposures, or social and sexual practices that can explain the high incidence of Kaposi's sarcoma among homosexuals has so far been inconclusive.[185,208] However, it does seem clear that Kaposi's sarcoma cells produce a number of cytokines that which may stimulate their own growth (autocrine effect),[211,276] and HIV-infected T cells release substances that also enhance the growth of Kaposi's sarcoma cells (paracrine effect).[210,278]

Clinical findings

Kaposi's sarcoma occurs in four distinct clinical forms: the chronic, the lymphadenopathic, the transplantation-associated, and the AIDS-related form.

Chronic Kaposi's sarcoma. In the chronic or classic form, the disease occurs primarily in males (90%) in late adult life (peak incidence, sixth or seventh decade). The disease is prevalent in certain parts of the world including Poland, Russia, Italy, and the central equatorial region of Africa. In the latter region it may account for up to 9% of all reported cancers. It is rare in the United States, accounting for only 0.02% of all cancers. This form also manifests a statistically significant association with either a second malignant tumor or altered immune state. A study from Memorial Hospital indicates that about one third of patients (34 of 92) with this form of Kaposi's sarcoma have or subsequently develop a second malignant tumor, and half of these neoplasms are of lymphoreticular origin including leukemia, lymphoma, and multiple myeloma.[299] Kaposi's sarcoma may also be associated with pure red cell aplasia[293] and autoimmune hemolytic anemia.[262,293] There is no association of this form of Kaposi's sarcoma with HIV-1, even in Africa.[186]

The disease commences with the development of multiple cutaneous lesions, usually on the distal portion of the lower extremity (Fig. 25-23). Less commonly the lesions occur on the upper extremity and rarely in a visceral organ in the absence of cutaneous manifestations. The initial lesion is a blue-red nodule, which is often accompanied by edema of the extremity. The latter sign has been interpreted by some as indicating deep soft tissue or lymphatic involvement by the tumor. The lesions slowly increase in size and number, spreading proximally and coalescing into plaques or polypoid growths that may resemble pyogenic granuloma. Occasional lesions may even ulcerate. In some patients, the early lesions regress, while others evolve so that many different stages of the disease are present at the same

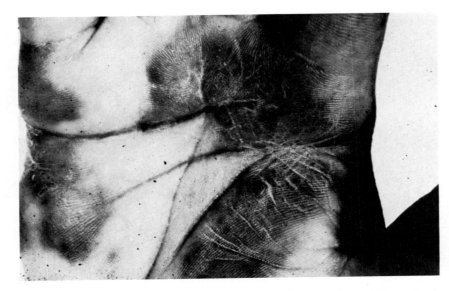

FIG. 25-23. Kaposi's sarcoma involving palm of hand. Lesions are elevated, hemorrhagic, and multifocal in distribution.

time. The course of the disease is characteristically prolonged.

Lymphadenopathic Kaposi's sarcoma. In contrast to the foregoing type, this form occurs primarily in young African children who present with localized or generalized lymphadenopathy with involvement of cervical, inguinal, and hilar lymph node chains and occasionally of ocular tissues and salivary gland. Skin lesions are usually sparse and, when they occur, develop more centrally than in the chronic form.[204] The course of the disease is fulminant, and this has been attributed to the greater tendency toward internal involvement. Preliminary evidence also suggests that this form is not associated with HIV-1 infection.[275]

Transplantation-associated Kaposi's sarcoma. The development of Kaposi's sarcoma among renal transplant patients is well established, although the actual incidence varies depending on the patient population, suggesting that genetic background influences the risk in the posttransplant setting as well. For example in Western countries the incidence of posttransplantation Kaposi's sarcoma has been estimated at less than 1%,[237,238] whereas in the Near East it approaches 4%. There are conflicting data as to whether the type of immunosuppression affects this risk.[290,305]

The disease develops several months to a few years after the transplant (average time, 16 months), and the extent of the disease can be correlated directly with the loss of cellular immunity as measured by response to PHA, Con A, PWM, and DNCB skin testing. In a few instances of transplantation-associated Kaposi's sarcoma, the tumor has occurred in a previous surgical site.[304]

The clinical course in this form of Kaposi's sarcoma is dependent both on the stage of the disease and the ability to successfully manipulate the dosage of immunosuppressives. In the experience cited by Qunibi et al.,[290] those patients with disease restricted to the skin who could tolerate a 50% reduction in the dosage of immunosuppression had a 100% response rate. However, those patients who develop organ or internal involvement succumb to their disease.

AIDS-related Kaposi's sarcoma. AIDS, caused by the human immunodeficiency virus (HIV-1), produces profound immunodeficiency and susceptibility to opportunistic infections and various tumors.[214] AIDS probably originated in Africa, where its epidemic proportions have been attributed both to heterosexual transmission and to transmission via contaminated medical equipment (e.g., syringes).[289] In the United States the majority of cases occur in the male homosexual population, although other risk groups, including intravenous drug users and hemophiliacs receiving factor VIII—enriched blood fractions, are also well recognized. Approximately 30% of patients with AIDS develop Kaposi's sarcoma, and in many instances diagnosis of the tumor leads to clinical recognition of the syndrome.[220] Kaposi's sarcoma, however, does not affect the known risk groups equally, and for this reason it is postulated that another agent alone or in concert with HIV-1 is responsible for the tumors.[197] Roughly 40% of homosexual patients with AIDS have developed Kaposi's sarcoma compared with less than 5% in the other recognized risk groups. It has only rarely occurred in transfusion recipients.[197,315] A number of epidemiological studies have, therefore, striven to identify social or sexual practices

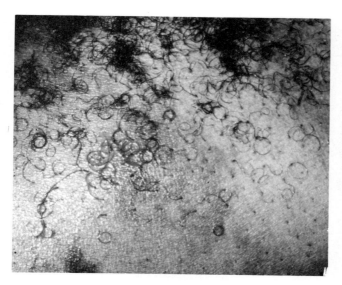

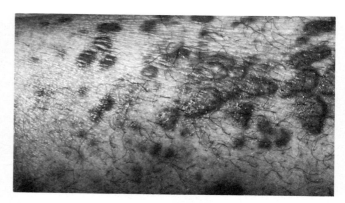

FIG. 25-25. Advanced stage of Kaposi's sarcoma in AIDS patient showing combination of patch, plaque, and nodular lesions. (Courtesy Dr. Abe Macher.)

FIG. 25-24. Early patch stage of Kaposi's sarcoma as seen in an AIDS patient. Lesion is flat and mottled. (Courtesy Dr. Abe Macher.)

within the homosexual group that may predispose them to develop Kaposi's sarcoma. In particular, some[185] but not all authors[208] have suggested that oral-anal contact may facilitate the transmission of a Kaposi's sarcoma agent.

In the AIDS syndrome, Kaposi's sarcoma develops in a young adult population (mean age, 39 years). Initially the lesions are small flat pink patches (Fig. 25-24) and only later acquire the classic blue-violet papular appearance (Fig. 25-25). They occur in almost any location, but predilection for lines of cleavage[229] and the tip of the nose has been noted.[301] About one half of patients have lymph node lesions and one third have gastrointestinal lesions as well as skin lesions.

Microscopic findings

There appears to be no fundamental difference in the appearance of Kaposi's sarcoma among the various clinical groups. However, in our experience, the early lesions of Kaposi's sarcoma are seen most commonly now in the AIDS patient, and the subtlety of changes in many cases presents an ongoing challenge to the surgical pathologist.

The earliest or *patch stage*[229] of Kaposi's sarcoma is a flat lesion characterized by a proliferation of miniature vessels surrounding larger ectatic vessels. A slightly more advanced patch lesion displays, in addition, a loosely ramifying network of jagged vessels in the upper dermis (Figs. 25-26 to 25-29). In some respects this stage resembles a well-differentiated angiosarcoma, except that the cells are so bland that they closely resemble normal capillary or lymphatic endothelium. There is also a sparse infiltrate of lymphocytes and plasma cells surrounding the patch lesion. The

histological changes seen in patch lesions have also been noted in clinically normal areas of skin in patients who have Kaposi's sarcoma elsewhere. This observation underscores the diffuseness of the disease process.[302]

The more advanced *plaque stage* of the disease produces a slight elevation of the skin, for at this point the vascular proliferation usually involves most of the dermis and may extend to the subcutis. A discernible, but relatively bland, spindle cell component, which is initially centered around the proliferating vascular channels, appears at this stage. In time the spindle cell foci coalesce and produce the classic nodular lesions of Kaposi's sarcoma (Fig. 25-30). Diagnosis of the well-established case is seldom difficult. Graceful arcs of spindled cells intersect one another in the manner of a well-differentiated fibrosarcoma (Fig. 25-31), but unlike fibrosarcoma, slitlike spaces containing erythrocytes separate the spindled cells and vascular channels (Fig. 25-32). In cross-section these arcs of spindled cells are equally diagnostic by virtue of the sievelike or honeycomb pattern they create (Fig. 25-33). Inflammatory cells (lymphocytes and plasma cells), hemosiderin deposits, and dilated vessels are commonly seen at the periphery of nodular lesions (Figs. 25-34 and 25-35). A rather characteristic, but probably not specific, feature of the well-established lesion is the presence of the hyaline globule. These PAS-positive, diastase-resistant spherules, measuring between 1 and 7 μ, may be located both intracellularly and extracellularly (Fig. 25-36). Some of the hyaline globules are effete erythrocytes, an idea which derives support from the finding of erythrocytes within phagolysosomes by ultrastructural analysis and by certain common histochemical features (positive for toluidine blue and endogenous peroxidase).[248]

Although the typical lesions of Kaposi's sarcoma are devoid of pleomorphism and a significant number of mitotic figures, histologically aggressive forms of Kaposi's sar-

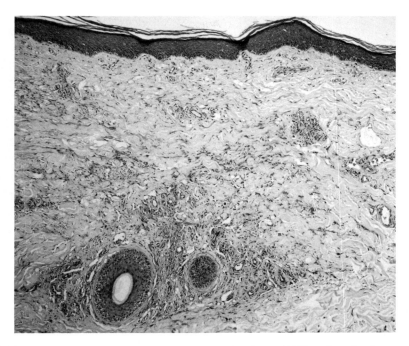

FIG. 25-26. Early lesion of Kaposi's sarcoma occurring in an AIDS patient. Lesions are flat or slightly elevated. (Hematoxylin-eosin stain; ×25.)

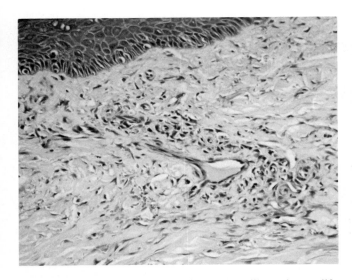

FIG. 25-27. Early lesion of Kaposi's sarcoma illustrating proliferation on miniature vessels around larger vessels. (Hematoxylin-eosin stain; ×250.)

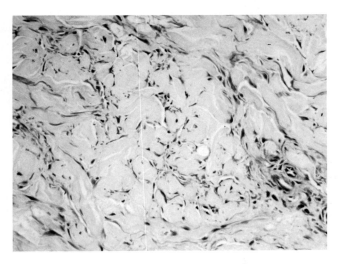

FIG. 25-28. Early lesion of Kaposi's sarcoma depicting jagged endothelial channels dissecting dermal collagen. (Hematoxylin-eosin stain; ×250.)

coma can be seen (Fig. 25-37). This may occur as a result of progressive histological dedifferentiation in otherwise typical cases. This phenomenon was observed in 5 of 14 autopsy cases reviewed by Cox and Helwig[199] and in two autopsy cases reported by Reed et al.[292] In our experience, poorly differentiated tumors may also arise ab initio and

seem to be more common in cases of Kaposi's sarcoma originating in Africa. In these tumors the cells not only appear more pleomorphic, but there may be a brisk level of mitotic activity. Kaposi's sarcoma, particularly in the setting of AIDS, may show transitional areas that appear more akin to angiosarcoma (Figs. 25-38 and 25-39). These areas

Text continued on p. 666.

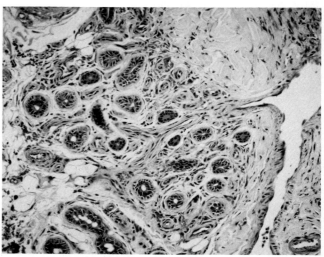

FIG. 25-29. Small vessels infiltrating adnexal structures in early lesion of Kaposi's sarcoma. (Hematoxylin-eosin stain; ×250.)

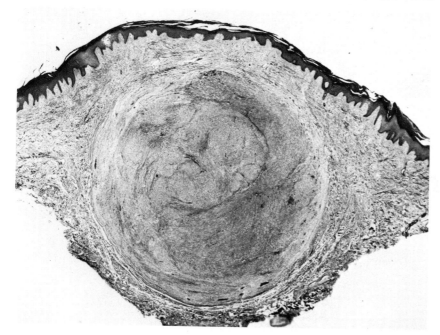

FIG. 25-30. Well-established lesion of Kaposi's sarcoma. Tumor is distinctly nodular. (Hematoxylin-eosin stain; ×25.)

FIG. 25-31. Kaposi's sarcoma illustrating monomorphic appearance of well-established lesion. (Hematoxylin-eosin stain; ×100.)

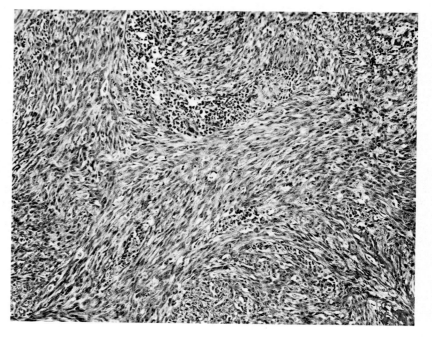

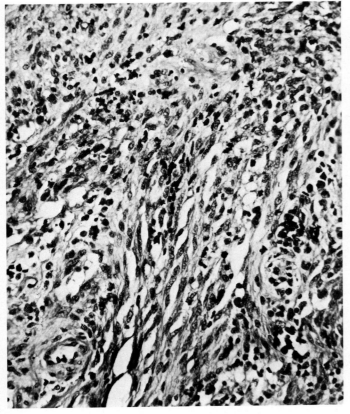

FIG. 25-32. Kaposi's sarcoma with typical slitlike vascular spaces as seen in longitudinal section. (Hematoxylin-eosin stain; ×250.)

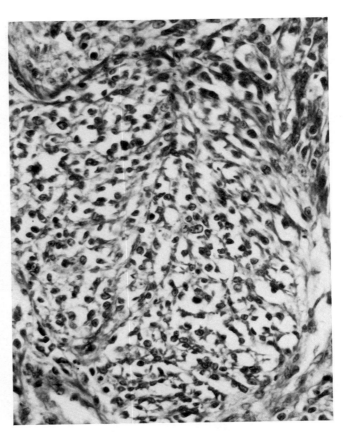

FIG. 25-33. Cross-sectional view of fascicle of Kaposi's sarcoma showing sievelike pattern. (Hematoxylin-eosin stain; ×250.)

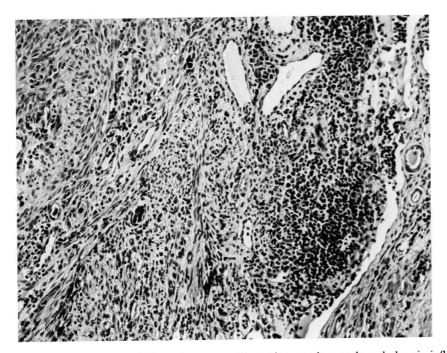

FIG. 25-34. Peripheral area of Kaposi's sarcoma illustrating ectatic vessels and chronic inflammatory cells. (Hematoxylin-eosin stain; × 160.)

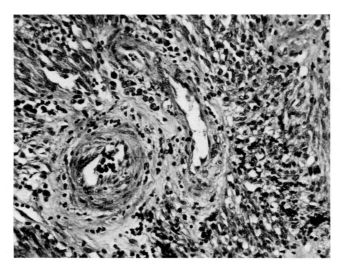

FIG. 25-35. Thick-walled vessels occasionally seen at periphery of lesions of Kaposi's sarcoma. (Hematoxylin-eosin stain; ×250.)

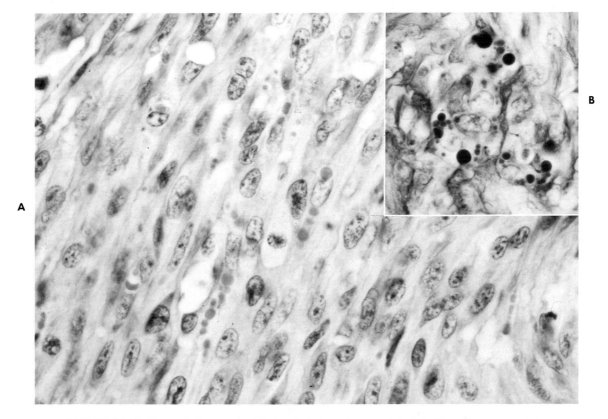

FIG. 25-36. Hyaline globules seen both intracellularly and extracellularly in Kaposi's sarcoma **(A).** Hyaline globules demonstrated in PAS staining following diastase digestion **(B).** (**A,** Hematoxylin-eosin stain; ×250; **B,** PAS; ×400.)

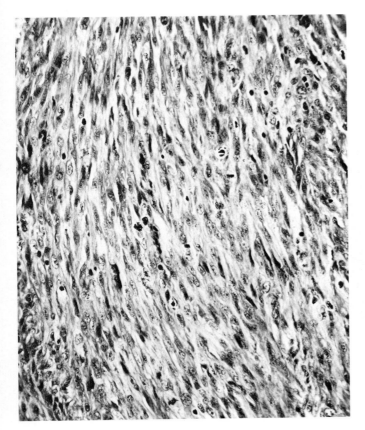

FIG. 25-37. Kaposi's sarcoma illustrating more cellularity, pleomorphism, and mitotic activity than the conventional case (see Fig. 25-10). (Hematoxylin-eosin stain; ×250.)

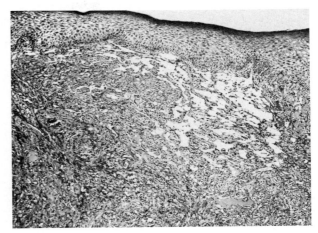

FIG. 25-38. Kaposi's sarcoma with transitional areas resembling angiosarcoma. (Hematoxylin-eosin stain; ×100.)

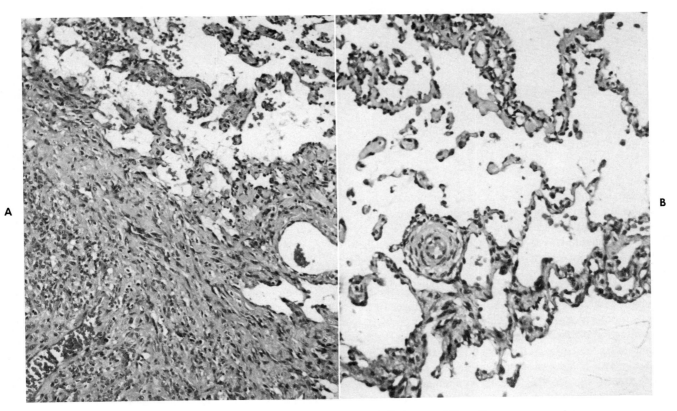

FIG. 25-39. High-power view of Fig. 25-16 showing spindled areas of Kaposi's sarcoma merging with angiomatous areas **(A),** which may have many of the features of angiosarcoma **(B).** (A and B, Hematoxylin-eosin stain; ×250.)

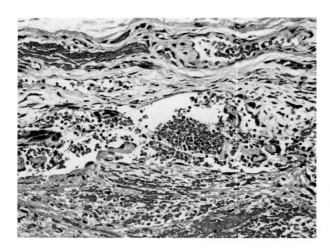

FIG. 25-40. Early Kaposi's sarcoma involving lymph node showing ectasia of subcapsular sinus and endothelial proliferation. (Hematoxylin-eosin stain; ×250.)

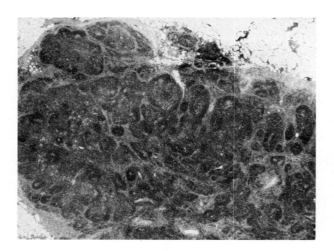

FIG. 25-41. Early Kaposi's sarcoma involving subcapsular sinus and interfollicular sinuses with overall preservation of lymph node structure. (Hematoxylin-eosin stain; ×15.)

may contain large ectatic vascular spaces similar to a hemangioma or lymphangioma and in addition possess papillary tufts lined by atypical endothelial cells (Fig. 25-39, *B*). The former feature was addressed in the literature, and such tumors were termed "lymphangioma-like Kaposi's sarcoma."[217]

Just as the early changes of Kaposi's sarcoma in the skin present a diagnostic challenge, so do early changes of this tumor in other organs. A particularly common problem is the evaluation of lymph nodes in the AIDS patient. Within lymph nodes the earliest changes may be represented by a mild angiectasia and proliferation of vessels in the subcapsular sinus (Fig. 25-40). The interfollicular sinuses are gradually involved and expanded (Figs. 25-41 and 25-42).

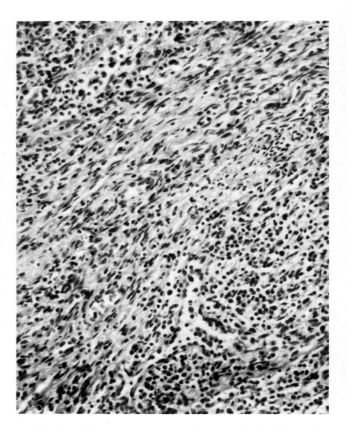

FIG. 25-42. High-power view of node in Fig. 25-18 showing interfollicular sinuses expanded by spindled cells of Kaposi's sarcoma. (Hematoxylin-eosin stain; ×160.)

The earliest stages may closely resemble the reactive lymph node condition known variously as nodal angiomatosis and vascular transformation of the subcapsular sinus, which occurs as a result of lymph node obstruction. Others have noted the similarity of these lymph nodes to Castleman's disease when the proliferating vessels are centered around the follicles.[235,300] Accurate diagnosis of these histologically ambiguous lymph nodes should include complete sectioning of the block. This tactic often reveals more solidly cellular spindled foci, which confirm the diagnosis.[235] Well-advanced cases of Kaposi's sarcoma involving lymph nodes do not present a problem of the same magnitude, for they show partial or complete lymph node effacement by a monotonous spindle cell proliferation (Fig. 25-43).

Special studies

Immunohistochemical studies have contributed significantly to our understanding of the histogenesis of this tumor. In the past, variable reporting of factor VIII-AG in this tumor led to controversy concerning its endothelial nature. However, factor VIII-AG has proved to be highly variable in malignant vascular tumors, may be differentially expressed depending on the type of endothelium, and is subject to a great variety of interpretations because of diffu-

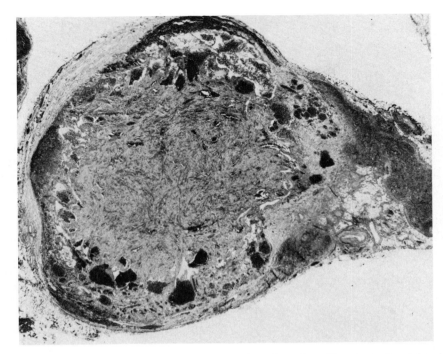

FIG. 25-43. Kaposi's sarcoma involving lymph node and causing effacement of nodal architecture. (Hematoxylin-eosin stain; ×15.)

Table 25-8. Histochemical and immunohistochemical staining of Kaposi's sarcoma

	Normal capillary	Normal lymphatic	Kaposi's sarcoma
Anti-factor VIII-AG[273]	+	+/−	−*
EN-4[245,246]	+	+	+
PAL-E[245,246]	+	−	− (Early lesions)
			+/− (Late lesion)
OKM5[296]	+	−	+*
Anti-E92[296]	+	−	+*
HC1[296]	+	−	+*
HLA/DR/Ia[184]	+	−	−*
Alkaline Phosphatase[184]	+++	−	−*
5' nucleotidase[184]	+	+++	+*
B721[303]	+	−	+

*Spindled cells of tumor.

sion artifact. The use of numerous monoclonal antibodies directed against various structural substances in the endothelial cell has provided the opportunity to circumvent these problems. Several groups have provided support for the endothelial nature of Kaposi's sarcoma using a number of monoclonal antibodies, but their findings have led to apparently contradictory conclusions as to whether Kaposi's sarcoma is derived from vascular or lymphatic endothelium (Table 25-8). Rutgers et al.[296] have concluded that the cells are more closely related to vascular endothelium because of immunostaining with three monoclonal antibodies (OKM5, anti-E92, and HCl), which react with capillary but not lymphatic endothelium. Scully et al.[303] likewise have documented immunoreactivity in Kaposi's sarcoma cells utilizing an antibody B721, which reacts with all vascular endothelium except for that of the renal glomerulus and sinusoids of the liver and spleen. Beckstead et al.,[184] on the other hand, argue for lymphatic endothelial differentiation because of the lack of HLA-DR/Ia and alkaline phosphatase and the intense 5' nucleotidase. Jones et al.[245,246] have illustrated that the immunoreactivity of the tumor varies with the type or stage of the disease, with the early patch stage having the immunological profile of a lymphatic tumor. These areas stain positively with a monoclonal antibody directed against all endothelium (EN-4) but do not stain with an antibody specific for vascular endothelium (PAL-E). More developed lesions, however, stain with EN-4 and are variable with PAL-E. Most recently Weich et al.[320] have proposed that the Kaposi's sarcoma cell may be closely related to a vascular smooth muscle cell since the tumors express mRNA for alpha smooth muscle actin.

Ultrastructural observations

Electron microscopy has traditionally supported the idea of the endothelial differentiation within these tumors. In the early lesions slender endothelial cells with oval nuclei and small nucleoli line slitlike lumina (Fig. 25-44). Few intercellular junctions are noted, and focally gaps may be

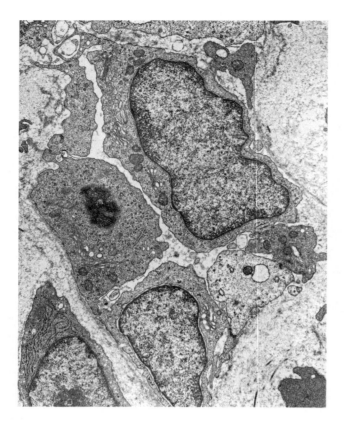

FIG. 25-44. Electron micrograph of Kaposi's sarcoma. Cells exhibit endothelial characteristics and are surrounded by fragmented basal lamina. Pericytes are absent or greatly reduced. (×9000.) (From *Am J Pathol* 111:62, 1983. Electron micrograph courtesy Dr. N. Scott McNutt.)

present between the cells. Fragmented basal lamina encircles the abluminal surface of the cells, and few if any pericytes are observed.[269] The latter observations seem to be more compatible with lymphatic than vascular differentiation. Advanced lesions not unexpectedly contain cells that have been variously described as "perithelial" or "fibroblastic," although immunohistochemical observations would indicate that these are actually modified endothelial cells. Ultrastructurally the spindled "perithelial" cells possess lysosomes and ferritin and appear to be actively phagocytic.

Differential diagnosis

As indicated, recognition of the early changes of Kaposi's sarcoma, especially in the AIDS patient, remains one of the most difficult diagnostic problems. The irregular infiltrative pattern of the endothelial cells in early lesions is more helpful in diagnosis than the degree of cytological atypia. However, the changes may be virtually indistinguishable from a well-differentiated angiosarcoma. An accurate clinical history becomes of paramount importance in establishing the diagnosis. In the well-advanced case, confusion

with a fibrosarcoma may occur. Features that distinguish a very cellular form of Kaposi's sarcoma from a fibrosarcoma include the presence of ectatic vessels and inflammatory cells at the periphery of the lesions, the more curvilinear fascicles, and the presence of hyaline globules.

Arteriovenous malformations may occasionally give rise to cutaneous lesions that clinically duplicate the picture of Kaposi's sarcoma. Such lesions have been termed "pseudo-Kaposi's sarcoma."[266] Histologically, these lesions consist of a proliferation of small capillary-sized vessels occasionally surrounded by extravasated erythrocytes and hemosiderin. Frank spindling and formation of slitlike lumina are not seen. Arteriographic studies documenting the presence of an underlying arteriovenous malformation and the clinical findings of a bruit in the area of the lesions provide additional contrasting points.

The spindle cell hemangioendothelioma (see Chapter 24) is frequently confused with Kaposi's sarcoma. Both the presence of cavernous vessels and the epithelioid endothelial cells (which are not seen in Kaposi's sarcoma) are the most reliable features for distinguishing the two tumors.

Behavior and treatment

The behavior of Kaposi's sarcoma is quite variable and is dependent on a number of interrelated factors such as the immunological competence of the host, the stage of the disease, and the presence or absence of opportunistic infections. In the chronic form of the disease, which occurs in more or less immunocompetent individuals who usually present with limited cutaneous disease, the disease-related mortality rate is between 10% and 20%. Even in patients in this group who die of their disease, the duration of the disease is between 8 and 10 years. However, an additional 25% of patients will die of a second malignant tumor.[281]

Patients with AIDS who develop Kaposi's sarcoma have a far more aggressive course. The overall mortality rate of patients with Kaposi's sarcoma and AIDS is 41%, within a relatively limited follow-up period, and is greatly influenced by the stage of the disease, presence of opportunistic infections, and presence of systemic symptoms.[274] Eighty percent of patients who remain without an opportunistic infection will be alive at 28 months compared with less than 20% with an opportunistic infection.[252]

Because of the relative paucity of cases of Kaposi's sarcoma in this country prior to the AIDS epidemic, there has been relatively little reported experience in the treatment of the disease. Surgery, formerly recommended, is no longer indicated apart from tissue diagnosis. The tendency toward multifocality even in the chronic form of the disease makes radiation or chemotherapy, or both, the preferred therapy. Staging of Kaposi's sarcoma patients (see box on p. 669) now provides a more uniform means of comparing treatment protocols. Stage I patients, usually examples of the chronic form of the disease, may be treated by local irra-

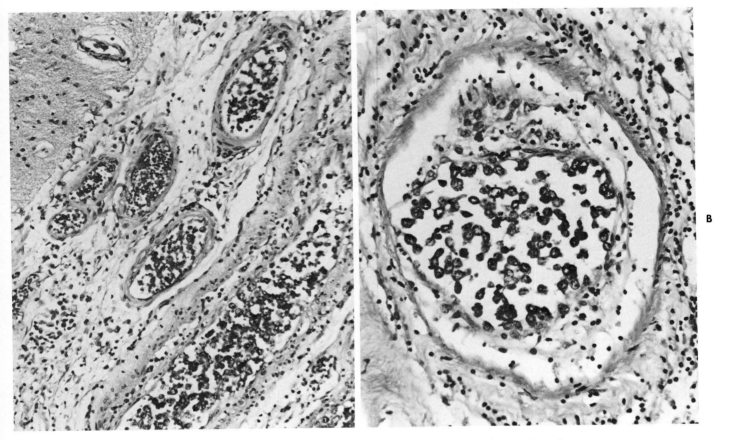

FIG. 25-45. Angiotropic lymphoma (proliferating angioendotheliomytosis) in a patient who presented with progressive neurological symptoms. **A,** At autopsy the tumor was restricted to vessels throughout the body. (×160.) **B,** Cells are primitive round cells with high nucleocytoplasmic ratio. (×400.)

Staging of Kaposi's sarcoma	
Stage I:	Cutaneous, locally indolent
Stage II:	Cutaneous, locally aggressive, with or without regional lymph nodes
Stage III:	Generalized mucocutaneous or lymph node involvement, or both
Stage IV:	Visceral involvement
Subtypes:	A. No systemic signs or symptoms B. Systemic signs: 10% weight loss or fever over 100° F orally unrelated to an identifiable source of infection lasting more than 2 weeks

diation.[252] Patients with stage III and IV disease, characteristic of AIDS-related Kaposi's sarcoma, require chemotherapy. Effective drugs in the treatment of this disease include etoposide, doxorubicin, bleomycin, vinblastine sulfate, interferon-alpha,[299,317] and zidovudine.

INTRAVASCULAR LYMPHOMATOSIS (ANGIOTROPIC LYMPHOMA)

Intravascular lymphomatosis, formerly called *proliferating angioendotheliomatosis,* is included in this chapter for historical interest only since it has been conclusively identified as a lymphoma rather than an endothelial tumor.

Originally described by Pfleger and Tappeiner,[334] this unusual tumor was formerly believed to be a diffuse neoplastic change of the endothelium throughout the body. Numerous recent reports attest to the fact that this tumor usually proves, in well-studied cases, to be a lymphoma with a predilection to involve the intravascular spaces.[323,324,326,328,336]

The disease occurs in adults and affects the sexes equally.

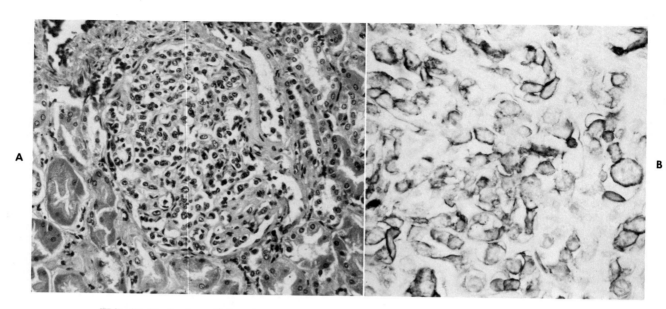

FIG. 25-46. Angiotropic lymphoma involving renal glomerular capillaries **(A)**. Malignant cells stained with antibody directed against leukocyte common antigen **(B)**. (A, ×250; B, peroxidase antiperoxidase technique, ×630.)

It begins with the development of multiple, indurated erythematous nodules or plaques of the skin, which bear a resemblance to erythema nodosum. Initially the general health of the patient is good, although occasionally fever and neurological signs are present. Histologically, the small vessels of the dermis and subcutis are filled with plump mononuclear cells, which occasionally appear to be in continuity with the endothelium (Figs. 25-45 and 25-46). The proliferating cells, accompanied by small fibrin thrombi, may virtually occlude small vessels. The cells have a high nucleocytoplasmic ratio, prominent nucleoli, and occasional mitotic figures. In those patients dying of the disease, neoplastic cells are found in vessels throughout the body, and in some instances they infiltrate the parenchyma of organs. In the past the mistaken assumption that these tumors were derived from endothelium and not lymphocytes is partly explained by the fact that there is minimal involvement of bone marrow, lymph nodes, and spleen. Studies allegedly reporting factor VIII-AG or Weibel-Palade bodies[340] in the tumor probably sampled adjacent reactive endothelium rather than tumor. Recent immunohistochemical studies clearly demonstrate that the tumors have the immunological profile of lymphomas,[323,324,336,342] the majority typing as B cell lymphomas,[323,328,336] others as T cell lymphomas,[336] and still others as lymphomas of mixed phenotype.[324] It has been suggested that these unusual lymphomas possess receptors causing them to home selectively to endothelium.[336] Because of the differences in treatment protocols, it is particularly important that these lesions be distinguished from a true soft tissue sarcoma.

REFERENCES
General

1. Alles JU, Bosslet K: Immunocytochemistry of angiosarcomas: a study of 19 cases with especial emphasis on the applicability of endothelial cell specific markers to routinely prepared tissues. *Am J Clin Pathol* 89:463, 1988.
2. Alpert LI, Benisch B: Hemangioendothelioma of the liver associated with microangiopathic hemolytic anemia. *Am J Med* 48:624, 1970.
3. Alrenga DP: Primary angiosarcoma of the liver: review article. *Int Surg* 60:198, 1975.
4. Ben-Ishak O, Auslander L, Rabison S, et al: Epithelioid angiosarcoma of the adrenal gland with cytokeratin expression: report of a case with accompanying mesenteric fibromatosis. *Cancer* 69:1808, 1992.
5. Ben-Ishak O, Kerner H, Brenner B, et al: Angiosarcoma of the colon developing in a capsule of a foreign body. *Am J Clin Pathol* 97:416, 1992.
6. Berry CL, Amerigo J: Blood group antigens in vascular tumors. *Virchows Arch (Pathol Anat)* 388:167, 1980.
7. Bricklin AS, Rushton HW: Angiosarcoma of venous origin arising in radial nerve. *Cancer* 39:1556, 1977.
8. Brown RW, Tornos C, Evans HL: Angiosarcoma arising from malignant schwannoma in a patient with neurofibromatosis. *Cancer* 70:1141, 1992.
9. Burgdorf WHC, Mukai K, Rosai J: Immunohistochemical identification of factor VIII-related antigen in endothelial cells of cutaneous lesions of alleged vascular nature. *Am J Clin Pathol* 75:167, 1981.
10. Byers RJ, McMahon RFT, Freemont AJ, et al: Epithelioid angio-

sarcoma arising in an arteriovenous fistula. *Histopathology* 21:87, 1992.

11. Chaudhuri B, Ronan SG, Manaligod JR: Angiosarcoma arising in a plexiform neurofibroma. *Cancer* 46:605, 1980.

12. Chen KTK, Hoffman KD, Hendricks EJ: Angiosarcoma following therapeutic irradiation. *Cancer* 44:2044, 1979.

13. Cohen PR, Rapini RP, Farhood AI: Expression of the human hematopoietic progenitor cell antigen CD34 in vascular and spindle cell tumors. *J Cutan Pathol* 20:15, 1993.

14. Curran KL, Kupchella CE, Tamburro CH: Urinary glycosaminoglycan patterns in angiosarcoma of the liver. *Cancer* 40:3050, 1977.

15. Davies JD, Rees GJG, Mera SL: Angiosarcoma in irradiated postmastectomy chest wall. *Histopathology* 7:947, 1983.

16. Dawson EK, McIntosh D: Granulation tissue sarcoma following long-standing varicose ulceration. *J R Coll Surg* 16:88, 1971.

17. DeYoung BR, Wick MR, Fitzgibbon JF, et al: CD31: an immunospecific marker for endothelial differentiation in human neoplasms. *Appl Immunohistochem* 1:97, 1993.

18. Eusebi V, Carcangiu ML, Dina R, et al: Keratin-positive epithelioid angiosarcoma of the thyroid: a report of four cases. *Am J Surg Pathol* 14:737, 1990.

19. Falk H, Thomas LB, Popper H, et al: Hepatic angiosarcoma associated with androgenic anabolic steroids. *Lancet* 2:1120, 1979.

20. Falk S, Krishnan J, Meis JM: Primary angiosarcoma of the spleen: a clinicopathologic study of 40 cases. *Am J Surg Pathol* 17:959, 1993.

21. Goette DK, Detlefs RL: Postirradiation angiosarcoma. *J Am Acad Dermatol* 12:922, 1985.

22. Gray MH, Rosenberg AE, Dickersin GR, et al: Cytokeratin expression in epithelioid vascular neoplasms. *Hum Pathol* 21:212, 1990.

23. Hayman J, Huygens H: Angiosarcoma developing around a foreign body. *J Clin Pathol* 36:515, 1983.

24. Hoch-Ligeti C: Angiosarcoma of liver associated with diethylstilbesterol. *JAMA* 240:1510, 1978.

25. Hudson CP, Hanno R, Callen JP: Cutaneous angiosarcoma in a site of healed herpes zoster. *Int J Dermatol* 23:404, 1984.

26. Jaffe EA: Endothelial cells and biology of factor VIII. *N Engl J Med* 296:377, 1977.

27. Jennings TA, Peterson L, Axiotis CA, et al: Angiosarcoma associated with foreign body material: a report of three cases. *Cancer* 62:2436, 1988.

28. Johnson WC: Pathology of cutaneous vascular tumors. *Int J Dermatol* 15:239, 1976.

29. Kauffman SL, Stout AP: Malignant hemangioendothelioma in infants and children. *Cancer* 14:1186, 1961.

30. Keane MM, Carney DN: Angiosarcoma arising from a defunctionalized arteriovenous fistula. *J Urol* 149:364, 1993.

31. Kuzu I, Bicknell R, Harris AL, et al: Heterogeneity of vascular endothelial cells with relevance to diagnosis of vascular tumors. *J Clin Pathol* 45:143, 1992.

32. Leake J, Sheehan MP, Rampling D, et al: Angiosarcoma complicating xeroderma pigmentosum. *Histopathology* 21:179, 1992.

33. Little D, Said JW, Siegel RJ, et al: Endothelial cell markers in vascular neoplasms: an immunohistochemical study comparing factor VIII-related antigen, blood group specific antigen, 6-keto-PGF1 alpha, and *Ulex europaeus* l lectin. *J Pathol* 149:89, 1986.

34. Mackay B, Ordonez NG, Huang W-L: Ultrastructural and immunocytochemical observations on angiosarcomas. *Ultrastruct Pathol* 13:97, 1989.

35. Maddox JC, Evans HL: Angiosarcoma of skin and soft tissue: a study of 44 cases. *Cancer* 48:1907, 1981.

36. Makk L, Delorme F, Creech J, et al: Clinical and morphologic features of hepatic angiosarcoma in vinyl chloride workers. *Cancer* 37:149, 1976.

37. Mandahl N, Jin Y, Heim S, et al: Trisomy 5 and loss of the Y chro-

mosome as the sole cytogenetic anomalies in a cavernous hemangioma/angiosarcoma. *Genes Chrom Cancer* 1:315, 1990.

38. Meis JM, Kindblom L-G, Enzinger FM: Angiosarcoma arising in von Recklinghausen's disease (NF1): report of five additional cases. *Mod Pathol* 7:8A, 1994.

39. Millstein DI, Chik-Kwun T, Campbell EW: Angiosarcoma developing in a patient with neurofibromatosis (von Recklinghausen's disease). *Cancer* 47:950, 1981.

40. Molina A, Bangs CD, Donlon T: Angiosarcoma of the scalp with a complex hypotetraploid karyotype. *Cancer Genet Cytogenet* 41:268, 1989.

41. Mukai K, Rosai J: Factor VIII-related antigen: an endothelial marker. In DeLellis RA, editor: *Diagnostic immunohistochemistry,* New York, 1984, Masson Publishing.

42. Nadji M, Gonzalez MS, Castro A, et al: Factor VIII-related antigen: an endothelial cell marker. *Lab Invest* 42:139A, 1980.

43. Ordonez NG, Batsakis JG: Comparison of *Ulex europaeus* I lectin and factor VIII-related antigen in vascular lesions. *Arch Pathol Lab Med* 108:129, 1984.

44. Parums DV, Cordell JL, Micklem K, et al: JC70: a new monoclonal antibody that detects vascular endothelium associated antigen on routinely processed tissue sections. *J Clin Pathol* 43:752, 1990.

45. Popper H, Thomas LB, Telles NC, et al: Development of hepatic angiosarcoma in man induced by vinyl chloride, Thorotrast, and arsenic. *Am J Pathol* 92:349, 1978.

46. Ramani P, Bradley NJ, Fletcher CDM: QBEND/10, a new monoclonal antibody to endothelium: assessment of its diagnostic utility in paraffin sections. *Histopathology* 17:237, 1990.

47. Sehested M, Hou-Jensen K: Factor VIII related–antigen as an endothelial marker in benign and malignant diseases. *Virchows Arch (Pathol Anat)* 391:217, 1981.

48. Sirgi KE, Wick MR, Swanson PE: B72.3 and CD34 immunoreactivity in malignant epithelioid soft tissue tumors: adjuncts in the recognition of endothelial neoplasms. *Am J Surg Pathol* 17:179, 1993.

49. Steiner GC, Dorfman HD: Ultrastructural study of hemangioendothelial sarcoma of bone. *Cancer* 29:122, 1972.

50. Stout AP: Hemangioendothelioma: a tumor of blood vessels featuring vascular endothelial cells. *Ann Surg* 118:445, 1943.

51. Suzuki Y, Hashimoto K, Crissman J, et al: The value of blood group–specific lectin and endothelial associated antibodies in the diagnosis of vascular proliferations. *J Cutan Pathol* 13:408, 1986.

52. Swanson PE, Wick MR: Immunohistochemical evaluation of vascular neoplasms. *Clin Dermatol* 9:243, 1991.

53. Traweek ST, Kandalaft PL, Mehta P, et al: The human progenitor cell antigen (CD34) in vascular neoplasia. *Am J Clin Pathol* 96:25, 1991.

54. Ulbright TM, Clark SA, Einhorn LH: Angiosarcoma associated with germ cell tumors. *Hum Pathol* 16:268, 1985.

55. Waldo ED, Vuletin JC, Kaye GI: The ultrastructure of vascular tumors: additional observations and a review of the literature. *Pathol Ann* 12:278, 1977.

56. Weiss SW, Nickoloff BJ: CD-34 is expressed by a distinctive cell population in peripheral nerve, nerve sheath tumors, and related lesions. *Am J Surg Pathol* 17:1039, 1993.

57. Weiss WM, Riles TS, Gouge TH, et al: Angiosarcoma at the site of a dacron vascular prosthesis: a case report and literature review. *J Vasc Surg* 14:87, 1991.

58. Wenig BM, Abbondanzo SL, Heffess CS: Epithelioid angiosarcoma of the adrenal glands: a clinicopathologic study of nine cases with a discussion of the implications of finding "epithelial-specific" markers. *Am J Surg Pathol* 18:62, 1994.

59. Wilkinson HA, Lucas JC, Foote FW: Primary splenic angiosarcoma. *Arch Pathol* 85:213, 1968.

60. Wilson-Jones E: Malignant vascular tumors. *Clin Exp Dermatol* 1:287, 1976.

61. Yonezawa S, Maruyama I, Sakae K, et al: Thrombomodulin as a marker for vascular tumors: comparative study with factor VIII and *Ulex europaeus* I lectin. *Am J Clin Pathol* 88:405, 1987.

Cutaneous angiosarcoma

62. Bardwil JM, Mocega EE, Butler JJ, et al: Angiosarcomas of the head and neck region. *Am J Surg* 116:548, 1968.
63. Burgoon CF, Sodenberg M: Angiosarcoma. *Arch Dermatol* 99:773, 1969.
64. Cardozo DW, Claud PL, Chen I, et al: Cystic pulmonary metastasis complicating angiosarcoma of the scalp. *Calif Med* 105:210, 1966.
65. Caro MR, Stubenrauch CH Jr: Hemangioendothelioma of the skin. *Arch Dermatol Syph* 51:295, 1945.
66. Farr HW, Carandang CM, Huvos AG: Malignant vascular tumors of the head and neck. *Am J Surg* 120:501, 1970.
67. Garrett MJ: Haemangiosarcoma: a case report. *Br J Dermatol* 1:193, 1959.
68. Girard C, Johnson WC, Graham JH: Cutaneous angiosarcoma. *Cancer* 26:868, 1970.
69. Haustein UJ-F: Angiosarcoma of the face and scalp. *Int J Dermatol* 30:851, 1991.
70. Hodgkinson DJ, Soule EH, Woods JE: Cutaneous angiosarcoma of the head and neck. *Cancer* 44:1106, 1979.
71. Holden CA, Jones EW: Angiosarcoma of the face and scalp. *J R Soc Med* (suppl 11) 78:30, 1985.
72. Holden CA, Spittle MF, Jones EW: Angiosarcoma of the face and scalp: prognosis and treatment. *Cancer* 59:1046, 1987.
73. Kanitakis J, Bendelac A, Chouvet B, et al: Hemangioendotheliome malin de la tete du sujet age: etude ultrastructurale et immunohistologique. *Ann Dermatol Venereol* 112:441, 1985.
74. Lane OG: Cutaneous angiosarcoma with metastasis. *Br J Cancer* 6:230, 1952.
75. McCarthy WD, Pack GT: Malignant blood vessel tumors. *Surg Gynecol Obstet* 91:465, 1950.
76. Muller R, Hajdu SI, Brennan MF: Lymphangiosarcoma associated with chronic filarial lymphedema. *Cancer* 59:174, 1987.
77. Newton JA, Apaull J, McGibbon DH, et al: Malignant angiosarcoma of the scalp: a case report with immunohistochemical studies. *Br J Dermatol* 112:97, 1985.
78. Reed RJ, Palomeque FE, Hairston MD III, et al: Lymphangiosarcomas of the scalp. *Arch Dermatol* 94:396, 1966.
79. Rosai J, Sumner HW, Kostianovsky M, et al: Angiosarcoma of the skin: a clinicopathologic and fine structural study. *Hum Pathol* 7:83, 1976.
80. Suurmond D: Haemangio-endothelioma (angioblastic sarcoma). *Br J Dermatol* 70:132, 1958.
81. Urbach F, Feineman L: Angiosarcoma. *Arch Dermatol* 99:774, 1969.
82. Watson WL, McCarthy WD: Blood and lymph vessel tumors. *Surg Gynecol Obstet* 71:56, 1940.
83. Weidman AI: Hemangioendothelioma of skin with metastasis to liver, lungs, and lymph nodes. *Arch Dermatol Syph* 62:655, 1950.
84. Wilson-Jones E: Malignant angioendothelioma of the skin. *Br J Dermatol* 76:21, 1964.

Angiosarcoma associated with lymphedema

85. Aird I, Weinbren K, Walter L: Angiosarcoma in a limb, the seat of spontaneous lymphedema. *Br J Cancer* 10:424, 1956.
86. Bachulis BL, Old JW, James AG: Postmastectomy lymphangiosarcoma in a patient with carcinoma of the rectum. *Am J Surg* 113:289, 1967.
87. Barnett WO, Hardy JD, Hendrix JH: Lymphangiosarcoma following postmastectomy lymphedema. *Ann Surg* 169:960, 1969.
88. Benda JA, Al-Jurf AS, Benson AB III: Angiosarcoma of the breast

following segmental mastectomy complicated by lymphedema. *Am J Clin Pathol* 87:651, 1987.
89. Boss JH, Urka J: Stewart-Treves syndrome: angiosarcoma in postmastectomy lymphedema associated with disseminated fibrinoid vascular lesions. *Am J Surg* 101:248, 1961.
90. Bowers WF, Shear EW, LeGolvan PC: Lymphangiosarcoma in the postmastectomy lymphedematous arm. *Am J Surg* 90:682, 1955.
91. Calnan J, Cowdell RH: Lymphangioendothelioma of the anterior abdominal wall: report of a case. *Br J Surg* 46:375, 1959.
92. Chen KTK, Gilbert EF: Angiosarcoma complicating generalized lymphangiectasia. *Arch Pathol Lab Med* 103:86, 1979.
93. Chu FCH, Treves N: The value of radiation therapy in postmastectomy lymphangiosarcoma. *Am J Roentgenol* 89:64, 1963.
94. Conte AJ, Rella AJ: Angiosarcoma in lymphedema following mastectomy. *N Y State J Med* 62:3966, 1962.
95. Cruse R, Fisher WC III, Usher FC: Lymphangiosarcoma in postmastectomy lymphedema: case report. *Surgery* 30:565, 1951.
96. Danese CA, Grishman E, Oh C, et al: Malignant vascular tumors of the lymphedematous extremity. *Ann Surg* 166:245, 1967.
97. Dembrow VD, Adair FE: Lymphangiosarcoma in the postmastectomy lymphedematous arm: a case report by a 10-year survivor treated by interscapulothoracic amputation and excision of local recurrence. *Cancer* 14:210, 1961.
98. Devi L, Bahuleyan CK: Lymphangiosarcoma of the lower extremity associated with chronic lymphedema of filarial origin. *Ind J Cancer* 14:176, 1977.
99. DiSimone RN, El-Mahdi AM, Hazra T, et al: The response of Stewart-Treves syndrome to radiotherapy. *Radiology* 97:121, 1970.
100. Doremus WP, Salvia GA: Lymphangiosarcoma in the postmastectomy lymphedematous arm. *Am J Surg* 96:576, 1958.
101. Dubin HU, Creehan EP, Headington JT: Lymphangiosarcoma and congenital lymphedema of the extremity. *Arch Dermatol* 110:608, 1974.
102. Eby CS, Brennan MJ, Fine G: Lymphangiosarcoma: a lethal complication of chronic lymphedema: report of two cases and review of the literature. *Arch Surg* 94:233, 1967.
103. Ende M: Lymphangiosarcoma: report of a case. *Pacif Med Surg* 74:80, 1966.
104. Ferraro LR: Lymphangiosarcoma in postmastectomy lymphedema: a case report. *Cancer* 3:511, 1950.
105. Finlay-Jones LR: Lymphangiosarcoma of the thigh: a case report. *Cancer* 26:722, 1970.
106. Fisher JH: Postmastectomy lymphangiosarcoma in the lymphedematous arm: a review of four cases. *Can J Surg* 8:350, 1965.
107. Fitzpatrick PJ: Lymphangiosarcoma and breast cancer. *Can J Surg* 12:172, 1969.
108. Francis KC, Lindquist HD: Lymphangiosarcoma of the lower extremity involved with chronic lymphedema. *Am J Surg* 100:617, 1967.
109. Frederici HH, Roberts SR: The fine structure of two postmastectomy angiosarcomas. *Lab Invest* 16:644A, 1967.
110. Froio GF, Kirkland WG: Lymphangiosarcoma in postmastectomy lymphedema. *Ann Surg* 135:421, 1952.
111. Fry WJ, Campbell DA, Coller FA: Lymphangiosarcoma in postmastectomy lymphedematous arm. *Arch Surg* 79:440, 1959.
112. Gray GF, Gonzalez-Licea A, Hartman WH, et al: Angiosarcoma in lymphedema: an unusual case of Stewart-Treves syndrome. *Bull Johns Hopkins Hosp* 119:117, 1968.
113. Hall-Smith SP, Haber H: Lymphangiosarcoma in postmastectomy lymphoedema (Stewart-Treves syndrome). *Proc R Soc Med* 47:174, 1954.
114. Herrmann JB, Ariel IM: Therapy of lymphangiosarcoma of the chronically edematous limb: 5-year cure of a patient treated by intraarterial radioactive yttrium. *Am J Roentgenol* 99:393, 1967.

115. Herrmann JB, Gruhn JG: Lymphangiosarcoma secondary to chronic lymphedema. *Surg Gynecol Obstet* 105:665, 1957.

116. Hillfinger MF, Eberle RD: Lymphangiosarcoma in postmastectomy lymphedema. *Cancer* 6:1192, 1953.

117. Hope-Stone HF, Bence EA: Lymphangiosarcoma occurring in association with lymphedema. *J Fac Radiol* 10:73, 1959.

118. Huey GR, Steham FB, Roth LM, et al: Lymphangiosarcoma of the edematous thigh after radiation therapy for carcinoma of the vulva. *Gynecol Oncol* 20:394, 1985.

119. Hume HA, Erb WH, Stevens LW: Lymphangiosarcoma following radical mastectomy. *Surg Gynecol Obstet* 116:117, 1963.

120. Jansey F, Szanto PB, Wright A: Postmastectomy lymphangiosarcoma in elephantiasis chirurgica: Stewart and Treves syndrome. *Q Bull Northwest Univ Med Sch* 31:301, 1957.

121. Jessner M, Zak FG, Rein CR: Angiosarcoma in postmastectomy lymphedema (Stewart-Treves syndrome). *Arch Dermatol* 65:123, 1952.

122. Kindblom L-G, Stenman G, Angervall L: Morphological and cytogenetic studies of angiosarcoma in Stewart-Treves syndrome. *Virchows Arch (Pathol Anat Histopathol)* 419:439, 1991.

123. Mackenzie DH: Lymphangiosarcoma arising in chronic congenital and idiopathic lymphoedema. *J Clin Pathol* 24:524, 1971.

124. Martin MB, Kon ND, Kawamoto EH, et al: Postmastectomy angiosarcoma. *Am J Surg* 50:541, 1984.

125. McWilliam LJ, Harris M: Histogenesis of postmastectomy angiosarcoma: an ultrastructural study. *Histopathology* 9:331, 1985.

126. Merrick T, Erlandson RA, Hajdu SI: Lymphangiosarcoma of a congenitally lymphedematous extremity. *Arch Pathol* 91:365, 1971.

127. Muller R, Hajdu SI, Brennan MF: Lymphangiosarcoma associated with chronic filarial lymphedema. *Cancer* 59:174, 1987.

128. Salm R: The nature of the so-called postmastectomy lymphangiosarcoma. *J Pathol Bacteriol* 85:445, 1963.

129. Schreiber H, Barry FM, Russell WC, et al: Stewart-Treves syndrome: a lethal complication of postmastectomy lymphedema and regional immune deficiency. *Arch Surg* 114:82, 1979.

130. Scott RB, Nydeck I, Conway H: Lymphangiosarcoma arising in lymphedema. *Am J Med* 18:1008, 1960.

131. Shirger A: Postoperative lymphedema: etiologic and diagnostic factors. *Med Clin North Am* 46:1045, 1962.

132. Silverberg SG, Kay S, Koss LG: Postmastectomy lymphangiosarcoma: ultrastructural observations. *Cancer* 27:100, 1971.

133. Sordillo EM, Sordillo PP, Hajdu SI, et al: Lymphangiosarcoma after filarial infection. *J Dermatol Surg Oncol* 7:235, 1981.

134. Sordillo PP, Chapman R, Hajdu SI, et al: Lymphangiosarcoma. *Cancer* 48:1674, 1981.

135. Stewart FW, Treves N: Lymphangiosarcoma in postmastectomy lymphedema. *Cancer* 1:64, 1949.

136. Taswell HF, Soule EH, Coventry MB: Lymphangiosarcoma in chronic lymphedematous extremities: report of 13 cases and review of the literature. *J Bone Joint Surg* 44A:277, 1962.

137. Toujas L, Ferrand B, Guelfi J, et al: Syndrome de Stewart-Treves: étude ultrastructurale d'un cas. *C R Assoc Anat* 139:1150, 1968.

138. Unruh H, Robertson DI, Karascwich E: Postmastectomy angiosarcoma: experience with three patients and electron microscopic observations in one. *Can J Surg* 22:556, 1979.

139. Woodward AH, Ivins JC, Soule EH: Lymphangiosarcoma arising in chronic lymphedematous extremities. *Cancer* 30:562, 1972.

140. Yap BS, Yap HY, McBride CM, et al: Chemotherapy for postmastectomy lymphangiosarcoma. *Cancer* 47:853, 1981.

141. Zdrojewski JF, Hodge SJ, Scheen SR, et al: Cutaneous angiosarcoma of the hip. *South Med J* 71:914, 1978.

Angiosarcoma of breast

142. Barber KW, Harrison EG, Clagett OT, et al: Angiosarcoma of the breast. *Surgery* 48:869, 1960.

143. Batchelor GH: Hemangioblastoma of the breast associated with pregnancy. *Br J Surg* 46:647, 1958.

144. Brown WG, Van Santen E: Haemangiosarcoma of the breast: a surgical pathology case report. *Med Rec Am (Houston)* 60:177, 1967.

145. Davis HL Jr, Skroch EE, Ramirez G, et al: Hemangiosarcoma of the breast. *Rocky Mt Med* 66:49, 1969.

146. Donnell RM, Rosen PP, Lieberman PH, et al: Angiosarcoma and other vascular tumors of the breast: pathologic analysis as a guide to prognosis. *Am J Surg Pathol* 5:629, 1981.

147. Dunegan LJ, Tobon H, Watson CG: Angiosarcoma of the breast: a report of two cases and a review of the literature. *Surgery* 79:57, 1976.

148. Edwards AT, Kellett HS: Hemangiosarcoma of breast. *J Pathol Bacteriol* 95:457, 1968.

149. Enticknap JB: Angioblastoma of the breast complicating pregnancy. *Br Med J* 2:51, 1946.

150. Gulesserian HP, Lawton RL: Angiosarcoma of the breast. *Cancer* 24:1021, 1969.

151. Horne WI, Percival WL: Hemangiosaroma of the breast. *Can J Surg* 18:81, 1975.

152. Kessler E, Kozenitsky IL: Haemangiosarcoma of breast. *J Clin Pathol* 24:530, 1971.

153. Khanna SK, Manchanda RL, Seigal RK, et al: Hemangioendothelioma (angiosarcoma) of the breast. *Arch Surg* 88:807, 1964.

154. MacKenzie DH: Angiosarcoma (hemangioblastoma) of the breast. *Br J Surg* 49:140, 1961.

155. Mallory TB, et al: Case records of the Massachusetts General Hospital: case 35321. *N Engl J Med* 241:241, 1949.

156. McClanahan BJ, Hogg L: Angiosarcoma of the breast. *Cancer* 7:586, 1954.

157. McDivitt RW, Stewart FW, Berg JW: Tumors of the Breast. Atlas of Tumor Pathology, Armed Forces Institute of Pathology, 1966, Fascicle 2, Second Series.

158. Merino MJ, Carter D, Berman M: Angiosarcoma of breast. *Am J Surg Pathol* 7:53, 1983.

159. Robinson JM, Castleman B: Benign metastasizing hemangioma. *Ann Surg* 104:453, 1936.

160. Shore JH: Hemangiosarcoma of the breast. *J Pathol Bacteriol* 74:289, 1957.

161. Steingaszner LC, Enzinger FM, Taylor HB: Hemangiosarcoma of the breast. *Cancer* 18:352, 1965.

162. Tibbs D: Metastasizing hemangiomata: a case of malignant hemangioendoethelioma. *Br J Surg* 40:465, 1953.

163. York NG: Malignant hemangioendothelioma of the breast. *Med J Aust* 2:1361, 1972.

Angiosarcoma of soft tissue

164. Fletcher CDM, Beham A, Bekir S, et al: Epithelioid angiosarcoma of deep soft tissue: a distinctive tumor readily mistaken for an epithelial neoplasm. *Am J Surg Pathol* 15:915, 1991.

165. Maiorana A, Fante R, Fano RA, et al: Epithelioid angiosarcoma of the buttock: case report with immunohistochemical study on the expression of keratin polypeptides. *Surg Pathol* 4:325, 1991.

Radiation-induced angiosarcoma

166. Cancellieri A, Eusebi V, Mambellin V, et al: Well-differentiated angiosarcoma of the skin following radiotherapy. *Pathol Res Pract* 187:301, 1991.

167. Edeiken S, Russo DP, Knecht J, et al: Angiosarcoma after tylectomy and radiation therapy for carcinoma of the breast. *Cancer* 70:644, 1992.

168. Givens SS, Ellerbroek NA, Butler JJ, et al: Angiosarcoma arising in an irradiated breast: a case report and review of the literature. *Cancer* 64:2214, 1989.

169. Moskaluk CA, Merino MJ, Danforth DN, et al: Low grade angiosarcoma of the skin of the breast: a complication of lumpectomy and radiation therapy for breast carcinoma. *Hum Pathol* 23:710, 1992.

170. Nanus DM, Kelsen D, Clark DGC: Radiation-induced angiosarcoma. *Cancer* 60:777, 1987.

171. Otis CN, Peschel R, McKhann C, et al: The rapid onset of cutaneous angiosarcoma after radiotherapy for breast cancer. *Cancer* 57:2130, 1986.

172. Paik HH, Komorowski R: Hemangiosarcoma of the abdominal wall following radiation therapy of endometrial carcinoma. *Am J Clin Pathol* 66:810, 1976.

173. Richards PG, Bessell EM, Goolden AWG: Spinal extradural angiosarcoma occurring after treatment for Hodgkin's disease. *Clin Oncol* 9:165, 1983.

174. Rubin E, Maddox WA, Mazur MT: Cutaneous angiosarcoma of the breast 7 years after lumpectomy and radiation therapy. *Radiology* 174:258, 1990.

175. Sessions SC, Smenk RD: Cutaneous angiosarcoma of the breast after segmental mastectomy and radiation therapy. *Arch Surg* 127:1362, 1992.

176. Shaikh NA, Beaconsfield T, Walker M, et al: Postirradiation angiosarcoma of the breast: a case report. *Eur J Surg Oncol* 14:449, 1988.

177. Stokkel MPM, Peterse HL: Angiosarcoma of the breast after lumpectomy and radiation therapy for adenocarcinoma. *Cancer* 69:1965, 1992.

178. Westerberg AH, Wiggers T, Henzen-Logmans SC, et al: Postirradiation angiosarcoma of the greater omentum. *Eur J Surg Oncol* 15:175, 1989.

179. Wovlov RB, Sato N, Azumi N, et al: Intraabdominal "angiosarcomatosis": report of two cases after pelvic irradiation. *Cancer* 67:2275, 1991.

Kaposi's sarcoma

180. Adlersberg R: Kaposi's sarcoma complicating ulcerative colitis: report of a case. *Am J Pathol* 54:143, 1970.

181. Aegerter EE, Peale AR: Kaposi's sarcoma: a critical survey. *Arch Pathol* 34:413, 1942.

182. Baddeley H: Kaposi sarcoma. *Proc R Soc Med* 67:866, 1974.

183. Becker SW, Thatcher HW: Multiple idiopathic hemorrhage sarcoma of Kaposi: historical review, nomenclature, theories relative to nature of disease with experimental studies of two cases. *J Invest Dermatol* 1:379, 1938.

184. Beckstead JH, Wood GS, Fletcher V: Evidence for the origin of Kaposi's sarcoma from lymphatic endothelium. *Am J Pathol* 119:294, 1985.

185. Beral V, Bull D, Darby S, et al: Risk of Kaposi's sarcoma and sexual practices associated with faecal contact in homosexual or bisexual men with AIDS. *Lancet* 339:632, 1992.

186. Biggar RJ, Melbye M, Kestems L, et al: Kaposi's sarcoma in Zaire is not associated with HTLV-III infection. *N Engl J Med* 311:1051, 1984.

187. Bisceglia M, Bosman C, Quirke P: A histologic and flow cytometric study of Kaposi's sarcoma. *Cancer* 69:793, 1992.

188. Bluefarb SM: *Kaposi's sarcoma.* Springfield, Ill., 1957, Charles C Thomas.

189. Bluefarb SM: Kaposi's sarcoma with extremity edema and ecchymosis. *JAMA* 204:747, 1968.

190. Borok T, Farina AT, Leider M: Radiotherapy for Kaposi's sarcoma. *J Dermatol Surg Oncol* 5:39, 1979.

191. Braddeley H, Bhana D: Lymphography in Kaposi sarcoma. *Clin Radiol* 22:291, 1971.

192. Browne SG: The hemorrhagic type of regression in Kaposi's sarcoma. *Arch Dermatol* 94:328, 1966.

193. Bryne JJ: Kaposi's sarcoma and its oral manifestations. *N Engl J Med* 266:337, 1962.

194. Cambardella RJ: Kaposi's sarcoma and its oral manifestations. *Oral Surg Oral Med Oral Pathol* 38:591, 1974.

195. Carey RW, Vickery AL: Kaposi's sarcoma, pulmonary nodules, septicemia, and disseminated intravascular coagulation. *N Engl J Med* 285:279, 1971.

196. Chor PJ, Santa Cruz DJ: Kaposi's sarcoma: a clinicopathologic review and differential diagnosis. *J Cutan Pathol* 19:6, 1992.

197. Cohn DL, Judson FN: Absence of Kaposi's sarcoma in hemophiliacs with the acquired immunodeficiency syndrome. *Ann Intern Med* 101:401, 1984.

198. Costa J, Rabson AS: Generalized Kaposi's sarcoma is not a neoplasm. *Lancet* 1:58, 1983.

199. Cox FH, Helwig EB: Kaposi's sarcoma. *Cancer* 12:289, 1959.

200. Dantzig PI: Kaposi sarcoma and polymyositis. *Arch Dermatol* 110:605, 1974.

201. Dayan AD, Lewis PD: Origin of Kaposi's sarcoma from the reticuloendothelial system. *Nature* 213:889, 1967.

202. D'Oliveria JJ, Oliveria TF: Kaposi's sarcoma in Bantu of Mozambique. *Cancer* 30:553, 1972.

203. Dorfman RF: Kaposi's sarcoma: the contribution of enzyme histochemistry to the identification of cell types. *Acta Unio Int Contra Cancrum* 18:464, 1962.

204. Dorfman RF: Kaposi's sarcoma with special reference to its manifestations in infants and children and to the concepts of Arthur Purdy Stout. *Am J Surg Pathol* (suppl) 10:68, 1986.

205. Dorfman RF: The ultrastructure of Kaposi's sarcoma. *Lab Invest* 13:939A, 1964.

206. Dutz W, Stout AP: Kaposi sarcoma in infants and children. *Cancer* 13:684, 1960.

207. Ecklung RE, Valatis J: Kaposi's sarcoma of lymph nodes. *Arch Pathol* 74:224, 1962.

208. Elford J, Tindall B, Sherkey T: Kaposi's sarcoma and insertive rimming (letter). *Lancet* 339:938, 1992.

209. Elmes BGT: Kaposi's sarcoma of lymph nodes: a report of two cases. *J Pathol Bacteriol* 67:610, 1954.

210. Ensoli B, Barillari G, Salahuddin SZ, et al: Tat protein of HIV-1 stimulates growth of cells derived from Kaposi's sarcoma: lesions of AIDS patients. *Nature* 345:84, 1990.

211. Ensoli B, Nakamura S, Salahuddin SZ, et al: AIDS-Kaposi's cells: long term culture with growth factor from retrovirus-infected CD4+T cells. *Science* 242:430, 1988.

212. Ettinger DS, Humphrey RL, Skinner MD: Kaposi's sarcoma associated with multiple myeloma. *Johns Hopkins Med J* 137:88, 1975.

213. Farman AG, Uys PB: Oral Kaposi's sarcoma. *Oral Surg Oral Med Oral Pathol* 39:288, 1975.

214. Fauci AS, Masur H, Gelmann EP, et al: The acquired immunodeficiency syndrome: an update. *Ann Intern Med* 102:800, 1985.

215. Fukunaga M, Silverberg S: Hyaline globules in Kaposi's sarcoma: a light microscopic and immunohistochemical study. *Mod Pathol* 4:187, 1991

216. Fukunaga M, Silverberg SG: Kaposi's sarcoma in patients with acquired immune deficiency syndrome: a flow cytometric DNA analysis of 26 lesions in 21 patients. *Cancer* 66:758, 1990.

217. Gange RW, Wilson-Jones E: Lymphangioma-like Kaposi's sarcoma: a report of 3 cases. *Br J Dermatol* 100:327, 1979.

218. Gellin GA: Kaposi's sarcoma: three cases of which two had unusual findings in association. *Arch Dermatol* 94:92, 1966.

219. Gilbert T, Evjy J, Edelstein L: Hodgkin's disease associated with Kaposi's sarcoma and malignant melanoma: case report of multiple primary malignancies. *Cancer* 28:293, 1971.

220. Giraldo G, Beth E, Buonaqurao FM: Kaposi's sarcoma: a natural model of interrelationships between viruses, immunologic responses,

genetics, and oncogenesis. *Antibiol Chemother* 32:1, 1984.

221. Giraldo G, Beth E, Coeur P, et al: Kaposi's sarcoma: a new model in the search for viruses associated with human malignancies. *J Natl Cancer Inst* 49:1495, 1972.

222. Giraldo G, Beth E, Huang ES: Kaposi's sarcoma and its relationship to cytomegalovirus (CMV). III. CMV DNA and CMV early antigens in Kaposi's sarcoma. *Int J Cancer* 26:23, 1980.

223. Giraldo G, Beth E, Kyalwazi SK: Etiological implications on Kaposi's sarcoma. *Antibiot Chemother* 29:12, 1981.

224. Goette KD, Odom RB: Kaposi sarcoma. *Arch Dermatol* 111:656, 1975.

225. Gokel JM, Kurzl R, Hubner G: Fine structure and origin of Kaposi's. *Pathol Eur* 11:45, 1976.

226. Goldblum OM, Kraus E, Bronner AK: Pseudo-Kaposi's sarcoma of the hand associated with an acquired iatrogenic arteriovenous fistula. *Arch Dermatol* 121:1038. 1985.

227. Gonzalez-Crussi F, Mossanen A, Robertson DM: Neurological involvement in Kaposi's sarcoma. *Can Med Assoc J* 100:481, 1969.

228. Gorham LW: Kaposi's sarcoma involving bone. *Arch Pathol* 76:456, 1963.

229. Gottlieb GJ, Ackerman AG: Kaposi's sarcoma: an extensively disseminated form in young homosexual men. *Hum Pathol* 13:882, 1982.

230. Grave GF: Kaposi sarcoma in African children. *Ann R Coll Surg Eng* 54:270, 1974.

231. Greenstein RH, Conston AS: Coexistent Hodgkin's disease and Kaposi's sarcoma: report of a case with unusual clinical features. *Am J Med Sci* 218:384, 1949.

232. Guarda LG, Silva EG, Ordonez HG, et al: Factor VIII in Kaposi's sarcoma. *Am J Clin Pathol* 76:197, 1981.

233. Haim S, Shafrir A, Better OS, et al: Kaposi's sarcoma in association with immunosuppressive therapy: report of two cases. *Israel J Med Sci* 8:1993, 1972.

234. Hardy MA, Goldfarb P, Levine S, et al: De novo Kaposi's sarcoma in renal transplantation: case report and brief review. *Cancer* 38:144, 1976.

235. Harris NL: Hypervascular follicular hyperplasia and Kaposi's sarcoma in patients at risk for AIDS. *N Engl J Med* 3120:462, 1984.

236. Harrison AC, Kahn LB: Myogenic cells in Kaposi's sarcoma: an ultrastructural study. *J Pathol* 124:157, 1978.

237. Harwood A: Kaposi's sarcoma in renal transplant patients. In *AIDS: The epidemic of Kaposi's sarcoma and opportunistic infections*. New York, 1984, Masson Publishing.

238. Harwood AR, Osoba D, Hofstader SL, et al: Kaposi's sarcoma in recipients of renal transplants. *Am J Med* 67:759, 1979.

239. Hashimoto K, Lever WF: Kaposi's sarcoma. *J Invest Dermatol* 43:539, 1964.

240. Hayes CW, Clark RM, Politano VA: Kaposi's sarcoma of the penis. *J Urol* 105:525, 1971.

241. Holecek MJ, Harwood AR: Radiotherapy of Kaposi's sarcoma. *Cancer* 41:1733, 1978.

242. Houston W, Pontin A, Kuhn T, et al: Kaposi's sarcoma of the penis. *Br J Urol* 47:315, 1975.

243. Huang E-S: Cytomegalovirus: its oncogenes and Kaposi's sarcoma. *Antibiot Chemother* 32:27, 1984.

244. Huang YQ, Li JJ, Rush MG, et al: HPV-16-related DNA sequences in Kaposi's sarcoma. *Lancet* 339:515, 1992.

245. Jones RR, Jones EW: The histogenesis of Kaposi's sarcoma. *Am J Dermatopathol* 8:369, 1986.

246. Jones RR, Spaull J, Spry C, et al: The histogenesis of Kaposi's sarcoma in patients with and without AIDS. *J Clin Pathol* 39:742, 1986.

247. Juhlin L: Kaposi's sarcoma after immunosuppressant therapy. *Acta Dermatol Venereol* 53:238, 1973.

248. Kao GF, Johnson FB, Sulica VI: The nature of the hyaline (eosinophilic) globules and vascular slits of Kaposi's sarcoma. *Am J Dermatopathol* 12:256, 1990.

249. Kaposi M: Idiopathisches multiples Pigmentsarkom der Haut. *Arch Dermatol Syph* 4:265, 1872.

250. Kiep O, Dahl O, Stenwig J: Association of Kaposi's sarcoma and prior immunosuppressive therapy: 5 year material of Kaposi's sarcoma in Norway. *Cancer* 42:2626, 1978.

251. Kostianovsky M, Lamy Y, Greco MA: Immunohistochemical and electron microscopic profiles of Kaposi's sarcoma and bacillary angiomatosis. *Ultrastruct Pathol* 16:629, 1992.

252. Krigel RL: Prognostic factors in Kaposi's sarcoma. In Friedman-Kien AE, Laubenstein LJ, editors: *AIDS: The epidemic of Kaposi's sarcoma and opportunistic infections*. New York, 1984, Masson Publishing.

253. Krown SE, Gold JMW, Niedzwiecki D, et al: Interferon-alpha with zidovudine safety, tolerance, and clinical and virologic effects in patients with Kaposi's sarcoma associated with the acquired immunodeficiency syndrome (AIDS). *Ann Intern Med* 112:812, 1990.

254. Laubenstein L: Staging and treatment of Kaposi's sarcoma in patients with AIDS. In Freidman-Kien AE, Laubenstein LJ, editors: *AIDS: the epidemic of Kaposi's sarcoma and opportunistic infections*. New York, 1984, Masson Publishing.

255. Law IP: Kaposi sarcoma and plasma cell dyscrasia. *JAMA* 229:1329, 1974.

256. Lee FD: A comparative study of Kaposi's sarcoma and granuloma pyogenicum in Uganda. *J Clin Pathol* 21:119, 1968.

257. Lee SCH, Moore OS: Kaposi's sarcoma of lymph nodes. *Arch Pathol* 80:651, 1965.

258. Levan NE, Korn CS: Tissue culture of Kaposi's sarcoma. *Arch Dermatol* 106:37, 1972.

259. Lo TCM, Salzman FA, Smedal MI, et al: Radiotherapy for Kaposi's sarcoma. *Cancer* 45:684, 1980.

260. Lothe F: Kaposi's sarcoma. *Acta Pathol Microbiol Scand* 161:1, 1963.

261. Lubin J, Rywlin AM: Lymphoma-like lymph node changes in Kaposi's sarcoma: two additional cases. *Arch Pathol* 92:338, 1971.

262. Maartensson J, Henrikson H: Immunohemolytic anemia in Kaposi's sarcoma with visceral involvement only. *Acta Med Scand* 150:175, 1954.

263. Maberry JD, Stone OJ: Kaposi's sarcoma with thymoma. *Arch Dermatol* 95:210, 1967.

264. MacKee GM, Cipollaryo AC: Idiopathic multiple hemorrhagic sarcoma. *Am J Cancer* 26:1, 1936.

265. Mariani G: *Arch Dermatol Syph* 98:267, 1909.

266. Marshall ME, Hatfield ST, Hatfield DR: Arteriovenous malformation simulating Kaposi's sarcoma (pseudo Kaposi's sarcoma). *Arch Dermatol* 121:99, 1985.

267. Mazzaferri EL, Penn GM: Kaposi's sarcoma associated with multiple myeloma. *Arch Intern Med* 122:521, 1968.

268. McCarthy WD, Pack GT: Malignant blood vessel tumors: a report of 56 cases of angiosarcoma and Kaposi's sarcoma. *Surg Gynecol Obstet* 91:465, 1950.

269. McNutt NS, Fletcher V, Conant MA: Early lesions of Kaposi's sarcoma in homosexual men: an ultrastructural comparison with other vascular proliferations in the skin. *Am J Pathol* 11:62, 1983.

270. Melnick PJ: Generalized primary angiosarcomatosis of lymph nodes. *Arch Pathol* 20:760, 1935.

271. Meyers DS, Jacobson VC: Multiple hemorrhagic sarcoma of Kaposi. *Am J Pathol* 3:321, 1927.

272. Miles SA, Martinez-Maza O, Rezai A, et al: Oncostatin M as a potent mitogen for AIDS-Kaposi's sarcoma-derived cells. *Science* 253:1432, 1992.

273. Millard PR, Heryet AR: An immunohistochemical study of factor

VIII–related antigen and Kaposi's sarcoma using polyclonal and monoclonal antibodies. *J Pathol* 146:31, 1985.

274. Mitsuyasu RT: Clinical variants and staging of Kaposi's sarcoma. *Semin Oncol* 14:13, (suppl 3), 1987.

275. Montagnier L: Personal communication.

276. Mottaz JH, Zelickson AS: Electron microscopic observations of Kaposi's sarcoma. *Acta Dermatol Venereol* 46:195, 1966.

277. Muggia FM: Treatment of classical Kaposi's sarcoma: a new look. In Friedman-Kien AE, Laubenstein LJ, editors: *AIDS: the epidemic of Kaposi's sarcoma and opportunistic infections*. New York, 1984, Masson Publishing.

278. Nakamura S, Salahuddin SZ, Biberfeld P, et al: Kaposi's sarcoma cells: long-term culture with growth factor from retrovirus-infected CD4+T-cells. *Science* 242:426, 1988.

279. Nickoloff BJ, Huang YQ, Li JJ, et al: Immunohistochemical detection of papillomavirus antigens in Kaposi's sarcoma. *Lancet* 339:548, 1992.

280. Niema M, Mustakallio KK: The fine structure of the spindle cell in Kaposi's sarcoma. *Acta Pathol Microbiol Scand* 63:567, 1965.

281. O'Brien PH, Brasfield RD: Kaposi's sarcoma. *Cancer* 19:1497, 1966.

282. O'Connell KM: Kaposi's sarcoma in lymph nodes: histological study of lesions from 16 cases in Malawi. *J Clin Pathol* 30:696, 1977.

283. Oettle AG: Kaposi's sarcoma in Africa. *Natl Cancer Inst Monographs* 7-10:281, 1961-62.

284. Olweny CLM, Kaddumkasa A, Atine I, et al: Childhood Kaposi's sarcoma: clinical features and therapy. *Br J Cancer* 33:555, 1976.

285. Olweny CLM, Masaba JP, Sikyewunda W, et al: Treatment of Kaposi's sarcoma with ICRD-159 (NSC-129943). *Cancer Treat Rep* 60:111, 1976.

286. Penn I: Kaposi's sarcoma in organ transplant recipient: report of 20 cases. *Transplantation* 27:8, 1979.

287. Pepler WJ: The origin of Kaposi's hemangiosarcoma: a histochemical study. *J Pathol Bacteriol* 78:553, 1959.

288. Pepler WJ, Theron JJ: An electron microscopy study of Kaposi's hemangiosarcoma. *J Pathol Bacteriol* 83:521, 1962.

289. Pilot P, Taelman H, Minlangu KB, et al: Acquired immunodeficiency syndrome in a heterosexual population in Zaire. *Lancet* 2:65, 1984.

290. Qunibi WY, Barri Y, Alfurayh O, et al: Kaposi's sarcoma in renal transplant recipients: a report of 26 cases from a single institution. *Transplant Proc* 25:1402, 1993.

291. Ramos CV, Taylor HB, Hernandez BA, et al: Primary Kaposi's sarcoma of lymph nodes. *Am J Clin Pathol* 66:998, 1976.

292. Reed WB, Kamath HM, Weiss L: Kaposi sarcoma with emphasis on the internal manifestations. *Arch Dermatol* 110:115, 1974.

293. Reynolds WA, Winkelman RK, Soule EH: Kaposi's sarcoma: a clinicopathologic study with particular reference to its relationship to the reticuloendothelial system. *Medicine* 44:419, 1965.

294. Roth JA, Schell S, Panzarino S, et al: Visceral Kaposi's sarcoma presenting as colitis. *Am J Surg Pathol* 2:209, 1978.

295. Rotman M, Rogow L, Rousis K: Radioisotope scanning of Kaposi's sarcoma: a modality for treatment. *Cancer* 33:58, 1974.

296. Rutgers JL, Wieczorek R, Bonetti F, et al: The expression of endothelial cell surface antigens by AIDS-associated Kaposi's sarcoma. *Am J Pathol* 122:493, 1986.

297. Rwomushana RJW, Bailey IC, Kyalwazi SK: Kaposi's sarcoma of the brain: a case report with necropsy findings. *Cancer* 36:1127, 1975.

298. Rywlin AM, Rosen L, Cabello B: Co-existence of Castleman's disease and Kaposi's sarcoma. *Am J Dermatopathol* 5:277, 1983.

299. Safai B, Johnson KG, Myskowski PL, et al: The natural history of Kaposi's sarcoma in the acquired immunodeficiency syndrome. *Ann Intern Med* 103:744, 1985.

300. Safai B, Miké V, Giraldo G, et al: Association of Kaposi's sarcoma with second primary malignancies: possible etiopathogenic implications. *Cancer* 45:1472, 1980.

301. Salahuddin SZ, Nakamura S, Bikerfeld P, et al: Angiogenic properties of Kaposi's sarcoma-derived cells after long term culture in vitro. *Science* 242:430, 1988.

302. Schwartz JL, Muhlbauer JE, Steiqbigel RT: Pre-Kaposi's sarcoma. *J Am Acad Dermatol* 11:377, 1984.

303. Scully PA, Steinman HK, Kennedy C, et al: AIDS-related Kaposi's sarcoma displays differential expression of endothelial surface antigens. *Am J Pathol* 130:244, 1988.

304. Shamroth JM, Ratanjee H, Kellen P, et al: Kaposi's sarcoma localized at the site of previous vascular surgery. *Arch Dermatol* 121:969, 1985.

305. Shmueli D, Sharpira Z, Yussim A, et al: The incidence of Kaposi's sarcoma in renal transplantation patients and its relation to immunosuppression. *Transplant Proc* 21:3209, 1989.

306. Siegal JH, Janis R, Alper JC, et al: Disseminated visceral Kaposi's sarcoma. *JAMA* 207:1493, 1969.

307. Slavin G, Cameron HM, Singh H: Kaposi's sarcoma in mainland Tanzania: a report of 117 cases, *Br J Cancer* 23:349, 1969.

308. Strachley CJ, Santos JI, Downey DM, et al: Kaposi's sarcoma in a renal transplant recipient. *Arch Pathol* 99:611, 1975.

309. Taylor JF, Templeton AC, Kyalwazi S, et al: Kaposi's sarcoma in pregnancy: two case reports. *Br J Surg* 58:577, 1971.

310. Taylor JF, Templeton AC, Vogel CL: Kaposi's sarcoma in Uganda: a clinicopathological study. *Int J Cancer* 8:122, 1971.

311. Taylor JF, Ziegler JL: Delayed cutaneous hypersensitivity reaction in patients with Kaposi's sarcoma. *Br J Cancer* 30:312, 1974.

312. Tedeschi CG: Some considerations concerning the nature of the so-called sarcoma of Kaposi. *Arch Pathol* 65:656, 1958.

313. Templeton AC: Studies in Kaposi's sarcoma: postmortem findings and disease patterns in women. *Cancer* 30:854, 1972.

314. Templeton AC, Bhanna D: Prognosis in Kaposi's sarcoma. *J Natl Cancer Inst* 55:1301, 1975.

315. Velez-Garcia E, Robles-Cardona N, Fradera J: Kaposi's sarcoma in transfusion-associated AIDS. *N Engl J Med* 312:648, 1985.

316. Vogel J, Hinrichs SH, Reynolds RK, et al: The HIV tat gene induces dermal lesions resembling Kaposi's sarcoma in transgenic mice. *Nature* 335:606, 1988.

317. Volberding P: Therapy of Kaposi's sarcoma with interferon. In Friedman-Kien AE, Laubenstein LJ, editors: *AIDS: the current epidemic of Kaposi's sarcoma and opportunistic infections*. New York, 1984, Masson Publishing.

318. Walter PR, Philippe EM, Nguemby-Mbina C, et al: Kaposi's sarcoma: presence of herpes-type virus particles in a tumor specimen. *Hum Pathol* 15:1145, 1984.

319. Warner TF, O'Loughlin S: Kaposi's sarcoma. *Lancet* 2:687, 1975.

320. Weich HA, Salahuddin SZ, Gill P, et al: AIDS-associated Kaposi's sarcoma-derived cells in long-term culture express and synthesize smooth muscle alpha-actin. *Am J Pathol* 139:1251, 1991.

321. Yokaiken RE: Features of the fine structure of Kaposi's sarcoma. *S Afr Med J* 36:989, 1962.

Intravascular lymphomatosis

322. Ansbacher L, Low N, Beck D, et al: Neoplastic angioendotheliosis, a clinicopathologic entity with multifocal presentation: case report. *J Neurosurg* 54:412, 1981.

323. Ansell J, Bhawan J, Cohen S, et al: Histiocytic lymphoma and malignant angioendotheliomatosis: one disease or two? *Cancer* 50:1506, 1982.

324. Bhawan J, Wolff SM, Ucci AA, et al: Malignant lymphoma and malignant angioendotheliomatosis: one disease. *Cancer* 55:570, 1985.

325. Braverman IM, Lerner AB: Diffuse malignant proliferation of vascular endothelium. *Arch Dermatol* 84:72, 1961.

326. Carroll TJ, Schelper RL, Goeken JA, et al: Neoplastic angioendotheliomatosis: immunopathologic and morphologic evidence for intravascular malignant lymphomatosis. *Am J Clin Pathol* 85:169, 1986.

327. Dolman CL, Sweeney VP, Magil A: Neoplastic angioendotheliosis: the case of the missed primary. *Arch Neurol* 36:5, 1979.

328. Ferry JA, Harris NL, Picker LJ, et al: Intravascular lymphomatosis (malignant angioendotheliomatosis): a B-cell neoplasm expressing surface homing receptors. *Mod Pathol* 1:444, 1988.

329. Haber H, Harris-Jones J, Wells A: Intravascular endothelioma (endothelioma in situ, systemic endotheliomatosis). *J Clin Pathol* 17:608, 1974.

330. Janda J, Vanek J: Systemic angioendotheliomatosis. *Zentralbl Allg Pathol* 122:351, 1978.

331. Keahey TM, Guerry DIV, Tuthill RJ, et al: Malignant angioendotheliomatosis proliferans treated with doxorubicin. *Arch Dermatol* 118:512, 1982.

332. Kurrein F: Systemic angioendotheliomatosis with metastasis. *J Clin Pathol* 29:323, 1975.

333. Person JR: Systemic angioendotheliomatosis: a possible disorder of circulating angiogenic factor. *Br J Dermatol* 96:326, 1977.

334. Pfleger L, Tappeiner J: Zur Kenntnis der systemisierten Endotheliomatose der cutanen Blutgefasse (Reticuloendotheliose?) *Hautarzt* 10:359, 1959.

335. Scott PWB, Silvers DN, Helwig EB: Proliferating angioendotheliomatosis. *Arch Pathol* 99:323, 1975.

336. Sheibani K, Battifora H, Winberg CD, et al: Further evidence that "malignant angioendotheliomatosis" is an angiotropic large-cell lymphoma. *N Engl J Med* 314:943, 1986.

337. Shiozaki H, Hoshino S, Oshimi K, et al: A case report of neoplastic angioendotheliosis which responded to a combination chemotherapy (CHOP). *J Jpn Soc Int Med* 73:374, 1983.

338. Vanek J: Intravasculřes Endotheliom. *Zentralbl Allg Pathol* 122:435, 1978.

339. Wells AL: Intravascular endothelioma (endothelioma in situ, systemic endotheliomatosis). *J Clin Pathol* 17:608, 1964.

340. Wick MR, Banks PM, McDonald TJ: Angioendotheliomatosis of the nose with fatal systemic dissemination. *Cancer* 48:2510, 1981.

341. Wick MR, Mills SE, Scheithauer BW, et al: Angioendotheliomatosis: an immunohistochemical reassessment. *Lab Invest* 52:75A, 1985.

342. Wrotnowski U, Mills SE, Cooper PH: Malignant angioendotheliomatosis: an angiotropic lymphoma? *Am J Clin Pathol* 3:244, 1985.

CHAPTER 26

TUMORS OF LYMPH VESSELS

NORMAL DEVELOPMENT AND ANATOMY OF THE LYMPHATIC SYSTEM

The lymphatic system, a diffuse network of endothelial channels, makes its appearance during the sixth week of human embryonic development. There is controversy as to whether it arises as an outgrowth from the venous system or differentiates de novo from adjacent mesenchyme. Proponents of the first theory include Sabin, who demonstrated numerous connections between lymphatics and veins by means of injection techniques in a series of graded pig embryos. She concluded that the lymphatic system arose as buds from the venous system. Others maintain that these connections between veins and lymphatics occur only after the lymphatics have been laid down and the system differentiates from mesenchyme. In either event the lymphatic system develops in close association with the venous system and parallels the venous drainage of an organ.

In the adult the lymphatics are an extensive unidirectional system of blunt-ending vessels that retrieve excess fluid from the interstitium, transport it to regional lymph nodes, and return it to the venous system by way of the thoracic duct. In addition, the lymphatics serve a special function in the absorption of protein and lipid from the liver and small intestine, respectively. These small vessels are nearly ubiquitous but are conspicuously absent in the brain, anterior chamber of the eye, and portions of organs served by an "open" or sinusoidal blood system such as bone marrow and red pulp of spleen. The smallest lymphatic vessels approximate the size of the blood capillary and are made up of fragile endothelial channels situated in a background of reticulum fibers and ground substance. Larger collecting channels contain, in addition, valves, muscle fibers, and elastic tissue, although the latter two are never developed to the extent observed in veins. At the level of the light microscope, the small lymphatics closely resemble the capillary and sometimes are only tentatively identified by the nature of their contents. However, fine structural analysis has documented rather significant differences. Although the basic conformation of the endothelial cell of the lymphatic system is similar to that of the blood capillary, it is invested

by neither a basement membrane nor pericytes. The former finding is also borne out by immunohistochemical analysis. Whereas antibodies to type IV collagen and laminin demonstrate a linear pattern of immunoreactivity around vascular capillary endothelium, it is lacking around lymphatic capillary endothelium.[1] Thus lymphatic endothelium is in direct contact with the interstitial space. This topographic relationship is believed important in the expeditious recovery of fluid because a basement membrane serves as a partial diffusion barrier. In addition, there are thin "anchoring filaments" that terminate directly on the abluminal surface of the cell membrane and probably serve to maintain patency of the lymphatics during periods of increased interstitial pressure. The intercellular contacts between lymphatic endothelia are quite variable. Although tight junctions (zonula adherens), macula adherens, and desmosomes are present, there are many areas of simple overlapping of cells with no junctions. This arrangement creates a "swinging door" effect so that fluid may passively enter the lymphatic space during periods of increased interstitial pressure. Pinocytotic vesicles, thin cytofilaments, modest numbers of mitochondria, and endoplasmic reticulum, similar to those in capillaries, are also present in lymphatic cells.

With the advent of numerous monoclonal antibodies directed against the structural components of endothelial cells, further differences between vascular and lymphatic capillary endothelium have been demonstrated, although the biochemical basis of these differences is not understood (see Chapter 23).[3,6]

LYMPHANGIOMAS

As with hemangiomas, it is often difficult to state whether lymphangiomas are true neoplasms, hamartomas, or lymphangiectasias. In actuality, this distinction is of little practical value because they are all benign lesions, and therapy is largely dictated by their location and clinical extent. Most authors regard lymphangiomas as malformations that arise from sequestrations of lymphatic tissue that fail to communicate normally with the lymphatic system (Fig. 26-1). These remnants may possess some capacity to pro-

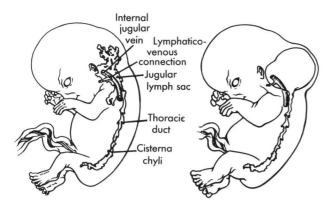

FIG. 26-1. Proposed mechanism for formation of lymphangioma. Lymphatic system in a normal fetus *(left)* with a patent connection between the jugular lymph sac and the internal jugular vein and a cystic hygroma from a failed lymphaticovenous connection *(right)*. (Modified from Chervenak FA et al: *N Engl J Med* 309:822, 1983.)

Table 26-1. Anatomical location of lymphangiomas (61 patients)*†

Anatomical location	Number
Head	35
Tongue	8
Cheek	7
Floor of mouth	7
Parotid	5
Other	8
Neck	25
Trunk and extremities	42
Axilla	15
Pectoral	10
Arm	6
Scapula	5
Other	7
Internal	6
Mediastinum	5
Abdomen	1

*Modified from Bill AH, Sumner DS: *Surg Gynecol Obstet* 120:79, 1965.
†The number of tumors is greater than 61 owing to the fact that large tumors were tabulated under several locations.

liferate, but more importantly they accumulate vast amounts of fluid; this accounts for their cystic appearance. The fact that most lymphangiomas become clinically manifest during childhood and develop in areas where the primitive lymph sacs occur (e.g., neck, axilla) provides presumptive evidence for this hypothesis. However, some early workers such as Goetsch[30] considered these lesions to be true neoplasms capable of locally aggressive behavior, while others have suggested that they arise when inflammation causes fibrosis and obstruction of lymphatic channels. Although it is probable that some lymphangiomas are acquired lesions arising on an obstructive basis following surgery, radiation, or infection in an affected part,[24,25,46] the majority seem to represent developmental lesions occurring relatively early in life.

Traditionally lymphangiomas have been divided into three groups.[4] The lymphangioma simplex or capillary lymphangioma is composed of small thin-walled lymphatics, whereas the cavernous lymphangioma consists of larger lymphatic channels with adventitial coats. The cystic lymphangioma or cystic hygroma is made up of large macroscopic lymphatic spaces that possess investitures of collagen and smooth muscle. Although this is the most widely used classification, it seems more appropriate to consider lymphangiomas as a single group of lesions for several reasons. First, the existence of the lymphangioma simplex must be questioned. We have never been completely convinced of their existence. Descriptions of such lesions may represent either early cavernous lymphangiomas or, alternatively, lymphangiectasia. Second, the distinction between cavernous and cystic lymphangiomas is often arbitrary. Some lymphangiomas have both cystic and cavernous components; this raises the possibility that the cystic

lymphangioma is merely a long-standing cavernous lymphangioma in which the cavernous spaces have been converted to cystic spaces. Bill and Sumner[13] suggest that histological differences are attributable to differences in anatomical location. Cystic lymphangiomas arise in areas such as the neck and axilla, where loose connective tissue allows for the expansion of the endothelium-lined channels; cavernous lymphangiomas develop in the mouth, lips, cheek, tongue, or other areas where dense connective tissue and muscle prevent expansion. We believe cystic and cavernous lymphangiomas are not sufficiently distinctive to be treated separately and have indicated significant differences only when applicable.

Clinical findings

Compared with hemangiomas, lymphangiomas are relatively rare. Anderson,[9] reviewing 768 benign tumors at Babies Hospital in New York over a 15-year period, identified only 48 lymphangiomas, and Bill and Sumner[13] estimated they accounted for 5 of 3000 admissions at Children's Orthopedic Hospital. Kindblom and Angervall[35] reported 100 lymphangiomas over a 5-year period at the Sahlgren Hospital. The sex incidence is roughly equal,[13,35] although a slight male predominance is often recorded. It is estimated that 50% to 65% of these tumors are present at birth, and as many as 90% may be manifest by the end of the second year of life.[13] In some series nearly one third were documented during adult life.[35] Those which present during adult life are the superficial cutaneous lymphangiomas (lymphangioma circumscriptum),[24,25,46,62] some of

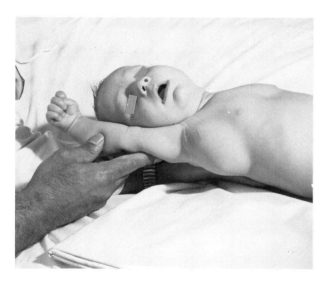

FIG. 26-2. Lymphangioma (cystic hygroma) of axilla.

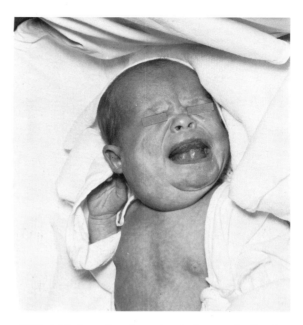

FIG. 26-3. Lymphangioma (cystic hygroma) of neck.

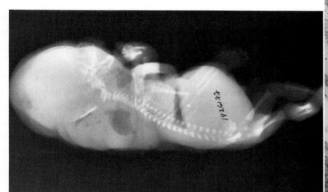

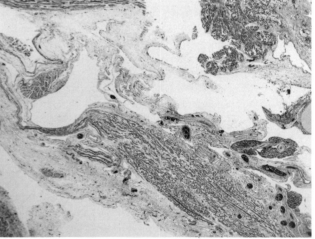

FIG. 26-4. **A,** Radiograph of a fetus with large cystic hygroma detected in utero by ultrasound. **B,** Section of cystic hygroma from fetus shown in **A.** (**B,** ×25.)

which may represent acquired lymphangiectasias and intraabdominal lymphangiomas that present after long symptom-free intervals. Lymphangiomas affect almost any part of the body served by the lymphatic system but show a predilection for the head, neck, and axilla (Figs. 26-2 and 26-3), sites that account for one half to three fourths of all lymphangiomas (Table 26-1). They also occur sporadically in various parenchymal organs including lung, gastrointestinal tract, spleen, liver, and bone. In the last three locations they occasionally signify the presence of diffuse or multifocal disease (see Lymphangiomatosis, below). Lymphangiomas also occur in association with hemangiomas in Maffucci's syndrome.[51]

The most common presentation of lymphangioma is that of a soft fluctuant mass that enlarges, remains static, or waxes or wanes during the period of clinical observation. In a few cases rapid enlargement can be related to an upper respiratory tract infection, which apparently causes obstruction in the lymphatics draining the tumor.

Lymphangioma (cystic hygroma) may also be detected

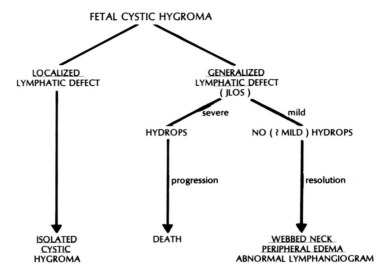

FIG. 26-5. Natural history of fetal nuchal cystic hygroma. A generalized lymphatic defect results from the jugular lymphatic obstruction sequence. Depending on the severity of the obstruction, varying degrees of hydrops are noted. (Modified from Chervenak FA et al: *N Engl J Med* 309:822, 1983.)

in utero by ultrasound (Fig. 26-4). Such cases merit special comment, since they have recently been shown to be associated with hydrops fetalis and Turner's syndrome, and also have a high death rate.[16,19] In the experience of Chervenak et al.[19] with 15 intrauterine cystic hygromas, 11 were associated with the cytogenetic findings of Turner's syndrome (45, X/O or 46,XO/46,XX). Thirteen of the fifteen had severe hydrops and none of the fifteen fetuses ultimately survived. Thus it seems that defects in the lymphatic as well as the vascular system comprise part of Turner's syndrome. The authors suggest that severe aberrations of the lymphatic system in this condition are incompatible with life, while milder forms are compatible with survival but give rise to webbing of the neck and edema of the hands and feet, which characterize the Turner's syndrome infantile phenotype (Fig. 26-5). Other syndromes may also be associated with fetal cystic hygroma, including Noonan's syndrome, familial pterygium colli, fetal alcohol syndrome, and several chromosomal aneuploidies.[27] Since aneuploidic conditions may recur in subsequent pregnancies, cytogenetic analysis of fetuses born with cystic hygroma is indicated.

Lymphangiomas of the head and neck

Lymphangiomas are most common in the neck, where they typically lie in the supraclavicular fossa of the posterior cervical triangle or extend toward the crest of the shoulder. Less frequently they are located in the anterior cervical triangle just below the angle of the jaw. Tumors in this location are the ones most apt to present with significant airway or feeding problems.[23] In about 10% of cases lymphangiomas of the neck extend into the mediastinum; this illustrates the need for preoperative chest radiographs prior to planning a surgical approach. Grossly, these tumors are unicystic or multicystic masses that involve the superficial soft tissue and tend to bulge outward rather than extend inward (Fig. 26-3). Consequently they usually do not compromise vital structures such as the trachea and esophagus unless they are quite large. In contrast to lymphangiomas of the neck, those involving the soft tissues of the lips, cheek, tongue, and mouth are usually of the cavernous type, frequently involve deep soft tissue structures, and cause functional impairment depending on their size.

Intraabdominal lymphangiomas

Intraabdominal tumors are quite rare (Fig. 26-6), as evidenced by the fact that Galifer et al.[28] have tabulated only 139 cases from the English literature. Although 60% are present in patients under the age of 5 years, a significant percentage do not become manifest until adult life. The most common location is the mesentery, followed by the omentum, mesocolon, and retroperitoneum (Table 26-2). In addition to a palpable mass, patients with tumors in the first three locations often develop symptoms of an acute condition in the abdomen caused by the common complications of intestinal obstruction, volvulus, and infarction. In fact, a provisional diagnosis of acute appendicitis is frequently entertained because of the common occurrence of right lower quadrant pain. In contrast, retroperitoneal tumors produce few acute symptoms but ultimately are diagnosed by virtue of a large palpable mass causing displacement of one or more organs. Most arise in the lumbar area and cause

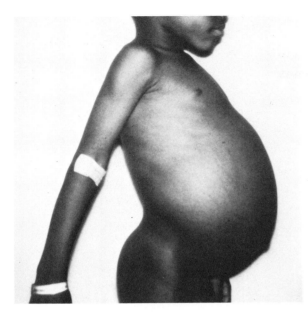

FIG. 26-6. Large intraabdominal lymphangioma.

Table 26-2. Location of intraabdominal lymphangiomas (139 cases)*

Anatomical location	No. cases	Percent
Mesentery	96	69
Jejunum	25	
Ileum	44	
Root of mesentery	5	
Not specified	22	
Omentum	21	15
Mesocolon	15	11
Retroperitoneum	7	5
TOTAL	139	100

*Modified from Galifer RB, et al: *Prog Pediatr Surg* 11:173, 1978.

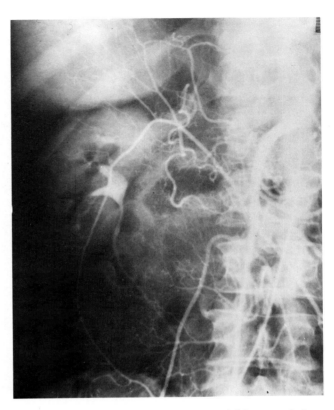

FIG. 26-7. Retroperitoneal lymphangioma visible as a soft tissue mass creating lateral deviation of ureter on intravenous pyelogram.

displacement of the kidney (Fig. 26-7), usually without urinary tract obstruction. Those arising in the superior portion of the retroperitoneum shift the pancreas and duodenum anteriorly.

In the past a preoperative diagnosis of abdominal lymphangioma was seldom made. With a combination of radiological studies, the diagnosis can usually be suspected.[38] Ultrasonography is useful in localizing and determining the cystic nature of the tumors. By arteriography, the lesions are poorly vascularized, and in a few reported cases connections between lower extremity lymphatics and the tumors can be demonstrated with lymphography. In CT scans the tumors appear as multiple, homogeneous, nonenhancing areas with variable attenuation values, depending on whether the fluid is chylous or serous.

Cutaneous lymphangiomas

Cutaneous lymphangiomas can be divided into superficial and deep forms.[25] The latter form is histologically and clinically identical to the usual cavernous lymphangioma and does not need additional elaboration (Fig. 26-8). The superficial intradermal form, sometimes referred to as *lymphangioma circumscriptum*,[25,46] has rather characteristic features. These lesions develop as multiple small vesicles or wartlike nodules that cover localized areas of skin (Fig. 26-9). However, in some cases large areas of the body are affected. Histologically, dilated irregular lymphatic channels fill the papillary dermis and protrude into the epidermis, giving the impression of being "intraepidermal." The overlying epidermis is acanthotic and thrown into papillae. Generally, the lesions are asymptomatic unless they become irritated. They may arise de novo or secondary to surgery or irradiation. In the latter setting some authors prefer to classify the lesions as "lymphangiectasis,"[24,25] although they are clinically and histologically indistinguishable from the de novo lesions.

Gross and microscopic findings

Lymphangiomas vary from well-circumscribed lesions made up of one or more large interconnecting cysts to ill-

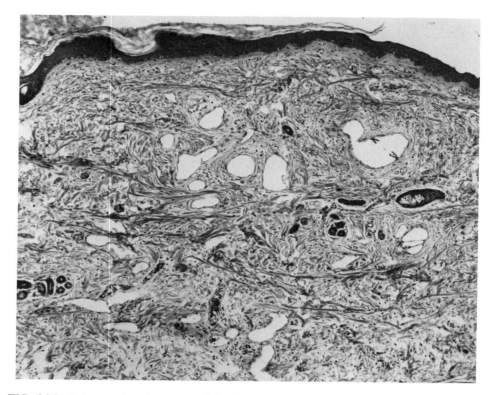

FIG. 26-8. Cutaneous lymphangioma of the deep type. Dilated lymphatic channels extend over large areas of skin and involve superficial as well as deep dermis. (×100.)

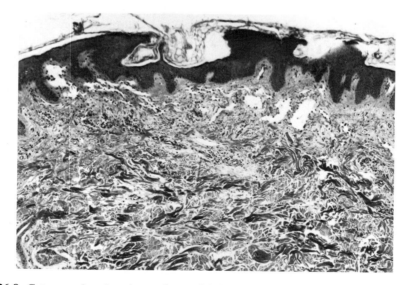

FIG. 26-9. Cutaneous lymphangioma of superficial type (lymphangioma circumscriptum). Lymphatic vessels are localized and restricted to superficial dermis.

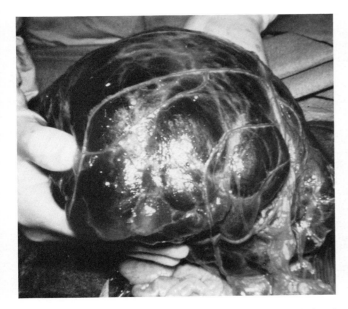

FIG. 26-10. Intraabdominal lymphangioma showing a lobulated cystic appearance. Dark discoloration is the result of secondary intralesional hemorrhage.

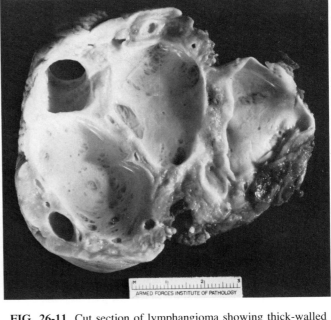

FIG. 26-11. Cut section of lymphangioma showing thick-walled cysts of various sizes.

defined, spongelike compressible lesions (Figs. 26-10 and 26-11) composed of microscopic cysts. The former are traditionally known as *cystic lymphangiomas (cystic hygroma),* while the latter are known as *cavernous lymphangiomas.* Tumors often combine features of both, and the differences between the two are offset by their overall similarities. Regardless of the size of the lymphatic spaces, both lesions are lined by attenuated endothelium resembling the normal lymphatic. Small lymphatic spaces have only an inconspicuous adventitial coat surrounding them, whereas large lymphatic spaces possess, in addition, fascicles of poorly developed smooth muscle (Figs. 26-12 and 26-13). The lymphatic spaces classically are filled with proteinaceous fluid containing lymphocytes, although occasionally erythrocytes may also be present. The stroma is composed of a delicate meshwork of collagen (Fig. 26-14) punctuated by small lymphoid aggregates (Fig. 24-15). Occasionally the lymphoid aggregates may become quite prominent, and such lesions have been descriptively termed "lymphangiolymphoma,"[35] an unfortunate choice of terms, since the lesions are not associated with nor do they progress to lymphomas. With repeated bouts of infection, the stroma of a lymphangioma becomes inflamed, edematous (Fig. 26-16), and ultimately fibrotic.

In most cases there is little difficulty in establishing the correct diagnosis. However, lymphangiomas with secondary hemorrhage are sometimes confused with cavernous hemangiomas. Histological features that favor the diagnosis

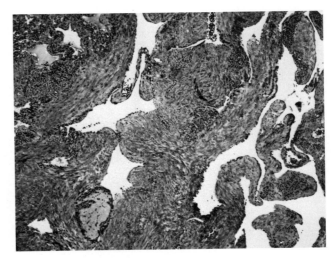

FIG. 26-12. Lymphangioma composed of predominantly thick-walled vessels with muscular coats. (×160.)

of lymphangioma over hemangioma include the presence of lymphoid aggregates in the stroma and more irregular lumina with widely spaced nuclei. Since lymphatic endothelium may express factor VIII–associated antigen as well as CD31 and occasionally may also bind *Ulex europaeus,*[78,81] immunohistochemical procedures are not an especially reliable means of separating hemangiomas from lymphangiomas. It has been our experience that if the di-

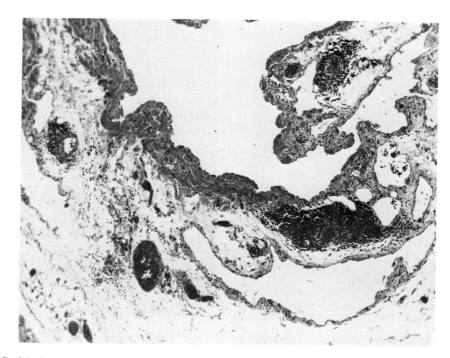

FIG. 26-13. Lymphangioma of omentum characterized by large lymphatics with muscle in their walls. (×160.)

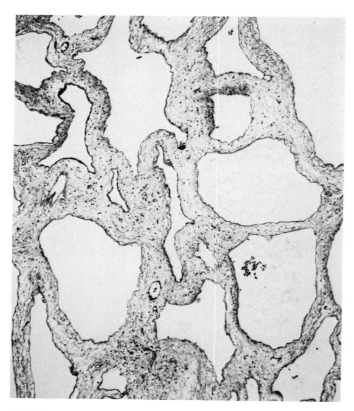

FIG. 26-14. Lymphangioma (cavernous type). Lymphatic vessels of irregular size and shape are embedded in loose collagenous matrix. (×160.)

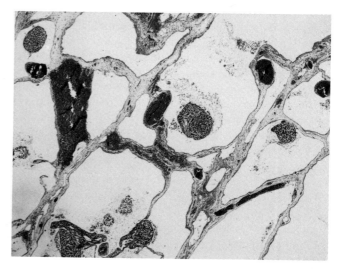

FIG. 26-15. Lymphangioma showing lymphoid aggregates in the walls. (×100.)

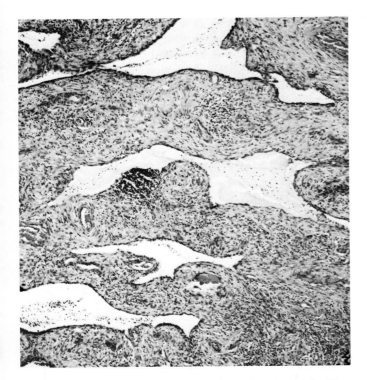

FIG. 26-16. Intraabdominal lymphangioma showing marked inflammatory changes in the stroma. Such tumors may be associated with symptoms of acute abdomen. (×160.)

agnosis cannot be readily made on routine hematoxylin and eosin-stained sections, it is doubtful that ancillary studies will help appreciably.

It is more important to distinguish an intraabdominal lymphangioma from a cystic form of mesothelioma or microcystic adenoma of the pancreas. The cystic mesothelioma presents as a multicystic mass that affects a large area of peritoneum and requires repeated surgery for control (see Chapter 30). The clinical extent of the lesion is at variance with the lymphangioma, which usually involves a localized area of peritoneum. Cystic mesotheliomas are composed of glandlike spaces that show greater variation in size than the vascular spaces of the lymphangioma. Moreover, there is a transition from normal or reactive mesothelium to the glandular spaces of the mesothelioma. However, out of context the cells may look surprisingly similar. The cells of mesothelioma possess numerous microvilli, whereas those of lymphangioma are smoothly contoured and resemble normal lymphatic endothelia. In ambiguous situations immunohistochemical procedures are an easy and reliable means of making this distinction since the cells of multicystic mesothelioma, like other mesothelial tumors but unlike lymphatic tumors, express cytokeratin and epithelial membrane antigen. Microcystic adenomas of the pancreas are composed of cystic spaces lined by cuboidal or low columnar epithelium (Fig. 26-17). The glandular spaces are more reg-

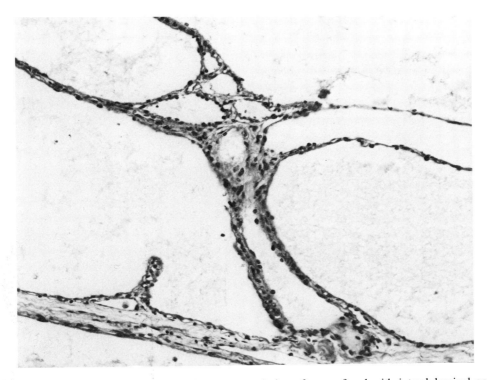

FIG. 26-17. Microcystic adenoma of pancreas, a lesion often confused with intraabdominal or retroperitoneal lymphangioma. Spaces are more regular in shape than in a lymphangioma and are lined by cuboidal epithelia, which overlie a fibrovascular stroma. (×250.)

ular in shape than in lymphangioma and rest on a stroma containing a rich network of small blood capillaries, a feature usually not encountered in lymphangiomas.

Behavior and treatment

Although lymphangioma is a benign lesion, it may cause significant morbidity because of its large size, critical location, or proclivity to become secondarily infected. Only rare cases are known to have regressed spontaneously,[42] and ultimately virtually all lesions require surgical treatment. The extent of the procedure should be dictated by the location and the desire to achieve a reasonable cosmetic result. For patients with lesions presenting early in life, the suggested time for surgery is between the ages of 18 and 24 months.[13] Usually cystic lymphangiomas are well circumscribed, are more amenable to complete excision, and are attended by a low rate of local recurrence. On the other hand, cavernous lymphangiomas in sites such as the tongue and palate have a tendency to insinuate themselves between muscle fibers, are difficult to excise, and are complicated by a high rate of local recurrence[13] and an incidence of nerve palsies of one third of the cases in one series.[23] A staged surgical excision is often required to eradicate these tumors. Sclerosing agents and radiotherapy have been employed in the past but should not be used as alternatives to surgery. In fact, it should be emphasized that there are cases of malignant transformations of previously irradiated lymphangioma[26] (see Chapter 25).

LYMPHANGIOMATOSIS

Lymphangioma affecting soft tissue or parenchymal organs in a diffuse or multifocal fashion is termed *lymphan-*

giomatosis. This extremely rare disease can be conceptualized as the lymphatic counterpart of angiomatosis (see Chapter 23). However, it should be emphasized that it is not always possible to clearly separate angiomatosis from lymphangiomatosis because overlapping occurs between the two. By convention the term *lymphangiomatosis* is reserved for cases showing predominantly, if not exclusively, lymphatic differentiation.

Like angiomatosis this disease occurs principally in children and rarely becomes manifest after the age of 20 years. The diagnosis of this condition at birth is uncommon because it seems that a latent period is required for these lesions to achieve sufficient size to become symptomatic. There is no sex predilection. The presenting symptoms are varied and depend on the site and extent of involvement. Over three fourths of patients have multiple bone lesions.* These well-delimited osteolytic lesions with a variable degree of sclerosis (Figs. 26-18 and 26-19) are usually asymp-

---

*References 64, 65, 69, 70, 72, 73, 77-83.

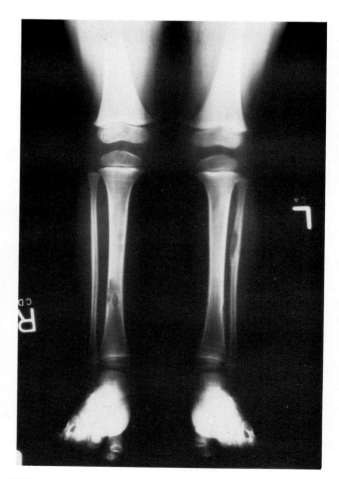

FIG. 26-19. Lymphangiomatosis (same case as Fig. 26-18) illustrating multiple, bilateral osteolytic lesions in long bones.

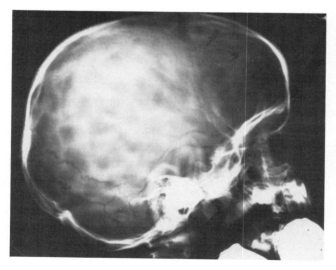

FIG. 26-18. Male child with lymphangiomatosis affecting multiple bones and soft tissue sites. Multiple osteolytic lesions are present in skull.

tomatic, are often discovered incidentally, and are frequently diagnosed as fibrous dysplasia or bone changes of hyperparathyroidism.[67] Acute symptoms more often relate to the presence of lymphangiomas in soft tissue, mediastinum, liver, spleen, or lung. The prognosis is determined by the extent of the disease.[78] Patients with liver, spleen, lung, and thoracic duct involvement usually have poor prognoses,[78,81,101] as the lesions tend to be diffuse and are not amenable to surgical excision. On the other hand, patients with skeletal involvement enjoy excellent prognoses because the bone lesions eventually stabilize in most cases. However, patients with lesions in the vertebrae may develop cord compression and ultimately die of their disease.[68] The diagnosis may be difficult to establish when only bone biopsy is undertaken. To the unsuspecting pathologist the bland dilated lymph channels devoid of cells may appear so innocuous as to be overlooked altogether, and more emphasis may be placed on the surrounding bone resorption and atrophy (Fig. 26-20). The attenuated lymphatic cells will show immunostaining rather consistently for factor VIII-associated antigen, CD31, occasionally with *Ulex europaeus*, and only weakly and focally for CD34.[78] Lesions involving soft tissue are recognized more easily. Some resemble lymphangiomas of the localized type; others consist of small ectatic lymph channels that seem to "dissect" through normal tissue in a permeative fashion (Fig. 26-21). The infiltrative appearance might suggest cancer on cursory inspection, although the lining cells resemble mature lymphatic endothelia. The appearance of these cases of lymphangiomatosis differs from that of angiomatosis in that the spaces are more irregular and seem to communicate with each other as if they represent a diffuse sinusoidal network. Unless secondary hemorrhage has ensued, they are filled with proteinaceous fluid and lymphocytes rather than blood.

LYMPHANGIOSARCOMA

Traditionally the lymphangiosarcoma is defined as a vascular sarcoma arising in the setting of chronic lymphedema.

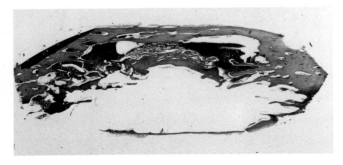

FIG. 26-20. Section of lymphangioma taken from rib in patient with lymphangiomatosis. Note delicate lining of lymphatic cells around defect (same case as Fig. 26-18).

Most cases occur in patients with postsurgical lymphedema, particularly as a result of radical mastectomy for breast carcinoma *(Stewart-Treves syndrome)*. However, they may develop in chronic lymphedema from almost any cause. Although the clinical setting suggests these tumors arise from proliferating lymphatic endothelium, it is difficult to separate them histologically from other forms of angiosarcomas; for this reason they are discussed collectively with angiosarcomas in Chapter 25.

LYMPHANGIOMYOMA AND LYMPHANGIOMYOMATOSIS

Lymphangiomyomatosis is a rare disease characterized by a proliferation of smooth muscle within the lymphatics and lymph nodes of the mediastinum, retroperitoneum, and often within the pulmonary parenchyma as well. Generally considered a multifocal malformation or hamartoma, it has variously been termed "intrathoracic angiomyomatous hyperplasia"[103] and "lymphangiopericytoma."[93] Localized lesions can be referred to as lymphangiomyoma, whereas extensive lesions involving large segments of the lymphatic chain with or without pulmonary involvement should be designated lymphangiomyomatosis.

Clinical findings

The disease occurs exclusively in females, usually during the reproductive years, with a mean age of about 40 years. A significant number of patients have taken oral contraceptives, but in view of the common usage of these products, it is difficult to know the significance of this observation. A unique patient with pulmonary and abdominal lymphangiomyomatosis occurring in association with a solitary fibrous tumor of the lung, cavernous hemangioma of the liver, meningioma, papillary thyroid carcinoma, and parathyroid adenoma was recently reported by Cagnano et al.[93] Progressive dyspnea is the most common symptom and can be related to the almost constant presence of chylous pleural effusion or to pulmonary involvement, which occurs in about half of the patients.[99,149] Other symptoms include pneumothorax and hemoptysis and, rarely, abdominal pain, chylous ascites,[110] and chyluria.[105,107]

Roentgenographic studies can be very helpful in diagnosing this condition. Lymphography indicates obstruction in the major lymphatic ducts (Fig. 26-22, *A*), ectatic lymph vessels distal to the obstruction, occasionally lymphatic-venous connections,[88] and general loss of lymph node architecture (Fig. 26-22, *B*). Chest roentgenograms demonstrate changes highly characteristic of this condition (Fig. 26-23). In the fully developed case a coarse reticular infiltrate with a bullous pattern is present throughout the lung. In contrast to chronic interstitial lung disease, the pulmonary volume is increased. Pulmonary function studies indicate airflow obstruction and markedly impaired gas exchange. The former defect results from poor communica-

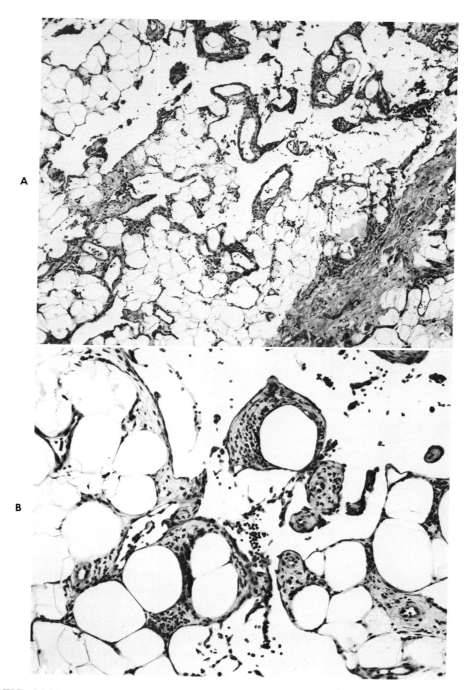

FIG. 26-21. Persistently recurring lymphangiomatosis of leg. Lymphatic channels diffusely involve soft tissue (**A**) and are composed of cells with little atypia (**B**). (**A,** ×60; **B,** ×160.)

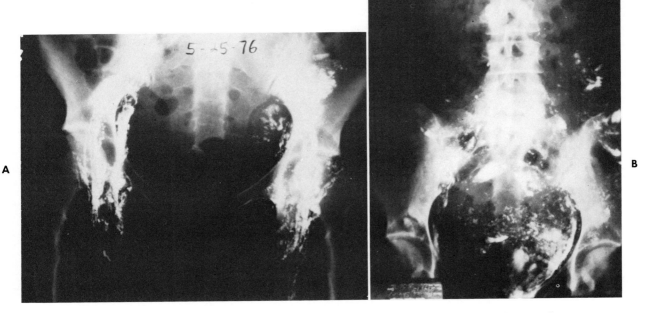

FIG. 26-22. Lymphangiogram of patient with lymphangiomyomatosis. **A,** Initial film shows markedly dilated lymphatic vessels suggesting proximal obstruction. **B,** Follow-up film (48 hours) shows amorphous collections of contrast material indicative of loss of normal lymph node architecture. (Courtesy Dr. Van Vliet, Grand Rapids, Michigan.)

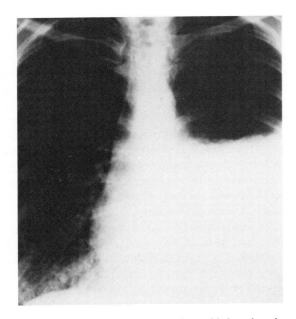

FIG. 26-23. Chest radiograph in a patient with lymphangiomyomatosis. Lung volume is unaltered despite extensive interstitial disease. Massive (chylous) effusion is present on left. (Courtesy Dr. Van Vliet, Grand Rapids, Michigan.)

tion of the emphysematous air spaces with the airways as a result of the proliferating muscle, whereas the latter defect is best explained by uneven ventilation or perfusion of the lung.[95]

Gross findings

At surgery these lesions are red to gray spongy masses that preferentially replace the thoracic duct and mediastinal lymph nodes (Fig. 26-24).[149] Less often they involve the retroperitoneal lymph nodes only, and in particularly dramatic cases the entire lymphatic chain from neck to inguinal region may be transformed into multiple confluent masses. Chylous effusion is encountered in the majority of cases, and in some instances the pleural surfaces are noted to "weep" fluid, suggesting the presence of numerous abnormal communications between the lymphatics and the pleural surface. When the process affects the lungs as well, the organ has a honeycomb appearance with formation of numerous blebs or bullae (Fig 26- 25).

Microscopic findings

The lymphangiomyoma has a remarkably uniform appearance. Smooth muscle cells are arranged in short fascicles around a ramifying network of endothelium-lined spaces (Figs. 26-26 and 26-27). The cells are plump with

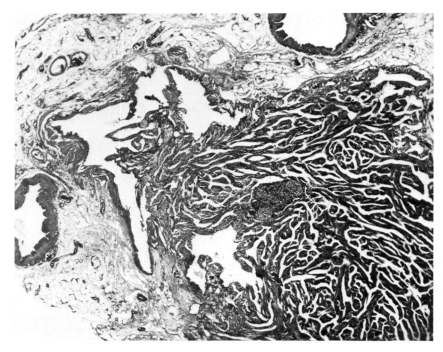

FIG. 26-24. Lymphangiomyomatosis involving large lymphatic channels. (×25.)

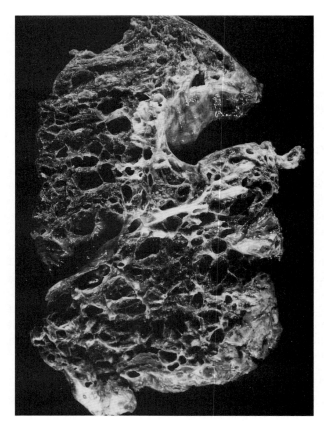

FIG. 26-25. Gross specimen of end stage of lymphangiomyomatosis.

abundant grainy eosinophilic cytoplasm and nuclei devoid of pleomorphism and mitotic activity (Fig. 26-27). Occasionally, foci of lymphocytes are scattered between the muscle cells; in many instances they represent vestiges of preexisting lymph nodes. The vascular spaces are usually empty but are sometimes filled with eosinophilic material containing fat droplets and occasional lymphocytes.

In the lung the pathological changes are quite extensive and severe. The primary lesion is that of a haphazard proliferation of smooth muscle cells, which surround arterioles, venules, and lymphatics (Figs. 26-28 and 26-29) and which diffusely thicken the alveolar septa (Fig. 26-30). Secondary changes ensue and include bulla formation as a result of air trapping by obstructed bronchioles and hemorrhage and hemosiderin deposition as a result of destruction of venules. Although the macroscopic appearance of honeycombing may initially suggest the diagnosis of end-stage interstitial fibrosis, the two lesions are quite different histologically. Lymphangiomyomatosis is characterized by an exclusive proliferation of smooth muscle cells that can be identified on a trichrome stain by their cytoplasmic fuchsinophilia. The muscle proliferation that accompanies end-stage interstitial fibrosis (muscular cirrhosis) is less striking and is always associated with areas of fibrosis.

Immunohistochemical findings

Muscle antigens can be localized within the unusual smooth muscle cells that characterize this condition, although smooth muscle actin is more consistently present

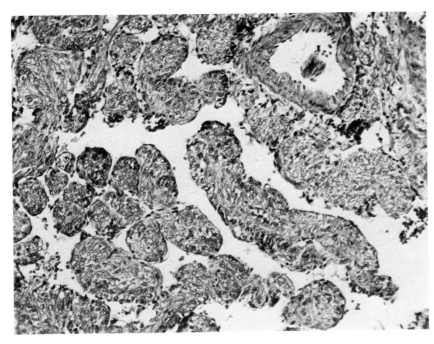

FIG. 26-26. Lymphangiomyoma illustrating classic "pericytoma" pattern. (×150.)

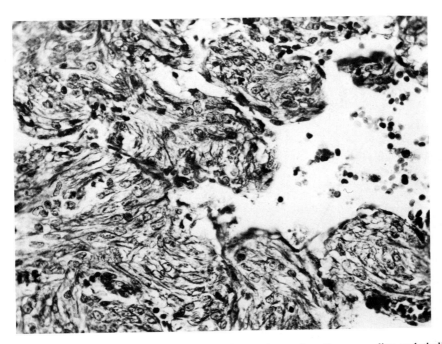

FIG. 26-27. Lymphangiomyoma depicting tufts of smooth muscle cells surrounding endothelium-lined spaces containing occasional lymphocytes.

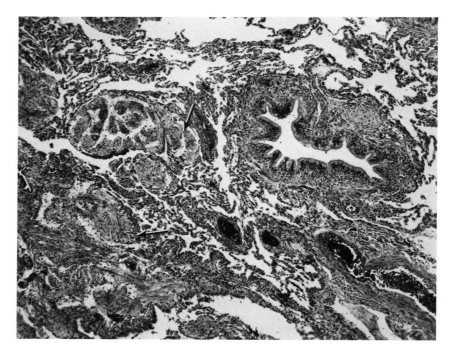

FIG. 26-28. Lymphangiomyomatosis involving lung and depicting perivascular proliferation of smooth muscle around lymphatics. (×60.)

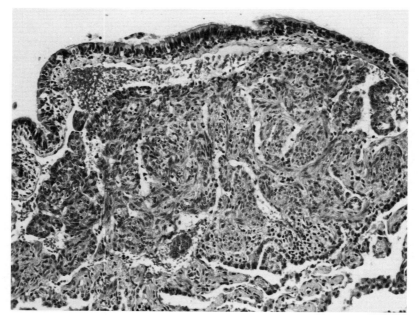

FIG. 26-29. Lymphangiomyomatosis of lung showing perivascular, submucosal location of lesion. (×250.)

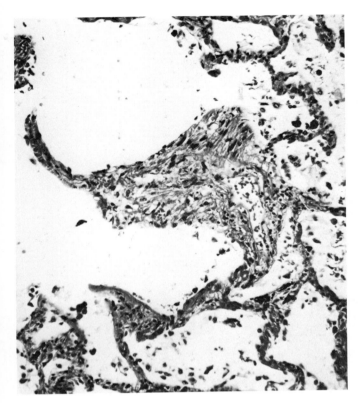

FIG. 26-30. Microscopic focus of lymphangiomyomatosis involving interalveolar septum. (×160.)

than desmin.[89,96,124,131,139] The muscle cells within lymphangiomyomatosis as well as those within angiomyolipoma, react with the antibody HMB45.[96] This unexpected pattern of staining more likely reflects cross-reactivity with an unrelated epitope, in our opinion, than the presence of a melanin precursor substance. Some have suggested that this antibody may be reacting with the electron-dense granules that have been identifed in the cytoplasm of the smooth muscle cells. Because of the sex-restricted nature of this condition and the fact that hormonal manipulation seems to affect the growth of lesions in some cases, there has been a great deal of interest in identifying hormone receptor substances within these lesions by both biochemical as well as immunohistochemical means. Some have reported nuclear estrogen or progesterone receptor protein[87,98,135] within these lesions by immunohistochemical procedures, whereas others have reported negative findings.[129] Actual measurements of receptor protein by biochemical methods have been minimally elevated.[87]

Ultrastructural findings

Several studies have confirmed the smooth muscle properties of the proliferating cells. The cells possess numerous myofilaments with dense bodies.[86,136,149] Additional features of smooth muscle differentiation include plicated nuclei, pinocytotic vesicles on the cell surface, and investiture by basal lamina. An unusual feature within these cells is the peculiar electron-dense granules containing a lamellar substructure.[106] Although the significance of these structures is not known, Chan et al.[96] postulate that they may be the source of the immunoreactivity with the HMB45 antibody. In one study of lung tissue, cells having the ultrastructural features of fibroblasts were identified in addition to typical smooth muscle cells. The authors suggest that the progenitor cell in the pulmonary lesion may be an interstitial cell.[113] The cells lining the slitlike spaces resemble normal endothelia. However, their discontinuous basal laminae and poorly formed intercellular attachments are more compatible with lymphatic than with vascular endothelium.[149]

Differential diagnosis

In the full-blown case there is rarely diagnostic difficulty. Problems arise in limited forms of the disease when only one or two lymph nodes in the mediastinum or retroperitoneum are examined. Partial replacement of a lymph node might initially suggest the diagnosis of metastatic leiomyosarcoma (Fig. 26-31). The most helpful histological feature is the consistent orientation of the smooth muscle cells around endothelial spaces (Fig. 26-31, B). Leiomyosarcomas show no predictable or consistent polarization toward vessels, and except in very well-differentiated cases they usually have more pleomorphism and mitotic activity. The presence of lipid droplets within the fluid bathing the smooth muscle cells in lymphangiomyomas is also very suggestive of the diagnosis. Since the smooth muscle cells of lymphangiomyomatosis react with HMB45 but conventional smooth muscle cells do not, this antibody can be used in making this distinction as well.

Rarely smooth muscle proliferations in the lung have features intermediate between a lymphangiomyomatosis and a metastatic well-differentiated leiomyosarcoma or so-called benign metastasizing leiomyoma. One such case was recently reported by Banner et al.,[85] and we have reviewed a similar case. In our case, hundreds of microscopic smooth muscle nodules were present throughout the lung but did not bear any consistent relationship to the lymphatics. They were composed of fusiform to spindled smooth muscle cells, only some of which had discernible linear striations. Follow-up information, indicating no apparent source for the tumor, strongly suggested a primary smooth muscle proliferation. Such cases deserve the closest scrutiny and careful clinical evaluation to rule out pulmonary metastasis of a well-differentiated smooth muscle tumor of gynecological, gastrointestinal, or retroperitoneal origin.

Behavior and treatment

The clinical course of patients with this disease is variable. Those having localized lesions may survive for long

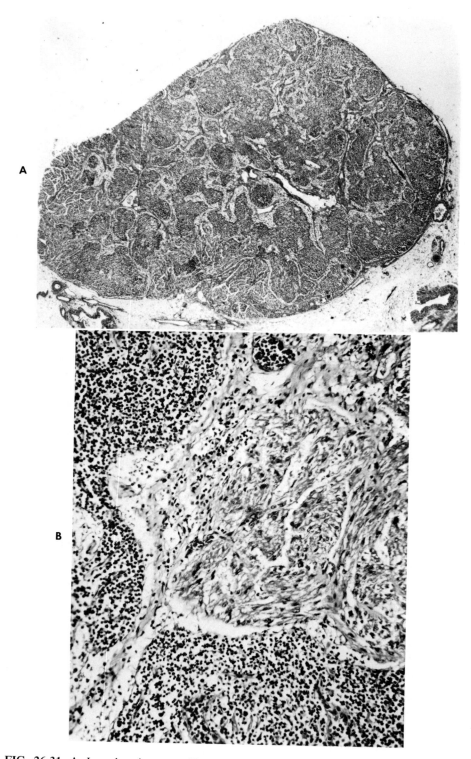

FIG. 26-31. A, Lymphangiomyoma illustrating partial and early involvement of subcapsular region and sinuses of lymph node. (×15.) **B,** High-power view illustrating well-differentiated nature of smooth muscle cells. (×160.)

periods following surgical excision. Patients with pulmonary involvement usually experience progressive pulmonary insufficiency and die of the disease within 1 to 10 years following diagnosis. Treatment of such patients is symptomatic. Obliteration of the pleural cavity by talc poudrage or instillation of nitrogen mustard prevents reaccumulation of chylous effusion,[120] and administration of medium-chain triglycerides reduces fluid and nutritional losses.[94] Low doses of irradiation to lung and mediastinum have resulted in long survival in two patients.[149] Both estrogen and progesterone receptor proteins have been detected in pulmonary or abdominal tissue in this disease.[90,125,142] Consequently there has been a growing interest in treating these patients with ablative or manipulative hormonal therapy. The most favorable results have been reported in women treated with high doses of medroxyprogesterone or oophorectomy, or both.* Very little response has been noted following tamoxifen (an estrogen antagonist) or androgen therapy.[125,144] In one dramatic case reported by Svendsen et al.,[142] a patient treated with medroxyprogesterone and oophorectomy became appreciably worse when tamoxifen was added to her regimen and again improved when it was discontinued.

DISCUSSION

There is still some lingering controversy as to whether lymphangiomyomatosis is part of the spectrum or a forme fruste of tuberous sclerosis. In support of their close relationship is the fact that about 1% of patients with tuberous sclerosis have pulmonary changes very similar to, if not identical to, lymphangiomyomatosis.[141,146,148] Second, re-

---

*References 84, 85, 90, 103, 114, 121, 136, 142.

nal angiomyolipomas, considered one of the hallmarks of tuberous sclerosis and occurring in about 80% of patients, have been documented in about 15% of patients with lymphangiomyomatosis.[127,145]

Those who doubt the relationship of the two diseases have emphasized minor histological and clinical differences. They state that the smooth muscle proliferation occurs preferentially around lymphatics in lymphangiomyomatosis, but around vessels in tuberous sclerosis.[141] This, they feel, accounts for the high incidence of chylothorax in the former but not in the latter. Other differences include the fact that lymphangiomyomatosis is not an inherited disease like tuberous sclerosis, is not associated with central nervous system lesions, and has never been documented in men.

Although the latter arguments seem to underscore significant differences between the two diseases, it should be emphasized that the majority of patients with tuberous sclerosis represent spontaneous mutations and, therefore, do not have affected family members.[101] Moreover, when pulmonary disease develops in tuberous sclerosis, over three quarters of the patients are females with minimal central nervous system symptoms.

It is our belief that overall the two diseases share more similarities than differences. In our experience there are in-

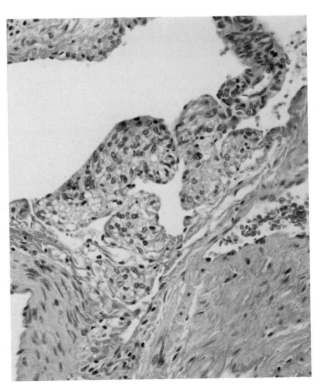

FIG. 26-33. High-power view of Fig. 26-32 showing smooth muscle proliferation surrounding lymphatic spaces of uterus. (×250.)

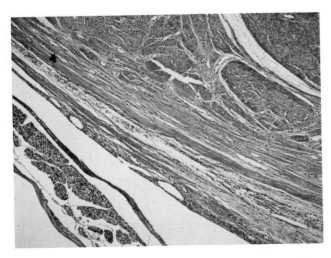

FIG. 26-32. Lymphangiomyomatosis involving subserosal lymphatics of the uterus in a patient with tuberous sclerosis. (×60.)

dubitable cases of tuberous sclerosis in which the pulmonary and extrapulmonary lesions are identical to those of lymphangiomyomatosis (Figs. 26-32 and 26-33). For these reasons we feel these two diseases are ends of a common spectrum.

REFERENCES
General

1. Barsky SH, Baker A, Siegel OP: Use of anti-basement membrane antibodies to distinguish blood vessel capillaries from lymphatic capillaries. *Am J Surg Pathol* 7:667, 1983.
2. Fraley EE, Weiss L: An electron microscopic study of lymphatic vessels in the penile skin of the rat. *Am J Anat* 109:85, 1961.
3. Knowles DM, Tolidjian B, Marboe C, et al: Monoclonal anti-human monocyte antibodies OKM1 and OKM5 possess distinctive tissue distributions including differential reactivity with vascular endothelium. *J Immunol* 132:2170, 1984.
4. Landing BH, Farber S: *Tumors of the cardiovascular system.* Atlas of Tumor Pathology. Armed Forces Institute of Pathology, 1956, Washington, D.C.
5. Leak LV, Burke JF: Fine structure of the lymphatic capillary and the adjoining connective tissue area. *Am J Anat* 118:785, 1966.
6. Schlingemann RO, Dingjan GM, Emeis JJ, et al: Monoclonal antibody PAL-E specific for endothelium. *Lab Invest* 52:72, 1985.

Lymphangioma

7. Alvich JP, Lepow HI: Cystic lymphangioma of hepatic flexure of colon: report of a case. *Ann Surg* 152:880, 1960.
8. Amos AS: Multiple lymphatic cysts of the mesentery. *Br J Surg* 46:588, 1958.
9. Anderson DH: Tumors of infancy and childhood. *Cancer* 4:890, 1951.
10. Barrana KG, Freeman NV: Massive infiltrating cystic hygroma of the neck in infancy. *Arch Dis Child* 48:523, 1973.
11. Beller AJ, Nach RL: Cystic lymphangioma of greater omentum. *Ann Surg* 132:287, 1950.
12. Berardi RS: Lymphangioma of the large intestine: report of a case and review of the literature. *Dis Colon Rectum* 17:265, 1974.
13. Bill AH, Sumner DS: A unified concept of lymphangioma and cystic hygroma. *Surg Gynecol Obstet* 120:79, 1965.
14. Bratu M, Brown M, Carter M, et al: Cystic hygroma of the mediastinum in children. *Am J Dis Child* 199:348, 1970.
15. Brindley GV, Brindley GV Jr: Lymphangioma of the mesentery. *Ann Surg* 127:907, 1948.
16. Byrne J, Blanc WA, Warburton D, et al: The significance of cystic hygroma in fetuses. *Hum Pathol* 15:61, 1984.
17. Cauwelaert V, Gruwez JA: Experience with lymphangioma. *Lymphology* 11:43, 1978.
18. Chait D, Yongers AJ, Beddoe GM, et al: Management of cystic hygromas. *Surg Gynecol Obstet* 139:55, 1974.
19. Chervenak FA, Isaacson G, Blakemore KJ: Fetal cystic hygroma: cause and natural history. *N Engl J Med* 309:822, 1983.
20. Corman ML, Haggitt RC: Lymphangioma of the rectum. *Dis Colon Rectum* 16:524, 1973.
21. Dische MR: Mediastinal lymphangioma with chylothorax in infancy: report of a case and review of the literature. *Am J Clin Pathol* 49:392, 1968.
22. Elliott RL, Williams RD, Bayles D, et al: Lymphangioma of the duodenum: case report with light and electron microscopic observation. *Ann Surg* 163:86, 1966.
23. Emery PJ, Bailey CM, Evans JNG: Cystic hygroma of the head and neck: a review of 37 cases. *J Laryngol Otol* 98:613, 1984.
24. Fisher I, Orkin M: Acquired lymphangioma (lymphangiectasis). *Arch Dermatol* 101:230, 1970.
25. Flanagan BP, Helwig EB: Cutaneous lymphangioma. *Arch Dermatol* 113:24, 1977.
26. Fonkalsrud EW: Surgical management of congenital malformation of the lymphatic system. *Am J Surg* 28:152, 1974.
27. Fryns JP, Kleczkowska K, Vandenberghe F, et al: Cystic hygroma and hydrops fetalis in dup(11p) syndrome. *Am J Med Genet* 22:287, 1985.
28. Galifer RB, Pous JG, Juskiewenski S, et al: Intraabdominal cystic lymphangiomas in childhood. *Prog Pediatr Surg* 11:173, 1978.
29. Gephart HR, Cherry JK: Omental lymphangioma masquerading as ascites. *Am J Surg* 115:861, 1968.
30. Goetsch E: Hygroma colli cysticum and hygroma axillare: pathologic and clinical study and report of 12 cases. *Arch Surg* 36:394, 1938.
31. Gross RE, Goeringer CF: Cystic hygroma of the neck. *Surg Gynecol Obstet* 69:48, 1939.
32. Harkins GA, Sabiston DC: Lymphangioma in infancy and childhood. *Surgery* 47:811, 1960.
33. Hilliard RI, McKendry JBJ, Phillips MJ: Congenital abnormalities of the lymphatic system: a new clinical classification. *Pediatrics* 86:988, 1990.
34. Kafka V, Novak K: Multicystic retroperitoneal lymphangioma in an infant appearing as an inguinal hernia. *J Pediatr Surg* 5:573, 1970.
35. Kindblom L-G, Angervall L: Tumors of lymph vessels. *Contemp Issues Surg Pathol* 18:163, 1991.
36. King DT, Duffy DM, Hirose PM, et al: Lymphangiosarcoma arising from lymphangioma circumscription. *Arch Dermatol* 115:969, 1976.
37. Kornfält R, Nilsson IM, Okmian L: Fibrinolysis in lymphangioma. *Acta Paediatr* 62:538, 1973.
38. Koshy A, Tandon RK, Kapur BML, et al: Retroperitoneal lymphangioma. *Am J Gastroenterol* 69:485, 1978.
39. Kutarna A: Value of lymphangiography in the diagnosis and treatment of lymphangioma. *Neoplasma* 22:81, 1975.
40. Leonidas JC, Brill PW, Bhan I, et al: Cystic retroperitoneal lymphangioma in infants and children. *Radiology* 127:203, 1978.
41. Marcus JB, Lynn JA: Ultrastructural comparison of an adenomatoid tumor, lymphangioma, hemangioma, and mesothelioma. *Cancer* 25:171, 1970.
42. Ngoc T, Ninh TX: Cystic hygroma in children: a report of 126 cases. *J Pediatr Surg* 9:191, 1974.
43. Owens FC, Franco-Jove D, Goldman ML, et al: Retroperitoneal lymphangioma: ultrasonic findings. *South Med J* 71:971, 1978.
44. Pachter MR, Lattes R: Mesenchymal tumors of the mediastinum. III. Tumors of lymph vascular origin. *Cancer* 16:108, 1963.
45. Palmer LC, Strauch WG, Welton WA: Lymphangioma circumscripta: a case with deep lymphatic involvement. *Arch Dermatol* 114:394, 1978.
46. Peachy RO, Limm CC, Whimster IW: Lymphangioma of skin: a review of 65 cases. *Br J Dermatol* 83:519, 1970.
47. Perkes EW, Haller JO, Kassner EG, et al: Mediastinal cystic hygroma in infants: two cases with no extension into the neck. *Clin Pediatr* 18:166, 1979.
48. Prioleau PG, Santa Cruz DJ: Lymphangioma circumscripta following radical mastectomy and radiation therapy. *Cancer* 42:1989, 1978.
49. Rauch RF: Retroperitoneal lymphangioma. *Arch Surg* 78:45, 1959.
50. Rekhi BM, Esselstyn CB, Levy I, et al: Retroperitoneal cystic lymphangioma: report of two cases and review of the literature. *Cleve Clin Q* 39:125, 1972.
51. Rosenquist GJ, Wolfe DC: Lymphangioma of bone. *J Bone Joint Surg* 34A:158, 1968.

52. Russell B, Pirdie RB: Lymphangioma circumscripta with involvement of deep lymphatics. *Br J Dermatol* 79:300, 1967.

53. Saijo M, Munro IR, Mancer K: Lymphangioma: a long-term follow-up study. *Plast Reconstr Surg* 56:642, 1975.

54. Seckler SG, Rubin H, Rabinowitz JG: Systemic cystic angiomatosis. *Am J Med* 37:976, 1964.

55. Singh S, Baboo M: Cystic lymphangioma in children: report of 32 cases including lesions at rare sites. *Surgery* 69:947, 1971.

56. Sun GC, Tang GK, Hill L: Mesenteric lymphangioma: a case report with transmission and scanning electron microscopic studies. *Arch Pathol Lab Med* 104:316, 1950.

57. Suringa DWR, Ackerman AB: Cutaneous lymphangiomas with dyschondroplasia (Maffucci's syndrome). *Arch Dermatol* 101:472, 1970.

58. Viar WN, Scott WF, Donald JM: Mesenteric cavernous lymphangioma: brief review and report of two cases. *Ann Surg* 153:157, 1961.

59. Wada A, Tateishi R, Terazawa T, et al: Lymphangioma of the lung. *Arch Pathol* 98:211, 1974.

60. Watson WL, McCarthy WD: Blood and lymph vessel tumors. *Surg Gynecol Obstet* 71:569, 1940.

61. Wayne ER, Burrington JD, Bailey WC, et al: Retroperitoneal lymphangioma: an unusual case of acute surgical abdomen. *J Pediatr Surg* 8:831, 1973.

62. Whimster IW: The pathology of lymphangioma circumscription. *Br J Dermatol* 10:35, 1974.

63. Witte MH, Witte CL: Lymphangiogenesis and lymphologic syndromes. *Lymphology* 19:21, 1986.

Lymphangiomatosis

64. Asch MJ, Cohen AH, Moore TC: Hepatic and splenic lymphangiomatosis with skeletal involvement. *Surgery* 76:334, 1974.

65. Bell A, Simon BK: Chylothorax and lymphangiomas of bone: unusual manifestation of lymphatic disease. *South Med J* 71:459, 1978.

66. Berberich FR, Bernstein ID, Ochs HD, et al: Lymphangiomatosis with chylothorax. *J Pediatr* 87:941, 1975.

67. Case records of the Massachusetts General Hospital. *N Engl J Med* 303:270, 1980.

68. Edwards WH, Thompson RC, Varsa EW: Lymphangiomatosis and massive osteolysis of the cervical spine: a case report and review of the literature. *Clin Orthop* 177:222, 1983.

69. Goldstein MR, Benchimol A, Cornerll W, et al: Chylopericardium with multiple lymphangiomas of bone. *N Engl J Med* 280:1034, 1969.

70. Gutierrez RM, Spjut HJ: Skeletal angiomatosis: report of three cases and a review of the literature. *Clin Orthop* 85:82, 1972.

71. Hamoudi A, Vassy L: Multiple lymphangioendothelioma of the spleen in a 12-year-old girl. *Arch Pathol* 99:605, 1975.

72. Harris R, Prandoni AS: Generalized primary lymphangiomas of bone: report of a case associated with congenital lymphedema of the forearm. *Ann Intern Med* 33:1302, 1950.

73. Hayes JT, Brody GL: Cystic lymphangiectasis of bone: a case report. *J Bone Joint Surg* 43A:107, 1961.

74. Jumbelic M, Feurstein IM, Dorfman HD: Solitary intraosseous lymphangioma. *J Bone Joint Surg* 66A:1479, 1984.

75. Miller SU, Preuett HJ, Long A: Fatal chylopericardium caused by hamartomatous lymphangiomatosis: case report and review of the literature. *Am J Med* 26:951, 1959.

76. Morphis LG, Arcinue FL, Krause JR: Generalized lymphangioma in infancy with chylothorax. *Pediatrics* 46:566, 1970.

77. Najman E, Fabecic-Sabadi V, Temmer B: Lymphangioma in the inguinal region with cystic lymphangiomatosis of bone. *J Pediatr* 71:561, 1967.

78. Ramani P, Shah A: Lymphangiomatosis: histologic and immunohistochemical analysis of four cases. *Am J Surg Pathol* 17:329, 1993.

79. Spjut HJ, Lindbom A: Skeletal angiomatosis: report of two cases. *Acta Pathol Microbiol Scand* 55:49, 1962.

80. Takamoto RM, Armstrong RC, Stanford W, et al: Chylothorax with multiple lymphangiomata of bone. *Chest* 59:687, 1971.

81. Tazelaar HD, Kerr D, Yousem SA, et al: Diffuse pulmonary lymphangiomatosis. *Hum Pathol* 24:1313, 1993.

82. Tsyb AF, Mukhamedzhanov IHK, Guseva LI: Lymphangiomatosis of bone and soft tissue (results of lymphangiographic examinations). *Lymphology* 16:181, 1983.

83. Tucker SM: Bilateral chylothorax with multiple osteolytic lesions: generalized abnormality of the lymphatic system. *Proc R Soc Med* 60:17, 1967.

Lymphangiomyoma and lymphangiomyomatosis

84. Adamson D, Heinrichs WL, Raybin DM, et al: Successful treatment of pulmonary lymphangiomyomatosis with oophorectomy and progesterone. *Am Rev Respir Dis* 132:916, 1985.

85. Banner AS, Carrington CB, Emory WB, et al: Efficacy of oophorectomy in lymphangioleiomyomatosis and benign metastasizing leiomyoma. *N Engl J Med* 305:204, 1981.

86. Basset F, Soler P, Marsac J, et al: Pulmonary lymphangiomyomatosis: three new cases studied with electron microscopy. *Cancer* 38:2357, 1976.

87. Berger U, Khaghani A, Pomerance A, et al: Pulmonary lymphangioleiomyomatosis and steroid receptors: an immunohistochemical study. *Am J Clin Pathol* 93:609, 1990.

88. Bhattacharyya AK, Balogh K: Retroperitoneal lymphangioleiomyomatosis: a 36-year benign course in a postmenopausal woman. *Cancer* 56:1144, 1985.

89. Bonetti F, Pea M, Martignoni G, et al: Cellular heterogeneity in lymphangiomyomatosis of the lung. *Hum Pathol* 22:727, 1991.

90. Brentani MM, Carvalho RR, Saldiva PH, et al: Steroid receptors in pulmonary lymphangiomyomatosis. *Chest* 85:96, 1984.

91. Burrell LST, Ross JM: A case of chylous effusion due to leiomyosarcoma. *Br J Tubercul* 31:38, 1937.

92. Bush JK, McLean RL, Sieker HO: Diffuse lung disease due to lymphangiomyoma. *Am J Med* 46:645, 1969.

93. Cagnano M, Benharroch D, Geffen DB: Pulmonary lymphangioleiomyomatosis: report of a case with associated multiple soft tissue tumors. *Arch Pathol Lab Med* 115:1257, 1991.

94. Calabrese PR, Frank HD, Taubin HL: Lymphangiomyomatosis with chylous ascites: treatment with dietary fat restriction and medium chain triglycerides. *Cancer* 4:895, 1977.

95. Carrington C, Cugell D, Gaensler E, et al: Lymphangioleiomyomatosis: physiologic-pathologic-radiologic correlations. *Am Rev Respir Dis* 116:977, 1977.

96. Chan JK, Tsang WY, Pau MY, et al: Lymphangiomyomatosis and angiomyolipoma: closely related entities characterized by hamartomatous proliferation of HMB-45 positive smooth muscle. *Histopathology* 22:445, 1993.

97. Collard M, Fievez M, Godart S, et al: The contribution of lymphangiography in the study of diffuse lymphangiomyomatosis. *Am J Roentgenol Rad Ther Nucl Med* 102:466, 1968.

98. Colley MH, Geppert E, Franklin WA: Immunohistochemical detection of steroid receptors in a case of pulmonary lymphangioleiomyomatosis. *Am J Surg Pathol* 13:803, 1989.

99. Cornog JL, Enterline HT: Lymphangiomyoma: a benign lesion of chyliferous lymphatics synonymous with lymphangiopericytoma. *Cancer* 19:1909, 1966.

100. Corrin B, Liebow AA, Friedman PJ: Pulmonary lymphangiomyomatosis. *Am J Pathol* 79:348, 1975.

101. Dawson J: Pulmonary tuberous sclerosis and its relationship to other forms of the disease. *Q J Med* 23:113, 1954.

102. Dwyer JM, Hickie JB, Garvan J: Pulmonary tuberous sclerosis. *Q J Med* 40:115, 1971.

103. Eliasson AH, Phillips YY, Tenholder MF: Treatment of lymphangioleiomyomatosis: a meta-analysis. *Chest* 96:1352, 1989.

104. Enterline HT, Roberts B: Lymphangiopericytoma. *Cancer* 8:582, 1955.

105. Frack MD, Simon L, Dawson BH: The lymphangiomyomatosis syndrome. *Cancer* 22:428, 1968.

106. Fukuda Y, Kawamoto M, Yamamoto A, et al: Role of elastic fiber degradation in emphysema-like lesions of pulmonary lymphangiomyomatosis. *Hum Pathol* 21:1252, 1990.

107. Gray SR, Carrington CB, Cornog JL: Lymphangiomyomatosis: report of a case with ureteral involvement and chyluria. *Cancer* 35:490, 1975.

108. Jao J, Gilbert ST, Messer R: Lymphangiomyoma and tuberous sclerosis. *Cancer* 29:1188, 1972.

109. Johnson SF, Davey DD, Cibull ML, et al: Lymphangioleiomyomatosis. *Am Surg* 59:395, 1993.

110. Joliat G, Stalder H, Kapanci Y: Lymphangiomyomatosis: a clinicoanatomical entity. *Cancer* 31:455, 1973.

111. Justin-Besancon L, Pequignot H, Galye JJ, et al: Lymphangiectasies pulmonaires diffuses acquises avec insuffisance respiratoire et chylothorax. *Arch Anat Pathol* 39:1179, 1963.

112. Kaku T, Toyoshima S, Enjoji M: Tuberous sclerosis with pulmonary and lymph node involvement: relationship to lymphangiomyomatosis. *Acta Pathol Jpn* 33:395, 1983.

113. Kane P, Lane B, Cordice J, et al: Ultrastructure of the proliferating cells in pulmonary lymphangiomyomatosis. *Acta Pathol Lab Med* 102:618, 1978.

114. Kitzsteiner KA, Mallen RG: Pulmonary lymphangiomyomatosis: treatment with castration. *Cancer* 46:2248, 1980.

115. Klein M, Kreiger O, Ruckser R, et al: Treatment of lymphangioleiomyomatosis by ovariectomy, interferon, alpha 2b, and tamoxifen: a case report. *Arch Gynecol Obstet* 252:99, 1992.

116. Lack EE, Dolan MF, Finisio J, et al: Pulmonary and extrapulmonary lymphangioleiomyomatosis: report of a case with bilateral renal angiomyolipomas, multifocal lymphangioleiomyomatosis, and a glial polyp of the endocervix. *Am J Surg Pathol* 10:650, 1986.

117. Laipply TC, Sherrick JC: Intrathoracic angiomyomatous hyperplasia associated with chronic chylothorax. *Lab Invest* 7:387, 1958.

118. Leeds SE, Benioff MA, Ortega P: Pulmonary lymphangiomyoma with renal angiolipomas. *Calif Med* 119:74, 1973.

119. Lie JT, Miller RD, Williams DE: Cystic disease of the lungs in tuberous sclerosis: clinicopathologic correlation, including body plethysmographic lung function tests. *Mayo Clin Proc* 55:547, 1980.

120. Lieberman J, Agliozzo CM: Intrapleural nitrogen mustard for treating chylous effusion of pulmonary lymphangioleiomyomatosis. *Cancer* 33:1505, 1974.

121. Logan RF, Fawcett IW: Oophorectomy for pulmonary lymphangioleiomyomatosis: a case report. *Br J Dis Chest* 79:98, 1985.

122. Luna CM, Gene R, Jolly EC, et al: Pulmonary lymphangiomyomatosis associated with tuberous sclerosis: treatment with tamoxifen and tetracycline-pleurodesis. *Chest* 88:473, 1985.

123. Malik SD, Pardee N, Martin CJ: Involvement of the lungs in tuberous sclerosis. *Chest* 58:538, 1970.

124. Matthews TJ, Hornall D, Sheppard MN: Comparison of the use of antibodies to alpha smooth muscle actin and desmin in pulmonary lymphangioleiomyomatosis. *J Clin Pathol* 46:479, 1993.

125. McCarty KS, Mossler JA, McLelland R, et al: Pulmonary lymphangiomyomatosis responsive to progesterone. *N Engl J Med* 303:1461, 1980.

126. Miller WR, Cornog JL Jr, Sullivan MA: Lymphangiomyomatosis: a clinical roentgenographic-pathologic syndrome. *Am J Roentgenol* 111:565, 1971.

127. Monteforte WJ, Kohnen PW: Angiomyolipomas in a case of lymphangiomyomatosis syndrome: relationship to tuberous sclerosis. *Cancer* 34:317, 1974.

128. Mori M, Ikeda T, Onoe T: Blastic Schwann cells in renal tumor of tuberous sclerosis complex. *Acta Pathol Jpn* 21:121, 1971.

129. Ohori NP, Yousem SA, Sonmez-Alpan E, et al: Estrogen and progesterone receptors in lymphangioleiomyomatosis, epithelioid hemangioendothelioma, and sclerosing hemangioma of the lung. *Am J Clin Pathol* 96:529, 1991.

130. Pachter MR, Lattes R: Mesenchymal tumors of the mediastinum. III. Tumors of lymph vascular origin. *Cancer* 16:108, 1963.

131. Peyrol S, Gindre D, Cordier AJF, et al: Characterization of the smooth muscle cell infiltrate and associated connective matrix of lymphangiomyomatosis: immunohistochemical and ultrastructural study of two cases. *J Pathol* 168:387, 1992.

132. Rienhoff MF, Shelley WM, Cornell WP: Lymphangiomatous malformation of the thoracic duct associated with chylous pleural effusion. *Ann Surg* 159:180, 1964.

133. Rosendal J: A case of diffuse myomatosis and cyst formation in the lung. *Acta Radiol* 23:138, 1942.

134. Sawicka EH, Morris AJR: A report of two long-surviving cases of pulmonary lymphangioleiomyomatosis and the response to progesterone therapy. *Br J Dis Chest* 79:400, 1985.

135. Schiaffino E, Tavani E, Dellafiore L, et al: Pulmonary lymphangiomyomatosis: report of a case with immunohistochemical and ultrastructural findings. *Appl Pathol* 7:265, 1989.

136. Silverstein EF, Ellis K, Wolff M, et al: Pulmonary lymphangiomyomatosis. *Am J Roentgenol* 120:832, 1974.

137. Sinclair W, Wright JL, Churg A: Lymphangioleiomyomatosis presenting in a postmenopausal woman. *Thorax* 40:475, 1985.

138. Sobonya RE, Quan SF, Fleishman JS: Pulmonary lymphangioleiomyomatosis: quantitative analysis of lesions producing airflow limitation. *Hum Pathol* 16:1122, 1985.

139. Steffelaar JW, Nijkamp DA, Hilvering C: Pulmonary lymphangiomyomatosis: demonstration of smooth muscle antigens by immunofluorescent technique. *Scand J Respir Dis* 58:103, 1977.

140. Stovin PGI: Pulmonary lymphangiomyomatosis syndrome. *J Pathol* 109:VII, 1973.

141. Stovin PGI, Lum LC, Flower CDR, et al: The lungs in lymphangiomyomatosis and in tuberous sclerosis. *Thorax* 30:497, 1975.

142. Svendsen TL, Viskum K, Hansborg N, et al: Pulmonary lymphangioleiomyomatosis: a case of progesterone receptor positive lymphangioleiomyomatosis treated with medroxyprogesterone, oophorectomy, and tamoxifen. *Br J Dis Chest* 78:264, 1984.

143. Taylor JR, Ryu J, Colby TV, et al: Lymphangioleiomyomatosis: clinical course in 32 patients. *N Engl J Med* 323:1254, 1990.

144. Tomasian A, Greenberg MS, Rumerman H: Tamoxifen for lymphangioleiomyomatosis. *N Engl J Med* 306:745, 1982.

145. Vadas G, Pare JA, Thurlbeck MW: Pulmonary and lymph node myomatosis: review of literature and report of case. *Can Med Assoc J* 96:420, 1967.

146. Valensi QJ: Pulmonary lymphangiomyoma, a probable forme fruste of tuberous sclerosis: a case report and survey of the literature. *Am Rev Respir Dis* 108:1411, 1973.

147. Vazquez JJ, Fernandez-Cuervo L, Fidalgo B: Lymphangiomyomatosis. *Cancer* 37:2321, 1976.

148. Vejlens G: Specific pulmonary alterations in tuberous sclerosis. *Acta Pathol Microbiol Scand* 18:317, 1941.

149. Wolff M: Lymphangiomyoma: clinicopathological study and ultrastructural confirmation of its histogenesis. *Cancer* 31:988, 1973.

CHAPTER 27

PERIVASCULAR TUMORS

In previous editions of this text we have discussed glomus tumor and hemangiopericytoma in separate chapters. However, as indicated in the recent classification of soft tissue tumors by the World Health Organization,[80] it is conceptually useful to place these tumors in the same category, since the cells within both tumors can be likened to cells that support or invest blood vessels (i.e., pericyte and glomus cell), in contrast to the much larger group of vascular lesions that display features of endothelial differentiation (e.g., hemangioma, lymphangioma, angiosarcoma). Glomus tumor and hemangiopericytoma are rather distinct lesions clinically and histologically, however.

GLOMUS TUMOR

Glomus tumor is a distinctive neoplasm the cells of which resemble the modified smooth muscle cells of the normal glomus body. It was originally considered a form of angiosarcoma, until Masson[54] published his classic paper on the subject in 1924. His work was based on observations of three patients who had experienced strikingly similar symptoms. Each suffered paroxysms of lancinating pain in the upper extremity, which abated abruptly following removal of a tumor. Masson compared the tumors to the normal glomus body and suggested that the lesion represented a hyperplasia or overgrowth of this structure. It is now well accepted that the tumor recapitulates the modified muscle cells found in this organ, although it is debatable, if not doubtful, that the majority represent hyperplasia of the structure.

The normal glomus body is a specialized form of arteriovenous anastomosis that serves in thermal regulation. It is located in the stratum reticularis of the dermis and is most frequently encountered in the subungual region, the lateral areas of the digits, and the palm.[62] According to Popoff,[62] the structure does not develop until several months after birth and gradually undergoes atrophy during late adult life. Although it may be damaged in certain disease states, there is evidence that it may regenerate, probably as a result of differentiation of perivascular cells. The glomus body is made up of an afferent arteriole, which is derived from the small arterioles supplying the dermis and which branches into two or four preglomic arterioles (Figs. 27-1 to 27-3). These arterioles are endowed with the usual complement of muscle cells and an internal elastic lamina, but they blend gradually into a thick-walled segment with an irregular lumen known as the Sucquet-Hoyer canal. This region is the arteriovenous anastomosis proper. It is lined by plump cuboidal endothelial cells, which in turn are surrounded by longitudinal and circular muscle fibers but no elastic tissue. Scattered throughout the muscle fibers are the rounded, epithelioid "glomus" cells. These canals drain into a series of thin-walled collecting veins. The entire glomic complex is encompassed by lamellated collagenous tissue containing small nerves and vessels.

Clinical findings

Glomus tumors are uncommon tumors with an estimated incidence of 1.6% in the five hundred consecutive soft tissue tumors reported from the Mayo Clinic.[69] The tumor is about equally common in both sexes, although there is a striking female predominance (3:1) among patients with subungual lesions.[9,69,74] The majority of glomus tumors are diagnosed during adult life (20 to 40 years of age), although often symptoms have been present for several years before actual diagnosis. The lesions develop as small blue-red nodules that are usually located in the deep dermis or subcutis of the upper or lower extremity. The single most common site is the subungual region of the finger, but other common sites include the palm, wrist, forearm, and foot. Glomus tumors rarely occur in the subcutaneous tissue near the tip of the spine, where they presumably arise from the glomus coccygeum (Fig. 27-4), although the precise criteria for the diagnosis of hyperplasia or neoplasia of the glomus body in this location are not clearly defined.[3,19] It is now recognized that the tumor may also develop in sites where the normal glomus body may be sparse or even absent. Unusual locations have included the patella,[66] chest wall, bone,[10,45,48,73] stomach,[6,27,38,39,81] colon,[8] nerve,[44] eyelid, nose (cited by Apfelberg), trachea,[41] and possibly mediastinum.[11] In our experience they have also occurred in the rectum, cervix, vagina, labia, and mesentery. Most glomus

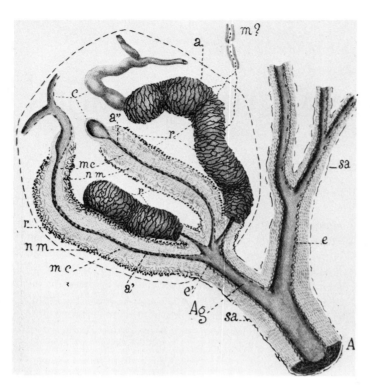

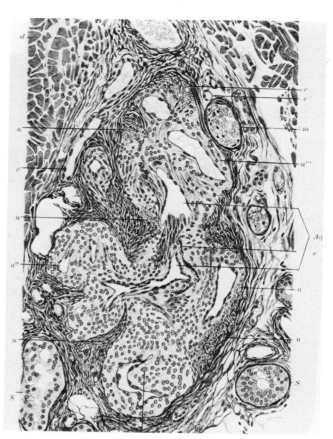

FIG. 27-1. Depiction of normal glomus body according to Masson. Afferent arteriole *(Ag)* gives rise to four preglomic arterioles, which blend with an irregular, thick-walled segment known as the Sucquet-Hoyer canal containing the arteriovenous anastomosis. It terminates in the collecting veins *(c)*. (From Masson P: *Lyon Chir* 21:257, 1924.)

FIG. 27-2. Graphic depiction of histological cross-section through glomus body according to Masson. Glomic arterioles of Sucquet-Hoyer canal *(a, a'', a' ")* contain glomus cells in their walls. Collecting veins are located at periphery *(c)*. Small nerves and collagen fibers encircle glomus body. (From Masson P: *Lyon Chir* 21:257, 1924.)

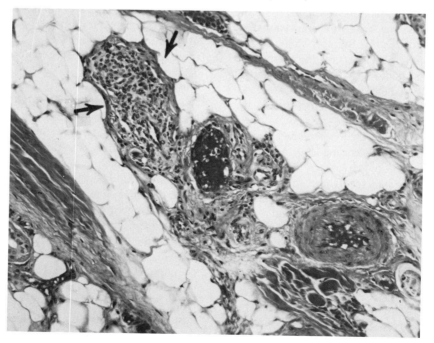

FIG. 27-3. Normal glomus body from foot. Arrows indicate Sucquet-Hoyer canal with glomus cells. (×160.)

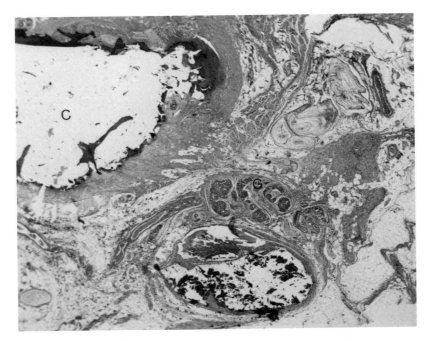

FIG. 27-4. Glomus coccygeum *(G)* located at ventral tip of coccyx *(C)*. Patient presented with pain and had dilated vessels containing glomus cells just beneath glomus body, raising the question of an early glomangioma arising in the glomus coccygeum. (×25.)

tumors are solitary lesions; however, in two large studies the incidence of multiple lesions was estimated to be just under 10%.[25,60] There are several striking instances of patients with multiple lesions.* These reports indicate certain differences between the solitary and multiple forms of the disease. Multiple glomus tumors occur more often during childhood, are rarely subungual, and are less likely to be painful or symptomatic. Histologically, they are usually poorly circumscribed tumors that resemble cavernous hemangiomas[21] (see discussion of glomangioma), in contrast to the ordinary glomus tumor, which is usually better circumscribed and more cellular. A few patients with multiple lesions have been known to have similarly affected family members or associated malformations[46]; this raises the possibility that certain cases are genetically determined. The report by Conant and Wiesenfeld[16] describing nine affected members in one family is compatible with an autosomal dominant mode of inheritance with incomplete penetrance.

The symptoms produced by glomus tumors are quite characteristic and often well out of proportion to the size of the neoplasm. Paroxysms of pain radiating away from the lesion are the most common complaint. These episodes can be elicited by changes in temperature, particularly exposure to cold, and tactile stimulation of even minor degree. In some patients the pain is accompanied by additional

signs of hypesthesia, muscle atrophy,[66] or osteoporosis of the affected part.[23,69] In unusual instances disturbances of autonomic function (e.g., Horner's syndrome) have been reported.[54] Although the mechanism of pain production has not been fully elucidated, the recent identification of nerve fibers containing immunoreactive substance P (a pain-associated vasoactive peptide) within glomus tumors suggests pain mediation through release of this substance.[43]

Gross findings

Grossly, the lesions are small blue-red nodules (usually measuring less than 1 cm) that are immediately apparent on clinical examination. Subungual lesions may be more difficult to detect, and care should be taken to look for ridging of the nail or discoloration of the nail bed. Radiographs are helpful when they demonstrate a small scalloped osteolytic defect with a sclerotic border[29] in the terminal phalanx, as this finding is highly characteristic of glomus tumor and epidermal inclusion cyst (Fig. 27-5). The more recent use of high-resolution MRI offers the promise of detecting extremely small soft tissue–based lesions.[35]

Microscopic findings

Glomus tumors show varying proportions of glomus cells, vascular structures, and smooth muscle tissue. According to the relative proportions, they have been divided into three groups: (1) glomus tumor proper, (2) glomangioma, and (3) glomangiomyoma. Although there is no sig-

*References 21, 33, 34, 46, 52, 55, 59, 72.

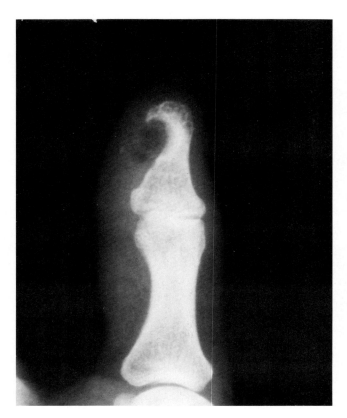

FIG. 27-5. Postoperative radiograph showing defect in distal phalanx created by subungual glomus tumor.

Table 27-1. Anatomical distribution of glomus tumors according to histological subtype (AFIP, 506 cases)

Anatomical location	Glomus tumor No. cases	%	Glomangioma No. cases	%	Glomangio- myoma No. cases	%
Upper extremity (finger)	176 (81)	34	45 (9)	9	16 (3)	3
Lower extremity	98	19	29	6	14	3
Head-neck	29	6	6	1	5	1
Trunk	24	5	8	2	0	0
Other (including gastrointestinal tract)	45	9	4	1	7	1
TOTAL	372	73	92	19	42	8

or eosinophilic cytoplasm (Fig. 27-9, *A*). The outlines of the cells are not fully appreciated in routine hematoxylin-eosin–stained sections, but can be accentuated with a periodic acid-Schiff stain or toluidine blue stain on 1-micron sections (Fig. 27-9, *B*). In these preparations a "chicken-wire" network of matrix material is present between the cells.

Only rarely do glomus cells deviate from the foregoing description, but when they do, alterations in either the nucleus or the cytoplasm may be seen. Large hyperchromatic nuclei (Fig. 27-10), probably representing a degenerative change analogous to that seen in some neurilemomas, may replace the typical round, regular nuclei. An even less common phenomenon is the acquisition of abundant granular, eosinophilic cytoplasm such that portions of the tumor appear "oncocytic"[68,71] (Fig. 27-11). Intravascular growth and signet-ring change of the cells have been noted in a multifocal gastric glomus tumor.[27]

Although the cells are regarded as variants of smooth muscle cells, the cytoplasm is usually devoid of glycogen, and there is only minimal fuchsinophilia observed on staining with the Masson trichrome stain, two features that contrast with the staining reactions of conventional smooth muscle cells. Peripherally the tumors possess an ill-defined rim of collagen containing small nerves and vessels. This rim seldom serves as a complete or totally confining capsule, since isolated nests of glomus cells can be identified outside its boundaries and occasionally in the walls of small vessels surrounding the main tumor mass (Fig. 27-12).

In contrast to the common form of glomus tumor, *glomangiomas* are less well circumscribed and constitute only about one fifth of the cases. Grossly and microscopically they resemble cavernous hemangiomas (Fig. 27-13). They are composed of gaping veins with small clusters of glomus cells in their walls (Figs. 27-13 and 27-14). Secondary thrombosis and phlebolith formation may occur within these lesions just as they would in an ordinary hemangioma.

nificant difference in the age incidence in these three groups, the location of the tumors varies (Table 27-1). Glomus tumors are most common in the upper extremity and show a marked predilection for the finger, particularly the subungual region. Glomangiomas predominate on the hand and forearm and are usually the type encountered in patients with multiple or familial lesions. Glomangiomyomas are nearly equally divided between the upper and lower extremities.

The common form of *glomus tumor* accounts for about three fourths of all cases in our material (Table 27-1). It is a well-circumscribed lesion consisting of tight convolutes of capillary-sized vessels surrounded by collars of glomus cells set in a hyalinized or myxoid stroma (Fig. 27-6). Rarely it occurs as a poorly circumscribed diffuse lesion (Fig. 27-7). Depending on the size of the nests of glomus cells, the tumor may have a highly vascular appearance reminiscent of a hemangiopericytoma or paraganglioma, or a cellular appearance suggestive of an epithelial tumor (Fig. 27-8). However, the glomus cell is quite distinctive, and its appearance is one of the most reliable means of distinguishing the tumor from others with similar growth patterns. The cell has a rounded, regular shape with a sharply punched-out rounded nucleus set off from the amphophilic

Text continued on p. 711.

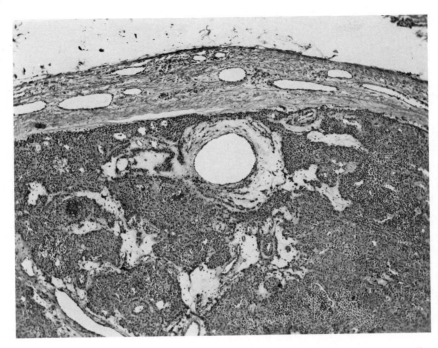

FIG. 27-6. Common form of glomus tumor showing dense fibrous pseudocapsule surrounding solid sheets of cells. (×15.)

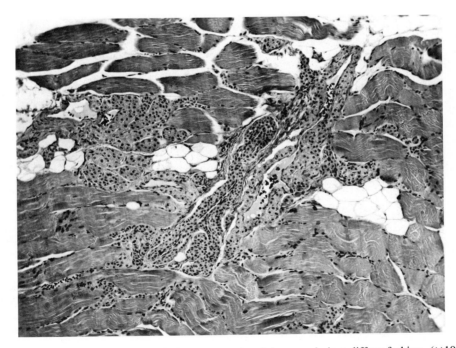

FIG. 27-7. Less common form of glomus tumor involving muscle in a diffuse fashion. (×100.)

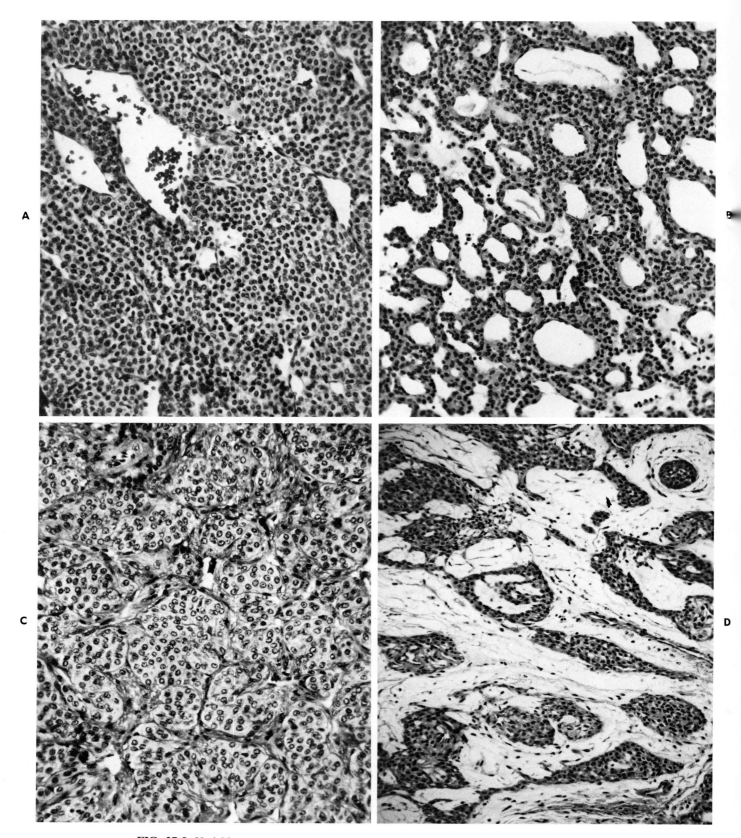

FIG. 27-8. Variable patterns within glomus tumors. Most tumors are composed of solid sheets of cells interrupted by vessels of varying sizes (**A** and **B**). Less often intricate vasculature with surrounding nests simulates the pattern of a paraganglioma (**C**). Myxoid change in stroma (**D**) is also a less frequent finding. (**A**, ×250; **B**, ×165; **C**, ×250; **D**, ×160.)

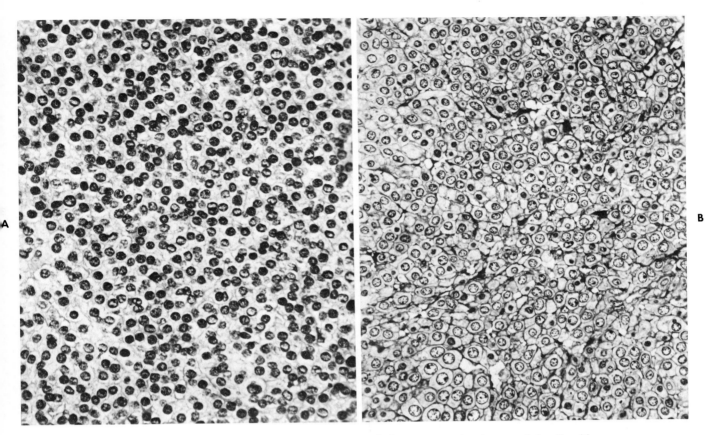

FIG. 27-9. A, Hematoxylin-eosin–stained section of glomus tumor showing rounded cells with punched-out nuclei and faintly staining cytoplasm. **B,** One-micron section stained with toluidine blue at same magnification as **A,** illustrating the "chickenwire" network of basal lamina material that encircles individual cells. (**A,** ×400; **B,** toluidine blue, ×400.)

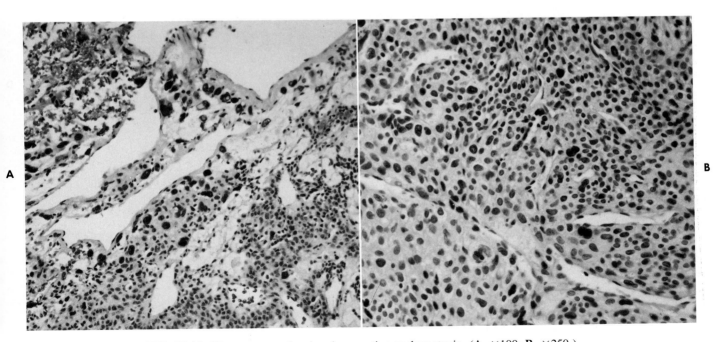

FIG. 27-10. Glomus tumor showing degenerative nuclear atypia. (**A,** ×100; **B,** ×250.)

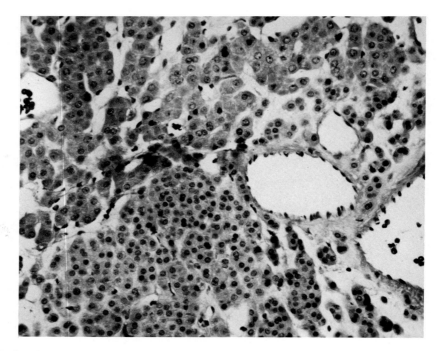

FIG. 27-11. Glomus tumor with cells having abundant granular eosinophilic cytoplasm resembling oncocytes. (×160.)

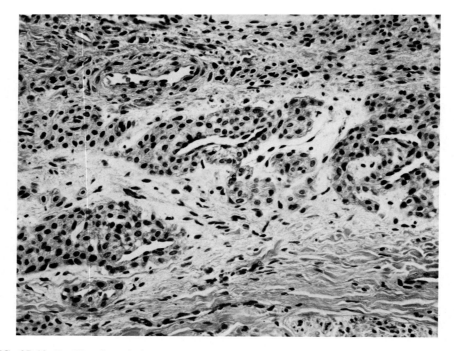

FIG. 27-12. Proliferation of glomus cells in vessels at periphery of glomus tumor. This feature may be very helpful in distinguishing solid forms of glomus tumors from adnexal tumors. (×250.)

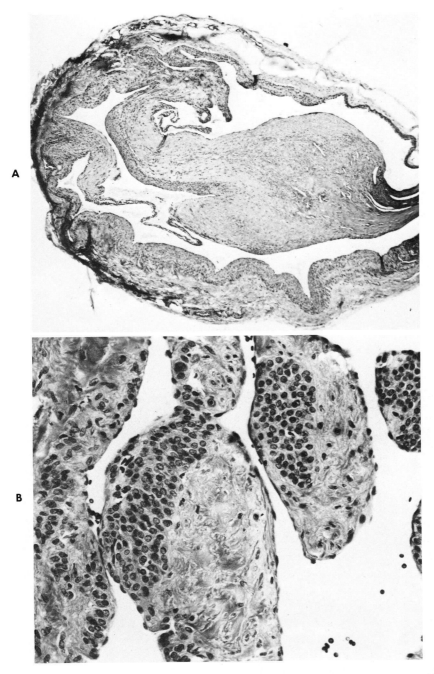

FIG. 27-13. Partially collapsed glomangioma illustrating dilated cavernous blood spaces **(A)** containing glomus cells in their walls **(B)**. **(A,** ×60; **B,** ×250.)

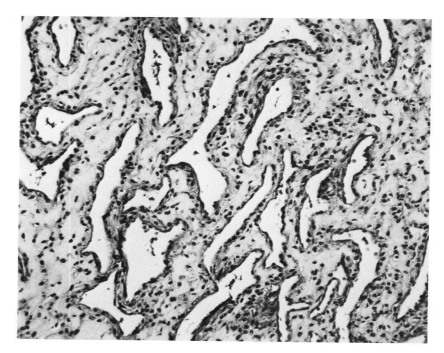

FIG. 27-14. Glomangioma with marked hyalinization. (×250.)

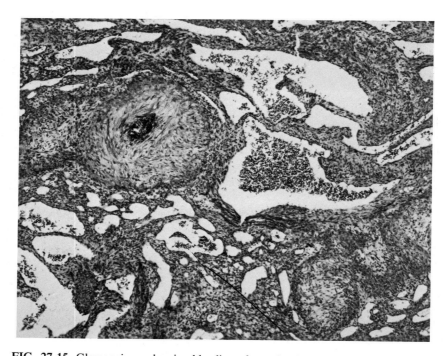

FIG. 27-15. Glomangioma showing blending of muscle of vessels with tumor. (×60.)

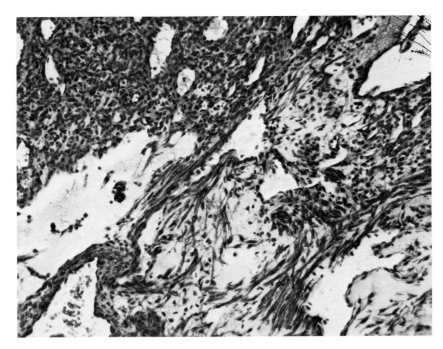

FIG. 27-16. Glomangiomyoma. Typical glomus cells undergo transition to smooth muscle *(right).* (×250.)

Glomangiomyomas account for less than 10% of all glomus tumors and, therefore, are the least frequent type. Their overall pattern may be identical to the ordinary glomus tumor or the glomangioma. However, in contrast to the foregoing types, there is a gradual transition from glomus cells to elongated, mature smooth muscle cells. This transition is most obvious in the region of large vessels, where the peripheral smooth muscle cells seem to blend with the tumor (Figs. 27-15 and 27-16).

Because glomus tumors are quite distinctive by virtue of their characteristic cells, location, and symptoms, errors in diagnosis are infrequent. Nonetheless, it has been our experience that very cellular glomus tumors are occasionally mistaken for adnexal tumors or less frequently intradermal nevi. In the former instance, it is important to note the intimate relationship of the cells around small vessels at the periphery of the tumor (Fig. 27-12) and the total lack of ductular differentiation or epithelial mucin production. Haupt et al.[30] have shown that the use of immunohistochemistry can reliably discriminate glomus tumors from solid forms of hidradenoma (the adnexal tumor most closely resembling a glomus tumor). Virtually all hidradenomas contained immunoreactive keratin, whereas none of the glomus tumors did. In addition hidradenomas frequently also express carcinoembryonic antigen and epithelial membrane antigen, two antigens not encountered in glomus tumor. Likewise, Kaye and Dehner[40] demonstrated that S-100 protein is a reliable marker in separating nevi from glomus tu-

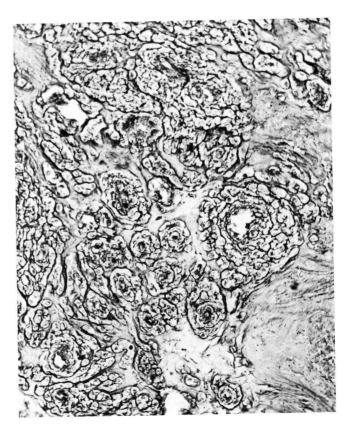

FIG. 27-17. Glomus tumor with delicate interstitial pattern of reticulin fibers. (Reticulin stain, ×245.)

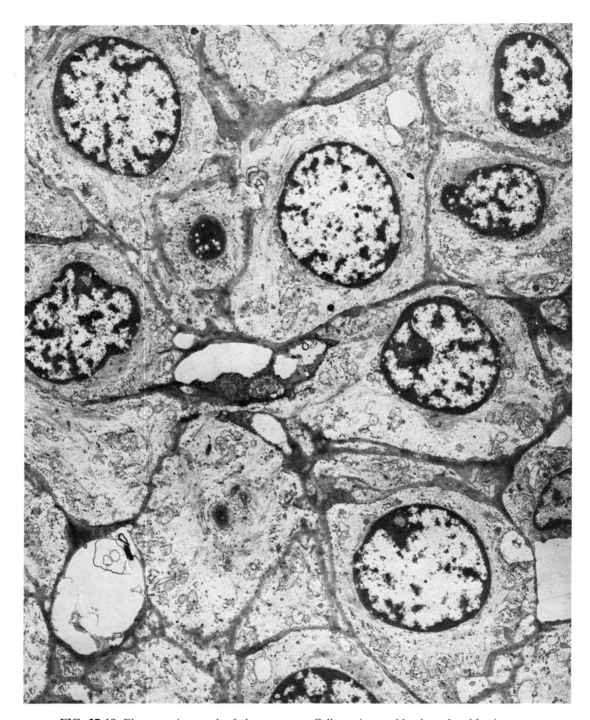

FIG. 27-18. Electron micrograph of glomus tumor. Cells are invested by dense basal lamina, possess pinocytotic vesicles along their surfaces, and contain cytoplasmic myofilaments with dense bodies. (Magnification reduced from 5000.) (Courtesy Department of Pathology, Veterans Administration Hospital, Hines, Illinois.)

mors. In the past, reticulin stain was often used to discriminate glomus tumors from epithelial ones because the former displayed a delicate interstitial pattern of fiber deposition (Fig. 27-17), in contrast to the latter. This staining technique, which is often difficult to perform and interpret, has been largely replaced by immunohistochemistry. Although electron microscopy can serve as a diagnostic adjunct, it is seldom needed given the rather typical features and reliability of immunohistochemistry in most cases.

Ultrastructural and immunohistochemical findings

Typically a glomus cell is a rounded or polygonal cell measuring 8 to 12 μ and having a rounded nucleus with occasional clefts and prominent nucleoli (Fig. 27-18). The cells are closely spaced and often interdigitate with each other along their short knobby processes. Their surfaces are invested by a relatively thick basal lamina. The cytoplasm contains modest numbers of mitochondria and endoplasmic reticulum but is most notable for the bundles of thin (8 nm) actinlike filaments that fill the cytoplasm. The bundles are well oriented, possess typical dense bodies, and occasionally terminate in dense attachment plaques on the cytoplasmic membrane. In those examples of glomus tumor having oncocytic features the cytoplasm is not surprisingly filled with numerous mitochondria, making it more difficult to identify microfilaments.[71]

Originally glomus cells were considered pericytes on the basis of certain morphological similarities noted in tissue culture.[58] However, as a result of the foregoing ultrastructural features,* the glomus tumor is generally considered more closely related to the smooth muscle cell. Certainly the quantity of myofilaments present in these cells exceeds that normally encountered in the pericyte, and the cell processes are less well developed than those of the latter cell.

Vimentin and muscle actin isoforms can be identified within nearly all glomus tumors.[27,30,60,63,67] Desmin is much more variable, however, and has been reported in no tumors[67] or the majority of tumors,[60,63] depending on the series. In concert with the ultrastructural features of the neoplasm, both laminin and type IV collagen, two constitutents of basal lamina, outline the cells or small groups of cells.[27] Nerve growth factor receptor and myelin-associated glycoprotein can be identified within some glomus tumors, although the meaning of these findings is not clear.[63]

Behavior and treatment

Although the question of "malignant transformation" of glomus tumor has been raised in the literature, this appears to be such a rare event that it can be dismissed from a practical point of view (see glomangiosarcoma, below). Essentially all glomus tumors are benign and are adequately treated by simple excision. Only 10% recur following con-

servative excision.[78] Infrequent cases of local recurrence probably represent persistence of tumor following inadequate excision or the infrequent benign glomus tumor growing in a diffuse or infiltrative fashion.[22,26,31,65] In one of the cases described by Rao and Weiss,[65] the glomus tumor was an integral part of an angiomatosis (diffuse form of hemangioma). In diffuse glomus tumor the extent of the excision should be gauged against the need for total control of the disease.

GLOMANGIOSARCOMA

Glomangiosarcomas are exceptionally rare lesions that contain areas of benign glomus tumor in association with areas of sarcoma. We have encountered four such cases out of several hundred glomus tumors at the AFIP, and others have been reported in the literature.[2,26] Three of our four cases involved the lower extremity, and two of the four cases involved muscle as well as subcutaneous tissue. None of our lesions metastasized, nor have any of those cited above. Therefore, it is difficult to accept them as malignant tumors in the fullest sense of the word. Histologically, all of our cases were characterized by sarcomatous areas that arose in the midst of areas of benign glomus tumor (Fig. 27-19). The malignant areas consist of short spindled cells having features somewhat intermediate between fibrosarcoma and leiomyosarcoma. Unlike leiomyosarcoma, the cells are short, stubby, and less well oriented. They display only a moderate degree of pleomorphism but usually ample mitotic activity. Ultrastructural study in one case demonstrated numerous well-oriented cytoplasmic myofilaments similar to those encountered in conventional leiomyosarcomas and prominent basal lamina. Therapy of these lesions has consisted of complete, but not necessarily wide, excision. To date this has proved to be adequate therapy, a finding that may be explained in part by the small size and relatively superficial location of the tumors.

A somewhat more controversial area has been the recognition and acceptance of malignant glomus tumors in which no benign component is present. Although theoretically such lesions should exist, there has not been any reliable way of recognizing them. Possibly the case reported by Lumley and Stansfeld[50] that produced metastasis is an example of this phenomenon, as are the two cases (cases 5 and 6) presented by Gould et al.[26] In the latter instances the presence of actin within one case and basal lamina in the other was construed by the authors as glomoid differentiation. Based on the photomicrographs of the lesions showing a relatively uniform round cell tumor without extensive necrosis, the diagnosis is tenable.

HEMANGIOPERICYTOMA

Hemangiopericytoma is a rather uncommon neoplasm that was first described and named by Stout and Murray[185] in 1942. In their original description the authors postulated

---

*References 28, 38, 56, 76, 77, 79.

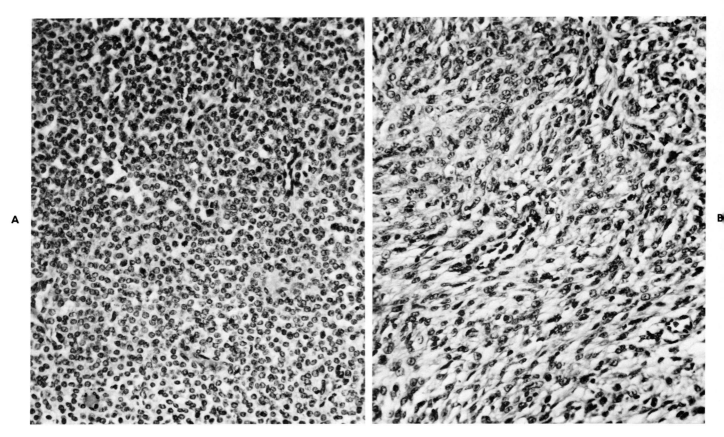

A																																																																																		B

FIG. 27-19. Glomangiosarcoma showing areas of typical glomus tumor **(A)** in association with spindled areas, which resemble an immature form of fibrosarcoma or leiomyosarcoma **(B).** (A and B, ×250.)

that the tumor was composed mainly of pericytes, a specific cell type first identified by Rouget[174] in 1873 and further defined by Zimmermann[201] in 1923 (Fig. 27-20). Stout and Murray postulated that this tumor was closely related to the glomus tumor but did not have its highly organized structure.[182,183] In subsequent years the clinical and morphological characteristics of hemangiopericytoma were more clearly defined, and its pericytic origin was confirmed ultrastructurally.

Pericytes are ubiquitous contractive, highly arborized cells that are normally arranged along capillaries and venules. They have multiple extensions that partly encircle the vascular channels regulating vascular caliber and modulating capillary blood flow and permeability (Fig. 27-20). The cells and their processes contain microfilaments, are enveloped by basal lamina, and stain positively for immunoreactive vimentin. They may act as phagocytic cells and are a potential source of fibroblasts, osteoblasts, and lipocytes.

Despite the great number of publications on hemangiopericytoma since its first description in 1942, diagnosis of

this tumor and prediction of its clinical behavior still cause considerable problems: pericytes, unlike most other mesenchymal cell types, lack readily identifiable cellular and immunohistochemical features, and under the light microscope are difficult to distinguish from endothelial cells, fibroblasts, and histiocytes. Therefore diagnosis of hemangiopericytoma rests mainly on recognition of its architectural pattern, and in the absence of an ultrastructural study, it is often difficult if not impossible to distinguish this tumor from other richly vascular neoplasms. As a result, some of these lesions have been mistakenly diagnosed as poorly differentiated hemangiopericytoma and have been reported as such in the literature, causing perhaps a malignant bias in the published survival rates.

An additional problem that frequently faces the pathologist is the difficulty of reliably predicting the biological behavior on the basis of the clinical and morphological parameters. There are obviously low-grade hemangiopericytomas that are readily cured by wide local excision and high-grade hemangiopericytomas that frequently recur and metastasize despite intensive therapy. But there are also

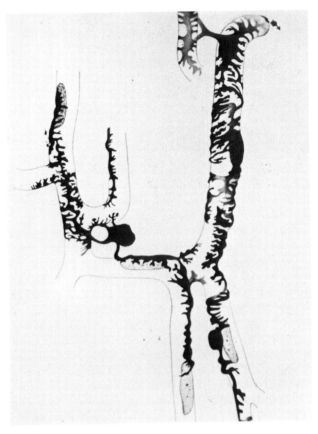

FIG. 27-20. Drawing of pericytes from Zimmermann's original description of these cells in 1923. Note the presence of multiple cytoplasmic processes. (From Zimmermann KW: *Z. Anat Entwicklungsg* 68:29, 1923.)

Table 27-2. Age distribution* of 105 patients with hemangiopericytoma

Age (years)	No. patients	Percent
0-9	1	1.0
10-19	4	4.0
20-29	20	19.0
30-39	13	12.5
40-49	23	22.0
50-59	20	19.0
60-69	14	13.0
70-79	9	8.5
80-89	1	1.0
TOTAL	105	100.0

*Median age, 45 years; range, 5½ to 80 years.

many borderline or intermediate forms in which accurate prediction of the clinical course is very difficult if not impossible. Furthermore, in rare instances prognosis is complicated by the fact that the primary tumor may exhibit a more benign appearance than the recurrent growth.

Clinical findings

Hemangiopericytoma is primarily a tumor of adult life with a median age of 45 years; it is rare in infants and children (Table 27-2). When it occurs in infants and children, it differs in several aspects from its adult counterpart and, therefore, will be discussed separately. The tumor occurs in both sexes with equal frequency. Tsuneyoshi et al.[192] report an incidence of 2.5% among 755 soft tissue sarcomas.

Most patients with this tumor complain of a slowly enlarging painless mass that usually has reached a fairly large size when treatment is sought. Tenderness and pain are infrequent and sometimes occur only during movement or exercise. Tumors in the pelvic fossa and the retroperitoneum may be associated with urinary retention, hydroureter, and hydronephrosis and rarely with constipation, abdominal distention, and vomiting. Except for one report of hemangiopericytoma in three members of one family, there is no evidence of increased familial incidence.[163]

Hypoglycemia has been noted in association with the tumor in several instances,[96,98,178] usually with large tumors located in the pelvis and retroperitoneum. In all of these cases blood sugar levels were restored to normal following complete or even partial removal of the tumor. Tumor assay for insulin in one of the cases gave negative results, however.[162] There is also one account in the literature in which hemangiopericytoma and hypoglycemia were associated with masculinization.[133]

Other manifestations of the disease, caused by the rich vascularity of hemangiopericytoma, are telangiectasia and elevated temperature of the overlying skin, unilateral varicose veins, and hemorrhoids, sometimes being associated with pulsation of the tumor and a distinct audible bruit. Because of these features some hemangiopericytomas were clinically mistaken for vascular malformations or aneurysms.

The clinical duration varies; most hemangiopericytomas are present for several months or even years before removal. One of our cases, a tumor of the left posterior thigh, was present for 15 years prior to operation; another was first noted at age 22 years and was surgically removed at age 52 years.[117] Stout and Cassel[184] report a hemangiopericytoma in a 92-year-old patient that allegedly had been present for 60 years. Among our consultation cases there is also a 104-year-old woman who developed a malignant lymphoma at the site of a hemangiopericytoma removed 10 years previously.

Anatomical location

The tumor is most common in the lower extremity, especially the thigh,[169] pelvic fossa,* and retroperito-

---

*References 109, 128, 143, 164, 171, 191, 195.

Table 27-3. Anatomical distribution of 106 cases with hemangiopericytoma

Anatomical site	No. patients	Percent
Head and neck	17	16.0
Trunk	15	14.2
Upper extremity	11	10.4
Lower extremity	37	34.9
Retroperitoneum, pelvis	26	24.5
TOTAL	106	100.0

neum.[82,112,202] Less frequently it affects the abdomen[97,168,184] and upper extremity. Among the 106 cases in our series,[117] 37 were in the lower limb and 26 were in the retroperitoneum and pelvis (Table 27-3). In the series reported by McMaster et al.,[151] the leading site was the thigh and inguinal region, with about one third of the cases occurring in these two locations. Most are deep seated, and the majority are found in muscle tissue. Dermal and subcutaneous hemangiopericytomas are much less common, especially if one excludes those occurring during infancy. We have also encountered two examples of intravascular hemangiopericytoma-like tumors.

Hemangiopericytomas in the region of the head pose special problems in diagnosis. The three major sites are the meninges, the nasal passages and paranasal sinuses, and the orbit.

Meningeal (cranial and intraspinal) hemangiopericytomas are indistinguishable under the light microscope, immunohistochemically, and ultrastructurally from hemangiopericytomas at other sites and are no longer considered variants of angioblastic meningioma.[107] They occur at a younger age than meningiomas, grow more often along the sinuses, bleed profusely at operation, and have a greater tendency to recur. They may metastasize to extracranial sites.[124,140,196] Guthrie et al.,[126] in a review of 44 cases of meningeal hemangiopericytomas, reported 5- and 15-year survival rates of 67% and 23%, respectively. Mena et al.,[152] in another large series, noted a recurrence rate of 60.6% and a metastatic rate of 23.4%.

Hemangiopericytomas of the nasal passages and paranasal sinuses differ slightly in their microscopic picture from those occurring elsewhere in the body. They tend to have cells with a greater amount of cytoplasm, vaguely reminiscent of glomus cells, have a more prominent spindle cell pattern, and are less vascular. Mitotic figures are absent or rare.[94,105,116,123,170] Because of these variations, the term "hemangiopericytoma-like tumors" was also used to describe these lesions.[103,104] Most hemangiopericytomas at this site behave in a benign manner. For example, in the study of Abdel-Fattah et al.,[82] 44 cases were described as benign and six as malignant. In another series of nine cases,[114] four recurred but none metastasized.

Orbital hemangiopericytomas are less common but are often difficult to distinguish from richly vascularized fibrous histiocytomas.[129,137,186] Croxatto and Font[106] reported a series of 30 cases with an 89% 5-year survival rate.

In addition, typical examples of primary hemangiopericytomas have been documented in the breast,[88,154,189] lung,[199] mediastinum,[146] uterus, ovary, and vagina,[125,131,177] and bone.[84,188]

Radiographic findings

Features seen on x-ray and CT scan are not specific, consisting merely of a well-circumscribed, radiopaque soft tissue mass, often displacing neighboring structures such as the urinary bladder, colon, and ureter.[118,132,150] Cystic changes are common, but calcification is rare and usually confined to large tumors of long duration.[85] In fact, speckled calcification in smaller tumors is suspect of a richly vascular synovial sarcoma, especially if the mass occurs in a young adult and is located near a large joint such as the knee.

Angiograms show a more characteristic picture, but they, too, are not sufficiently typical to permit unequivocal diagnosis. They show evidence of rapid circulation indicated by a richly vascular mass with dilatation of the arteries and a diffuse capillary blush or opacification in the arterial phase (Fig. 27-21) and a dense uniform tumor stain and dilatation of the draining vessels in the vicinity of the tumor in the venous phase. Early visualization of veins, suggesting an arteriovenous shunt, is occasionally noted.[90,136,141-143,187,198] Microangiographic studies of hemangiopericytoma have been carried out by Angervall et al.[87]

Gross findings

Hemangiopericytoma usually presents as a solitary well-circumscribed to fairly well-circumscribed mass covered by a thin, richly vascular pseudocapsule. It averages 4 to 8 cm in diameter, but lesions as small as 1 cm and as large as 21 cm have been seen in our series. There are also several reports in the literature of very large hemangiopericytomas, including one measuring 23 cm in greatest diameter.[88,121,128,155,169] On cut section the tumor is gray-white to red-brown, with a variable number of dilated vascular spaces and not infrequently areas of hemorrhage and cystic degeneration. Necrosis is common in malignant forms of hemangiopericytoma.

Microscopic findings

Characteristically the tumor consists of tightly packed cells around ramifying thin-walled, endothelium-lined vascular channels ranging from small capillary-sized vessels to large gaping sinusoidal spaces (Figs. 27-22 to 27-26). The cells have round to oval nuclei measuring 7 to 13 μ in diameter and moderate amounts of cytoplasm with ill-defined borders. In some cases there are also focal spindle cell ar-

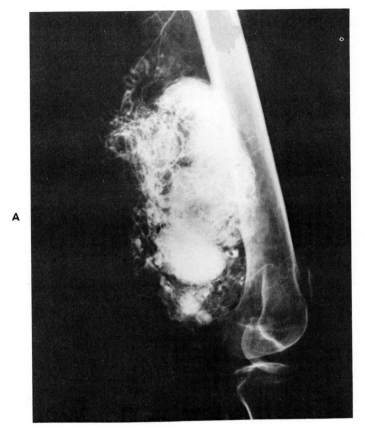

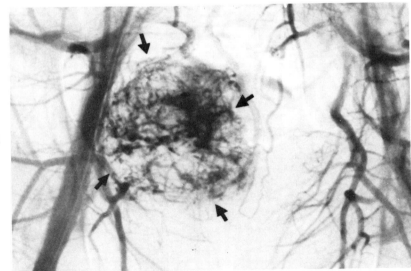

FIG. 27-21. **A,** Angiogram of hemangiopericytoma of left lower thigh showing capillary blush and tortuous veins draining the tumor. **B,** Angiogram of hemangiopericytoma in pelvic fossa distinctly outlining the tumor *(arrows).* (From Enzinger FM, Smith BH: *Hum Pathol* 7:61, 1976.)

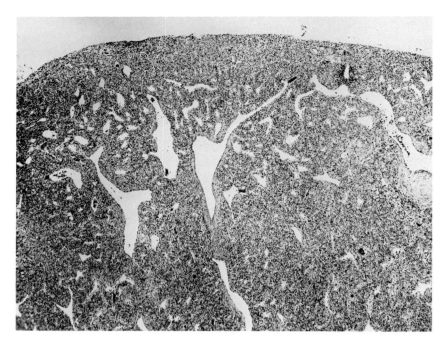

FIG. 27-22. Hemangiopericytoma. Low-power picture showing circumscription of the lesion and characteristic vascular pattern consisting of anastomosing vessels of varying calibers. (×30.)

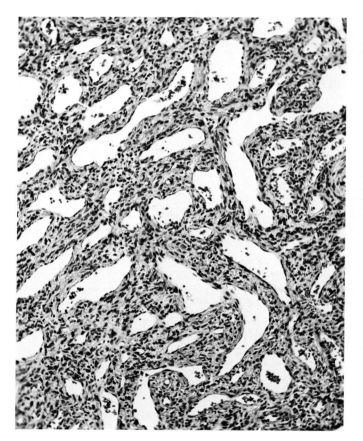

FIG. 27-23. Hemangiopericytoma showing richly vascular pattern consisting of thin-walled vessels lined by a single layer of flattened endothelial cells. (×130.)

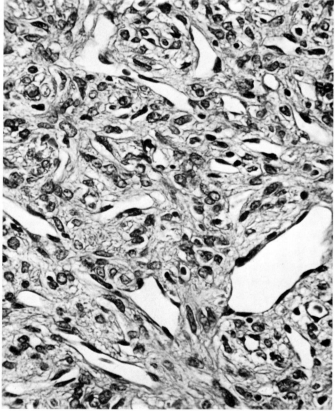

FIG. 27-24. Hemangiopericytoma. Dilated sinusoidal vascular channels surrounded by tumor cells with indistinct cellular outlines. (×440.)

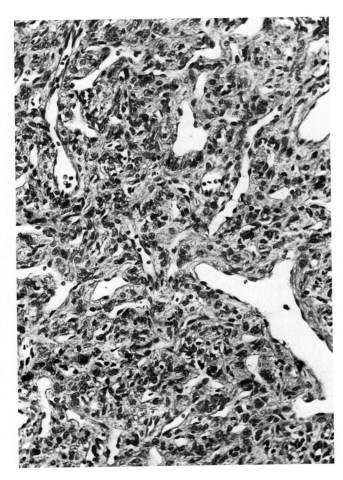

FIG. 27-25. Hemangiopericytoma. Gaping vascular channels, lined by a single layer of endothelium, are surrounded by haphazardly arranged tumor cells with oval nuclei and indistinct cytoplasm. (×260.) (From Enzinger FM, Smith BH: *Hum Pathol* 7:61, 1976.)

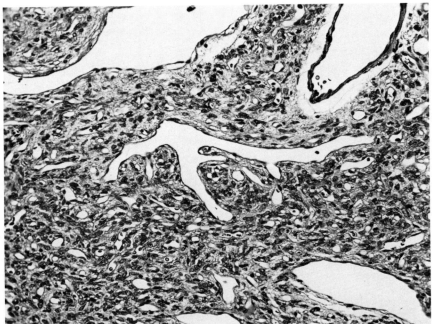

FIG. 27-26. Hemangiopericytoma. Branching vessels show the typical "antler" or "staghorn" configuration. (×195.) (From Enzinger FM, Smith BH: *Hum Pathol* 7:61, 1976.)

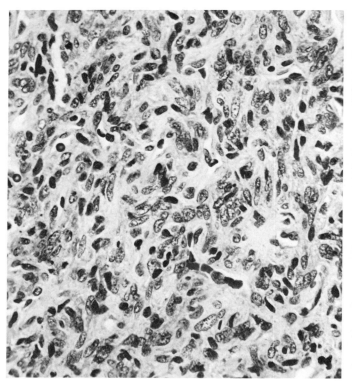

FIG. 27-27. Solid portions of hemangiopericytoma. Narrow vascular channels are compressed by the surrounding tumor cells. (×400.)

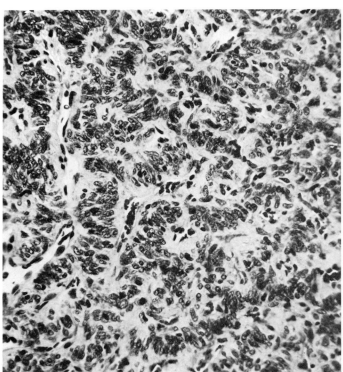

FIG. 27-28. Hemangiopericytoma. Palisading of nuclei between vascular channels gives the false impression of a neural tumor. (×250.)

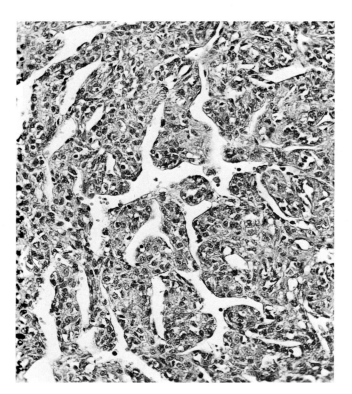

FIG. 27-29. Malignant hemangiopericytoma with a prominent vascular pattern and immature-appearing tumor cells. (×195.)

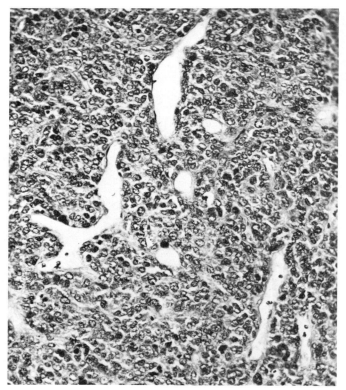

FIG. 27-30. Malignant hemangiopericytoma. Note hypercellularity and pleomorphism of tumor cells. Ten or more mitotic figures per 10 HPF were counted in this case. (×180.)

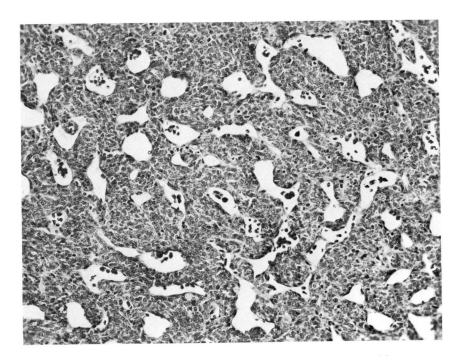

FIG. 27-31. Malignant hemangiopericytoma showing prominent cellularity and immature appearance of the tumor cells. (×145.) (From Enzinger FM, Smith BH: *Hum Pathol* 7:61, 1976.)

eas, but the spindle cells are never arranged in long bundles or fascicles as in fibrosarcoma or synovial sarcoma. There are also solid cellular areas (Fig. 27-27) and sometimes focal palisading reminiscent of neural tumor (Fig. 27-28). Focal smooth muscle differentiation has been observed but is rare.[110] The number of mitotic figures varies and is a helpful criterion in predicting the clinical behavior: fewer than two or three mitotic figures per 10 high power fields (HPF) are a prognostically favorable feature. Four or more mitotic figures per 10 HPF are usually indicative of a rapidly growing tumor capable of recurrence and metastasis. The latter tumors also tend to be more cellular, with a slight to moderate degree of cellular pleomorphism and occasional areas of necrosis and hemorrhage (Figs. 27-29 to 27-31). Cellular pleomorphism and mitotic activity, however, are uncommon in hemangiopericytomas of the nasal passages and the paranasal sinuses.

Degeneration of tumor tissue, accompanied by a marked decrease in cellularity and a striking increase in the amount of interstitial mucoid material, is a common feature that has led repeatedly to a mistaken diagnosis of myxoid liposarcoma despite the absence of lipoblasts and a plexiform capillary pattern (Figs. 27-32 and 27-33). Scattered lymphocytes and mast cells are quite common, but foam cells, fat cells, and lipomatous areas are rare.[190] Focal cartilaginous metaplasia is another rare feature and, if present, should raise the question of a mesenchymal chondrosarcoma.

The intervening vascular channels form a continuous ramifying vascular network that shows a striking variation in caliber. As a rule, the dilated branching vessels divide and communicate with vessels of small or minute size that may be partly compressed and obscured by the surrounding cellular proliferation. Typically, the dividing sinusoidal vessels have a "staghorn" or "antlerlike" configuration. Vessels with thick muscular coats are rare. Like other richly vascular tumors, the entire neoplasm functions as an arteriovenous shunt, causing increased venous pressure, marked vascular dilatation at the periphery of the tumor and surrounding areas, and increased oxygen saturation in the veins draining the tumor.[131] The presence of dilated vessels next to the tumor not infrequently leads to massive hemorrhage during surgical excision, a feature that must be taken into consideration when planning therapy.

Unlike hemangioendotheliomas and angiosarcomas, the constituent vessels are lined by a single layer of attenuated endothelial cells surrounded by a basal lamina, which in most but not all cases is clearly outlined with reticulin preparation and with PAS staining (Fig. 27-34). Reticulin and collagen fibers also enmesh the individual tumor cells, but the amount of reticulin and collagen varies substantially from case to case; fibrosis may be diffuse, localized, or nodular or may be confined to the immediate perivascular zone, sometimes with marked hyalinization and narrowing and partial obstruction of the vascular lumina (Figs. 27-35 and 27-36).

Hemangiopericytoma tends to be well circumscribed,

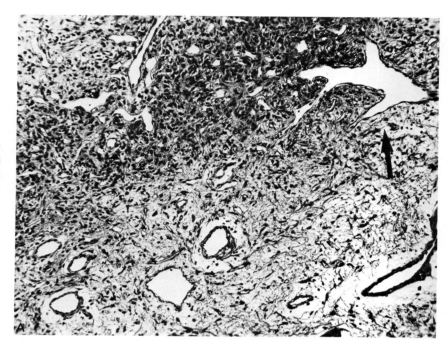

FIG. 27-32. Transition between typical hemangiopericytoma pattern and myxoid area. Note "staghorn" configuration of dilated sinusoidal vessel *(arrow).* (×110.) (From Enzinger FM, Smith BH: *Hum Pathol* 7:61, 1976.)

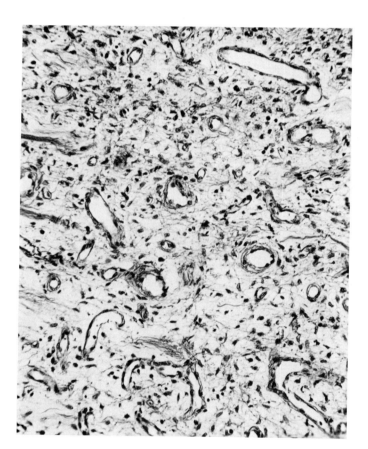

FIG. 27-33. Myxoid portion of hemangiopericytoma superficially resembling a myxoid liposarcoma. (×165.) (From Enzinger FM, Smith BH: *Hum Pathol* 7:61, 1976.)

with superficial lobulation caused by retraction of the tumor surface at the sites where the feeder vessels enter the neoplasm. Sometimes small satellite nodules become separated from the main tumor mass and are found within or outside the pseudocapsule (Fig. 27-37). Tissue culture studies show a mixed cell population consisting of large flattened cells and stellate cells, which are presumably endothelial cells and pericytes, respectively.[119,147,195]

Immunohistochemical findings

The cells of hemangiopericytoma contain vimentin as the sole intermediate filament, but the intensity of staining varies considerably from tumor to tumor. The cells also react with factor XIIIa and HLA-DR antigen[157] and, similar to other vascular tumors, stain positively with QBEND10 (CD34).[91] In contrast to the endothelial cells lining the interspersed vascular channels, the cells of hemangiopericytoma do not stain for factor VIII–related antigen, *Ulex europaeus* I lectin, or alpha-smooth muscle actin. Immunostaining for desmin, myoglobin, low- and high-molecular cytokeratin, and epithelial membrane antigen is negative.[154,157,166,175] Prominent desmin expression, however, was observed in a hemangiopericytoma of the thyroid that showed features of both hemangiopericytoma and smooth muscle tumor. Dictor et al.,[110] who described this case, named these hybrid cells "myopericytes," in analogy to myofibroblasts. Positive staining for various neural markers such as S-100 protein, Leu-7, and myelin-associated glycoprotein, is an unusual and unexplained finding that was noted in our material and some of the reported cases.[107,166]

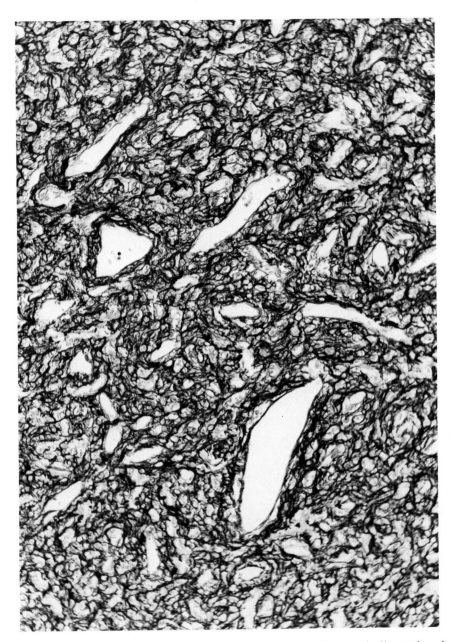

FIG. 27-34. Hemangiopericytoma. Reticulin preparation reveals dense reticulin meshwork surrounding vessels and tumor cells. (×230.) (From Enzinger FM, Smith BH: *Hum Pathol* 7:61, 1976.)

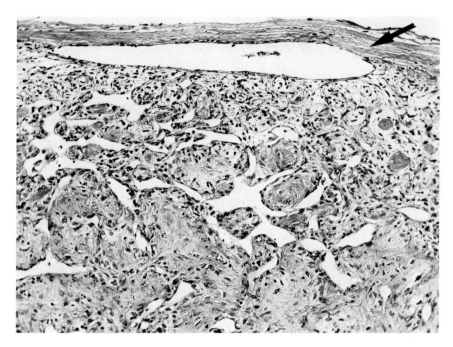

FIG. 27-35. Peripheral portion of hemangiopericytoma showing, in addition to the typical vascular pattern, dense fibrosis of the tumor matrix and marked dilatation of a subcapsular vascular channel *(arrow)*, probably the result of an arteriovenous shunt within the tumor. (×30.) (From Enzinger FM, Smith BH: *Hum Pathol* 7:61, 1976.)

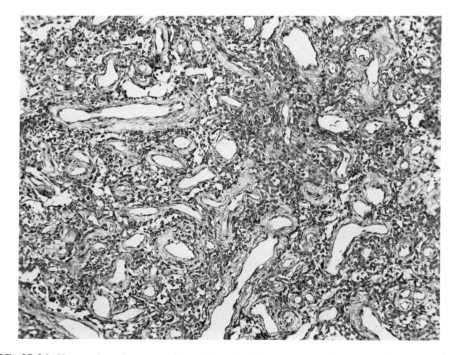

FIG. 27-36. Hemangiopericytoma with perivascular fibrosis and marked thickening of the basal laminae. (×110.) (From Enzinger FM, Smith BH: *Hum Pathol* 7:61, 1976.)

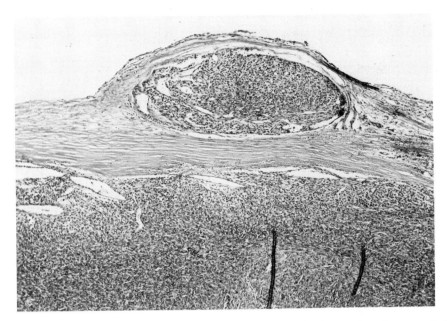

FIG. 27-37. Isolated tumor nodule within the fibrous capsule of a hemangiopericytoma. (×50.)

Ultrastructural findings

Numerous ultrastructural studies have established the predominantly pericytic nature of the tumor: like normal pericytes the cells of hemangiopericytoma surround endothelium-lined vascular spaces and possess large round or ovoid nuclei and pale-staining cytoplasm with few organelles but numerous elongated cytoplasmic extensions, being in close contact with the adjacent vascular channels. The organelles consist of profiles of rough-surfaced endoplasmic reticulum with few ribosomes, rod-shaped or oval mitochondria, and small bundles of microfilaments. Pinocytotic vesicles constitute a common and conspicuous feature, but desmosomes are poorly developed and rare. Characteristically, the individual cells are separated from the adjacent endothelial cells by a distinct, sometimes multilayered basal lamina and from one another by a continuous or discontinuous basal lamina or deposits of basal lamina-like material, as well as variable amounts of ground substance and collagen[94,102,145,167] (Fig. 27-38). In addition to the pericytic cells there are histiocyte-like cells and myoid cells; the latter are intermediate in appearance between pericytes and smooth muscle cells and contain bundles of microfilaments, focal condensations, and attachment plates.[108,127,147,156,159]

Cytogenetic analysis

Multiple chromosome abnormalities have been observed, including translocation t(12;19)[180] and t(13;22).[149]

INFANTILE HEMANGIOPERICYTOMA

Although this tumor is usually described together with adult hemangiopericytoma, it deserves separate consideration because of its different histological picture and clinical behavior. According to our cases, these lesions mostly occur in infants during the first year of life and, like juvenile hemangiomas, are mostly located in the subcutis and oral cavity. Tumors in older children and deep-seated tumors in the muscle, the mediastinum, and the abdomen have also been described.[89,115,138] Alpers et al.[86] reported an infantile hemangiopericytoma of the tongue and sublingual region that was discovered at birth, grew in an infiltrative manner, and recurred rapidly after local excision. After 30 months the child was well with no evidence of further recurrence or metastasis. All lesions in our cases have been solitary, but there are rare accounts of patients with multiple lesions.*

Microscopically, infantile hemangiopericytoma bears a close resemblance to the adult type, but many lesions, especially superficial ones, are multilobulated, often with distinct intravascular and perivascular satellite nodules outside the main tumor mass (Fig. 27-40, *A*) and frequent endovascular growth (Fig. 27-40, *B*). There is often increased mitotic activity and focal necrosis, features that indicate a poor prognosis in adult-type hemangiopericytoma but generally do not with the infantile form. Judging from our cases

---

*References 92, 99, 111, 130, 144, 176, 193.

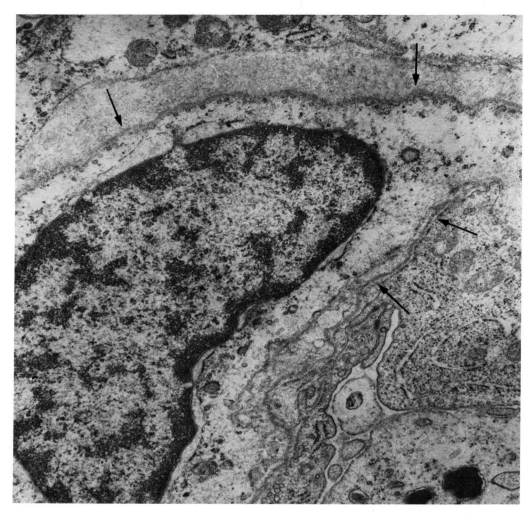

FIG. 27-38. Ultrastructure of hemangiopericytoma showing paucity of organelles, pinocytotic vesicles, and distinct basal laminae *(arrows).* (×14,970.) (From Tavassoli FA, Weiss SW: *Am J Surg Pathol* 5:745, 1981.)

and the literature, most of these tumors tend to follow a benign clinical course, are curable by local excision, or, as reported by Chen et al.,[101] may regress spontaneously. In rare instances, however, there may be local infiltrative growth or recurrence and even metastasis.[89,138] Deep-seated lesions and those occurring in older children seem to pursue a more aggressive clinical course than superficial ones occurring during the first years of life.[86,89] The hemangiopericytoma-like pattern found in lobular or tufted hemangioma—a variant of lobular capillary hemangioma marked by dermal or subcutaneous capillary or vascular lobules—infantile myofibromatosis, and infantile fibrosarcoma must be distinguished from that of infantile hemangiopericytoma (see Chapters 11, 12, and 23).

Differential diagnosis

The distinction of hemangiopericytoma from other neoplasms with prominent vascular patterns may cause considerable difficulties, but most hemangiopericytomas can be identified by their uniform cellular and vascular pattern and the dense reticulin meshwork that surrounds the individual tumor cells. Among the many tumors that may mimic hemangiopericytoma, benign and malignant fibrous histiocytoma, synovial sarcoma, and mesenchymal chondrosarcoma are the most important. Careful sampling of the tumor will reveal the correct diagnosis in most of these tumors.

Fibrous histiocytoma, particularly its deep subcutaneous form, usually displays a more prominent and more uniform

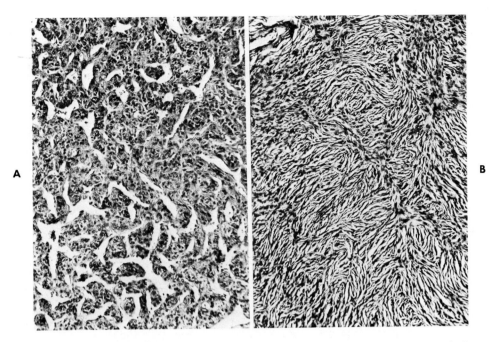

FIG. 27-39. Hemangiopericytoma displaying in different portions of the same tumor a typical vascular pattern (**A**) and a distinct storiform pattern (**B**). (**A** and **B**, ×90.)

spindle cell pattern than hemangiopericytoma, often with a distinct storiform arrangement of the tumor cells. There are, however, occasional examples of this tumor in which distinction may be exceedingly difficult (Fig. 27-39). For unknown reasons most of these hybrid tumors seem to occur in the soft tissues of the orbit. A focal vascular pattern reminiscent of hemangiopericytoma is also seen in occasional examples of malignant fibrous histiocytoma.

Synovial sarcoma exhibits in about 10% to 20% of cases a distinctive but focal hemangiopericytoma pattern. This pattern, however, does not show the broad range in the caliber of the vascular channels and is almost always associated with distinct spindle cell and sometimes myxoid, hyalinized, and calcified areas. Moreover, the presence of a focal biphasic or glandular pattern or positive staining for immunoreactive cytokeratin permits an unequivocal diagnosis of synovial sarcoma. According to Nemes,[157] the absence of factor XIIIa–positive cells is also helpful in differential diagnosis. Clinical findings suggesting synovial sarcoma include a tumor that is painful, multinodular or multilobulated, and located near a large joint (especially the knee) in a patient between 12 and 35 years of age (see Chapter 29).

Mesenchymal chondrosarcoma simulates the features of hemangiopericytoma in the closely packed small cell areas but is readily recognizable by the presence of islets of well-differentiated cartilage or, much less frequently, bone. Ill-

defined foci of immature cartilage may also be present within the small cell component (see Chapter 35).

Juxtaglomerular tumors that occur in young persons, secrete renin, and cause hypertension may also be misinterpreted as hemangiopericytomas,[122,161,172,194] especially those very rare examples that occur in extrarenal locations such as the retroperitoneum. In most of these neoplasms large epithelioid cells and thick-walled vessels are present; moreover, some contain PAS-positive renin crystals.

Other benign and malignant neoplasms that may cause difficulties in diagnosis include juvenile hemangioma, glomus tumor, angiosarcoma, vascular forms of leiomyoma and leiomyosarcoma, stromal sarcoma, malignant peripheral nerve sheath tumor (malignant schwannoma), mesothelioma, and liposarcoma.

Discussion

The difficulties of reaching an accurate diagnosis and predicting the clinical behavior have been repeatedly stressed in the literature, and, not surprisingly, the reported data as to the relative incidence of low- and high-grade hemangiopericytomas vary considerably. In fact, some cases cannot be assigned to either group, making it necessary to establish a borderline or intermediate group of hemangiopericytomas in which a reliable prediction of the biological potential is not possible.

Based on an analysis of our cases,[117] however, a malig-

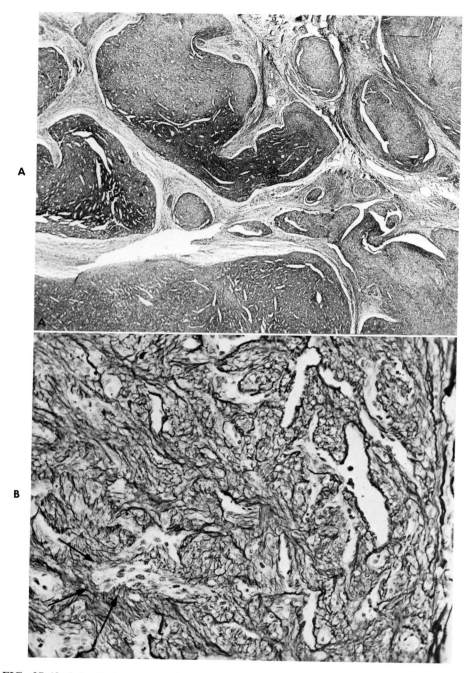

FIG. 27-40. Infantile hemangiopericytoma showing the typical multilobular arrangement of the tumor cells (**A**) and intravascular endothelial proliferation (**B**) suggesting a transition between hemangiopericytoma and hemangioendothelioma *(arrows)*. (**A**, ×22; **B**, reticulin preparation, ×180.) (From Enzinger FM, Smith BH: *Hum Pathol* 7:61, 1976.)

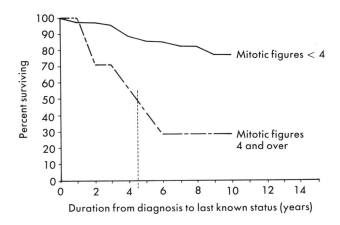

FIG. 27-41. Chart showing actuarial survival rate in hemangiopericytoma and relative survival by degree of mitotic figures. Mitotic figures and necrosis are the two most important criteria in distinguishing benign from malignant hemangiopericytoma. (From Enzinger FM, Smith BH: *Hum Pathol* 7:61, 1976.)

nant clinical course is associated with large size of the tumor (greater than 5 cm), increased mitotic rate (four or more mitotic figures per 10 HPF) (Fig. 27-41), a high degree of cellularity, immature and pleomorphic tumor cells, and foci of hemorrhage and necrosis. McMaster et al.,[151] in a review of 60 cases from the files of the Mayo Clinic, used similar but less stringent criteria for malignant behavior: either a slight degree of anaplasia and one mitotic figure per 10 HPF or a moderate degree of cellular anaplasia and one mitotic figure per 20 HPF. Cellular anaplasia and mitotic activity, however, are not always reliable clues to the malignant potential, and we have seen cases without these features that have metastasized.[158,181] There may also be a relationship between anatomic site and behavior; hemangiopericytomas in the nasal passages, paranasal sinuses, and breast seem to pursue a much more favorable clinical course than those in the meninges and other sites.[88,103,104,123] Assessment of the proliferating cell nuclear antigen (PCNA) may be another predictor of proliferative activity and, hence, clinical behavior[200]; but judging from a single report, DNA flow cytometry seems to be of little value in this regard.[120]

In our series of 93 cases of hemangiopericytoma with follow-up information, 16 (17.2%) tumors metastasized. In the literature, however, the metastatic rate ranges from as little as 11.7%[179] to 56.5%,[160] probably reflecting variations in histological diagnosis and therapy. Usually metastasis becomes apparent within a period of 5 years after the initial diagnosis, but late metastases occurring 10 or more years after the initial diagnosis are not uncommon. The lung and the skeleton are the most frequent metastatic sites. Lymph node metastasis is rare. Recurrence is an ominous sign, and most recurrent tumors develop metastases at a later date. For example, in the Tsuneyoshi et al.[192] series of 19 malignant hemangiopericytomas, 11 recurred and nine of the 11 died of metastasis. Examples of tumors that recurred 15 or more years after the initial excision are on record.[168,190]

Therapy

Complete local excision seems to be the primary treatment for tumors having a uniform histological picture with no or minimal mitotic activity and without cellular pleomorphism or areas of necrosis or hemorrhage. Radical surgery, with or without adjunctive radiotherapy, is required in less well-differentiated hemangiopericytomas. In fact, in these cases postoperative radiation therapy[113,135,139,153,181] seems to have some advantage over chemotherapy.[95,100,197] For example, Mira et al.[153] reported a satisfactory response to preoperative embolization, surgical removal, and radiation with complete regression in 47% of 29 patients. Response was best with dosages of more than 35 Gy and tumors measuring less than 5 cm. In all cases of hemangiopericytoma surgical removal is facilitated if the afferent vessels are ligated during the initial stage of the operation or by preoperative embolization.[179] This not only reduces the size of the tumor but also minimizes the danger of operative hemorrhage. Reduction in size of the tumor may also be accomplished by preoperative radiotherapy. There is also some information that chemotherapy may effect partial or complete remisson in metastatic hemangiopericytomas.[95,100,197]

REFERENCES
Glomus tumor

1. Adair FE: Glomus tumor: a clinical study with a report of ten cases. *Am J Surg* 25:1, 1954.
2. Aiba M, Hirayama A, Kuramochi S: Glomangiosarcoma in a glomus tumor: an immunohistochemical and ultrastructural study. *Cancer* 61:1467, 1988.
3. Albrecht S, Zbieranowski I: Incidental glomus coccygeum: when a normal structure looks like a tumor. *Am J Surg Pathol* 14:922, 1990.
4. Anagostou CD, Papademetriou DG, Toumazani MN: Subcutaneous glomus tumors. *Surg Gynecol Obstet* 136:945, 1973.
5. Apfelberg DB, Teasler JL: Unusual locations and manifestations of glomus tumors (glomangiomas). *Am J Surg* 116:62, 1968.
6. Appleman HD, Helwig EB: Glomus tumors of the stomach. *Cancer* 23:203, 1969.
7. Bailey OT: The cutaneous glomus and its tumors—glomangiomas. *Am J Pathol* 11:915, 1935.
8. Barua R: Glomus tumor of the colon: first reported case. *Dis Colon Rectum* 31:138, 1988.
9. Beaton LI, Davis L: Glomus tumor: report of three cases: analysis of 271 recorded cases. *Q Bull Northwest U Med Sch* 15:245, 1941.
10. Bergstrand H: Multiple glomic tumors. *Am J Cancer* 29:470, 1937.

11. Brindley GV: Glomus tumor of the mediastinum. *J Thorac Surg* 18:417, 1949.

12. Brooks JJ, Miettinen M, Virtanen I: Desmin immunoreactivity in glomus tumors. *Am J Clin Pathol* 87:292, 1987.

13. Brown H: Glomus tumors. *Br Med J* 1:799, 1973.

14. Camirand P, Giroux JM: Subungual glomus tumor: radiological manifestations. *Arch Dermatol* 102:677, 1970.

15. Carroll RE, Berman AT: Glomus tumors of the hand: review of the literature and report of 28 cases. *J Bone Joint Surg* 54A:691, 1972.

16. Conant MA, Wiesenfeld SL: Multiple glomus tumors of the skin. *Arch Dermatol* 103:481, 1971.

17. Curr JF: Arteriovenous aneurysm due to glomangioma. *J R Coll Surg Edinb* 19:374, 1974.

18. Dervan PA, Tobbia IN, Casey M, et al: Glomus tumours: an immunohistochemical profile of 11 cases. *Histopathology* 14:483, 1989.

19. Duncan L, Halverson J, DeSchryver-Kecskemeti K: Glomus tumor of the coccyx: a curable cause of coccygodynia. *Arch Pathol Lab Med* 115:78, 1991.

20. Ekestrom S: A comparison between glomus tumor and angioleiomyoma. *Acta Pathol Microbiol Scand* 27:86, 1950.

21. Eyster WH, Montgomery H: Multiple glomic tumors. *Arch Dermatol Syph* 62:893, 1950.

22. Faggioli GL, Bertoni F, Stella A, et al: Multifocal diffuse glomus tumor: a case report of glomangiomyoma and review of the literature. *Int Angiol* 7:281, 1988.

23. Freier DT, Lindenauer SM: Subcutaneous glomus tumor. *Am J Surg* 120:359, 1970.

24. German WM: Glomus tumor of triceps muscle. *Am J Clin Pathol* 15:199, 1945.

25. Goodman TF, Abele DC: Multiple glomus tumors: a clinical and electron microscopic study. *Arch Dermatol* 103:11, 1971.

26. Gould EW, Manivel JC, Albores-Saavedra J, et al: Locally infiltrative glomus tumors and glomangiosarcomas: a clinical, ultrastructural, and immunohistochemical study. *Cancer* 65:310, 1990.

27. Haque S, Modlin IM, West AB: Multiple glomus tumors of the stomach with intravascular spread. *Am J Surg Pathol* 16:291, 1992.

28. Harris M: Ultrastructure of a glomus tumor. *J Clin Pathol* 24:520, 1971.

29. Harris WR: Erosion of bone produced by glomus tumor. *Can Med Assoc J* 70:684, 1954.

30. Haupt HM, Stern JB, Berlin SJ: Immunohistochemistry in the differential diagnosis of nodular hidradenoma and glomus tumor. *Am J Dermatopathol* 14:310, 1992.

31. Hayes MM, Van der Westhuizen N, Holden GP: Aggressive glomus tumor of the nasal region: report of a case with multiple local recurrences. *Arch Pathol Lab Med* 117:649, 1993.

32. Ho KL, Pak MSY: Glomus tumor of the coccygeal region: case report. *J Bone Joint Surg* 62A:141, 1980.

33. Hollingsworth JR, Ochsner JL: A multifocal diffuse glomus tumor. *Am Surg* 38:161, 1972.

34. Horton C, Maquire C, Nicholas G, et al: Glomus tumors: an analysis of 25 cases. *Arch Surg* 71:712, 1955.

35. Idy-Peretti I, Cermakova E, Dion E, et al: Subungual glomus tumor: diagnosis based on high-resolution MR images. *Am J Roentgenol* 159:1351, 1992.

36. Jackson H, Balkin R: Glomus tumors (angiomyoneuromas): a clinical and pathologic report of an unusual case. *Arch Surg* 53:100, 1946.

37. Jepson RP, Harris JD: Glomus tumors. *Med J Aust* 2:252, 1970.

38. Kanwar YS, Manaligod JR: Glomus tumor of the stomach: an ultrastructural study. *Arch Pathol* 99:392, 1975.

39. Kay S, Callahan WP, Murray MR, et al: Glomus tumors of the stomach. *Cancer* 4:726, 1951.

40. Kaye VM, Dehner LP: Cutaneous glomus tumor: a comparative immunohistochemical study with pseudoangiomatous intradermal melanocytic nevi. *Am J Dermatopathol* 13:2, 1991.

41. Kim YI, Kim JH, Sub JS, et al: Glomus tumor of the trachea: report of a case with ultrastructural observation. *Cancer* 15:881, 1989.

42. King ES: Glomus tumor. *Aust N Z J Surg* 23:280, 1954.

43. Kishimoto S, Nagatani H, Miyashita A, et al: Immunohistochemical demonstration of substance P–containing nerve fibres in glomus tumours. *Br J Dermatol* 113:213, 1985.

44. Kline SC, Moore JR, deMente SH: Glomus tumor originating within a digital nerve. *J Hand Surg* 15:98, 1990.

45. Kobayashi Y, Kawaguchi T, Imoto K, et al: Intraosseous glomus tumor in the sacrum: a case report. *Acta Pathol Jpn* 40:858, 1990.

46. Kohout E, Stout AP: The glomus tumor in children. *Cancer* 14:555, 1961.

47. Krishna B, Kacker SK: Glomangioma of external ear. *J Laryngol* 83:83, 1969.

48. Lattes R, Bull DC: A case of glomus tumor with primary involvement of bone. *Ann Surg* 127:187, 1948.

49. Lehman W, Kraisal C: Glomus tumor within bone. *Surgery* 25:1181, 1949.

50. Lumley JSP, Stansfeld AG: Infiltrating glomus tumor of lower limb. *Br Med J* 1:484, 1972.

51. MacKenzie DH: Intraosseous glomus tumors. *J Bone Joint Surg* 44B:648, 1962.

52. Maley ED, MacDonald CJ: Bilateral subungual glomus tumors. *Plast Reconstr Surg* 55:488, 1975.

53. Mason ML, Weil A: Tumor of a subcutaneous glomus. *Surg Gynecol Obstet* 58:807, 1934.

54. Masson P: Le glomus neuromyarterieal des regions tactiles et ses tumeurs. *Lyon Chir* 21:257, 1924.

55. McEvoy BF: Multiple hamartomatous glomus tumors of the skin. *Arch Dermatol* 104:188, 1971.

56. Miettinin M, Lehto V-P, Virtanen I: Glomus tumor cells: Evaluation of smooth muscle and endothelial cell properties. *Virchows Arch (Cell Pathol)* 43:139, 1983.

57. Mullis WF, Rosato FE, Rosato EF, et al: The glomus tumor. *Surg Gynecol Obstet* 135:705, 1972.

58. Murad J, Von Haam Z, Murthy MSN: The ultrastructure of hemangiopericytoma and a glomus tumor. *Cancer* 22:1239, 1968.

59. Murray MR, Stout AP: The glomus tumor: investigation of its distribution and behavior and the identity of its "epithelioid" cell. *Am J Pathol* 18:183, 1942.

60. Nuovo MA, Grimes MM, Knowles DM: Glomus tumors: clinicopathologic and immunohistochemical analysis of forty cases. *Surg Pathol* 3:31, 1990.

61. Oberdalhoff H, Schutz W: Pathogenesis of multiple glomus tumors. *Chirurg* 22:145, 1951.

62. Popoff NW: The digital vascular system with reference to the state of the glomus in inflammation, arteriosclerotic gangrene, thromboangiitis obliterans, and supernumerary digits in man. *Arch Pathol* 18:295, 1934.

63. Porter PG, Bigler SA, McNutt M, et al: The immunophenotype of hemangiopericytoma and glomus tumors with special reference to muscle protein expression: an immunohistochemical study and review of the literature. *Mod Pathol* 4:46, 1991.

64. Raisman V, Mayer L: Tumors of the neuromyarterial glomus: report of cases. *Arch Surg* 30:929, 1935.

65. Rao VK, Weiss SW: Angiomatosis of soft tissue: an anlaysis of the histologic features and clinical outcome in 51 cases. *Am J Surg Pathol* 16:764, 1992.

66. Riveros M, Pack GT: The glomus tumors: report of 20 cases. *Ann Surg* 133:394, 1951.

67. Schurch W, Skalli O, Lagace R, et al: Intermediate filament proteins and actin isoforms as markers for soft tissue tumor differenti-

ation and origin. III. Hemangiopericytomas and glomus tumors. *Am J Pathol* 136:771, 1990.

68. Shin DLH, Park SS, Lee JH, et al: Oncocytic glomus tumor of the trache. *Chest* 98:1021, 1990.

69. Shugart RR, Soule EH, Johnson EW: Glomus tumor. *Surg Gynecol Obstet* 117:334, 1963.

70. Siegel MW: Intraosseous glomus tumor: a case report. *Am J Orthop* 9:68, 1967.

71. Slater DN, Cotton DWK, Azzopardi JG: Oncocytic glomus tumour: a new variant. *Histopathology* 11:523, 1987.

72. Sluiter JT, Postma C: Multiple glomus tumors of the skin. *Acta Derm-Venerol* 39:98, 1959.

73. Smyth M: Glomus cell tumors in the lower extremity: report of two cases. *J Bone Joint Surg* 53A:157, 1971.

74. Stout AP: Tumors of the neuromyoarterial glomus. *Am J Cancer* 24:255, 1935.

75. Tanaka S, Takeuchi S: Glomus tumor of the stomach. *Jpn J Cancer Clin* 20:708, 1974.

76. Tarnowski WM, Hashimoto K: Multiple glomus tumors: an ultrastructural study. *J Invest Dermatol* 52:474, 1969.

77. Toker C: Glomangioma: An ultrastructural study. *Cancer* 23:487, 1969.

78. Tsuneyoshi M, Enjoji M: Glomus tumor: a clinicopathologic and electron microscopic study. *Cancer* 50:1601, 1982.

79. Venkatachalam MA, Greally JG: Fine structure of glomus tumor: similarity of glomus cells to smooth muscle. *Cancer* 23:1176, 1969.

80. Weiss SW, Sobin LH: *WHO classification of soft tissue tumours.* Berlin, 1994, Springer Verlag.

81. West AB, Buckley PJ: Mantle zone lymphoma in a gastric glomus tumor. *Cancer* 70:2246, 1992.

Hemangiopericytoma

82. Abdel-Fattah HM, Adams GL, Wick MR: Hemangiopericytoma of the maxillary sinus and skull base. *Head Neck* 12:77, 1990.

83. Ackerman LV, Warren S: Hemangiopericytoma of retroperitoneal space. *J Mo Med Assoc* 45:380, 1948.

84. Adler CP, Trager D: Malignant hemangiopericytoma: a soft tissue and bone tumor. *Z Orthop* 127:611, 1989.

85. Alpern MB, Thorsen MK, Kellman GM, et al: CT appearance of hemangiopericytoma. *J Comput Assist Tomogr* 10:264, 1986.

86. Alpers CE, Rosenau W, Finkbeiner WE, et al: Congenital (infantile) hemangiopericytoma of the tongue and the sublingual region. *Am J Clin Pathol* 81:377, 1984.

87. Angervall L, Kindblom LG, Nielsen JM, et al: Hemangiopericytoma: a clinicopathologic, angiographic and microangiographic study. *Cancer* 42:2412, 1978.

88. Arias-Stella J Jr, Rosen PP: Hemangiopericytoma of the breast. *Mod Pathol* 1:98, 1988.

89. Atkinson JB, Mahour GH, Isaacs H Jr, et al: Hemangiopericytoma in infants and children: a report of six patients. *Am J Surg* 148:372, 1984.

90. Ayella RJ: Hemangiopericytoma: a case report with arteriographic findings. *Radiology* 97:611, 1970.

91. Aziza J, Mazerolles C, Selves J, et al: Comparison of the reactivities of monoclonal antibodies QBEND10 (CD34) and BNH9 in vascular tumors. *Appl Immunohistochem* 1:51, 1993.

92. Baker DL, Oda D, Myall RW: Intraoral infantile hemangiopericytoma: literature review and addition of a case. *Oral Surg Oral Med Oral Pathol* 73:596, 1992.

93. Batsakis JG, Jacobs JB, Templeton AC: Hemangiopericytoma of the nasal cavity: electron optic study and clinical correlations. *J Laryngol Otol* 97:361, 1983.

94. Battifora H: Hemangiopericytoma: ultrastructural study of five cases. *Cancer* 31:1418, 1973.

95. Beadle GF, Hillcoat BL: Treatment of advanced malignant heman-

giopericytoma with combination adriamycin and DTIC: a report of four cases. *J Surg Oncol* 22:167, 1983.

96. Benn JJ, Firth RG, Sonksen PH: Metabolic effect of an insulin-like factor causing hypoglycemia in a patient with haemangiopericytoma. *Clin Endocrinol* 32:769, 1990.

97. Binder SC, Wolfe HJ, Deterling RA: Intra-abdominal hemangiopericytoma: report of four cases and review of the literature. *Arch Surg* 107:536, 1973.

98. Bommer G, Altenähr F, Kühnau J Jr, et al: Ultrastructure of hemangiopericytoma associated with paraneoplastic hypoglycemia. *Z Krebsforsch* 85:231, 1976.

99. Brandeis WE, Bolkenius M, Daum R, et al: Das Hemangiopericytom im Kindesalter. *Z Kinderchirurg* 39:51, 1984.

100. Bredt AB, Serpick AA: Metastatic hemangiopericytoma treated with vincristine and actinomycin D. *Cancer* 24:266, 1969.

101. Chen KT, Kassel SH, Medrano VA: Congenital hemangiopericytoma. *J Surg Oncol* 31:127, 1986.

102. Chomette G, Auriol M, Tereau Y: Hémangiopéricytome malin: A propos de l'analyse ultrastructurale et histoenzymologique d'une observation. *Ann Anat Pathol (Paris)* 23:41, 1978.

103. Compagno J: Hemangiopericytoma-like tumors of the nasal cavity: a comparison with hemangiopericytoma of soft tissues. *Laryngoscope* 88:460, 1978.

104. Compagno J, Hyams J: Hemangiopericytoma-like intranasal tumors: a clinicopathologic study of 23 cases. *Am J Clin Pathol* 66:672, 1976.

105. Conley JJ, Clairmont AA, Eberle RC: Hemangiopericytoma. *Arch Otolaryngol* 103:374, 1977.

106. Croxatto JO, Font RL: Hemangiopericytoma of the orbit: a clinicopathologic study of 30 cases. *Hum Pathol* 13:199, 1982.

107. d'Amore ESG, Manivel JG, Sung JH: Soft tissue and meningeal hemangiopericytomas: an immunohistochemical and ultrastructural study. *Hum Pathol* 21:414, 1990.

108. Dardick I, Hammar SP, Scheithauer BW: Ultrastructural spectrum of hemangiopericytoma: a comparative study of fetal, adult and neoplastic pericytes. *Ultrastruct Pathol* 13:111, 1989.

109. DeVilliers DR, Farman J, Campbell JAH: Pelvic haemangiopericytoma: preoperative arteriographic demonstration. *Clin Radiol* 18:318, 1967.

110. Dictor M, Elner A, Andersson T, et al: Myofibromatosis-like hemangiopericytoma metastasizing as differentiated vascular smooth muscle and myosarcoma: myopericytes as a subset of "myofibroblasts." *Am J Surg Pathol* 16:1239, 1992.

111. Dingham RO: Hemangiopericytoma: report of two cases, one of congenital origin. *Plast Reconstr Surg* 21:399, 1958.

112. Douglas JL, Mitchell R, Short DW: Retroperitoneal haemangiopericytoma. *Br J Surg* 53:31, 1966.

113. Dube VE, Paulson JF: Metastatic hemangiopericytoma cured by radiotherapy. *J Bone Joint Surg* 56A:833, 1974.

114. Eichhorn JH, Dickersin GR, Bhan AK, et al: Sinonasal hemangiopericytoma: a reassessment with electron microscopy, immunohistochemistry, and long-term follow-up. *Am J Surg Pathol* 14:856, 1990.

115. Eimoto T: Ultrastructure of an infantile hemangiopericytoma. *Cancer* 40:2161, 1977.

116. Eneroth CM, Fluur E, Soderberg G, et al: Nasal hemangiopericytoma. *Laryngoscope* 80:17, 1970.

117. Enzinger FM, Smith BH: Hemangiopericytoma: an analysis of 106 cases. *Hum Pathol* 7:61, 1976.

118. Fink HE, Oberman H: Hemangioendothelial cell sarcoma and hemangiopericytoma. *Am J Roentgenol* 89:155, 1963.

119. Fisher ER, Kaufman N, Mason EJ: Hemangiopericytoma: histologic and tissue culture studies. *Am J Pathol* 28:653, 1952.

120. Fletcher CDM, Camplejohn RS: DNA flow cytometry in haemangiopericytomas is of no prognostic value (abstract). *J Pathol* 151:31A, 1987.

121. Gensler S, Caplan LH, Laufman H: Giant benign hemangiopericytoma functioning as an arteriovenous shunt. *JAMA* 198:203, 1966.

122. Gherardi G, Arya S, Hickler RB: Juxtaglomerular body tumor: a rare occult, but curable cause of lethal hypertension. *Hum Pathol* 5:236, 1974.

123. Gill BS, Mehra YN: Haemangiopericytoma in nasal cavity. *J Laryngol Otol* 82:839, 1968.

124. Goellner JR, Laws ER Jr, Soule EH, et al: Hemangiopericytoma of the meninges: Mayo Clinic experience. *Am J Clin Pathol* 70:375, 1978.

125. Greene RR, Gerbie AB, Gerbie MV, et al: Hemangiopericytomas of the uterus. *Am J Obstet Gynecol* 106:1020, 1970.

126. Guthrie BL, Ebersold MJ, Scheithauer BW, et al: Meningeal hemangiopericytoma: histopathologic features, treatment, and long-term follow-up of 44 cases. *Neurosurgery* 25:514, 1989.

127. Hahn MJ, Dawson R, Esterly JA, et al: Hemangiopericytoma: an ultrastructural study. *Cancer* 31:255, 1973.

128. Hakala RT, Page D, Fleischli DJ: Paravesical hemangiopericytoma. *J Urol* 103:436, 1970.

129. Haney RF: Hemangiopericytoma of the orbit. *Arch Ophthalmol (Chicago)* 71:206, 1964.

130. Hayes MM, Dietrich BE, Uys CJ: Congenital hemangiopericytomas of skin. *Pediatr Dermatopathol* 8:148, 1986.

131. Hiura M, Nogawa T, Nagai N, et al: Vaginal hemangiopericytoma: a light microscopic and ultrastructural study. *Gynecol Oncol* 21:376, 1985.

132. Hoeffel JC, Chardot C: Radiologic patterns of hemangiopericytoma of the leg. *Am J Surg* 123:591, 1972.

133. Howard JW, Davis PL: Retroperitoneal hemangiopericytoma associated with hypoglycemia and masculinization. *Del Med J* 31:29, 1959.

134. Iwaki T, Fukui M, Takeshita I, et al: Hemangiopericytoma of the meninges: a clinicopathologic and immunohistochemical study. *Clin Neuropathol* 7:93, 1988.

135. Jääskeläinen J, Servo A, Maltia M, et al: Intracranial hemangiopericytoma: radiology, surgery, radiotherapy and outcome. *Surg Neurol* 23:227, 1985.

136. Jaffe J: Hemangiopericytoma: angiographic findings. *Br J Radiol* 33:614, 1960.

137. Jakobiec FA, Howard GM, Jones IS, et al: Hemangiopericytoma of the orbit. *Am J Ophthalmol* 78:816, 1974.

138. Jenkins JJ III: Case 7, congenital malignant hemangiopericytoma. *Pediatr Pathol* 7:119, 1987.

139. Jha N, McNeese M, Barkley HT Jr, et al: Does radiotherapy have a role in hemangiopericytoma management? Report of 14 new cases and review of the literature. *Int J Radiol Oncol Biol Phys* 13:1399, 1987.

140. Kastendieck H, Kloppel G, Altenähr E: Morphologie und klinische Bedeutung des meningealen Hämangioperizytoms. *Z Krebsforsch* 85:287, 1976.

141. Kato N, Kato S, Ueno H: Hemangiopericytoma: characteristic features observed by magnetic resonance imaging angiography. *J Dermatol* 17:701, 1990.

142. Kaude JV, Moccia WA, Wertman DE, et al: Pelvic hemangiopericytoma: ultrasonic findings and comparison with angiography. *Fortschr Geb Roentgenstr Nuklearmed* 132:347, 1980.

143. Kaude JV, Tylen U: Angiographische Symptomatic des Hämangiopericytoms. *Radiologie* 11:345, 1971.

144. Kauffman SL, Stout AP: Hemangiopericytoma in children. *Cancer* 13:695, 1960.

145. Kishikawa M, Tsuda N, Fujii H: Ultrastructural study of hemangiopericytoma and hemangioendothelioma. *J Electron Micr* 24:134, 1975.

146. Koo BC, Smith RR, Morgan RJ, et al: Computed mediastinal hemangiopericytoma: computed tomography correlation. *J Comput Tomogr* 9:253, 1985.

147. Kuhn C III, Rosai J: Tumors arising from pericytes: ultrastructure and organ culture of a case. *Arch Pathol* 88:653, 1969.

148. Leu HJ: Hämangioperizytom. *Zentralbl Allg Pathol* 125:139, 1981.

149. Limon J, Rao U, Dal Cin P, et al: Translocation t(13;22) in hemangiopericytoma. *Cancer Genet Cytogenet* 21:309, 1986.

150. Lorigan JG, David CL, Evans HL, et al: The clinical and radiologic manifestations of hemangiopericytoma. *AJR Am J Roentgenol* 153:345, 1989.

151. McMaster MJ, Soule EH, Ivins JC: Hemangiopericytoma: a clinicopathologic study and long-term follow-up of 60 patients. *Cancer* 36:2232, 1975.

152. Mena H, Ribas JL, Pezeshkpour GH, et al: Hemangiopericytoma of the central nervous system: a review of 94 cases. *Hum Pathol* 22:84, 1991.

153. Mira JG, Chu FC, Fortner JG: The role of radiotherapy in the management of malignant hemangiopericytoma: report of eleven new cases and review of the literature. *Cancer* 39:1254, 1977.

154. Mittal KR, Gerald W, True LD: Hemangiopericytoma of the breast: report of a case with ultrastructural and immunohistochemical staining. *Hum Pathol* 17:1181, 1986.

155. Morris P, Stahl R, Liriano E, et al: Giant retroperitoneal pelvic hemangiopericytoma. *J Cardiovasc Surg* 32:778, 1991.

156. Murad TM, Von Haam E, Murthy MSN: Ultrastructure of a hemangiopericytoma and a glomus tumor. *Cancer* 22:1239, 1968.

157. Nemes Z: Differentiation markers in hemangiopericytoma. *Cancer* 69:133, 1992.

158. Neumann H: Morphologie und Klinik des Hämangioperizytoms: Eine Analyse von 84 Fällen mit einem eigenen Beitrag. *Pathologe* 4:64, 1983.

159. Nunnery EW, Kahn LB, Reddick RL, et al: Hemangiopericytoma: a light microscopic and ultrastructural study. *Cancer* 47:906, 1981.

160. O'Brien P, Brasfield RD: Hemangiopericytoma. *Cancer* 18:249, 1965.

161. Ohmori H, Motoi M, Sato H, et al: Extrarenal renin-secreting tumor associated with hypertension. *Acta Pathol Jpn* 27:567, 1977.

162. Paullada JJ, Lisci-Gramilla A, Gonzales-Angulo A, et al: Hemangiopericytoma associated with hypoglycemia. *Am J Med* 44:990, 1968.

163. Plukker JT, Koops HS, Molenaar I, et al: Malignant hemangiopericytoma in three kindred members of one family. *Cancer* 61:841, 1988.

164. Poole RR, Barry JM, Carey TC: Hemangiopericytomas in male pelvis. *Urology* 14:167, 1979.

165. Popoff NA, Malinin TI, Rosomoff HL: Fine structure of intracranial hemangiopericytoma and angiomatous meningioma. *Cancer* 34:1187, 1974.

166. Porter PL, Bigler SA, McNutt M, et al: The immunophenotype of hemangiopericytomas and glomus tumors with special reference to muscle protein expression: an immunohistochemical study and review of the literature. *Mod Pathol* 4:46, 1991.

167. Ramsey HJ: Fine structure of hemangiopericytoma and hemangioendothelioma. *Cancer* 19:2005, 1966.

168. Rew DA, Allen JP: Late recurrence of an abdominal hemangiopericytoma. *J R Soc Med* 80:552,1989.

169. Reynolds FC, Lansche WE: Hemangiopericytoma of the lower extremity. *J Bone Joint Surg* 40A:921, 1958.

170. Rhodes RE Jr, Brown HA, Harrison EG Jr: Hemangiopericytoma of the nasal cavity: review of the literature and report of three cases. *Arch Otolaryngol* 79:505, 1964.

171. Roberts DI: Pelvic hemangiopericytoma. *Urology* 9:684, 1977.

172. Robertson PW, Klidjian A, Harding LK, et al: Hypertension due to renin-secreting renal tumor. *Am J Med* 43:963, 1967.

173. Rosai J: Vascular neoplasms. *Am J Surg Pathol* 10:26, 1986.

174. Rouget C: Mémoire sur le développement, la structure, et propriétés physiologiques des capillaires sanguins et lymphatiques. *Arch Physiol Norm Pathol* 5:603, 1873.

175. Schürch W, Skalli O, Lagacér, et al: Intermediate filament proteins

and actin isoforms as markers for soft tissue tumor differentiations and origin. III. Hemangiopericytomas and glomus tumors. *Am J Pathol* 136:771, 1990.

176. Seibert JJ: Multiple congenital hemangiopericytomas of the head and neck. *Laryngoscope* 88:1006, 1978.

177. Silverberg SG, Willson MA, Board JA: Hemangiopericytoma of the uterus: an ultrastructural study. *Am J Obstet Gynecol* 110:397, 1971.

178. Simon R, Greene RC: Perirenal hemangiopericytoma: a case associated with hypoglycemia. *JAMA* 189:155, 1964.

179. Smullens SN, Scotti D, Osterholm JL, et al: Preoperative embolization of retroperitoneal hemangiopericytomas as an aid in their removal. *Cancer* 50:1870, 1982.

180. Sreekantaiah C, Bridge JA, Rao UN, et al: Clonal chromosomal abnormalities in hemangiopericytoma. *Cancer Genet Cytogenet* 54:173, 1991.

181. Staples JJ, Robinson RA, Wen BC, et al: Hemangiopericytoma: the role of radiotherapy. *Int J Radiat Oncol Biol Phys* 19:445, 1990.

182. Stout AP: Hemangiopericytoma: a study of 25 new cases. *Cancer* 2:1027, 1949.

183. Stout AP: Tumors featuring pericytes: glomus tumor and hemangiopericytoma. *Lab Invest* 5:217, 1956.

184. Stout AP, Cassel C: Hemangiopericytoma of omentum. *Surgery* 13:578, 1943.

185. Stout AP, Murray MR: Hemangiopericytoma: a vascular tumor featuring Zimmermann's pericytes. *Ann Surg* 116:26, 1942.

186. Sullivan TJ, Wright JE, Wulc AE, et al: Haemangiopericytoma of the orbit. *Aust N Z J Ophthalmol* 20:325, 1992.

187. Sutton D, Pratt AE: Angiography of hemangiopericytoma. *Clin Radiol* 18:324, 1967.

188. Tang JS, Gold RH, Mirra JM, et al: Hemangiopericytoma of bone. *Cancer* 62:848, 1988.

189. Tavassoli FA, Weiss S: Hemangiopericytoma of the breast. *Am J Surg Pathol* 5:745, 1981.

190. Theunissen PH, Ariëns AT, Pannebakker MA, et al: Spätrezidiv eines Hämangioperizytoms mit lipomatöser Komponente. *Pathologe* 11:346, 1990.

191. Trulock TS, Gould RA, Glenn JF: Massive pelvic hemangiopericytoma. *J Urol* 127:1197, 1982.

192. Tsuneyoshi M, Daimaru Y, Enjoji M: Malignant hemangiopericytoma and other sarcomas with hemangiopericytoma-like pattern. *Pathol Res Pract* 178:446, 1984.

193. Tulenko JF: Congenital hemangiopericytoma: case report. *Plast Reconstr Surg* 41:276, 1968.

194. Warshaw BL, Anand SK, Olsen DL, et al: Hypertension secondary to a renin-producing juxtaglomerular tumor. *J Pediatr* 94:247, 1979.

195. Wilbanks GD, Szymanska Z, Miller AW: Pelvic hemangiopericytoma: report of four patients and review of the literature. *Am J Obstet Gynecol* 123:555, 1975.

196. Winek RR, Scheithauer BW, Wick MR: Meningioma, meningeal hemangiopericytoma (angioblastic meningioma), peripheral hemangiopericytoma and acoustic schwannoma: a comparative immunohistochemical study. *Am J Surg Pathol* 13:251, 1989.

197. Wong PP, Yagoda A: Chemotherapy of malignant hemangiopericytoma. *Cancer* 41:1256, 1978.

198. Yaghmai I: Angiographic manifestations of soft-tissue and osseous hemangiopericytomas. *Radiology* 126:653, 1978.

199. Yousem SA, Hochholzer L: Primary pulmonary hemangiopericytoma. *Cancer* 59:549, 1987.

200. Yu CCW, Hall PA, Fletcher CDM, et al: Haemangiopericytoma: the prognostic value of immunohistochemical staining with a monoclonal antibody to proliferating cell nuclear antigen (PCNA). *Histopathology* 19:29, 1991.

201. Zimmermann KW: Der feinere Bau der Blutkapillaren. *Zeitschr Anat Entwicklungsg* 68:29, 1923.

202. Zirkin RM: Retroperitoneal hemangiopericytoma. *Int Surg* 62:395, 1977.

CHAPTER 28

BENIGN TUMORS AND TUMORLIKE LESIONS OF SYNOVIAL TISSUE

The synovial membrane forms the lining of the joints, tendons, and bursae. In addition, its cells synthesize hyaluronate, a major component of synovial fluid, and facilitate the exchange of substances between blood and synovial fluid.[2] The synovial membrane varies considerably in appearance, depending on local mechanical factors and the nature of the underlying tissue. For instance, the synovial surface of joints subjected to high pressure is flat and acellular, whereas joints under less stress have a redundant surface lined by cells that resemble cuboidal or columnar epithelium.[5] Unlike epithelial lining cells, the synovial cells do not rest on a basal lamina but blend with the underlying stromal elements,[2] occasionally forming only an incomplete layer at the surface. Thus joint fluid and blood vessels may come in close contact with each other, a relationship that probably enhances solute exchange between the two compartments. On electron microscopic studies the synovial membrane is composed of two cell types.[2,7] Type A cells are characterized by long filopodia, which extend upward and form a ramifying feltwork of overlapping processes devoid of junctional attachment.[2] In addition, they have a prominent Golgi apparatus, numerous vacuoles containing granular material, mitochondria, and pinocytotic vesicles. Under appropriate conditions these cells may engage in phagocytosis. Type B cells are reminiscent of fibroblasts in their ultrastructural profile. They lack elaborate cytoplasmic processes and instead have a well-developed rough endoplasmic reticulum. Although seemingly different, these cells probably represent functional modulations of the same cell because transitional forms are often seen.[7] Synovial cells can also be characterized by means of monoclonal antibodies, although it is not yet possible to clearly relate a given antigenic phenotype with a given ultrastructural appearance. This is partly explained by the fact that when analyzed outside their normal milieu, the cells may assume an altered appearance. It is also possible that a given antigenic phenotype may be associated with a range of morphological appearances. In any event, it appears that a significant proportion of cells lining the intimal surface of joints express antigens commonly associated with cells of the monocyte-macrophage series.[3,6] Synovial cells have provisionally been classified into three types by Burmester et al.[3] Type I cells are characterized by Ia antigens, Fc receptors, and five different monocyte differentiation antigens, and by the property of phagocytosis. Type II cells have Ia antigens but no Fc receptors or monocyte differentiation antigens, and they are also not phagocytic. Type III cells express fibroblastic but few monocytic antigens and unlike the first two cell types possess a proliferative capacity.

A number of benign tumors and tumorlike lesions arise from the synovium such as chondroma of tendon sheath, fibroma of tendon sheath, synovial chondromatosis, and synovial hemangioma, yet only the giant cell tumor is considered prototypical. This tumor is the most common benign tumor of tendon sheath and synovium and, moreover, is the only one that generally recapitulates the appearance of the normal synovial cell. It is occasionally referred to as "benign synovioma,"[51] an unfortunate term that connotes to many a benign form of synovial sarcoma. In actuality, giant cell tumors share few similarities with synovial sarcomas. In the localized form they occur principally on the digits and sometimes in an intraarticular location, locations where synovial sarcomas are rarely found. Histologically, the cellular polymorphism of the giant cell tumor is greater than that of the synovial sarcoma, and the rare giant cell form of malignant fibrous histiocytoma (malignant giant cell tumor of soft parts) more closely resembles malignant giant cell tumors of soft parts than synovial sarcomas. It is therefore preferable to consider giant cell tumors as a distinct subset of synovial-based lesions and not as benign analogues of synovial sarcoma.

In the past century concepts concerning the pathogenesis of these lesions have undergone constant revision. The earliest descriptions of the giant cell tumor of tendon sheath indicate that it was considered a sarcoma until the classic description by Heurteux,[30] in which he suggested it was benign and proposed the term *myeloma of tendon sheath*. Subsequent writers have emphasized the presence of foam cells within these lesions and have consequently grouped these tumors with true xanthomas occurring in the setting of hyperlipidemia (Chapter 13). Giant cell tumors, however, almost always arise in normolipemic persons and bear only a superficial similarity to tendinous xanthomas.

The most significant contribution to the understanding of giant cell tumors was made by Jaffe et al.,[32] who regarded the synovium of tendon sheath, bursa, and joint as an anatomical unit that could give rise to a common family of lesions including the giant cell tumor of tendon sheath (nodular tenosynovitis), localized and diffuse forms of pigmented villonodular synovitis, and rare examples of extraarticular pigmented villonodular synovitis arising from bursae pigmented villonodular bursitis. The differences in clinical extent and growth, they maintained, were influenced by anatomical location. Lesions of the joints tended to expand inward and grow along the joint surface as the path of least resistance. Tumors of tendon sheath of necessity grew outward, molded and confined by the shearing forces of the tendon. At present there has been no improvement of their elegant unifying concept. On the other hand, their hypothesis that such lesions are reactive processes arising as a result of chronic inflammation is probably incorrect. The preponderance of evidence indicates these are neoplastic. Observations that trauma precedes about half of cases, that some cases are multifocal,[20,26] and that similar lesions have been induced following intraarticular injections of blood in experimental animals,[31,52] seem offset by recent cytogenetic studies indicating a clonal abnormality (trisomy 7) in these lesions, a finding which speaks strongly to a neoplastic process.[25,44] However, these cytogenetic data must be reconciled with molecular diagnostic studies which indicate that by X chromosome inactivation analysis the lesions are polyclonal[45]; this might be explained by contamination of cellular isolates by normal cells and by the fact that random reactivation of the X chromsome may occur in neoplasms. A neoplastic origin is also supported by the fact that these lesions are all capable of a certain degree of autonomous growth. All demonstrate a respectable rate of local recurrence, which is affected by the clinical extent of the disease and the ease of surgical removal. Host factors may also affect the clinical behavior, as recently abnormalities of cellular immunity have been observed.[36] Moreover, there are exceedingly rare cases of giant cell tumors that have given rise to metastatic disease; one case reported by Carstens and Howell[18] was of the localized type, and a second, which we reviewed, was of the diffuse type. For these reasons we employ the term *tenosynovial giant cell tumor* over many other terms in the literature and divide the tumors into localized and diffuse forms, depending on their growth characteristics. The histological features

also vary slightly between the two forms. The localized type primarily affects the digits and arises from the synovium of tendon sheath or interphalangeal joint. The diffuse form occurs in areas adjacent to large weight-bearing joints such as the knee and ankle and in many instances represents extraarticular extension of pigmented villonodular synovitis. A small number of cases of diffuse giant cell tumors have no intraarticular components and probably take origin from bursae associated with large joints. Pigmented villonodular synovitis restricted to the joint proper is not specifically discussed in this chapter; the reader is referred to several excellent works on the subject in the literature.[11,16,28,32,35]

TENOSYNOVIAL GIANT CELL TUMOR, LOCALIZED TYPE (NODULAR TENOSYNOVITIS)

The localized form of giant cell tumor is characterized by a discrete proliferation of rounded synovial-like cells accompanied by a variable number of multinucleated giant cells, inflammatory cells, siderophages, and xanthoma cells. This tumor was first described by Chassaignac,[19] who referred to it as a "cancer of tendon sheath." It subsequently has been designated by others as fibrous histiocytoma of synovium,[33] pigmented nodular synovitis,[38] and nodular tenosynovitis,[12,32] all of which serve to underscore the lack of agreement concerning its basic nature and line of differentiation.

Clinical findings

The giant cell tumor may occur at any age, but it is most common between the ages of 30 and 50 years. The sex ratio is skewed toward females.[33,37,51] The tumors occur predominantly on the hand, where they represent the most common neoplasm of that region[33] (Figs. 28-1 and 28-2). Less common sites include the feet, ankles, and knees. In the experience of Jones et al.[33] at the Mayo Clinic, 91 of 118 cases occurred on the finger, 14 on the knee, 1 on the hip, and 4 collectively on the palm, wrist, or foot. Finger lesions are typically located adjacent to the interphalangeal joint, although other sites may also be affected. Jaffe et al.[32] originally commented on the preferential location of these tumors for the flexor surface, yet subsequent workers have shown that the lesions may be more evenly distributed between flexor and extensor tendons.[25,33] In some they may even be found in a lateral or circumferential location.

The tumors develop gradually over a long period and often remain the same size for several years. On physical examination they are fixed to deep structures but are usually not attached to skin unless the lesion occurs in the distal portion of the fingers where skin is closely related to tendon. Serum cholesterol levels are normal. Antecedent trauma occurs in a variable number of patients, but its association with the lesions may be fortuitous. Radiographic studies usually document a circumscribed soft tissue mass in about half of the patients and occasionally various de-

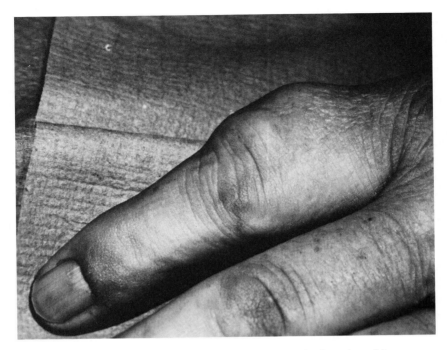

FIG. 28-1. Localized giant cell tumor involving proximal portion of finger.

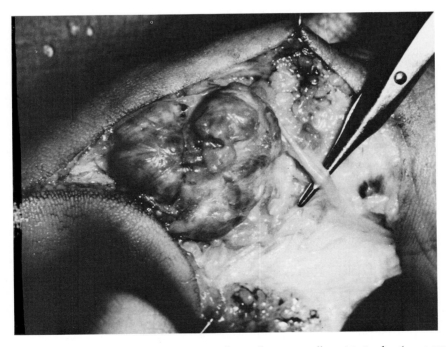

FIG. 28-2. Localized giant cell tumor. Lobulated mass is present adjacent to tendon (same case as Fig. 28-1).

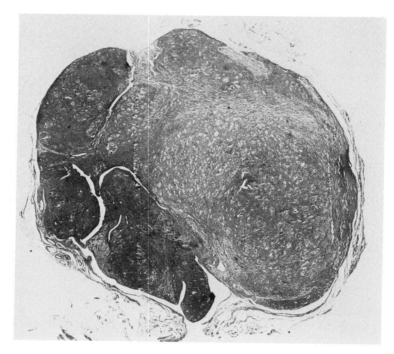

FIG. 28-3. Localized giant cell tumor illustrating early stage of lesion. Tumor compresses synovium to form deep grooves or clefts within substance of tumor. (×14.)

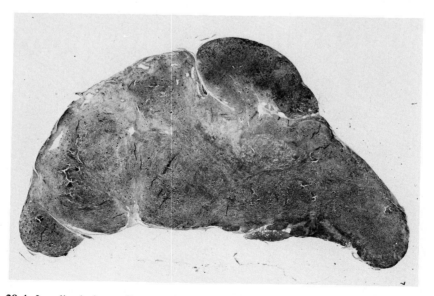

FIG. 28-4. Localized giant cell tumor illustrating later stage of lesion. Deep synovial clefts are obliterated and replaced by fibrous bands that impart a vague lobular pattern to tumor. Concave surface at bottom is created by underlying tendon. (×16.)

generative changes of the adjacent joint.[33] In only a small portion of patients, however, does cortical erosion of bone occur. According to Jones et al.,[33] this was observed in 10% of patients, but it was present in almost half of those reported by Fletcher and Horn.[23] Our experience parallels that of Jones, although obviously the incidence of bone changes is influenced by the selection of patients receiving radiographic studies and by the location of the tumors. It has been suggested that giant cell tumors of the feet more frequently produce changes because the dense ligaments of that region are more likely to prevent outward growth of the tumors.[23]

Gross findings

Giant cell tumors are circumscribed lobulated masses that occasionally possess shallow grooves along their deep surfaces created by the underlying tendons[51] (Figs. 28-3 and 28-4). They are usually relatively small, ranging in size from 0.5 to 3 or 4 cm in diameter. Those on the feet are usually larger and more irregular in shape than those on the hands. On cut section the tumors have a mottled appearance consisting of a pink-gray background flecked with yellow or brown, depending on the amount of lipid and hemosiderin.

Microscopic findings

In the experience of Wright,[51] who has studied the evolution of these tumors, the earliest lesion is a villous structure that projects into the synovial space of the tendon sheath. Limited space prevents continued growth into the cavity so that ultimately the tumor grows outward in a cauliflower fashion and compresses synovial-lined clefts into its substance. At the stage at which most lesions are surgically excised, they are exophytic masses attached to tendon sheath and have smooth but lobulated contours. They are partially invested by a dense collagenous capsule that penetrates the tumors, dividing them into vague nodules (Fig. 28-4). The capsule is not totally confining, as isolated nests of tumor can be identified outside its bounds, especially at the deep margin where tumor blends with synovial membrane.

The appearance of the giant cell tumor varies depending on the proportion of mononuclear cells, giant cells, and xanthoma cells, and the degree of collagenization (Figs. 28-5 to 28-9). Most tumors are moderately cellular and are composed of sheets of rounded or polygonal cells (Fig. 28-6), which blend with hypocellular collagenized zones in which the cells appear slightly spindled. Cleftlike spaces

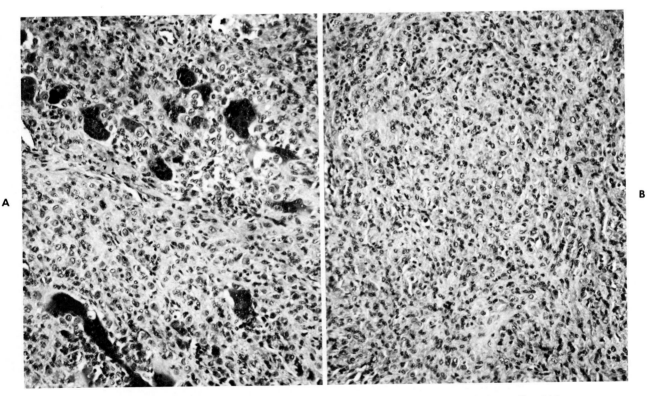

FIG. 28-5. Localized form of giant cell tumor showing variation in number of giant cells within same tumor. Some areas (**A**) have numerous giant cells, whereas others (**B**) have none. Predominant cell is rounded and resembles a synovial cell or histocyte. (**A** and **B**, ×160.)

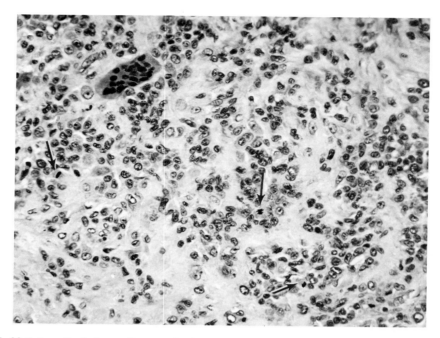

FIG. 28-6. Localized giant cell tumor. Basic cell is relatively uniform but may display occasional mitotic figures *(arrows)*. (×250.)

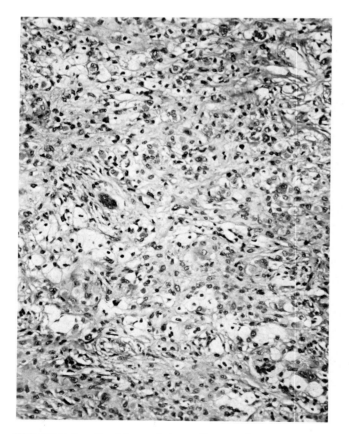

FIG. 28-7. Localized form of giant cell tumor showing focal collections of xanthoma cells. (×160.)

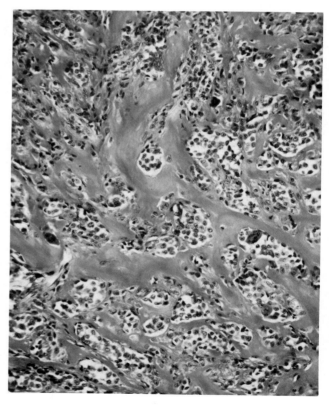

FIG. 28-8. Hyalinization within a localized giant cell tumor. (×160.)

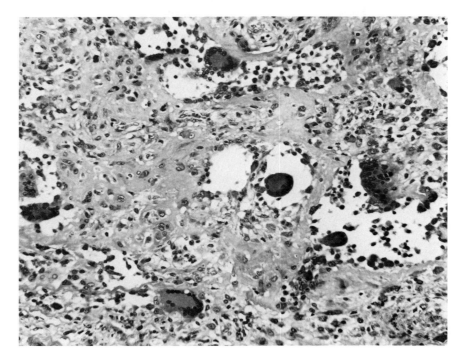

FIG. 28-9. Pseudoglandular or alveolar spaces within a localized giant cell tumor. (×160.)

are occasionally present (Fig. 28-9). Some probably represent synovial-lined spaces, whereas others are artificial spaces caused by shrinkage and loss of cellular cohesion. Multinucleated giant cells are scattered randomly throughout the lesions. In the typical case they are relatively numerous but become sparse in highly cellular lesions, particularly recurrent ones. These cells, which form by fusion of the more prevalent mononuclear cells, have a variable number of nuclei ranging from as few as 3 or 4 to 50 to 60. Xanthoma cells are also frequent, tend to be located geographically within these tumors, and often contain fine hemosiderin granules (Fig. 28-7). Cartilaginous and osseous metaplasias are a rare focal finding in these tumors.

The diagnosis of giant cell tumor per se is rarely difficult, but the evaluation of certain atypical features can be problematic. For instance, the presence of mitotic figures occasionally leads to a mistaken diagnosis of cancer (Fig. 28-6). However, this feature occurs in over half of the half of the cases,[51] and in our experience is a focal phenomenon within benign giant cell tumors. Rao and Vigorita[43] documented 3 or more mitotic figures per 10 high-power fields in over 10% of their cases. Although it may indicate an actively growing lesion that is likely to recur, we have no evidence to suggest that such lesions metastasize. In about 1% to 5% of cases tumor thrombi are observed in small veins draining these lesions (Fig. 28-10). Likewise, this feature does not correlate with the ability to produce metastasis based on preliminary follow-up information in our cases. In fact, because of the extreme rarity of metastasizing forms of giant cell tumor,

it is justifiable to adopt a conservative approach in the interpretation of these atypical features.

Differential diagnosis

Occasionally benign lesions located in the vicinity of tendon sheath may be confused with giant cell tumors. These include foreign body granulomas, necrobiotic granulomas, tendinous xanthomas, and fibromas of tendon sheath. Granulomatous lesions, however, are less localized and have a greater complement of inflammatory cells. Necrobiotic granulomas are characterized by cores of degenerating collagen rimmed by histiocytes and a prominent zone of proliferating capillaries. Giant cells are usually scarce or nonexistent. The distinction of giant cell tumor with a prominent xanthomatous component and tendinous xanthoma formerly represented a problem in differential diagnosis. As a result of the recognition and early treatment of hyperlipidemia, this is seldom a practical problem for the surgical pathologist today. In contrast to giant cell tumors, tendinous xanthomas arising in the setting of hyperlipidemia are often multiple and occur within the tendon proper (Chapter 13). Histologically, they consist almost exclusively of xanthoma cells with only a few multinucleated giant cells and chronic inflammatory cells. "Cholesterol clefts" are characteristic of tendinous xanthomas but are usually absent in giant cell tumors. Finally, fibromas of tendon sheath may bear some similarity to hyalinized forms of giant cell tumor. In general, their cells appear fibroblastic, and their stroma are more uniformly hyalinized. In rare instances fibromas of tendon sheath may evolve by way of sclerosis in

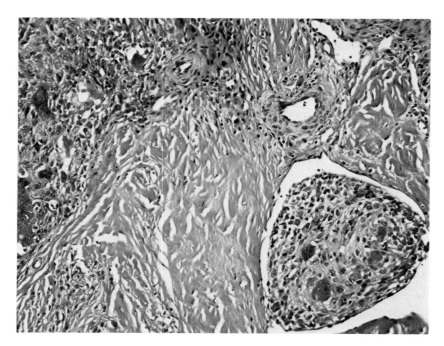

FIG. 28-10. Focus of tumor within a vein in a localized giant cell tumor. This feature does not necessarily indicate cancer. (×160.)

a preexisting giant cell tumor so that it is possible to encounter lesions combining features of both. Occasionally epithelioid sarcomas with numerous giant cells can mimick a giant cell tumor. The relatively monomorphic population of cells and strong and diffuse expression of keratin distinguish it from giant cell tumor.

Ultrastructural, enzymatic, cell marker, and ploidy studies

In most ultrastructural studies, the cells of these tumors have been compared with normal synovium,[9,21] and the existence of both types of synovial cells has been used by some as support for a reactive process.[9] Most cells within these tumors have abundant cytoplasm and elongated cell processes. A smaller number have well-developed endoplasmic reticulum.

Both enzymatic and cell marker studies have supported the hypothesis that the cells are most closely related to monocytes and macrophages. They possess acid phosphatase, beta glucuronidase, alpha-naphthyl acetate esterase,[48,50] and the following cell surface markers:[48] HLA-A, B, C, HLA-DR, LCA, Leu-M3, and Leu-3. Wood et al.[50] have suggested osteoclastic lineage on the basis of these findings, an interpretation formerly suggested by Carstens[17] on the basis of ultrastructural observations.

DNA ploidy analysis of a small group of tenosynovial giant cell tumors indicates that diploid patterns are invariably present in the localized forms and in pigmented villonodular synovitis, whereas nearly half of diffuse tenosynovial giant cell tumors are aneuploid. The last group also

displays a higher proliferation index than the former two groups, a findng that the authors believe reflects rapid uncontrolled growth.[8]

Behavior and treatment

Giant cell tumors are benign lesions that nonetheless possess a capacity for local recurrence. In our cases this occurs in about 10% to 20% of cases, a rate roughly in accordance with that reported by others.[33,38,43] Wright[51] reported a recurrence rate of 44% and indicated that extended follow-up data on outpatients account for the higher rate.[51] Recurrences seem to develop more often in very cellular lesions with increased mitoses[51] and in patients who have simple enucleations, since microscopic residua are invariably left behind at the deep margin. Local excision with a small cuff of normal tissue is usually considered adequate therapy, even for those lesions with increased cellularity and mitotic activity. Most will be cured by this approach, and more extended surgery can always be planned at a later time for persistently recurring lesions.

TENOSYNOVIAL GIANT CELL TUMOR, DIFFUSE TYPE (PROLIFERATIVE SYNOVITIS, FLORID SYNOVITIS, EXTRAARTICULAR PIGMENTED VILLONODULAR SYNOVITIS, PIGMENTED VILLONODULAR BURSITIS)

This form of giant cell tumor can be regarded as the soft tissue counterpart of diffuse pigmented villonodular synovitis of the joint space. In most instances this lesion prob-

Table 28-1. Anatomical distribution of diffuse giant cell tumor of tendon sheath (AFIP, 40 patients)

Location	No. cases
Knee	15
Ankle and foot	12
Wrist	5
Finger	3
Elbow	2
Hip and sacroiliac region	2
Toe	1
TOTAL	40

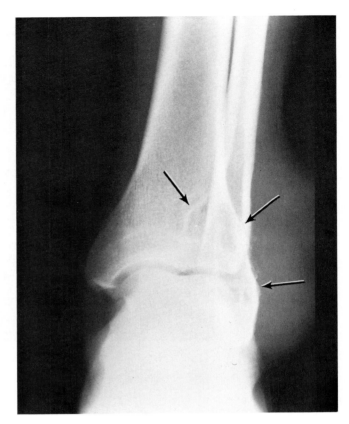

FIG. 28-11. Radiograph of a diffuse form of giant cell tumor. Large soft tissue mass is present in ankle region and has caused secondary destruction of distal tibia and fibula *(arrows)*. Minimal changes in joint space suggest tumor probably arose in an extraarticular location.

ably represents extraarticular extension of a primary intraarticular process, a contention supported by the similarity in age, location, clinical presentation, and symptoms between the two processes. In rare instances this disease may reside completely outside a joint, in which case its origin must be ascribed to synovium of bursa or tendon sheath. In his original description of villonodular synovitis, Jaffe described four extraarticular cases (pigmented villonodular bursitis), two arising from the popliteal bursa, one from the bursa anserina, and one from the ankle bursa.[32] Additional cases have been reported in the thigh by Peterson et al.[40] and Probst[42] and in the groin (apparently arising from the iliopectineal bursa).[49] One of 34 cases of pigmented villonodular synovitis reported by Atmore et al.[11] was extraarticular in location, and several of the cases reported by Arthaud[10] would probably also qualify as diffuse forms of giant cell tumor. In many instances it may be difficult to clearly define the origin of the tumor. Therefore we have employed the term *tenosynovial giant cell tumor of the diffuse type* when there is a poorly confined soft tissue mass with or without involvement of the adjacent joint.

In comparison with localized giant cell tumor, this form is rather uncommon and displays certain clinical differences. There is a tendency for the lesions to occur in young persons. About half of the patients in our cases are diagnosed prior to the age of 40 years, a mean incidence quite similar to that of pigmented villonodular synovitis. Females are affected slightly more often than males. Typically symptoms are of relatively long duration, often several years, and include pain and tenderness in the affected extremity. The additional presence of joint effusion, hemarthrosis, limitation of joint motion, and locking signify articular involvement in most cases. Its anatomical distribution parallels that of pigmented villonodular synovitis and includes the knee followed by the ankle and foot (Table 28-1). Uncommon locations are the finger, elbow, toe, and temporomandibular and sacroiliac areas. Radiographically, a soft tissue mass is usually evident and may be accompanied by osteoporosis, widening of the joint space, and cortical erosion of the adjacent bone (Fig. 28-11). Arteriogra-

phy may suggest cancer because of increased vascularity and early filling to the venous system.

At surgery the lesions are large, firm or spongelike, multinodular masses. Color varies from white to yellow or brown, although usually staining with hemosiderin is less evident than in their articular counterparts and they usually do not have grossly discernible villous patterns (Figs. 28-12 and 28-13).

In contrast to localized giant cell tumors, this form is not surrounded by a mature collagenous capsule, but instead it grows in expansive sheets (Figs. 28-14 and 28-15), which are interrupted by cleftlike or pseudoglandular spaces (Fig. 28-16). Many of the spaces represent residual synovial membrane, while others are probably artifactual. The predominant cell is rounded or polygonal. Its cytoplasm may be clear or deeply brown when ladened with hemosiderin (Fig. 28-15, *B*). Gradual transition between these cells, spindled cells (Fig. 28-17), and xanthoma cells (Fig. 28-18) is common, and in some tumors the diagnosis of xanthoma may be suggested. Multinucleated giant cells and chronic inflammatory cells are intermingled so that the net

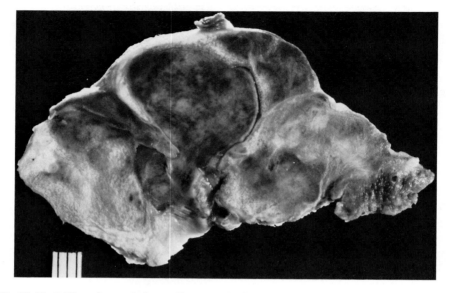

FIG. 28-12. Diffuse form of giant cell tumor. Lesion has multinodular appearance with variegated color. Shaggy villous projections, typical of pigmented villonodular synovitis, are not seen.

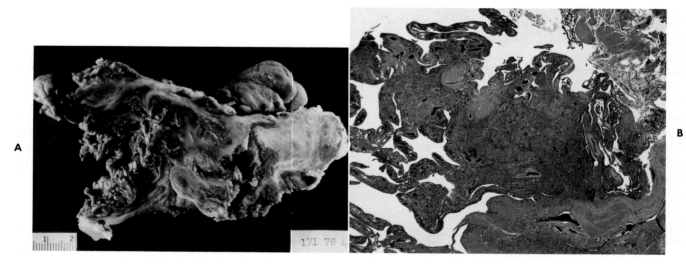

FIG. 28-13. Intraarticular form of diffuse form of giant cell tumor to contrast with extraarticular form shown in Fig. 28-12. Note shaggy villous appearance in the gross (**A**) and microscopic (**B**) specimens. (**B**, ×25.)

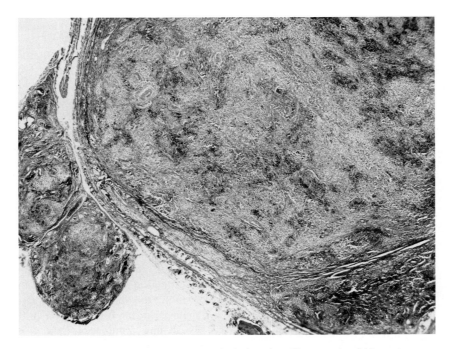

FIG. 28-14. Diffuse form of giant cell tumor depicting sheetlike growth within main tumor mass and small secondary nodules. (×15.)

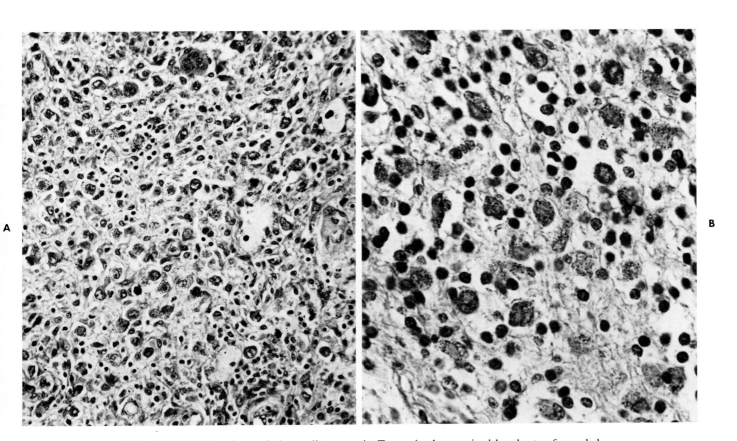

FIG. 28-15. Diffuse form of giant cell tumor. **A,** Tumor is characterized by sheets of rounded synovial-like cells, along with occasional xanthoma cells, inflammatory cells, and giant cells. (×250.) **B,** Basic cell often has hemosiderin-laden cytoplasm. (×350.)

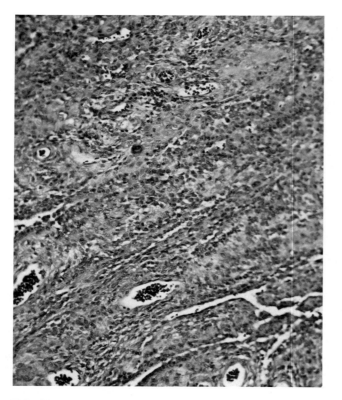

FIG. 28-16. Pseudoglandular spaces within diffuse form of giant cell tumor. (×250.)

effect is that of a highly polymorphic population of cells. However, in general, giant cells are less numerous than in localized tumors. In cellular areas the collagenous stroma is delicate and inconspicuous (Fig. 28-15, *A*), whereas in hypocellular areas the tumor may be quite hyalinized (Fig. 28-19).

These lesions usually present greater diagnostic problems than their localized counterparts. The pronounced cellularity, coupled with the clinical findings of an extensive, destructive mass is likely to lead to a diagnosis of cancer. Particular problems arise in the very early lesions consisting of a monomorphic population of rounded cells with a high nuclear cytoplasmic ratio and brisk mitotic rate (Figs. 28-20 to 28-22). Focal necrosis may be present if torsion of a pedunculated tumor nodule has occurred (Fig. 28-20). In such cases attention should be paid to the synovial-based location and to the apparent maturation of these tumor nodules at their periphery (Fig. 28-22). In the peripheral zones the cells acquire a more prominent, slightly xanthomatous-appearing cytoplasm (Fig. 28-22, *B*). Additional sections occasionally will disclose focal giant cells, and iron staining may identify modest amounts of hemosiderin not discernible in routine sections. In more advanced lesions consisting of the classic polymorphic cellular population, other problems in differential diagnosis occur. For example, the pseudoglandular spaces are often misinterpreted as glandular spaces of a synovial sarcoma or the alveolar spaces of a

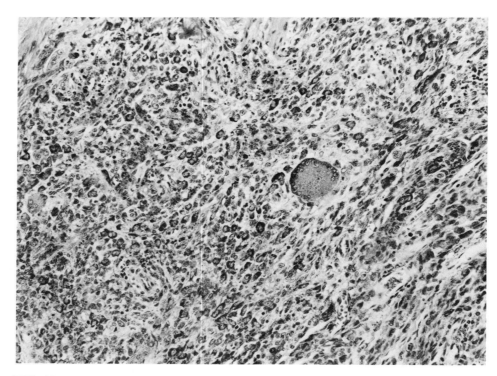

FIG. 28-17. Diffuse form of giant cell tumor showing blending of rounded cells with spindled cells. Tumor is deeply pigmented from intracellular hemosiderin deposits. (×160.)

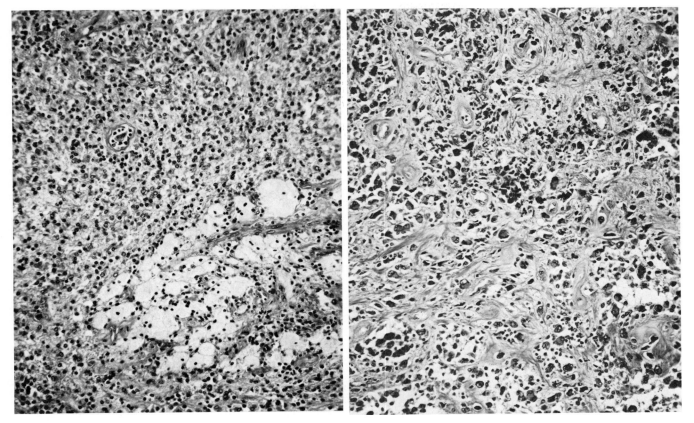

FIG. 28-18. Focal xanthomatous change within a diffuse giant cell tumor.

FIG. 28-19. Hyalinization within a diffuse giant cell tumor. (×250.)

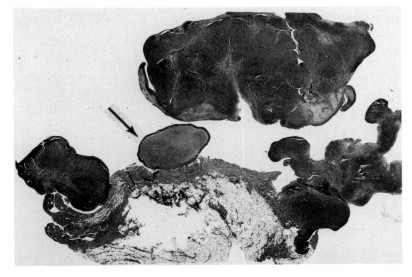

FIG. 28-20. Early stage of diffuse intraarticular giant cell tumor. Note necrosis of one of the nodules *(arrow)* due to torsion of the tumor on its stalk. (×15.)

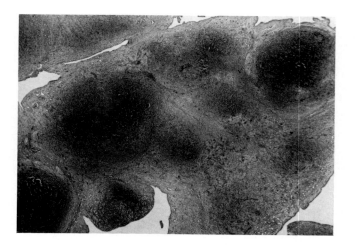

FIG. 28-21. Early stage of diffuse giant cell tumor (same case as Fig. 28-20). The lesion has a distinctly nodular architecture. (×60.)

rhabdomyosarcoma. The giant cell tumor shows a great variation in type and arrangement of cells. Its geographical pattern of xanthomatous regions alternating with cellular hyalinized regions contrasts with the more uniform spindled appearance of most synovial sarcomas and the primitive round cells of childhood rhabdomyosarcomas. Diffuse giant cell tumors with prominent xanthomatous components must also be separated from inflammatory or xanthomatous forms of *malignant fibrous histiocytoma* (Chapter 15). The latter, however, usually occur in the retroperitoneum and contain xanthomatous areas and spindled areas resembling the conventional forms of malignant fibrous histiocytoma. Moreover, most inflammatory forms of malignant fibrous histiocytoma have a predominantly acute inflammatory background, which contrasts with the modest number of chronic inflammatory cells that are present in giant cell tumors.

Behavior and treatment

Although there is a great deal of literature concerning the behavior and treatment of pigmented villonodular synovi-

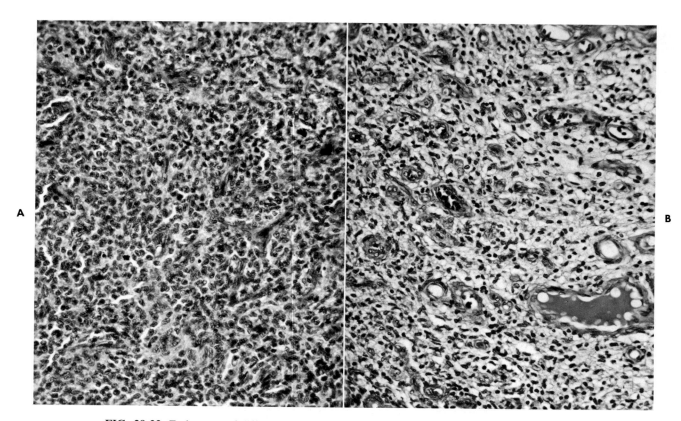

FIG. 28-22. Early stage of diffuse giant cell tumor (same case as Fig. 28-20). The centers of the nodules shown in Fig. 28-21 are composed of rather primitive cells with a high mitotic rate **(A)**. At the periphery of the nodules the cells have smaller nuclei and more cytoplasm, which appears slightly xanthomatous **(B)**. There is also ingrowth of capillaries in these zones. (**A** and **B**, ×250.)

tis, there are few data concerning extraarticular forms of the disease. Preliminary follow-up information in our cases indicates that 40% to 50% of patients develop local recurrence. Recurrence rates in pigmented villonodular synovitis have been reported as 25% by Schwartz et al.[46] and 46% by Byers et al.[16] Recurrences in pigmented villonodular synovitis can be correlated with location in the knee and incomplete excision, with a cumulative probability of recurrence of 15% at 5 years and 35% at 25 years.[46] We have also reviewed one example of a diffuse recurrent giant cell tumor arising from the foot that metastasized to the lung after several years (Figs. 28-23 to 28-24). This case, however, appears to be unique, because metastases have not been observed in the collective experiences of others. Thus from a practical point of view, these lesions should be regarded as locally aggressive, but nonmetastasizing, lesions. Therapy should be based on a desire to remove the tumor as completely as possible without producing severe disability for the patient. Although wide excision or amputation is the best choice for local control of disease, it obviously implies significant morbidity, especially for lesions located adjacent to major joints. Less radical excision, therefore, can be justified in these cases. Although radiotherapy has been endorsed for treatment of surgically unresectable villonodular synovitis,[29] there is no recorded experience concerning its use in this form of the disease.

MALIGNANT GIANT CELL TUMOR OF TENDON SHEATH

Malignant giant cell tumors of tendon sheath comprise a rare group of tumors the existence of which has been doubted by some and the diagnosis of which is very difficult. The belief that giant cell tumor is an inflammatory condition has led to the foregone conclusion by some that malignant forms of this disease do not exist. Others have accepted any sarcoma that contains giant cells arising in the vicinity of tendon as a "malignant giant cell tumor of tendon sheath."[38] Consequently, malignant giant cell tumors of tendon sheath as reported in the literature constitute a variety of lesions, including clear cell sarcoma,[3] fibrosarcoma, epithelioid sarcoma,[13] and malignant fibrous histiocytoma. Still others have implied that diffuse forms of giant cell tumors, which behave in a locally aggressive fashion and ultimately require amputation, be considered malignant, although the morphological appearance may remain unaltered in the course of the disease. Although each of these approaches has its validity, we have generally reserved the designation of malignant giant cell tumor of tendon sheath for lesions in which benign giant cell tumor coexists with frankly malignant areas or, alternatively, when the original lesion was typical of benign giant cell tumor and the recurrence appeared malignant.

Defined in this fashion, true malignant giant cell tumors

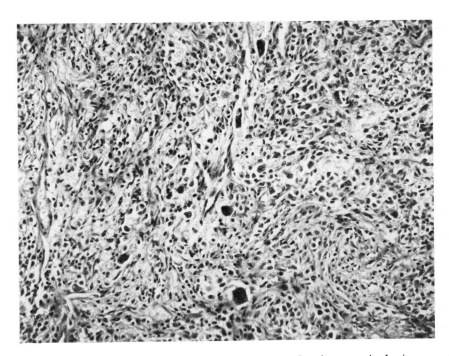

FIG. 28-23. Diffuse form of giant cell tumor of foot that produced metastasis. Lesion was characterized by bland proliferation of mononuclear and giant cells. Pulmonary metastasis is shown in Fig. 28-24.

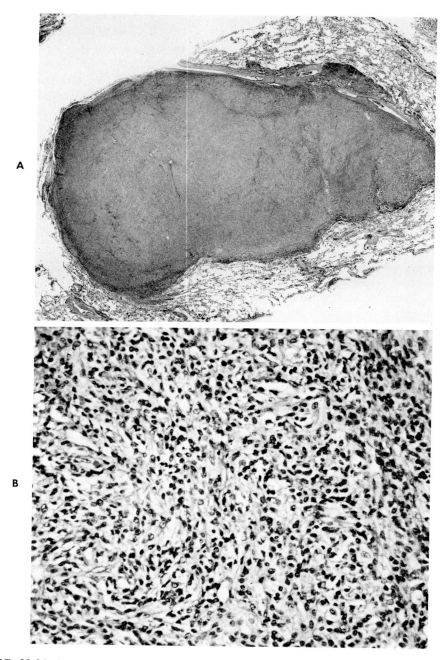

FIG. 28-24. A, Pulmonary metastasis from diffuse form of giant cell tumor of foot (same case as Fig. 28-10). (×15.) **B,** Tumor was essentially identical to original tumor except it had fewer giant cells.

of tendon sheath are an extremely rare group of tumors and are far outnumbered by benign giant cell tumors or even tumors with atypical features. They occur in the distal extremities, and histologically they bear a close similarity to malignant fibrous histiocytoma (Fig. 28-25) except they usually are less pleomorphic. Giant cells are usually less numerous than in the benign forms, and the mononuclear

cells are large with prominent nucleoli and abundant cytoplasm. Both typical and atypical mitotic figures are present throughout the tumor in contrast with the focal distribution in benign lesions. There is little stromal collagen, and the tumors grow in cellular sheets or large nodules that may have focal hemorrhages and necrosis.

There are no collective data on the behavior of these tu-

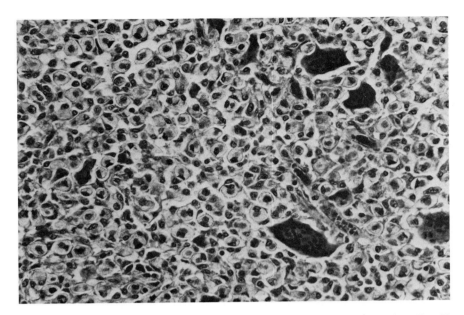

FIG. 28-25. Malignant giant cell tumor of tendon sheath as shown on histological studies. Tumor was characterized by sheets of round cells devoid of intervening stroma. (×250.)

mors. They are certainly locally aggressive lesions, but the frequency with which they produce metastasis is not known. Their distal location probably confers on them a better prognosis than might be anticipated from the histological appearance. The case reported by Carstens and Howell[18] seems to be an acceptable example of malignant giant cell tumor that repeatedly recurred over a period of 20 years and ultimately gave rise to numerous local metastases on the same extremity. However, the recent case reported by Nielsen and Kiaer[39] is probably better interpreted as an intraarticular sarcoma with giant cells rather than a malignant form of tenosynovial giant cell tumor, since no benign component was identified. Wide excision or amputation of true malignant forms of tenosynovial giant cell tumors is indicated.

MISCELLANEOUS CONDITIONS RESEMBLING DIFFUSE GIANT CELL TUMOR

Occasionally reactive synovial lesions may mimic the appearance of a diffuse giant cell tumor, particularly of the intraarticular type (pigmented villonodular synovitis). Perhaps the most common condition that produces this mimicry is intraarticular hemorrhage. Long known to be associated with synovitis in hemophiliacs, intraarticular hemorrhage can give rise to hyperplastic changes of the synovium consisting of villous change and large deposits of hemosiderin.[59,60] However, only in the early stages of chronic hemarthrosis are the lesions reminiscent of pigmented villonodular synovitis. In the late stage the synovium is flattened and the subjacent tissue markedly fibrotic. A second, but less well-recognized, condition is the synovitis associated with failed orthopedic prosthetic devices.[54-56,62,63] Collectively termed "detritic synovitis," these lesions are characterized by villous hyperplasia of the synovium (Fig. 28-26). The subsynovial space is infiltrated with histiocytes, multinucleated giant cells, and variable numbers of chronic inflammatory cells. The prosthetic material can be detected under polarized light as weakly birefringent intracellular or extracellular spicules (Fig. 28-27, A). Usually it can also be stained with oil red O, but it requires a long incubation period (up to 48 hours) (Fig. 28-27, B).[51] These reactions can occur with polyethylene and silicone rubber devices and possibly also methylmethacrylate, which is used as a cement in metal prostheses. In addition, histiocytic reactions in the lymph nodes draining the regions of prosthetic devices have been reported.[53,57] Finally, we reviewed synovial tissue from a patient with alpha-mannosidase deficiency who developed a bilateral destructive synovitis of the ankle region.[61] The hyperplastic villous-appearing synovium was infiltrated with clear-appearing histiocytes containing PAS-positive, diastase-resistant material (Fig. 28-28) representing partially degraded oligosaccharides within lysosomes (Fig. 28-29). Although definitive diagnosis requires an adequate clinical history with confirmatory biochemical data, the presence of a systemic disease was suspected because of the bilaterally symmetrical distribution of the lesions, a distribution seldom encountered in pigmented villonodular synovitis.

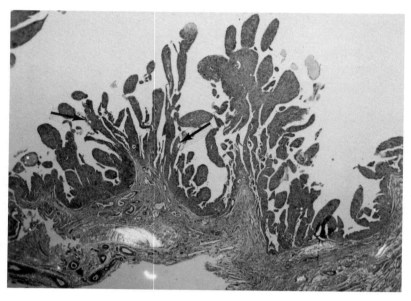

FIG. 28-26. Detritic synovitis showing villous configuration of synovium. Graft material is visible as birefringent particles in this partially polarized view. (×15.)

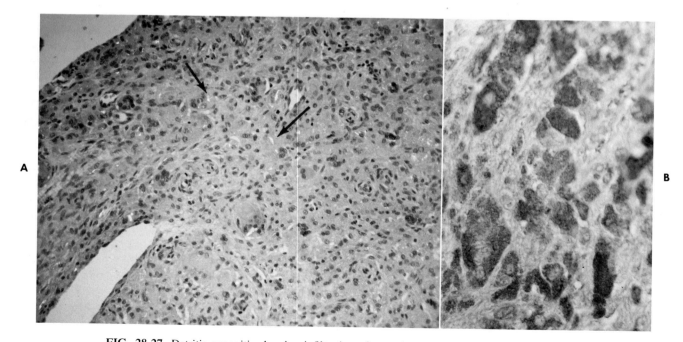

FIG. 28-27. Detritic synovitis showing infiltration of synovium with histiocytes and giant cells. Foreign material can be seen as birefringent spicules within cells **(A)**. Foreign material also stains following prolonged incubation with oil red O. (Oil Red O; ×250.)

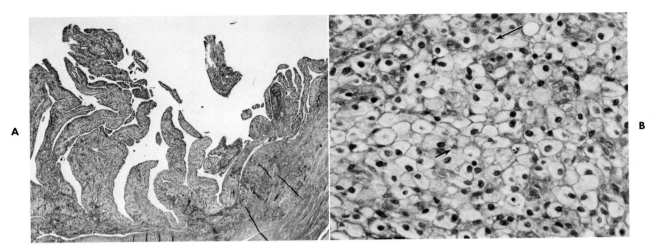

FIG. 28-28. Synovitis due to alpha-mannosidase deficiency. At low power, lesion superficially resembles a pigmented villonodular synovitis **(A)**. At high power, infiltrate consists of clear-appearing histocytes containing PAS-positive, diastase-resistant bodies representing partially degraded oligosaccharides *(arrows)*. (**A,** ×5, **B,** ×250.) (From Weiss SW, Kelly WD: *Am J Surg Pathol* 7:487, 1983.)

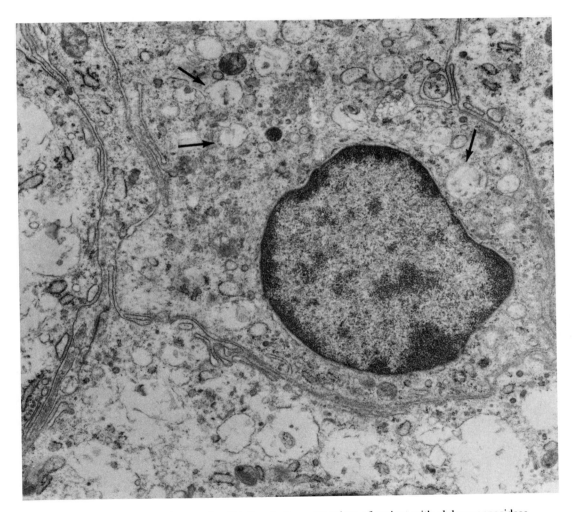

FIG. 28-29. Electron micrograph of histiocyte from synovium of patient with alpha-mannosidase deficiency. Oligosaccharide is represented by granuloamorphous material within lysosomes *(arrow)*. (×5775.) (From Weiss SW, Kelly WD: *Am J Surg Pathol* 7:487, 1983.)

REFERENCES
General

1. Adam WS: Fine structure of synovial membrane: phagocytosis of colloidal carbon from the joint cavity. *Lab Invest* 15:680, 1966.
2. Barland P, Novikoff AB, Hamerman D: Electron microscopy of the human synovial membrane. *J Cell Biol* 14:207, 1962.
3. Burmester GR, Dimitriu-Bona A, Waters SJ, et al: Identification of three major synovial lining cell populations by monoclonal antibodies directed to Ia antigens and antigens associated with monocytes/macrophages and fibroblasts. *Scand J Immunol* 17:69, 1983.
4. Ghadially FN, Roy S: *Ultrastructure of synovial joints in health and disease*. London, 1969, Butterworth.
5. Lever JD, Ford EHR: Histological, histochemical, and electron microscopic observations on synovial membrane. *Anat Rec* 132:525, 1958.
6. Palmer DG, Selvendran Y, Allen C, et al: Features of synovial membrane identified with monoclonal antibodies. *Clin Exp Immunol* 59:529, 1985.
7. Schmidt D, Mackay B: Ultrastructure of human tendon sheath and synovium: implication for tumor histogenesis. *Ultrastruct Pathol* 3:269, 1982.

Giant cell tumor of tendon sheath

8. Abdul-Karim FW, El-Naggar A, Joyce MJ, et al: Diffuse and localized tenosynovial giant cell tumor and pigmented villonodular synovitis: a clinicopathologic and flow cytometric DNA analysis. *Hum Pathol* 23:729, 1992.
9. Alguacil-Garcia A, Unni KK, Goellner JR: Giant cell tumor of tendon sheath and pigmented villonodular synovitis: an ultrastructural study. *Am J Clin Pathol* 69:6, 1978.
10. Arthaud JB: Pigmented nodular synovitis: report of 11 lesions in non-articular locations. *Am J Clin Pathol* 58:511, 1972.
11. Atmore WG, Dahlin DC, Ghormley RK: Pigmented villonodular synovitis: a clinical and pathologic study. *Minn Med* 39:196, 1956.
12. Baes H, Tanghe W: Nodular tenosynovitis. *Dermatologica* 149:149, 1974.
13. Barnard JDW: Pigmented villonodular synovitis in the temporomandibular joint: a case report. *Br J Oral Surg* 13:183, ç1975.
14. Bliss BO, Reed RJ: Large cell sarcomas of tendon sheath: malignant giant cell tumors of tendon sheath. *Am J Clin Pathol* 49:776, 1968.
15. Brown-Crosby E, Inglis A, Bullough PG: Multiple joint involvement with pigmented villonodular synovitis. *Radiology* 122:671, 1977.
16. Byers PD, Cotton RE, Deacon OW, et al: The diagnosis and treatment of pigmented villonodular synovitis. *J Bone Joint Surg* 50B:290, 1968.
17. Carstens PHB: Giant cell tumors of tendon sheath: an electron microscopic study of 11 cases. *Arch Pathol* 102:99, 1978.
18. Carstens PHB, Howell RS: Malignant giant cell tumor of tendon sheath. *Virchows Arch (Pathol Anat)* 382:237, 1979.
19. Chassaignac CME: Cancer de la gaine des tendons. *Gaz Hosp Civ Milit* 47:185, 1852.
20. Crosby EB, Inglis A, Bullough PG: Multiple joint involvement with pigmented villonodular synovitis. *Radiology* 122:671, 1977.
21. Eisenstein R: Giant cell tumor of tendon sheath. *J Bone Joint Surg* 50A:476, 1968.
22. Eisig S, Dorfman HD, Cusamano RJ, et al: Pigmented villonodular synovitis of the termporomandibular joint: case report and review of the literature. *Oral Surg Oral Med Oral Pathol* 73:328, 1992.
23. Fletcher AG, Horn RC: Giant cell tumors of tendon sheath origin. *Ann Surg* 133:374, 1951.
24. Fletcher JA, Henkle C, Atkins L, et al: Trisomy 5 and trisomy 7 are nonrandom aberrations in pigmented villonodular synovitis: confirmation of trisomy 7 in uncultured cells. *Genes Chromosom Cancer* 4:264, 1992.
25. Galoway JDB, Broders AC, Ghormley RK: Xanthoma of tendon sheaths and synovial membranes: a clinical and pathologic study. *Arch Surg* 40:485, 1940.
26. Geweiler JA, Wilson JW: Diffuse biarticular pigmented villonodular synovitis. *Radiology* 93:845, 1969.
27. Ghadially FN, Ailsby RL, Young NK: Ultrastructure of the haemophilic synovial membrane and electron probe x-ray analysis of hemosiderin. *J Pathol* 120:201, 1976.
28. Ghadially FN, Lalonde JA, Dick CE: Ultrastructure of pigmented villonodular synovitis. *J Pathol* 127:19, 1979.
29. Granowitz SP, D'Antonio J, Mankin HJ: The pathogenesis and long-term end results of pigmented villonodular synovitis. *Clin Orthop* 114:335, 1976.
30. Heurteux MA: Myelome des gaines tendineuses. *Arch Gen Med* 167:40, 160, 1891.
31. Hoaglund FT: Experimental hemarthrosis. *J Bone Joint Surg* 49:285, 1967.
32. Jaffe HL, Lichtenstein L, Sutro CJ: Pigmented villonodular synovitis, bursitis, and tenosynovitis: a discussion of the synovial and bursal equivalents of the tenosynovial lesions commonly denoted as xanthoma, xanthogranuloma, giant cell tumor, or myeloplaxoma of the tendon sheath, with some consideration of the tendon sheath lesion itself. *Arch Pathol* 31:731, 1941.
33. Jones FE, Soule EH, Coventry MB: Fibrous histiocytoma of synovium (giant cell tumor of tendon sheath, pigmented nodular synovitis). *J Bone Joint Surg* 51A:76, 1969.
34. Kahn LB: Malignant giant cell tumor of the tendon sheath. *Arch Pathol* 95:203, 1973.
35. Kindblom LG, Gunterberg B: Pigmented villonodular synovitis involving bone. *J Bone Joint Surg* 60A:830, 1978.
36. Kinsella TD, Vasey F, Ashworth MA: Perturbations of humoral and cellular immunity in a patient with pigmented villonodular synovitis. *Am J Med* 58:444, 1975.
37. Mason ML, Woolston WH: Isolated giant cell xanthomatic tumors of the fingers and hand. *Arch Surg* 15:499, 1927.
38. Myers BW, Masi AT, Feigenbaum SL: Pigmented villonodular synovitis and tenosynovitis: a clinical epidemiologic study of 166 cases and literature review. *Medicine* 59:223, 1980.
39. Nielsen AL, Kiaer T: Malignant giant cell tumor of synovium and locally destructive pigmented villonodular synovitis: ultrastructural and immunohistochemical study and review of the literature. *Hum Pathol* 20:765, 1989.
40. Peterson LFA, Johnson EW Jr, Woolner LB: Extraarticular pigmented villonodular synovitis of the knee: report of a case. *Am J Clin Pathol* 30:158, 1958.
41. Pignatti G, Mignani G, Bacchini, et al: Case report 590: diffuse pigmented villonodular synovitis with a cartilaginous component. *Skel Radiol* 19:65, 1990.
42. Probst FP: Extraarticular pigmented villonodular synovitis affecting bone: the role of angiography as an aid in its differentiation from similar bone-destroying conditions. *Radiologe* 13:436, 1973.
43. Rao AS, Vigorita VJ: Pigmented villonodular synovitis (giant cell tumor of the tendon sheath and synovial membrane): a review of eighty-one cases. *J Bone Joint Surg* 66A:76, 1984.
44. Ray RA, Morton CC, Lipinski KK, et al: Cytogenetic evidence of clonality in a case of pigmented villonodular synovitis. *Cancer* 67:121, 1991.
45. Sakkers RJ, de Jong D, van der Heul RO: X-chromosome inactivation in patients who have pigmented villonodular synovitis. *J Bone Joint Surg* 73A:1532, 1991.

46. Schwartz HS, Unni KK, Pritchard DJ: Pigmented villonodular synovitis: a retrospective review of affected large joints. *Clin Orthop* 247:243, 1989.
47. Shrikhande SS, Sampat MB: Nonarticular villous synovitis. *Indian J Cancer* 3:92, 1976.
48. Ushijima M, Hashimoto H, Tsuneyoshi M, et al: Giant cell tumor of the tendon sheath (nodular tenosynovitis): a study of 207 cases to compare the large joint group with the common digit group. *Cancer* 57:875, 1986.
49. Weisser JR, Robinson DW: Pigmented villonodular synovitis of iliopectineal bursa: a case report. *J Bone Joint Surg* 33A:988, 1951.
50. Wood GS, Beckstead JH, Kempson RL, et al: Giant cell tumor of tendon sheath (GCTTS) phenocyte of monocyte/macrophage lineage. *Lab Invest* 54:71A, 1986.
51. Wright CJE: Benign giant cell synovioma. *Br J Surg* 38:257, 1951.
52. Young JM, Hudacek AG: Experimental production of pigmented villonodular synovitis in dogs. *Am J Pathol* 30:799, 1954.

Miscellaneous conditions resembling diffuse giant cell tumors

53. Alboraes-Saavedra J, Vuitch LF, Delgado R, et al: Sinus histiocytosis of pelvic lymph nodes after hip replacement: a histiocytic proliferation induced by cobalt-chromium and titanium. *Am J Surg Pathol* 18:83, 1994.
54. Christie AD, Weinberger KA, Dietrich M: Silicone lymphadenopathy and synovitis: complications of silicone elastomer finger joint prostheses. *JAMA* 237:1463, 1977.
55. Ewald FC, Sledge CB, Corson JM, et al: Giant cell synovitis associated with failed polyethylene patellar replacements. *Clin Orthop* 15:213, 1976.
56. Gordon M, Bullough PG: Synovial and osseous inflammation in failed silicone-rubber prostheses: a report of six cases. *J Bone Joint Surg* 64A:574, 1982.
57. Gray MH, Talbert ML, Talbert WM, et al: Changes seen in lymph nodes draining sites of large joint prosthesis. *Am J Surg Pathol* 13:1050, 1989.
58. Johnson FB: Personal communication, 1984.
59. Rodnan GP, Brower TD, Hellstroma HR, et al: Post-mortem examination of an elderly severe hemophiliac, with observations on the pathologic findings in hemophilic joint disease. *Arthritis Rheum* 2:152, 1959.
60. Stein H, Duthie RB: Pathogenesis of chronic haemophilic arthropathy. *J Bone Joint Surg* 63B:601, 1981.
61. Weiss SW, Kelly WD: Bilateral destructive synovitis associated with alpha-mannosidase deficiency. *Am J Surg Pathol* 7:487, 1983.
62. Worsing RA, Engber WD, Lange TA: Reactive synovitis from particulate silastic. *J Bone Joint Surg* 64A:581, 1982.
63. Yamashina M, Moatamed F: Periarticular reactions to microscopic erosion of silicone-polymer implants. *Am J Surg Pathol* 9:215, 1985.

CHAPTER 29

SYNOVIAL SARCOMA

Synovial sarcoma is a clinically and morphologically well-defined entity that has been described extensively in the literature. It occurs primarily in the paraarticular regions of the extremities, usually in close association with tendon sheaths, bursae, and joint capsules. It is uncommon, however, in joint cavities. On rare occasions it is encountered in areas without any apparent relationship to synovial structures, such as the tongue, parapharyngeal region, or abdominal wall.

Its existence and its microscopic resemblance to normal synovium were recognized early in the literature, but its origin from preformed synovial tissues has never been fully substantiated. In 1927 Smith[131] coined the term *synovioma,* and in 1936 Knox[66] suggested the name *synovial sarcoma.* Earlier cases, dating back to the turn of the nineteenth century, were designated variously as *adenosarcoma, perithelial sarcoma, synovial sarcoendothelioma, sarcomesothelioma,* and *mesothelioma of joints.*[70] Stuer (1893),[135] and Lejars and Rubens-Duval (1910)[73] are usually credited with the first accurate descriptions of this neoplasm. In some of the earlier reports, however, tumorlike inflammatory processes and benign giant cell tumors were not always clearly distinguished from synovial sarcomas. Also, in some of the more recent reports[46,128] the collective term *tendosynovial sarcoma* was used for a heterogenous group of neoplasms that includes, in addition to synovial sarcoma, epithelioid sarcoma, clear cell sarcoma, and chordoid sarcoma.

At the AFIP, during a 10-year period, we saw 345 examples of synovial sarcoma, making it the fourth most common type of sarcoma in our material after malignant fibrous histiocytoma, liposarcoma, and rhabdomyosarcoma. The reported data as to the frequency of this tumor vary: Pack and Ariel[113] observed an incidence of 8.4% among all malignant tumors of soft somatic tissues studied at Memorial Hospital. Others reported an incidence of 5.6%,[143] 6.9%,[120] and 10%[14] among soft tissue sarcomas; Hampole and Jackson[49] calculated an average incidence of 2.75 per 100,000 population based on a study carried out in Saskatchewan, Canada.

The criteria for histological diagnosis vary in different institutions, but several basic and closely interrelated types are recognized: the classic *biphasic type,* with distinct epithelial and spindle cell components in varying proportions; the *monophasic fibrous type,* a fibrosarcoma-like spindle cell tumor without any demonstrable epithelial component; and, at the other extreme of the morphological spectrum, the *monophasic epithelial type.* The biphasic and monophasic fibrous types are about equally common, but positive identification of the latter requires immunohistochemical demonstration of cytokeratin or epithelial membrane antigen. The monophasic epithelial type is difficult to distinguish from carcinoma but usually can be recognized by the presence of a small or minute focus of fibrosarcoma-like spindle cells. Synovial sarcoma may also present as a poorly differentiated small cell neoplasm in which the distinction between epithelial and spindle cell elements is largely obscured.

CLINICAL FINDINGS
Age and sex incidence

Synovial sarcoma is most prevalent in adolescents and young adults between 15 and 40 years of age. In our series of 345 cases the median age was 26.5 years; 90% of the affected patients were under 50 years of age, and 72% were under 40 years of age. There are no newborns among our cases, but there are several children 10 years of age or younger, including a 1-year-old child with a tumor of the elbow region and a 2-year-old child with a tumor of the knee (Fig. 29-1). Similar cases of synovial sarcoma in children have been reported in the literature, including rare examples in newborns.* In the Cadman et al.[14] series the median age at time of operation was 31.3 years, with 83.6% of the patients being between 10 and 50 years of age. In Geiler's review of 418 synovial sarcomas from the literature,[39,40] the average age of the patients was 35 years. In his series only 17 of the cases (2.6%) occurred in children under 10 years of age.

Males are more often affected than females; the average

---

*References 21, 56, 69, 72, 126, 142.

757

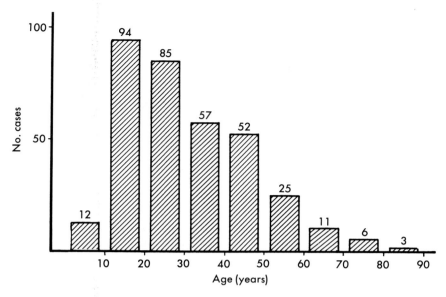

FIG. 29-1. Age distribution of 345 cases of synovial sarcoma reviewed at the AFIP during a 10-year period. The tumor may occur at any age, but it is rare in patients younger than 10 years and older than 60 years.

male to female ratio is 1.2:1. Neither in our series nor in the literature is there evidence of a predilection for any particular race. About 10% of our cases affected blacks.

Clinical complaints

The most typical presentation is that of a palpable deep-seated swelling or mass associated with pain or tenderness in slightly more than half of cases. Less frequently, pain or tenderness is the only manifestation of the disease. There may be minor limitation of motion, but severe functional disturbance or weight loss is seldom encountered, and when it occurs, it is nearly always associated with poorly differentiated tumors of long duration and large size. The exact cause of the comparatively high incidence of pain or tenderness remains unknown, but there is no evidence that an inflammatory process ever precedes the onset of the tumor. Other clinical complaints are rare and are related to the location of the tumor: patients with synovial sarcomas in the hypopharynx, for instance, often suffer from difficulties in swallowing and breathing and not infrequently have alteration or loss of voice.[118] Secondary involvement of nerves may cause projected pain, numbness, and paresthesia. Synovial sarcoma of the hand may lead to carpal tunnel syndrome.[148]

The preoperative duration of symptoms varies considerably. Generally, the tumor grows slowly and insidiously, often giving a false impression as to the degree of malignancy and delaying diagnosis and therapy. In the majority of cases the duration ranges from 2 to 4 years, but there are also cases in which a slow-growing mass or pain at the tumor site has been noted for as long as 20 years prior to operation. Not infrequently these cases are wrongly diagnosed initially as arthritis, synovitis, or bursitis.

Trauma

The question remains unsettled whether or not trauma contributes to the development of synovial sarcoma. Although the majority of patients fail to give a definite history of antecedent trauma, there are patients with such a history in our cases and in the literature. Most of these sustained a minor or major injury during athletic or recreational activities such as football, basketball, or riding a bicycle. The interval between the episode of trauma and onset of the tumor varies considerably, ranging from a few weeks to as long as 15 years. There are cases in the literature with an even longer interval: Vincent,[147] for example, described a 60-year-old man who had suffered an injury of the right hip at age 20 years and 40 years later developed a synovial sarcoma in the same location. In some cases trauma may be merely a coincidence related to the predominance of synovial sarcomas in the extremities, as suggested by reports of patients who suffered injury *after* the presence of a mass had been noted.[48] We have never seen a radiation-induced synovial sarcoma, but one such case, a synovial sarcoma of the neck, has been documented.[99]

Anatomical location

Synovial sarcomas occur predominantly in the extremities, where they tend to arise in the vicinity of large joints, especially the knee region (Table 29-1). They are intimately

Table 29-1. Synovial sarcoma (AFIP, 345 cases)

Anatomical location	No. cases	Percent
Head-neck	31	9.0
Neck (12)		
Pharynx (7)		
Larynx (7)		
Trunk	28	8.1
Chest (10)		
Abdominal wall (9)		
Upper extremities	80	23.2
Forearm-wrist (24)		
Shoulder (22)		
Elbow-upper arm (20)		
Hand (14)		
Lower extremities	206	59.7
Thigh-knee (102)		
Foot (45)		
Lower leg-ankle (33)		
Hip-groin (22)		
TOTAL	345	100.0

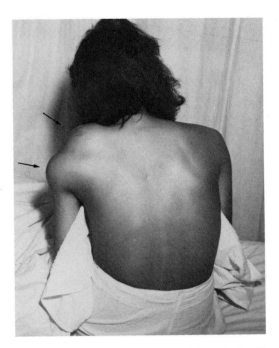

FIG. 29-2. Biphasic synovial sarcoma of the left shoulder *(arrows)* in a 24-year-old woman; the patient died of pulmonary metastasis 24 months after removal of the tumor by forequarter amputation. Note the large size and multinodular character of the growth.

related to tendons, tendon sheaths, and bursal structures, usually just beyond the confines of the joint capsule; less frequently they are attached to fascial structures, ligaments, aponeuroses, and interosseous membranes. They are definitely rare within joint cavities, and according to our material and most reviews, intraarticular synovial sarcomas amount to fewer than 5% of all cases.[32,87]

Among the reviewed AFIP cases, 83% were located in the extremities, with 60% in the lower extremities and 23% in the upper extremities. Nine percent of the cases were situated in the region of the head and neck, and 8.1% were in the region of the trunk (Table 29-1). The actual incidence of synovial sarcomas in the regions of the head and neck and trunk is probably much lower, since the AFIP material contains a disproportionately greater number of cases at unusual locations. In fact, in most accounts 85% to 95% of the cases are present in the extremities, and only 5% to 15% manifest in the head and neck region and the trunk, including the abdominal wall and retroperitoneum[101,120,129,150] (Fig. 29-2).

In the extremities the single most common site is the knee region, closely followed by the lowermost portion of the thigh; no less than one third of cases affect this general area. Next in frequency are the regions of the ankle and foot, elbow, upper arm, and shoulder. Surprisingly, few synovial sarcomas occur in the fingers and toes. Even less common are apparently primary intravascular synovial sarcomas, as reported by Miettinen et al.[94] and Shaw and Lais.[127]

Synovial sarcoma of the head and neck

Since the first description of this tumor by Pack and Ariel,[113] the occurrence of synovial sarcoma in the head and neck region has drawn considerable attention, and approximately 70 cases have been reported in the literature, mostly case reports.* The majority of these tumors seem to originate within the paravertebral connective tissue spaces and manifest as solitary retropharyngeal or parapharyngeal masses near the carotid bifurcation. Additional cases in this general area have been reported in the soft palate,[86] tongue,[51,104,109] maxillofacial region,[110] angle of the mandible,[57] sternoclavicular region,[85] scapular region,[75] and esophagus.[5] Most occur in young adults, but sporadic cases in children, including a 15-month-old patient, have been reported.[74] Because of the unusual location, synovial sarcomas in this region are often misdiagnosed.

In our series of 24 cases,[118] 13 were located in the hypopharyngeal or retropharyngeal region, 3 in the region of the hyoid bone, 1 in the mastoid area, and 7 in various other portions of the anterior and posterior neck (Fig. 29-3). Another AFIP report described 11 synovial sarcomas from the orofacial region.[130] Wide surgical excision and long-term follow-up is important. In the series reported by Amble et al.[4] 4 of 9 patients who were followed for more than 5 years died of their disease.

*References 9, 12, 36, 44, 50, 59, 68, 76, 97, 100.

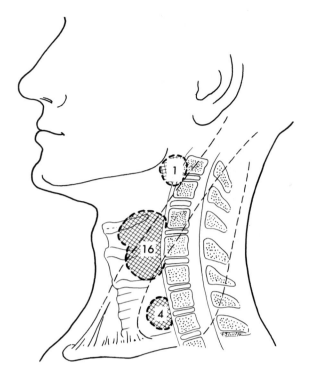

FIG. 29-3. Anatomical distribution of 21 synovial sarcomas of the neck, an unusual location for this tumor. Most of these neoplasms manifest as retropharyngeal or parapharyngeal masses that cause difficulties in breathing or swallowing.

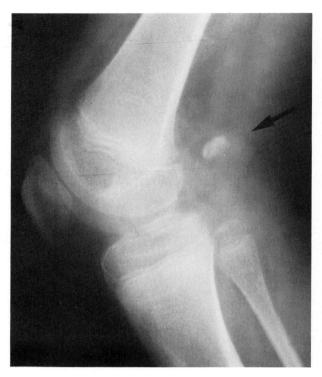

FIG. 29-4. Roentgenograph of a synovial sarcoma originating in the popliteal fossa. Note focal calcification of the tumor (arrow), a feature that is present in about 20% of cases.

Synovial sarcoma of the abdominal wall

This is another curious and uncommon site of this tumor; only 2.6% of all synovial sarcomas observed during a 10-year period were situated in this particular region. Like synovial sarcomas at other sites, these neoplasms are usually deep seated, occur on both the left and right sides, and are more common in the lower half of the abdomen. In the absence of any other synovial structures in this region, bursal origin has been claimed,[10] but we have never observed remnants of normal synovial or bursal structures in these tumors or, for that matter, in the abdominal wall, although two of our cases arose within appendectomy scars. Fetsch and Meis,[33] who reviewed 27 cases culled from the AFIP material, noted a large number of cystic tumors among their cases. The age and sex incidence of these tumors as well as their behavior corresponds to that of synovial sarcomas at other sites.*

RADIOGRAPHIC FINDINGS

Roentgenographs may be of considerable help in reaching a clinical or preoperative diagnosis of synovial sarcoma.

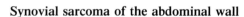

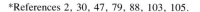

*References 2, 30, 47, 79, 88, 103, 105.

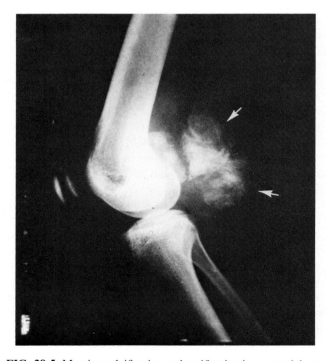

FIG. 29-5. Massive calcification and ossification in a synovial sarcoma of the popliteal fossa (arrows). In general, tumors with extensive calcification carry a better prognosis than those without.

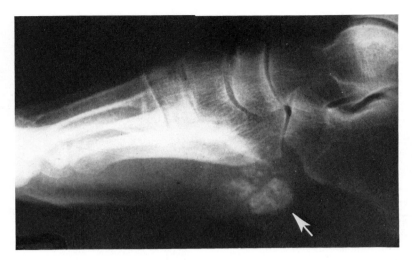

FIG. 29-6. Roentgenograph of a synovial sarcoma of the planta pedis showing extensive calcification of the tumor tissue *(arrow).*

In fact, in several of our patients a clinical diagnosis of synovial sarcoma was suggested solely on the basis of the roentgenographic examination. The majority of synovial sarcomas present on x-ray films as round or oval, more or less lobulated swellings or masses of moderate density, usually located in close proximity to a large joint. The underlying bone tends to be uninvolved, but in about 15% to 20% of the cases there is a periosteal reaction, superficial bone erosion, or invasion. Massive bone destruction is rare, and is mostly caused by poorly differentiated synovial sarcomas of long duration and large size.[20,52,116,133,134] In the Cadman et al.[14] series 10.6% of the tumors invaded the adjacent bone. Likewise, in Strickland and Mackenzie's series[134] 18 of 65 cases showed some alteration of bone, mostly pressure atrophy and periosteal proliferation.

The most striking radiological characteristic, found in 15% to 20% of synovial sarcomas, is the presence of multiple small spotty radiopacities caused by focal calcification and, less frequently, bone formation.[89,123,146,150] In most instances these changes consist merely of fine stippling, but in some cases large portions of the tumor are marked or even outlined by radiopaque masses (Figs. 29-4 to 29-6). Confusion with other tumors is possible, but radiopacities are rarely observed in liposarcoma, extraskeletal myxoid chondrosarcoma, or rhabdomyosarcoma, and their irregular contours help to distinguish them from pheboliths of hemangioma. Extraskeletal osteosarcoma is generally encountered in patients older than 50 years. Angiographic studies of synovial sarcoma usually reveal a prominent vascularity not only of the primary tumor but also of the metastases (Fig. 29-7).[108]

CT scans and MRI have become valuable tools in deter-

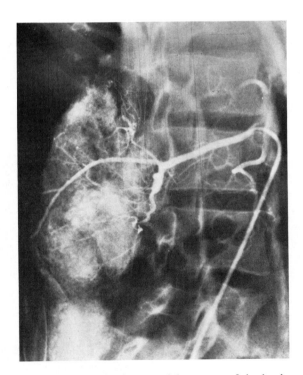

FIG. 29-7. Angiogram of a synovial sarcoma of the lumbar region displaying the prominent vascularity of synovial sarcoma as well as dense areas of calcification.

mining the site of origin and extent of the lesion. Like conventional x-rays, they show a paraarticular heterogenous septated mass, often with associated calcification or bone erosion, but do not provide a specific or diagnostic picture.[83,102]

GROSS FINDINGS

The gross appearance varies considerably depending on the rate of growth as well as the location of the tumor. Slow-growing lesions tend to be sharply circumscribed, round, or multilobular, and, as a result of compression of adjacent tissues by the expansively growing tumor, are completely or partially invested by a smooth glistening pseudocapsule. Cyst formation may be prominent, and occasional examples may present as multicystic masses (Figs. 29-8 to 29-10). Most of the tumors are firmly attached to surrounding tendons, tendon sheaths, or the exterior wall of the joint capsule, and not infrequently portions of these structures adhere to the gross specimen. On palpation they are either soft or firm, depending on their collagen content. On section they are yellow to gray-white. They may attain a size of 15 cm or more, but in the average case they measure 3 to 5 cm in greatest diameter. Very small lesions, measuring less than 1 cm in greatest dimension, are present in our material. As already mentioned, calcification is common but rarely is a discernible gross feature. Less well differentiated and more rapidly growing examples of synovial sarcoma tend to be poorly circumscribed and commonly exhibit a rather variegated and often friable or shaggy appearance, frequently with multiple areas of hemorrhage, necrosis, and cyst formation. Markedly hemorrhagic tumors have been confused for angiosarcomas or even organizing hemangiomas.

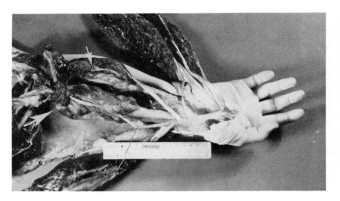

FIG. 29-8. Synovial sarcoma of the forearm in an 18-year-old male. The patient died of lung and bone metastases 1 year after treatment by amputation. Note multinodular growth of tumor along flexor tendon *(arrows).*

MICROSCOPIC FINDINGS

Unlike most other types of sarcomas, the tumor is composed of two morphologically different types of cells that form a characteristic biphasic pattern: *epithelial cells,* resembling those of carcinoma, and fibrosarcoma-like *spindle cells,* sometimes incorrectly designated as *stromal cells.* Transitional forms between epithelial and spindle cells sug-

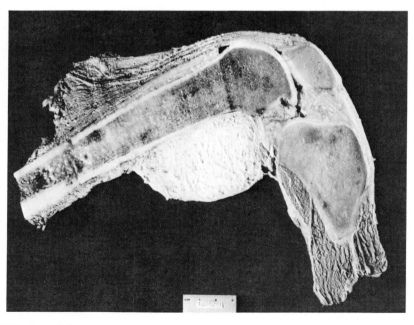

FIG. 29-9. Synovial sarcoma of the lower thigh and popliteal region, the most common single location of this neoplasm.

gest a close generic relationship, a relationship that is also supported by tissue culture, ultrastructural findings, and particularly immunohistochemical findings.[3,106] Depending on the relative prominence of the two cellular elements and the degree of differentiation, synovial sarcomas form a continuous morphological spectrum and can be broadly classified into (1) the *biphasic type,* with distinct epithelial and spindle cell components in varying proportions, (2) the *monophasic fibrous type,* (3) the rare *monophasic epithelial type,* and (4) the *poorly differentiated type.*

Biphasic synovial sarcoma

This type—the classic type of synovial sarcoma—is generally readily recognizable by the coexistence of morphologically different but histogenetically related epithelial cells and fibroblast-like spindle cells.

The epithelial cells are characterized by large, round or oval, vesicular nuclei and abundant pale-staining cytoplasm with distinctly outlined cellular borders. The cells are cuboidal to tall and columnar, and are disposed in solid cords, whorls, or nests, or they border irregular pseudoglandular, cleftlike or cystlike spaces that contain granular or homogeneous eosinophilic secretions (Figs. 29-11 to 29-14). The cleftlike spaces lined by epithelial cells must be distinguished from cleftlike artifacts that are the result of tissue shrinkage. Outpouchings of the cystlike spaces into the surrounding uninvolved tissue may wrongly suggest origin within a bursa, particularly because some of these spaces are lined by a single layer of epithelial cells bearing a close resemblance to normal synovium (Fig. 29-15).

Not infrequently cuboidal or flattened epithelial cells also cover small villous or papillary structures and bear a vague

resemblance to a papillary carcinoma. A diagnosis of squamous cell carcinoma may also be suggested by focal squamous metaplasia, including the occasional formation of squamous pearls and keratohyalin granules (Figs. 29-16 and 29-17).

The surrounding spindle cell or fibrous component consists mostly of well-oriented, rather plump, spindle-shaped cells of uniform appearance with small amounts of indistinct cytoplasm and oval dark-staining nuclei. Generally the cells form solid, compact sheets that are virtually indistinguishable from fibrosarcoma, except perhaps for the absence of long sweeping fascicles or a herringbone pattern, a more irregular nodular arrangement, a greater amount of nuclear chromatin, and fewer mitotic figures (Figs. 29-18 to 29-21). Mitotic figures in synovial sarcoma occur in both epithelial and spindle-shaped cells, but as a rule only the poorly differentiated forms of the tumor exhibit more than two mitotic figures per 1 HPF. Occasionally there is palisading of the nuclei, but in contrast to leiomyosarcomas and malignant schwannomas, this feature is confined to a tiny portion of the tumor.

Commonly the cellular portions of synovial sarcoma alternate with less cellular areas that are markedly altered by collagen deposition, myxoid change, or calcification. The collagen may be diffusely distributed and hyalinized or may form narrow bands or plaquelike masses that are associated at times with a markedly thickened basement membrane separating epithelial and spindle cell elements. The myxoid areas are generally less conspicuous and tend to occupy only a small, ill-defined portion of the tumor.[63]

Calcification with or without ossification is another diagnostically important and characteristic feature that is

Text continued on p. 769.

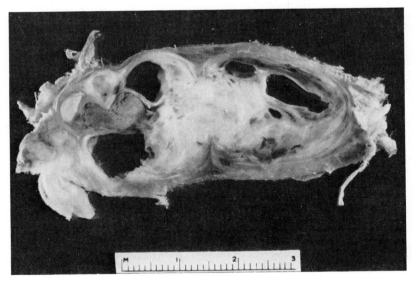

FIG. 29-10. Multicystic synovial sarcoma of the knee region.

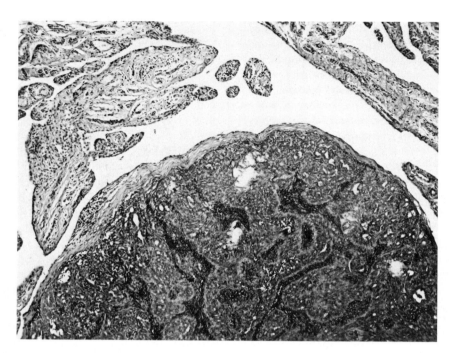

FIG. 29-11. Biphasic synovial sarcoma growing within a synovium-lined space and closely associated with synovial villi. (×45.)

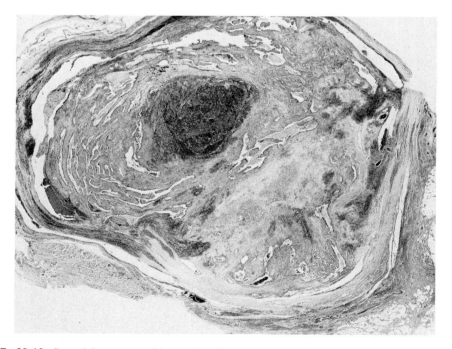

FIG. 29-12. Synovial sarcoma with a well-differentiated biphasic tumor at the periphery and a poorly differentiated tumor at the center of the neoplasm. (×9.)

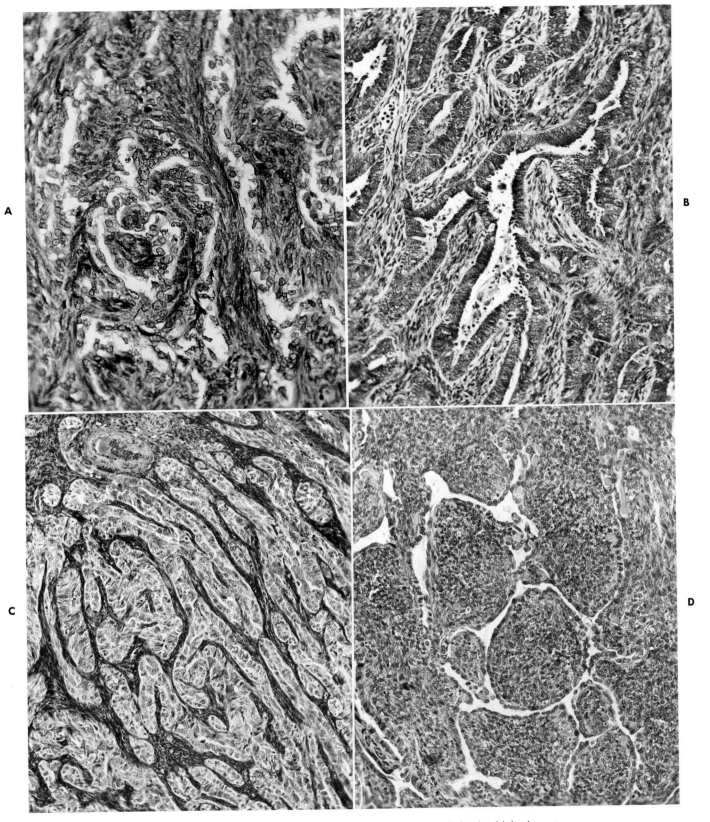

FIG. 29-13. A to **D,** Examples of typical synovial sarcomas with distinctive biphasic pattern: columnar, or cuboidal epithelial, cells surrounded by fibrosarcoma-like spindle cell elements. (**A,** ×160; **B,** ×145; **C,** ×115; **D,** ×180.)

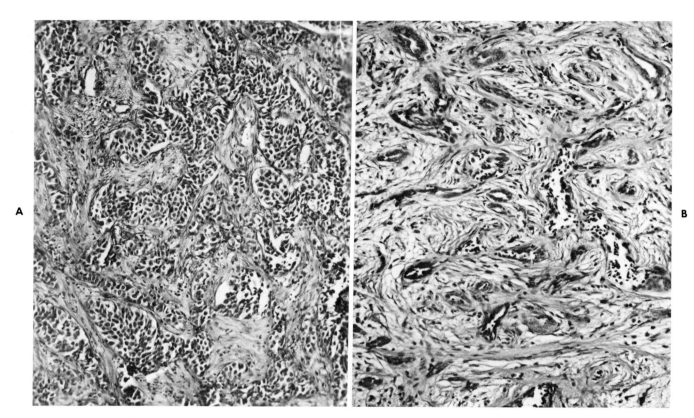

FIG. 29-14. Synovial sarcoma lacking the characteristic spindle cell component (**A**). The diagnosis or synovial sarcoma was confirmed by the presence of a distinctive biphasic pattern in other portions of the tumor (**B**). (**A**, ×110; **B**, ×160.)

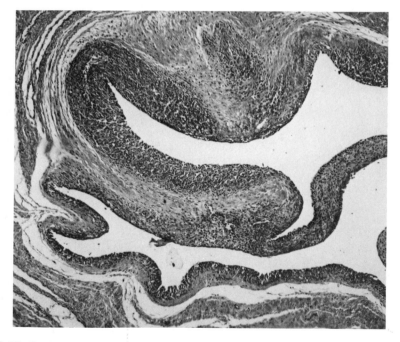

FIG. 29-15. Cystic portion of an otherwise typical biphasic synovial sarcoma. The cystic areas are part of the tumor rather than evidence of bursal origin. (×40.)

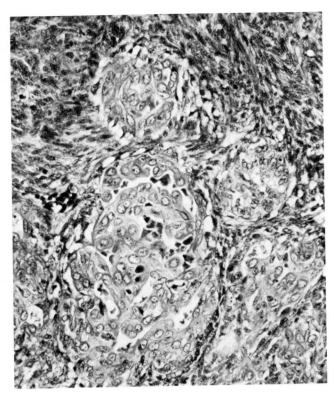

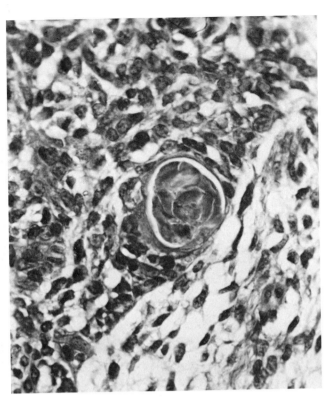

FIG. 29-16. Synovial sarcoma with biphasic pattern and focal squamous differentiation of the epithelial component. (×225.)

FIG. 29-17. Synovial sarcoma with squamous differentiation and squamous pearl formation, a rare feature of this tumor. (×250.)

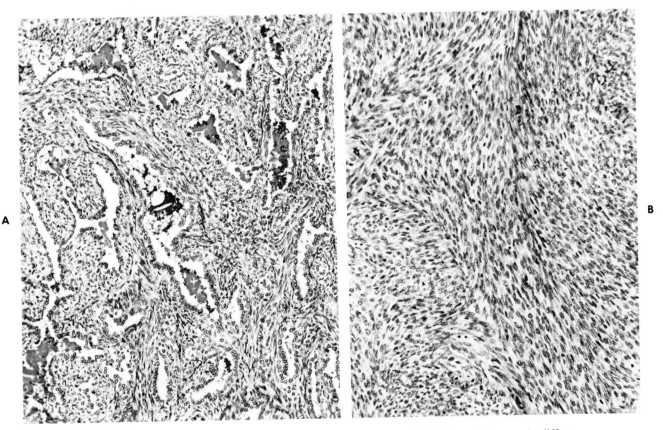

FIG. 29-18. Synovial sarcoma showing biphasic (A) and monophasic fibrous (B) areas in different portions of the same tumor. The fibrosarcomatous areas by themselves are difficult to distinguish from those of a fibrosarcoma except for cytokeratin expression in the spindle cells. (A and B, ×130.)

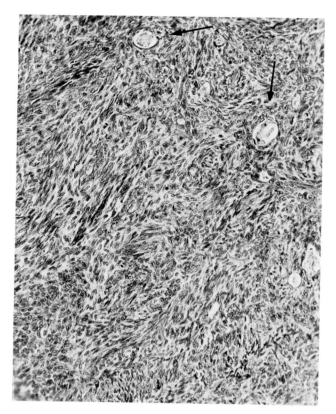

FIG. 29-19. Predominantly fibrous-type synovial sarcoma with scattered pseudoglandular structures *(arrows)*. (×130.)

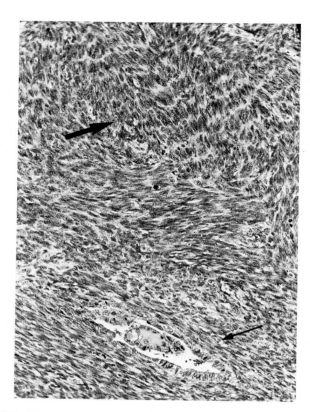

FIG. 29-20. Synovial sarcoma with foci of palisading *(thick arrow)* and pseudoglandular differentiation *(thin arrow)*. (×90.)

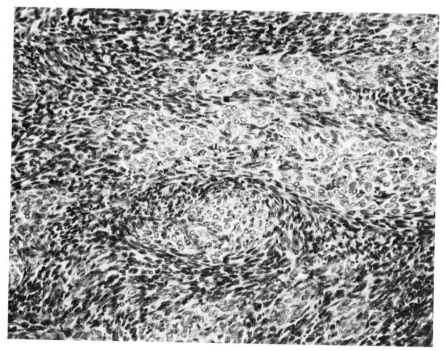

FIG. 29-21. Transition between pale-staining epithelial and dark-staining spindle cell elements in synovial sarcoma. (×160.)

present to a varying degree in about 20% of synovial sarcomas. It may be inconspicuous and consist merely of a few small irregularly distributed spherical concretions, or it may be extensive and occupy a large portion of the neoplasm.[96,123,146] In general, calcification is preceded by hyalinization and is more pronounced at the periphery of the tumor than at its center. Rarely chondroid changes are present, nearly always together with focal calcification and ossification (Figs. 29-22 to 29-26).

Mast cells are yet another typical feature of synovial sarcoma; they show no particular arrangement but are more numerous in the spindle cell than in the epithelial portions of the neoplasm. Inflammatory elements and multinucleated giant cells are rare, although Wright[149] and Geiler[39] describe giant cell forms of synovial sarcoma.

The degree of vascularity varies: in some cases it is a dominant feature and there are numerous dilated vascular spaces resembling hemangiopericytoma; in others there are merely a few scattered vascular structures. Vascular invasion is not uncommon and constitutes a prognostically unfavorable sign. Secondary changes such as hemorrhage are most prominent in poorly differentiated tumors. Scattered lipid macrophages, siderophages, multinucleated giant cells, and deposits of cholesterol may be present but are much less conspicuous in synovial sarcoma than in synovitis (Figs. 29-27 and 29-28).

Monophasic fibrous synovial sarcoma

The monophasic fibrous form of synovial sarcoma is a relatively common neoplasm, the existence of which has been confirmed not only by the presence of tumors with only a minute focus of epithelial differentiation but also by positive immunostaining of some or most of the spindle cells for keratin and epithelial membrane antigen (Figs. 29-29 to 29-32 and 29-43) and by ultrastructural features, such as occasional intercellular spaces with filopodia.[67] Since this type is closely related to the biphasic type and merely represents one extreme of its morphological spectrum, the discussed morphological parameters of the spindle cell portion of the biphasic type, such as cellular appearance, hyalinization, myxoid change, mast cell infiltrate, and focal calcification, apply equally to the monophasic fibrous type.[81] There is also no evidence that the clinical manifestations of the monophasic fibrous type of synovial sarcoma differ significantly from those of the biphasic type.

Text continued on p. 774.

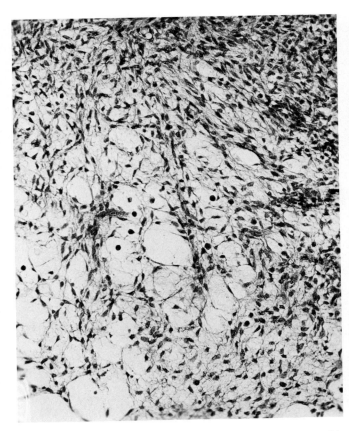

FIG. 29-22. Synovial sarcoma showing loosely textured myxoid microcystic alterations of the spindle cell areas. (×165.)

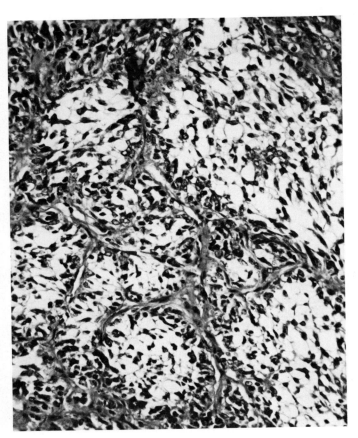

FIG. 29-23. Poorly differentiated synovial sarcoma with myxoid change in one portion of the tumor. (×250.)

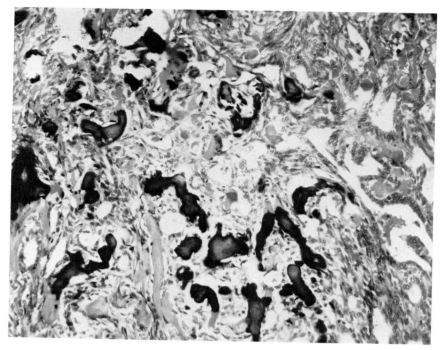

FIG. 29-24. Calcification originating from the hyalinized stroma of biphasic synovial sarcoma. (×160.)

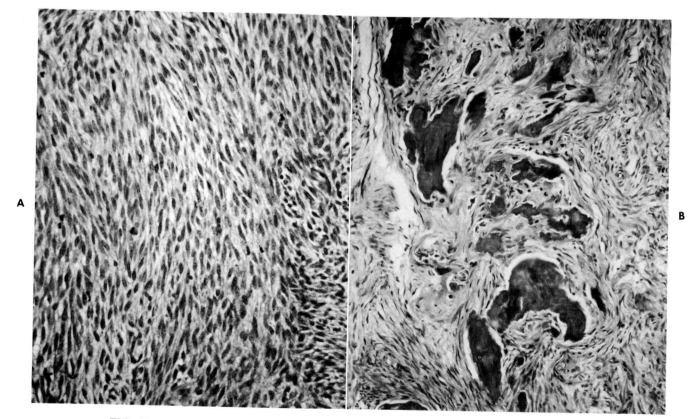

FIG. 29-25. Monophasic fibrous type of synovial sarcoma (**A**) with extensive calcification in one portion of the tumor (**B**). (**A** and **B**, ×160.)

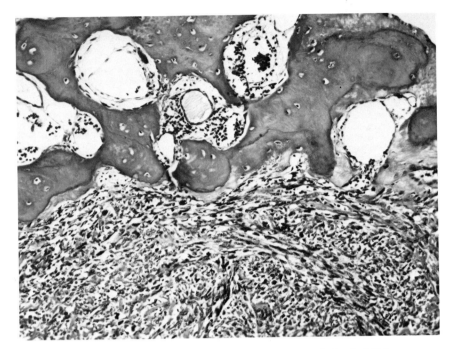

FIG. 29-26. Synovial sarcoma with osseous metaplasia. (×160.)

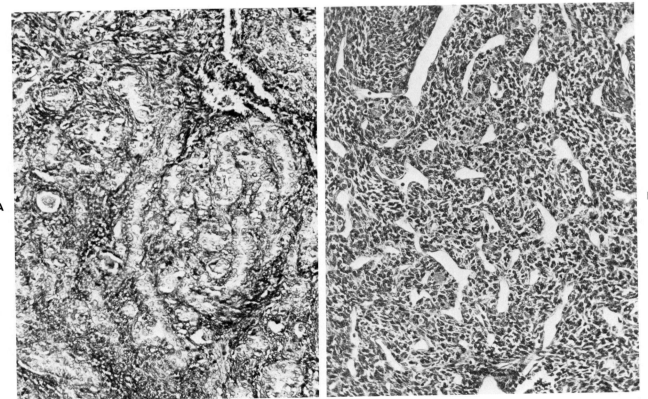

FIG. 29-27. Synovial sarcoma with biphasic **(A)** and hemangiopericytoma-like **(B)** areas, a common finding in less well-differentiated portions of this tumor. (**A** and **B**, ×165.)

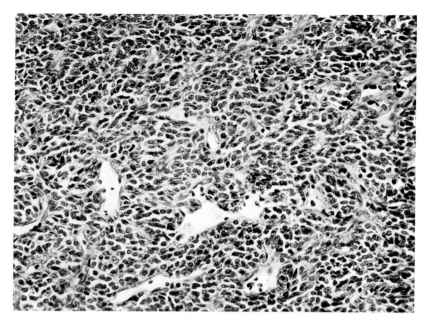

FIG. 29-28. Synovial sarcoma with distinct hemangiopericytoma pattern. (×165.)

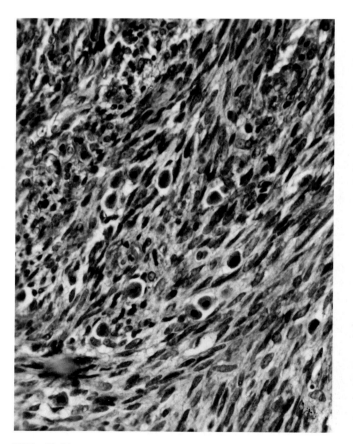

FIG. 29-29. Monophasic fibrous synovial sarcoma with prominent mast cell infiltrate confirmed by cytokeratin positivity of the tumor cells. (×160.)

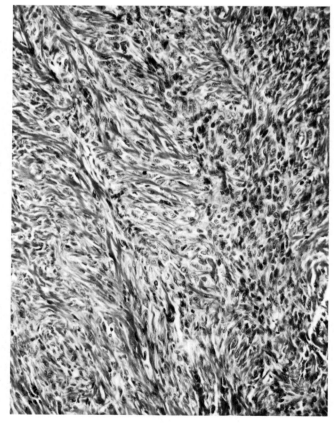

FIG. 29-30. Monophasic fibrous synovial sarcoma. (×160.)

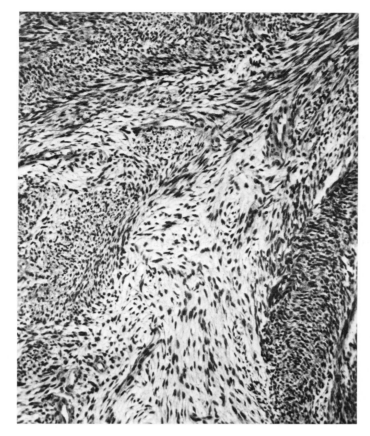

FIG. 29-31. Monophasic fibrous synovial sarcoma with myxoid change in the spindle cell areas. (×160.)

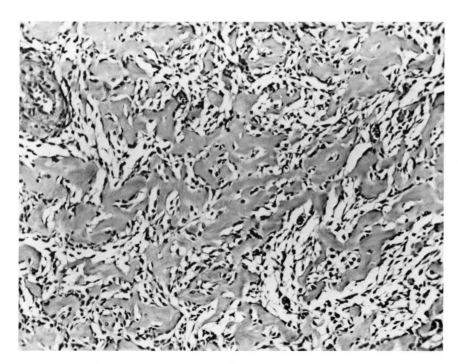

FIG. 29-32. Focal hyalinization and myxoid change in monophasic fibrous synovial sarcoma. (×140.)

Monophasic epithelial synovial sarcoma

What has been said about the diagnosis of the monophasic fibrous type of synovial sarcoma applies also to this rarely recognized neoplasm. In our experience it is often extremely difficult to render this diagnosis with any degree of certainty, especially when a host of other, more frequently occurring epithelial and mesenchymal neoplasms may display almost identical microscopic features. Differential diagnosis includes not only many metastatic and adnexal carcinomas but also malignant melanoma, malignant epithelioid schwannoma, and epithelioid sarcoma. We have encountered several likely tumors of this type, but all of these had minute foci of spindle cell differentiation, and essentially and strictly speaking were biphasic synovial sarcomas with an exceptionally prominent epithelial pattern. Farris and Reed[31] and Majeste and Beckman[84] described examples of this histological type as "monophasic glandular synovial sarcoma and carcinoma of the soft tissues" and as "synovial sarcoma with an overwhelming epithelial component," respectively. The latter tumor also displayed a distinct spindle cell pattern in a small portion of the tumor. Obviously, as with the monophasic fibrous type, other features must be weighed in making this diagnosis, such as the age of the patient, the location of the tumor, and the presence of mast cells, calcifications, and PAS-positive material within the cells or within minute intercellular spaces. It must be emphasized that neither the large size of a tumor nor its long duration and staining characteristics can be relied on to rule out metastatic carcinoma (Figs. 29-33 and 29-34).

Poorly differentiated synovial sarcoma

Drawing a sharp line between well-differentiated and poorly differentiated synovial sarcomas is for obvious reasons not always possible, but separation of these tumors is of practical importance not only because the poorly differentiated type poses a special problem in diagnosis but also because it behaves more aggressively and metastasizes in a significantly greater percentage of cases. The incidence of the poorly differentiated type among synovial sarcomas is difficult to estimate, but in one of our studies almost 20% were of this type.[28] Microscopically they are largely composed of solidly packed oval or spindle-shaped cells of small size that seem to be intermediate in appearance between epithelial and spindle cells, often with very little evidence of differentiation, simulating small cell carcinoma or angiosarcoma. There are also cases with well-differentiated and poorly differentiated areas in the same neoplasm (see Figs. 29-12 and 29-27). Recognition is based on the presence of occasional, sometimes rather vague biphasic areas that may be discernible only with the help of reticulin and immunohistochemical preparations and the presence of a richly vascular pattern with dilated thin-walled vascular spaces resembling those of malignant hemangiopericytoma. In fact, it appears that a high percentage of sarcomas interpreted as malignant hemangiopericytomas is actually poorly differentiated synovial sarcomas. The prominent pericytoma pattern of many of these tumors also assists in distinguishing them from neuroepithelioma or extraskeletal Ewing's sarcoma. Neuroepithelioma, in particular, may be simulated by the occasional perivascular arrangement of the tumor cells in a rosettelike manner. The cells of poorly differentiated synovial sarcoma may or may not stain positively for cytokeratin or epithelial membrane antigen (Figs. 29-35 to 29-37).

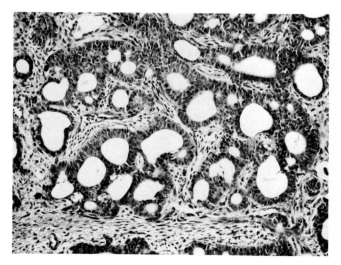

FIG. 29-33. Monophasic epithelial-type synovial sarcoma. Other portions of this tumor displayed a distinct biphasic pattern. (×160.)

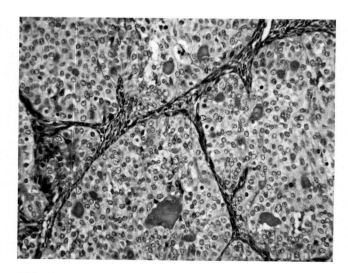

FIG. 29-34. Monophasic epithelial type of synovial sarcoma with a poorly developed spindle cell pattern. (×160.)

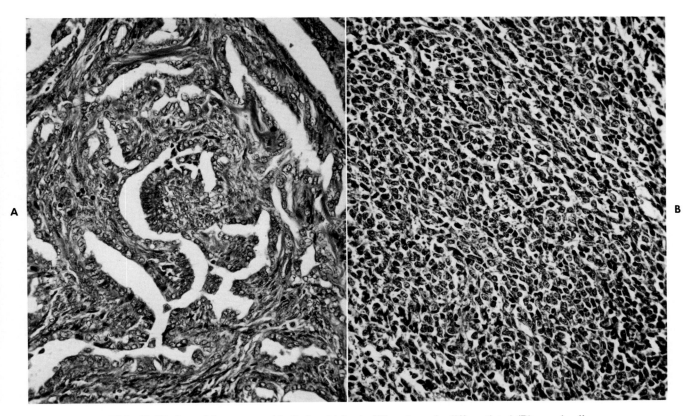

FIG. 29-35. Synovial sarcoma with distinct biphasic **(A)** and poorly differentiated **(B)** round cell areas. (×250.)

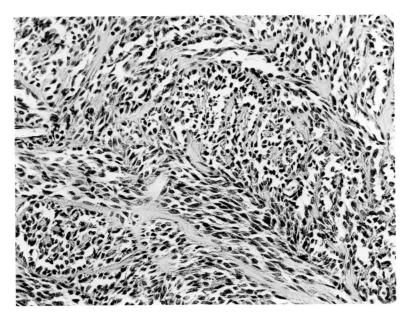

FIG. 29-36. Poorly differentiated synovial sarcoma composed of plump spindle cell elements suggesting early epithelial differentiation. (×130.)

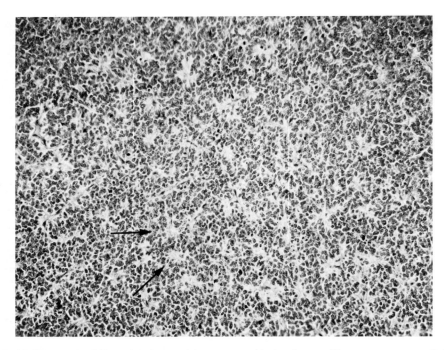

FIG. 29-37. Poorly differentiated synovial sarcoma with focal rosettelike structures superficially resembling a neuroepithelioma. The diagnosis is based on the presence of a typical biphasic pattern in another portion of this neoplasm. (×100.)

Special staining procedures

Two distinctive types of mucinous material are present in synovial sarcoma. Secretions within the epithelial cells, intracellular clefts, and pseudoglandular spaces stain positively with the PAS, colloidal iron, alcian blue, and mucicarmine stains. The staining characteristics of the mucinous secretions remain unaltered after treatment of the secretions with diastase and hyaluronidase, but in general and in distinction to adenocarcinomas, the mucinous material is more conspicuous within the intracellular clefts and pseudoglandular spaces than within the secreting epithelial cells (Fig. 29-38). Katenkamp and Stiller[61] noted that this material loses its staining ability with alcian blue at pH 5.7 and between 0.2 and 0.45 magnesium chloride concentration. Buonassisi and Ozzello,[13] using tissue cultures, identified the mucinous material as chondroitin sulfate B and heparin-related glycosaminoglycans. Nakamura et al.[107] analyzed six synovial sarcomas and found, in addition to hyaluronic acid, chondroitin sulfate, and heparatin sulfate, sialic acid in the epithelial elements. Sialic acid was absent in the spindle cell areas. In contrast to mesothelioma, granular intracellular glycogen that stains positively for PAS is never a striking feature of synovial sarcoma.

The second type of mucinous material, stromal or mesenchymal mucin, which is elaborated by the spindle cells, also stains positively for colloidal iron and alcian blue stains, but it is weakly carminophilic and stains negatively with the PAS preparation. It is present within the interstices of the spindle cell or fibrosarcoma-like areas and the loosely textured myxoid portions of the tumor. This material is rich in hyaluronic acid and, like other mesenchymal mucins, is completely removed by prior treatment of the secretions with hyaluronidase. It does not stain below 0.45 magnesium chloride concentration.[61,119] PAS and alcian blue preparations—as well as various metachromatic stains and naphthol AS-D chloroacetate esterase—are also useful in the identification of the mast cell infiltrate. Pisa et al.[114] demonstrated alkaline and acid phosphatase and ATPase in the epithelial cells, but not in the spindle cells, of synovial sarcoma.

Reticulin preparation may unmask the biphasic pattern in those tumors in which it is not clearly discernible with the hematoxylin-eosin preparation; the absence or paucity of reticulin fibers in the epithelial portions of the tumor helps to set them apart from the surrounding spindle cell areas (Figs. 29-39 to 29-41).

Immunohistochemical findings

Both the epithelial and spindle cell elements of synovial sarcoma show reactivity for low- and high-molecular-weight cytokeratins and, less intensely, for epithelial membrane antigen.[1,17-19,34,112,122] Positive immunostaining for keratin is demonstrable in nearly all biphasic synovial sarcomas and in many tumors of the monophasic fibrous type.

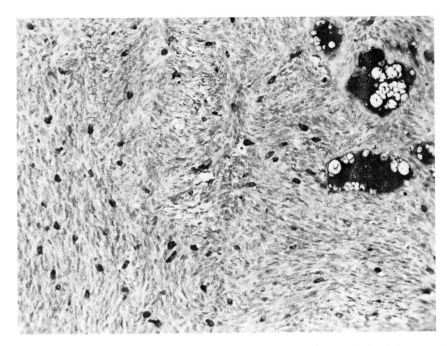

FIG. 29-38. Synovial sarcoma showing PAS-positive material in the pseudoglandular spaces and scattered PAS-positive mast cells in the spindle cell areas. The mucinous material within the pseudoglandular spaces is indistinguishable in its staining characteristics from the epithelial mucin of adenocarcinoma. (×180.)

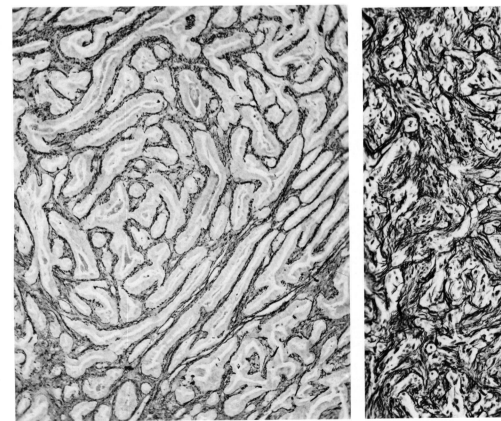

FIG. 29-39. Reticulin stain outlining the epithelial component of an unusually well-differentiated synovial sarcoma. (Same case as in Fig. 29-13, C.) (×75.)

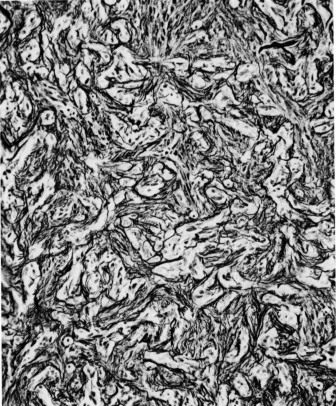

FIG. 29-40. Reticulin preparation of synovial sarcoma with sharply delineated biphasic pattern.

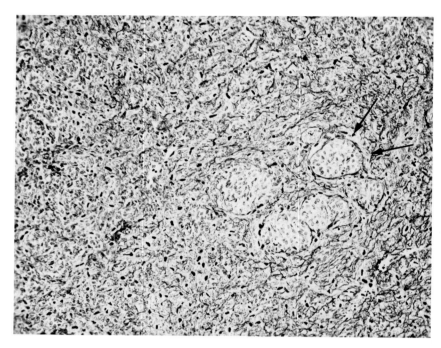

FIG. 29-41. Poorly differentiated synovial sarcoma in which the presence of a biphasic pattern is unmasked by the reticulin stain. (×120.)

The keratin polypeptides have a wide range of varying specificity: according to Miettinen,[91] synovial sarcoma shares keratin 8 and 18 with other spindle cell sarcomas, but keratin 7 and 19 and desmoplakin seem to be specific to this tumor. The intensity of staining is more pronounced in the epithelial than the spindle cell component, and is greatly improved by prior trypsinization of the sections; sometimes, especially in tumors of the monophasic type, only a few isolated cells may express the antigen, making it necessary to stain and examine multiple sections from different portions of the tumor[45,92,93,138] (Figs. 29-42 and 29-43). Vimentin is readily demonstrable in the spindle cells but is usually absent in the epithelial cells. Normal nonneoplastic synovial cells and the cells of tenosynovial giant cell tumor (nodular tenosynovitis) stain for vimentin but not for keratin or epithelial membrane antigen. Synovial sarcoma may also stain for Leu-7[1] and S-100 protein.[35,126]

Ultrastructural findings

The biphasic tumors are composed of epithelial and spindle cells with transitional forms between the two cell types. The epithelial cells have sharply defined ovoid nuclei with narrow and dense rims of chromatin and abundant cytoplasm containing mitochondria, a prominent Golgi complex, rare paranuclear aggregates of intermediate filaments, lysosomes, and smooth and rough endoplasmic reticulum, sometimes arranged in stacked arrays. On rare occasions tonofilaments are found in the epithelial cells, especially in

the areas of squamous metaplasia. Frequently, the epithelial cells are disposed in clusters or glandlike structures, with microvilli or villous filopodia on the surfaces facing the intercellular or pseudoglandular spaces. Many of the spaces contain electron-dense mucinous material. In contrast to the cells of normal synovium, the epithelial cells are interconnected by junctional complexes, zonulae adherentes, or desmosome-like structures. The fibroblast-like spindle cells have irregularly outlined nuclei, marginated chromatin, and small nucleoli. The cytoplasm contains mitochondria and a prominent Golgi apparatus, but there is less cytoplasm and a less well-developed rough endoplasmic reticulum than that of typical fibroblasts. A continuous basal lamina, a structure that is absent in normal synovium, often separates the epithelial clusters and glandlike structures from the surrounding spindle-shaped cells* (Fig. 29-44).

The ultrastructural features of the monophasic fibrous type are indistinguishable from those of the spindle cell areas of the biphasic type. There are, however, identifying features of early epithelial differentiation, such as intercellular or cleftlike spaces of varying size bordered by multiple microvilli, as well as poorly developed junctions or desmosome-like structures. In addition, there are occasional cell clusters similar to those seen in the biphasic type. There is no distinct basal lamina but there are occasional frag-

---

*References 8, 26, 38, 64, 78, 80, 98, 115, 125, 140.

ments of basal lamina or condensed ground substance at the cell surfaces.[25,34,67,90] Tsuneyoshi et al.[143] described the presence of membrane-bound secretory granules and tubulated bodies containing filamentous structures.

Cytogenetic findings

The chromosome pattern may be helpful in identifying the tumor. According to Turc-Carel et al.[145] and oth-

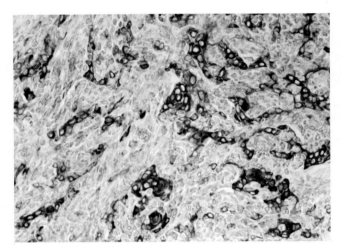

FIG. 29-42. Biphasic synovial sarcoma showing immunostaining for keratin in most of the epithelial cells and occasional spindle cells. (×160.)

ers,[22,24,65,77] the cells of synovial sarcoma show a characteristic balanced translocation between chromosomes X and 18, t(X;18)(p11.2;q11.2) in the majority of cases. The translocation is usually the only abnormality, and occurs in synovial sarcomas of both the biphasic and monophasic fibrous type, as well as in poorly differentiated synovial sarcomas.

DIFFERENTIAL DIAGNOSIS

Separating synovial sarcoma from other neoplasms may be difficult, and in some instances a reliable diagnosis is not possible without immunohistochemical examination. In general, biphasic types of synovial sarcoma cause few problems in diagnosis, especially if the tumor, like most synovial sarcomas, is located in the extremities near a large joint and occurs in a young adult.

Epithelioid sarcoma has an age incidence similar to that of synovial sarcoma and similar ultrastructural features, but most of these tumors occur in the hand or forearm, either in the dermis or in association with tendons, often with ulceration of the overlying skin. In general the tumors show a distinct multinodular pattern with central necrosis of the tumor nodules and deep eosinophilia of the tumor cells. Unlike synovial sarcoma there is neither intracellular mucin formation nor a clear demarcation between epithelial and spindle cells. Both epithelial and spindle cells, however, stain for cytokeratin and vimentin, and there is a close ultrastructural resemblance between these tumors.[37] In fact, Schiffman[124] reported the occurrence of epithelioid sarcoma

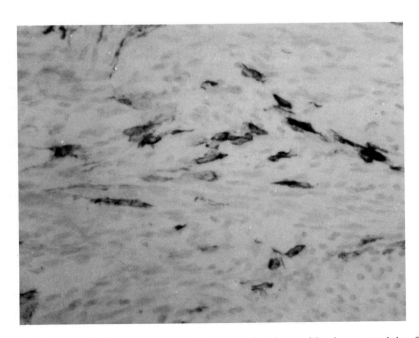

FIG. 29-43. Monophasic fibrous-type synovial sarcoma showing positive immunostaining for keratin in the spindle cells. (×250.)

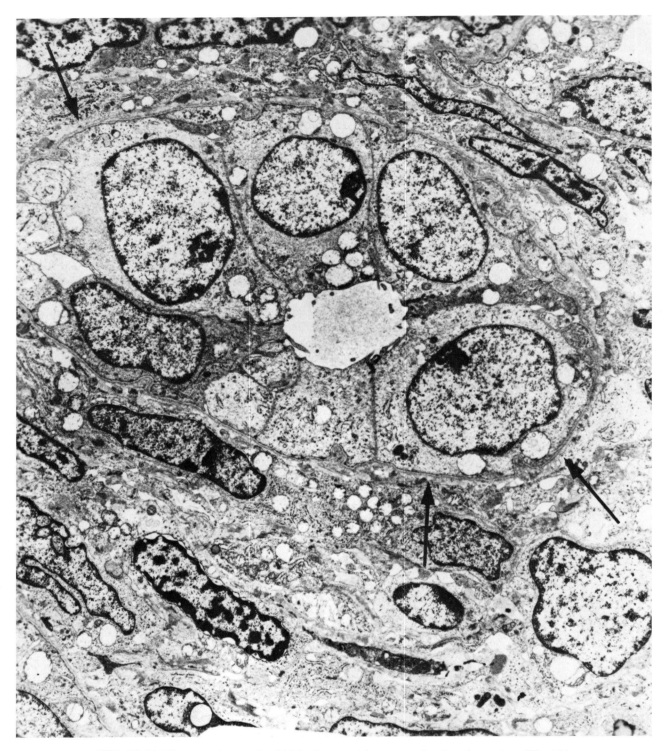

FIG. 29-44. Electron micrograph of biphasic synovial sarcoma showing short microvilli within the small pseudoglandular space and separation of the epithelial and fibroblast-like spindle cell elements by a distinct basal lamina *(arrows)*. (Courtesy Dr. R.F. Armstrong, Victoria Hospital, London, Canada.)

and synovial sarcoma in the same knee (see Chapter 38).

Clear cell sarcoma (malignant melanoma of soft parts) is recognizable by its nestlike pattern, pale-staining nuclei with prominent nucleoli, occasional multinucleated giant cells, and, in most cases, abundant intracellular glycogen. The cells do not stain for cytokeratin but in the majority of cases contain cells that stain for S-100 protein and melanin. Premelanosomes are usually demonstrable ultrastructurally.

Malignant peripheral nerve sheath tumor (malignant schwannoma) may bear a close resemblance to the monophasic fibrous type of synovial sarcoma, but there is no evidence that synovial sarcoma arises in a large nerve or neurofibroma or in a patient with neurofibromatosis. *Glandular malignant peripheral nerve sheath tumor (glandular malignant schwannoma)*, a very rare neoplasm, usually can be recognized by the presence of intestinal-type epithelium with goblet cells, the occasional association with rhabdomyosarcomatous elements (Triton tumor), and the occurrence in patients with manifestations of neurofibromatosis. S-100 protein preparations do not help in differential diagnosis, since cells positive for S-100 protein are occasionally also encountered in the spindle cell portions of synovial sarcomas.

Monophasic fibrous synovial sarcoma can be distinguished from *fibrosarcoma* by its frequent location near large joints, its irregular and often multilobular growth pattern, the plump appearance of the nuclei, and the focal whorled arrangement of the spindle cells. In general, mitotic figures are less common than in fibrosarcoma. Additional factors suggesting synovial sarcoma are the presence of mast cells, foci of calcification, and, most importantly, the demonstration of cytokeratin in the tumor cells.

Distinction of purely epithelial forms of synovial sarcoma from *adnexal or metastatic carcinoma* is virtually impossible in the absence of a focal biphasic pattern. Fortunately, most of these tumors, when carefully sampled, have focal spindle cell areas that are sufficiently characteristic to allow a specific diagnosis. *Eccrine spiradenoma* and other forms of adnexal tumors, *carcinosarcoma*, and various types of *metastatic carcinomas* have also been mistaken for biphasic synovial sarcoma.

DISCUSSION
Recurrence and metastasis

Although recent achievements in therapy have lowered the incidence of recurrence and metastasis, the overall long-term outlook of synovial sarcoma is still rather bleak, and depends largely on the type of therapy. As one would expect, the outlook is poorest in cases treated merely by local excision with inadequate margins and without any supplementary therapy. In these cases, recurrence rates as high as 70% and 83%[4,89] are given. With more adequate surgical excision or with adjunctive radiotherapy the recurrence rates range from as low as 28%[82] to 36%.[28] Patients with more than one recurrence are not rare, and among our cases there are some with four, five, and even six recurrences over a period of several years.

Although the recurrent growth usually manifests within the first 2 years after initial therapy, this is not true in all instances. Among synovial sarcomas that we have seen on consultation, there were no less than eight that recurred more than 10 years after the first treatment, including three with recurrent growth at 15, 17, and 21 years. Likewise, Sutro[139] observed a synovial sarcoma that recurred after 35 years.

Metastatic lesions develop in about half of cases, but many make their appearance many years after the initial diagnosis. As in other types of sarcoma, the principal sites of metastasis are the lung, followed by the lymph nodes and the bone marrow. In our cases[28] the lung was involved in 94% of patients with metastasis and the lymph nodes in 21%; similarly, in the series of Ryan et al.,[121] the lung was affected in 94% of cases and the lymph nodes in 10%.

There are numerous accounts of late metastasis, as well as long periods of survival after metastasis. At the AFIP there are cases in which lung metastases appeared as late as 15 and 17 years after the initial therapy and cases in which the patient survived 10 years or more after evidence of metastasis was first noted. Thunold and Bang[141] observed a woman who had a calcified synovial sarcoma removed at age 14 years and developed lung metastasis 26 years later at age 40 years. On the other hand, there are rare instances in which pulmonary metastasis is already present at the time of or prior to the initial diagnosis. Microscopically, the metastatic lesions are largely similar to the primary neoplasm, but metastases of biphasic tumors often exhibit a more prominent spindle cell pattern than the primary lesion, a lesser degree of cellular differentiation, and increased mitotic activity.

Prognosis

Reported 5-year survival rates of synovial sarcoma range from 36%[41] to 64%[45] and 82% in heavily calcified tumors (Table 29-2); 10-year survival rates range from 20%[111] to 38%.[132] The differences in the 5- and 10-year survival rates reflect the relatively high incidence of late metastases.

Features influencing prognosis

Several clinical and microscopic factors influence the length of survival. Major clinical factors associated with a more favorable clinical course are young age of the patient (15 years or younger), tumor size smaller than 5 cm, and distal rather than proximal location in the extremities.[132] Earlier detection and therapy may explain the better prognosis of patients with pain[113] and tumors located in the head and neck region.[118]

There is still no agreement as to the prognostic signifi-

Table 29-2. Synovial sarcoma: reported 5-year survival rates

Authors	Percent
Varela-Duran and Enzinger (1982)*	82
Tsuneyoshi et al. (1983)	51
Soule (1986)	55
Golouh et al. (1990)	64
Schmidt et al. (1991)†	63
Oda et al. (1993)	54

*Heavily calcified synovial sarcomas.

†Synovial sarcomas of children and adolescents (7-year survival rates).

Table 29-3. Synovial sarcoma*

Favorable prognostic factors
  Young age (<15 years)
  Distal limb
  Tumor smaller than 5 cm
  Biphasic histological pattern (?)
  Marked calcification and ossification
  Euploidy
Unfavorable prognostic factors
  Older than 20 years
  Proximal limb
  Large tumor size (5 cm or larger)
  Monophasic fibrous pattern (?)
  Poorly differentiated pattern
  High mitotic rate (>10/10 HPF)
  High nuclear grade
  Aneuploidy
  Extensive necrosis
  Vascular invasion
  Marginal excision

*References 11, 27-29, 45, 111, 117, 151.

cance of the microscopic subtype. In some studies[28,82,126] there is virtually no difference between predominantly epithelial and spindle cell tumors, but most record a worse prognosis for tumors of the monophasic fibrous type.* Oda et al.[111] add rhabdoid cells and a high nuclear grade as unfavorable factors. Synovial sarcomas with extensive calcification and ossification seem to fare best, and of 32 such cases in our material, 82% of the patients survived 5 years.[146] Prognosis is least favorable for the poorly differentiated (small cell) type of synovial sarcoma. There is little information in regard to DNA analysis, but El-Naggar et al.[27] found 67% of 46 synovial sarcomas to be diploid and 33% aneuploid. Patients with diploid neoplasms had a significant survival advantage over those with aneuploid tumors. In our series there is also an inverse correlation between survival rates and mitotic activity, incidence of necrosis, and vascular invasion. This was also noted by others,[98,117] who concluded that survival rates were significantly lower in patients with tumors having a high mitotic rate (more than 10 or 15 mitoses per 10 HPF) and extensive tumor necrosis (Table 29-3).

Therapy

There is no general agreement as to the best type of therapy. Simple local excision without ancillary therapy, however, is clearly incapable of checking the growth and spread of the tumor; consequently, most reviewers recommend prompt drastic surgical measures as the therapy of choice. These include radical local excision, often with removal of an entire muscle or muscle group, and amputation, depending mainly on the size of the tumor and its location. Because radical local excision is often impossible with tumors situated near a large joint—the favored location of synovial sarcoma—adjunctive radiotherapy, in addition to local excision of the tumor, is favored over amputation.[62] Suit et al.,[136,137] using high dosages of cobalt or electron-beam radiation, reported that 10 of 15 synovial sarcomas did not

*References 11, 29, 45, 101, 143, 151.

exhibit local, regional, or distant growth 24 months or more after therapy, even after simple excision of the neoplasm. Excision and radiotherapy seem to be particularly suitable for neoplasms of small size, but amputation may still be the optimal therapy for very large and otherwise unresectable synovial sarcomas.

Radiation of regional lymph nodes is preferable to resection, but it should be limited to those cases with clear evidence of lymph node enlargement. Shiu et al.[128] reported a 35% 5-year survival rate with wedge or segmental resection of solitary or multiple pulmonary metastases. There is still inadequate information as to the efficacy of present-day chemotherapy in the treatment of synovial sarcomas. Ryan et al.[121] report a 50% complete or partial response rate to chemotherapy of metastatic synovial sarcomas, but emphasize that the response was of short duration, with recurrence of metastases within less than 1 year. Nonetheless, in prognostically unfavorable cases of synovial sarcoma, multidrug chemotherapy may be attempted in the hope of preventing or suppressing metastases. There is no evidence that therapy influences the morphological picture.

DIFFERENTIATION

There is still considerable debate as to the exact line of differentiation. The cells of synovial sarcoma differ in several aspects from normal synovium, and synovial sarcoma is not known to ever arise within a benign synovial lesion such as villonodular synovitis, giant cell tumor of tendon sheath, or benign synovioma. In fact, benign biphasic synovioma, if it exists, must be an exceedingly rare neoplasm that is difficult to distinguish from an early and extremely well-differentiated synovial sarcoma or an unusual form of adnexal tumor.

Potential sources of synovial sarcoma are (1) normal non-neoplastic synovium of joints, tendon sheaths, or bursae, (2) specialized forms of mesenchymal tissue (so-called arthrogenous mesenchyme); or (3) primitive mesenchyme or ordinary fibrous connective tissue analogue to the synovial membrane formation in traumatic or occupational bursae (synovial metaplasia). Points *in favor of* origin from preformed synovium—or arthrogenous mesenchyme—are the long-established predilection of synovial sarcomas for the vicinity of large joints, an area where the majority of tendon sheaths and bursal structures are congregated, and the undeniable microscopic resemblance between tumor tissue and normal and hyperplastic synovium. In this regard it is also of interest that epithelial transformation of human synovial tissue was observed in tissue culture,[17] and that Ghadially and Roy[43] were able to produce synovial sarcoma–like neoplasms in rats with injections of 9,10-dimethyl-1,2-benzanthracene (DMBA) into the joint cavity. Evidence *against* origin from preformed synovial cells, however, is the relative scarcity of synovial sarcomas within joint cavities[32,87] and the presence of these tumors in locations in which normal synovial structures are rare or nonexistent, as in the tonsillar fossa, parapharyngeal region, and abdominal wall. Origin in a synovial bursa has been recorded,[23] but it is not always easy to distinguish between a synovial sarcoma arising within a preformed bursa and a well-differentiated synovial sarcoma having a well-differentiated multicystic pattern. Objections against origin from the synovial lining cells have also been raised on histochemical and ultrastructural grounds. Normal, nonneo-plastic, synovial and subsynovial cells (1) react only with vimentin but not with cytokeratin or epithelial membrane antigens, (2) display different cytoplasmic bindings for lectins, and (3) lack, under the electron microscope, microvilli or filopodia, tight junctions, or demosome-like structures and basal lamina.[8,18,19,42,95] In fact, on the strength of these findings some reviewers believe that the term *synovial sarcoma* should be abandoned and the terms *connective tissue carcinosarcoma* or *soft tissue carcinoma* used instead.[23,42,95] This uncertainty as to the exact line of differentiation is also reflected in the new edition of the World Health Organization Soft Tissue Classification, in which synovial sarcoma is placed among the "miscellaneous soft tissue tumors."

Although the final answer to this question is still pending, it is conceivable and even likely that synovial sarcoma, like most other types of malignant mesenchymal tumors, arises from primitive mesenchyme, or so-called arthrogenous mesenchyme, rather than preformed synovial cells in an environment that induces or promotes epithelial cellular differentiation reminiscent but not typical of functioning synovial tissue. For this reason, and in view of the fact that at least 90% of synovial sarcomas arise near a large joint, it seems best to retain for the time being the conventional term *synovial sarcoma*.

Except for the S-100 positivity of some synovial sarcomas and the spindle cell pattern there is very little that would give support to neural origin of synovial sarcoma, as suggested by Ichinose et al.[53-55] The frequent history of pain and the rare attachment of synovial sarcoma to a large nerve may very well be due to the predilection of this tumor for the periarticular areas of the extremities.

REFERENCES

1. Abenoza P, Manivel JC, Swanson PE, et al: Synovial sarcoma: Ultrastructural study and immunohistochemical analysis by a combined peroxidase-antiperoxidase/avitin-biotin-peroxidase complex procedure. *Hum Pathol* 17:1107, 1986.
2. Al-Dewachi HS, Sangai BC, Zakaria MA: Synovial sarcoma of the abdominal wall: a case report and study of its fine structure. *J Surg Oncol* 18:335, 1981.
3. Alvarez-Fernandez E, Escalona-Zapata J: Monophasic mesenchymal synovial sarcoma: its identification by tissue culture. *Cancer* 47:628, 1981.
4. Amble FR, Olsen KD, Nascimento AG, et al: Head and neck synovial sarcoma. *Otolaryngol Head Neck Surg* 107:631, 1992.
5. Amr SS, Shihabi NK, Al Hajj H: Synovial sarcoma of the esophagus. *Am J Otolaryngol* 5:266, 1984.
6. Ariel IM, Pack GT: Synovial sarcoma. Review of 25 cases. *N Engl J Med* 268:1272, 1963.
7. Attie JN, Steckler RM, Platt N: Cervical synovial sarcoma. *Cancer* 25:758, 1970.
8. Barland P, Novikoff AB: Electron microscopy of human synovial membrane. *J Cell Biol* 14:207, 1962.
9. Batsakis JG, Nishiyama RH, Sullinger GD: Synovial sarcomas of the neck. *Arch Otolaryngol* 85:327, 1967.
10. Berkheiser SW: Synovioma-like tumor (synovial sarcoma) of the abdominal wall: report of a case. *Ann Surg* 135:114, 1952.
11. Buck P, Mickelson MR, Bonfiglio M: Synovial sarcoma: a review of 33 cases. *Clin Orthop* 156:211, 1981.
12. Bukachevsky RP, Pincus RL, Shechtman FG, et al: Synovial sarcoma of the head and neck. *Head Neck* 14:44, 1992.
13. Buonassisi V, Ozzello L: Sulfated mucopolysaccharide reproduction by synovial sarcoma cells in vivo and in tissue culture. *Cancer Res* 33:874, 1973.
14. Cadman NL, Soule EH, Kelly PJ: Synovial sarcoma: an analysis of 134 tumors. *Cancer* 18:613, 1965.
15. Cagle LA, Mirra JM, Storm FK, et al: Histologic features relating to prognosis in synovial sarcoma. *Cancer* 59:1810, 1987.
16. Cameron HU, Kostuik JP: A long-term follow-up of synovial sarcoma. *J Bone Joint Surg* 56B:613, 1974.
17. Castor CW, Prince RK, Dorstewitz EL: "Epithelial transformation" of human synovial connective tissue cell. Cytologic and biochemical consequences. *Proc Soc Exp Biol* 108:574, 1961.
18. Corson JM, Weiss LM, Banks-Schlegel SP, et al: Keratin proteins and carcinoembryonic antigen in synovial sarcomas: an immunohistochemical study of 24 cases. *Hum Pathol* 15:615, 1984.
19. Corson JM, Weiss LM, Banks-Schlegel SP, et al: Keratin proteins in synovial sarcoma. *Am J Surg Pathol* 7:107, 1983.

20. Craig RM, Pugh DG, Soule EH: The roentgenologic manifestations of synovial sarcoma. *Radiology* 65:837, 1955.

21. Crocker DW, Stout AP: Synovial sarcoma in children. *Cancer* 12:1123, 1959.

22. Dal Cin P, Rao U, Jani-Sait S, et al: Chromosomes in the diagnosis of soft tissue tumors. I. Synovial sarcoma. *Mod Pathol* 5:357, 1992.

23. Dardick I, Ramjohn S, Thomas MJ, et al: Synovial sarcoma: interrelationship of the biphasic and monophasic subtypes. *Pathol Res Pract* 187:871, 1991.

24. DeLeeuw B, Berger W, Sinke RJ, et al: Identification of a yeast artificial chromosome (YAC) spanning the synovial sarcoma-specific t(x;18)(p11.2;q11.2) breakpoint. *Genes Chromosom Cancer* 6:182, 1993.

25. Dickersin GR: Synovial sarcoma: a review and update, with emphasis on the ultrastructural characterization of the nonglandular component. *Ultrastruct Pathol* 15:379, 1991.

26. Dische FE, Darby AJ, Howard ER: Malignant synovioma: electron microscopical findings in three patients and review of the literature. *J Pathol* 124:149, 1978.

27. El-Naggar AK, Ayala AG, Abdul-Karim FW, et al: Synovial sarcoma. A DNA flow cytometric study. *Cancer* 65:2295, 1990.

28. Enzinger FM: Recent trends in soft tissue pathology. In *Tumors of bone and soft tissue.* Eighth Annual Clinical Conference on Cancer, 1963. University of Texas M.D. Anderson Hospital and Tumor Institute. Chicago, 1965, Year Book Medical Publishers, pp 315-332.

29. Evans HL: Synovial sarcoma: a study of 23 biphasic and 17 probable monophasic examples. *Pathol Annu* 15:309, 1980.

30. Faerber EN, Leonidas JC, Bhan I: Synovial sarcoma of the anterior abdominal wall. *Mt Sinai J Med* (NY) 51:705, 1984.

31. Farris KB, Reed RJ: Monophasic, glandular, synovial sarcomas and carcinomas of the soft tissues. *Arch Pathol Lab Med* 106:129, 1982.

32. Fetsch JF, Meis JM: Intraarticular synovial sarcoma. Personal communication, 1993.

33. Fetsch JF, Meis JM: Synovial sarcoma of the abdominal wall. *Cancer* 72:469, 1993.

34. Fisher C: Synovial sarcoma: Ultrastructural and immunohistochemical features of epithelial differentiation in monophasic and biphasic tumors. *Hum Pathol* 17:996, 1986.

35. Fisher C, Schofield JB: S-100 protein positive synovial sarcoma. *Histopathology* 19:375, 1991.

36. Fisher RM, Spiro OC: Cervical synovial sarcoma in a young boy. *S Afr Med J* 48:2181, 1974.

37. Gabbiani G, Fu YS, Kaye GI et al: Epithelioid sarcoma: a light and electron microscopic study suggesting a synovial origin. *Cancer* 30:486, 1972.

38. Gabbiani G, Kaye GI, Lattes R, et al: Synovial sarcoma: electron microscopic study of a typical case. *Cancer* 28:1031, 1971.

39. Geiler G: *Die Synovialome: Morphologie und Pathogenese.* Berlin, 1961, Springer-Verlag.

40. Geiler G: Gelenktumoren, in Spezielle pathologische Anatomie. Doerr W, Seifert G., vol. 18, Berlin-Heidelberg, 1984, Springer Verlag, pp 647.

41. Gerner RE, Moore G: Synovial sarcoma. *Ann Surg* 181:22, 1975.

42. Ghadially FN: Is synovial sarcoma a carcinosarcoma of connective tissue? *Ultrastruct Pathol* 11:147, 1987.

43. Ghadially FN, Roy S: Experimentally produced synovial sarcomas. *Cancer* 19:1901, 1966.

44. Golomb HM, Gorny J, Powell W, et al: Cervical synovial sarcoma at the bifurcation of the carotid artery. *Cancer* 35:483, 1975.

45. Golouh R, Vuzevski V, Bracko M, et al: Synovial sarcoma: a clinicopathologic study of 36 cases. *J Surg Oncol* 45:20, 1990.

46. Hajdu SI, Shiu MH, Fortner JG: Tendosynovial sarcoma: a clinicopathological study of 136 cases. *Cancer* 39:1201, 1977.

47. Hale JE, Calder I: Synovial sarcoma of the abdominal wall. *Br J Cancer* 24:471, 1970.

48. Hamperl H: Malignes Synovialom und Trauma. *Zentralbl Chir* 94:889, 1969.

49. Hampole MK, Jackson BA: Analysis of 25 cases of malignant synovioma. *Can Med Assoc J* 99:1025, 1968.

50. Harrison EG, Marden-Black B, Devine KD: Synovial sarcoma primary in the neck. *Arch Pathol* 71:137, 1961.

51. Holtz F, Magielski JE: Synovial sarcomas of the tongue base: the seventh reported case. *Arch Otolaryngol* 111:271, 1985.

52. Horowitz AL, Resnick D, Watson RC: The roentgen features of synovial sarcomas. *Clin Radiol* 24:481, 1973.

53. Ichinose H, Derbes VJ, Hoerner HE: Cutaneous pain without tumor: a manifestation of occult synovioma. *Cutis* 21:74, 1978.

54. Ichinose H, Hoerner HE, Derbes VJ: Minute synovial sarcoma in the occult nonpalpable phase. A case report. *J Bone Joint Surg* 60A:836, 1978.

55. Ichinose H, Powell L, Hoerner HE, et al: The potential histogenetic relationship of the peripheral nerve to synovioma. *Cancer Res* 39:4270, 1979.

56. Israels SJ, Chan HS, Daneman A, et al: Synovial sarcoma in childhood. *AJR Am J Roentgenol* 142:803, 1984.

57. Jacobs LA, Weaver AW: Synovial sarcoma of the head and neck. *Am J Surg* 128:527, 1974.

58. Jaffe HL, Lichtenstein L: Synovial sarcoma (synovioma). *Bull Hosp Joint Dis* 2:3, 1941.

59. Jernstrom P: Synovial sarcoma of the pharynx. *Am J Clin Pathol* 24:957, 1954.

60. Joensson G: Malignant tumors of the skeletal muscles, fasciae, joint capsules, tendon sheaths, and serous bursae. *Acta Radiol* (Suppl) 36:1, 1938.

61. Katenkamp D, Stiller D: Synovial sarcoma of the abdominal wall: light microscopic, histochemical and electron microscopic investigations. *Virchows Arch (Pathol Anat)* 388:349, 1980.

62. Kaufman J, Tsukada Y: Synovial sarcoma with brain metastases: report of a case responding to supervoltage irradiation and review of the literature. *Cancer* 38:96, 1976.

63. King ES: Tissue differentiation in malignant synovial tumors. *J Bone Joint Surg* 34B:97, 1952.

64. Klein W, Huth F: The ultrastructure of malignant synovioma. *Beitr Path* 153:194, 1974.

65. Knight JC, Reeves BR, Kearney L, et al: Localization of the synovial sarcoma t(x;18)(p11.2;q11.2) breakpoint by fluorescence in situ hybridization. *Hum Mol Genet* 1:633, 1992.

66. Knox LC: Synovial sarcoma. Report of three cases. *Am J Cancer* 28:461, 1936.

67. Krall RA, Kostianovsky M, Patchefsky AS: Synovial sarcoma: a clinical, pathological, and ultrastructural study of 26 cases supporting the recognition of a monophasic variant. *Am J Surg Pathol* 5:137, 1981.

68. Krugman ME, Rosin HD, Toker C: Synovial sarcoma of the head and neck. *Arch Otolaryngol* 98:53, 1973.

69. Kuhl J, Kuhner U, Wunsch PH: Synovialsarkom im Kindesalter: Probleme der Therapie und prognostische Faktoren. *Z Kinderchirurg* 27:9, 1979.

70. Lauche A: Zur Kenntnis von Pathologie und Klinik der Geschwülste mit Synovialmembran-artigem Bau (Synovialome oder synoviale Endothelio-Fibrome und–Sarkome). *Frankf Ztschft Path* 59:1, 1947-1948.

71. Lawrence RR: Monophasic synovial sarcoma: a case report. *Plast Reconstr Surg* 36:325, 1965.

72. Lee SM, Hajdu SI, Exelby PR: Synovial sarcomas in children. *Surg Gynecol Obstet* 138:701, 1974.

73. Lejars F, Rubens-Duval H: Les sarcomes primitifs des synoviales articulaires. *Rev Chir (Paris)* 41:751, 1910.

74. Lenoir P, Ramet J, Goosens A, et al: Retropharyngeal synovial sarcoma in an infant: report of a case and of its response to chemotherapy; review of the literature. *Pediatr Hematol Oncol* 8:45, 1991.

75. Letts H, Singh I: Synovial sarcoma in the scapular region of a 12-year-old child: a case report. *Pediatrics* 41:1004, 1968.

76. Liebman EP, Harwick RD, Ronis ML, et al: Synovial sarcoma of the cervical area. *Laryngoscope* 84:889, 1974.

77. Limon J, Mrozek K, Mandahl N, et al: Cytogenetics of synovial sarcoma: presentation of ten new cases and review of the literature. *Genes Chromosom Cancer* 3:338, 1991.

78. Lombardi L, Rilke F: Ultrastructural similarities and differences of synovial sarcoma, epithelioid sarcoma and clear cell sarcoma of tendons and aponeuroses. *Ultrastruct Pathol* 6:209, 1984.

79. Lord GA, Goodale F: Synovial sarcoma arising in the anterior abdominal wall. *Arch Surg* 81:1020, 1960.

80. Luse SA: A synovial sarcoma studied by electron microscopy. *Cancer* 13:312, 1960.

81. Mackenzie DH: Monophasic synovial sarcoma—a histological entity? *Histopathology* 1:51, 1977.

82. Mackenzie DH: Synovial sarcoma. A review of 58 cases. *Cancer* 19:169, 1966.

83. Mahajan H, Lorigan JG, Shirkhoda A: Synovial sarcoma: MR imaging. *Magn Reson Imaging* 7:211, 1989.

84. Majeste RM, Beckman EN: Synovial sarcoma with an overwhelming epithelial component. *Cancer* 61:2527, 1988.

85. Marsh HO, Shellito JG, Callahan WP: Synovial sarcoma of the sternoclavicular region. *J Bone Joint Surg* 45A:151, 1963.

86. Massarelli G, Tanda F, Salis B: Synovial sarcoma of the soft palate: report of a case. *Hum Pathol* 9:341, 1978.

87. McKinney CD, Mills SE, Fechner RE: Intraarticular synovial sarcoma. *Am J Surg Pathol* 16:1017, 1992.

88. Mehrotra S, Gupta A, Mital V: Synovial sarcoma of the anterior abdominal wall. *J Indian Med Assoc* 64:146, 1975.

89. Menendez LR, Brien E, Brien WW: Synovial sarcoma: a clinicopathologic study. *Orthop Rev* 21:465, 1992.

90. Mickelson MR, Brown GA, Maynard JA, et al: Synovial sarcoma: an electron microscopic study of monophasic and biphasic forms. *Cancer* 45:2109, 1980.

91. Miettinen M: Keratin subsets in spindle cell sarcomas: keratins are widespread but synovial sarcoma contains a distinctive keratin polypeptide pattern and desmoplakins. *Am J Pathol* 138:505, 1991.

92. Miettinen M, Lehto VP, Virtanen I: Keratin in the epithelial-like cells of classical biphasic synovial sarcoma. *Virchows Arch (Cell Pathol)* 40:157, 1982.

93. Miettinen M, Lehto VP, Virtanen I: Monophasic synovial sarcoma of spindle-cell type: epithelial differentiation as revealed by ultrastructural features, content of prekeratin and binding of peanut agglutinin. *Virchows Arch (Cell Pathol)* 44:187, 1983.

94. Miettinen M, Santavirta S, Slatis, P: Intravascular synovial sarcoma. *Hum Pathol* 18:1075, 1987.

95. Miettinen M, Virtanen I: Synovial sarcoma—a misnomer. *Am J Pathol* 117:18, 1984.

96. Milchgrub S, Ghandur-Mnaymneh L, Dorfman HD, et al: Synovial sarcoma with extensive osteoid and bone formation. *Am J Surg Pathol* 17:357, 1993.

97. Miller LH, Santa Ella-Latimer L, Miller TH: Synovial sarcoma of the larynx. *Trans Am Acad Ophthalmol Otolaryngol* 80:448, 1975.

98. Mirra JM, Wang S, Bhuta S: Synovial sarcoma with squamous differentiation of its mesenchymal glandular elements: a case report with light-microscopic, ultramicroscopic and immunologic correlation. *Am J Surg Pathol* 8:791, 1984.

99. Mischler NE: Synovial sarcoma of the neck associated with previous head and neck radiation therapy. *Arch Otolaryngol* 104:482, 1978.

100. Mitcherling JJ, Collins EM, Tomich CE, et al: Synovial sarcoma of the neck. Report of a case. *J Oral Surg* 34:64, 1976.

101. Moberger G, Nilsonne U, Friberg S: Synovial sarcoma. *Acta Orthop Scand (Suppl)* 111:3, 1968.

102. Morton MJ, Berquist TH, McLeod RA, et al: MR imaging of synovial sarcoma. *Am J Roentgenol* 156:337, 1991.

103. Moses R, Chomet B, Gibbel M: Synovial sarcoma occurring in the anterior abdominal wall. *Am J Surg* 97:120, 1959.

104. Moussavi H, Ghodsi S: Synovial sarcoma of the tongue: report of a case. *J Laryngol Otol* 88:795, 1974.

105. Murphy E, Margarit E: Synovial sarcoma of the anterior abdominal wall. *Ann Surg* 168:928, 1968.

106. Murray MR, Stout AP, Pogogeff IA: Synovial sarcoma and normal synovial tissue cultivated in vitro. *Ann Surg* 120:843, 1944.

107. Nakamura T, Nakata K, Hata S, et al: Histochemical characterization of mucosubstances in synovial sarcoma. *Am J Surg Pathol* 8:429, 1984.

108. Nogel P, Mockwitz J: Angiographische Befunde bei einem Synovialsarkom. *Fortschr Roentgenstr* 118:219, 1973.

109. Novotny GM, Fort TC: Synovial sarcoma of the tongue. *Arch Otolaryngol* 94:77, 1971.

110. Nunez-Alonso C, Gashti EN, Christ ML: Maxillofacial synovial sarcoma: light and electron microscopic study of two cases. *Am J Surg Pathol* 3:23, 1979.

111. Oda Y, Hashimoto H, Tsuneyoshi M, et al: Survival in synovial sarcoma: a multivariate study of prognostic factors with special emphasis on the comparison between early death and long-term survival. *Am J Surg Pathol* 17:35, 1993.

112. Ordonez NG, Mahfouz SM, Mackay B: Synovial sarcoma: an immunohistochemical and ultrastructural study. *Hum Pathol* 21:733, 1990.

113. Pack GT, Ariel IM: Synovial sarcoma (malignant synovioma): a report of 60 cases. *Surgery* 28:1047, 1950.

114. Pisa R, Bonetti F, Chilosi M, et al: Synovial sarcoma enzyme histochemistry of a typical case. *Virchows Arch (Pathol Anat)* 398:67, 1982.

115. Povysil C: Synovial sarcoma with squamous metaplasia. *Ultrastruct Pathol* 7:207, 1984.

116. Raben M, Calabrese A, Higinbotham NL, et al: Malignant synovioma. *Am J Roentgenol* 93:145, 1965.

117. Rööser B, Willen H, Huguson A, et al: Prognostic factors in synovial sarcoma. *Cancer* 63:2182, 1989.

118. Roth JA, Enzinger FM, Tannenbaum M: Synovial sarcoma of the neck: a follow-up study of 24 cases. *Cancer* 35:1243, 1975.

119. Roy S, Ghadially FN: Synthesis of hyaluronic acid by synovial cells. *J Pathol Bacteriol* 93:555, 1967.

120. Russell WO, Cohen J, Enzinger F, et al: A clinical and pathological staging system for soft tissue sarcomas. *Cancer* 40:1562, 1977.

121. Ryan JR, Baker LH, Benjamin RS: The natural history of metastatic synovial sarcoma: experience of the Southwest Oncology group. *Clin Orthop* 164:257, 1982.

122. Salisbury JR, Isaacson PG: Synovial sarcoma: an immunohistochemical study. *J Pathol* 147:49, 1985.

123. Salzer-Kuntschik M: Malignes Synovialom des linken Oberschenkels mit knoechernen Ausdifferenzierungen. *Verh Dtsch Ges Pathol* 58:276, 1974.

124. Schiffman R: Epithelioid sarcoma and synovial sarcoma in the same knee. *Cancer* 45:158, 1980.

125. Schmidt D, Mackay B: Ultrastructure of human tendon sheath and synovium: implications for tumor histogenesis. *Ultrastruct Pathol* 3:269, 1982.

126. Schmidt D, Thum P, Harms D, et al: Synovial sarcoma in children and adolescents: a report from the Kiel Pediatric Tumor Registry. *Cancer* 67:1667, 1991.

127. Shaw GR, Lais CJ: Fatal intravascular synovial sarcoma in a 31-year-old woman. *Hum Pathol* 24:809, 1993.

128. Shiu MH, McCormack PM, Hajdu SI, et al: Surgical treatment of tendosynovial sarcoma. *Cancer* 43:889, 1979.

129. Shmookler BM: Retroperitoneal synovial sarcoma: a report of four cases. *Am J Clin Pathol* 77:686, 1982.

130. Shmookler BM, Enzinger FM, Brannon RB: Orofacial synovial sarcoma: a clinicopathologic study of 11 new cases and review of the literature. *Cancer* 50:269, 1982.

131. Smith LW: Synoviomata. *Am J Pathol* 3:355, 1927.

132. Soule EH: Synovial sarcoma. *Am J Surg Pathol* 10 (Suppl I):78, 1986.

133. Stephan G, Dörken H: Röntgendiagnostik und Klinik des malignen Synovialoms—Beobachtungen bei 31 Patienten. *Fortschr Roentgenstr* 116:62, 1972.

134. Strickland B, Mackenzie DH: Bone involvement in synovial sarcoma. *J Fac Radiologists (London)* 10:64, 1959.

135. Stuer J: Eine ungenwöhnliche Geschwulst der Ellbogengelenksgegend. *Inaug Diss Wuerzburg,* 1893.

136. Suit HD, Russell WO, Martin RG: Management of patients with sarcoma of soft tissue in an extremity. *Cancer* 31:1247, 1973.

137. Suit HD, Russell WO, Martin RG: Sarcoma of soft tissue: clinical and histopathological parameters and response to treatment. *Cancer* 35:1478, 1975.

138. Sumitomo M, Hirose T, Kudo E, et al: Epithelial differentiation in synovial sarcoma: correlation with histology and immunophenotypic expression. *Acta Pathol Jpn* 39:381, 1989.

139. Sutro CJ: Synovial sarcoma of the soft parts in the first toe: recurrence after 35 years' interval. *Bull Hosp Joint Dis* 37:105, 1976.

140. Taxy JB, Battifora H: The electron microscope in the study and diagnosis of soft tissue tumors. In *Diagnostic electron microscopy,* New York, 1980, John Wiley & Sons, p 135.

141. Thunold J, Bang G: Synovial sarcoma: a case report. *Acta Orthop Scan* 47:231, 1976.

142. Tillotson JF, McDonald JR, Janes JM: Synovial sarcomata. *J Bone Joint Surg* 33A:459, 1951.

143. Tsuneyoshi M, Yokoyama K, Enjoji M: Synovial sarcoma: a clinicopathologic and ultrastructural study of 42 cases. *Acta Pathol Jpn* 33:23, 1983.

144. Turc-Carel C, Dal Cin P, Limon J, et al: Involvement of chromosome X in primary cytogenetic change in human neoplasia: nonrandom translocation in synovial sarcoma. *Proc Natl Acad Sci U S A* 84:1981, 1987.

145. Turc-Carel C, Dal Cin P, Limon J, et al: Translocation X;18 in synovial sarcoma. *Cancer Genet Cytogenet* 23:9, 1986.

146. Varela-Duran J, Enzinger FM: Calcifying synovial sarcoma. *Cancer* 50:345, 1982.

147. Vincent RG: Malignant synovioma. *Ann Surg* 152:777, 1960.

148. Weiss AP, Steichen JB: Synovial sarcoma causing carpal tunnel syndrome. *J Hand Surg* 17:1024, 1992.

149. Wright CJ: Malignant synovioma. *J Pathol Bacteriol* 64:585, 1962.

150. Wright PH, Sim FH, Soule EH, et al: Synovial sarcoma. *J Bone Joint Surg* 64A:112, 1982.

151. Zito RA: Synovial sarcoma: an Australian series of 48 cases. *Pathology* 16:45, 1984.

CHAPTER 30

MESOTHELIOMA

Since Wagner et al.[153] demonstrated in 1960 a high incidence of mesothelioma among asbestos workers in the Cape Province of South Africa, mounting attention has been paid to this tumor, and numerous reports and reviews of mesothelioma have appeared in the medical literature. Mesothelioma is by no means a new disease, having been recognized as a distinctive clinicopathological entity since the second half of the nineteenth century.[53,58,64] Sporadic reports of this neoplasm have been recorded in the literature under various synonyms such as endothelioma,[36] papillomatosis,[168] and carcinosarcoma.[18] Adami (1908)[2] is usually credited with coining the term *mesothelioma* and Klemperer and Rabin (1931)[235] with distinguishing and defining its epithelial and fibrous types.

The marked proliferation of reported cases in the medical literature is not only a reflection of widespread interest in the disease and its etiology—and the evolution of more specific diagnostic criteria—but undoubtedly is also due to an actual increase in its rate of occurrence over the past decades. Whitwell and Rawcliffe[162] were able to identify in their material only 12 cases from 1955 to 1963 but 38 cases from 1964 to 1970. Similarly, Newhouse and Thompson[110] encountered 10 cases prior to 1950 and 40 cases from 1951 to 1964. This steady increase in the number of newly observed cases parallels and follows the steep rise in the output and use of asbestos fibers in industrial countries during the first half of this century. Because there is a 20- to 40-year time lag between exposure to asbestos and development of the disease, this trend is likely to persist for several more years. However, the recent worldwide reduction in the industrial and commercial use of asbestos fibers is bound to cause the incidence of malignant mesothelioma to decrease, probably in the late 1990s or at the beginning of the next century.[8]

Mesothelioma is a tumor of adult life that mainly affects persons older than 50 years and is slightly more common in men than in women. It arises from the mesothelial cells or the underlying mesenchymal cells of serosal surfaces, and is about five times more common in the pleural than in the peritoneal cavity. Not infrequently it involves both pleura and peritoneum as the result of direct extension through the diaphragm. It also occurs as a primary tumor in the pericardium[46] and tunica vaginalis testis,[175,179,202] but the incidence at those two sites is less than 5% of all cases. Data as to incidence vary considerably, but the annual incidence of diffuse mesothelioma in the adult male population of the United States is estimated to be between 7 and 13 per million.[138] Similarly, the reported incidence of asbestos exposure in patients with mesothelioma varies greatly, ranging from as little as 20% to as much as 99%. The incidence is much higher in men than in women and higher with peritoneal than pleural involvement.

The prognosis differs slightly according to type. It is grave with the diffuse epithelial and biphasic types and even less favorable with the fibrous (sarcomatoid) type; nearly all patients with these tumors die of complications caused by the primary neoplasm within 12 to 18 months after diagnosis. Metastases do occur but usually at a late stage of the disease. There is still no effective mode of therapy, but multiagent chemotherapy, in addition to surgery, seems to alleviate symptoms and prolong survival.

HISTOLOGICAL CLASSIFICATION

Three histological types of diffuse mesothelioma are usually distinguished: (1) epithelial, (2) fibrous (sarcomatoid), and (3) biphasic or mixed, showing both epithelial and fibrous features in close association. Epithelial and biphasic types of diffuse mesothelioma display a wide range of growth patterns and cellular compositions, and vary from well-differentiated tubulopapillary forms, which are readily recognizable, to poorly differentiated types consisting merely of solid nests and sheets of tumor cells that may be uniform in appearance or may show considerable cellular pleomorphism. As with synovial sarcoma, recognition of the fibrous or sarcomatoid type also may pose considerable diagnostic problems, often requiring immunohistochemical analysis.

There is only limited information as to the incidence and distribution of the various types. Among *diffuse mesotheliomas,* the epithelial type is by far the most common. For example, in the study by Leigh et al.[88] of 746 diffuse peritoneal mesotheliomas, 44% were of the epithelial type, 22% of the biphasic or mixed type, and 9% of the fibrous (sarcomatous) type, but in 25% there was no agreement among the reviewers as to the exact histological type. In the earlier series of Kannerstein and Churg,[73] 75.6% of 82 cases were of the epithelial type, 22% of the biphasic or mixed type, and 4% of the fibrous type. Other studies report a similar distribution of the various types but with a substantial divergence in the incidence of the fibrous type.[154] Localized mixed or biphasic types are extremely rare, and only a few of these cases have been reported.[42a,251] Some of these are perhaps early forms of the diffuse type.

Additional histological types that belong in this group of tumors are (1) the *well-differentiated papillary mesothelioma*, a tumor of intermediate malignancy; (2) the rare *multicystic peritoneal mesothelioma*, a tumor that is frequently mistaken for lymphangioma; and (3) the *benign mesothelioma of the genital tract*, a neoplasm that is often referred to as *adenomatoid tumor* in order to clearly distinguish it from malignant diffuse mesotheliomas occurring in the same locations. *Localized fibrous tumor of the pleura and peritoneum (localized fibrous mesothelioma)* is also included in the classification of mesothelial tumors, but this tumor is now generally considered to be of fibroblastic rather than mesothelial origin.

DIFFUSE MESOTHELIOMA
Clinical findings

Diffuse mesothelioma is mainly found in adults between 45 and 75 years of age, regardless of whether it originates in the pleural, pericardial, or peritoneal cavity or the scrotum. Data as to the sex incidence vary considerably; however, in most reviews, especially those with a large number of industrial workers, men outnumber women by a considerable margin.[3,6,73,100] Mesotheliomas in children are rare, but typical examples are present among our cases and are recorded in the literature.[11,21,54,77] Among the 13 cases collected by Grundy and Miller,[62] 10 were of the fibrous or fibrous-papillary type and 3 were of the undifferentiated type. Only 2 of the 13 occurred in children younger than 10 years of age.

The clinical symptoms differ substantially and depend on the primary location of the neoplasm. *Diffuse pleural mesothelioma* usually manifests with chest pain, shortness of breath, and significant weight loss over a short period; it may also cause chronic cough, fever, and radiating pain in the shoulder or arm. Physical examination usually reveals decreased chest excursion, diminished or absent breath sounds, and, in virtually all patients, evidence of serous or hemorrhagic pleural effusion that accumulates rapidly and requires frequent aspirations. Pulmonary osteoarthropathy with arthritic pain and clubbing of the fingers or toes is encountered in 5% to 10% of cases, but it is much less common with diffuse mesothelioma than with the localized fibrous tumor of the pleura. Laboratory studies are not helpful in diagnosis, but in some instances the blood studies may show leukocytosis and anemia, or there may be a high platelet count with thromboembolic episodes and pulmonary embolism.[107]

Patients with *diffuse peritoneal mesothelioma* usually give a history of nagging or burning abdominal or epigastric pain, which tends to be more severe after meals. The pain is often accompanied by constipation, anorexia, nausea, or vomiting. Palpation of the abdomen discloses marked distention, increased density, and at times an ill-defined mass. Ascites is often demonstrable; it may be massive and frequently persists despite repeated paracenteses. Regional lymph nodes may be palpable and on biopsy may show evidence of metastatic disease.[164] In some cases peritoneoscopy is helpful in diagnosis.[22,104] Pericardial mesotheliomas tend to be associated with pericardial effusion, arrhythmia, or cardiac failure[144]; mesotheliomas of the tunica vaginalis are usually marked by a hydrocele or a scrotal mass.[72]

Radiographic findings

Roentgenographic and CT examinations in patients with *diffuse pleural mesothelioma* show a rather distinct picture, but it rarely permits an unequivocal diagnosis. The outstanding features are marked effusion, sometimes with compression of the adjacent lung and atelectasis, diffuse or irregular nodular thickening of the pleura or interlobular fissure, and, not infrequently, an intrathoracic mass. Less commonly there is widening or displacement of the mediastinum and a nodular infiltrate of the pulmonary parenchyma and pneumothorax secondary to invasion of the underlying visceral pleura and lung. Pulmonary fibrosis, however, is usually less severe than with asbestosis or carcinoma.[91]

X-ray films and CT scans of *diffuse peritoneal mesothelioma* show thickening of the visceral and parietal peritoneums and omentum or multiple small nodules, often together with ascites, signs of gastrointestinal tract dysfunction, and intestinal obstruction. There may also be pleural plaques in patients with asbestosis. Magnetic resonance imaging or ultrasonography may be superior to CT scan in demonstrating peritoneal masses, especially in the presence of ascites.*

Pleural and ascitic fluid

Examination of the pleural or ascitic fluid shows it to be viscid and amber-colored or frankly hemorrhagic with demonstrable malignant cells in slightly more than half of the cases. For example, in the series by Wanebo et al.[155] pleural fluid was studied in 35 diffuse mesotheliomas, but in

---

*References 14, 119, 125, 138, 161, 167.

only 15 were the cells recognized as malignant and in 5 as characteristic of mesothelioma. Markedly elevated levels of hyaluronic acid have been observed in a high percentage of cases, but this is also seen, although much less frequently, in carcinomas and sarcomas.* Azumi et al.,[13] using a hyaluronate binding probe, found significant staining for hyaluronate in 26 of 33 mesotheliomas but only 3 of 37 adenocarcinomas.

Needle biopsy

Needle biopsy guided by ultrasonography or CT scan is diagnostic in only a small percentage of cases, and thoracotomy and open biopsy may be necessary to establish the diagnosis. In many cases, however, needle biopsy in combination with immunocytochemical studies and electron microscopic examinations of the biopsy material may permit a firm diagnosis of mesothelioma (see Tables 30-1, 30-2, and 30-3).[146,149]

Mesothelioma and asbestos exposure

Although the association between pulmonary asbestosis and carcinoma was established in the early 1930s, the causal relationship between asbestos exposure and mesothelioma was not recognized until 1960, when Wagner et al.[153] gave a detailed account of 47 cases of diffuse mesothelioma observed within a 5-year period in the asbestos regions of South Africa. In 1964 Selikoff et al.[129] published their report on "asbestos exposure and neoplasia" in insulation workers of the New York area. Since publication of these reports, numerous studies carried out in England,[109,110] Scotland,[102] South Africa,[153,160] Canada,[99-101] the United States,[74,128,129] and other parts of the world have confirmed the observations of Wagner and colleagues, and have demonstrated an increased incidence of mesothelioma not only among asbestos miners but also among industrial workers with a prolonged history of asbestos exposure.

Selikoff et al.,[132] in their classic study of 17,800 asbestos insulation workers, found that in 2271 consecutive deaths there were 175 mesotheliomas plus a large number of pulmonary carcinomas and carcinomas at other sites. In fact, in their series, cancer was responsible for 44% of all deaths, as compared with an expected rate of 19%. Of the 175 cases of mesothelioma, 63 (36%) involved the pleura and 112 (64%) the peritoneum; most became apparent 25 to 40 years after the worker had started employment and been exposed to asbestos. This time lag between exposure and emergence of symptoms serves to explain not only the rarity of mesothelioma in young persons but also the surge in its incidence following a period in which the output and use of asbestos has risen tremendously, especially in highly industrialized countries.

Exposure to asbestos is an occupational hazard not only in the mining and milling industries but also in the process of manufacturing, repairing, installing (and removing) asbestos products such as thermal and electrical insulations, floor and ceiling tiles, automobile brake and clutch linings, cement tiles and pipes, and numerous other applications. Domestic exposure appears to be of lesser significance but has been observed in one or more relatives of asbestos workers, as well as in persons and even animals living in the vicinity of asbestos mines and industries. It is notable, however, that the risk of developing mesothelioma varies greatly with the duration and intensity of exposure and also with the type of asbestos and dimension of asbestos fibers: the risk is greatest with crocidolite, the blue asbestos mined in the Cape Province of South Africa and parts of Australia. The risk is less with amosite and least with chrysotile, the white asbestos that is found chiefly in Canada and Russia and amounts to more than 95% of the asbestos used commercially. Exposure to more than one type of fiber is common, however, and it has been suggested that the cancerogenicity of chrysotile is due to contamination with noncommercial amphiboles such as actinolite, tremolite, and anthophyllite.[31]

The risk of developing mesothelioma seems to be enhanced with thin straight fibrils of submicroscopic dimensions—as found in crocidolite—that reach the peripheral portions of the lung and penetrate tissues more readily.[121] After inhalation the fibrils are capable of passage into the pleural cavity. They may also be able to penetrate the bowel wall and migrate to the peritoneum, as suggested by animal experiments.[118,152] Occasionally they are carried to regional lymph nodes and other tissues such as the pancreas, liver, and kidney.[86] The curlier fibrils of chrysotile are probably less penetrating and are more readily removed by macrophages and lymphatics.[40]

Most of the asbestos fibers in the body are too small to be visualized with the light microscope, but they are readily recognized in the lung as "asbestos bodies," asbestos fibers coated with acid mucopolysaccharides and hemosiderin granules. These segmented "nail-headed," golden-brown structures, however, are difficult to distinguish from the ferruginous structures formed about a nonasbestos core, such as iron, talc, mica, carbon, and rutile. Assisting in the distinction of these fibers are the thin, transparent, usually straight central core of asbestos, the refractile yellow core of talc and mica, and the black core of iron and rutile.[35,43] Examination with the electron and scanning microscopes reveals that most ferruginous bodies seem to possess asbestos cores. Asbestos bodies are markedly increased in many construction workers and in patients with asbestosis or mesothelioma. The number of fibers seems to parallel the degree of exposure.[6,31,34,123]

A more efficient way of demonstrating and counting ferruginous bodies is the examination of lung juice smear,[162] and particularly digestion of wet lung tissue with sodium

---

*References 30, 44, 55, 61, 68, 79, 108, 116.

hypochlorite and membrane filtration. Using the latter method Smith and Naylor[137] found ferruginous bodies in 100% of consecutive autopsies, regardless of the cause of death. Likewise, Churg[31] found asbestos bodies in nearly all of the cases examined, but he noted a considerable increase in concentration in workers in certain asbestos-related occupations and in patients with mesothelioma. Counts of asbestos fibers with the electron microscope are even more reliable than those with tissue digestion.[12] Electron diffraction patterns and especially energy-dispersive x-ray spectroscopy have been shown to be useful for diagnosis and for distinguishing the various types of asbestos.[31,122]

Although measures have been taken in recent years to reduce asbestos exposure of industrial workers and the general population, it is likely—considering the long latent period of the disease—that the high incidence of mesothelioma will continue over the coming years. At particular risk are those who have been exposed to asbestos for several years, either as workers in the asbestos industry or as persons living in an asbestos-contaminated urban or industrial atmosphere. Also at risk are workers engaged in the demolition of buildings or refitting of ships containing asbestos packings around boilers and furnaces. With short or less intensive exposure the incidence of mesothelioma is lower and the adverse effects are more delayed.[128] Smoking does not seem to enhance the risk of developing the disease.

Detailed descriptions of the prevalence of mesothelioma and the risk and environmental aspects of asbestos exposure were given in a review by Kannerstein et al. in 1978,[74] Selikoff and Hammond in 1979,[131] and Craighead in 1982, 1987, and 1989.[38,39,41]

Other possible causes of mesothelioma such as nonasbestos fibers, chronic inflammation, scarring, and radiation were discussed by Peterson et al.[115] and Hillerdal and Berg.[67] A markedly increased incidence of diffuse mesothelioma has also been observed in two small Anatolian villages of central Turkey, where the soil contains large amounts of erionite, a hydrated aluminum silicate of the zeolite family of minerals.[90]

Classification of asbestos

Amphiboles
Crocidolite (blue asbestos)
Amosite
Anthophyllite
Tremolite
Actinolite

Serpentines
Chrysotile (white asbestos)

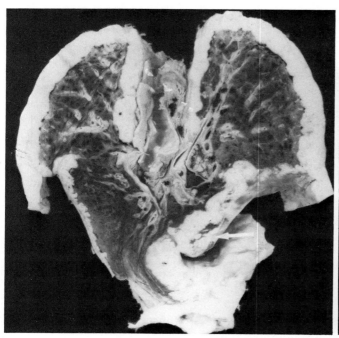
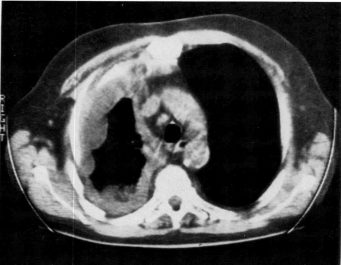

FIG. 30-1. A, Diffuse mesothelioma *(arrow)* encasing and compressing both lungs of a 63-year-old man. **B,** CT scan of diffuse pleural mesothelioma showing complete encasement of the right lung by tumor tissue.

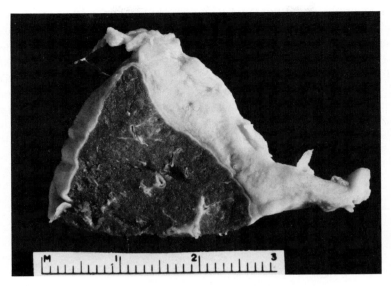

FIG. 30-2. Diffuse epithelial mesothelioma of the serosal surface of the spleen in 70-year-old woman. The tumor also encased the intestines and caused massive ascites.

Gross findings

Initially the disease is characterized by numerous small nodules or plaques covering visceral and parietal serosal surfaces. At a later stage the individual nodules fuse and form a diffuse, sheetlike thickening, frequently encasing and compressing the lungs or the intestines and sometimes the liver and spleen (Figs. 30-1 and 30-2). In the thoracic cavity the growth tends to be rather uniform but often is more pronounced in the serosal coverings of the lower lobe and diaphragm; in the peritoneum involvement is usually more variable, and the diffuse or multinodular growth is often associated with large localized masses or a conglomerate of variably sized tumor nodules (Fig. 30-3). Massive involvement of the omentum is a common occurrence that may simulate clinically the presence of a solitary localized neoplasm. The final stages of the disease are marked by massive encasement of the viscera with matting of the affected structures, commonly causing complete obliteration of the pleural or peritoneal cavity, and severe and often fatal functional disturbances. In many cases the tumor tissue invades the adjacent lung or viscera, but in general, invasion is more superficial than deep and is confined to the immediate subserosal tissues. Not infrequently the tumor extends through the chest or abdominal wall along a needle biopsy tract or a scar from a previous excision—a complication that must be given consideration when planning thoracoscopy, peritoneoscopy, or needle biopsy or when aspirating fluid for cytological examination or relief of symptoms. (See Fig. 30-8.)

The excised tissue varies greatly in appearance and may be firm and rubbery or soft and gelatinous; on section it is

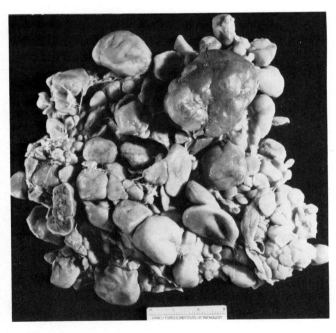

FIG. 30-3. Peritoneal mesothelioma presenting as a conglomerate of variably sized tumor nodules.

generally gray-white and glistening, frequently with foci of hemorrhage or necrosis.

Microscopic findings

Although no two mesotheliomas are exactly alike and there is often a striking variation in different portions of the same neoplasm, most diffuse mesotheliomas are of the *epithelial type* and can be readily identified by their characteristic tubulopapillary pattern. This pattern consists of papillary structures, branching tubules, and glandlike acinar and cystic spaces lined by rather uniform cuboidal or flattened epithelial-like cells with vesicular nuclei, one or two inconspicuous nucleoli, and abundant eosinophilic cytoplasm with distinct cytoplasmic borders (Figs. 30-4 to 30-6). Mitotic figures are absent or rare in well-differentiated neoplasms, but they may be numerous in poorly differen-

tiated ones. The surrounding matrix varies from myxoid to dense fibrous with or without hyalinization.

In addition to the typical tubulopapillary and tubuloglandular pattern, some tumors are composed of small uniform cells arranged in a delicate lacelike pattern (Figs. 30-7 and 30-8) and others contain sheets of vacuolated cells vaguely reminiscent of liposarcoma (Fig. 30-9). Still others are marked by cleftlike structures to large, irregular, cystic spaces lined by a single layer of flattened epithelial cells

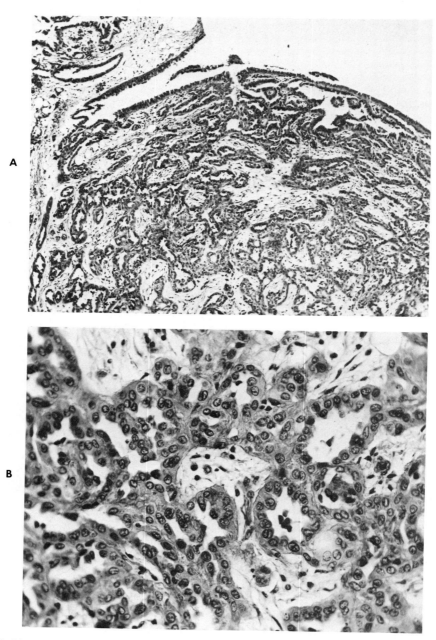

FIG. 30-4. Diffuse mesothelioma of the epithelial type showing the characteristic tubulopapillary pattern **(A)** composed of tumor cells with large rounded, fairly uniform nuclei and deeply eosinophilic cytoplasm in a glandlike arrangement **(B).** (**A,** ×65; **B,** ×350.)

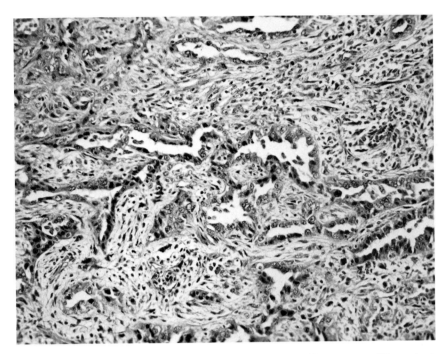

FIG. 30-5. Diffuse epithelial mesothelioma showing a tubulopapillary pattern. The patient, a 47-year-old man, had associated hypoglycemia. (×250.)

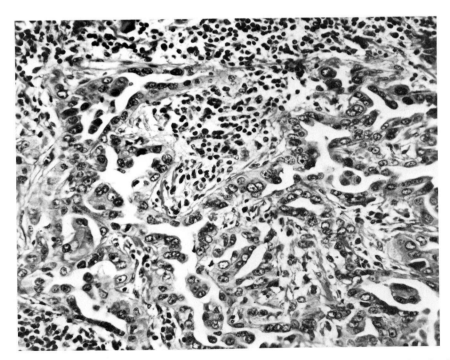

FIG. 30-6. Diffuse epithelial mesothelioma of pleura with papillary infoldings into the glandlike spaces. (×250.)

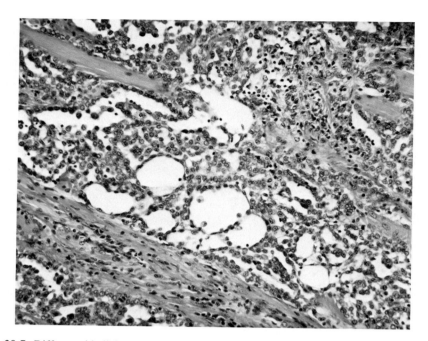

FIG. 30-7. Diffuse epithelial mesothelioma displaying uniformity of tumor cells and a microcystic growth pattern. (×160.)

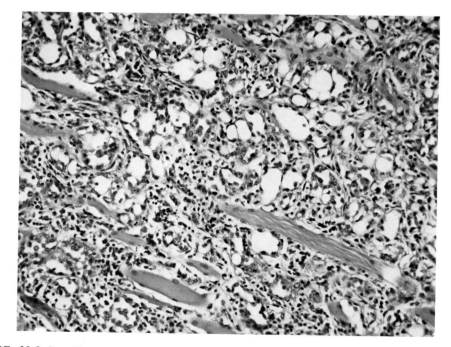

FIG. 30-8. Lacelike growth of diffuse epithelial mesothelioma occurring in the thoracotomy scar of the chest wall in a 61-year-old man. (×160.)

(Figs. 30-10 and 30-11). In some of these cases fusion or rupture of the cystic spaces leads to the formation of large mucin-filled pools; in others the cystic structures are filled or replaced by multiple papillary projections with fibrous cores that bear a close resemblance to papillary carcinoma (Fig. 30-12).

There are also less well-differentiated epithelial mesotheliomas in which the tubulopapillary pattern is largely inconspicuous or absent, and the tumor consists merely of small round or polygonal cells that are disposed in a linear or cordlike pattern or in clusters and solid nests and sheets (Figs. 30-13 and 30-14). In these areas some cells may possess a perinuclear clear zone or may show varying degrees of vacuolization resembling a clear cell tumor (Fig. 30-15). Associated with these changes is often a striking loss of cellular cohesion, with rounded or polygonal cells freely floating in the mucinous pools or dispersed in a loosely textured, myxoid stroma. This loss of cellular cohesion constitutes a frequent and useful feature in the differential diagnosis of mesothelioma (Figs. 30-16 and 30-17). There are also sporadic tumors consisting of scattered nests of small hyperchromatic cells that have been classified as *small cell mesotheliomas*.[95] Calcospherites or psammoma bodies occur in approximately 5% of mesotheliomas, notably in those of the tubulopapillary type.

The second type, the *fibrous* or *sarcomatoid type* of diffuse mesothelioma, may be difficult to diagnose and is apt to be confused with fibrosarcoma, malignant fibrous histiocytoma, or malignant hemangiopericytoma. As a rule, however, there are well-oriented, spindle-shaped, fibroblast-like cells with nuclear hyperchromatism, pleomorphism, and occasional giant cells associated with areas of dense fibrosis, hyalinization, and necrosis (Fig. 30-18).

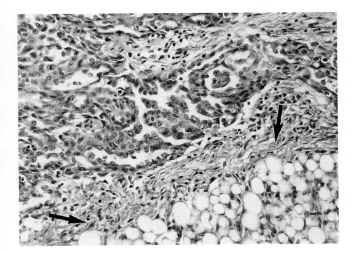

FIG. 30-9. Diffuse epithelioid mesothelioma showing both a distinct tubulopapillary pattern and a sheet of large vacuolated cells resembling lipoblasts *(arrows)*. (×250.)

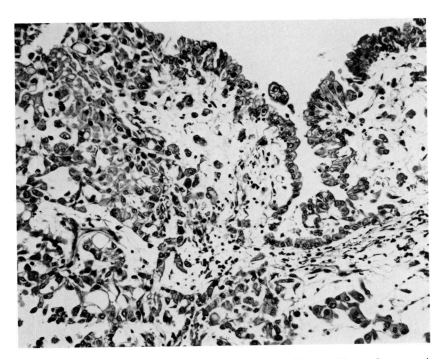

FIG. 30-10. Diffuse epithelial mesothelioma of the pleura in a 63-year-old man. Large cystic space is lined by a single layer of mesothelial cells that blend with less well-differentiated portions of the tumor. (×160.)

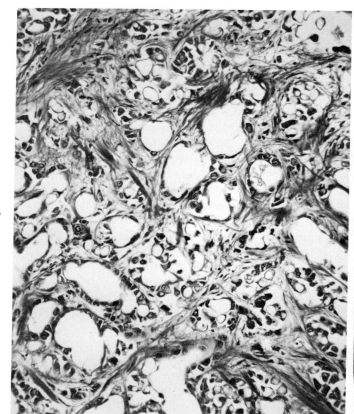

A

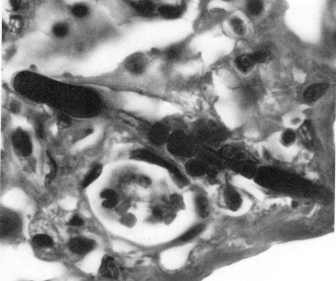

FIG. 30-11. Diffuse pleural mesothelioma in a patient who had been an asbestos miner for 14 years. **A,** Irregular cystic spaces lined by a single layer of mesothelial cells. (×160.) **B,** Ferruginous (asbestos) body from the adjacent lung. (×1000.)

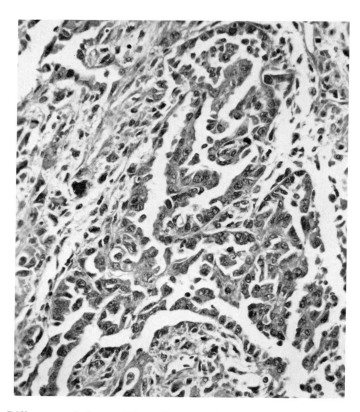

FIG. 30-12. Diffuse mesothelioma of the peritoneum with infoldings and papillary projections of mesothelial cells. (×250.)

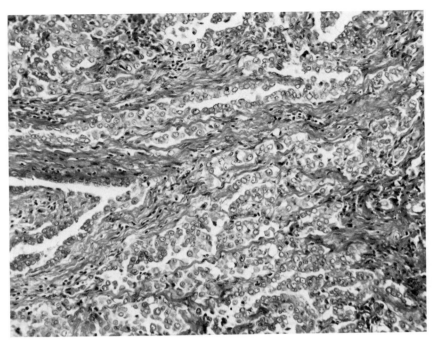

FIG. 30-13. Solid cordlike arrangement of mesothelial cells in a diffuse epithelial mesothelioma of peritoneum. (×160.)

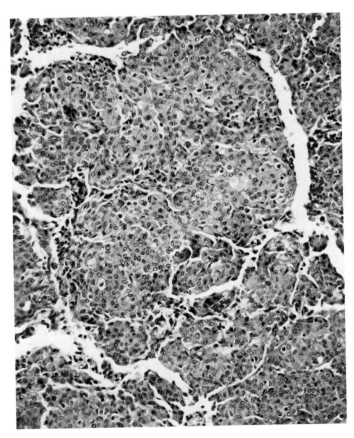

FIG. 30-14. Solid mass of mesothelial cells in a diffuse pleural mesothelioma of a former asbestos miner (same case as in Fig. 30-11). (×160.)

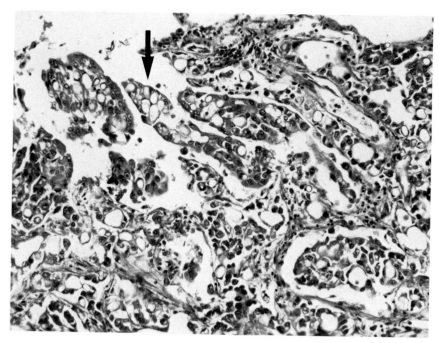

FIG. 30-15. Diffuse peritoneal mesothelioma composed of solid nests of tumor cells showing focal vacuolization *(arrow)*. (×160.)

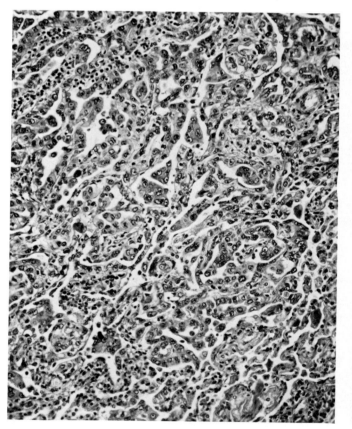

FIG. 30-16. Diffuse mesothelioma composed of irregular, randomly arranged tubulopapillary structures and small nests of tumor cells. The patient had severe hypoglycemia preoperatively. (×160.)

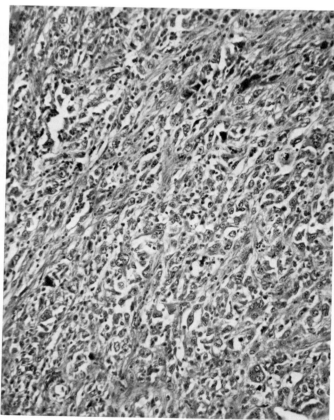

FIG. 30-17. Diffuse epithelial mesothelioma made up of loosely arranged, poorly differentiated, round or polygonal cells. Other portions of this tumor showed a well-differentiated tubulopapillary pattern (same case as in Fig. 30-6). (×160.)

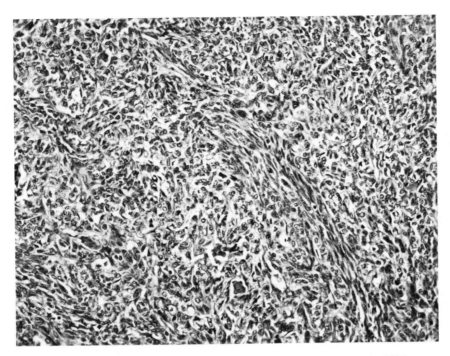

FIG. 30-18. Fibrous (sarcomatoid) type of diffuse mesothelioma. (×160.)

The presence of some of these fibrosing areas may cause confusion with a reactive fibrosing process, but the cellular atypia and increased mitotic activity will aid in the differential diagnosis. There also may be a focal whorled, storiform, or pericytoma pattern, but we have never encountered the herringbone pattern of fibrosarcoma or the prominent palisading of malignant schwannoma. The term *desmoplastic diffuse mesothelioma* has been applied to richly collagenous tumors of this type, which bear some resemblance to the malignant form of localized fibrous tumor. Despite the extensive desmoplasia in these cases, the clinical course is that of a highly malignant neoplasm.[27] Osseous or cartilaginous metaplasia in some cases may raise the question of chondrosarcoma or osteosarcoma.[169] Foci of epithelial differentiation are rare in the sarcomatoid type of diffuse mesothelioma and may be found only after careful scrutiny of multiple sections. In the absence of such areas, diagnosis rests mainly on the presence of the diffuse and pleomorphic spindle cell pattern and the characteristic immunohistochemical and ultrastructural findings.

The third type, the *mixed* or *biphasic type* of diffuse mesothelioma, can be identified in most instances without much difficulty. This type often bears a striking resemblance to synovial sarcoma and consists of a mixture of epithelial and sarcomatous components. It differs, however, from most biphasic synovial sarcomas by the absence of intracellular mucin that stains positively for PAS (Fig. 30-19). The fibrous matrix of the biphasic type can be distinguished from that of the purely epithelial type by its greater cellularity and more irregular pattern. As in synovial sarcoma, there are also tumors in which most of the cells are intermediate in appearance between epithelial and fibrous elements. As in the diffuse fibrous type, osseous and cartilaginous differentiation occurs occasionally[169] (Fig. 30-20). Several investigators have noted the prevalence of the mixed type among patients with an occupational history of asbestos exposure.[100] There is some question as to whether localized forms of epithelial or biphasic mesothelioma exist, but one such tumor in the peritoneum—with an uneventful 10-year follow-up—has been depicted in the World Health Organization classification of soft tissue tumors and others have been described in the literature.[42a, 251]

Staining characteristics

Special stains are helpful in the diagnosis of mesothelioma and particularly in the differentiation of this tumor from adenocarcinoma. As in normal mesothelium, the occasional mucin droplets that are present in the tumor cells stain positively with the alcian blue and colloidal iron (AMP) stains and lose their staining characteristics or stain less intensely after treatment of the sections with hyaluronidase. Unlike adenocarcinoma—and many synovial sarcomas—however, the mucin droplets do not stain with the PAS preparation after diastase digestion. Glycogen granules that are positive for PAS and sensitive to diastase digestion are present in the cytoplasm of many tumor cells, how-

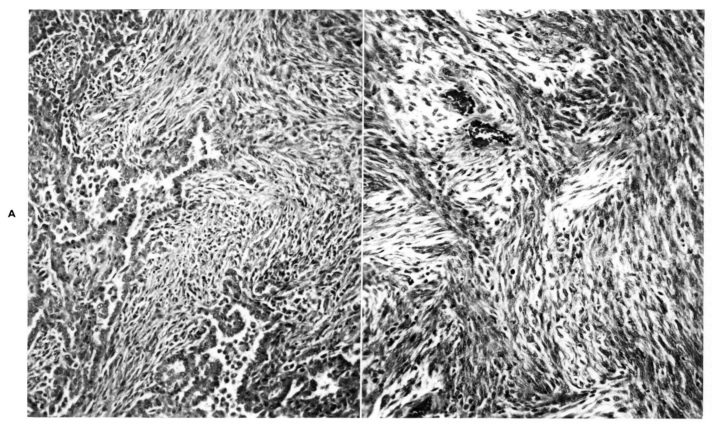

FIG. 30-19. Mixed-type peritoneal mesothelioma with biphasic area **(A)** and partly myxoid spindle cell area **(B)**. (**A** and **B**, ×160.)

Table 30-1. Differential diagnosis of mesothelioma and adenocarcinoma based on intracellular mucin*

Stain	Malignant epithelial mesothelioma	Adenocarcinoma
PAS†	−	+
PAS-diastase	−	+
Alcian blue	+	+
Alcian blue-hyaluronidase	−+	+

*Including mucin within acinar spaces.
†Intracellular, PAS-positive glycogen granules are present in many epithelial and biphasic mesotheliomas.
−, Negative staining; +, positive staining; −+, negative or positive staining.

Table 30-2. Differential diagnosis of mesothelioma and adenocarcinoma based on immunohistochemistry*

Markers or antibodies	Malignant mesothelioma	Adenocarcinoma
Vimentin	+++	+
Cytokeratin	+++	+++
Epithelial membrane antigen	++	++
Carcinoembryonic antigen	0-+	+++ !
Leu-M1	0-+	+++ !
Ber-EP4	0-+	++
B72.3	+	+++ !
MFG2	+	++

*References 15, 16, 20, 24, 57, 105, 134, 135, 145, 148, 154, 159, 165, 169a.
0- +++, Intensity of immunoreactivities.

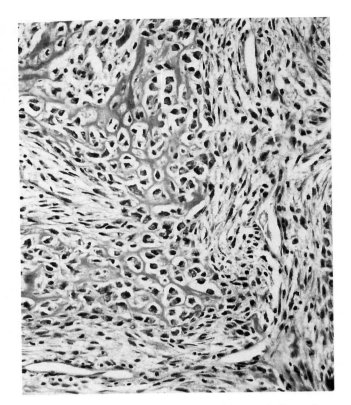

FIG. 30-20. Malignant fibrous (sarcomatoid) mesothelioma showing focal osteoid differentiation. (×250.) (From Youssm SA, Hochholzer L: *Arch Pathol Lab Med* 111:63, 1987.)

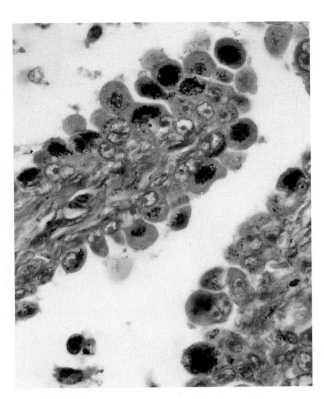

FIG. 30-21. Intracellular PAS-positive glycogen granules in a diffuse epithelioid mesothelioma. (×350.)

ever[20,52,136] (Fig. 30-21). Many of the intracellular droplets accept the mucicarmine stain and are metachromatic with the toluidine blue and thionin preparations. Unfortunately, mucin droplets that stain positively for alcian blue (and negatively for PAS) are rare or entirely absent in at least half of cases, especially in tumors that are less well differentiated (Table 30-1).

The stromal mucin outside the tumor cells stains with alcian blue but is removed by hyaluronidase, a finding that mesothelioma shares with other sarcomas and that is of little significance in reaching a diagnosis. Reticulin preparations show varying amounts of reticulin fibrils between tumor cells, and sometimes are helpful in bringing out a hidden biphasic pattern in malignant mesotheliomas of the fibrous (sarcomatoid) type.

Immunohistochemical findings

Immunostaining is indispensable for the diagnosis of mesothelioma. Most diffuse epithelial and biphasic mesotheliomas—and many diffuse fibrous (sarcomatoid) mesotheliomas—stain positively for high- and low-molecular-weight cytokeratins and to a lesser extent for epithelial membrane antigen, and hence these stains are of little help

in differential diagnosis from adenocarcinoma* (Figs. 30-22 and 30-23). Unlike adenocarcinoma, carcinoembryonic antigen is rare to absent in mesothelioma. Vimentin immunoreactivity is more often expressed by mesothelioma than adenocarcinoma.[24,32,70] Many other markers have been used in an effort to discriminate between these two tumors: Leu-M1 antigen, B72.3, Ber-EP4, and HMFG-2 have been shown to be much less common in mesothelioma than carcinoma, and used in combination will reduce the risk of false-negative results and permit a reliable diagnosis† (Table 30-2). Monoclonal antibodies against mesothelial membrane antigen (ME1, ME2)[139] and against K1, in cryostat sections, have been reported to stain positively in mesotheliomas and to be absent in adenocarcinomas.[29]

Ultrastructural findings

Although mesotheliomas share some ultrastructural similarities with adenocarcinoma, they can be distinguished by the presence of abundant long, slender, sometimes tortu-

---

*References 15, 17, 37, 69, 71, 94, 114, 141, 158, 195.
†References 15, 16, 57, 134, 135, 145, 148, 159, 165.

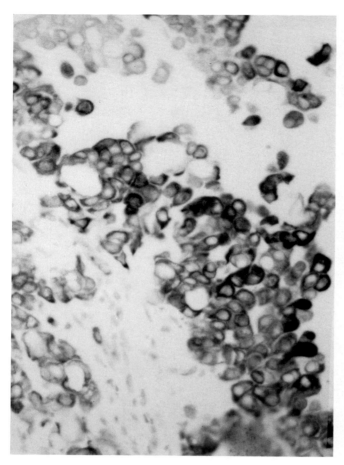

FIG. 30-22. Diffuse mesothelioma demonstrating positive immunostaining for polyclonal cytokeratin. (×250.)

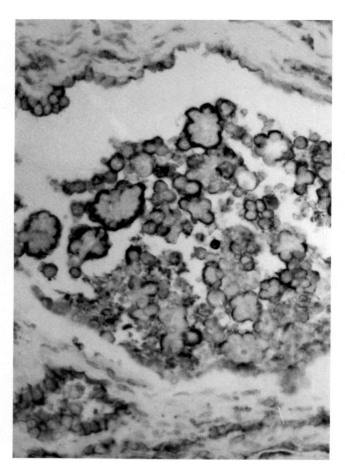

FIG. 30-23. Diffuse mesothelioma expressing immunoreactivity for epithelial membrane antigen. (×250.)

ous microvilli having a bushlike or shaggy appearance (Fig. 30-24). The microvilli are found on the free surfaces of the tumor cells as well as in intracellular and intercellular lumina. The microvilli of adenocarcinoma are also located on the surface and inside cells but are generally much shorter, less numerous, and have a more clublike appearance.[26a,157,158] These differences are also readily discernible with the scanning electron microscope.[49,140,156] The cells of mesothelioma are further marked by large nuclei with prominent nucleoli, a moderate number of mitochondria enveloped by rough endoplasmic reticulum, and, frequently, glycogen granules and bundles of intermediate filaments. There are smooth-surfaced intracellular vacuoles, but the Golgi apparatus and the associated smooth endoplasmic reticulum are rather inconspicuous. Suzuki et al.[143] observed rare lysosomes and osmiophilic lamellar structures in occasional tumor cells. Basal laminae are present but are often interrupted or incomplete. There are also junctional structures or desmosomes between adjoining cells and intermediate filaments or tonofilaments that are often limited

to the apical portion of the cell or arranged circumferentially around the nucleus. There are no ultrastructural differences between pleural and peritoneal mesotheliomas.*

Examination of the biphasic or mixed type of mesothelioma discloses a similar picture, but there are, in addition, fibroblast or myofibroblast-like cells with elongated nuclei and abundant rough endoplasmic reticulum and myofilaments with dense body formations and whorled aggregates of perinuclear intermediate filaments.[19] Transitional forms between the epithelial and fibrous cells are not uncommon and can be recognized by the presence of intercellular microcavities with microvilli.[140] The latter feature has also been encountered in diffuse (sarcomatoid) fibrous mesothelioma.

The extracellular spaces contain collagen fibers and colloidal iron-positive material, especially in close contact with the microvilli. None of the ultrastructural studies revealed asbestos fibers within the tumor cells, even in those

---

*References 26a, 80, 82, 143, 156, 157.

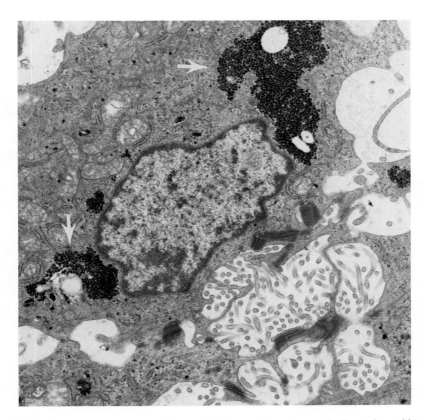

FIG. 30-24. Electron microscopic picture of diffuse peritoneal mesothelioma in a 66-year-old woman. Note intracellular and intercellular lumina with multiple slender microvilli and intracellular deposits of glycogen *(arrows)*. (×26,400.) (Courtesy Dr. Frederic I. Volini, West Suburban Hospital, Oak Park, Illinois.)

Table 30-3. Differential diagnosis of mesothelioma and adenocarcinoma based on ultrastructural findings*

Ultrastructural features	Malignant mesothelioma	Adenocarcinoma
Microvilli	+++	+-++
	Long, slender, "bushy"	Short, blunt, clublike
Desmosomes	++	+-++
Intermediate filaments	+-+++	0-+
Basement membranes	++	++
Glycogen	++	0-+

*References 26a, 143, 156, 157.
0- +++, Range and prominence of reported ultrastructural features.

cases in which they were readily demonstrable in the surrounding pulmonary parenchyma.

Cytometric and cytogenetic findings

Cytometric studies seem to be of little use diagnostically, except that most malignant mesotheliomas are diploid whereas most adenocarcinomas are aneuploid. Burmer et al.[25] conducted a flow cytometric analysis of 46 cases and found 65% to be diploid and 35% aneuploid. In a similar study, El-Naggar et al.[50] found 78% of malignant mesotheliomas to be diploid. Other investigators[56,60,103] achieved similar results; they also showed that aneuploidy of mesothelial cells in effusion specimens clearly indicates malignancy. Gibas et al.[60] found clonal abnormalities in more than half of their patients.

DIFFERENTIAL DIAGNOSIS
Mesothelial hyperplasia

It is not always possible to separate well-differentiated epithelial mesothelial neoplasms from reactive mesothelial proliferations on the basis of a small biopsy specimen, but in general, reactive or inflammatory mesothelial proliferations are limited to the serosal surfaces, where they may form small papillary structures, usually with gradual transitions between normal and hyperplastic mesothelium. These proliferations may also take the form of small, isolated cellular aggregates within the cul-de-sac, hernial sac,

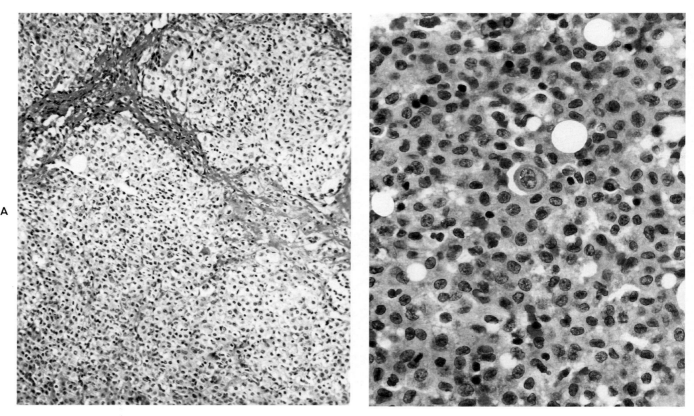

FIG. 30-25. Reactive mesothelial proliferation in hernial sac **(A)** (×160) and pericardium **(B).** (×250.) Note uniformity of cells and absence of supporting stroma.

hydrocele, and other open or closed outpouchings of the abdominal, pleural, or pericardial cavity. The cells of these aggregates are usually held together by fibrinous material and are associated with a variable number of inflammatory elements. Mesothelial proliferations of this kind are also marked by the great uniformity of the constituent cells, the absence of mitotic figures and necrosis, the coexpression of vimentin and keratin, and the absence of immunostaining for p53 protein.[26a] In occasional benign cases, there may be slight cellular pleomorphism and rare mitoses.[96] Reactive hyperplastic mesothelial proliferations tend to occur in younger persons than does mesothelioma, and there is generally a history of chronic infection or therapeutic radiation (Fig. 30-25, A and B).

Rosai and Dehner[126] described similar mesothelial hyperplasias in hernial sacs; they occurred mostly in the inguinal region of children and followed hernial incarceration or some other mechanical injury. The lesions were marked by nodular proliferations of atypical mesothelial cells associated with fibrin deposits and inflammatory, vascular, and fibroblastic elements. Since we have seen similar proliferations as a response to contamination by talc, examination under polarized light is advisable, even if there is no history of previous abdominal surgery.

Reactive fibroblastic proliferation, as in visceral or parietal pleural fibrosis, is also likely to be mistaken for diffuse mesothelioma, especially its sarcomatoid or desmoplastic type.[42] The benign nature of the lesion usually can be identified by the lack of significant cellular pleomorphism, areas of necrosis, as well as invasion of adjacent structures such as the contiguous lung and the chest wall.[51,96]

Still another and rare lesion mimicking a metastatic mesothelioma or carcinoma is a benign proliferation of mesothelial cells in mediastinal lymph nodes that was described in two patients by Brooks et al.[23]

Adenocarcinoma

Distinction of diffuse mesothelioma from adenocarcinoma and other primary or metastatic epithelial neoplasms is the most difficult problem in diagnosis. Adenocarcinomas and particularly peripheral pulmonary carcinomas may show extensive pleural involvement and may be composed of large cells bearing a close resemblance to mesothelioma (pseudomesotheliomatous carcinoma[47]). These tumors, however, arise invariably within the pulmonary parenchyma, a feature that may be evident on CT scan. Moreover, in contradistinction to mesothelioma, the intracellular mucin produced by many of these tumors stains well with PAS and in most instances the cells stain positively with anti-CEA, Leu-1, and other markers. This also applies to metastases of occult carcinomas of the breast, ovary, and other visceral organs, which are usually multiple and involve both lungs. Obviously a detailed clinical history may prove most helpful in some of these cases. Tables 30-1, 30-2, and 30-3 provide guidelines for the tinctorial and immunohistochemical differentiation of epithelial and mixed mesotheliomas from primary and metastatic adenocarcinomas.

Prognosis and therapy

The outlook is grave, and most patients with diffuse mesothelioma die of the disease within 1 or 2 years. Walz and Koch[154] reported a median survival period of 13 months, with a 2-year survival rate of 29% and a 5-year survival rate of only 4%. Survival rates vary slightly according to tumor type. Oels et al.[111] noted an average survival period of 18 months for patients with diffuse epithelial mesothelioma, 5 months for those with the biphasic type, and 4 months for those with the diffuse fibrous (sarcomatoid) type. Survival periods are equally short or even shorter in diffuse fibrous (sarcomatoid) mesothelioma with extensive desmoplasia. In fact, in the series reported by Cantin et al.,[27] metastases occurred more frequently in desmoplastic than nondesmoplastic diffuse fibrous mesotheliomas. As the disease progresses, symptoms become increasingly severe, and many patients die of respiratory failure or intestinal obstruction. Additional complications are caused by extension of the tumor into neighboring tissues, such as the lung, chest wall, diaphragm, intestinal wall, or retroperitoneum, and by recurrence, sometimes along a needle tract of a previous aspiration or needle biopsy or the scar of a previous excision. Metastases do occur but at a relatively late stage of the disease. Kannerstein and Churg[73] reported metastases in 18 of 50 autopsy cases. In their series the most common sites of metastasis were the regional lymph nodes, especially those in the mediastinum, abdomen, and supraclavicular region, and the liver, lungs, adrenal glands, and bone marrow. Sometimes lymph node metastases are the first manifestation of the disease.[142] Blood-borne metastases are more commonly associated with fibrous (sarcomatoid) forms of diffuse mesothelioma than with any other microscopic types.[162]

As is evident from the survival rates, treatment is rarely effective, although remissions have been achieved in some instances. Diffuse pleural mesothelioma is surgically treated by parietal pleurectomy or decortication, but necessarily resection is often incomplete and incapable of preventing continued growth.[65] Diffuse peritoneal mesotheliomas are usually unresectable, unless the tumors are partially localized, as is often the case with predominantly fibrous mesotheliomas of the peritoneal cavity. Radiation has been given alone or in addition to surgery, but many believe that the tumor is insensitive to radiation.*

There is also little information as to the efficacy of chemotherapy, but palliation, remissions, and improved survivals rates have been observed with various chemotherapeutic agents such as cyclophosphamide, methotrexate, 5-fluorouracil, cisplatin, and especially doxorubicin.† The available data are insufficient to adequately assess the effect of chemotherapy, and longer, carefully controlled studies on a larger number of cases are needed for reliable evaluation of the optimal type of therapy.

WELL-DIFFERENTIATED PAPILLARY MESOTHELIOMA

This is a rare mesothelial tumor of borderline malignancy that is marked by single layer of well-differentiated flattened or cuboidal mesothelial cells lining a delicate to coarse papillary fibrous core (Fig. 30-26). The lesions may be localized or multifocal and are primarily located in the peritoneum, with a predilection for the omentum, mesentery, and pelvis; they may also arise from the spermatic cord (tunica vaginalis testis) and the surfaces of the testis. Many are incidental findings at surgical exploration or autopsy. The staining and electron microscopic features of the lining cells are typical of well-differentiated mesothelial cells.[174,177,180] Rarely, the features of papillary mesothelioma may be associated with those of an adenomatoid tumor.[205] As with malignant mesothelioma, negative staining of the cells with PAS after diastase digestion and the results of immunohistochemical studies, especially carcino-

---

*References 82, 85, 87, 92, 97, 124.
†References 4, 7, 9, 28, 63, 93, 166.

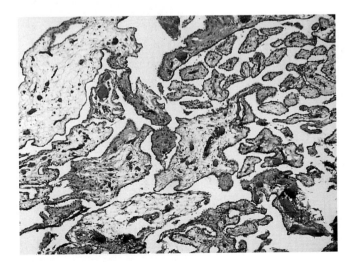

FIG. 30-26. Well-differentiated papillary mesothelioma showing a single layer of uniform mesothelial cells covering a fibrous to myxoid papillary core. (×160.)

embryonic antigen and Leu-M1, help to distinguish the lesion from surface papillary carcinoma.[136,163,178]

While most of these tumors, especially those that are small and localized, are benign and cured by local excision, some recur, often after many years, or progress to malignant mesothelioma with occasional distant metastases.[72,120,170,179] The malignant variants usually can be recognized by their solid or infiltrative growth, cellular atypia, high mitotic rate and necrosis. There are occasional cases with a history of asbestos exposure.[172,175]

MULTICYSTIC PERITONEAL MESOTHELIOMA

This term has been used to describe another unusual mesothelial lesion that seems to be related to the well-differentiated papillary mesothelioma, and that deserves separate consideration because of its characteristic histological picture and its benign behavior. In the past this lesion was often confused with cystic lymphangioma, with mesenteric lymphatic cyst in basal cell nevus syndrome, or, despite its different clinical course, with diffuse mesothelioma or even a disseminated form of mucin-producing adenocarcinoma. Plaut[192] and much later Rhind and Wright[193] and others[182,188,194,195] documented such lesions and suggested their mesothelial origin, but only in recent years was the mesothelial origin confirmed by immunohistochemical and ultrastructural studies.[191,196]

Multicystic peritoneal mesothelioma occurs chiefly in adults, with a predilection for young and middle-aged women. It is usually noted because of vague lower abdominal pain or symptoms suggesting partial intestinal obstruction, such as distension, nausea, or vomiting. Exploratory laparotomy reveals a characteristic picture; numerous thin-walled transparent cysts are unevenly distributed in the serosal and subserosal tissues of the parietal and visceral peritoneum of the abdomen and pelvis, often forming multicystic masses. The cysts measure from a few millimeters in diameter to several centimeters and contain clear serous fluid (Fig. 30-27). Occasionally, there are also multiple filamentous and stringlike adhesions between the peritoneum, intestines, and viscera.[185,186,189,190,198] Rhind and Wright's[193] patient had massive ascites but was well 4 years after onset of symptoms.

Microscopic examination discloses one or more variously sized, rounded or irregularly shaped cystic spaces lined by a single layer of flattened or cuboidal mesothelial cells, sometimes displaying a brush border. Less commonly the cells are plump and protrude into the lumen in a hobnail or even papillary pattern. Focal squamous metaplasia is occasionally seen. The cystic spaces are separated by loose, edematous tissue often containing chronic inflammatory cells, fibrin deposits, and sometimes entrapped mesothelial cells resembling infiltrating carcinoma. Transition between multicystic mesothelioma and adenomatoid tumor has been observed (Figs. 30-28 and 30-29).[198] The secreted material within the spaces stains positively with alcian blue and colloidal iron but negatively with PAS. Similarly staining ma-

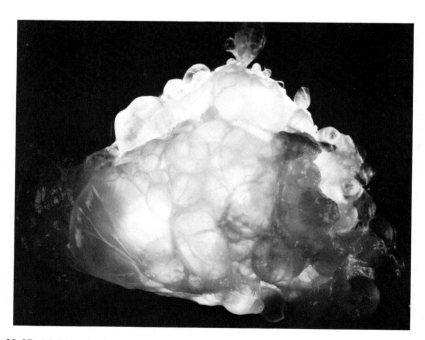

FIG. 30-27. Multicystic peritoneal mesothelioma consisting of multiple transparent, fluid-filled cysts.

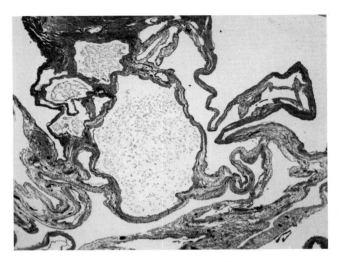

FIG. 30-28. Multicystic peritoneal mesothelioma mimicking a cystic lymphangioma. (×65.)

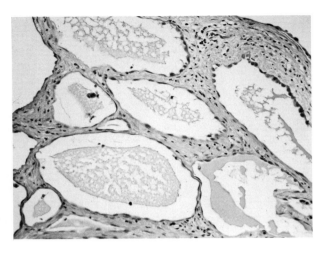

FIG. 30-29. Multicystic peritoneal mesothelioma. The cysts are lined by flattened and cuboidal mesothelial cells. (×100.)

terial is found as a thin coating on the luminal surfaces of the tumor cells and rarely as small droplets intracellularly.

Like other forms of mesothelioma the lining cells stain positively for immunoreactive cytokeratin and epithelial membrane antigen,[177] a feature that rules out cystic lymphangioma (Fig. 30-30). Moreover, cystic lymphangioma occurs chiefly in male children and adolescents and microscopically is characterized by stromal aggregates of lymphocytes, an endothelial lining that sometimes but not always stains positively with factor VIII–related protein, and that is often surrounded by a layer of smooth muscle tissue.

Other conditions that must be considered in differential diagnosis include reactive mesothelial proliferations, well-differentiated papillary mesothelioma, and ovarian and extraovarian serous or papillary carcinomas[171,173,176,197] and endometriosis.

Electron microscopic studies carried out by Moore et al.[191] and Mennemeyer and Smith[190] revealed the ultrastructural characteristics of mesothelial cells, especially slender microvilli on the luminal surfaces of the lining cells, well-developed basal laminae, and tight desmosomal junctions. There are also numerous intracytoplasmic filaments, ovoid mitochondria, and prominent rough-surfaced endoplasmic reticulum (Figs. 30-31 and 30-32).

The clinical course is largely that of a benign lesion. Among 25 cases with follow-up information reported by Weiss and Tavassoli,[198] 21 were alive, 2 died of other causes, and two died of the disease. The 2 patients who died were an infant who had a mixture of cystic and diffuse epithelial mesothelioma and a 47-year-old man who refused therapy and died 12 years after the detection of the

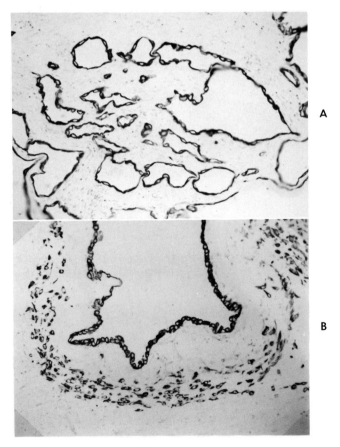

FIG. 30-30. A, Multicystic peritoneal mesothelioma showing immunostaining for cytokeratin (same case as Fig. 30-29). (×60.) The lining cells as well as subjacent fibroblast-like cells are immunoreactive for cytokeratin **(B).** (×160.)

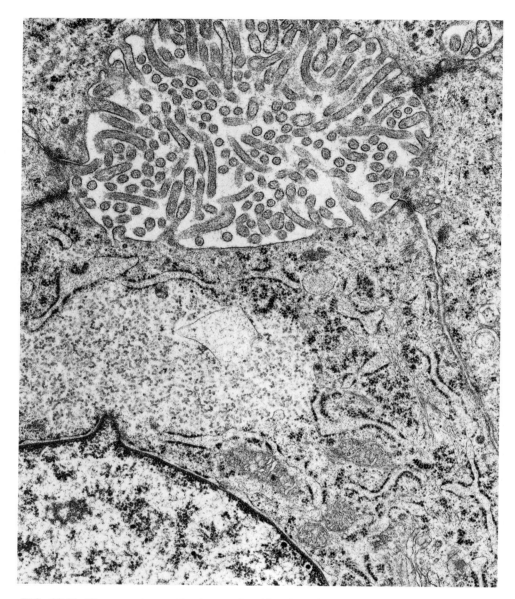

FIG. 30-31. Electron microscopic picture of multicystic peritoneal mesothelioma showing intercellular space with numerous slender microvilli and deposits of intracellular glycogen. (From Mennemeyer R, Smith M: *Cancer* 44:692, 1979.)

abdominal mass. The appropriate therapy seems to be total surgical excision for localized lesions and subtotal resection or debulking procedures for more extensive lesions.[198] Sometimes the large number of lesions and their small size may preclude complete resection, with further spread and recurrence years after the initial excision. The pathogenesis of the lesion is not clear. Certainly the multiplicity of lesions, their spread and recurrence, and the reported transitions toward adenomatoid tumor are more in keeping with a neoplasm than a reactive process. Development of the lesion following asbestos exposure must be extremely rare,

but one such lesion in a man has been reported.[187] Although diffuse epithelial mesothelioma may present at times as a multicystic growth, it usually can be identified by its less uniform gross appearance, its greater cellularity, and its cellular pleomorphism.

BENIGN MESOTHELIOMA OF THE GENITAL TRACT (ADENOMATOID TUMOR)

This is still another type of mesothelioma, which is apparently confined to the genital tract. It occurs in both sexes; in men it affects the epididymis, testicular tunic, and sper-

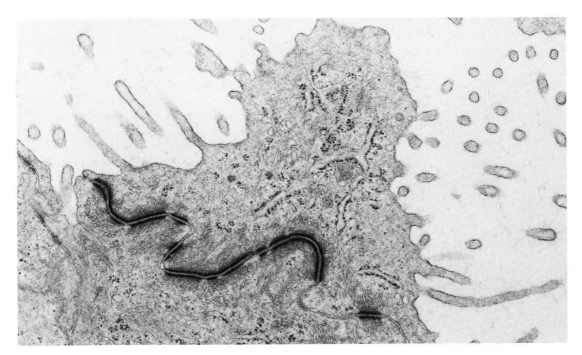

FIG. 30-32. Electon microscopic picture of multicystic peritoneal mesothelioma with short microvilli, prominent tight desmosomal junction, and converging microfilaments. (From Mennemeyer R, Smith M: *Cancer* 44:692, 1979.)

matic cord; in women it arises in the uterus, fallopian tubes, and rarely the ovary. Its mesothelial origin, first suggested by Masson et al.[212] in 1942, is now firmly established, but the earlier noncommittal term *adenomatoid tumor,* coined by Golden and Ash[204] in 1945, is still widely employed in order to clearly distinguish this tumor from the rare papillary mesothelioma of the tunica vaginalis and ovary. The clinical course is uneventful, and local resection is adequate therapy.

Clinical findings

In general, the tumor presents as a small indurated mass or swelling that is painless and nontender. It is usually an incidental finding at routine examination, surgery for some other cause (hysterectomy), or autopsy. It rarely occurs before the age of 20 years and is chiefly encountered in patients between 30 and 60 years of age. Its most common site is the epididymis, especially its lower pole, followed in frequency by the uterus (near the cornua of the uterine fundus),[206] fallopian tube,[220] and testicular tunic and rarely the ovary or the spermatic cord.[189,197] Craig and Hart[201] described an extragenital example of this tumor, but in this case it is difficult to rule out a benign mesothelial proliferation or an epithelial type of mesothelioma. The tumor is usually solitary, but multiple nodular lesions have been observed. A small number of these lesions in the scrotum are associated with hydroceles. There are no systemic changes. Kannerstein and Lustig,[208] however, described one patient with this tumor who had bilateral gynecomastia and a positive Aschheim-Zondek pregnancy test that reverted to normal after removal of the tumor.

Pathological findings

Gross examination reveals a firm mass generally measuring less than 2 cm in greatest dimension. The mass is well circumscribed with a smooth, moist, glistening, yellow-gray cut surface. On microscopic examination the tumor possesses a variable structural pattern ranging from irregularly arranged, dilated tubular channels and glandlike spaces lined by flattened or cuboidal cells to solid nests and strands of plump cells having abundant eosinophilic cytoplasm (Fig. 30-33). As in other types of mesothelioma, desquamated cells are often present within the dilated spaces. Lee et al.[209] distinguished canalicular, tubular, and plexiform patterns. The fibrous stroma may be sparse or abundant and may contain aggregates of lymphocytes. The smooth muscle component, which is present and even conspicuous in some cases, is most likely residual. It was also interpreted as an inherent part of the tumor and was cited as evidence for its origin in the müllerian duct. This theory of origin is not supported by several electron microscopic studies,[203,210,211,215,218] which disclosed the characteristic fea-

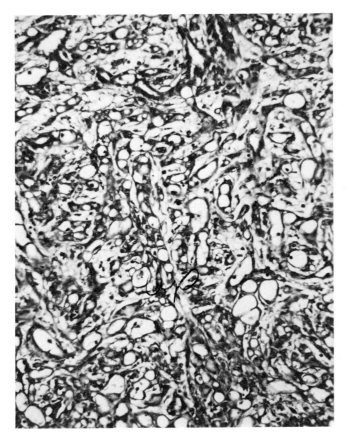

FIG. 30-33. Benign mesothelioma of the genital tract (adenomatoid tumor) showing characteristic tubular pattern. (×160.)

tures of mesothelial cells, including long, bushy microvilli on the luminal surfaces and intercellular spaces, irregular cytoplasmic protrusions, and desmosomes, often associated with tonofibrils. Like mesothelial cells at other sites, the cells stain positively with cytokeratin and do not stain with factor VIII and *Ulex europaeus* antibodies.[200,214,217] The latter stains are positive in histiocytoid (epithelioid) hemangioma of the testis, a tumor that must be distinguished from richly vascular variants of adenomatoid tumor.[199]

The tumor is benign, and there is no evidence of malignant transformation. It is important to distinguish it from papillary mesothelioma of the genital tract, especially that of the tunica vaginalis testis.[76,117,179]

LOCALIZED (SOLITARY) FIBROUS TUMOR OF THE PLEURA AND PERITONEUM (FIBROUS MESOTHELIOMA)

Although the exact origin of this tumor is still debated, most reviewers believe that it arises from submesothelial fibrous connective tissue and should be classified as a variant of fibroma *(localized fibrous tumor of the pleura and peritoneum, subserosal fibroma)*. There are also those who

favor origin from modified mesothelial cells and prefer a diagnosis of fibrous mesothelioma. A fibrous tissue origin is supported by the fact that the tumor is frequently covered by an intact layer of mesothelial cells, that it lacks mesothelial features in tissue culture and ultrastructural studies, and that there is no evidence of intracellular cytokeratin or EMA on immunohistochemical studies.[227,231,244] Origin from modified mesothelial cells, on the other hand, is difficult to rule out, in view of the characteristic locations of the tumor and the established potential of mesothelial cells to differentiate along epithelial and fibroblastic lines.[225,233,243,248,249]

Since the first report of this entity by Klemperer and Rabin[235] in 1931, it has been shown that localized fibrous tumor is found much more frequently in the pleural than the abdominal cavity but that it is much less common at both sites than the diffuse type of mesothelioma.[155] Rare intrapulmonary, mediastinal, nasal, nasopharyngeal, and hepatic forms of the tumor have also been described.[230,234,236,250,253] There is still little information as to the actual incidence of the lesion; it is relatively rare, and Okike et al.[242] found only 2.8 cases per 100,000 registrations at the Mayo Clinic.

There are benign and malignant forms of the tumor (fibrosarcoma of the pleura and peritoneum), the benign variant being three to four times as common as the malignant one.[223,227] There is no clear relationship to asbestos exposure, but rare instances of this association have been described.[242,246]

Clinical findings

Localized fibrous tumor (fibrous mesothelioma) principally affects older persons between the fourth and seventh decades of life and, unlike diffuse mesothelioma, is slightly more common in women than men. It tends to be asymptomatic, and in most patients its existence is discovered during routine x-ray examination or for some other reasons unrelated to the disease. It may also cause minor symptoms such as vague pleuritic pain, chronic cough, and shortness of breath, but these symptoms are mostly associated with tumors of larger size. Arthritic pain and clubbing of the fingers (osteoarthropathy) occur in about 10% of cases and, in fact, are more common in the localized than in the diffuse type. It is of interest that these changes recede within a few months after removal of the tumor and come back when it recurs. Pleural effusion, as well as chest pain and dyspnea, is more commonly associated with the malignant than the benign variant of the tumor.[227]

Hypoglycemia

Although hypoglycemia has been observed with diffuse mesotheliomas, it more commonly is associated with solitary fibrous tumors of the pleura and peritoneum, especially those of large size.[48,241] It occurs in about 5% of cases, is

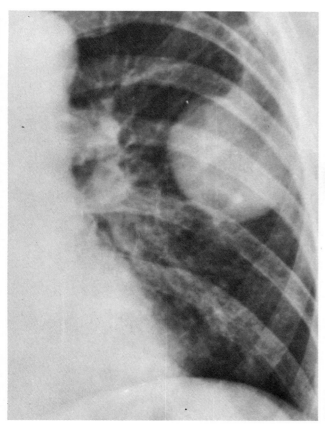
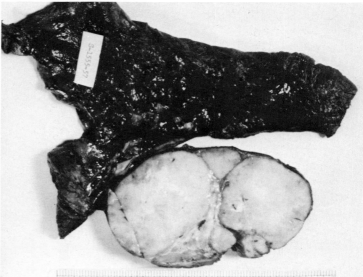

FIG. 30-34. **A,** Radiograph of localized fibrous tumor of the pleura (localized fibrous mesothelioma) showing sharply circumscribed mass in left pleural space. **B,** Gross specimen of localized fibrous mesothelioma (subserosal fibroma) showing attachment to the right lung.

more common in females than males, and sometimes is the first manifestation of the disease; according to England et al.[227] it is more frequently associated with tumors in the right than the left hemithorax. Typical symptoms range from profuse sweating, headaches, and restlessness to disorientation, convulsions, and coma. One of our patients with hypoglycemia suffered "4 strokes" within 4 consecutive days; another became manic, with psychotic manifestations and a fasting blood sugar level as low as 18 mg/dl. Kniznik et al.[83] reported a 58-year-old patient with severe hypoglycemia who had a localized fibrous tumor (fibrous mesothelioma) in the pleural space that measured 28 cm in greatest diameter. Hypoglycemia, of course, is not a specific feature of this tumor and mesothelioma; it occurs also in association with fibrosarcoma, hemangiopericytoma, and other nonpancreatic mesenchymal and epithelial neoplasms. The exact physiological mechanism remains obscure; release of insulin-like substances by the tumor, inhibition of gluconeogenesis, pressure on splanchnic nerves, and excessive consumption of glucose have been mentioned among the possible causes. In most patients the hypoglycemic episodes are effectively treated by surgical removal of the tumor.

Radiographic findings

Roentgenographic and CT examination usually reveals the presence of a solitary rounded, sharply outlined, homogenous density or mass in the pleural or peritoneal cavity. The mass may be sessile or pedunculated and may shift its position in different postures.[240,242] Sometimes the tumor is evidenced merely as an ovoid thickening of an interlobular fissure (Fig. 30-34, *A*).

Pathological findings

Grossly the tumor manifests as a solitary localized mass that is attached with a richly vascularized pedicle or a broad base to the visceral or parietal pleura or the peritoneum and that is covered by a smooth glistening capsule (Fig. 30-34, *B*). The tumor arises more commonly from the visceral than the parietal pleura and in about half of cases is attached to the serosa by a single pedicle. On the average it measures 5 to 6 cm in diameter, but examples measuring as large as

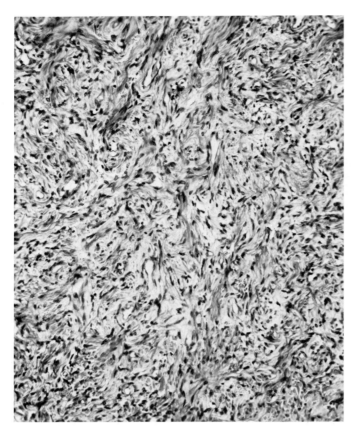

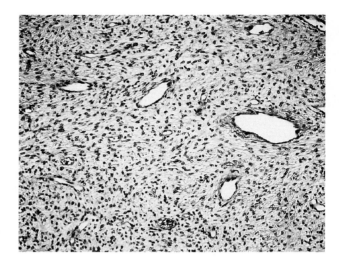

FIG. 30-36. Myxoid portion of a localized fibrous tumor of the pleura (fibrous mesothelioma) with gaping vascular spaces (same tumor as Fig. 30-37). (×160.)

FIG. 30-35. Localized fibrous tumor of the pleura (localized fibrous mesothelioma) composed of spindle cells forming collagen and mucoid material. (×160.)

20 to 30 cm in diameter and filling the entire hemithorax have been described. The largest tumor in the series of England et al.[227] measured 39 cm in greatest diameter. The cut surface has a uniform or nodular, firm, gray-white appearance or shows a variegated picture with alternating firm and soft myxoid areas, sometimes with cystic spaces and areas of hemorrhage and necrosis.

Under the microscope most of the tumors are composed of uniform collagen-forming spindle cells, which are arranged in interlacing fascicles and show no or minimal mitotic activity (Fig. 30-35). Some show associated myxoid changes or extensive fibrosis and hyalinization, often with wirelike bundles of collagen and, rarely, with focal calcification. Not infrequently, richly and poorly cellular myxoid or hyalinized areas are present in different portions of the same neoplasm (Figs. 30-36 and 30-37). Many tumors are covered by an intact layer of mesothelial cells, and some contain entrapped alveolar or bronchial epithelium at the serosal attachment sites that may be mistaken for an epithelial component (Fig. 30-38). The vascularity varies from narrow vascular clefts that may mimic mesothelium-lined

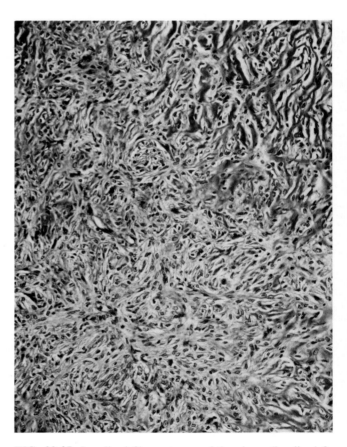

FIG. 30-37. Localized fibrous tumor of the pleura (localized fibrous mesothelioma) with focal hyalinization. (×160.)

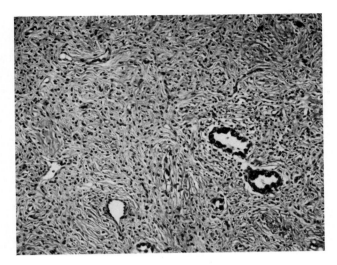

FIG. 30-38. Localized fibrous tumor of the pleura (localized fibrous mesothelioma) with entrapped alveolar structures. (×160.)

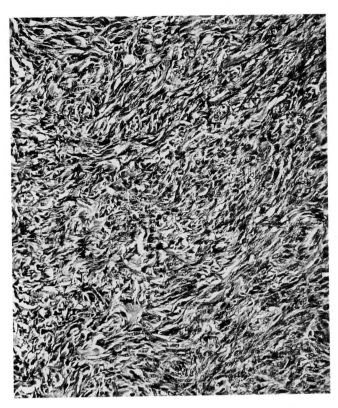

FIG. 30-39. Malignant localized fibrous tumor of the pleura exhibiting increased cellularity and cellular pleomorphism. (×160.)

spaces to gaping and branching vascular channels virtually indistinguishable from those of hemangiopericytoma.

The malignant variants can be recognized by their greater cellularity, cellular pleomorphism, and increased mitotic activity, usually more than four mitotic figures per 10 HPF[227] (Fig. 30-39). In fact, without immunohistochemical examination, this tumor may be difficult to distinguish from sarcomatoid or desmoplastic mesotheliomas.[27] It does not show, however, the herringbone pattern of fibrosarcoma.

Immunohistochemical studies reveal no evidence of mesothelial differentiation; the tumor cells are negative for anticytokeratin and epithelial membrane antigen, but stain with antibodies against vimentin and, occasionally, muscle-specific actin.[224,225,227,228,244] By contrast, the nonneoplastic fibroblast-like subserosal cells of fibrous pleural plaques and pleural scars stain positively for cytokeratin.[19,51,105]

Ultrastructurally, the tumors consist of fibroblast-like spindle cells with rough endoplasmic reticulum, cytoplasmic filaments, multiple elongated or pseudopod-like processes, and occasional primitive junctions but without microvilli, glycogen, basal laminae, or tonofilaments.[222,224,225,231] None of the reviewers found any clearcut ultrastructural evidence of mesothelial differentiation. Only Kawai et al.[233] reported "minimal differentiation toward mesothelial cells." Others favored a "subset of mesothelioma" because of the presence of plump cytoplasmic processes and tight intercellular junctions.[225,243]

Clinical course and prognosis

The prognosis of the localized fibrous tumor of the pleura and peritoneum (localized fibrous mesothelioma) varies greatly, and careful microscopic examination in regard to cellularity, pleomorphism, and mitotic activity is necessary in all cases for reliable prediction of the clinical course. The data regarding the incidence of malignancy show a wide range: in the series of Okike et al.[242] only 8 of 60 cases were malignant. But in the large series of England et al.,[227] 39 of 169 cases with follow-up information did not respond to therapy; they were nonresectable or recurrent and developed metastases. Morphologically benign lesions merely require complete local resection, which may include in some cases segmental resection or even lobectomy. Malignant fibrous tumors, particularly nonpedunculated ones, are in need of a more radical therapy similar to that outlined under diffuse malignant mesotheliomas.

REFERENCES
Diffuse mesothelioma

1. Ackerman LV: Tumors of the retroperitoneum, mesentery, and peritoneum. In *Atlas of tumor pathology,* Armed Forces Institute of Pathology, 1954, sec VI, fascicles 23 and 24, Washington, DC.

2. Adami JG: *Principles of pathology,* Philadelphia, 1908, Lea & Febiger.

3. Adams VI, Unni KK: Diffuse mesothelioma of pleura: diagnostic criteria based on autopsy study. *Am J Clin Pathol* 82:15, 1984.

4. Adams VI, Unni KK, Muhm JR, et al: Diffuse mesothelioma of pleura: diagnosis and survival in 92 cases. *Cancer* 58:1540, 1986.

5. Aisner J, Wiernik PH: Malignant mesothelioma: current status and future prospects. *Chest* 74:438, 1978.

6. Antman KH: Clinical presentation and natural history of benign and malignant mesothelioma. *Semin Oncol* 8:313, 1981.

7. Antman KH, Blum RH, Greenberger JS, et al: Multimodality therapy for malignant mesothelioma based on a study of natural history. *Am J Med* 68:356, 1980.

8. Antman KH, Corson JM: Benign and malignant mesothelioma. *Clin Chest Med* 6:127, 1985.

9. Antman KH, Pomfret EA, Aisner J, et al: Peritoneal mesothelioma: natural history and response to chemotherapy. *J Clin Oncol* 1:386, 1983.

10. Arai H, Endo M, Sasai Y, et al: Histochemical demonstration of hyaluronic acid in a case of pleural mesothelioma. *Am Rev Respir Dis* 111:699, 1975.

11. Armstrong GR, Raafat F, Ingram L, et al: Malignant peritoneal mesothelioma in childhood. *Arch Pathol Lab Med* 112:1159, 1988.

12. Ashcroft T, Heppleston AG: The optical and EM determination of pulmonary asbestos fiber concentration and its relation to the human pathological reaction. *J Clin Pathol* 26:224, 1973.

13. Azumi N, Underhill CB, Kagan E, et al: A novel biotinylated probe specific for hyaluronate: its diagnostic value in diffuse malignant mesothelioma. *Am J Surg Pathol* 16:116, 1992.

14. Banner MP, Gohel VK: Peritoneal mesothelioma. *Radiology* 129:637, 1978.

15. Battifora H, Kopinski MI: Distinction of mesothelioma from adenocarcinoma: an immunohistochemical approach. *Cancer* 55:1679, 1985.

16. Bedrossian CW, Bonsib S, Moran C: Differential diagnosis between mesothelioma and adenocarcinoma: a multimodal approach based on ultrastructure and immunocytochemistry. *Semin Diagn Pathol* 9:124, 1992.

17. Blobel GA, Moll R, Franke WW, et al: The intermediate filament cytoskeleton of malignant mesotheliomas and its diagnostic significance. *Am J Pathol* 121:235, 1985.

18. Boehme M: Primäres Sarcocarcinom der Pleura. *Virchows Arch (Pathol Anat)* 81:181, 1880.

19. Bolen JW, Hammar SP, McNutt MA: Reactive and neoplastic serosal tissue: a light microscopic, ultrastructural, and immunocytochemical study. *Am J Surg Pathol* 10:34, 1986.

20. Bollinger DJ, Wick MR, Dehner LP, et al: Peritoneal malignant mesothelioma versus serous papillary adenocarcinoma: a histochemical and immunohistochemical comparison. *Am J Surg Pathol* 13:659, 1989.

21. Brenner J, Sordillo PP, Magill GB: Malignant mesothelioma in children: report of seven cases and review of the literature. *Med Pediatr Oncol* 9:367, 1981.

22. Brenner J, Sordillo PP, Magill GB, et al: Malignant peritoneal mesothelioma. Review of 25 patients. *Am J Gastroenterol* 75:311, 1981.

23. Brooks JS, Livolsi VA, Pietra GG: Mesothelial cell inclusions in mediastinal lymph nodes mimicking metastatic carcinoma. *Am J Clin Pathol* 93:741, 1990.

24. Brown RW, Clark GM, Tandon AK, et al: Muliple marker immunohistochemical phenotypes distinguishing malignant pleural mesothelioma from pulmonary adenocarcinoma. *Hum Pathol* 24:347, 1993.

25. Burmer GC, Rabinovitch PS, Kulander BG, et al: Flow cytometric analysis of malignant pleural mesotheliomas. *Hum Pathol* 20:777, 1989.

26a. Burns TR, Greenberg SD, Mace ML, et al: Ultrastructural diagnosis of epithelial malignant mesothelioma. *Cancer* 56:2036, 1985.

26b. Cayle PT, Brown RW, Lebovitz RM: p53 immunostaining in the differentiation of reactive processes from malignancy in pleural biopsy specimens. *Hum Pathol* 25:443, 1994.

27. Cantin R, Al-Jabi M, McCaughey WT: Desmoplastic diffuse mesothelioma. *Am J Surg Pathol* 6:215, 1982.

28. Casey Jones DE, Silver D: Peritoneal mesotheliomas. *Surgery* 86:560, 1979.

29. Chang K, Pai LH, Pass H, et al: Monoclonal antibody K1 reacts with epithelial mesothelioma but not with lung adenocarcinoma. *Am J Surg Pathol* 16:259, 1992.

30. Chiu B, Churg A, Tengblad A, et al: Analysis of hyaluronic acid in the diagnosis of malignant mesothelioma. *Cancer* 54:2195, 1984.

31. Churg A: Fiber counting and analysis in the diagnosis of asbestos-related disease. *Hum Pathol* 13:381, 1982.

32. Churg A: Immunohistochemical staining for vimentin and keratin in malignant mesothelioma. *Am J Surg Pathol* 9:360, 1985.

33. Churg J, Rosen SH, Moolten S: Histological characteristics of mesothelioma associated with asbestos. *Ann N Y Acad Sci* 132:614, 1965.

34. Churg A, Sakoda N, Warnock ML: A simple method for preparing ferruginous bodies for electron microscopic examination. *Am J Clin Pathol* 68:513, 1977.

35. Churg A, Warnock ML, Green N: Analysis of the cores of ferruginous (asbestos) bodies from the general population. *Lab Invest* 40:31, 1975.

36. Clarkson FA: Primary endothelioma of the pleura. *Can Med Assoc J* 4:192, 1914.

37. Corson JM, Pinkus GS: Mesothelioma: Profile of keratin proteins and carcinoembryonic antigen: an immunoperoxidase study of 20 cases and comparison with pulmonary adenocarcinoma. *Am J Pathol* 108:80, 1982.

38. Craighead JE: Current pathogenetic concepts of diffuse malignant mesothelioma. *Hum Pathol* 18:544, 1987.

39. Craighead JE: The epidemiology and pathogenesis of malignant mesothelioma. *Chest* 96:925, 1989.

40. Craighead JE, Abraham JL, Churg A, et al: The pathology of asbestos-associated diseases of the lung and pleural cavities: diagnostic criteria and proposed grading schema. *Arch Pathol Lab Med* 106:544, 1982.

41. Craighead JE, Mossman BT: The pathogenesis of asbestos-associated diseases. *N Engl J Med* 306:1446, 1982.

42. Crotty TB, Colby TV, Gay PC, et al: Desmoplastic malignant mesothelioma masquerading as sclerosing mediastinitis: a diagnostic dilemma. *Hum Pathol* 23:79, 1992.

42a. Crotty TB, Myers JL, Katzenstein AA, et al: Localized malignant mesothelioma: a clinicopathologic and flow cytometric study. *Am J Surg Pathol* 18:357, 1994.

43. Crouch E, Churg A: Ferruginous bodies and the histologic evaluation of dust exposure. *Am J Surg Pathol* 8:109, 1984.

44. Dahl IMS, Laurent TC: Concentration of hyaluronan in the serum of untreated cancer patients with special reference to patients with mesothelioma. *Cancer* 62:326, 1988.

45. Dardick I, Al-Jabi M, Elliot WT, et al: Diffuse epithelial mesothelioma – a review of the ultrastructural spectrum. *Ultrastruct Pathol* 11:503, 1987.

46. Dawe CJ, Wood DA, Mitchell S: Diffuse fibrous mesothelioma of the pericardium. *Cancer* 6:794, 1953.

47. Dessy E, Pietra GG: Pseudomesotheliomatous carcinoma of lung. An immunohistochemical and ultrastructural study of three cases. *Cancer* 68:1747, 1991.

48. Devroede GJ, Tirol AF: Giant pleural mesothelioma associated with hypoglycemia and hyperthyroidism. *Am J Surg* 116:130, 1968.

49. Dionne PG, Wang NS: A scanning electron microscopic study of diffuse mesothelioma and some lung carcinomas. *Cancer* 40:707, 1977.

50. El-Naggar AK, Ordonez NG, Garnsey L, et al: Epithelioid pleural mesothelioma and pulmonary adenocarcinoma. A comparative DNA flow cytometric study. *Hum Pathol* 22:972, 1991.

51. Epstein JI, Budin RE: Keratin and epithelial membrane antigen immunoreactivity in nonneoplastic fibrous pleural lesions: implications for the diagnosis of desmoplastic mesothelioma. *Hum Pathol* 17:514, 1986.

52. Fisher ER, Hellstrom HR: The periodic acid–Schiff reaction as an aid in the identification of mesothelioma. *Cancer* 13:837, 1960.

53. Fisher-Wasels B: Ueber die primaeren malignen Geschwülste der Serosadeckzellen. *Z Krebsforsch* 37:22, 1932.

54. Fraire AE, Greenberg SD, Buffler P, et al: Mesothelioma of childhood. *Cancer* 62:838, 1988.

55. Frebourg T, Lerebours G, Delpech B, et al: Serum hyaluronate in malignant pleural mesothelioma. *Cancer* 59:2104, 1987.

56. Frierson HF, Mills SE, Legier JF: Flow cytometric analysis of ploidy in immunohistochemically confirmed examples of malignant mesothelioma. *Am J Clin Pathol* 90:240, 1988.

57. Gaffey MJ, Mills SE, Swanson PE, et al: Immunoreactivity for BER-EP4 in adenocarcinomas, adenomatoid tumors, and malignant mesotheliomas. *Am J Surg Pathol* 16:593, 1992.

58. Geschickter CF: Mesothelial tumors. *Am J Cancer* 26:378, 1936.

59. Ghosh AK, Gatter KC, Dunnill MS, et al: Immunohistological staining or reactive mesothelium, mesothelioma, and lung carcinoma with a panel of monoclonal antibodies. *J Clin Pathol* 40:19, 1987.

60. Gibas Z, Li FP, Antman KH, et al: Chromosome changes in malignant mesothelioma. *Cancer Genet Cytogenet* 20:191, 1986.

61. Gotteherer A, Taryle DA, Reed CE, et al: Pleural fluid analysis in malignant mesothelioma: prognostic implications. *Chest* 100:1003, 1991.

62. Grundy GW, Miller RW: Malignant mesothelioma in childhood: report of 13 cases. *Cancer* 30:1216, 1972.

63. Hamm-Antman KH: Malignant mesothelioma. *N Engl J Med* 4:200, 1980.

64. Herzog F: Ein Fall von maligner Deckzellengeschwulst des Peritoneums. *Zieglers* 58:390, 1914.

65. Hilaris BS, Nori D, Kwong F, et al: Pleurectomy and postoperative radiation in the treatment of malignant pleural mesothelioma. *Int J Radiat Oncol Biol Phys* 10:325, 1984.

66. Hillerdal G: Malignant mesothelioma 1982: review of 4710 published cases. *Br J Dis Chest* 77:321, 1983.

67. Hillerdal G, Berg J: Malignant mesothelioma secondary to chronic inflammation and old scars. *Cancer* 55:1968, 1985.

68. Hillerdal G, Lindqvist U, Engström-Laurent A: Hyaluronan in pleural effusions and in serum. *Cancer* 67:2410, 1991.

69. Holden J, Churg A: Immunohistochemical staining for keratin and carcinoembryonic antigen in the diagnosis of malignant mesothelioma. *Am J Surg Pathol* 8:277, 1984.

70. Jasani B, Edwards RE, Thomas ND, et al: The use of vimentin antibodies in the diagnosis of malignant mesothelioma. *Virchows Arch (Pathol Anat)* 406:441, 1985.

71. Kahn HJ, Thorner PS, Yeger H, et al: Distinct keratin patterns demonstrated by immunoperoxidase staining of adenocarcinomas, carcinoids, and mesotheliomas using polyclonal and monoclonal antikeratin antibodies. *Am J Clin Pathol* 86:566, 1986.

72. Kamiya M, Elmoto T: Malignant mesothelioma of the tunica vaginalis. *Pathol Res Pract* 186:680, 1990.

73. Kannerstein M, Churg J: Peritoneal mesothelioma. *Hum Pathol* 8:83, 1977.

74. Kannerstein M, Churg J, Magner D: Histochemistry in the diagnosis of malignant mesothelioma. *Ann Clin Lab Sci* 3:207, 1973.

75. Kannerstein M, Churg J, McCaughey WTE: Asbestos and mesothelioma: a review. *Pathol Annu* 13:81, 1978.

76. Kasdon EJ: Malignant mesothelioma of the tunica vaginalis testis. *Cancer* 23:1144, 1969.

77. Kauffman SL, Stout AP: Mesothelioma in children. *Cancer* 17:539, 1964.

78. Kawai T, Suzuki M, Kageyama K: Reactive mesothelial cells and mesothelioma of the pleura. *Virchows Arch (Pathol Anat)* 393:251, 1981.

79. Kawai T, Suzuki M, Shinmai M, et al: Glycosaminglycans in malignant diffuse mesothelioma. *Cancer* 56:567, 1985.

80. Kay S, Silverberg SG: Ultrastructural studies of a malignant fibrous mesothelioma of the pleura. *Arch Pathol* 92:449, 1971.

81. Klima M, Gyorkey F: Benign pleural lesions and malignant mesothelioma. *Virchows Arch (Pathol Anat)* 376:181, 1977.

82. Klima M, Spjut HJ, Seybold WD: Diffuse malignant mesothelioma. *Am J Clin Pathol* 65:583, 1976.

83. Kniznik DO, Roncoroni AJ, Rosenberg M, et al: Giant fibrous pleural mesothelioma associated with myocardial restriction and hypoglycemia. *Respiration* 37:346, 1979.

84. Krumhaar D, Lange S, Hartmann C, et al: Follow-up study of 100 malignant pleural mesotheliomas. *Thorac Cardiovasc Surg* 33:272, 1985.

85. Kucuksu N, Thomas W, Ezdinli EZ: Chemotherapy of malignant diffuse mesothelioma. *Cancer* 37:1265, 1976.

86. Langer AM, Selikoff IJ, Sastre A: Chrysotile asbestos in the lungs of persons in New York City. *Arch Environ Health* 22:348, 1971.

87. Legha SS, Muggia FM: Pleural mesothelioma: clinical features and therapeutic impressions. *Ann Intern Med* 87:613, 1977.

88. Leigh J, Rogers AJ, Ferguson DA, et al: Lung asbestos fiber content and mesothelioma cell type, site, and survival. *Cancer* 68:135, 1991.

89. Lerner HJ, Schoenfeld DA, Martin A, et al: Malignant mesothelioma: The Eastern Cooperative Oncology Group (ECOG) experience. *Cancer* 52:1981, 1983.

90. Lilis R: Fibrous zeolites and endemic mesothelioma in Cappadocia, Turkey. *J Occup Med* 23:548, 1981.

91. Libshitz HI: Malignant pleural mesothelioma: the role of computed tomography. *J Comput Tomogr* 8:15, 1984.

92. Loosli H, Hurlimann J: Immunohistochemical study of malignant diffuse mesotheliomas of the pleura. *Histopathology* 8:793, 1984.

93. Markman M, Cleary S, Pfeifle C, et al: Cisplatin administered by the intracavitary route as treatment for malignant mesothelioma. *Cancer* 58:18, 1986.

94. Marschall RJ, Herbert A, Braye SG, et al: Use of antibodies to carcinoembryonic antigen and human milk fat globule to distinguish carcinoma, mesothelioma, and reactive mesothelium. *J Clin Pathol* 37:1215, 1984.

95. Mayall FG, Gibbs AR: The histology and immunohistochemistry of small cell mesothelioma. *Histopathology* 20:47, 1992.

96. McCaughey WT, Colby TV, Battifora H, et al: Diagnosis of diffuse malignant mesothelioma: experience of a US/Canadian mesothelioma panel. *Mod Pathol* 4:342, 1991.

97. McCormack P, Nagasaki F, Hilaris B, et al: Surgical treatment of pleural mesothelioma. *J Thorac Cardiovasc Surg* 84:834, 1982.

98. McDonald AD, Harper A, El-Attar OA, et al: Epidemiology of primary malignant mesothelial tumors in Canada. *Cancer* 26:914, 1970.

99. McDonald AD, Magner D, Eyssen G: Primary malignant mesothelial tumors in Canada, 1960-1968: a pathological review by the mesothelioma panel of the Canadian Tumor Reference Centre. *Cancer* 31:869, 1973.

100. McDonald JC, Armstrong B, Case B, et al: Mesothelioma and asbestos fiber type. *Cancer* 63:1544, 1989.

101. McDonald JC, Liddel FDK: Mortality in Canadian miners and millers exposed to chrysotile. *Ann N Y Acad Sci* 330:1, 1979.

102. McEwen J, Finlayson A, Mair A, et al: Mesothelioma in Scotland. *Br Med J* 4:575, 1970.

103. Mellin W, Brockman M, Sawal O, et al: DNA-Bildzytometrie maligner Pleuramesotheliome. *Verh Dtsch Ges Pathol* 75:481, 1991.

104. Moertel CG: Peritoneal mesothelioma. *Gastroenterology* 63:346, 1972.

105. Montag AG, Pinkus GS, Corson JM: Immunoreactivity for keratin proteins in sarcomatoid diffuse malignant mesothelioma: a diagnostic discriminant among malignant spindle cell tumors. *Lab Invest* 52:44A, 1985.

106. Montag AG, Pinkus GS, Corson JM: Keratin protein immunoreactivity of sarcomatoid and mixed types of diffuse malignant mesothelioma: an immunoperoxidase study of 30 cases. *Hum Pathol* 19:336, 1988.

107. Nakano T, Fujii J, Tamura S: Thrombocytosis in patients with malignant pleural mesothelioma. *Cancer* 58:1699, 1986.

108. Nakano T, Fujii J, Tamura S, et al: Glycosaminoglycans in malignant pleural mesothelioma. *Cancer* 57:106, 1986.

109. Newhouse ML, Berry G: Patterns of mortality in asbestos factory workers in London. *Ann N Y Acad Sci* 330:53, 1979.

110. Newhouse ML, Thompson H: Mesothelioma of pleura and peritoneum following exposure to asbestos in the London area. *Br J Ind Med* 22:261, 1965.

111. Oels HC, Harrison EG Jr, Carr DT: Diffuse malignant mesothelioma of the pleura. *Chest* 60:564, 1971.

112. O'Hara CJ, Corson JM, Pinkus GS, et al: ME1. A monoclonal antibody that distinguishes epithelial-type malignant mesothelioma from pulmonary adenocarcinoma and extrapulmonary malignancies. *Am J Pathol* 136:421, 1990.

113. Ordonez NG: The immunohistochemical diagnosis of mesothelioma: differentiation of mesothelioma and lung adenocarcinoma. *Am J Surg Pathol* 13:276, 1989.

114. Otis CN, Carter D, Cole S, et al: Immunohistochemical evaluation of pleural mesothelioma and pulmonary adenocarcinoma. A biinstitutional study of 47 cases. *Am J Surg Pathol* 11:445, 1987.

115. Peterson JT, Greenberg SD, Buffler PA: Non–asbestos-related malignant mesothelioma: a review. *Cancer* 54:951, 1984.

116. Pettersson T, Frosth B, Riska H, et al: Concentration of hyaluronic acid in pleural fluid as a diagnostic aid for malignant mesothelioma. *Chest* 94:1037, 1988.

117. Pizzolato P, Lamberty J: Mesothelioma of spermatic cord: electron microscopic and histochemical characteristics of its mucopolysaccharides. *Urology* 8:403, 1976.

118. Pooley FD, Clark N: Fiber dimensions and aspect ratio of crocidolite, chrysotile, and amosite particles detected in lung tissue specimens. *Ann N Y Acad Sci* 330:711, 1979.

119. Raptopoulos V: Peritoneal mesothelioma. *Crit Rev Diagn Imaging* 24:293, 1985.

120. Riddell RH, Goodman MJ, Moossa AR: Peritoneal malignant mesothelioma in a patient with recurrent peritonitis. *Cancer* 48:134, 1981.

121. Rogers AJ, Leigh J, Berry G, et al: Relationship between lung asbestos fiber type and concentration and relative risk of mesothelioma. *Cancer* 67:1912, 1991.

122. Roggli VL, McGavran MH, Subach J, et al: Pulmonary asbestos counts and electron probe analysis of asbestos body cores in patients with mesothelioma: a study of 25 cases. *Cancer* 50:2423, 1982.

123. Roggli VL, Pratt PC, Brody AR: Asbestos content of lung tissue in asbestos-associated diseases: a study of 110 cases. *Br J Ind Med* 43:18, 1986.

124. Rogoff EE, Hilaris BS, Huvos AG: Long-term survival in patients with malignant peritoneal mesothelioma treated with irradiation. *Cancer* 32:656, 1973.

125. Ros PR, Yushok TJ, Buck JL, et al: Peritoneal mesothelioma: radiologic appearances correlated with histology. *Acta Radiol* 32:355, 1991.

126. Rosai J, Dehner LP: Nodular mesothelial hyperplasia in hernia sacs: a benign reactive condition simulating a neoplastic process. *Cancer* 35:165, 1975.

127. Rose RG, Palmer JD, Lougheed MN: Treatment of peritoneal mesothelioma with radioactive colloidal gold. *Cancer* 8:478, 1955.

128. Seidman H, Selikoff IJ, Hammond EC: Short-term asbestos work exposure and long-term observation. *Ann N Y Acad Sci* 330:61, 1979.

129. Selikoff IJ, Churg J, Hammond EC: Asbestos exposure and neoplasia. *JAMA* 188:22, 1964.

130. Selikoff IJ, Churg J, Hammond EC: Relation between exposure to asbestos and mesothelioma. *N Engl J Med* 272:560, 1965.

131. Selikoff IJ, Hammond EC: Health hazards of asbestos exposure. *Ann N Y Acad Sci* 330:1, 1979.

132. Selikoff IJ, Hammond EC, Seidman H: Mortality experience of insulation workers in the United States and Canada. *Ann N Y Acad Sci* 330:91, 1979.

133. Sheibani K, Battifora H, Burke JS, et al: Leu-M1 antigen in human neoplasms: an immunohistologic study of 400 cases. *Am J Surg Pathol* 10:227, 1986.

134. Sheibani K, Esteban JM, Bailey A, et al: Immunopathologic and molecular studies as an aid to the diagnosis of malignant mesothelioma. *Hum Pathol* 23:107, 1992.

135. Sheibani K, Shin SS, Kezirian J, et al: Ber-EP4 antibody as a discriminant in the differential diagnosis of malignant mesothelioma versus adenocarcinoma. *Am J Surg Pathol* 15:779, 1991.

136. Silcocks PB, Herbert A, Wright DH: Evaluation of PAS-diastase and carcinoembryonic antigen staining in the differential diagnosis of malignant mesothelioma. *J Pathol* 149:133, 1986.

137. Smith MJ, Naylor B: A method for extracting ferruginous bodies from sputum and pulmonary tissue. *Am J Clin Pathol* 58:250, 1972.

138. Spirtas R, Beebe GW, Connelly RR, et al: Recent trends in mesothelioma incidence in the United States. *Am J Ind Med* 9:397, 1986.

139. Stahel RA, O'Hara CJ, Waibel R, et al: Monoclonal antibodies against mesothelial membrane antigen discriminate between malignant mesothelioma and adenocarcinoma. *Int J Cancer* 41:218, 1988.

140. Stoebner B, Bernaudin JF, Nebut M, et al: Contribution of electron microscopy to the diagnosis of pleural mesothelioma. *Ann N Y Acad Sci* 330:751, 1979.

141. Strickler JG, Herndier BG, Rouse RV: Immunohistochemical staining in malignant mesotheliomas. *Am J Clin Pathol* 88:610, 1987.

142. Sussman J, Rosai J: Lymph node metastasis as the initial manifestation of malignant mesothelioma: report of six cases. *Am J Surg Pathol* 14:819, 1990.

143. Suzuki Y, Churg J, Kannerstein M: Ultrastructure of human malignant diffuse mesothelioma. *Am J Pathol* 85:241, 1976.

144. Sytman AL, MacAlpin RN: Primary pericardial mesothelioma: report of two cases and review of literature. *Am Heart J* 81:760, 1971.

145. Szpak CA, Johnston WW, Roggli V, et al: The diagnostic distinction between malignant mesothelioma of the pleura and adenocarcinoma of the lung as defined by monoclonal antibody (B72.3). *Am J Pathol* 122:252, 1986.

146. Tao LC: Aspiration biopsy cytology of mesothelioma. *Diagn Cytopathol* 5:14, 1989.

147. Thompson ME, Bromberg PA, Amenta JS: Acid mucopolysaccharide determination: a useful adjunct for the diagnosis of malignant mesothelioma with effusion. *Am J Clin Pathol* 52:335, 1969.

148. Tuttle SE, Lucas JG, Bucci DM, et al: Distinguishing malignant mesothelioma from pulmonary adenocarcinoma: an immunohistochemical approach using a panel of monoclonal antibodies. *J Surg Oncol* 45:72, 1990.

149. VonHoff DD, LiVolsi V: Diagnostic reliability of needle biopsy of the parietal pleura. *Am J Clin Pathol* 64:200, 1975.

150. Wagner JC: Epidemiology of diffuse mesothelial tumors: evidence of an association from studies in South Africa and United Kingdom. *Ann N Y Acad Sci* 132:575, 1965.

151. Wagner JC: Mesothelioma and mineral fibers. *Cancer* 57:1905, 1986.

152. Wagner JC, Berry G, Timbrell V: Mesotheliomata in rats after inoculation with asbestos and other materials. *Br J Cancer* 28:173, 1973.

153. Wagner JC, Sleggs AC, Marchand P: Diffuse pleural mesothelioma and asbestosis exposure in the Northwestern Cape Province. *Br J Ind Med* 17:260, 1960.

154. Walz R, Koch HK: Malignant pleural mesothelioma: some aspects of epidemiology, differential diagnosis, and prognosis: histological and immunohistochemical evaluation and follow-up of mesotheliomas diagnosed from 1964 to January 1985. *Pathol Res Pract* 186:124, 1990.

155. Wanebo HJ, Martini N, Melamed MR, et al: Pleural mesothelioma. *Cancer* 38:2481, 1976.

156. Wang N: Electron microscopy in the diagnosis of pleural mesotheliomas. *Cancer* 31:1046, 1973.

157. Warhol MJ: The ultrastructural localization of keratin proteins and carcinoembryonic antigen in malignant mesotheliomas. *Am J Pathol* 116:385, 1984.

158. Warhol MJ, Hickey WF, Corson JM: Malignant mesothelioma: ultrastructural distinction from adenocarcinoma. *Am J Surg Pathol* 6:307, 1982.

159. Warnock ML, Stoloff A, Thor A: Differentiation of adenocarcinoma of the lung from mesothelioma: periodic acid–Schiff, monoclonal antibodies B72.3 and Leu-M1. *Am J Pathol* 133:30, 1988.

160. Webster I: Mesotheliomatous tumors in South Africa: pathology and experimental pathology. *Ann N Y Acad Sci* 132:623, 1965.

161. Wechsler RJ, Rao VM, Steiner RM: The radiology of thoracic malignant mesothelioma. *Crit Rev Diagn Imaging* 20:283, 1984.

162. Whitwell F, Rawcliffe RM: Diffuse malignant pleural mesothelioma and asbestos exposure. *Thorax* 26:6, 1971.

163. Wick MR, Loy T, Mills ES, et al: Malignant epithelioid pleural mesothelioma versus peripheral pulmonary adenocarcinoma: a histochemical, ultrastructural, and immunohistologic study of 103 cases. *Hum Pathol* 21:759, 1990.

164. Winslow DJ, Taylor HB: Malignant peritoneal mesotheliomas. *Cancer* 13:127, 1960.

165. Wirth PR, Legier J, Wright GL: Immunohistochemical evaluation of seven monoclonal antibodies for differentiation of pleural mesothelioma from lung adenocarcinoma. *Cancer* 67:655, 1991.

166. Yap BS, Benjamin RS, Burgess MA, et al: The value of Adriamycin in the treatment of diffuse malignant pleural mesothelioma. *Cancer* 42:1692, 1978.

167. Yeh HC, Chahinian P: Ultrasonography and computed tomography of peritoneal mesothelioma. *Radiology* 135:705, 1980.

168. Yoshida T: Gleichzeitige Papillomatose der Pleura und des Peritoneums, zugleich ein Beitrag zur Frage des primären Carcinoms der serösen Häute. *Virchows Arch (Pathol Anat)* 299:363, 1937.

169. Yousem SA, Hochholzer L: Malignant mesotheliomas with osseous and cartilaginous differentiation. *Arch Pathol Lab Med* 111:62, 1987.

169a. Zeng L, Fleury-Feith J, Monnet I, et al: Immunocytochemical characterization of cell lines from human malignant mesothelioma: characterization of human mesothelioma cell lines by immunocytochemistry with a panel of monoclonal antibodies. *Hum Pathol* 25:227, 1994.

Well-differentiated papillary mesothelioma

170. Burrig KF, Pfitzer P, Hort W: Well-differentiated papillary mesothelioma of the peritoneum: a borderline mesothelioma. *Virchows Arch (Pathol Anat)* 417:1443, 1990.

171. Chen KTK, Flam MS: Peritoneal papillary serous carcinomas with long-term survival. *Cancer* 58:1371, 1986.

172. Daya D, McCaughey WT: Well-differentiated papillary mesothelioma of the peritoneum: a clinicopathologic study of 22 cases. *Cancer* 65:292, 1990.

173. Foyle A, Al-Jabi M, McCaughey WT: Papillary peritoneal tumors in women. *Am J Surg Pathol* 5:241, 1981.

174. Goepel JR: Benign papillary mesothelioma of peritoneum: a histological, histochemical, and ultrastructural study of six cases. *Histopathology* 5:21, 1981.

175. Grove A, Lidang-Jensen M, Donna A: Mesothelioma of the tunica vaginalis testis and hernial sacs. *Virchows Arch (Pathol Anat)* 415:283, 1989.

176. Kannerstein M, Churg J: Papillary tumors of the peritoneum in women: mesothelioma or papillary carcinoma. *Am J Obstet Gynecol* 127:306, 1977.

177. Lovell FA, Cranston PE: Well-differentiated papillary mesothelioma of the peritoneum. *Am J Radiol* 155:1245, 1990.

178. Mikuz G, Höpfel-Kreiner I: Papillary mesothelioma of the tunica vaginalis propria testis. *Virchows Arch (Pathol Anat)* 396:231, 1982.

179. Mills SE, Andersen WA, Fechner RE, et al: Serous surface papillary carcinoma: a clinicopathologic study of 10 cases and comparison with stage III-IV ovarian carcinoma. *Am J Surg Pathol* 12:827, 1988.

180. Swerdlow M: Mesothelioma of the pelvic peritoneum resembling papillary cystadenocarcinoma of the ovary. *Am J Obstet Gynecol* 77:197, 1959.

181. Wick MR, Mills SE, Dehner LP, et al: Serous papillary carcinoma arising from peritoneum and ovaries: a clinicopathologic and immunohistochemical comparison. *Int J Gynecol Pathol* 8:179, 1989.

Multicystic peritoneal mesothelioma

182. Ball NJ, Urbanski SJ, Green FH, et al: Pleural multicystic mesothelial proliferation: the so-called multicystic mesothelioma. *Am J Surg Pathol* 14:375, 1990.

183. Bell DA, Scully RE: Serous borderline tumors of the peritoneum. *Am J Surg Pathol* 14:230, 1990.

184. Canty MD, Williams J, Volpe RJ, et al: Benign cystic mesothelioma in a male. *Am J Gastroenterol* 85:311, 1990.

185. Carpenter HA, Lancaster JR, Lee RA: Multilocular cysts of the peritoneum. *Mayo Clin Proc* 57:634, 1982.

186. Katsube Y, Mukai K, Silverberg SG: Cystic mesothelioma of the peritoneum: a report of five cases and review of the literature. *Cancer* 50:1615, 1982.

187. Kjellvold K, Nesland JM, Holm R, et al: Multicystic peritoneal mesothelioma. *Pathol Res Pract* 181:767, 1986.

188. Krieger JS, Fisher ER, Richards MR: Multiple mesothelial cysts of the peritoneum. *Am J Surg* 84:328, 1952.

189. McFadden DE, Clement PB: Peritoneal inclusion cysts with mural mesothelial proliferation. A clinicopathologic analysis of six cases. *Am J Surg Pathol* 10:844, 1986.

190. Mennemeyer R, Smith M: Multicystic, peritoneal mesothelioma: a report with electron microscopy of a case mimicking intraabdominal cystic hygroma (lymphangioma). *Cancer* 44:692, 1979.

191. Moore JH, Crum CP, Chandler JG, et al: Benign cystic mesothelioma. *Cancer* 45:2395, 1980.

192. Plaut A: Multiple peritoneal cysts and their histogenesis. *Arch Pathol* 5:754, 1928.

193. Rhind JA, Wright CJE: Mesothelioma of the peritoneum: report of a case and review of the literature. *Br J Surg* 36:359, 1949.

194. Ross MJ, Welch WR, Scully RE: Multilocular inclusion cysts (so-called cystic mesothelioma). *Cancer* 64:1336, 1989.

195. Schneider V, Partridge JR, Gutierrez F, et al: Benign cystic mesothelioma involving the female genital tract: report of four cases. *Am J Obstet Gynecol* 145:355, 1983.

196. Sienkowski IK, Russell AJ, Dilly SA, et al: Peritoneal cystic mesothelioma: an electron microscopic and immunohistochemical study of two male patients. *J Clin Pathol* 39:440, 1986.

197. Truong LD, Maccato ML, Awalt H, et al: Serous surface carcinoma of the peritoneum: a clinicoapthologic study of 22 cases. *Hum Pathol* 21:99, 1990.

198. Weiss SW, Tavassoli FA: Multicystic mesothelioma: an analysis of pathologic findings and biologic behavior in 37 cases. *Am J Surg Pathol* 12:737, 1988.

Benign mesothelioma of the genital tract (adenomatoid tumor)

199. Banks ER, Mills SE: Histiocytoid (epithelioid) hemangioma of the testis: the so-called vascular variant of an "adenomatoid tumor." *Am J Surg Pathol* 14:584, 1990.

200. Barwick KW, Madri JA: An immunohistochemical study of adenomatoid tumors utilizing keratin and factor VIII antibodies: evidence for a mesothelial origin. *Lab Invest* 47:276, 1982.

201. Craig JR, Hart WR: Extragenital adenomatoid tumor: evidence for the mesothelial theory of origin. *Cancer* 43:1678, 1979.

202. Eimoto T, Inoue I: Malignant fibrous mesothelioma of the tunica vaginalis. *Cancer* 39:2059, 1977.

203. Ferenczy A, Fenoglio J, Richart RM: Observations on benign mesothelioma of the genital tract: a comparative ultrastructural study. *Cancer* 30:244, 1972.

204. Golden A, Ash JE: Adenomatoid tumors of the genital tract. *Am J Pathol* 21:63, 1945.

205. Hanrahan JB: A combined papillary mesothelioma and adenomatoid tumor of the omentum: report of a case. *Cancer* 16:1497, 1963.

206. Horn RC Jr, Lewis GC Jr: Mesothelioma of the female genital tract: review of the literature and report of five cases involving the uterus. *Am J Clin Pathol* 21:251, 1951.

207. Jablokow VR, Jagatic J, Rubnitz ME: Adenomatoid tumors of the genital tract: report of 12 cases and review of the literature. *J Urol* 95:573, 1966.

208. Kannerstein M, Lustig M: The adenomatoid tumor of the genital tract. *J Newark Beth Israel Hosp* 13:25, 1962.

209. Lee MJ Jr, Dockerty MB, Thompson GJ, et al: Benign mesotheliomas (adenomatoid tumors) of genital tract. *Surg Gynecol Obstet* 91:221, 1950.

210. Mackay B, Bennington JL, Skoglund RW: The adenomatoid tumor: fine structural evidence for a mesothelial origin. *Cancer* 27:109, 1971.

211. Marcus JB, Lynn JA: Ultrastructural comparison of an adenomatoid tumor, lymphangioma, hemangioma, and mesothelioma. *Cancer* 25:171, 1970.

212. Masson P, Riopelle JL, Simard LC: Le mesotheliome benin de la sphere genitale. *Rev Can Biol* 1:720, 1942.

213. Mostofi FK, Price EB: Tumors of the male genital system. In *Atlas of tumor pathology*, Armed Forces Institute of Pathology, 1973, pp 79-80, Washington, DC.

214. Said JW, Nash G, Lee M: Immunoperoxidase localization of keratin proteins, carcinoembryonic antigen, and factor VIII in adenomatoid tumors: evidence of mesothelial derivation. *Hum Pathol* 13:1106, 1982.

215. Salazar H, Kanbour A, Burgess F: Ultrastructure and observation on the histogenesis of mesotheliomas, adenomatoid tumors, of the female genital tract. *Cancer* 29:141, 1972.

216. Söderström KO: Origin of adenomatoid tumor: a comparison between the structure of adenomatoid tumor and epididymal duct cells. *Cancer* 49:2349, 1982.

217. Stephenson TJ, Mills PM: Adenomatoid tumours: an immunohistochemical and ultrastructural appraisal of their histogenesis. *J Pathol* 148:327, 1986.

218. Taxy JB, Battifora H, Oyasu R: Adenomatoid tumors: a light-microscopic, histochemical, and ultrastructural study. *Cancer* 34:306, 1974.

219. Tuttle JP, Rous SN, Harrold MW: Mesotheliomas of the spermatic cord. *Urology* 10:466, 1976.

220. Youngs LA, Taylor HB: Adenomatoid tumors of the uterus and fallopian tube. *Am J Clin Pathol* 48:537, 1967.

Localized (solitary) fibrous tumor of the pleura and peritoneum (fibrous mesothelioma)

221. Briselli M, Mark EJ, Dickersin GR: Solitary fibrous tumors of the pleura: eight new cases and review of 360 cases in the literature. *Cancer* 47:2678, 1981.

222. Bürrig KF, Kastendieck H: Ultrastructural observations on the histogenesis of localized fibrous tumors of the pleura (benign mesothelioma). *Virchows Arch (Pathol Anat)* 403:413, 1984.

223. Dalton WT, Zolliker AS, McCaughey WT, et al: Localized primary tumors of the pleura: an analysis of 40 cases. *Cancer* 44:1465, 1979.

224. Dervan PA, Tobin B, O'Connor M: Solitary (localized) fibrous mesothelioma: evidence against mesothelial origin. *Histopathology* 10:867, 1986.

225. Doucet J, Dardick I, Srigley JR, et al: Localized fibrous tumour of serosal surfaces: imunohistochemical and ultrastructural evidence for a type of mesothelioma. *Virchows Arch (Pathol Anat)* 409:349, 1986 .

226. El-Naggar A, Ward RN, Ro JY: Fibrous tumor with hemangiopericytic pattern: so-called localized fibrous tumor of pleura. *Lab Invest* 56:21A, 1987.

227. England DM, Hochholzer L, McCarthy MJ: Localized benign and malignant fibrous tumor of the pleura: a clinicopathologic review of 223 cases. *Am J Surg Pathol* 13:640, 1989.

228. Epstein JI, Budin RE: Keratin and epithelial membrane antigen immunoreactivity in nonneoplastic fibrous pleural lesions: implications for the diagnosis of desmoplastic mesothelioma. *Hum Pathol* 17:514, 1986.

229. Foster EA, Ackerman LV: Localized mesotheliomas of the pleura: the pathologic evaluation of 18 cases. *Am J Clin Pathol* 34:349, 1960.

230. Goodlad JR, Fletcher CD: Solitary fibrous tumour at unusual sites: analysis of a series. *Histopathology* 19:515, 1991.

231. Hernandez FJ, Fernandez BB: Localized fibrous tumors of pleura: a light and electron-microscopic study. *Cancer* 34:1667, 1974.

232. Janssen JP, Wagenaar SJ, Van der Borsch JM, et al: Benign localized mesothelioma of the pleura. *Histopathology* 9:309, 1986.

233. Kawai T, Mikata A, Torikata C, et al: Solitary (localized) pleural mesothelioma: a light and electron-microscopic study. *Am J Surg Pathol* 2:365, 1978.

234. Kim H, Damjanov I: Localized fibrous mesothelioma of the liver: report of a giant tumor studied by light and electron microscopy. *Cancer* 52: 1662, 1983.

235. Klemperer P, Rabin CB: Primary neoplasms of the pleura: a report of five cases. *Arch Pathol* 11:385, 1931.

236. Kottke-Marchant K, Hart WR, Broughan T: Localized fibrous tumor (localized fibrous mesothelioma) of the liver. *Cancer* 64:1096, 1989.

237. Lee KS, Im JG, Choe KO, et al: CT findings in benign fibrous mesothelioma of the pleura: pathologic correlation in nine patients. *Am J Roentgenol* 158:983, 1993.

238. Mandal AK, Rozer MA, Salem FA, et al: Localized benign mesothelioma of the pleura associated with a hypoglycemic episode. *Arch Intern Med* 143:1608, 1983.

239. Masson EA, MacFarlane IA, Graham D, et al: Spontaneous hypoglycemia due to pleural fibroma: role of insulin-like growth factors. *Thorax* 46:930, 1991.

240. Mendelson DS, Meary E, Buy JN, et al: Localized fibrous pleural mesothelioma: CT findings. *Clin Imaging* 15:105, 1991.

241. Nelson R, Burman SO, Kiani R, et al: Hypoglycemic coma associated with benign pleural mesothelioma. *J Thorac Cardiovasc Surg* 69:306, 1975.

242. Okike N, Bernatz PE, Woolner LB: Localized mesothelioma of the pleura: benign and malignant variants. *J Thorac Cardiovasc Surg* 75:363, 1978.

243. Osamura RY: Ultrastructure of a localized fibrous mesothelioma of the pleura: report of a case with histogenetic considerations. *Cancer* 39:139, 1977.

244. Said JW, Nash G, Banks-Schlegel S, et al: Localized fibrous mesothelioma: an immunohistochemical and electron microscopic study. *Hum Pathol* 15:440, 1984.

245. Scharifker D, Kaneko M: Localized fibrous "mesothelioma" of pleura (submesothelial fibroma): a clinicopathologic study of 18 cases. *Cancer* 43:627, 1979.

246. Shabanah FH, Sayegh SF: Solitary (localized) pleural mesothelioma: report of two cases and review of the literature. *Chest* 60:558, 1971.

247. Steinetz C, Clarke R, Jacobs GH, et al: Localized fibrous tumor of the pleura: correlation of histopathological, immunohistochemical, and ultrastructural features. *Pathol Res Pract* 186:344, 1990.

248. Stout AP, Himadi GM: Solitary (localized) mesothelioma of the pleura. *Ann Surg* 133:50, 1951.

249. Stout AP, Murray MR: Localized pleural mesothelioma: investigation of its characteristics and histogenesis by the method of tissue culture. *Arch Pathol* 34:951, 1942.

250. Witkin GB, Rosai J: Solitary fibrous tumor of the mediastinum: a report of 14 cases. *Am J Surg Pathol* 13:547, 1989.

251. Yesner R, Hurwitz A: Localized pleural mesothelioma of epithelial type. *J Thorac Surg* 26:325, 1953.

252. Young RH, Clement PB, McCaughey WT: Solitary fibrous tumors ("fibrous mesotheliomas") of the peritoneum. *Arch Pathol* 114:493, 1990.

253. Yousem SA, Flynn SD: Intrapulmonary localized fibrous tumor: intraparenchymal so-called localized fibrous mesothelioma. *Am J Clin Pathol* 89:365, 1988.

CHAPTER 31

BENIGN TUMORS OF PERIPHERAL NERVES

Despite the common nature of peripheral nerve tumors, they continue to pose problems in classification and nomenclature. Virchow's original classification emphasized the relationship of these tumors to the neuron proper by dividing the tumors into true and false neuromas. True neuromas exhibited neuronal differentiation and were a heterogenous group of lesions that included what would now be called traumatic neuroma and ganglioneuroma. False neuromas were nerve sheath tumors such as neurofibroma and neurilemoma. The latter group has gradually been accepted as the more common and significant group of peripheral nerve tumors and forms the principal focus of this chapter. Ganglioneuroma, although also of peripheral nerve origin, is discussed with tumors of autonomic nerves because it arises in association with autonomic ganglia.

Both neurofibroma and neurilemoma contain cells most closely related to the normal Schwann cell. Acceptance of this point has in part resulted from our expanded understanding of the function of the Schwann cell. Not only does this cell serve to produce and maintain myelin, but it can also, under certain circumstances, produce collagen.[18,21] Thus, in a sense, the potentiality expressed by the normal Schwann cell is paralleled by that of the cells of nerve sheath tumors.[20] Because neurofibroma and neurilemoma are closely related neoplasms, some authors support a unified system of classification and refer to both by a common designation.[66,105,118] However, we have retained a divisional approach for several reasons (Table 31-1). It is true, of course, that some nerve sheath tumors defy precise classification. We have seen neurilemomas with a plexiform pattern, and there are cutaneous neurofibromas that have areas indistinguishable from neurilemoma. Such tumors are rare, and most can be classified along the guidelines discussed in this chapter. Ultrastructurally the tumors are different. Neurilemoma contains a more homogenous population of cells, whereas neurofibroma contains a mixture of cell types. Recent emphasis on specialized cells, too, may help distinguish neurofibroma. Other reasons for distinguishing the tumors are practical. As pointed out in scholarly papers by Geschickter[75] and Stout,[106] the two tumors occur in different clinical settings. In contrast to neurilemoma, neurofibroma occurs in younger persons, has a slightly different anatomical distribution, and has a significant association with von Recklinghausen's disease. In this disease there is a definite risk of malignant transformation for neurofibroma, a phenomenon almost never encountered in neurilemoma.

In addition to the nerve sheath tumors, we have included in this chapter some pseudotumorous lesions of nerve (e.g., traumatic neuroma, Morton's neuroma, nerve sheath ganglion) and two rare tumors, extracranial meningioma and pigmented neuroectodermal tumor of infancy. The last two tumors are difficult to classify and are included because of their usually benign behavior and presumed neural crest origin.

EMBRYOGENESIS AND NORMAL ANATOMY

The peripheral nervous system can be defined simplistically as nervous tissue outside the brain and spinal cord. It is an extensive system that includes somatic and autonomic nerves, end organ receptors, and supporting structures. It develops when axons lying close to one another grow out from the neural tube and are gradually invested with Schwann cells. The origin of Schwann cells has been debated. Some maintain they arise directly from the neural tube, whereas others insist they arise from the neural crest, a group of cells that lie lateral to the neural tube and beneath the ectoderm of the developing embryo. Most evidence to date supports neural crest derivation.[1] The major peripheral nerve trunks form by fusion and division of segmental spinal nerves and therefore often contain mixtures of sensory, motor, and autonomic elements. Precise identification of these elements is not always possible solely on morphological grounds. As the peripheral nerves form, the Schwann cells migrate peripherally from the spinal ganglia, orient themselves parallel to the axons, and encase them with their cytoplasm. In myelinated fibers only one axon segment is encased by one Schwann cell, and synthesis and spiraling of the schwannian plasma membrane around the axon create the myelin sheath. However, discontinuities of

Table 31-1. Comparison of neurilemoma and neurofibroma

	Neurilemoma	Neurofibroma
Peak age	20 to 50 years	20 to 40 years; younger age in neurofibromatosis
Common locations	Cutaneous nerves of head, neck, flexor surfaces of extremities; less often mediastinum and retroperitoneum	Cutaneous nerves; deep nerves and viscera affected also in neurofibromatosis
Histological appearance	Encapsulated tumor composed of Antoni A and B areas; rarely plexiform growth pattern	Localized, diffuse, or plexiform tumor that is usually not encapsulated
Degenerative changes	Common	Occasional
S-100 protein immunostaining	Intense and relatively uniform staining in a given lesion	Variable staining of cells in a given lesion
Occurrence in neurofibromatosis 1 (von Recklinghausen's disease)	Uncommon	Plexiform neurofibroma or multiple neurofibromas characteristic of disease
Malignant transformation	Extremely rare	Rare in solitary form; more common in neurofibromatosis

the myelin sheath exist at those points where adjacent Schwann cells meet but where there is no lamination of the plasma membrane (nodes of Ranvier). In nonmyelinated nerves several axon segments are ensheathed by a common Schwann cell. However, they are not enclosed beyond the initial stage of enfolding and therefore are invested with only a single or at most a few layers of schwannian plasma membrane. In humans the process of myelination commences in the eighteenth week of intrauterine life, is usually advanced by birth, and continues for several years postnatally.[1]

In the fully developed nerve a layer of connective tissue or epineurium surrounds the entire nerve trunk (Fig. 31-1). This structure varies in size depending of the location of the nerve and is composed of a mixture of collagen and elastic fibers along with mast cells. Several nerve fascicles lie within the confines of the epineurium, and each, in turn, is surrounded by a well-defined sheath known as the perineurium. These small nerve fascicles anticipate the subsequent division of the nerve into smaller branches, and for this reason the terms *epineurium* and *perineurium* can be used interchangeably when referring to small nerves. The smallest connective tissue unit of the nerve is the endoneurium, an intricate network of collagen, blood vessels, and fibroblasts encircling individual nerve fibers.

Considerable emphasis has recently been placed on the nature of the perineurium.[17] The outer portion of the perineurium consists of layers of connective tissue, while the inner portion is represented by a multilayered, concentrically arranged sheath of flattened cells.[24] These cells, which are best defined by electron microscopy and immunohistochemistry, have been termed *perineural fibroblasts* and *perineural epithelium*.[24] They are continuous with the pia-

arachnoid of the central nervous system and appear to be important in maintaining a diffusion barrier for the peripheral nerve. Although formerly considered to be derived from the neural crest, recent evidence indicates that these cells originate from fibroblasts and hence are derivatives of mesenchyme as opposed to the neural crest.[16] In contrast to Schwann cells, perineural cells do not express S-100 protein but do express epithelial membrane antigen, an immunophenotypic profile identical to pia-arachnoid cells. Ultrastructurally they form close junctions with each other and possess basal lamina along the endoneurial and perineurial aspects of the cell,[24] features not encountered in the ordinary fibroblast and Schwann cell. The cytoplasm is rather poor in organelles except for the prominent, well-aligned pinocytotic vesicles along their surface and occasional myofilaments. Peculiar acellular whorled structures, known as *Renaut's bodies,* are occasionally found directly beneath the perineurium. Their significance is unknown. Despite the undoubted importance of the investing connective tissue, the critical supporting element is the Schwann cell. It provides mechanical protection for the axon, produces and maintains the myelin sheath, and serves as a tube to guide regenerating nerve fibers. By light microscopy it is difficult to distinguish this cell from a fibroblast because their nuclei look so similar. However, by electron microscopy a Schwann cell is easily identified by its intimate relationship to its axons and by a continuous basal lamina that coats the surface of the cell facing the endoneurium. Current evidence suggests that the Schwann cell synthesizes this basal lamina[24] and is also capable of synthesizing collagen precursors.[18,20] Except for occasional 10-nm fibrils, microtubules, and mitochondria, other cytoplasmic organelles are not especially prominent except during periods of increased

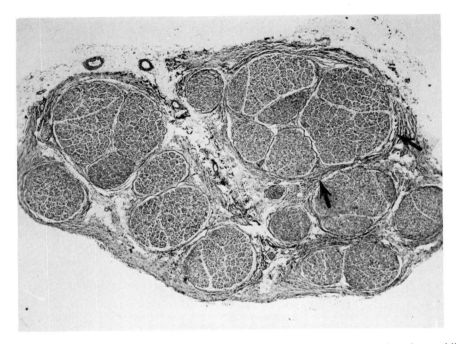

FIG. 31-1. Normal sciatic nerve in cross-section. Entire nerve is surrounded by epineurium, while smaller nerve fascicles are encompassed by perineurium *(arrows).* (×6.)

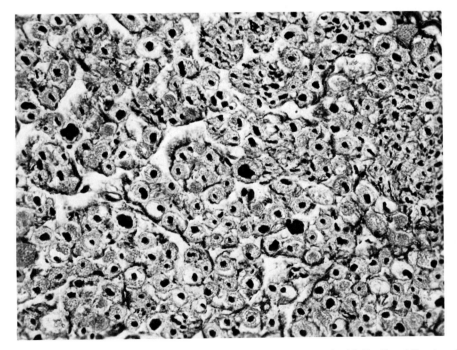

FIG. 31-2. Normal peripheral nerve cut in cross-section and stained with Bodian (silver) stain. Individual axons stain positively; surrounding myelin sheath does not stain. Thickness of axons and myelin sheath varies and determines conduction speed. (×400.)

metabolism (e.g., myelin synthesis).[19] Pi granules, flattened lamellations of osmiophilic material, are occasionally present in a perinuclear location, but their significance is unknown. In routine preparations it is difficult to separate the axon from the myelin sheath. This distinction, however, is easily accomplished with special stains. Silver stains selectively stain the axon (Fig. 31-2), whereas stains such as Luxol fast blue stain myelin. With these stains the variation in diameter of axon and myelin sheath can be appreciated. In general, moderate or heavily myelinated fibers correspond to sensory and motor fibers with fast conduction speeds, whereas lightly myelinated or unmyelinated fibers correspond to autonomic fibers with slower conduction speeds.[19] Ultrastructurally the cytoplasm of the axon is characterized by numerous cytoplasmic filaments, slender mitochondria, and a longitudinally oriented endoplasmic reticulum. Nissl substance, a feature of the nerve cell body, is not present in the axoplasm. In addition, small vesicles are occasionally observed; they may represent packets of neurotransmitter substance en route to the nerve terminal.

TRAUMATIC (AMPUTATION) NEUROMA

Traumatic neuroma is an exuberant but nonneoplastic proliferation of a nerve occurring in response to injury or surgery. Under ideal circumstances the ends of a severed nerve reestablish continuity by an orderly growth of axons from proximal to distal stump through tubes of proliferating Schwann cells. However, if close apposition of the ends of nerve is not maintained or if there is no distal stump, a disorganized proliferation of the proximal nerve gives rise to a neuroma. Symptomatic neuromas are usually the result of surgery, notably amputation. Occasionally other surgical procedures such as cholecystectomy[31] have been incriminated in their pathogenesis. A rare form of traumatic neuroma is seen in rudimentary (supernumerary) digits that undergo autoamputation in utero. These lesions appear as raised nodules on the ulnar surface of the proximal fifth finger. They contain a disordered proliferation of nerves similar to a conventional traumatic neuroma (Fig. 31-3).[11,33]

Clinically neuroma presents as a firm nodule that is occasionally tender or painful. Strangulation of the proliferating nerve by scar tissue, local trauma, and infection have all been invoked as possible explanations of the pain. Grossly the lesions are circumscribed, white-gray nodules located in continuity with the proximal end of the injured or transected nerve. They consist of a haphazard proliferation of nerve fascicles, including axons with their investitures of myelin, Schwann cells, and fibroblasts. The fascicles are usually less well myelinated than the parent nerve and are embedded in a background of collagen (Fig. 31-4). The participation of all elements of the nerve fascicles distinguishes this lesion from neurofibroma. In areas where the fascicles are small and the matrix is poorly collagenized and highly myxoid, similarity to neurofibroma may be quite striking (Fig. 31-5).

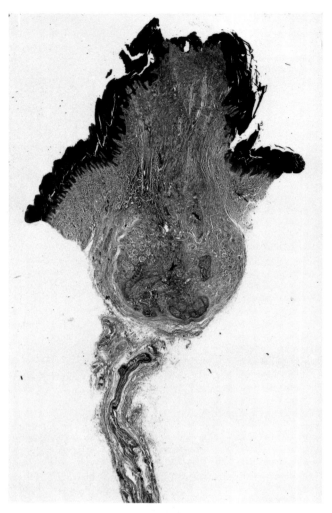

FIG. 31-3. Rudimentary digit that underwent autoamputation in utero and showed areas of traumatic neuroma. (×15.)

Treatment of these lesions is, in part, prophylactic. After traumatic nerve injury, an attempt should be made to reappose the ends of the severed nerve so that regeneration of the proximal end will proceed down the distal trunk in an orderly fashion. Injection of the proximal nerve trunk with various solutions (formaldehyde, gentian violet) at the time of surgery to prevent neuroma formation has generally fallen into disrepute. Once a neuroma has formed, removal is indicated when it becomes symptomatic or when it must be distinguished from recurrent tumor in a patient who has had cancer-related surgery.[26] Simple excision of the lesion and re-embedding the proximal nerve stump in an area away from the old scar constitute the conventional therapy.

MUCOSAL NEUROMA

This form of neuroma involves the mucosal surfaces of the lips, mouth, eyelids, and intestines in patients with type

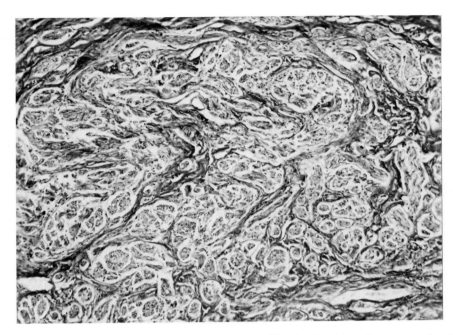

FIG. 31-4. Traumatic neuroma composed of small proliferating fascicles of nerve enveloped in collagen. (×100.)

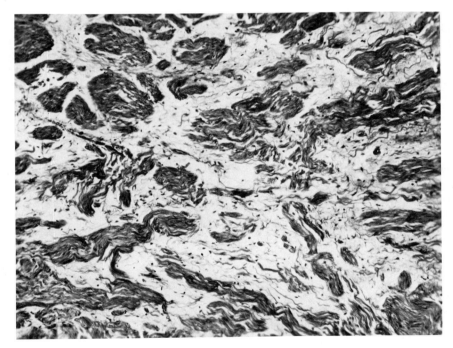

FIG. 31-5. Myxoid areas within a traumatic neuroma superficially resembling a neurofibroma. (×100.)

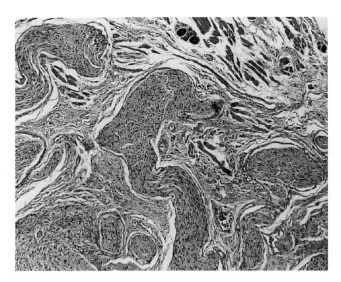

FIG. 31-6. Mucosal neuroma from patient with multiple endocrine neoplasia type IIb. Irregular, convoluted nerves with prominent perineurium lie within submucosal tissue. (×100.)

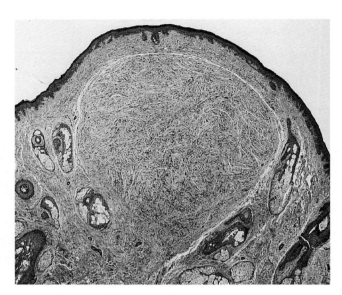

FIG. 31-7. Palisaded encapsulated neuroma. (×15.)

IIb multiple endocrine neoplasia characterized by bilateral pheochromocytoma, C cell hyperplasia and medullary carcinoma of the thyroid, and parathyroid hyperplasia.[36] The lesions are notable for the irregular, tortuous bundles of nerve having a prominent perineurium that lie scattered throughout the submucosa of the oral cavity (Fig. 31-6). In the gastrointestinal tract the myenteric autonomic nerves appear hyperplastic and contain increased numbers of neurons.[35]

PACINIAN NEUROMA

Pacinian neuroma refers to a localized hyperplasia of the pacinian corpuscles that occurs following trauma and commonly produces pain.[37-39] Typically it develops on the digits, where it produces a localized mass either attached to the nerve by a slender stalk or as a nodule beneath the epineurium. Histologically it consists of an increased number of mature pacinian corpuscles associated with small nerves.

PALISADED ENCAPSULATED NEUROMA (SOLITARY CIRCUMSCRIBED NEUROMA)

Although this lesion was described over two decades ago by Reed et al.,[44] its acceptance as a distinct entity was slow because of uncertainty as to its overlap with the common neurilemoma. It has rather distinct clinical features, which, in concert with its appearance, warrant a separate term.[40-43] The palisaded encapsulated neuroma develops as a small asymptomatic nodule in the area of the face of adult patients and affects the sexes equally. Affected patients do not display manifestations of neurofibromatosis 1 or multiple endocrine neoplasia type IIb. Histologically it is com-

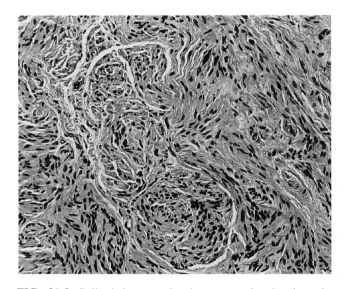

FIG. 31-8. Palisaded encapsulated neuroma showing irregular bundles of nerves containing both nerve and nerve sheath cells. (×160.)

posed of one or more circumscribed or encapsulated nodules that occupy the deep dermis and subcutaneous tissues (Fig. 31-7). In some cases the nodules may form clublike extensions into the subcutaneous tissue.[41] They consist of a solid proliferation of Schwann cells and lack the variety of stromal changes (e.g., myxoid change, hyalinization) that may be encountered in neurilemoma and neurofibroma (Fig. 31-8). Although superficially these neuromas may resemble neurilemoma, particularly if minor degrees of nu-

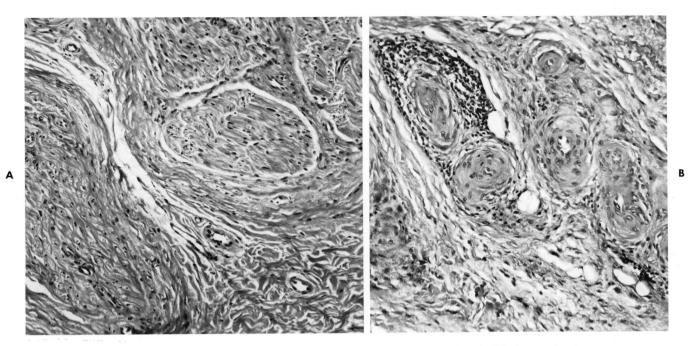

FIG. 31-9. Morton's neuroma. Dense perineural (**A**) and perivascular fibrosis (**B**) characterize the lesion. (**A** and **B**, ×250.)

clear palisading are noted, they differ by the presence of axons, best demonstrated with silver stains, that traverse the lesion in close association with the Schwann cells. Neurilemomas may contain axons, but these are typically located peripherally immediately beneath the capsule. In most instances simple excision of these lesions has proved curative.

MORTON'S NEUROMA (MORTON'S TOE, MORTON'S METATARSALGIA)

Morton's neuroma is not a true tumor but rather a fibrosing process of the plantar digital nerve, which results in paroxysmal pain in the sole of the foot, usually between the heads of the third and fourth metatarsals and less often between the second and third. The pain typically commences with exercise, is alleviated by rest, and may radiate into the toes or leg. In some cases a small area of point tenderness can be defined, although generally no mass can be palpated. The condition is almost always unilateral. Because women are affected more often than men, the wearing of ill-fitting high-heeled shoes has been incriminated in the pathogenesis of this condition. Lesions histologically similar to Morton's neuroma are sometimes seen adjacent to nerves in the hand, where they are undoubtedly related to chronic occupational or recreational injury. At surgery the characteristic lesion is a firm fusiform enlargement of the plantar digital nerve at its bifurcation point. In advanced cases the nerve may be firmly attached to the adjacent bursa and soft tissue. Although grossly the lesion resembles a traumatic neuroma or neurofibroma, it is quite different histologically. Proliferative changes characterize traumatic neuromas, whereas degenerative changes are the hallmark of Morton's neuroma. Edema and fibrosis occur within the nerve (Fig. 31-9). Hyalinization of endoneurial vessels may also be present in some cases. Elastic fibers are diminished within the center of the lesions but are increased at its periphery, where they have a bilaminar appearance similar to the elastic fibers within elastofibroma.[11] As the lesion progresses, the fibrosis becomes marked and envelops the epineurium and perineurium in a concentric fashion and may even extend into the surrounding tissue. Pathogenetically the changes have been explained by compression of the neurovascular bundles by the adjacent metatarsal heads. Whether the injury is primarily neural or is mediated via vascular ischemia is not resolved. Although conservative measures such as wearing of orthopedic footwear have been used, the most successful therapy consists of removal of the affected nerve segment.

GANGLIONEUROMA

Because of the overlap between this tumor and primitive neuroblastic tumors, ganglioneuroma is discussed in Chapter 33.

NERVE SHEATH GANGLION

Rarely ganglia occur in intraneural locations. Such lesions present as tender masses with pain or numbness in

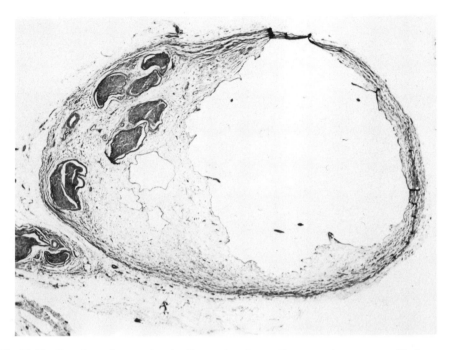

FIG. 31-10. Ganglion of nerve sheath. Connective tissue of nerve undergoes myxoid change and cystification. (×25.)

the distribution of the affected nerve. The majority of these lesions are located within the external popliteal nerve[48] at the head of the fibula, which suggests that a particular type of injury or irritation leads to their development. The nerve displays a localized swelling that corresponds to myxoid change with secondary cyst formation. In some cases, however, the unlined cysts may dominate the histological picture and cause marked displacement of the nerve fascicles toward one side of the sheath (Fig. 31-10). This lesion, like its soft tissue counterpart, represents a degenerative process rather than a neoplasm. The myxoid zones within these lesions have unfortunately led to some confusion with the so-called nerve sheath myxoma. This entity is a true neoplasm of probable Schwann cell origin and is quite distinct from nerve sheath ganglion (see discussion of neurothekeoma, below). Therapy of nerve sheath ganglion consists of local excision, although decompression is acceptable if integrity of the nerve is threatened.

NEUROMUSCULAR HAMARTOMA (NEUROMUSCULAR CHORISTOMA; BENIGN TRITON TUMOR)

Tumors composed of skeletal muscle and neural elements are collectively referred to as *Triton tumors* in accord with an early hypothesis concerning their histogenesis (Chapter 32). The best recognized of these mosaic tumors is the malignant schwannoma with rhabdomyoblastic differentiation (malignant Triton tumor), although combinations such as rhabdomyosarcoma with ganglion cells (ectomesenchymoma) also occur. Benign Triton tumors are extremely rare and are represented principally by the neuromuscular hamartoma or choristoma. The high level of differentiation of these lesions suggests they are hamartomas or choristomas rather than tumors and possibly occur when primitive mesenchyme of developing limb buds is included within the nerve sheath. Of the eight cases reviewed from the literature all occurred in very young children and developed as masses within various large nerve trunks, particularly the brachial and sciatic. A recent case described by O'Connell and Rosenberg[54] presented as multiple lesions outside nerve. Because of their strategic locations, neurological symptoms are quite prominent. The tumors are multinodular masses subdivided by fibrous bands into smaller nodules or fascicles. Each fascicle is composed of highly differentiated skeletal muscle fibers that vary in size but are often larger than normal. Intimately associated with the skeletal muscle and sharing the same perimysial sheath are both small myelinated and nonmyelinated nerves (Fig. 31-11). At times the fibrous component surrounding the lesions may be so dense and cellular as to suggest the diagnosis of a fibromatosis replacing muscle and nerve. Follow-up information in our cases as well as those in the literature supports their benignity. Even incomplete excision has resulted in amelioration of symptoms and progressive decrease in

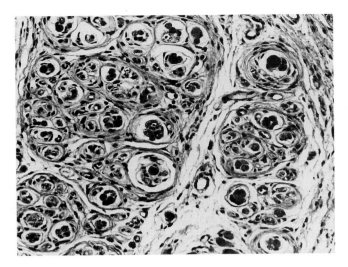

FIG. 31-11. Neuromuscular hamartoma composed of short bundles of mature nerve and muscle. (×250.) (From Markel SF, Enzinger FM: *Cancer* 49:140, 1982.)

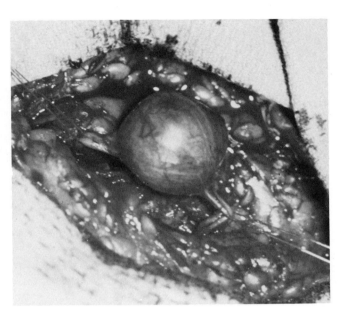

FIG. 31-12. Neurilemoma arising as an eccentric growth from nerve.

size. Therefore, after correct diagnosis, treatment should be conservative and aimed primarily at maintaining the integrity of the nerve.

NEURILEMOMA (BENIGN SCHWANNOMA)

Neurilemoma, also referred to as *schwannoma, neurinoma,* and *perineural fibroblastoma,* is an encapsulated nerve sheath tumor consisting of two components: a highly ordered cellular component (Antoni A area) and a loose myxoid component (Antoni B area). The presence of encapsulation and the two types of Antoni areas plus uniformly intense immunostaining for S-100 protein[13] distinguish neurilemoma from neurofibroma.

Clinical findings

Neurilemomas occur at all ages but are most common in persons between the ages of 20 and 50 years.[75] They affect the sexes in roughly equal numbers. The tumors have a predilection for the head, neck, and flexor surfaces of the upper and lower extremities.[106] Consequently the spinal roots and the cervical, sympathetic, vagus, peroneal, and ulnar nerves are most commonly affected. Deeply situated tumors predominate in the posterior mediastinum and the retroperitoneum. Neurilemomas almost always occur as solitary lesions but in unusual instances are multiple or occur in the setting of von Recklinghausen's disease (neurofibromatosis 1).[85,106] In Stout's scholarly review[106] of neurilemoma, 18% (nine cases) had evidence of neurofibromatosis 1. These figures, coupled with our own experience, suggest that this association is more than fortuitous.

Neurilemoma is a slowly growing tumor that is usually present several years before diagnosis. When it involves small nerves, this tumor is freely movable except for a single point of attachment. In larger nerves the tumor is movable except along the long axis of the nerve where the attachment restricts mobility. Pain and neurological symptoms are uncommon unless the tumor becomes large. In some instances the patient is vaguely aware that the tumor waxes and wanes in size,[106] a phenomenon that might be related to fluctuations in the amount of cystic change in the lesion. Deep neurilemomas are symptomatic by virtue of their larger size and impingement on neighboring structures. Of particular significance is the posterior mediastinal neurilemoma, which often originates from or extends into the vertebral canal. Such lesions, termed *dumbbell tumors,*[132] pose difficult problems in management because patients may develop profound neurological difficulties.

Gross findings

Because these tumors arise within nerve sheaths, they are surrounded by a true capsule consisting of the epineurium. Depending on the size of the involved nerve, the appearance of the tumor will vary. Tumors of small nerves may resemble neurofibromas by virtue of their fusiform shape, and they often eclipse or obliterate the nerve of origin. In larger nerves the tumors present as eccentric masses over which the nerve fibers are splayed (Fig. 31-12).

On cut section these tumors have a pink, white, or yellow appearance and usually measure less than 5 cm (Fig. 31-13). Tumors in the retroperitoneum and mediastinum may be considerably larger. As a result, these tumors are more likely to manifest secondary degenerative changes

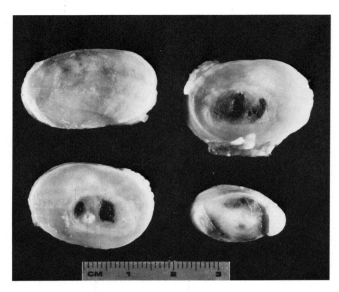

FIG. 31-13. Multiple transverse sections through a neurilemoma. Tumors are well circumscribed and commonly display foci of hemorrhage and cyst formation.

such as cystification and calcification (see discussion of ancient schwannoma, below).

Microscopic findings

Most neurilemomas are uninodular masses surrounded by fibrous capsules consisting of epineurium and residual nerve fibers (Fig. 31-14). Neurites are generally not demonstra-

ble within the substance of the tumor. In rare cases the neurilemoma may arise intradermally (Fig. 31-15) or, as mentioned above, manifest as a plexiform or multinodular growth (Figs. 31-16 and 31-17) similar to a plexiform neurofibroma.

The hallmark of a neurilemoma is the pattern of alternating Antoni A and B areas (Fig. 31-18). The relative amounts of these two components vary, and they may either blend imperceptibly or change abruptly. Antoni A areas are composed of compact spindle cells that usually have twisted nuclei, indistinct cytoplasmic borders, and occasionally clear intranuclear vacuoles (Lochkern). They are arranged in short bundles or interlacing fascicles (Figs. 31-19 and 31-20). In highly differentiated Antoni A areas there may be nuclear palisading, whorling of the cells (similar to meningioma), and Verocay bodies (Fig. 31-20), formed by two compact rows of well-aligned nuclei separated by fibrillary cell processes. Mitotic figures are occasionally present but can usually be dismissed if the lesion otherwise has all the hallmarks of neurilemoma. S-100 protein, an acidic protein common to supporting cells of the central and peripheral nervous system, can be demonstrated in neurilemomas,[7,12,13] particularly in the Antoni A areas.

Antoni B areas are far less orderly and less cellular. The spindled or oval cells are arranged haphazardly within the loosely textured matrix, which is punctuated by microcystic change, inflammatory cells, and delicate collagen fibers (Fig. 31-21). The large, irregularly spaced vessels that are very characteristic of neurilemoma become most conspicuous in the hypocellular Antoni B areas. Their gaping tortuous lumina are often filled with thrombus material in vari-

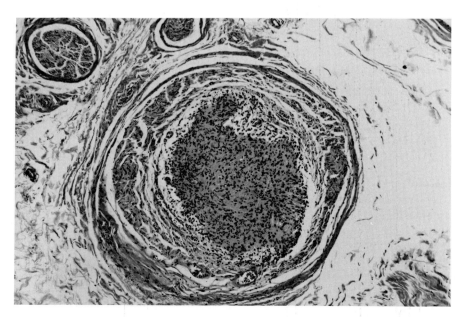

FIG. 31-14. Microscopic neurilemoma discovered incidentally. Tumor arose in central portion of nerve and flattened residual nerve and sheath around itself as a capsule. (×60.)

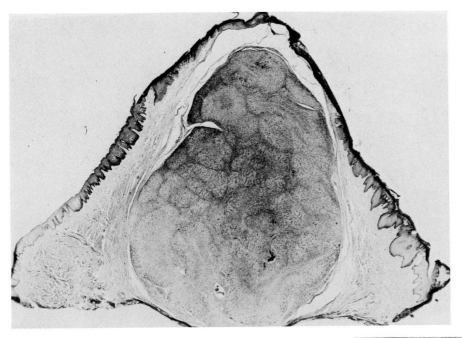

FIG. 31-15. Unusual example of neurilemoma occurring in an intradermal location. (×9.)

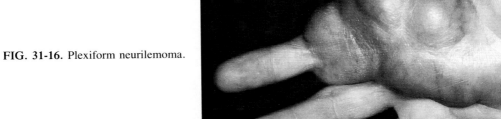

FIG. 31-16. Plexiform neurilemoma.

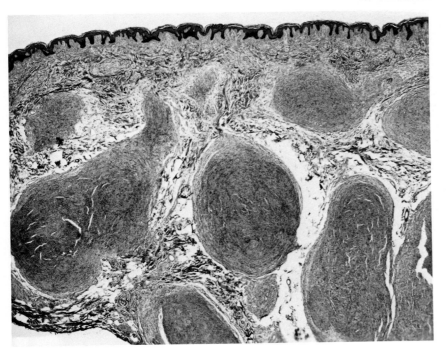

FIG. 31-17. Very rare example of neurilemoma characterized by intradermal growth and a plexiform growth pattern. Plexiform neurilemomas do not appear to have significant association with neurofibromatosis 1. (×15.)

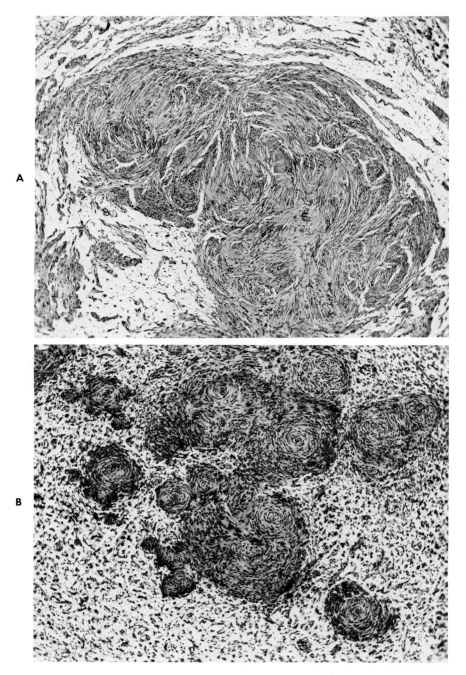

FIG. 31-18. Two examples of neurilemomas showing sharp partitioning of tumor into cellular Antoni A and myxoid Antoni B areas. Cellular zones have a vague fascicular pattern **(A)** or a whorled configuration **(B)**. (**A**, ×50; **B**, ×80.)

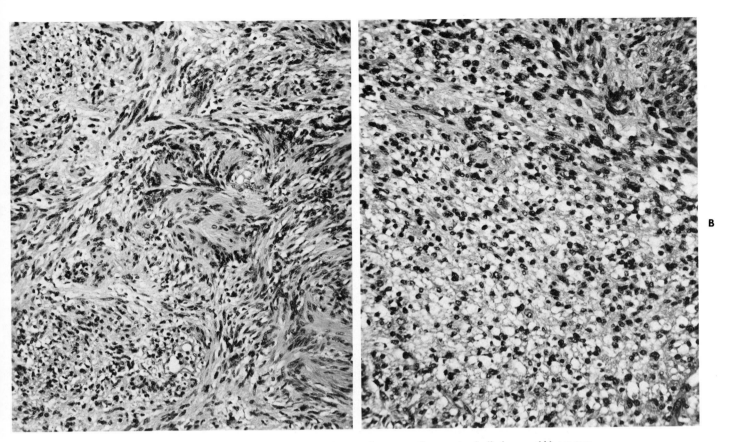

B

FIG. 31-19. Variation of Antoni A areas of a neurilemoma. Compact spindled areas **(A)** are typical, but these are often degenerative changes including vacuolar changes of the cytoplasm and loss of cellular cohesion **(B)**. **(A** and **B,** ×160.)

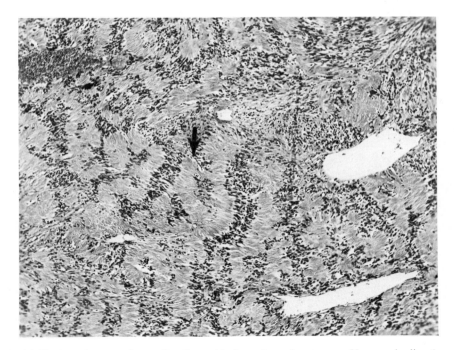

FIG. 31-20. Prominent nuclear palisading with formation of numerous Verocay bodies *(arrow)* within a neurilemoma. (×80.)

ous stages of organization, and their walls are thickened by dense fibrosis. Glands and benign epithelial structures may occur within neurilemomas (Fig. 31-22). Judging from the number and type of glands this seems to represent true epithelial differentiation within the tumor rather than entrapment or induced proliferation of normal structures.[62,74] However, on occasion, neurilemomas may develop cystic

spaces lined by Schwann cells that assume a rounded or epithelioid appearance. This change may be confused with true epithelial differentiation (Figs. 31-23 to 31-25). Such tumors have been referred to as *pseudoglandular schwannoma*. Rarely neurilemomas contain a significant population of small lymphocyte-like Schwann cells (Fig. 31-26), which are arranged around collagen nodules forming giant

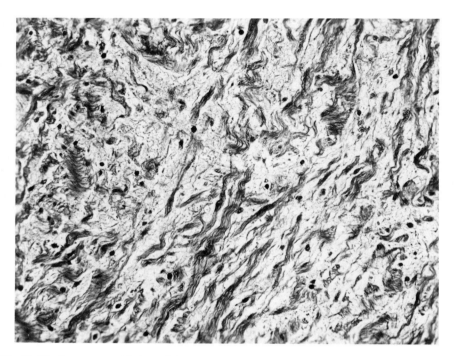

FIG. 31-21. Loose myxoid Antoni B area of neurilemoma. Note similarity to neurofibroma. (×250.)

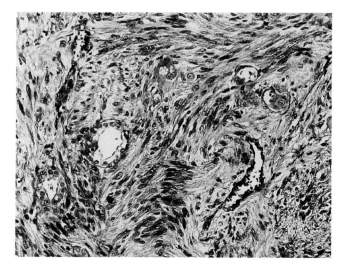

FIG. 31-22. Neurilemoma with benign glands and squamous islands. (×250.)

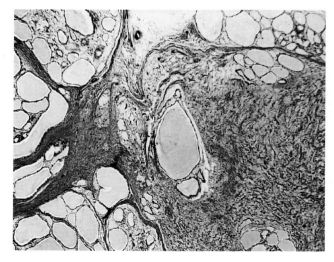

FIG. 31-23. Neurilemoma with cystic spaces resembling glands or dilated lymphatics. (×60.)

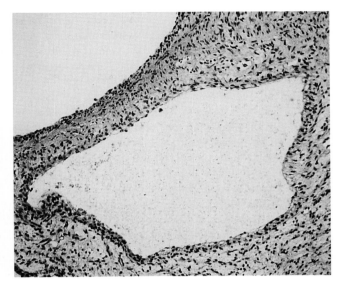

FIG. 31-24. High-power view of Fig. 31-23 showing that cystic spaces are not lined by endothelium but by flattened Schwann cells. (×250.)

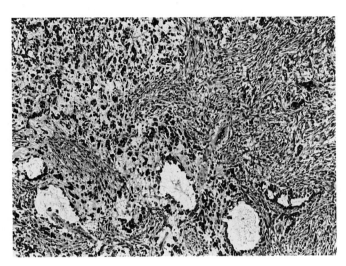

FIG. 31-25. Pseudoglandular neurilemoma. The Schwann cells focally show epithelioid change and appear to line irregular spaces. (×100.)

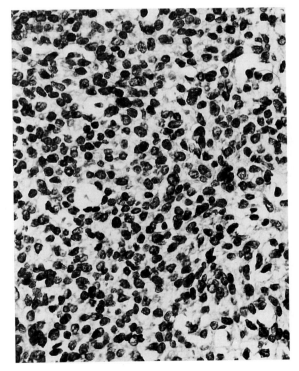

FIG. 31-26. Small, rounded lymphocyte-like Schwann cells within neurilemoma. (×250.)

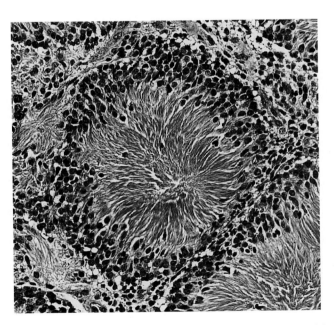

FIG. 31-27. Giant rosette within neurilemoma formed by radial arrangement of Schwann cells around collagen core. (×160.)

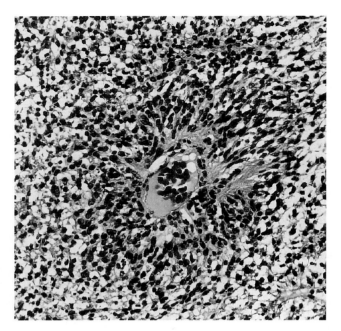

FIG. 31-28. Perivascular rosette within a neurilemoma. (×160.)

rosettes (Fig. 31-27) or around vessels forming perivascular rosettes (Fig. 31-28).[76]

Ultrastructural and immunohistochemical findings

The electron microscope has provided some of the best evidence in support of the separate nature of the neurilemoma and neurofibroma. In contrast to neurofibroma, which contains a mixture of cell types, neurilemoma consists almost exclusively of Schwann cells.[5,147] These cells have attenuated cell processes that emanate from the cell body and lie in undulating layers adjacent to the cell body.[70,97,107,110,147] Basal lamina consisting of electron-dense material (measuring approximately 50 nm) coats the surface of the Schwann cell and lies in redundant stacks between the cells along with typical and long-spacing collagen (Fig. 31-29). The cytoplasm of the Schwann cell contains a flattened, occasionally invaginated nucleus, microfibrils, occasional lysosomes, and scattered mitochondria. In Antoni B areas the Schwann cells possess increased numbers of lysosomes and myelin figures and have only a fragmented basal lamina, suggesting that these are degenerated Antoni A areas.

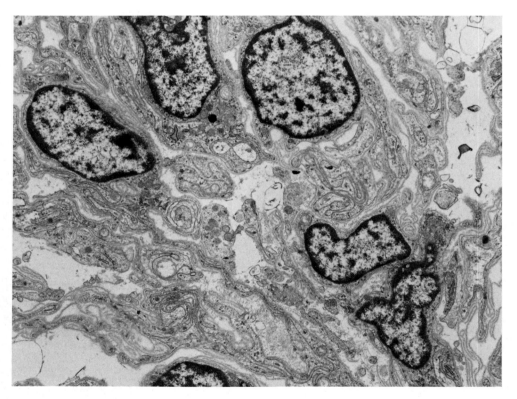

FIG. 31-29. Electron micrograph of neurilemoma. Cells give off long cytoplasmic processes, which lie in layers adjacent to the cell body and are invested by well-formed continuous basal lamina. (From Taxy JB, Battifora H: The electron microscope in the diagnosis of soft tissue tumors. In Trump B, Jones RT, editors: *Diagnostic electron microscopy,* New York, 1980, John Wiley & Sons.)

In concert with ultrastructural observations, most cells within neurilemomas have the antigenic phenotype of Schwann cells. S-100 protein is strongly expressed by most cells of neurilemomas (Fig. 31-30), in contrast to the cells of neurofibromas, which variably express the antigen. Leu-7 and occasionally glial fibrillary acidic protein are present within these tumors. Although the expression of S-100 protein is somewhat diminished in the Antoni B areas, immunostaining for this protein is so consistent and of such intensity that it serves as an important diagnostic tool. In our experience it is most valuable in diagnosing severely degenerated neurilemomas in which the amount of myxoid change or fibrosis obscures the neoplastic nature of the lesion altogether. It usually also distinguishes deeply situated neurilemomas from well-differentiated leiomyosarcomas. This important differential point is especially difficult in biopsy material from large intraabdominal or retroperitoneal masses. The difficulty can be further compounded by the fact that both neurilemomas and leiomyosarcomas can display equivalent degrees of nuclear palisading. Whereas S-100 protein immunostaining is nearly always observed in neurilemomas, it is seldom observed in leiomyosarcomas in our experience. Additional helpful stains include the Masson trichrome stain to document the presence or absence of longitudinal striations. Immunostaining for myelin proteins has also been used to identify benign and malignant Schwann cell tumors, but results have been variable[3,4,223] (see also Chapter 32).

Degenerated neurilemoma (ancient schwannoma)

Ancient schwannomas are neurilemomas that display pronounced degenerative changes.[57,65] These are usually large tumors of long duration, and a significant percentage are located in deep structures such as the retroperitoneum.[65] Degenerative changes include cyst formation, calcification, hemorrhage, and hyalinization (Figs. 31-31 to 31-35). The tumor itself is usually infiltrated by large numbers of siderophages and histiocytes. One of the most treacherous aspects of this tumor is the degree of nuclear atypia encountered. The Schwann cell nuclei are large, hyperchromatic, and often multilobed but lack mitotic figures (Figs. 31-34 and 31-35). These tumors behave as ordinary neurilemomas; therefore the nuclear atypia can be regarded as a purely degenerative change.

Cellular schwannoma

First described in 1969 by Harkin and Reed[6] and later by Woodruff et al.,[116] the cellular schwannoma has become a well-recognized variant of schwannoma[73,89,114] which, because of its cellularity, mitotic activity, and occasional presence of bone destruction, is diagnosed as malignant in over one fourth of cases.[114] Defined as a neurilemoma composed predominantly or exclusively of Antoni A areas that lack Verocay bodies, it occurs in a similar age group as classic neurilemoma but tends to develop more often in deep structures such as the posterior mediastinum and retroperitoneum. Only about one fourth develop in the deep soft tissues of the extremities. It may present as a palpable asymptomatic mass noted radiographically or as a mass producing neurological symptoms. Like classic schwannomas, the lesions appear circumscribed, if not encapsulated. Microscopically they are characterized by Antoni A areas,

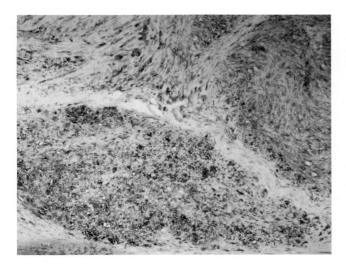

FIG. 31-30. Neurilemoma showing diffuse intense immunostaining for S-100 protein. (Anti-S-100 protein, peroxidase-antiperoxidase, ×75.)

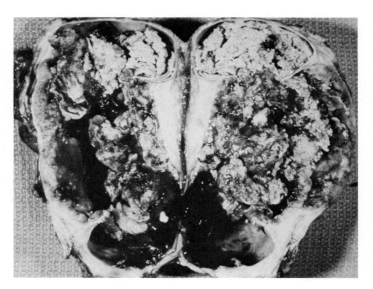

FIG. 31-31. Gross specimen of neurilemoma of retroperitoneum showing extensive degenerative changes (ancient neurilemoma). Tumors are characterized by areas of old and new hemorrhage, cyst formation, and calcification.

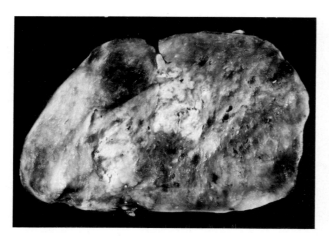

FIG. 31-32. Degenerated neurilemoma of retroperitoneum showing large flecks of calcification.

which dominate the histological picture but may be seen juxtaposed to small zones of Antoni B areas. In addition to short intersecting fascicles and whorls of Schwann cells, the Antoni A areas may display long, sweeping fascicles of Schwann cells sometimes arranged in a herringbone fashion (Fig. 31-36). The presence of this pattern often suggests the diagnosis of fibrosarcoma or leiomyosarcoma to those unfamiliar with cellular schwannoma. Mitotic activity may be observed but usually is low (less than 4/10 HPF).[114] Focal areas of necrosis can be seen in up to 10% of cases. The cells fringing the necrotic zones, however, are differentiated Schwann cells and lack the hyperchromatism and anaplasia so typically encountered around the areas of zonal necrosis in malignant nerve sheath tumors. Like classic neurilemomas, cellular schwannoma displays diffuse, intense immunoreactivity for S-100 protein.

Important factors that should suggest a benign diagnosis include cellularity that is disproportionately high compared with the levels of mitoses and atypia, sharp circumscription if not encapsulation, perivascular hyalinization, occasionally minute focal Antoni B areas, and invariably strong, diffuse immunoreactivity for S-100 protein. We believe that staining for S-100 protein is an invaluable adjunct in making this diagnosis, particularly if one is dealing with material obtained by small needle biopsies of large retroperitoneal or mediastinal masses. In fact, it has been our approach not to make a diagnosis of malignancy on the basis of needle biopsies of differentiated spindle cell tumors having a herringbone pattern if staining for S-100 protein is strongly positive. There is a good possibility that such lesions are cellular schwannomas, and such a diagnosis may be better made on the basis of an incisional biopsy.

Although initial skepticism was expressed about the biological behavior of cellular schwannoma with some suggesting that it was, in fact, a low-grade malignant periph-

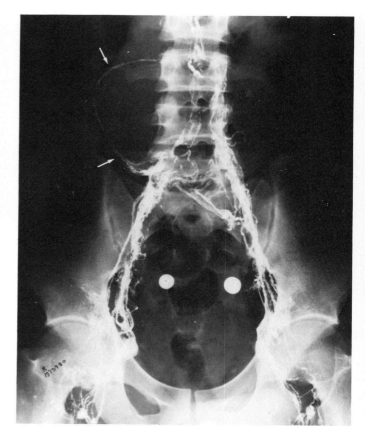

FIG. 31-33. Large retroperitoneal neurilemoma creating deviation of lymphatics on lymphangiogram (arrows).

eral nerve sheath tumor, several recent large studies with extended follow-up information[73,89,114] have reaffirmed the initial findings of Woodruff et al.[116] Over 100 cases have been reported, with nearly one third having follow-up periods of more than 5 years. Less than 5% of patients have developed recurrences, and none has developed metastatic disease. In most cases reported by White et al.,[114] treatment was conservative and consisted of surgical excision only. That these truly represent variants of neurilemoma is indicated not only by histological but also cytogenetic similarities.[89]

Plexiform neurilemoma

About 5% of neurilemomas grow in a plexiform or multinodular pattern, which may or may not be apparent macroscopically (Figs. 31-16 and 31-17). Patients with these tumors do not differ significantly from patients with the ordinary form of neurilemoma. Of the approximately 50 cases reported in the literature, only 2 have had neurofibromatosis.[72,83,86] Thus, this lesion does not carry the same implications as plexiform neurofibroma. In our experience, plexiform neurilemomas have a tendency to be extremely cellular and to lack significant Antoni B zones. This feature,

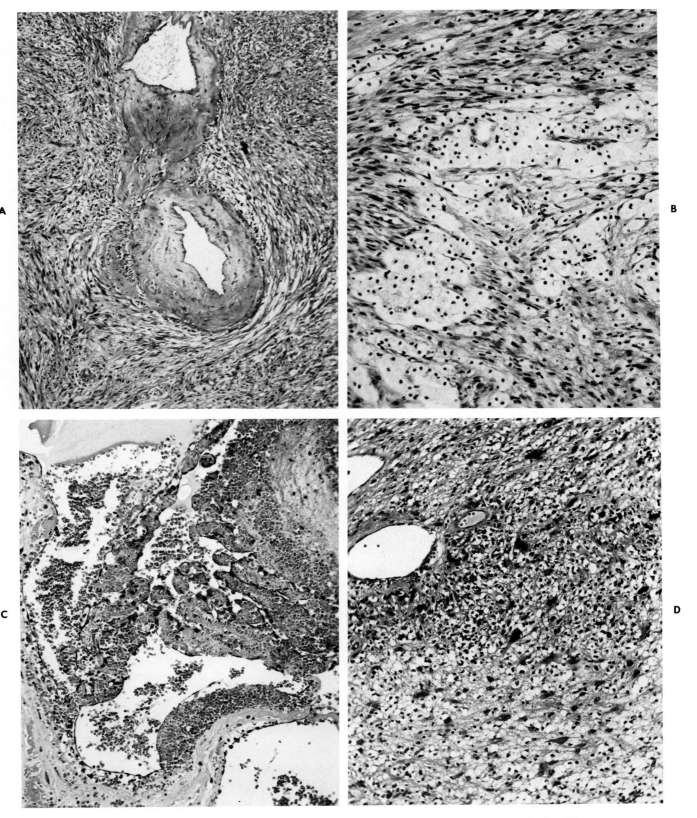

FIG. 31-34. Degenerative change within a neurilemoma, including perivascular hyalinization (**A**), xanthomatous infiltration (**B**), gaping vessels with organizing thrombus (**C**), and degenerative nuclear atypia (**D**). (**A**, ×160; **B**, ×250; **C**, ×160; **D**, ×145.)

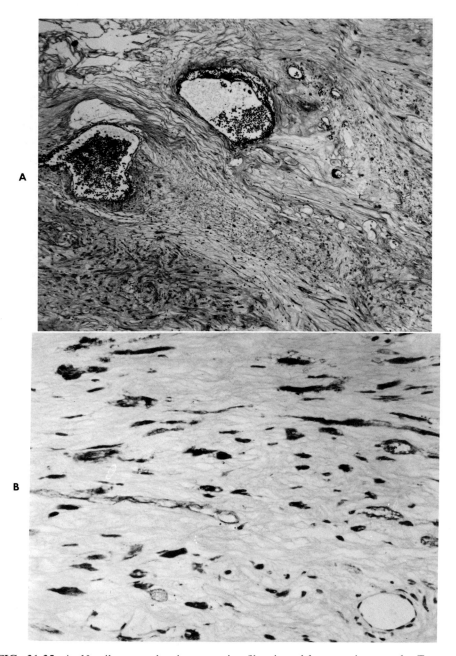

FIG. 31-35. A, Neurilemoma showing extensive fibrosis and large gaping vessels. Tumor was confused with old organized hematoma. B, Immunostaining confirmed the presence of S-100 protein positive cells throughout lesion. (A, ×100; B, anti-S-100 protein, peroxidase-antiperoxidase, ×250.)

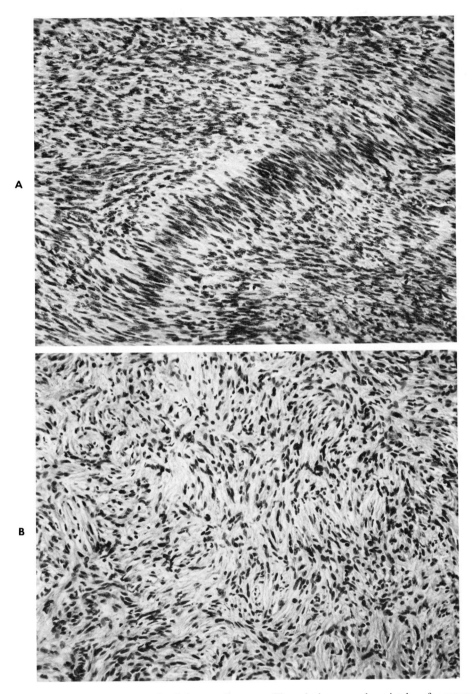

FIG. 31-36. Two examples of cellular neurilemoma. These lesions may be mistaken for sarcomas because they are composed predominantly of highly cellular Antoni A areas with hyperchromatic nuclei. (**A** and **B**, ×160.)

coupled with their plexiform growth, not infrequently suggests the possibility of malignancy supervening on a plexiform neurofibroma.

Discussion

Neurilemomas behave in a benign fashion. In Stout's series of 50 cases[106] none recurred after simple or even incomplete excision. Malignant change is exceedingly rare and from a practical point of view can be discounted. Of the well over one thousand neurilemomas we have seen, there has been only one instance of true malignant transformation. In that case the original tumor had the features of a classic neurilemoma, whereas the recurrent tumor, eight years later, had areas of malignancy. The patient later succumbed to metastatic disease. Isolated case reports of this phenomenon also exist. The case reported by Carstens and Schrodt[63] seems to be a unique and acceptable example of malignant transformation of a neurilemoma. The tumor, an encapsulated mass of the hand of several years' duration, contained, in addition to typical Antoni A and B areas, a malignant focus resembling a neuroblastoma. More recently, Hanada et al.[78] and Rasbridge et al.[96] have reported malignant transformation in 2 cases of neurilemoma. It is difficult to exclude an unusually cellular schwannoma from the illustrations in the first case. In the second case malignancy is clearly depicted, but the administration of radiation 2 years prior to the diagnosis of malignancy leaves open the possibility of a postirradiation sarcoma with an unusually short latency period.[96] Other reports allegedly documenting this transformation are less convincing. As pointed out by Stout,[106] most of the early reports[61,67,71,77,81] do not clearly distinguish between neurofibromas and neurilemomas. Other recent reports either fail to make this distinction[66] or report cases occurring in the setting of neurofibromatosis 1,[91] which are probably neurofibromas that have undergone malignant change. The treatment of neurilemomas is simple excision. However, incomplete excision is certainly warranted for those lesions in which complete excision would cause significant and permanent damage to the adjacent nerve.

NEURILEMOMATOSIS (SCHWANNOMATOSIS) AND MULTIPLE LOCALIZED NEURILEMOMAS

In rare instances neurilemomas may occur multifocally and assume one of two forms. In the first form, known as *neurilemomatosis,* patients present with hypacusia and multiple cutaneous neurilemomas along with a variety of intracranial tumors (meningioma, glioma, astrocytoma, neurilemoma). This disease does not occur on a familial basis and therefore appears distinct from both forms of neurofibromatosis.[120,121] In the second form, patients develop multiple cutaneous neurilemomas, often along the course of a given nerve, but do not develop intracranial lesions.[119] In order to separate this form from the first type, the term

multiple localized neurilemomas has been used. It is not yet clear whether these two forms are part of the same syndrome or distinct entities.[119]

LYMPH NODE NEURILEMOMA

The so-called *lymph node neurilemoma* described in previous editions of this book is a distinctive spindle cell tumor showing nuclear palisading and containing dense collagen bundles (amianthoid fibers). The cells comprising these tumors appear to be modified smooth muscle cells rather than Schwann cells, and probably arise from similar cells that normally reside in some lymph node chains. This tumor is currently termed *palisaded myofibroblastoma,* or *intranodal spindle cell tumor with amianthoid fibers,* and is discussed more completely elsewhere (see Chapter 18).

MELANOTIC SCHWANNOMA

A very rare form of pigmented neural tumor commonly arising from the sympathetic nervous system was described in 1934 by Millar[130] as *malignant melanotic tumor of ganglion cells,* discussed under the term *melanocytic schwannoma* by Fu et al.,[125] and recently redesignated *psammomatous melanotic schwannoma* by Carney, who noted its association with the Carney complex.[122] Based on our experience[123] and that in the literature, the lesion is a distinctive neoplasm of adult life that differs substantially from classic schwannoma despite the similarity in names. The tumor arises commonly from the spinal or autonomic nerves near the midline. However, a number of cases have been reported in the stomach as well as bone and soft tissue. Unusual sites include the heart, bronchus, liver, and skin.[122] Over half of patients with the tumor have evidence of Carney's syndrome (myxomas, spotty pigmentation, and endocrine overactivity producing Cushing's syndrome), and in these patients the tumor typically develops at an earlier age (average, 22.5 years) than those without the syndrome (average, 33.2 years).[122] About 20% of patients will have multiple tumors, and in such patients there is an even higher probability that other manifestations of Carney's complex will be present.[122] The symptoms related specifically to the tumor depend on its location and rate of growth, but most commonly are pain and neurological symptoms in the affected part. Most striking is a case reported by Fu et al.,[125] in which the patient lost sympathetic nerve function in the ipsilateral lower extremity. In one of our cases, a well-encapsulated lesion of the mediastinum, the patient was symptom-free, and the lesion was detected on a routine chest radiograph. The tumors are usually circumscribed or encapsulated and vary from black-brown to grey-blue in color. It is often difficult to make out cellular detail in these tumors because of the heavy pigment deposits. Usually there are at least focal areas having little or no pigment, so that the character of the cells can be evaluated. The cells vary in shape from polygonal to spindled and blend gradu-

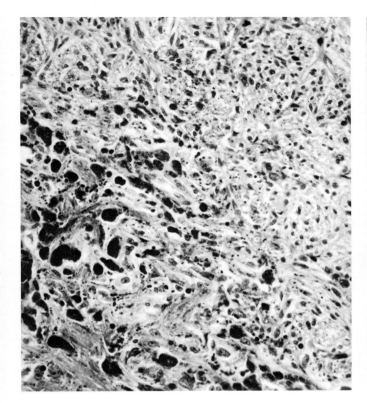

FIG. 31-37. Melanocytic schwannoma showing pigmented spindled areas adjacent to nonpigmented areas. (×250.)

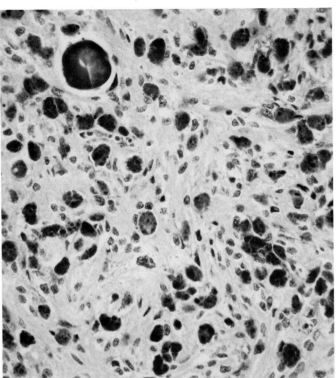

FIG. 31-38. Melanocytic schwannoma showing numerous pigmented cells and calcific spherules resembling psammoma bodies. (×250.)

ally from one to another (Figs. 31-37 and 31-38). This feature, coupled with the ill-defined borders of the cytoplasm, often imparts a syncytial quality to the tumors that is somewhat reminiscent of a neurilemoma. Likewise, the nuclei may display clear intranuclear vacuoles typical of Schwann cells. Nuclear chromatism may be marked, and the nucleoli are often quite prominent. Occasionally there is a vague palisading or formation of whorled structures such that the tumor resembles a neurilemoma or neurofibroma. Ganglion cell differentiation has not been observed in our material, although in the original case, attenuated cytoplasmic processes led Millar[130] to conclude that the tumor cells were ganglionic. Psammoma bodies are present in a majority of cases in our experience, although Carney noted them in all of his cases but cited that extensive sampling was necessary to document them in some cases.[122]

The melanin pigment may be coarsely clumped or finely granular and varies from area to area. Tinctorially it is similar to dermal melanin and stains positively for Fontana's stain and negatively for iron and PAS. On immunohistochemical studies, these tumors strongly express S-100 protein and a melanoma-associated antigen (HMB-45). Ultrastructurally there is a spectrum of maturation, including

premelanosomes and melanosomes, which leads one to conclude that the pigment is synthesized by the tumor cell.[129] Except for the presence of melanosomes, the cells resemble Schwann cells with elaborate cytoplasmic processes that interdigitate or spiral in the manner of mesaxons. The biological behavior of these tumors is difficult to predict. Most are characterized by slow growth in the absence of metastasis, although four tumors reported by Carney (13%) produced metastasis.[122] He concluded that neither tumor size nor ploidy predicted metastatic potential. In our experience we have generally designated those lesions with significant mitotic activity as malignant. When metastases develop they, too, abound with melanin pigment.

SOLITARY NEUROFIBROMA

Solitary neurofibroma is a localized neurofibroma that, by definition, occurs in a patient who does not have neurofibromatosis 1. Its exact incidence is unknown because of the difficulty in excluding the diagnosis of neurofibromatosis 1 in some persons such as the very young, in whom the initial presentation of the disease may be a solitary neurofibroma, or patients who have no affected family members. Despite these problems, it appears that cases of solitary neurofibroma outnumber those of neurofibromatosis 1. In the series by Geschickter[75] about 90% of neurofibromas were of the solitary type, while the remainder were found in the setting of neurofibromatosis 1. Thus it is clear that the presence of a solitary neurofibroma does not establish the diagnosis of neurofibromatosis 1.

Clinical findings

Solitary neurofibromas, like their inherited counterparts, affect the sexes equally. Most develop in persons between the ages of 20 and 30 years.[75] Because the majority are superficial lesions of the dermis or subcutis, they are found evenly distributed over the body surface. They grow slowly as painless nodules and produce few symptoms. Grossly

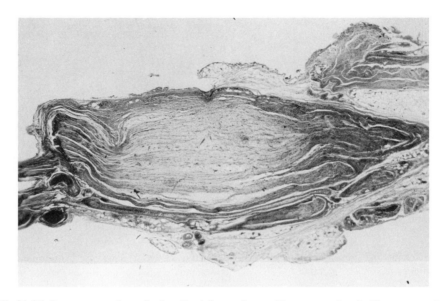

FIG. 31-39. Low-power view of a localized form of neurofibroma causing fusiform expansion of a subcutaneous nerve. Normal nerve is seen at far end of the field. (×4.)

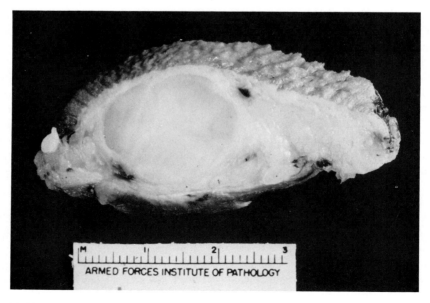

FIG. 31-40. Localized form of neurofibroma occurring within the subcutis. Note circumscribed appearance of the tumor.

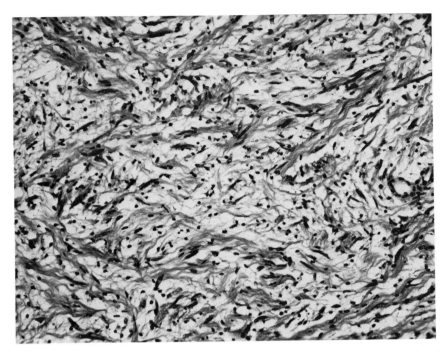

FIG. 31-41. Typical appearance of a neurofibroma consisting of Schwann cells associated with wire-like collagen fibrils and modest amounts of stromal mucosubstances. (×160.)

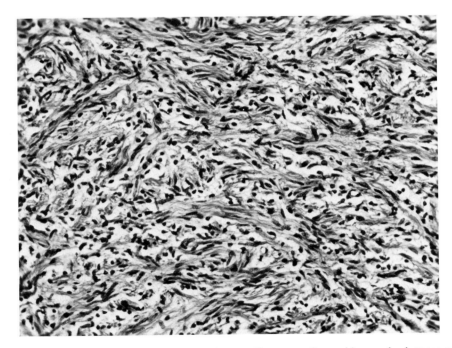

FIG. 31-42. Cellular form of neurofibroma. Note small amount of myxoid ground substance compared with that in Fig. 31-44. (×225.)

they are white-gray tumors that lack the secondary degenerative changes common to neurilemomas. If they arise in major nerves, they expand the structure in a fusiform fashion, and normal nerve can be seen entering and exiting from the mass (Fig. 31-39). If such a lesion remains confined by the epineurium, it possesses a true capsule. However, more commonly these tumors arise in small nerves and readily extend into soft tissue. Such tumors appear circumscribed but are nonencapsulated (Fig. 31-40).

Microscopic findings

Histologically the neurofibroma varies, depending on its content of cells, mucin, and collagen (Figs. 31-41 to 31-46). In its most characteristic form the neurofibroma contains interlacing bundles of elongated cells having wavy,

dark-staining nuclei. The cells are intimately associated with wirelike strands of collagen, and small to moderate amounts of mucoid material separate the cells and collagen. The stroma of the tumor is dotted with occasional mast cells, lymphocytes, and rarely xanthoma cells (Fig. 31-46). Less frequently the neurofibroma is very cellular and consists of Schwann cells set in a more uniform collagen matrix devoid of mucosubstances (Fig. 31-42). In such tumors the cells may be arranged in fascicles, whorls, or even a storiform pattern. In certain respects these cellular neurofibromas may resemble Antoni A areas of a neurilemoma. Unlike in neurilemoma, they are not encapsulated and lack a clear partition into two zones. Moreover, small neurites can usually be demonstrated throughout these tumors. Least commonly these tumors are highly myxoid and easily confused with myxomas; this form of neurofibroma usually occurs on the extremities. These hypocellular neoplasms contain pools of acid mucopolysaccharide with widely spaced Schwann cells (Fig. 31-44). In contrast to the cells of myxoma, the cells of neurofibroma usually have a greater degree of orientation. The vascularity is also more prominent, and with careful searching features of specific differentiation (e.g., Wagner-Meissner bodies) may be found. Recently we reviewed one unique neurofibroma with focal rosettes and mucin-producing glands (Fig. 31-47). Neurofibromas having areas of rhabdomyoma have been reported.[55,58] S-100 protein can be identified within these tumors but in our experience is not as striking as in neurilemoma (Fig. 31-48).

In addition to the spectrum of conventional neurofibromas, there are several unusual types discussed in this chapter that are of interest principally to the pathologist.

Pacinian neurofibroma

Although conventional neurofibroma may contain occasional structures that resemble the specialized tactile

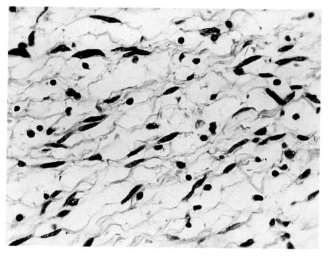

FIG. 31-43. Neurofibroma showing the irregular spindled shape of tumor cells. (×400.)

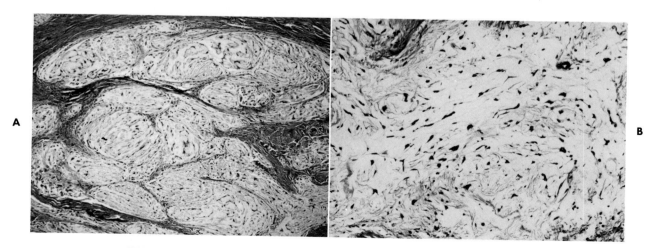

FIG. 31-44. Neurofibroma showing extreme myxoid change. (A, ×60; B, ×160.)

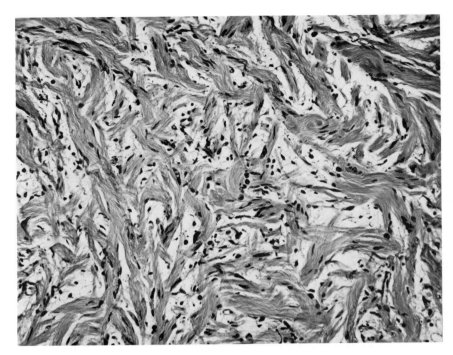

FIG. 31-45. Hyalinized form of neurofibroma showing many thick collagen bundles. (×160.)

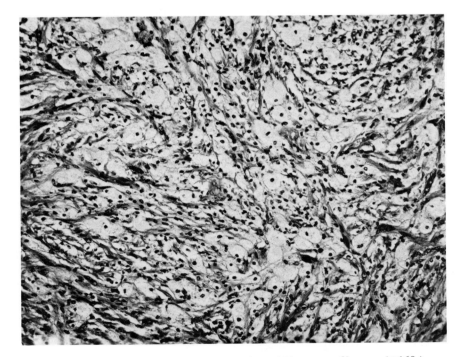

FIG. 31-46. Xanthomatous change occurring within a neurofibroma. (×160.)

(Wagner-Meissner body) or pressure (pacinian corpuscle) receptors, it is highly unusual to find a neurofibroma in which these elements predominate (Fig. 31-49). The so-called pacinian neurofibroma[92,93] described by Prichard and Custer[92] contains a plethora of structures that resemble normal pressure receptors. These tumors have been reported in adolescents and adults in such sites as the hand, foot, and buttock. None of the patients had neurofibromatosis 1. The paucity of cases prevents any meaningful analysis of these points. Although by convention these tumors have been considered neurofibromas, in some instances the overall pattern is suggestive of neurilemoma. Those resembling

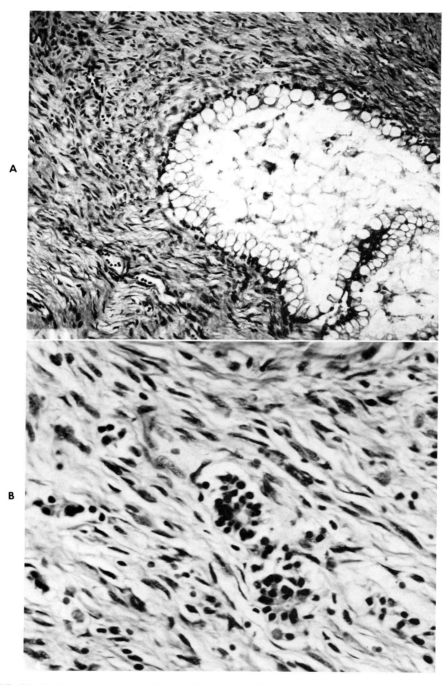

FIG. 31-47. A unique example of neurofibroma in which mature mucus-secreting glands (A) and rosettes (B) were present. (A, ×160; B, ×400.)

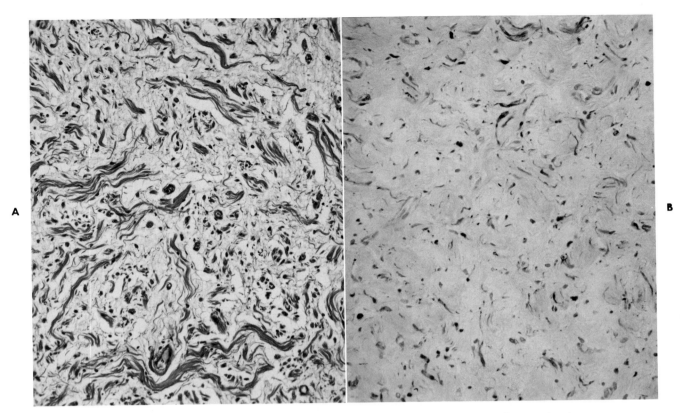

FIG. 31-48. **A,** Neurofibroma. **B,** Immunostaining for S-100 protein in neurofibroma showing heterogeneity with respect to immunoreactivity. (**A,** ×250; **B,** anti-S-100 protein, peroxidase-antiperoxidase, ×250.)

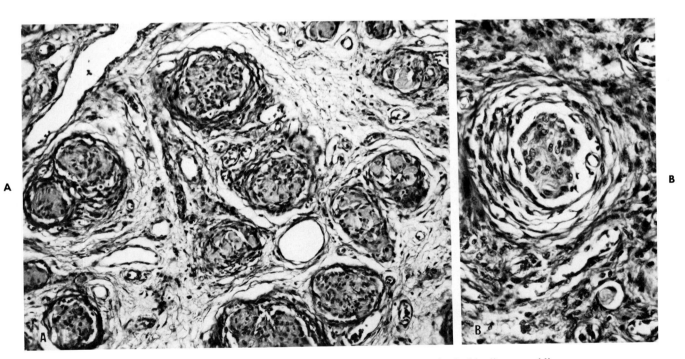

FIG. 31-49. **A,** Pacinian neurofibroma characterized by numerous spherical bodies resembling rudimentary pressure receptors (pacinian corpuscles). (×160.) **B,** High-power view of pacinian body with central zone of polygonal cells flanked by peripheral zone of concentrically flattened cells. (×250.)

neurofibromas consist of sheets of rounded or oval Schwann cells, which gradually become transformed into the lamellar pacinian bodies. In other tumors the pacinian bodies stand in sharp contrast to the surrounding meshlike background similar to the juxtaposition of Antoni A and B ar-

eas in neurilemoma. The variation in the pacinian bodies has been compared to the stages of differentiation of the normal pacinian corpuscle. Those resembling the early pacinian corpuscle consist of balls or nests of rounded cells containing small central cores of elongated cells. Others

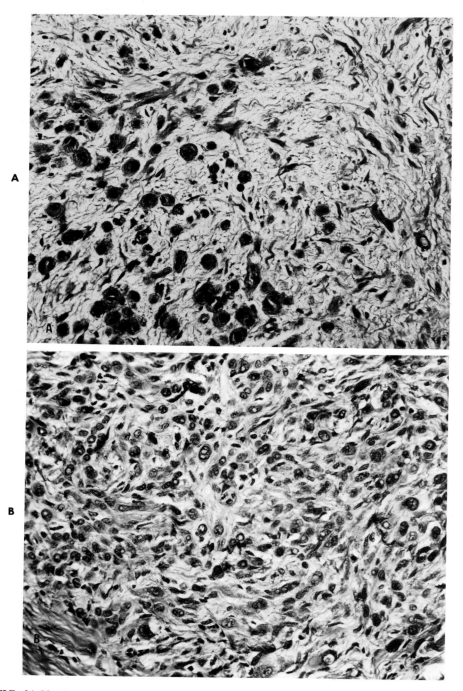

FIG. 31-50. Two examples of epithelioid neurofibroma. **A,** Tumor blends with areas resembling a more conventional neurofibroma. (×160.) **B,** Most portions of the tumor had an epithelioid appearance but it arose as a cutaneous mass in a patient with von Recklinghausen's disease. (×250.)

contain a predominance of elongated cells arranged in lamellae and separated by delicate collagen fibrils. In these structures the resemblance to the normal pacinian corpuscle is more obvious. One ultrastructural study of this tumor suggests the cells resemble the perineural epithelial cell.[111] However, the tumor, as depicted, appears to be a neurofibroma with Wagner-Meissner bodies rather than pacinian bodies. Pacinian neuroma differs from this tumor by the presence of perfectly formed, albeit larger, pacinian bodies.

Epithelioid neurofibroma

Histogenetically this tumor can be thought of as a neurofibroma in which the epithelial potential of the neural crest is expressed. This tumor, like pacinian neurofibroma, is quite rare. Its scarcity, coupled with the diagnostic problems it poses, accounts for the fact that it has received little attention in the literature. In our opinion, it can only be reliably and consistently recognized when it arises within a nerve or when it merges with an area of typical neurofibroma. The "epithelial" area of this tumor is usually quite cellular and has only a modest matrix of collagen and mucosubstances. The small, rounded Schwann cells have variably staining cytoplasm and are arranged in compact nests or short cords (Fig. 31-50). Despite the "epithelial" features of these cells, their borders are seldom as distinct as those of a true epithelial neoplasm, and there is usually a greater amount of interstitial collagen between groups of cells and especially between individual cells. S-100 protein can be demonstrated within the epithelioid Schwann cells as well as the spindled ones.

Pigmented neurofibroma

Because the neural crest gives rise to both Schwann cells and melanocytes, it is not surprising that some nerve sheath tumors may show evidence of melanocytic differentiation. Although most of these pigmented tumors have been classified as solitary forms of neurofibromas, it is clear that melanin production may occur in the neurofibromas of neurofibromatosis 1 as well as in neurilemomas. In most cases the pigment is present only microscopically within occasional cells so that the tumor does not appear grossly black (Fig. 31-51). The pigment possesses the tinctorial and ultrastructural features of dermal melanin.

Discussion

Although solitary neurofibromas do not carry the same incidence of malignant change as their inherited counterparts, the exact risk is unknown but it is probably quite small. Simple excision of these tumors is considered adequate therapy.

NEUROFIBROMATOSIS

Neurofibromatosis, also named *von Recklinghausen's disease* for the man who described the disease in 1882, was formerly considered a single disease but is now known to

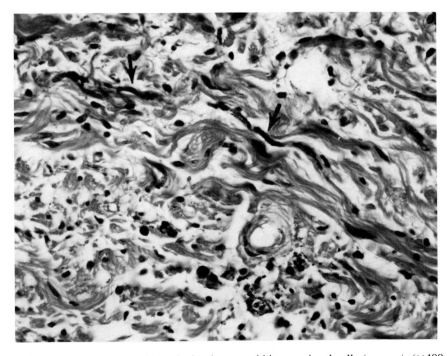

FIG. 31-51. Neurofibroma with melanin pigment within occasional cells *(arrows)*. (×400.)

be two clinically and genetically distinct diseases. The more common disease, formerly known as the peripheral form of neurofibromatosis, is now designated *neurofibromatosis 1*, whereas the less common disease, formerly known as the central form, is now designated *neurofibromatosis 2 (bilateral acoustic neurofibromatosis)*.

Neurofibromatosis 1

Neurofibromatosis 1 is a common genetic disease that affects one in every 2500 to 3000 live births,[128] and it accounts for one admission out of 3100 at the Mayo Clinic.[135] It is inherited as an autosomal dominant with a high rate of penetrance. Because only half of the patients with this disease have affected family members, the remainder of the patients obviously represent new mutations. The mutation rate, estimated at 10^{-4} per gamete per generation, is among the highest for a dominantly inherited trait.

Neurofibromatosis 1 is associated with deletions, insertions, or mutations in the neurofibromatosis 1 gene,[143] a tumor suppressor gene located in the pericentromeric region of chromosome 17.[133] Spanning a distance of 300 kb and containing within it three additional genes, it is one of the largest human genes identified to date. It encodes a protein known as neurofibromin, which localizes to the microtubular system and is ubiquitously distributed in all tissues. Although the function of neurofibromin is not fully defined, it is somewhat homologous with the family of GAP proteins (GTPase activating protein) which are believed to be important in the control of cell growth through their down-regulation of the ras gene product.

Diagnostic criteria for neurofibromatosis 1*
Neurofibromatosis 1 is diagnosed in an individual with two or more of the following signs or factors: • Six or more café-au-lait macules over 5 mm in greatest diameter in prepubertal individuals, and over 15 mm in greatest diameter in postpubertal individuals • Two or more neurofibromas of any type or one plexiform neurofibroma • Freckling in the axillary or inguinal region • Optic glioma • Two or more Lisch nodules (iris hamartomas) • A distinctive osseous lesion such as sphenoid dysplasia or thinning of long bone cortex with or without pseudoarthrosis • A first-degree relative (parent, sibling, or offspring) with neurofibromatosis 1 by the above criteria
*From National Institutes of Health Consensus Development Conference Statement, vol 6(12), July 13-15, 1987.

Clinical findings. Clinically there are a number of signs and symptoms that characterize this disease. In order to make the diagnosis, two or more of the cardinal features of the disease must be present (see the accompanying box).

In the typical patient, neurofibromatosis 1 becomes evident within the first few years of life, when café-au-lait

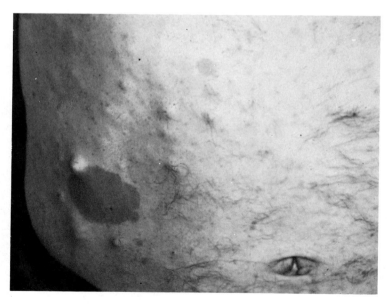

FIG. 31-52. Café-au-lait spot. These pigmented lesions usually herald the onset of neurofibromatosis 1. They are usually multiple, occur on unexposed surfaces, and typically are several centimeters in diameter.

spots develop. These pigmented macular lesions resemble freckles, especially in the early stage when they are small. Typically they become much larger and darker in color with age and occur mainly on unexposed surfaces of the body (Fig. 31-52). One of the most characteristic locations for these spots is the axilla (axillary freckle sign). Pathologically they are characterized by an increase in melanin pigment in the basal layer of the epidermis. The pigment may be present in the form of giant melanosomes (macromelanosomes), a feature that has been used as a means of histologically distinguishing them from other pigmented lesions[146] (e.g., freckle, lesions of Albright's disease). However, it has been emphasized that the giant granules are not invariably found[170]; their presence may be a function of the age of the lesion. It has been suggested that in adults only lesions greater than 1.5 cm be considered café-au-lait spots for purposes of diagnosis.[128] Because the number of café-au-lait spots increases with age and over 90% of patients with neurofibromatosis have these lesions, their number serves as a useful guideline in making the diagnosis. Not only do these lesions herald the onset of the disease, but in older patients they often give some indication as to the form and severity of the disease.[128] For instance, patients with few café-au-lait spots tend to have either (1) late onset of palpable neurofibromas, (2) localization of neurofi-

bromas to one segment of the body, or (3) neurofibromatosis 2.

The neurofibromas, the hallmark of the disease, make their appearance during childhood or adolescence after the café-au-lait spots. The time course varies greatly; some tumors emerge at birth, and others appear during late adult life (Fig. 31-53). They may be found in virtually any location and in unusual instances may be restricted to one area of the body (segmental neurofibromatosis).[128,153] Unusual symptoms have been related to the presence of these tumors in various organs, including the gastrointestinal tract,[144] appendix,[152] larynx,[159] blood vessels,[141,165,168] and heart.[161] The tumors are usually slowly growing lesions. Acceleration of their growth rate has been noted during pregnancy and at puberty. Sudden increase in the size of one lesion should always raise the question of malignant change.

In addition to peripheral neurofibromas, patients with neurofibromatosis 1 may also develop central nervous system tumors that include optic nerve glioma, astrocytoma, and a variety of heterotopias. Acoustic neuroma, the hallmark of neurofibromatosis 2, is virtually never encountered in neurofibromatosis 1. Unusual "bright lesions" may be detected by T2-weighted MRI in the brain of up to 50% of children with neurofibromatosis 1, although the precise nature and significance of these lesions is unknown.

Pigmented hamartomas of the iris (Lisch nodules) are present in over 90% of patients with neurofibromatosis 1 (Figs. 31-54 and 31-55).[162] These asymptomatic lesions are not present in normal individuals or in those with neurofibromatosis 2. Although they cannot be correlated with other

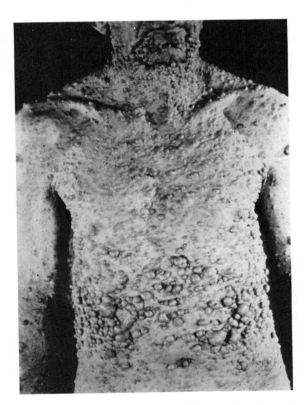

FIG. 31-53. Male patient with neurofibromatosis of long duration.

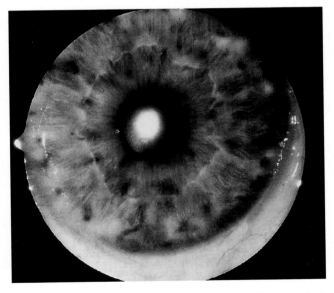

FIG. 31-54. Lisch nodule in a patient with neurofibromatosis 1. Pigmented areas are seen as dark zones within the iris.

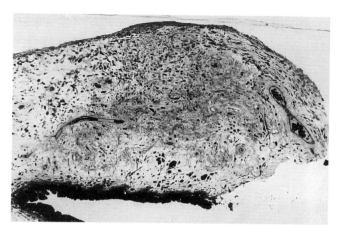

FIG. 31-55. Lisch nodule showing collections of pigment within the iris. (×25.)

specific manifestations of neurofibromatosis 1, they are extremely helpful in establishing the diagnosis.

Skeletal abnormalities occur in almost 40% of patients with this disease.[135,138,164,177] They include erosive defects secondary to impingement by soft tissue tumors as well as primary defects. These include scalloping of the vertebra, congenital bowing of long bones with pseudoarthrosis, unilateral orbital malformations, and cystic osteolytic lesions. In the past the intraosseous cystic lesions were believed to be skeletal neurofibromas. However, the majority of such lesions have a histological appearance similar to a nonossi-

fying fibroma or fibrous cortical defect. They are characterized by fascicles of fibroblasts arranged in short intersecting fascicles (sometimes in a storiform pattern) and punctuated with occasional giant cells.

Gynecomastia may develop in young men with neurofibromatosis. Histologically it does not have the appearance of true gynecomastia and thus has been termed *pseudogynecomastia*. The breast stroma is hyalinized and contains small nerve fibers and fibroblasts, some of which may be multinucleated. In addition to these well-recognized signs and symptoms, the disease may also be associated with diverse symptoms not clearly referable to the presence of tumors. They include disorders of growth, sexual maturation and mentation,[138] and abnormalities of the lung.[150,164,175] Certain tumors, including neurilemoma,[84,106] pheochromocytoma,[138] ganglioneuroma, nephroblastoma,[173] and leukemia[139,151] have been reported in this disease.

Pathological findings. Several types of neurofibromas occur in this disease, and they may be distinguished on the basis of their gross and microscopic appearances.

Localized neurofibroma. Localized neurofibroma is the most common type encountered in this disease, but it is histologically the least characteristic because essentially identical lesions occur on a solitary basis outside neurofibromatosis 1. These tumors are typically located in the dermis and subcutis but may be located in deep soft tissue as well. These tumors are larger than solitary neurofibromas. Large pendulous tumors of the skin are often alluded to as *fibroma molluscum*. Histologically these tumors are no different from solitary neurofibromas and embrace a spectrum from

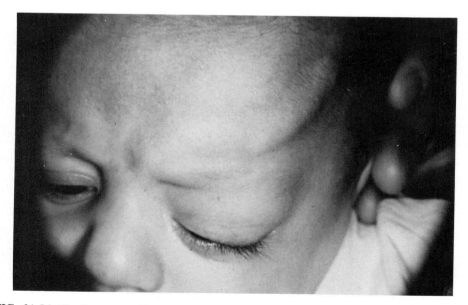

FIG. 31-56. Plexiform neurofibroma occurring in the subcutis of the scalp and involving the upper eyelid. Note irregular tortuous contour of tumor. Lesions of this type are virtually pathognomonic of neurofibromatosis 1.

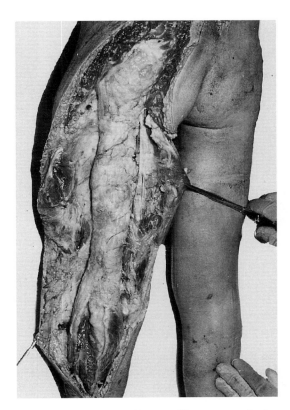

FIG. 31-57. Plexiform neurofibroma of lower extremity in patient with neurofibromatosis 1.

highly cellular to highly myxoid tumors. Malignant degeneration may occur but is more common in deeply situated lesions. The presence of mitotic activity is required in order to document malignant change because nuclear pleomorphism can be seen in benign lesions.

Plexiform neurofibroma. Plexiform neurofibroma is virtually pathognomonic of this disease,[2,6] provided that the definition of a plexiform neurofibroma is stringent (Figs. 31-56 to 31-61). Plexiform neurofibromas essentially always develop in early childhood, often before the cutaneous neurofibromas have fully developed. Those plexiform neurofibromas involving an entire extremity give rise to the condition known as *elephantiasis neuromatosa,* in which the extremity is enlarged. The overlying skin is loose, redundant, and hyperpigmented, while the underlying bone may be hypertrophied, a phenomenon probably related to the increased vascular supply to the limb (Fig. 31-60).

Macroscopically plexiform neurofibromas are large lesions that affect large segments of a nerve, distorting it and contorting it into a "bag of worms" (Figs. 31-58 and 31-59). Smaller lesions, which simply have a plexiform pattern when viewed microscopically rather than macroscopically, should not be interpreted as plexiform neurofibromas for purposes of establishing the diagnosis of neurofibromatosis 1.

Microscopically the lesion consists of a tortuous mass of expanded nerve branches, which are seen cut in various planes of section. Occasionally the cells spill out of the nerves into soft tissue. In these cases, the plexiform neurofibroma is embedded in a backdrop of neurofibromatous tissue. In the early stages the nerves may simply have an in-

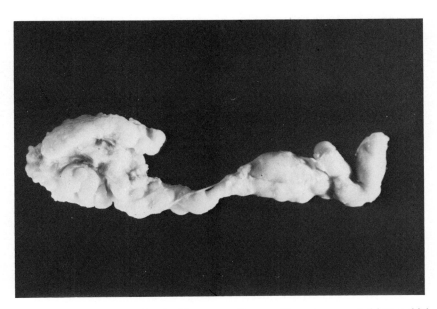

FIG. 31-58. Gross appearance of a plexiform neurofibroma. Nerve is converted into a thick convoluted mass, which has been likened to a "bag of worms."

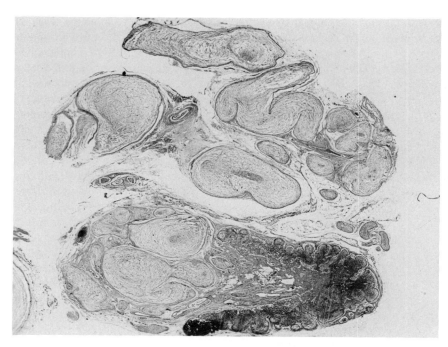

FIG. 31-59. Plexiform neurofibroma involving nerve and extending into the hilum of a lymph node. Apparent lymph node involvement does not indicate malignancy but simply reflects the diffuseness of the process. (×5.)

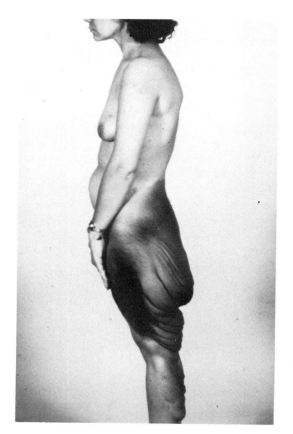

FIG. 31-60. Patient with neurofibromatosis 1 and large neurofibroma of leg resulting in elephantiasis neuromatosa.

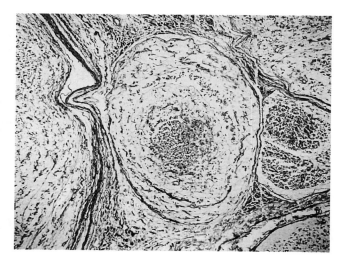

FIG. 31-61. Plexiform neurofibroma showing expansion of endoneurium by myxoid ground substance. (×100.)

crease in the endoneurial matrix material, resulting in wide separation of the small nerve fascicles (Fig. 31-61). In late stages the nerve fibers are replaced by a proliferation of isolated Schwann cells interspersed with thick wavy collagen bundles. With special stains, small axons can be demonstrated within the tumors. As in other neurofibromas, nuclear pleomorphism is sometimes encountered. It is the presence of mitotic figures, however, that is indicative of malignant change.

Electron microscopy of these lesions has documented the participation of several cell types.[110,137,147] The predominant cell is the Schwann cell, which is surrounded by basal lamina (Fig. 31-62). These cells may invest small axons, spiral around themselves, or lie singly in the matrix. A significant number of fibroblasts are also present; these are distinguished from Schwann cells by their prominent endoplasmic reticulum and their lack of basal lamina. It has been suggested that these lesions are really hamartomas because of the polymorphic population of cells. Although the early lesions have many of the features of a hyperplastic process, the advanced lesions manifest a capacity of autonomous growth and malignant transformation, characteristics of a true neoplasm.

Diffuse neurofibroma. Diffuse neurofibroma is an un-

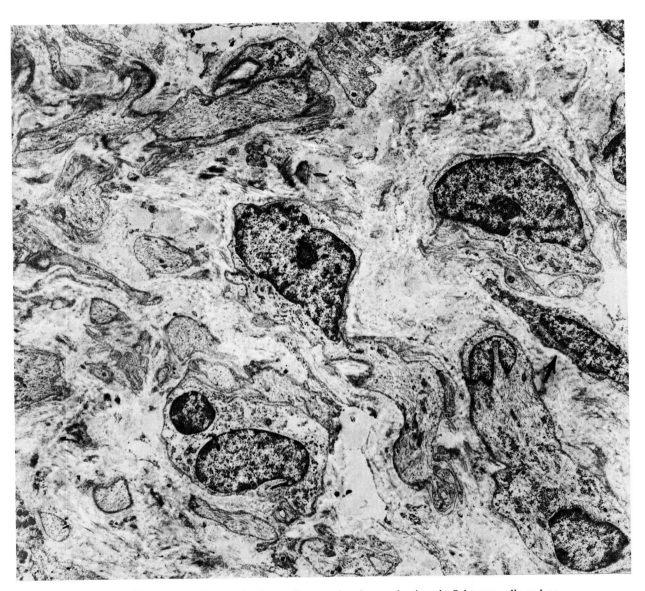

FIG. 31-62. Electron micrograph of neurofibroma showing predominantly Schwann cells and occasional fibroblasts *(arrow).* (×5775.)

common but distinctive form of neurofibroma that occurs principally in children and young adults. Some have termed these lesions *paraneurofibroma*[11] to indicate the extension of the tumor beyond the confines of the perineurium. It is not yet clear how often this tumor is associated with neurofibromatosis. In our cases, at least 10% of patients with this lesion also have neurofibromatosis. This probably represents a very low estimate of the incidence because the young age of patients with diffuse neurofibroma often precludes a reliable diagnosis of neurofibromatosis.

Clinically this tumor is most common in the head and neck region and presents as a plaquelike elevation of the skin. On cut section, the entire subcutis between superficial fascia and dermis is thickened by firm, grayish tissue (Fig. 31-63). As its name implies, this form of neurofibroma is ill-defined and spreads extensively along connective tissue septa and between fat cells. Despite its infiltrative growth, it does not destroy but rather envelops the normal structures it encompasses in much the same fashion as dermatofibrosarcoma protuberans (Figs. 31-64 and 31-65). It differs from the conventional neurofibroma in that it has a very uniform matrix of fine fibrillary collagen. The Schwann cells, which lie suspended in the matrix, are usually less elongated than those of conventional neurofibroma and have short fusiform or even round contours (Figs. 31-66 to 31-70). The sheets of tumor contain clusters of Meissner body-like structures, a characteristic feature of this lesion that serves to distinguish it from the superficial aspect

of dermatofibrosarcoma protuberans (Fig. 31-66). Some diffuse neurofibromas consist of a rather complex arrangement of several mesenchymal elements in addition to the neurofibromatous tissue (Fig. 31-68). These tumors, which seem to be more common in neurofibromatosis, consist of neurofibromatous tissue admixed with mature fat or large ectatic vessels. The latter structures at times may be so striking as to eclipse the neural component and can result in the erroneous impression of exuberant granulation tissue. Rarely nuclear palisading is present in diffuse neurofibromas (Fig. 31-69).

In our experience, malignant transformation rarely occurs in diffuse neurofibroma. We have seen only one acceptable case of diffuse neurofibroma undergo malignant change.

Discussion. Unlike solitary neurofibromas, those encountered in neurofibromatosis may cause significant morbidity. The large number of lesions usually makes surgical therapy impossible. Therefore surgery has traditionally been reserved for lesions that are large, painful, or located in strategic areas where continued expansion would compromise organ function.[131] Even after attempted complete excision of these lesions, clinical recurrences occasionally develop, a phenomenon related to the ill-defined nature of the tumors. A problem of greater importance is that of malignant transformation. The exact incidence is difficult to determine and has been estimated at 2% to 29% of patients with the disease.[134,138,145,160,169] The often-quoted frequency of 13%[145] is too high an estimate in our opinion

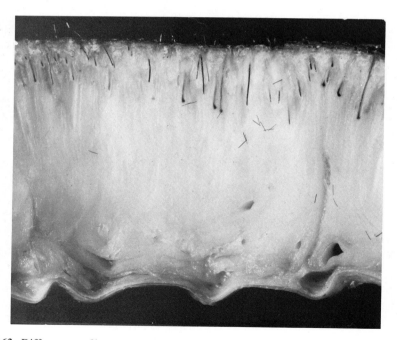

FIG. 31-63. Diffuse neurofibroma presenting as an ill-defined expansion of the subcutaneous region of scalp.

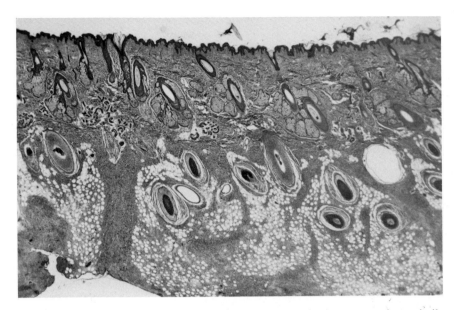

FIG. 31-64. Diffuse neurofibroma with extensive permeation of subcutaneous tissue similar to a dermatofibrosarcoma protuberans. (×15.)

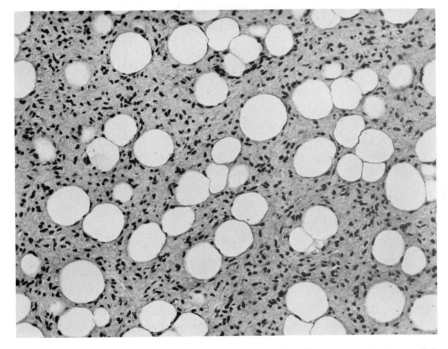

FIG. 31-65. Diffuse neurofibroma involving subcutaneous fat. Pattern is reminiscent of the pattern of infiltration of a dermatofibrosarcoma protuberans. (×150.)

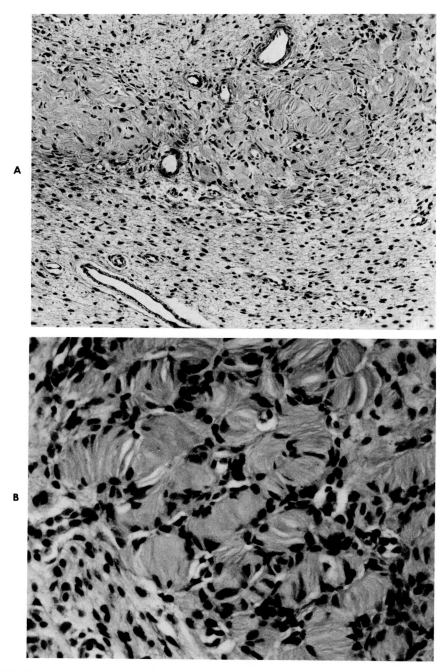

FIG. 31-66. **A,** Diffuse neurofibroma showing the fine fibrillary collagenous background punctuated with Wagner-Meissner bodies. (×165.) **B,** Wagner-Meissner bodies within a diffuse neurofibroma. (×400.)

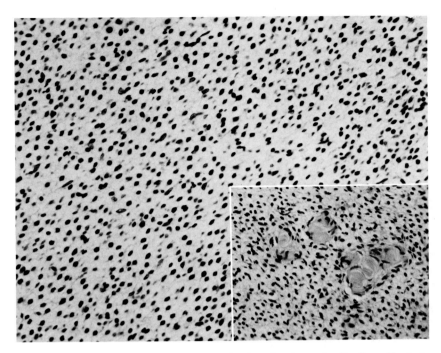

FIG. 31-67. Diffuse neurofibroma consisting predominantly of round cells. Inset illustrates occasional Wagner-Meissner bodies found in the tumor. (×160; *inset,* ×160.)

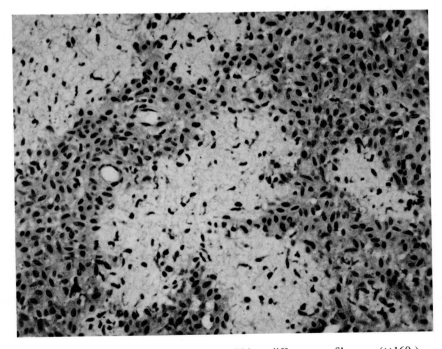

FIG. 31-68. Myxoid and cellular areas within a diffuse neurofibroma. (×160.)

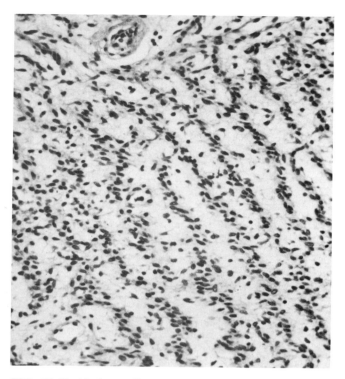

FIG. 31-69. Nuclear palisading within a diffuse neurofibroma. (×160.)

because it is based on ascertainment of cases reported in the literature. The true incidence is probably closer to the lower figure of 2%.[138] This supposition is reinforced by the follow-up study of a nationwide cohort of 212 Danish patients with neurofibromatosis.[172] Nine of the 212 patients developed a sarcoma of nerve or soft tissue origin, and 16 developed a glioma. Most malignant tumors occurred in the proband group (84 patients), who, by definition, required hospitalization and were probably more severely affected by the disorder. The authors suggest that the natural history of neurofibromatosis may be more accurately reflected by the majority of patients, relatives of the probands (128 patients), who did not require hospitalization and whose prognosis may have been better than previously thought. Both groups, however, had decreased survival rate after 40 years when compared with the general population.

In our experience, the patients at greatest risk to develop sarcomas are those who have had the disease for many years.[142] Over three fourths of patients with neurofibromatosis and malignant schwannoma have had the disease 10 years or longer, and only rarely do sarcomas complicate the course of patients who have had the disease less than 5 years. Typically, patients developing sarcomas present with rapid enlargement or pain in a preexisting neurofibroma. Both symptoms, especially the former, should always lead to biopsy. Once malignant change has supervened, the ther-

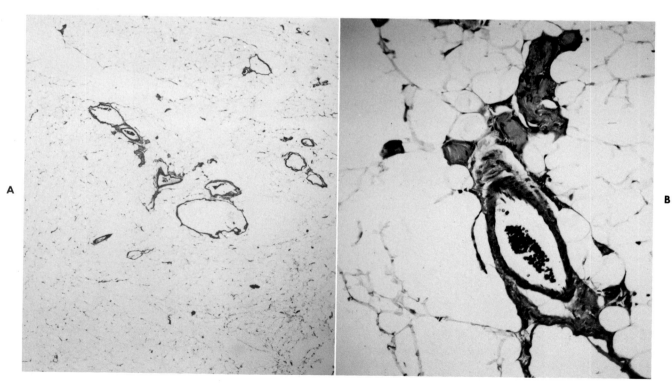

FIG. 31-70. A, Diffuse neurofibroma with extensive fatty overgrowth. B, Wagner-Meissner bodies within the fat identify the neural nature of the lesion. (A, ×25; B, ×250.)

apy should consist of radical local excision or amputation. Unfortunately, the prognosis for patients developing malignant schwannomas in this setting is quite poor, with fewer than 20% surviving 5 years[142] (Chapter 32).

Neurofibromatosis 2 (bilateral acoustic neurofibromatosis)

Neurofibromatosis 2 is a far rarer disease than neurofibromatosis 1, affecting one in 50,000 persons. Like neurofibromatosis 1, this disease is inherited as an autosomal dominant with a high rate of penetrance (95%). The gene, localized to chromosome 22, encodes a protein known as merlin, which is homologous to the moesin-ezrine-radixin proteins that play a role in the binding of the cell membrane to intracellular matrix.

The disease usually has its onset in adolescence or early adult life, with the development of tinnitus or hearing loss due to the presence of bilateral acoustic neuromas. Although café-au-lait spots and neurofibromas may occur in neurofibromatosis 2, they are usually few in number. In addition to acoustic neuromas, other central nervous system tumors occur commonly, including schwannomas of other cranial nerves, meningioma, and ependymoma. Diagnostic criteria are listed in the accompanying box.

PERINEURIOMA

Perineurioma is a rare soft tissue tumor composed of cells resembling those of the normal perineurium. It was first described in 1978 by Lazarus and Trombetta[181] on the basis of ultrastructural findings. Although a number of cases have been reported recently,[178,179,182,185,186] the tumor has been slow to gain wide recognition and acceptance because of the lack of clear-cut criteria for diagnosis. Furthermore, tumors that have been identified as perineuriomas have had varying histological appearances with considerable overlap with neurofibroma, indicating that it is not possible to consistently recognize these tumors on the basis of light microscopy alone. Rather, it requires light microscopy with either ultrastructural or immunohistochemical confirmation.

From acceptable reported cases, the tumor appears to be a rare, deeply situated soft tissue mass primarily found in women. Histologically it resembles neurofibroma except that the cells tend to be arranged in short fascicles, often in a storiform pattern (Fig. 31-71). Earlier cases reported as storiform perineural fibroma may represent examples of this tumor. Highly cellular lesions may suggest the diagnosis of cellular schwannoma or transitional meningioma,[186] whereas hyalinized lesions have been compared with the so-called childhood fibrous tumor with psammoma bodies. The diagnosis of perineurioma is confirmed by identification of a predominant population of cells that have the ultrastructural or immunophenotypic features of perineural cells. The cells have elongated processes invested by basal lamina and containing surface-oriented pinocytotic vesicles. They express epithelial membrane antigen but lack S-100 protein. To date, all reported cases have had a benign course.

Diagnostic criteria for neurofibromatosis 2*

Neurofibromatosis 2 is diagnosed in an individual who has the following:
1. Bilateral eighth nerve masses seen with appropriate imaging techniques (e.g., CT scan or MRI)

or

2. A first-degree relative with neurofibromatosis 2 and either
   a. unilateral eighth nerve mass, or
   b. two of the following:
      neurofibroma
      meningioma
      glioma
      schwannoma
      juvenile posterior subcapsular lenticular opacity

*From National Institutes of Health Consensus Development Conference Statement, vol 5(12), July 13-15, 1987.

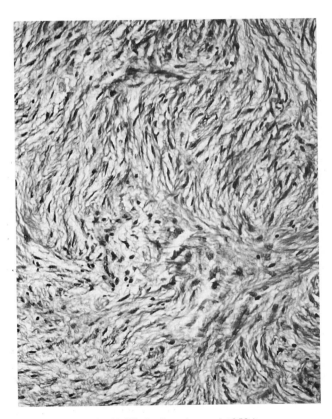

FIG. 31-71. Perineurioma. (×250.)

GRANULAR CELL TUMOR

Although considered a tumor of uncertain lineage in our first edition, the overwhelming evidence supports neural differentiation of the granular cell tumor. However, it is sufficiently distinctive in appearance to be separated from neurofibroma and neurilemoma. Muscle origin, an early concept proposed by Abrikossoff[187] in 1926, is no longer regarded as a likely possibility and, for this reason, the noncommittal term *granular cell tumor* is preferred over *granular cell myoblastoma*. Other synonyms emphasizing the neural origin of the tumor are *granular cell neuroma*,[206] *granular cell neurofibroma*,[207] and *granular cell schwannoma*.[208] Reactive granular lesions at sites of trauma are a separate and unrelated entity.[241] The lesion is fairly common; for example, Vance and Hudson[249] found one case among 346 surgical specimens. Neural origin is strongly supported by the close association of the tumor cells with nerves and the results of the histochemical and electron microscopic studies.

Granular cell tumor generally occurs as a small, poorly circumscribed nodule that may be solitary or multiple and always pursues a benign clinical course. Malignant granular cell tumor is a well-established but extremely rare entity that is found in approximately 1% to 2% of all granular cell tumors. Because it poses a difficult diagnostic problem, it is discussed under a separate heading.

Clinical findings

Granular cell tumor is rarely diagnosed prior to microscopic examination of the biopsy or excised specimen and, in many instances, is an incidental finding during a routine physical or an examination for some other cause. It occurs in patients of any age, but is most common in persons in the fourth, fifth, and sixth decades of life and is rare in children.[230] It is about twice as common in women as in men. In some but not all reviews, African-American patients outnumber whites by a considerable margin.[211] In one series, for example, two thirds of the patients were African-Americans.[244]

As a rule, the lesion manifests as a solitary painless nodule located in the dermis or subcutis, and, less frequently, in the submucosa, smooth muscle, or striated muscle. It is also found in the internal organs, particularly the larynx, bronchus, stomach, and bile duct. Usually the nodule is smaller than 3 cm and has been noted for less than 6 months.

Approximately 10% to 15% of patients with granular cell tumor have lesions at multiple sites, frequently involving the subcutis, submucosa, and one or more visceral structures. The number of lesions varies greatly from patient to patient, but as many as 50 separate nodules have been counted in some cases. Multiple lesions may appear synchronously or over a period of many years. Increased familial incidence is extremely uncommon, but it has been reported.[195,225] Yet there is no record in the literature or in our cases of multiple (or solitary) granular cell tumors occurring in a patient with the stigmata of neurofibromatosis.

Granular cell tumor may arise at virtually any site. In our cases it is most common in the tongue, followed by the anterior and posterior chest wall and the upper limbs. Fewer cases are situated in the neck, breast, and lower limbs. In the Strong et al.[246] series, the three common sites are the head and neck (especially the tongue), the chest wall, and the arm. Additional cases are located in the larynx, stomach, vulva, and anogenital region. Other reports give essentially the same anatomical distribution,[209,244,248] including a small number of cases in the upper respiratory tract[202] and intestines.[215,234]

Pathological findings

Granular cell tumors tend to be poorly circumscribed; consequently, the tumor is usually removed together with portions of the adjacent adipose tissue or muscle. In the majority of cases, the nodule measures less than 3 cm in diameter, and on cut section it is characteristically pale yellow-tan or yellow-gray.

Under the microscope it consists of rounded or polygonal cells of uniform character, with small, centrally placed vesicular nuclei and coarsely granular eosinophilic cytoplasm (Figs. 31-72 to 31-74). Not infrequently there are, in addition, larger intracytoplasmic particles of similar eosinophilic material that are surrounded by a clear zone.

Longitudinal or cross-striations are absent. The nuclei vary little in size and shape, but occasional areas may exhibit mild to moderate degrees of nuclear pleomorphism. In these cases, however, pleomorphism is unassociated with increased mitotic activity. Smaller cells containing coarse particles that are strongly positive for PAS are interspersed between the granular cells (interstitial cells, angulate body cells) (Fig. 31-75). In one of our cases we found an intracellular asteroid body (Fig. 31-76).

The growth pattern varies; the cells tend to be disposed in ribbons or nests divided by slender fibrous connective tissue septa or in large sheets without any particular cellular arrangement. Older lesions frequently exhibit marked desmoplasia, and some of these can be identified only by the presence of a few scattered nests of granular cells within a dense mass of collagen (Fig. 31-77).

About two thirds of the nodules are located in the dermal, subcutaneous, or submucosal tissues. Some of these are associated with marked acanthosis or pseudoepitheliomatous hyperplasia of the overlying squamous epithelium, a striking feature that has repeatedly caused this process to be mistaken for squamous cell carcinoma (Fig. 31-78).[236] In one reported case such a lesion was interpreted as a laryngeal carcinoma and treated by laryngectomy.[249] Similarly, in one of our cases a small granular cell tumor of the tongue with pseudoepitheliomatous hyperplasia was mistaken for a squamous cell carcinoma.

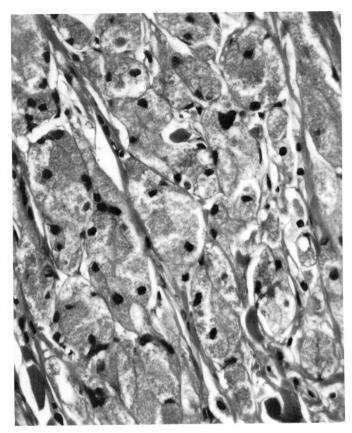 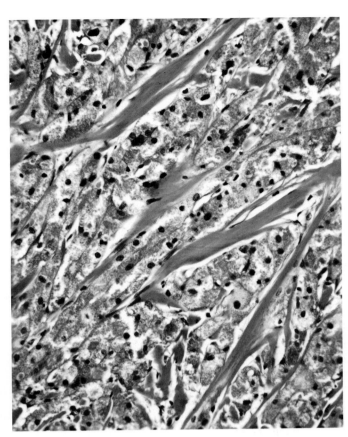

FIG. 31-72. Granular cell tumor consisting of polygonal cells with coarsely granular cytoplasm and pyknotic nuclei. (×400.)

FIG. 31-73. Granular cell tumor. Nests of granular cells separated by bundles of mature collagen. (×250.)

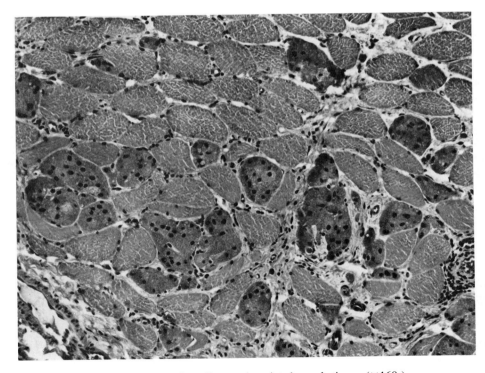

FIG. 31-74. Granular cell tumor in striated muscle tissue. (×160.)

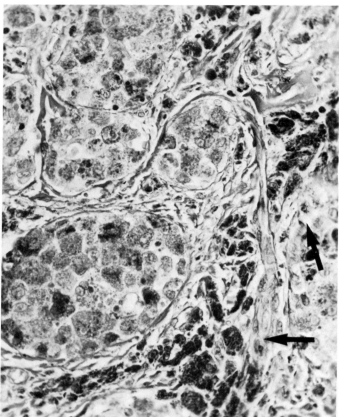

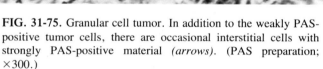

FIG. 31-75. Granular cell tumor. In addition to the weakly PAS-positive tumor cells, there are occasional interstitial cells with strongly PAS-positive material *(arrows)*. (PAS preparation; ×300.)

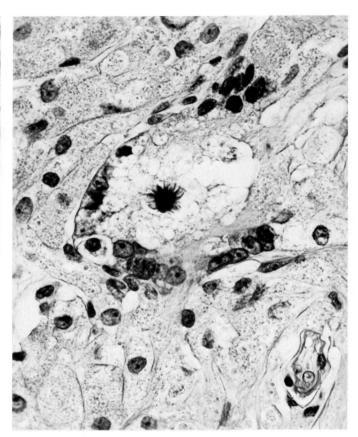

FIG. 31-76. Granular cell tumor with distinct asteroid body in one of the granular cells. (×575.)

Another important, histogenetically significant feature is the close association between granular cells and peripheral nerves. Frequently the granular cells encompass small nerves or replace them almost entirely and are recognizable only by the residual neurites that can be demonstrated with the Bodian method or similar silver preparations (Fig. 31-79). At times clusters of granular cells are also surrounded by circumferentially arranged spindle cells in the manner of perineurium (Fig. 31-80).

Less frequently the granular cells involve or replace the musculature; they grow along the muscle fibers or even seem to extend within the sarcolemmal sheath. They may also be found in smooth muscle tissue, fibrous tissue such as tendons, fasciae, or ligaments, and, rarely, small lymphoid aggregates or even lymph nodes, a feature that should not be confused with lymph node metastasis (Fig. 31-81).

Unlike the cells of most benign and malignant muscle tumors, the granular cells do not contain glycogen. They stain weakly with PAS preparation both before and after diastase digestion and assume a red-brown color with the trichrome stain. Pearse[232] and others[188,193,194,242,252] have given detailed accounts of the various histochemical staining reactions.

Immunohistochemical investigation reveals positive staining for S-100 protein (Fig. 31-82), neuron-specific enolase, laminin, and various myelin proteins. The cells do not react with antibodies for neurofilament proteins or glial fibrillary acidic protein (GFAP).[221,223,228] According to Nathrath and Remberger,[229] the interstitial cells stain for myelin protein.

Ultrastructurally, granular cell tumor shows a highly characteristic picture that has been well described in the literature.* Typically the intracellular granules consist of membrane-bound, presumably autophagic vacuoles that contain cellular debris, including mitochondria, myelin figures, fragmented rough endoplasmic reticulum, and, according to some authors, myelinated and nonmyelinated axonlike structures (Figs. 31-83 and 31-84). There are also

---

*References 189, 199, 208, 211, 213, 214, 222, 237, 243, 244, 250, 252.

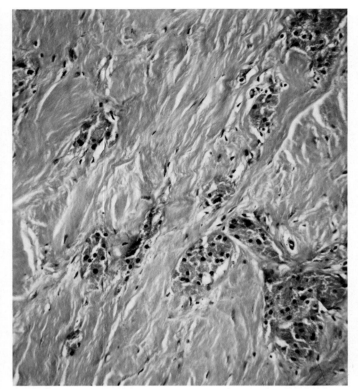

FIG. 31-77. Granular cell tumor with marked desmoplasia. (×160.)

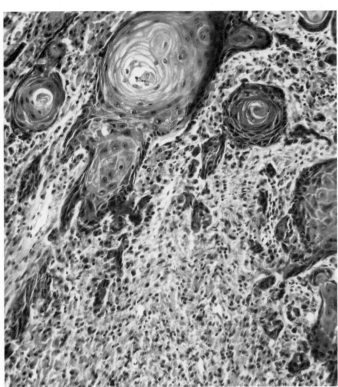

FIG. 31-78. Granular cell tumor with pseudoepitheliomatous hyperplasia, a frequent feature that has been mistaken for squamous cell carcinoma. (×160.)

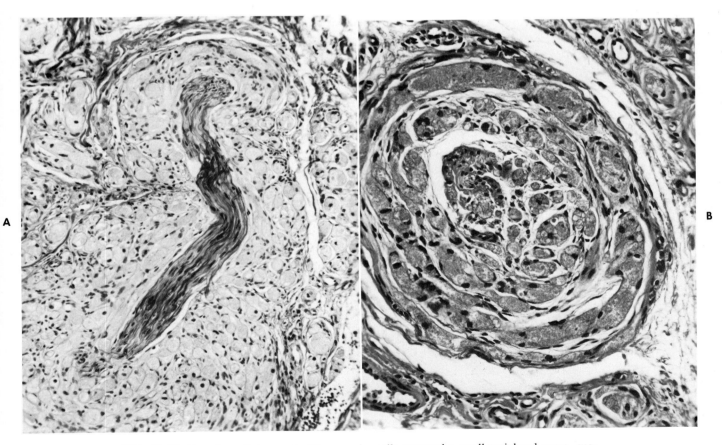

FIG. 31-79. Granular cell tumor. **A,** The granular cells surround a small peripheral nerve, suggesting nerve sheath origin. (×160.) **B,** Concentric arrangement of granular cells about a remnant of a small peripheral nerve. The patient, a 12-year-old boy, had lesions on both arms. (×250.)

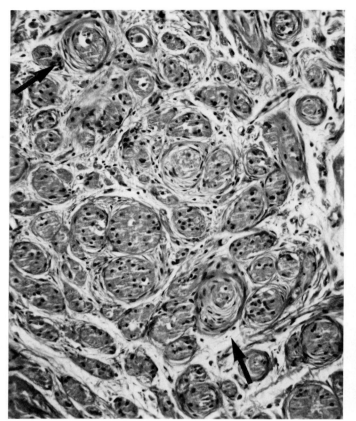

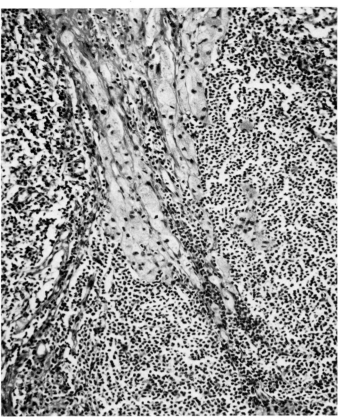

FIG. 31-80. Granular cell tumor. Circumferentially arranged spindle cells about nests of granular cells, reminiscent of a neuroma *(arrows).* (×160.)

FIG. 31-81. Granular cells in regional lymph node, a feature that may be confused with lymph node metastasis of malignant granular cell tumor. (×160.)

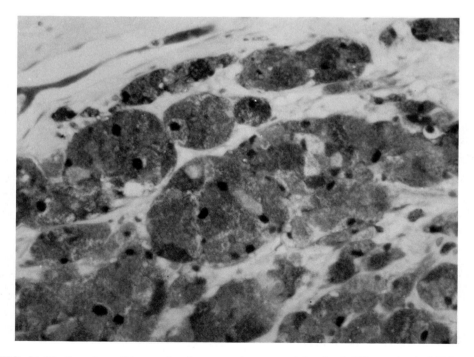

FIG. 31-82. Granular cell tumor showing strong immunostaining for S-100 protein. (×160.)

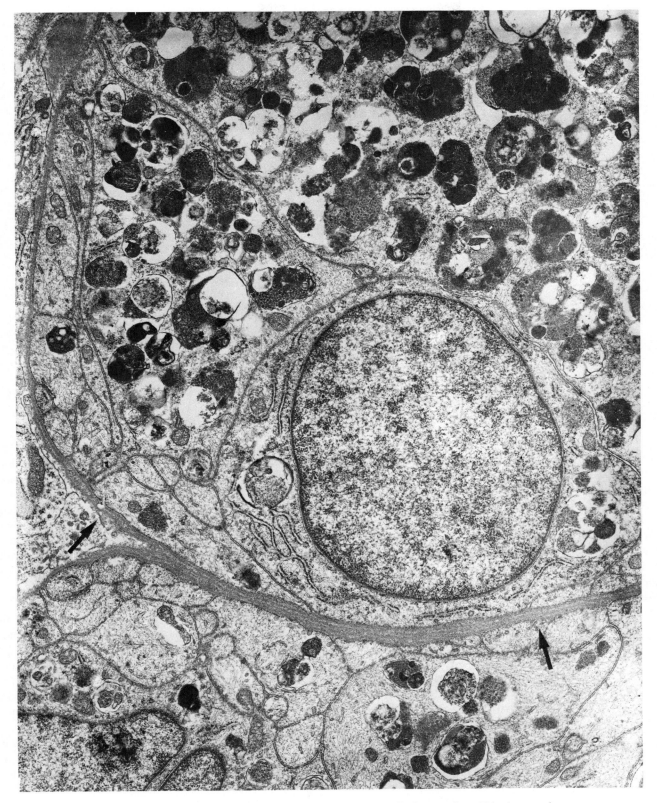

FIG. 31-83. Ultrastructure of granular cell tumor. Large autophagic granules within the cytoplasm of the tumor cell surrounded by a distinct basal lamina *(arrows)*. (Courtesy Dr. Zelma Molnar, Veterans Administration Hospital, Hines, Illinois.)

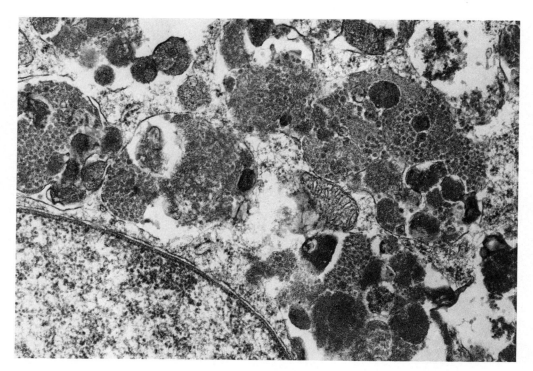

FIG. 31-84. Large vacuoles containing finely granular structures and small masses of electron-dense material.

smaller interstitial cells with angulated bodies containing packets of parallel microtubules (Fig. 31-85), microfilaments, and lipid material as well as cells with multiple cytoplasmic processes, partly surrounded by incomplete basal laminae.

Bhawan et al.[197] pointed out the resemblance between inclusions in the interstitial cells and the phagocytized breakdown products found in Gaucher-like cells.

Christ and Ozzello[201] demonstrated distinct myofilaments in the cytoplasm of benign granular cell tumor of the urinary bladder in a 23-year-old woman. This tumor, however, may represent granular changes in a leiomyoma.

Differential diagnosis

Benign and malignant granular cell tumors are strikingly similar in histological appearance. In fact, some metastasizing granular cell tumors are virtually indistinguishable from the benign type, even if the sections of the primary tumor are examined in retrospect. In most cases, however, there are subtle histological differences that aid in diagnosis; for example, malignant granular cell tumors tend to be slightly more cellular, and the cells are smaller and often assume a more elongated appearance. There is also increased mitotic activity, but mitotic figures are never numerous, and 2 or more mitotic figures/10 HPF should raise the suspicion of malignancy.

The problem of diagnosis is further complicated by the fact that cellular variability or cellular pleomorphism alone is not always a reliable diagnostic criterion and occasionally may be seen in portions of a perfectly benign granular cell tumor. Clinical features that support a malignant diagnosis are a history of local recurrence, rapid recent growth, and large size of the tumor. Tumors measuring 5 cm or more in diameter are more likely malignant than smaller ones, although a few of the reported malignant granular cell tumors were less than 3 cm in diameter.[279]

Differentiation from other benign neoplasms should not be too difficult. The coarsely granular cytoplasm and the absence of cross-striations and glycogen distinguish benign granular cell tumor from rhabdomyoma; the absence of lipid droplets distinguishes it from hibernoma and fibroxanthoma. Awareness of the frequent association of dermal granular cell tumor and marked acanthosis of the overlying squamous epithelium will prevent a mistaken diagnosis of squamous cell carcinoma.

Finally, reactive changes that occur in association with surgical trauma or other types of injury may stimulate a benign granular cell tumor. The granular cell in these lesions tends to be associated with inflammatory elements and areas of necrosis and stains more intensely with the alcian blue stain and PAS preparation (see also Chapter 13). It also lacks the ribbonlike or nestlike cellular orientation of

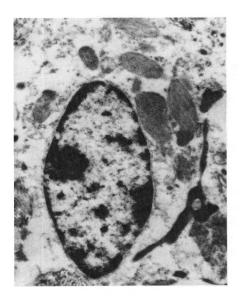

FIG. 31-85. Angulated bodies in interstitial cell of granular cell tumor. (×7800.)

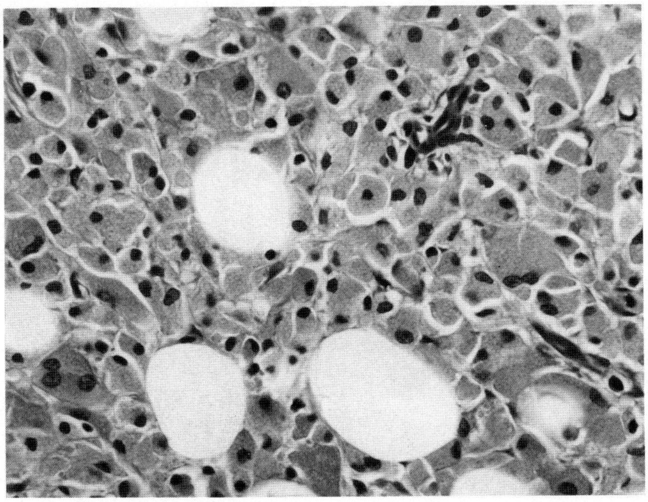

FIG. 31-86. Granular cell reaction to epoxy polymer for prosthetic replacement of hip joint. (×160.)

granular cell tumors. Sobel and Churg,[242] who gave a detailed account of this lesion, found several examples in the scar of cesarean sections. Massive granular reaction to epoxy polymer may also occur near prosthetic joint replacements (Fig. 31-86) (see also Chapter 13).

Differentiation

Most of the earlier accounts of granular cell tumor concurred with Abrikossoff's opinion[187] that the lesion most likely shows muscle differentiation and is best classified as granular cell myoblastoma.[202,216,218,230,232] It was soon recognized, however, that the lesion arises not only in muscle but also more frequently in other tissues and that in many instances there is a close relationship between granular cells and peripheral nerves.[191,193,194,236] This was first pointed out by Feyrter[197,207] in 1935 (granular cell neuroma) and later by Fust and Custer[209,210] in 1948 (granular cell neurofibroma). More recently the concept of neural differentiation found strong support in the electron microscopic findings; chiefly on this basis Fisher and Wechsler[208] favored Schwann cell lineage and proposed the term *granular cell schwannoma*. Others agreed with their concept[205,216,234] and suggested that the granular cells are Schwann cells altered by a lysosomal defect.[211]

Schwann cell origin is further supported by the positive staining of cytoplasm and nuclei for S-100 protein,* especially since S-100 protein is absent in perineural cells or endoneural fibroblasts. Additional staining of the granular cells for myelin proteins (PO and P2) and myelin-associated

glycoproteins suggests that the granules are myelin or myelin breakdown products[223,239] as was originally suggested by Fisher and Wechsler.[208] The angular bodies in the interstitial cells are not marked by antibodies to S-100 protein, but they are positive on staining with antibodies to myelin protein.[223]

Additional evidence for neural origin is the presence of residual axons in many granular cell tumors, the sporadic occurrence of the tumor in cranial, autonomic, and peripheral nerves, and, as in neurofibromatosis, the development of multiple tumors in different portions of the body and, very rarely, in two generations of the same family.[195,216,225,235]

Prognosis

Excluding malignant examples of the tumor, recurrence is rare. Six of 92 cases recurred in the series reported by Strong et al.[246]; one of them recurred after 10 years. We have no detailed follow-up data, but the recurrence rate seems to be even lower in our cases. Therefore local surgical excision should be curative in nearly all cases.

CONGENITAL (GINGIVAL) GRANULAR CELL TUMOR

This term, as well as its synonyms *congenital epulis, congenital granular cell myoblastoma,* and *granular cell fibroblastoma,* has been applied to a variant of granular cell tumor that is indistinguishable in its structure and staining characteristics from this tumor but differs by its exclusive occurrence in infants at or immediately after birth, and by its characteristic location in the labial aspect of the dental

*References 13, 190, 197, 225, 229, 238.

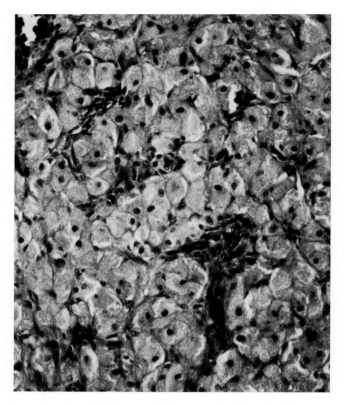

FIG. 31-87. Congenital granular cell tumor of the upper jaw in a 5-month-old girl. Note the increased vascularity compared to adult granular cell tumor. (×160.)

ridge, with a predilection for the upper jaw. It also differs from adult granular cell tumors by its prominent vascularity, the presence of scattered remnants of odontogenic epithelium, and the strong phosphatase activity of the tumor cells. Moreover, it lacks interstitial cells with angulate bodies and does not show immunostaining for laminin or S-100 protein (Fig. 31-87).[236,257,261] About 10% of these lesions are multiple, and approximately 90% afflict girls.[253,260,266] Characteristically, the condition manifests as a protruding, round or ovoid nodule that is covered by a smooth mucosal surface and is firmly attached to the gum by a broad base or infrequently by a pedicle. Ulceration of the mucosa is uncommon, and microscopically there is no evidence of pseudoepitheliomatous hyperplasia of the overlying squamous epithelium.[260] Like other forms of granular cell tumor, the nodules are small and average 1 to 2 cm in greatest diameter.

There is usually no further growth after birth, and there is no tendency toward local recurrence. In fact, even without therapy, most congenital granular cell tumors cease to grow or regress spontaneously. In Cussen and MacMahon's case,[255] for instance, the lesion almost completely disappeared after 4 months and could no longer be detected af-

ter 3 years. Lack et al.[260] also report that lesions treated later in the neonatal period were smaller and exhibited some evidence of involution. There is no record of a malignant counterpart of this tumor.

The exact nature of this condition is still not clear, and there is little support for origin from odontogenic epithelial cells. Like histiocytes, many of the cells contain neutral fat and lysosomal particles possess ruffled borders with small irregular extensions or filopodia, and lack basal laminae.

MALIGNANT GRANULAR CELL TUMOR

Although in the earlier literature a variety of malignant soft tissue tumors had been labeled as malignant granular cell tumors, this diagnosis should be restricted to neoplasms that are similar in histological appearance to benign granular cell tumors but can be separated on the basis of cellular pleomorphism, mitotic activity, and, most importantly, biological behavior; that is, their capacity to produce metastases. In particular, the term should not be applied to alveolar soft part sarcoma (organoid malignant granular cell myoblastoma) or to granular forms of sarcomas derived from muscle or vascular tissues.[282]

Judging from our cases and the literature, the tumor is exceedingly rare, only 1% to 2% of all granular cell tumors. Ravich et al.[283] are usually credited with the first account of this entity. It occurred in the wall of the urinary bladder of a 31-year-old woman who died of metastatic disease 17 months after the tumor was removed surgically and diagnosed as a malignant granular cell tumor. Since their report, about 25 additional cases have been described.[203,267,289]

Clinical findings

In nearly all aspects, the malignant tumors are indistinguishable from the benign granular cell tumors except they have never been observed in infants or children and most are larger and usually measure more than 4 cm in greatest diameter. A history of long clinical duration and recent rapid growth has been observed in some cases, suggesting the possibility of malignant transformation from a preexisting benign granular cell tumor, analogous to the malignant transformation of neurofibromas. One of the reported malignant granular cell tumors allegedly had been present for 50 years[277]; another arose in the radial nerve.[289] Still another developed in the back of a 36-year-old man; he and his father had multiple granular cell tumors.[217]

Pathological findings

The gross and microscopic appearances of the neoplasm, like its clinical picture, bear a close resemblance to those of the benign type. The tumor is generally poorly circumscribed, extends into the neighboring tissues, and has a pale yellow-gray cut surface. On the average, however, it is larger and measures 4 to 10 cm in greatest diameter. Ma-

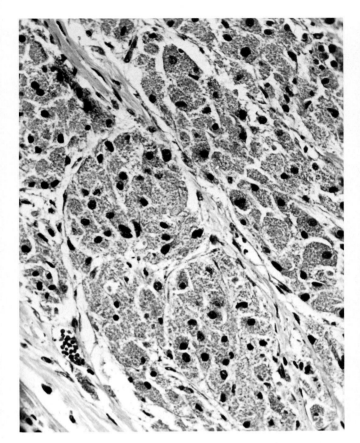

FIG. 31-88. Malignant granular cell tumor of the right arm in a 65-year-old woman. The patient died of multiple metastatic lesions to the lung. (×265.)

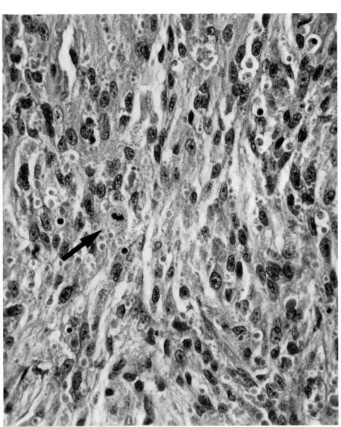

FIG. 31-89. Malignant granular cell tumor arising in the right arm of a 12-year-old boy. Note spindle cell pattern, coarsely granular cytoplasm, and mitotic figure *(arrow)*. (×400.)

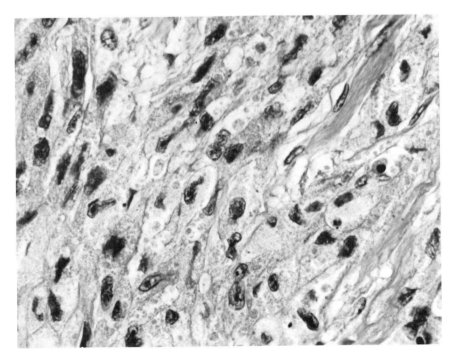

FIG. 31-90. Malignant granular cell tumor of the chest wall. The tumor shows a striking variation in size and shape of the nuclei and a coarsely granular cytoplasm. (×600.)

lignant granular cell tumors as small as 1.5 cm have also been observed.[279] The histological picture tends to be less uniform, and the cells show a greater variability in shape and size, including spindle cells and cells with large hyperchromatic nuclei (Figs. 31-88 to 31-90). The mitotic activity varies. It may be minimal or absent, as in Mackenzie's case,[279] but usually the tumor can be recognized by its increased mitotic activity (2 or more mitotic figures/10 HPF).

Necrosis may be a conspicuous feature in some tumors. In one case reported by Ross et al.,[285] portions of the tumor displayed a storiform pattern. Vascular invasion is uncommon in the primary tumor but is encountered not infrequently in metastatic lesions. The ultrastructural features and the various staining reactions, including the immunohistochemical characteristics, are similar to those of the benign type.[267,279,287]

Differential diagnosis

Distinction from other malignant tumors is readily accomplished if attention is paid to the usual location of the tumor in the subcutis, the eosinophilic and uniformly granular appearance of the constituent cells, and the absence of a richly vascular endocrine or organoid growth pattern as in alveolar soft part sarcoma or paraganglioma. In some instances less well-differentiated and smaller cells are present, but these are never as numerous as in typical cases

of embryonal rhabdomyosarcoma, and there are no cytoplasmic cross-striations or glycogen. Spindle cell areas may be found occasionally, but these are less regular and less conspicuous than those of the granular variant of leiomyosarcoma. The differential diagnosis between benign and malignant granular cell tumor is discussed with the benign type.

Discussion

Because the diagnosis is rarely made in the absence of recurrence or metastasis, determination of the biological behavior and efficacy of therapy is difficult. Typically the malignant form of granular cell tumor recurs before it metastasizes, usually within a period of less than one year. Metastasis occurs through the lymphatics and the bloodstream, and both lymph node metastases and metastases to the lung, liver, and bone are common. The interval between excision of the primary tumor and metastasis is quite variable, but in most cases it takes several years before the metastatic lesions become apparent. In fact, in one of the two cases described by Crawford and De Bakey,[203] the tumor metastasized 14 years after the initial excision.

Treatment (radical surgical therapy, roentgenotherapy, and chemotherapy) has been largely ineffective.[286,305] Mackenzie's patient[279] received a total of 5770 rad of radiotherapy, but the tumor continued to grow and produced metastases. In the case of Steffelaar et al.,[286] a metastasiz-

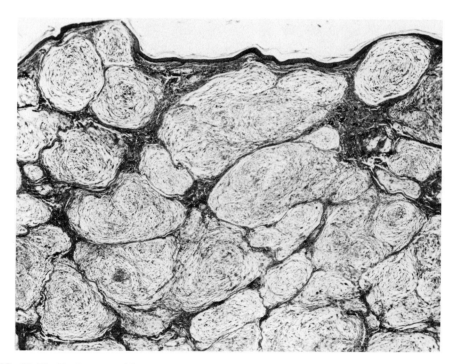

FIG. 31-91. Benign myxoid tumor of nerve sheath, also called *nerve sheath myxoma*. Tumors have a distinct multinodular or septate appearance. (×25.)

ing tumor from the thoracic wall, there was no response to chemotherapy (Adriamycin and vincristine).

NEUROTHEKEOMA (NERVE SHEATH MYXOMA)

In 1969, Harkin and Reed[6] described an unusual myxoid tumor of probable nerve sheath origin under the term *myxoma of nerve sheath*. Its distinctive appearance led them to provisionally separate it from variants of neurofibroma. More recently Gallager and Helwig[295] reported 53 similar cases under the name *neurothekeoma* to stress its nerve sheath origin, and still others have utilized the term *bizarre cutaneous neurofibromas*.[296] The tumor mistakenly described as *pacinian neurofibroma* by MacDonald and Wilson-Jones[297] is also an example of this tumor. We believe these tumors are most closely related to neurofibroma. These tumors usually arise during childhood and early adult life and have a predilection for the upper portion of the body such as the head, neck, and shoulder. Mucous membranes are rarely involved. They are situated in the dermis and subcutis and in an exceptional instance occur in deep soft tissue. Histologically the tumor is divided into distinct lobules by fibrous connective tissue (Figs. 31-91 to 31-93). Each lobule consists of a myxoid matrix which may consist of either hyaluronic acid[295] or sulfated acid mucins (Fig. 31-92).[298] Usually the cells display little pleomorphism and minimal numbers of mitotic figures. Benign giant cells are occasionally present within the lobules, and rarely neurites can be identified among the tumor cells. Although most tumors are quite myxoid, some tumors are more cellular, with nuclear atypia and mitoses. Known as *cellular neurothekeoma*,[293,294] they may be mistaken for sarcoma to those unfamiliar with the basic architectural pattern of the tumor.

Neurothekeoma is usually regarded as a variant of a nerve sheath tumor because of its overall histological similarity to a neurofibroma and its infrequent origin from a nerve (Fig. 31-94). Some have recently questioned this concept, however, and have suggested that there may be two different lesions or subtypes included under this term.[293,294] Evidence in support of two different subtypes is mounted by the observation that S-100 protein is usually easily demonstrated within highly myxoid neurothekeomas but not within the more cellular forms.

The differential diagnosis of this unusual tumor includes notably focal mucinosis, myxoid malignant fibrous histiocytoma, and myxoid neurofibroma. Focal mucinosis does not display the degree of circumscription, lobulation, or cellularity seen in neurothekeoma. Myxoid malignant fibrous histiocytomas are poorly circumscribed, more pleomorphic lesions with a more elaborate and organized vasculature and no septations. Moreover, most develop as large, deeply situated tumors in adults in contrast to neurothekeoma, which occurs principally in the superficial soft tissues of young individuals. Distinction of this tumor from neurofibroma is more of an academic point, since they are probably related. In general the multinodularity and the whorled arrangement

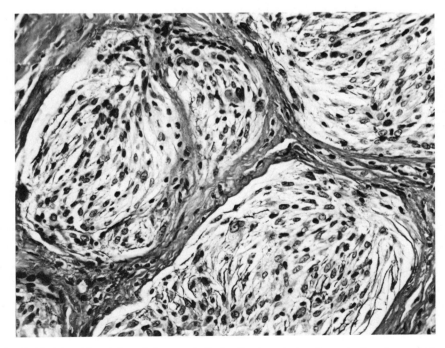

FIG. 31-92. Myxoid nodules of plump spindled cells characterize the majority of myxoid tumors of nerve sheath. (×250.)

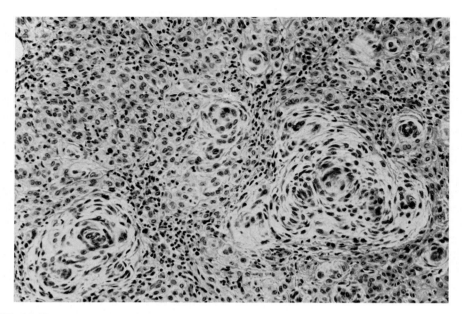

FIG. 31-93. Myxoid tumor of nerve sheath (neurothekeoma) with areas simulating a "histiocytic" tumor. (×160.)

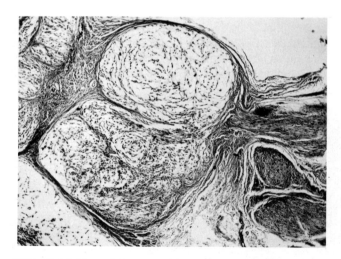

FIG. 31-94. Neurothekeoma arising from a nerve. (×25.)

of the cells of neurothekeoma contrasts with most neurofibromas. Rarely the tumor recurs.

EXTRACRANIAL MENINGIOMA

Extracranial meningiomas are rare tumors that occur in the skin or soft tissue of the scalp or along the vertebral axis. By definition they are not associated with an underlying meningioma of the neuraxis, and extracranial extension of an intracranial tumor should always be considered before accepting a meningioma in soft tissue or skin as a primary tumor at that site. Although all true extracranial

meningiomas probably arise from ectopic arachnoid lining cells, their precise presentation and localization suggest at least two different pathogenetic mechanisms.[299]

One form of extracranial meningioma, termed type I by Lopez et al.,[299] occurs in children and young adults and usually is present at birth. The lesions are situated in the skin of the scalp, forehead, and paravertebral areas and, as a result, may be mistaken clinically for cutaneous lesions, including epidermal inclusion cyst, skin tag, and nevus. The pathogenesis is probably similar to that of meningocele and is believed to be the result of abnormalities of neural tube closure with relocation of meningeal tissue in the surrounding skin and subcutis (Fig. 31-95). This proposal explains the congenital nature of the type I tumor and its distribution, which coincides with that of meningocele. The similarity of this tumor to meningocele is heightened by its histological appearance. Although some consist of solid, isolated nests of meningothelial cells in the skin, others may contain a rudimentary stalk or cystic cavity (Fig. 31-96). Such lesions occupy an intermediate position in the spectrum between meningocele and extracranial meningioma and have been named *meningeal hamartomas*. Type I meningioma is benign, although persistence of a connection with the central nervous system can lead to postoperative meningitis or neurological deficits.

The second form of extracranial meningioma (type II) (Fig. 31-97) may occur at any age, but adults are usually affected. These tumors are situated in the vicinity of the sensory organs (eye, ear, nose) or along the paths of the cranial and spinal nerves. Symptoms associated with the tu-

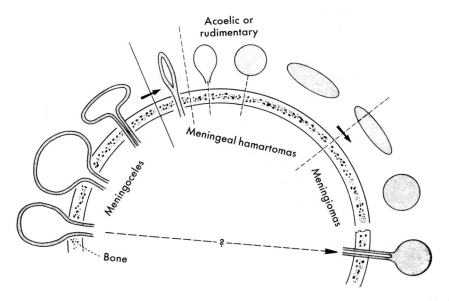

FIG. 31-95. Histogenesis of cutaneous meningiomas. Diagram showing possible relationship between meningoceles, meningeal hamartomas, and type I extracranial meningiomas. The first retain their connections with the central nervous system and are predominantly cystic, whereas the last two lose the connections and are solid. (From Lopez DA, et al: *Cancer* 34:728, 1974.)

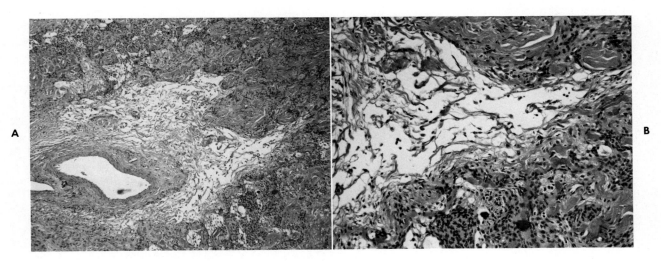

FIG. 31-96. Type I ectopic meningioma from a child showing partially cystic central area. (**A**, ×60; **B**, ×250.)

mor are related to its size, location, and growth rate. Histologically, these lesions are indistinguishable from the ordinary intracranial meningioma. The solid nests of meningothelial cells are arranged in sheets or whorls and occasionally are punctuated by psammoma bodies (Fig. 31-98). In addition to surgical removal, appropriate studies to exclude an intracranial component are recommended for these more deeply situated tumors.

GLIAL HETEROTOPIAS

Like ectopic meningeal rests, ectopic deposits of glial tissue occur occasionally on the scalp. Over the years they have been designated by a variety of names, including nasal glioma, glial hamartoma, and heterotopic glial tissue.[301] The common presentation of a glial heterotopia is that of a polypoid mass at the root of the nose or to one side of the bridge of the nose in an infant, which grows in a commen-

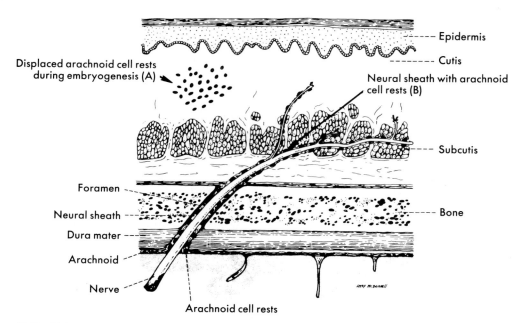

- - - Epidermis

- - - - Cutis

Displaced arachnoid cell rests
during embryogenesis (A)

Neural sheath with arachnoid
cell rests (B)

- - - Subcutis

Foramen

Neural sheath

Dura mater

Arachnoid

Nerve

- - - Bone

Arachnoid cell rests

FIG. 31-97. Primary cutaneous meningiomas. Diagram shows two possible origins of primary cutaneous meningiomas. Type I (A) may result from abnormalities of neural tube closure with resultant ectopic arachnoid cell rests. Type II (B), which occurs in adults and follows the distribution of the sensory organs and nerves, probably is derived from arachnoid rests in nerve sheaths. (From Lopez DA, et al: *Cancer* 34:728, 1974.)

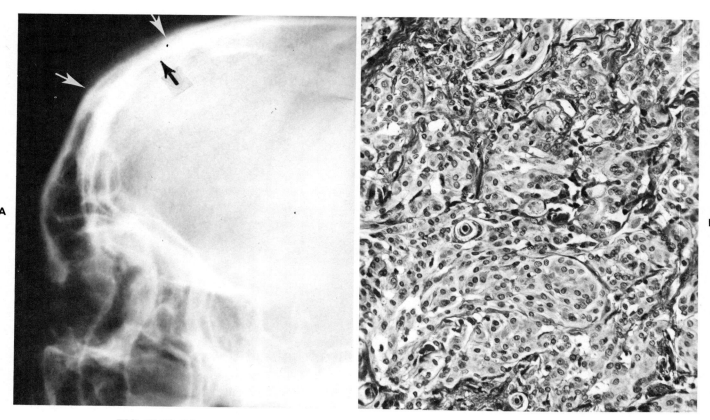

A

B

FIG. 31-98. Primary cutaneous meningioma of the frontal area of the scalp. **A,** Radiograph demonstrates extracranial location of frontal mass. Outer table of skull is partly eroded between white arrows, while inner table is intact *(black arrow).* **B,** Tumor consists of whorls of plump epithelioid cells indistinguishable from cells of intracranial form of meningioma. (×250.)

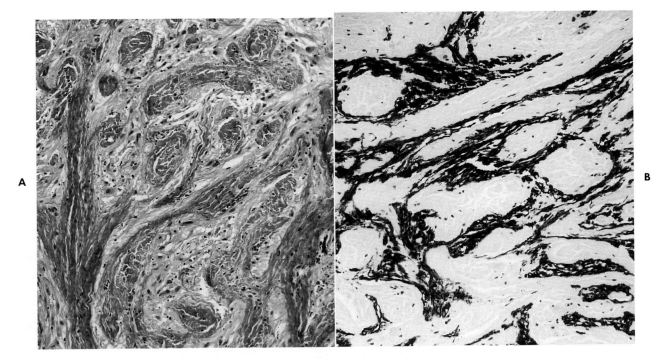

FIG. 31-99. A, Glial heterotopia showing lightly staining glial tissue interspersed between collagen *(dark areas).* (×160.) **B,** Immunostaining for glial fibrillary acidic protein highlights glial tissue against negatively staining backdrop of collagen. (×160.)

surate fashion with the infant. In most cases, the lesions lack a communication with the brain. However, in the few that do communicate with the brain, the connection occurs through the cribriform plate such that rhinorrhea may be an accompanying symptom. Histologically the lesions consist of mats of mature glial tissue which, in addition to astrocytes, may also contain neurons (Fig. 31-99). Although most glial heterotopias may be viewed as variants of encephalocele, in which the communication with the brain is lost, we have recently encountered two cases of glial heterotopias on the chest wall of adults, suggesting that other pathogenetic mechanisms allow for the development of these unusual lesions.

MELANOTIC NEUROECTODERMAL TUMOR OF INFANCY (RETINAL ANLAGE TUMOR, MELANOTIC PROGONOMA)

First described in 1918 by Krompecher, this rare tumor of disputed histogenesis has been referred to as *congenital melanocarcinoma, melanotic adamantinoma, retinal anlage tumor, melanotic progonoma,* and *pigmented epulis of infancy.* Although most current studies support a neural crest origin of this tumor, there is little evidence that the tumor specifically represents retinal anlage. Therefore, we prefer the less fanciful term *melanotic neuroectodermal tumor of infancy.*

Clinical findings

The tumor usually develops during the first year of life and presents as a protruding mass in the upper or lower jaw. The skin or mucosa is tightly stretched over the lesion, but it is rarely if ever ulcerated. Radiographically, the tumor is a cystic radiolucent lesion with a capacity for local destruction and displacement of the developing teeth (Fig. 31-100). Patients with this tumor in unusual sites such as the anterior fontanelle, epididymis,[308,309,326] mediastinum,[319] and brain[324] develop symptoms referable to those sites. The few cases reported in the uterus[322] and shoulder[318] and those in adults[317] should be disregarded because they represent different lesions altogether. However, we have encountered one example of this tumor in the soft tissues of the extremity, and it has also been reported in long bone.

Gross and microscopic findings

Grossly, the tumor ranges in color from slate gray to blue-black, depending on the amount of melanin pigment. It is composed of irregular alveolar spaces lined by cuboidal cells containing varying amounts of melanin pigment (Fig. 31-101). In addition, small, round, less well differentiated cells resembling those of neuroblastoma lie within the alveolar space or as isolated nests within a fibrous stroma. Neurofibrillary material, resembling glial tissue, may be seen in association with these cells within the spaces. In two exceptional cases, glial tissue was found outside the epithelial islands. One case was a tumor arising in the brain in which the entire stroma was glial,[324] and the second was a tumor arising in a glial heterotopia of the oropharynx.[315]

The cuboidal cells have the electron microscopic features of epithelial and melanocytic cells.[306] They are bounded by basal laminae and elaborately interdigitate laterally with neighboring cells, forming desmosomes. Both mature and immature melanosomes similar to those of melanocytes and

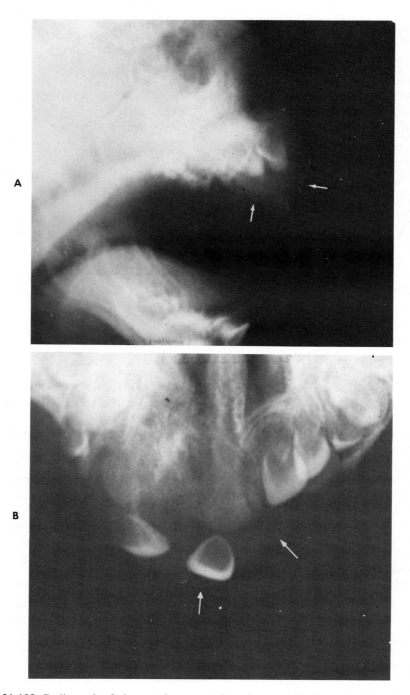

FIG. 31-100. Radiograph of pigmented neuroectodermal tumor of infancy (retinal anlage tumor) occurring in the maxilla. Tumor is represented by vaguely outlined soft tissue mass *(arrows)* with destruction of maxilla **(A)** and displacement of teeth **(B)**.

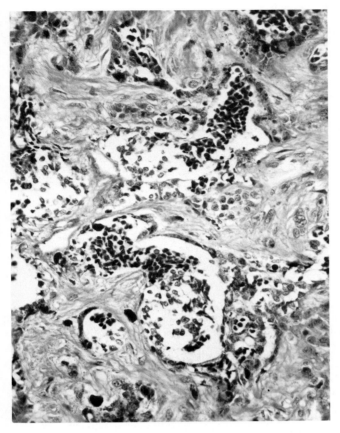

FIG. 31-101. Pigmented neuroectodermal tumor of infancy showing flattened pigmented epithelial cells lining alveolar spaces. Immature, nonpigmented rounded cells lie clumped within the spaces. (×160.)

melanoma cells are present within the cytoplasm. Functionally they share certain properties of the melanocyte in that melanization of these cells may be increased by agents that induce similar changes in melanocytes of animals.[306] Immunohistochemically the cuboidal cells express cytokeratin and a melanoma-associated antigen (HMB-45). Neuron specific enolase, Leu-7, and synaptophysin are variably present in the epithelial cells as well as the small neuroblastic element.

The rounded, less well-differentiated cells contain few organelles but are believed to be neuroblastic by virtue of their elongated cell processes, dense core vesicles,[306] and intracytoplasmic neurofilamentous material.[306,310] Their association with glial-like areas and, in one case, with ganglioneuromatous areas[306] provides further support for this contention.

Discussion

Traditionally this tumor has been considered benign. However, in a recent large series from the AFIP, nearly half of those with follow-up information recurred, and 5% to 10% of cases reported in the literature have produced metastasis.[306,312,316] One case, a stillborn, was noted to have multiple metastases at delivery.[316] A second case, a tumor of the epididymis, produced micrometastases in regional lymph nodes,[312] and two others metastasized as primitive neuroblastic tumors devoid of melanin.[306,312] Although metastasis is a relatively uncommon event, attempts to eradicate the tumor at the time of initial surgery should be endorsed. Unfortunately it has not been possible to predict recurrence or metastasis in this disease by conventional parameters or by utilization of more sophisticated techniques such as flow cytometry.

The histogenesis of this tumor has been controversial. The concepts of a congenital melanoma and an odontogenic tumor are now obsolete for various reasons. The former does not account for the primitive neuroblastic component, and the latter does not take into consideration tumors in sites where there are no odontogenic rests. To date the most appealing theory is that the tumor is derived from neural crest.[304,306] This concept allows latitude in the distribution of the lesions, accounts for the presence of pigmented and neuroblastic elements, and explains the rare tumor associated with increased levels of vanillylmandelic acid.[304,306] It does not seem necessary to specifically compare this tumor with developing retina; in fact, the embryological evidence against this has been extensively summarized.[304] It seems more probable that this tumor merely reflects a primitive stage or degree of differentiation common to many types of pigmented neuroepithelium.

REFERENCES
General

1. Asbury AK, Johnson PC: Pathology of peripheral nerve. In *Major problems in pathology,* vol 9, Philadelphia, 1978, WB Saunders Co.

2. Burger PC, Vogel FS: Peripheral nerve. In *Surgical pathology of the nervous system,* New York, 1975, John Wiley & Sons, Chap 9, p 537.

3. Clark HB, Minesky JJ, Agrawal D, et al: Myelin basic protein and P2 protein are not immunohistochemical markers for Schwann cell neoplasms: a comparative study using antisera to S-100, P2, and myelin basic proteins. *Am J Pathol* 121:96, 1985.

4. Dobersen MJ, Gascon P, Trost S, et al: Murine monoclonal antibodies to the myelin-associated glycoprotein react with large granular lymphocytes of human blood. *Proc Natl Acad Sci* 82:552, 1985.

5. Erlandson RA, Woodruff JM: Peripheral nerve sheath tumors. *Cancer* 49:273, 1982.

6. Harkin JC, Reed RJ: Tumors of the peripheral nervous system. In *Atlas of tumor pathology,* 1969, Armed Forces Institute of Pathology, second series, fascicle 3, Washington, DC.

7. Kahn H, Marks A, Thom H, et al: Role of antibody to S-100 protein in diagnostic pathology. *Am J Clin Pathol* 79:341, 1983.

8. Nakajima T, Watanaba S, Soto Y, et al: An immunoperoxidase study of S-100 protein distribution in normal and neoplastic tissues. *Am J Surg Pathol* 6:715, 1982.

9. Ortiz-Hidalgo C, Weller RO: Peripheral nervous system. In Sternberg SS, editor: *Histology for pathologists,* New York, 1992, Raven Press.

10. Reed RJ: Cutaneous manifestations of neural crest disorders (neurocristopathies). *Int J Dermatol* 16:807, 1977.

11. Reed RJ, Harkin JC: Supplemental tumors of the peripheral nervous system. In *Atlas of tumor pathology,* 1983, Armed Forces Institute of Pathology, Washington, DC.

12. Steffansson K, Wollmann R, Jerkovic M: S-100 protein in soft tissue tumors derived from Schwann cells and melanocytes. *Am J Pathol* 106:261, 1982.

13. Weiss SW, Langloss JM, Enzinger FM: The role of the S-100 protein in the diagnosis of soft tissue tumors with particular reference to benign and malignant Schwann cell tumors. *Lab Invest* 49:299, 1983.

14. Woodruff JM: Tumors and tumorlike conditions of the peripheral nerve. In Ninfo V, Chung EB, Cavazzana AO, editors: *Tumors and tumorlike lesions of soft tissue,* New York, 1991, Churchill Livingstone.

Embryogenesis and normal anatomy

15. Babel J, Bischoff A, Spoendlin H: *Ultrastructure of the peripheral nervous system and sense organs,* St. Louis, 1970, Mosby, p 24.

16. Bunge MB, Wood PM, Tynan LB, et al: Perineurium originates from fibroblasts: demonstration in vitro with a retroviral marker. *Science* 243:229, 1989.

17. Burkel WE: The histological fine structure of perineurium. *Anat Rec* 158:177, 1967.

18. Church RL, Tanzer M, Pfeiffer SE: Collagen and procollagen production by a clonal line of Schwann cells. *Proc Natl Acad Sci* 70:1943, 1973.

19. Elvin LG: The structure and composition of motor, sensory, and autonomic nerves and nerve fibers. In Bourne GH, editor: *The structure and function of nervous tissue. Structure I.* New York, 1968, Academic Press, vol 1, p 325.

20. Murray MR, Stout AP: Demonstration of the formation of reticulin by schwannian tumor cells in vitro. *Am J Pathol* 18:585, 1942.

21. Nathaniel EJH, Pease DC: Collagen and basement membrane formation by Schwann cells during nerve regeneration. *J Ultrastruct Res* 9:550, 1963.

22. Ochoa J, Mair WGP: The normal sural nerve in man. I. Ultrastructure and numbers of fibers and cells. *Acta Neuropathol (Berl)* 13:197, 1969.

23. Ochoa J, Mair WGP: The normal sural nerve in man. II. Changes in axons and Schwann cells due to aging. *Acta Neuropathol (Berl)* 13:217, 1969.

24. Shantha TR, Bourne GH: The perineural epithelium—a new concept. In Bourne GH, editor: *The structure and function of nervous tissue. Structure I.* New York, 1968, Academic Press, vol 1, p 379.

25. Thomas PK: The connective tissue of peripheral nerve: an electron microscopic study. *J Anat* 97:35, 1963.

Traumatic (amputation) neuroma

26. Boldrey F: Amputation neuroma in nerves implanted in bone. *Ann Surg* 118:1052, 1943.

27. Cieslak AK, Stout AP: Traumatic and amputation neuromas. *Arch Surg* 53:646, 1946.

28. Das Gupta TW, Brasfield RD: Amputation neuromas in cancer patients. *NY J Med* 69:2129, 1969.

29. Haymaker W: The pathology of peripheral nerve injuries. *Milit Surg* 102:448, 1948.

30. Huber CC, Lewis LD: Amputation neuroma: their development and prevention. *Arch Surg* 1:85, 1920.

31. Hume RH, Buxton RW: Post cholecystectomy amputation neuroma. *Am Surg* 20:698, 1954.

32. Lassmann H, Ammerer HP: Schwann cells and perineurium in neuroma: some morphological aspects. *Virchows Arch (Cell Pathol)* 15:313, 1974.

33. Shapiro L, Juhlin E, Brownstein MH: Rudimentary polydactyly: an amputation neuroma. *Arch Dermatol* 108:223, 1973.

34. Snyder CC, Knowles RP: Traumatic neuromas. *J Bone Joint Surg* 47A:641, 1965.

Mucosal neuroma

35. Carney JA, Hayles AB: Alimentary tract manifestations of multiple endocrine neoplasia, type 2b. *Mayo Clin Proc* 52:543, 1977.

36. Williams ED, Pollack DJ: Multiple mucosal neuromata with endocrine tumors: a syndrome allied to von Recklinghausen's disease. *J Pathol* 91:71, 1966.

Pacinian neuroma

37. Fletcher CDM, Theaker JM: Digital Pacinian neuroma: a distinctive hyperplastic lesion. *Histopathology* 15:249, 1989.

38. Hart WR, Thompson NW, Hildreth DH, et al: Hyperplastic pacinian corpuscles: a cause of digital pain. *Surgery* 70:730, 1971.

39. Schuler FA III, Adamson JE: Pacinian neuroma: an unusual cause of finger pain. *Plast Reconstr Surg* 62:576, 1978.

Palisaded encapsulated neuroma

40. Albrecht S, Kahn HJK, From L: Palisaded encapsulated neuroma: an immunohistochemical study. *Mod Pathol* 2:403, 1989.

41. Argenyi ZB, Cooper PH, Santa Cruz D: Plexiform and other unusual variants of palisaded encapsulated neuroma. *J Cutan Pathol* 20:34, 1993.

42. Dakin MC, Leppard B, Theaker JM: The palisaded encapsulated neuroma (solitary circumscribed neuroma). *Histopathology* 20:405, 1992.

43. Fletcher CDM: Solitary circumscribed neuroma of the skin (so-called palisaded, encapsulated neuroma): a clinicopathologic and immunohistochemical study. *Am J Surg Pathol* 13:574, 1989.

44. Reed RJ, Fine RM, Meltzer HD: Palisaded encapsulated neuromas of the skin. *Arch Dermatol* 106:865, 1972.

Morton's neuroma

45. Lassmann G, Lassmann H, Stockinger L: Morton's metatarsalgia: light and electron microscopic observations and their relations to entrapment neuropathies. *Virchows Arch (Pathol Anat)* 370:307, 1976.

46. Reed RJ, Bliss BO: Morton's neuroma. Regressive and productive intermetatarsal elastofibrositis. *Arch Pathol* 95:123, 1973.

47. Scotti TM: The lesion of Morton's metatarsalgia (Morton's toe). *Arch Pathol* 63:91, 1957.

Nerve sheath ganglion

48. Barrett R, Cramer F: Tumors of the peripheral nerves and so-called ganglia of the peroneal nerve. *Clin Orthop* 27:135, 1963.

49. Cobb CA III, Moiel RN: Ganglion of the peroneal nerve: report of two cases. *J Neurosurg* 41:255, 1974.

50. Gurdjian ES, Larsen RD, Lindner DW: Intraneural cyst of the peroneal and ulnar nerves: report of two cases. *J Neurosurg* 23:76, 1965.

Neuromuscular hamartoma (neuromuscular choristoma; benign Triton tumor)

51. Bonneau R, Brochu P: Neuromuscular choristoma: a clinicopathologic study of two cases. *Am J Surg Pathol* 7:521, 1983.

52. Louhimo I, Rapola J: Intraneural muscular hamartoma: report of two cases in small children. *J Pediatr Surg* 7:696, 1972.

53. Markel SF, Enzinger FM: Neuromuscular hamartoma: a benign "Triton tumor" composed of mature neural and striated muscle elements. *Cancer* 49:140, 1982.

54. O'Connell JX, Rosenberg AE: Multiple cutaneous neuromuscular choristomas: report of a case and a review of the literature. *Am J Surg Pathol* 14:93, 1990.

55. Orlandi E: Sopra un caso di rhabdomioma del nervo ischiatico. *Arch Sci Med (Torino)* 19:113, 1895.

56. Zwick DL, Livingston K, Clapp L: Intracranial nerve rhabdomyoma/choristoma in a child: a case report and discussion of possible histogenesis. *Hum Pathol* 20:390, 1989.

Neurilemoma (benign schwannoma)

57. Ackerman LV, Taylor FH: Neurogenous tumors within the thorax. *Cancer* 4:669, 1951.

58. Azzopardi JG, Eusebi V, Tison V, et al: Neurofibroma with rhabdomyomatous differentiation: benign "Triton" tumor of the vagina. *Histopathology* 7:561, 1983.

59. Barbosa J, Hansen LS: Solitary multilobular schwannoma of the oral cavity. *J Oral Med* 39:231, 1984.

60. Bird CC, Willis RA: The histogenesis of pigmented neurofibromas. *J Pathol* 97:631, 1969.

61. Brandes WW: A malignant neurinoma (schwannoma) with epithelial elements. *Arch Pathol* 16:649, 1933.

62. Brooks JJ, Draffen RM: Benign glandular schwannoma. *Arch Pathol Lab Med* 116:192, 1992.

63. Carstens H, Schrodt G: Malignant transformation of a benign encapsulated neurilemoma. *Am J Clin Pathol* 51:144, 1969.

64. Chandra S, Jerva MJ, Clemis JD: Ultrastructural characteristics of human neurilemoma cell nuclei. *Cancer Res* 35:2000, 1975.

65. Dahl I: Ancient neurilemoma (schwannoma). *Acta Pathol Microbiol Scand* 85A(6):812, 1977.

66. Das Gupta TK, Brasfield RD, Strong EW, et al: Benign solitary schwannomas (neurilemomas). *Cancer* 24:355, 1979.

67. Denecke K: Uber zwei Falle von metastasierenden Neurinomen des Magendarmkanals. *Beitr Path Anat* 89:242, 1932.

68. Dible JH: Verocay bodies and pseudomeisserian corpuscles. *Pathol Bacteriol* 85:425, 1963.

69. Dinakar I, Rao SB: Neurilemomas of peripheral nerves. *Int Surg* 55:15, 1971.

70. Fisher ER, Vuzevski VD: Cytogenesis of schwannoma (neurilemoma), neurofibroma, dermatofibroma, and dermatofibrosarcoma as revealed by electron microscopy. *Am J Clin Pathol* 49:141, 1968.

71. Fittipaldi C: Contributo allo studio dei neurinomi. *Riv Patol Nerve Ment* 39:521, 1932.

72. Fletcher CDM, Davies SE: Benign plexiform (multinodular) schwannoma: a rare tumor unassociated with neurofibromatosis. *Histopathology* 19:971, 1986.

73. Fletcher CDM, Davies SE, McKee PH: Cellular schwannoma: a distinct pseudosarcomatous entity. *Histopathology* 11:21, 1987.

74. Fletcher CDM, Madziwa D, Heyderman E, et al: Benign dermal schwannoma with glandular elements—true heterology or a local "organizer" effect? *Clin Exp Dermatol* 11:475, 1986.

75. Geschickter CF: Tumors of the peripheral nerves. *Am J Cancer* 25:377, 1935.

76. Goldblum JR, Beals TF, Weiss SW: Neuroblastoma-like neurilemoma. *Am J Surg Pathol* 18:266, 1994.

77. Gulcke N: Zur Klinik des Neurinomas. *Arch Klin Chir* 142:478, 1926.

78. Hanada M, Tanaka T, Kanayama S, et al: Malignant transformation of intrathoracic ancient neurilemoma in a patient without Von Recklinghausen's disease. *Acta Pathol Jpn* 32:527, 1982.

79. Helanin SS: Peculiar connective tissue tumor of the hair scalp (tactile corpuscle neurinoma). *Acta Pathol Scand* 24:299, 1947.

80. Hill RP: Neuroma of Wagner-Meissner tactile corpuscles. *Cancer* 4:879, 1951.

81. Hume GH: Cases of tumour of nerve trunks. *Lancet* 2:654, 1891.

82. Hybbinette CH: Solitary benign nerve sheath tumors around the knee joint: report of four cases. *Acta Orthop Scand* 44:296, 1973.

83. Iwashita T, Enjoji M: Plexiform neurilemoma: a clincopathologic and immunohistochemical analysis of 23 tumors from 20 patients. *Virchows Arch (Pathol Anat)* 422:305, 1986.

84. Izumi AK, Rosato FE, Wood MG: Von Recklinghausen's disease associated with multiple neurilemomas. *Arch Dermatol* 104:172, 1971.

85. Jacoby LB, Pulaski K, Rouleau GA, et al: Clonal analysis of human meningiomas and schwannomas. *Cancer Res* 50:6783, 1990.

86. Kao GF, Laskin WB, Olsen TG: Solitary cutaneous plexiform neurilemoma (schwannoma): a clinicopathologic, immunohistochemical, and ultrastructural study of 11 cases. *Mod Pathol* 2:20, 1989.

87. Katz DR: Neurilemoma with calcerosiderotic nodules. *Isr J Med Sci* 10:1156, 1974.

88. Livingstone K: Tumors of peripheral nerves. *Surg Clin North Am* 27:554, 1947.

89. Lodding L, Kindblom L-G, Angervall L, et al: Cellular schwannoma: a clinicopathologic study of 29 cases. *Virchows Arch (Pathol Anat)* 416:237, 1990.

90. Mandybur TI: Melanotic nerve sheath tumors. *J Neurosurg* 41:187, 1974.

91. Murray MR, Stout AP: Schwann cells versus fibroblasts as the origin of the specific nerve sheath tumor. *Am J Pathol* 16:41, 1940.

92. Prichard RW, Custer RP: Pacinian neurofibroma. *Cancer* 5:297, 1952.

93. Prose PH, Gherardo GJ, Coblenz A: Pacinian neurofibroma. *AMA Arch Dermatol* 76:65, 1957.

94. Raimondi AJ, Beckman F: Perineurial fibroblastomas: their fine structure and biology. *Acta Neuropathol (Berl)* 8:1, 1967.

95. Ramzy I: Benign schwannoma: demonstration of Verocay bodies using fine needle aspiration. *Acta Cytol* 21:316, 1977.

96. Rasbridge SA, Browse NL, Tighe JR, et al: Malignant nerve sheath tumor arising in a benign ancient schwannoma. *Histopathology* 14:525, 1989.

97. Razzuk MA, Urschel HC, Martin JA, et al: Electron microscopical observations on mediastinal neurilemoma, neurofibroma, and ganglioneuroma. *Ann Thorac Surg* 15:73, 1973.

98. Regan JF, Juler GL, Schmutzer KJ: Retroperitoneal neurilemoma. *Am J Surg* 134:140, 1977.

99. Saxen E: Tumours of tactile end-organs. *Acta Pathol Microbiol Scand* 25:66, 1948.

100. Schochet SS Jr, Barret DA II: Neurofibroma with aberrant tactile corpuscles. *Acta Neuropathol (Berl)* 28:161, 1974.

101. Sian CS, Ryan SF: The ultrastructure of neurilemoma with emphasis on Antoni B tissue. *Hum Pathol* 12:145, 1981.

102. Sobel HJ, Marquet E, Schwarz R: Is schwannoma related to granular cell myoblastoma? *Arch Pathol* 95:396, 1973.

103. Stener B, Angervall L, Nilsson L, et al: Angiographic and histological studies of the vascularization of peripheral nerve tumors. *Clin Orthop* 66:113, 1969.

104. Stenman G, Kindblom LG, Johansson M, et al: Clonal chromosome abnormalities and in vitro growth characteristics of classical and cellular schwannomas. *Cancer Genet Cytogenet* 57:121, 1991.

105. Stochdorph O: Uber Gewebsbilder von Tumoren der peripheren Nerven. *Acta Neuropathol (Berl)* 4:245, 1965.

106. Stout AP: The peripheral manifestations of specific nerve sheath tumor (neurilemoma). *Am J Cancer* 24:751, 1935.

107. Sun CN, White HJ: An electron microscopic study of a schwannoma with special reference to banded structures and peculiar membranous multiple-chambered spheroids. *J Pathol* 114:13, 1974.

108. Vilanova JR, Burgos-Bretones JJ, Alvarez JA, et al: Benign schwannomas: a histopathological and morphometric study. *J Pathol* 137:281, 1982.

109. Virchow R: *Die krankhaften Geschwulste*. Bd3. Berlin, 1863, August Hirschwald.

110. Waggener JD: Ultrastructure of benign peripheral nerve sheath tumors. *Cancer* 19:699, 1966.

111. Weiser G: An electron microscope study of "pacinian neurofibroma." *Virchows Arch (Pathol Anat)* 366:331, 1975.

112. Whitaker WG, Droulias C: Benign encapsulated neurilemoma: a report of 76 cases. *Am Surg* 42:675, 1976.

113. White NB: Neurilemomas of the extremity. *J Bone Joint Surg* 49A:1605, 1967.

114. White W, Shiu MH, Rosenblum MK, et al: Cellular schwannoma: a clinicopathologic study of 57 patients and 58 tumors. *Cancer* 66:1266, 1990.

115. Winkelmann RK, Johnson LA: Cholinesterases in neurofibromas. *Arch Dermatol* 85:106, 1962.

116. Woodruff JM, Godwin TA, Erlandson RA, et al: Cellular schwannoma: a variety of schwannoma sometimes mistaken for a malignant tumor. *Am J Surg Pathol* 5:733, 1981.

117. Woodruff JM, Marshall ML, Godwin TA, et al: Plexiform (multinodular) schwannoma: a tumor simulating the plexiform neurofibroma. *Am J Surg Pathol* 7:691, 1983.

118. Zulch KI: *Brain tumors: their biology and pathology*. New York, 1962, Springer-Verlag.

Neurilemomatosis (schwannomatosis)

119. Buenger KM, Porter NC, Dozier SE, et al: Localized multiple neurilemomas of the lower extremity. *Cutis* 51:36, 1993.

120. Purcell SM, Dixon SL: Schwannomatosis: an unusual variant of neurofibromatosis or a distinct clinical entity? *Arch Dermatol* 125:390, 1989.

121. Shishibo T, Niimura M, Ohtsuka F, et al: Multiple cutaneous neurilemomas as a skin manifestation of neurilemomatosis. *J Am Acad Dermatol* 10:744, 1984.

Melanotic schwannoma

122. Carney JA: Psammomatous melanotic schwannoma: a distinctive heritable tumor with special associations including cardiac myxoma and the Cushing syndrome. *Am J Surg Pathol* 14:206, 1990.

123. Font R, Enzinger FM: Unpublished observations.

124. Font RL, Truong LD: Melanotic schwannoma of soft tissues: electron microscopic observations and review of the literature. *Am J Surg Pathol* 8:129, 1984.

125. Fu YS, Kaye GI, Lattes R: Primary malignant melanocytic tumors of the sympathetic ganglia with an ultrastructural study of one. *Cancer* 36:2029, 1975.

126. Killeen RM, Davy CL, Bauserman SC: Melanocytic schwannoma. *Cancer* 62:174, 1988.

127. Krausz T, Azzopardi JG, Pearse E: Malignant melanoma of the sympathetic chain: with consideration of pigmented nerve sheath tumors. *Histopathology* 8:881, 1984.

128. Lowman RM, LiVolsi VA: Pigmented (melanotic) schwannomas of the spinal canal. *Cancer* 46:391, 1980.

129. Mennenmeyer RP, Hammar SP, Tytus JS, et al: Melanotic schwannomas: clinical and ultrastructural studies of three cases with evidence of intracellular melanin synthesis. *Am J Surg Pathol* 3:3, 1979.

130. Millar WG: A malignant melanotic tumor of ganglion cells arising from thoracic sympathetic ganglion. *J Pathol Bacteriol* 35:351, 1932.

Neurofibromatosis 1 and 2

131. Adkins JC, Ravitch MM: The operative management of von Recklinghausen's neurofibromatosis in children, with special reference to lesions of the head and neck. *Surgery* 82:342, 1977.

132. Akwari OE, Payne WAS, Onofrio BM, et al: Dumbbell neurogenic tumors of the mediastinum. *Mayo Clin Proc* 53:353, 1978.

133. Barker D, Wright E, Nguyen L, et al: Gene for von Recklinghausen neurofibromatosis is in the pericentromeric region of chromosome 17. *Science* 236:1100, 1987.

134. Brasfield RD, Das Gupta TK: Von Recklinghausen's disease: a clinicopathological study. *Ann Surg* 175:86, 1972.

135. Canale DJ, Bebin J: Von Recklinghausen disease of the nervous system. In Vinken PJ, Bruyn GW, editors: *Handbook of clinical neurology*, vol 14, p 132, New York, 1972, American Elsevier Publishers.

136. Charache H: Multiple neurofibroma with sarcomatous transformation and skeletal involvement. *Arch Dermatol Syph* 40:185, 1939.

137. Chino F, Tsuruhara T: Electron microscopic study of von Recklinghausen's disease. *Jpn J Med Sci* 21:249, 1968.

138. Crowe FW, Schull WJ, Neel JV: *A clinical, pathological, and genetic study of multiple neurofibromatosis*, Springfield, Illinois, 1956, Charles C Thomas.

139. Fraumeni JF: Neurofibromatosis and childhood leukemia. *Br Med J* 4:489, 1971.

140. Friedman JM, Fialkow PJ, Greene CL, et al: Probable clonal origin of neurofibrosarcoma in a patient with hereditary neurofibromatosis. *J Natl Cancer Inst* 69:1289, 1982.

141. Greene J, Fitzwater J, Burgess J: Arterial lesions associated with neurofibromatosis. *Am J Clin Pathol* 62:481, 1974.

142. Guccion JG, Enzinger FM: Malignant schwannoma associated with von Recklinghausen's neurofibromatosis. *Virchows Arch (Pathol Anat)* 383:43, 1979.

143. Gutmann DH, Collins FS: Recent progress toward understanding the molecular biology of von Recklinghausen's neurofibromatosis. *Ann Neurol* 31:555, 1992.

144. Hochberg FH, DaSilva AB, Galdabini J, et al: Gastrointestinal involvement in von Recklinghausen's neurofibromatosis. *Neurology* 24:1144, 1974.

145. Hosoi K: Multiple neurofibromatosis (von Recklinghausen's disease) with special reference to malignant transformation. *Arch Surg* 22:258, 1931.

146. Jimbow K, Szabo G, Fitzpatrick TB: Ultrastructure of giant pigmented granules (macromelanosomes) in the cutaneous pigmented macules of neurofibromatosis. *J Invest Dermatol* 61:300, 1973.

147. Lassmann H, Jurecka W, Lassmann W, et al: Different types of benign nerve sheath tumors: light microscopy, electron microscopy, and autoradiography. *Virchows Arch (Pathol Anat)* 375:197, 1977.

148. Lichtenstein BW: Neurofibromatosis (von Recklinghausen's disease of nervous system): analysis of a total pathologic picture. *Arch Neurol Psychiatr* 62:822, 1949.

149. Martuza RL, Eldridge R: Neurofibromatosis 2 (bilateral acoustic neurofibromatosis). *N Engl J Med* 318:684, 1988.

150. Massaro D, Katz S, Mathews MJ, et al: Von Recklinghausen's neurofibromatosis associated with cystic lung disease. *Am J Med* 38:233, 1965.

151. McEvoy MW, Mann JR: Neurofibromatosis with leukemia. *Br Med J* 3:641, 1971.

152. Merck C, Kindblom LG: Neurofibromatosis of the appendix in von Recklinghausen's disease. *Acta Pathol Microbiol Scand* 83A:623, 1975.

153. Miller RM, Sparkes RS: Segmental neurofibromatosis. *Arch Dermatol* 113:837, 1977.

154. Minor CL, Koop CE: Experiences with the management of plexiform neurofibroma. *Pediatrics* 24:482, 1959.

155. Mulvihill JJ, Parry DM, Sherman JL, Pikus A, et al: Neurofibromatosis 1 (Recklinghausen disease) and neurofibromatosis 2 (bilateral acoustic neurofibromatosis). *Ann Intern Med* 113:39, 1990.

156. National Institutes of Health: *Neurofibromatosis: National Institutes of Health consensus development conference statement.* Bethesda, Maryland, July 13-15, 1987, U.S. Department of Health and Human Services, 6(12), pp 1-9.

157. Nicholls EM: Somatic variation and multiple neurofibromatosis. *Hum Hered* 19:473, 1969.

158. Nurnberger F, Muller G, Rockert H: Zur Ultrastruktur des Neurofibroms. *Arch Klin Exp Derm* 237:796, 1970.

159. Pleasure J, Geller SA: Neurofibromatosis in infancy presenting with congenital stridor. *Am J Dis Child* 113:390, 1967.

160. Preston FW, Walsh WS, Clarke TS: Cutaneous neurofibromatosis (von Recklinghausen's disease). *Arch Surg* 64:13, 1952.

161. Pung S, Hirsch EF: Plexiform neurofibromatosis of the heart and neck. *Arch Pathol* 59:341, 1955.

162. Riccardi VM: Von Recklinghausen neurofibromatosis. *N Engl J Med* 305:1617, 1981.

163. Rodriguez HA, Berthrong M: Multiple primary intracranial tumors in von Recklinghausen's neurofibromatosis. *Arch Neurol* 14:467, 1966.

164. Sagel SS, Forrest JV: Interstitial lung disease in neurofibromatosis. *South Med J* 68:647, 1975.

165. Salyer WR, Salyer DC: The vascular lesions of neurofibromatosis. *Angiology* 25:510, 1974.

166. Sane S, Yunis E: Subperiosteal or cortical cyst and intramedullary neurofibromatosis: uncommon manifestations of neurofibromatosis. *J Bone Joint Surg* 53:1194, 1971.

167. Schenkein I, Bueker ED, Helson L, et al: Increased nerve-growth stimulating activity in disseminated neurofibromatosis. *N Engl J Med* 290:613, 1974.

168. Schorn D, Griessel PJ, Ziady F: Neurofibromatosis with renovascular hypertension. *S Afr Med J* 48:1537, 1974.

169. Scott OLS: Disease of the skin. In Sorsby A, editor: *Clinical genetics,* London, 1953, Butterworth & Co, p 580.

170. Silvers DN, Greenwood RS, Helwig EG: Café-au-lait spots without giant pigment granules: occurrence in suspected neurofibromatosis. *Arch Dermotol* 110:87, 1974.

171. Snyder SH: Nerve growth factor in neurofibromatosis (letter). *N Engl J Med* 290:626, 1974.

172. Sorensen SA, Mulvihill JJ, Nielsen A: Long-term follow-up of von Recklinghausen neurofibromatosis: survival and malignant neoplasms. *N Engl J Med* 314:1010, 1986.

173. Stay EJ, Vawter G: The relationship between nephroblastoma and neurofibromatosis (von Recklinghausen's disease). *Cancer* 39:2550, 1977.

174. Wander JV, Das Gupta TK: Neurofibromatosis. *Curr Probl Surg* 14:1, 1977.

175. Webb WR, Goodman PC: Fibrosing alveolitis in patients with neurofibromatosis. *Radiology* 122:289, 1977.

176. Weber K, Braun-Falco O: Zur Ultrastruktur der Neurofibromatose. *Hautarzt* 23:116, 1972.

177. Zorab P, Edwards H: Spinal deformity in neurofibromatosis. *Lancet* 2:823, 1972.

Perineurioma

178. Ariza A, Bilbao JM, Rosai J: Immunohistochemical detection of epithelial membrane antigen in normal perineurial cells and perineurioma. *Am J Surg Pathol* 12:678, 1988.

179. Carneiro F, Brandao O, Correia AC, et al: Spindle cell tumor of the breast. *Ultrastruct Pathol* 15:335, 1991.

180. Erlandson RA: The enigmatic perineurial cell and its participation in tumors and in tumorlike entities. *Ultrastruct Pathol* 15:335, 1991.

181. Lazarus SS, Trombetta LD: Ultrastructural identification of a benign perineurial cell tumor. *Cancer* 41:1823, 1978.

182. Ohno T, Park P, Akai M, et al : Ultrastructural study of a perineurioma. *Ultrastruct Pathol* 5:495, 1988.

183. Theaker JM, Fletcher CDM: Epithelial membrane antigen expression by the perineurial cell: further studies of peripheral nerve lesions. *Histopathology* 14:581, 1989.

184. Theaker JM, Gatter KC, Puddle J: Epithelial membrane antigen expression by the perineurium of peripheral nerve and in peripheral nerve tumors. *Histopathology* 13:171, 1987.

185. Tsang WYW, Chan JKC, Chow LTC, et al: Perineurioma: an uncommon soft tissue neoplasm distinct from localized hypertrophic neuropathy and neurofibroma. *Am J Surg Pathol* 16:756, 1992.

186. Weidenheim KM, Campbell WG: Perineurial cell tumor: Immunohistochemical and ultrastructural characterization: relationship to other peripheral nerve tumors with a review of the literature. *Virchows Arch (Pathol Anat)* 408:375, 1986.

Granular cell tumor

187. Abrikossoff A: Ueber Myome ausgehened von der quergestreiften willkuerlichen Muskulatur. *Virchows Arch (Pathol Anat)* 260:215, 1926.

188. Alkek DS, Johnson WC, Graham JH: Granular cell myoblastoma, a histological and enzymatic study. *Arch Dermatol* 98:543, 1968.

189. Aparicio SR, Lumsden CE: Light- and electron-microscopic studies on the granular cell myoblastoma of the tongue. *J Pathol* 97:339, 1969.

190. Armin A, Connelly EM, Rowden G: An immunoperoxidase investigation of S-100 protein in granular cell myoblastomas: evidence for Schwann cell derivation. *Am J Clin Pathol* 79:37, 1983.

191. Ashburn LL, Rodger RC: Myoblastomas, neural origin. Report of six cases, one with multiple tumors. *Am J Clin Pathol* 22:440, 1952.

192. Azzopardi JG: Histogenesis of granular cell "myoblastoma." *J Pathol Bacteriol* 71:85, 1956.

193. Bangle R: A morphologic and histochemical study of granular cell myoblastoma. *Cancer* 5:950, 1952.

194. Bangle R Jr: An early granular cell myoblastoma confined within a small peripheral myelinated nerve. *Cancer* 6:790, 1953.

195. Baraf CS, Bender B: Multiple cutaneous granular cell myoblastoma. *Arch Dermatol* 89:243, 1964.

196. Bedetti CD, Martinez AJ, Beckford NS, et al: Granular cell tumors arising in myelinated peripheral nerves: light and electron microscopy and immunoperoxidase study. *Virchows Arch (Pathol Anat)* 402:175, 1983.

197. Bhawan H, Malhorta R, Naik DR: Gaucherlike cells in granular cell tumor. *Hum Pathol* 14:730, 1983.

198. Buley ID, Gatter KC, Kelly PMA, et al: Granular cell tumours revisited: an immunohistological and ultrastructural study. *Histopathology* 12:263, 1988.

199. Carstens PH: Ultrastructure of granular cell myoblastoma. *Acta Pathol Microbiol Scand* 78:685, 1970.

200. Chimelli L, Symon L, Scaravilli F: Granular cell tumor of the fifth cranial nerve. Further evidence for Schwann cell origin. *J Neuropathol Exp Neurol* 43:634, 1984.

201. Christ ML, Ozzello L: Myogenous origin of a granular cell tumor of the urinary bladder. *Am J Clin Pathol* 56:736, 1971.

202. Compagno J, Hyams VJ, Ste-Marie P: Benign granular cell tumors of the larynx: a review of the 36 cases with clinicopathologic data. *Ann Otol Rhinol Laryngol* 84:308, 1975.

203. Crawford ES, De Bakey ME: Granular cell myoblastoma: two unusual cases. *Cancer* 6:786, 1953.

204. Dhillon AP, Rode J: Immunohistochemical studies of S-100 protein and other neural characteristics expressed by granular cell tumour. *Diagn Histopathol* 6:23, 1983.

205. Eberle R, Conley J: Granular cell schwannoma (myoblastoma). *Arch Otolaryngol (Chicago)* 88:174, 1968.

206. Feyrter F: Ueber die granularen neurogenen Gewachse. *Beitr Pathol Anat* 110:181, 1949.

207. Feyrter F: Ueber die granularen Neurome (sogenannte Myoblastome). *Virchows Arch (Pathol Anat)* 322:66, 1952.

208. Fisher ER, Wechsler H: Granular cell myoblastoma—a misnomer: EM and histochemical evidence concerning its Schwann cell derivation and nature (granular cell schwannoma). *Cancer* 15:936, 1962.

209. Fust JA, Custer RP: Granular cell "myoblastoma" and granular cell neurofibromas: separation of the neurogenous tumors from the myoblastoma group. *Am J Pathol* 24:674, 1948.

210. Fust JA, Custer RP: On the neurogenesis of so-called granular cell myoblastoma. *Am J Clin Pathol* 19:522, 1949.

211. Garancis JC, Komorowski RA, Kuzma JF: Granular cell myoblastoma. *Cancer* 25:542, 1970.

212. Gifford RPM, Birch HW: Granular cell myoblastoma of multicentric origin involving the vulva. *Am J Obstet Gynecol* 117:184, 1973.

213. Goodman MD, Cooper PH: Granular cell tumor (myoblastoma) of the stomach. Case report with ultrastructural findings and review of the literature. *Am J Dig Dis* 17:1117, 1972.

214. Haisken W, Langer E: Die submikroscopische Struktur des sogenanten Myoblastenmyoms. *Frankf Z Path* 71:600, 1962.

215. Horn RC Jr, Stout AP: Granular cell myoblastoma. *Surg Gynecol Obstet* 76:315, 1943.

216. Hurlbut WE: Multiple granular cell schwannomas. *Arch Dermatol* 103:557, 1971.

217. Khansur T, Balducci L, Tavassoli M: Identification of desmosomes in the granular cell tumor: implications in histologic diagnosis and histogenesis. *Am J Surg Pathol* 9:898, 1985.

218. Klemperer P: Myoblastoma of the striated muscle. *Am J Cancer* 20:324, 1934.

219. Krouse TB, Mobini J: Multifocal granular cell myoblastoma: report of a case involving trachea, stomach, and anterior abdominal wall. *Arch Pathol* 96:95, 1973.

220. Lack EE, Worsham GF, Callihan MD, et al: Granular cell tumor: a clinicopathologic study of 110 patients. *J Surg Oncol* 13:301, 1980.

221. Miettinen M, Lehtonen E, Lehtola H, et al: Histogenesis of granular cell tumour: an immunological and ultrastructural study. *J Pathol* 142:221, 1984.

222. Moscovic EA, Azar HA: Multiple granular cell tumors ("myoblastomas"): case report with electron microscopic observations and review of the literature. *Cancer* 20:2032, 1967.

223. Mukai M: Immunohistochemical localization of S-100 protein and peripheral nerve myelin proteins (P2 protein and PO protein) in granular cell tumors. *Am J Pathol* 112:139, 1983.

224. Murphy GH, Dockerty MB, Broders AC: Myoblastoma. *Am J Pathol* 25:1157, 1949.

225. Murray DE, Seaman E, Ultzinger W: Granular cell myoblastomas in successive generations. *J Surg Oncol* 1:193, 1969.

226. Murray R: Cultural characteristics of three granular cell myoblastomas. *Cancer* 4:857, 1951.

227. Naidech JH, Axelrod RD, Seliger G: Granular cell tumor (myoblastoma) of the stomach. *Am J Roentgenol* 113:254, 1971.

228. Nakazato Y, Ishizeki J, Takahashi K, et al: Immunohistochemical localization of S-100 protein in granular cell myoblastoma. *Cancer* 49:1624, 1982.

229. Nathrath WBJ, Remberger K: Immunohistochemical study of granular cell tumours. Demonstration of neuron specific enolase, S-100 protein, laminin, and alpha-1-antichymotrypsin. *Virchows Arch A Pathol Anat Histopathol* 408:421, 1986.

230. Papageorgiou S, Litt JZ, Pomeranz JR: Multiple granular cell myoblastomas in children. *Arch Dermatol* 96:168, 1967.

231. Paskin DL, Hull JD: Granular cell myoblastoma. A comprehensive review of 15 years' experience. *Ann Surg* 175:501, 1972.

232. Pearse AGE: The histogenesis of granular cell myoblastoma. *J Pathol Bacteriol* 62:351, 1950.

233. Pour P, Althoff J, Cardesa A: Granular cells in tumors and in non-tumorous tissue. *Arch Pathol* 95:135, 1973.

234. Propst A, Weiser G: Das granulare Neuron Feyrters. *Wien Klin Wochenschr* 83:31, 1971.

235. Rao TV, Puri R, Reddy GNN: Intracranial trigeminal nerve granular cell myoblastoma: case report. *J Neurosurg* 59:706, 1983.

236. Ratzenhofer M: Granulaere falsche Neurome (sog. Myoblastenmyome) und sekundaere Wucherung de Deckepithels. *Virchows Arch (Pathol Anat)* 320:138, 1951.

237. Save-Soderbergh J: Basal lamina in granular cell tumors. *Hum Pathol* 6:637, 1975.

238. Seo IS, Azarelli B, Warner TF, et al: Multiple visceral and cutaneous granular cell tumors: ultrastructural and immunocytochemical evidence of Schwann cell origin. *Cancer* 53:2104, 1984.

239. Smolle J, Konrad K, Kerl H: Granular cell tumors contain myelin-associated glycoprotein: an immunohistochemical study using Leu-7 monoclonal antibody. *Virchows Arch A Pathol Anat Histopathol* 406:1, 1985.

240. Sobel HJ: Granular cell myoblastoma: an electron-microscopic and cytochemical study illustrating the genesis of granules and aging of myoblastoma cells. *Am J Pathol* 65:59, 1971.

241. Sobel HJ, Arvin E, Marquet E, et al: Reactive granular cell in sites of trauma. *Am J Clin Pathol* 61:223, 1974.

242. Sobel HJ, Churg J: Granular cells and granular cell lesions. *Arch Pathol* 77:132, 1974.

243. Sobel HJ, Marquet E, Schwarz R: Is schwannoma related to granular cell myoblastoma? *Arch Pathol* 95:396, 1973.

244. Sobel HJ, Schwarz R, Marquet E: Light and electron microscopic study of the origin of granular cell myoblastoma. *J Pathol* 109:101, 1973.

245. Stefansson K, Wollmann RL: S-100 protein in granular cell tumors (granular cell myoblastoma). *Cancer* 49:1834, 1982.

246. Strong EW, McDivitt RW, Brasfield RD: Granular cell myoblastoma. *Cancer* 25:415, 1970.

247. Toto PD, Restarski J: Histogenesis of the granular-cell myoblastoma. *Oral Surg Oral Med Oral Pathol* 24:384, 1967.

248. Tsuneyoshi M, Enjoji M: Granular cell tumor: a clinicopathological study of 48 cases. *Fukuoka Acta Medica* 69:495, 1978.

249. Vance S, Hudson R: Granular cell myoblastoma. *Am J Clin Pathol* 52:208, 1969.

250. Weiser G: Granularzelltumor (Granulares Neuron Feyrter) und Schwannsche Phagen: Electronenoptische Untersuchung von 3 Faellen. *Virchows Arch (Pathol Anat)* 380:49, 1978.

251. White SW, Gallager RL, Rodman OG: Multiple granular-cell tumors. *J Dermatol Surg Oncol* 6:57, 1980.

252. Whitten JB: The fine structure of an intraoral granular-cell myoblastoma. *Oral Surg Oral Med Oral Pathol* 26:202, 1968.

Congenital (gingival) granular cell tumor

253. Bhaskar SN, Akamine R: Congenital epulis (congenital granular cell fibroblastoma). *J Oral Surg* 8:517, 1955.

254. Costas JB, DiPiramo S: Congenital epulis (congenital granular-cell fibroblastoma). *Oral Surg Oral Med Oral Pathol* 26:497, 1968.

255. Cussen LJ, MacMahon RA: Congenital granular cell myoblastoma. *J Pediatr Surg* 10:249, 1975.

256. Fuhr AH, Krogh PHJ: Congenital epulis of the newborn: centennial review of the literature and a report of a case. *J Oral Surg* 30:30, 1972.

257. Ganley CJ, El Attar AM: Congenital myoblastoma of the newborn. *Oral Surg Oral Med Oral Pathol* 20:645, 1965.

258. Henefer EP, Abaza NA, Anderson SP: Congenital granular cell epulis: report of a case. *Oral Surg Oral Med Oral Pathol* 47:515, 1979.

259. Koppang HS: Congenital gingival granular-cell myoblastoma. *Oral Surg Oral Med Oral Pathol* 34:98, 1972.

260. Lack E, Crawford BE, Worsham GF, et al: Gingival granular cell tumors of the newborn (congenital "epulis"): a clinical and pathologic study of 21 patients. *Am J Surg Pathol* 5:37, 1981.

261. Lack EE, Perez-Atayde AR, McGill TJ, et al: Gingival granular cell tumor of the newborn (congenital "epulis"): ultrastructural observations relating to histogenesis. *Hum Pathol* 13:686, 1982.

262. Lifshitz MS, Flotte TJ, Greco MA: Congenital granular cell epulis. Immunohistochemical and ultrastructural observations. *Cancer* 53:1845, 1984.

263. Matthews JB, Mason GI: Oral granular cell myoblastoma: an immunohistochemical study. *J Oral Pathol* 11:343, 1982.

264. Slootweg P, de Wilde P, Vooijs P, et al: Oral granular cell lesions. An immunohistochemical study with emphasis on intermediate-sized filament proteins. *Virchows Arch (Pathol Anat)* 402:35, 1983.

265. Tucker JC, Rusnock EJ, Azumi N: Gingival granular cell tumors of the newborn: an ultrastructural and immunohistochemical study. *Arch Pathol Lab Med* 114:895, 1990.

266. Volkmann J: Myoblastenmyom: Eine stelene angeborene Oberkiefergeschwulst bei einem Neugeborenen. *Zentralbl Chir* 56:2982, 1929.

Malignant granular cell tumor

267. Al-Sarraf M, Loud A, Vaitkevicius V: Malignant granular cell tumor. *Arch Pathol* 91:550, 1971.

268. Bussany-Caspari W, Hammar CH: Zur Malignitaet der sogenannten Myoblastenmyome. *Zentralbl Allg Pathol* 98:401, 1958.

269. Cadotte M: Malignant granular cell myoblastoma. *Cancer* 33:1417, 1974.

270. Donhuijsen K, Samtleben W, Leder LD, et al: Malignant granular cell tumor. *J Cancer Res Clin Oncol* 95:93, 1979.

271. Dunnington JH: Granular cell myoblastoma of the orbit. *Arch Ophthalmol* 40:14, 1948.

272. Finkel G, Lane B: Granular cell variant of neurofibromatosis: ultrastructure of benign and malignant tumors. *Hum Pathol* 13:959, 1982.

273. Gamboa LG: Malignant granular cell myoblastoma. *Arch Pathol* 60:663, 1955.

274. Harrer WV, Patchefsky AS: Malignant granular cell myoblastoma of the posterior mediastinum. *Chest* 61:95, 1972.

275. Hunter DT, Dewar JP: Malignant granular cell myoblastoma: report of a case and review of the literature. *Am Surg* 26:554, 1960.

276. Kindblom LG, Olsson KM: Malignant granular cell tumor: a clinicopathologic and ultrastructural study of a case. *Pathol Res Pract* 172:384, 1981.

277. Krieg AF: Malignant granular cell myoblastoma: a case report. *Arch Pathol* 74:251, 1962.

278. Kubacz GJ: Malignant granular cell myoblastoma: report of a case. *Aust NZ J Surg* 40:291, 1971.

279. Mackenzie DH: Malignant granular cell myoblastoma. *J Clin Pathol* 20:739, 1967.

280. Madhavan M, Aurora AL, Sen SB: Malignant granular cell myoblastoma. *Indian J Cancer* 11:360, 1974.

281. McWilliam LJ, Harris M: Granular cell angiosarcoma of the skin: histology, electron microscopy, and immunohistochemistry of a newly recognized tumor. *Histopathology* 9:1205, 1985.

282. Nistal M, Paniagua R, Pizazo ML, et al: Granular changes in vascular leiomyosarcoma. *Virchows Arch (Pathol Anat)* 386:239, 1980.

283. Ravich A, Stout AP, Ravich RA: Malignant granular cell myoblastoma involving the urinary bladder. *Ann Surg* 121:361, 1945.

284. Robertson AJ, McIntosh W, Lamont P, et al: Malignant granular cell tumor (myoblastoma) of the vulva. Report of a case and review of the literature. *Histopathology* 5:69, 1981.

285. Ross RC, Miller TR, Foote FW: Malignant granular cell myoblastoma. *Cancer* 5:112, 1952.

286. Steffelaar JW, Nap M, van Haelst UJGM: Malignant granular cell tumor: report of a case with special reference to carcinoembryonic antigen. *Am J Surg Pathol* 6:665, 1982.

287. Svejda J, Horn V: Disseminated granular-cell pseudotumor: so-called metastasizing granular cell myoblastoma. *J Pathol Bacteriol* 76:343, 1958.

288. Tyagi SP, Khan MH, Tyagi N: Malignant granular cell tumor. *Indian J Cancer* 15:77, 1978.

289. Usui M, Ishii S, Yamawaki S, et al: Malignant granular cell tumor of the radial nerve: an autopsy observation with electron microscopic and tissue culture studies. *Cancer* 39:1547, 1977.

Neurothekeoma (nerve sheath myxoma)

290. Angervall L, Kindblom L, Haglid K: Dermal nerve sheath myxoma. *Cancer* 53:1752, 1984.

291. Aronson PJ, Fretzin DF, Potter BS: Neurothekeoma of Gallager and Helwig (dermal nerve sheath myxoma variant): report of a case with electron microscopic and immunohistochemical studies. *J Cutan Pathol* 12:506, 1985.

292. Barnhill RL, Dickersin GR, Nickeleit V, et al: Studies on the cellular origin of neurothekeoma: clinical, light microscopic, immunohistochemical, and ultrastructural observations. *J Am Acad Dermatol* 25:80, 1991.

293. Barnhill RL, Mihm MC Jr: Cellular neurothekeoma: a distinctive variant of neurothekeoma mimicking nevomelanocytic tumors. *Am J Surg Pathol* 14:113, 1990.

294. Calonje E, Wilson-Jones E, Smith NP, et al: Cellular "neurothekeoma": an epithelioid variant of pilar leiomyoma? Morphological and immunohistochemical analysis of a series. *Histopathology* 20:397, 1992.

295. Gallager RL, Helwig EB: Neurothekeoma: a benign cutaneous tumor of nerve sheath origin. *Am J Clin Pathol* 74:759, 1980.

296. King D, Barr R: Bizarre cutaneous neurofibromas. *J Cutan Pathol* 7:21, 1980.

297. MacDonald DM, Wilson-Jones E: Pacinian neurofibroma. *Histopathology* 1:247, 1977.

298. Pulitzer DR, Reed RJ: Nerve sheath myxoma. *Am J Dermatopathol* 7:409, 1985.

Extracranial meningioma

299. Lopez DA, Silvers DN, Helwig EB: Cutaneous meningiomas: a clinicopathologic study. *Cancer* 34:728, 1974.

300. Theaker JM, Fleming KA: Meningioma of the scalp: a case report with immunohistochemical features. *J Cutan Pathol* 14:49, 1987.

Glial heterotopias

301. Orkin M, Fisher I: Heterotopic brain tissue (heterotopic neural rest). *Arch Dermatol* 94:699, 1966.

302. Rios JJ, Diaz-Cano SL, Rivera-Hueto F, et al: Cutaneous ganglion cell choristoma. *J Cutan Pathol* 18:469, 1991.

Melanotic neuroectodermal tumor of infancy

303. Allen M, Harrison W, Jahrsdoerfer R: Retinal anlage tumors. *Am J Clin Pathol* 51:309, 1969.

304. Borello ED, Gorlin RJ: Melanotic neuroectodermal tumor of infancy: a neoplasm of neural crest origin. *Cancer* 19:196, 1966.

305. Cutler LS, Chaudhry AP, Topazian R: Melanotic neuroectodermal tumor of infancy: an ultrastructural, literature review, and reevaluation. *Cancer* 48:257, 1981.

306. Dehner LP, Sibley RK, Sauk JJ, et al: Malignant melanotic neuroectodermal tumor of infancy: a clinical, pathologic, ultrastructural, and tissue culture study. *Cancer* 43:1389, 1979.

307. Dooling EC, Chi JeG, Gilles FH: Melanotic neuroectodermal tumor of infancy: its histological similarities to fetal pineal gland. *Cancer* 39:1535, 1977.

308. Duckworth R, Seward GR: Amelanotic ameloblastic odontoma. *Oral Surg Oral Med Oral Pathol* 19:73, 1965.

309. Eaton WL, Ferguson JP: A retinoblastic teratoma of the epididymis. *Cancer* 9:718, 1956.

310. Frank GL, Koten HE: Melanotic hamartoma ("retinal anlage tumor") of the epididymis. *J Pathol Bacteriol* 93:549, 1967.

311. Hayward AF, Fickling BW, Lucas RB: An electron microscope study of a pigmented tumor of the jaw of infants. *Br J Cancer* 23:702, 1969.

312. Johnson RE, Scheithauer BW, Dahlin DC: Melanotic neuroectodermal tumor of infancy. *Cancer* 52:661, 1983.

313. Kapadia SH, Frisman DM, Hitchcock CL, et al: Melanotic neuroectodermal tumor of infancy. *Am J Surg Pathol* 17:566, 1993.

314. Koudstall J, Oldhoff J, Panders AK, et al: Melanotic neuroectodermal tumor of infancy. *Cancer* 22:151, 1968.

315. Lee SC, Henry MM, Gonzalez-Crussi F: Simultaneous occurrence of melanotic neuroectodermal tumor and brain heterotopia in the oropharynx. *Cancer* 38:249, 1976.

316. Lindahl F: Malignant melanotic progonoma: one case. *Acta Pathol Microbiol Scand* 78A:532, 1970.

317. Lurie HI: Congenital melanocarcinoma, melanocytic adamantinoma, retinal anlage tumor, progonoma, and pigmented epulis of infancy: summary and review of the literature and report of the first case in an adult. *Cancer* 14:1090, 1961.

318. Lurie HI, Isaacson C: A melanotic progonoma in the scapula. *Cancer* 14:1088, 1961.

319. Misugi K, Okajima H, Newton WA, et al: Mediastinal origin of a melanotic progonoma or retinal anlage tumor: ultrastructural evidence for neural crest origin. *Cancer* 18:477, 1965.

320. Navas Palacios JJ: Malignant melanotic neuroectodermal tumor: light and electron microscopic study. *Cancer* 46:529, 1980.

321. Pettinato G, Manivel C, d'Amore ESG, et al: Melanotic neuroectodermal tumor of infancy: an immunohistochemical study. *Histopathology* 12:425, 1988.

322. Schulz DM: A malignant melanotic neoplasm of the uterus resembling the retinal anlage tumor. *Am J Clin Pathol* 28:524, 957.

323. Stirling RW, Powell G, Fletcher CDM: Pigmented neuroectodermal tumor of infancy: an immunohistochemical study. *Histopathology* 12:425, 1988.

324. Stowens D, Lin TH: Melanotic progonoma of the brain. *Hum Pathol* 5:105, 1974.

325. William AO: Melanotic ameloblastoma ("progonoma") of infancy showing osteogenesis. *J Pathol Bacteriol* 93:545, 1967.

326. Zone RM: Retinal analage tumor of the epididymis: a case report. *J Urol* 103:106, 1970.

CHAPTER 32

MALIGNANT TUMORS OF THE PERIPHERAL NERVES

MALIGNANT PERIPHERAL NERVE SHEATH TUMOR

In previous editions of this text, we have used the term *malignant schwannoma* to refer to sarcomas that arise from nerve or display features of neural differentiation. This term, however, has two major shortcomings. It implies that all such tumors exhibit Schwann cell differentiation when, in fact, such tumors can recapitulate the appearance of any cell of the nerve sheath, including the Schwann cell, perineural fibroblast, or fibroblast. Thus, they range in appearance from tumors that are indistinguishable from fibrosarcoma to tumors in which the cells display many of the features of Schwann cells. Second, the term *malignant schwannoma* potentially conveys the erroneous impression that such tumors develop in neurilemoma (benign schwannoma), a phenomenon that is rare. Thus, the term *malignant peripheral nerve sheath tumor (MPNST)* is preferred for most spindle cell sarcomas arising from nerve or neurofibroma, or showing nerve sheath differentiation. This term has been recently adopted by the World Health Organization Committee for the Classification of Soft Tissue Tumors. Although primitive neuroectodermal tumors also arise from peripheral nerves, they are considered along with neuroblastic tumors and Ewing's sarcoma in Chapter 33.

The diagnosis of MPNST is one of the most difficult and elusive diagnoses in soft tissue diseases because of the lack of standardized diagnostic criteria. Although there is general agreement that if a sarcoma arises from a peripheral nerve or a neurofibroma it can usually be considered an MPNST,* there is less agreement about the diagnostic criteria for tumors occurring outside these settings. As a result, the incidence of this sarcoma is uncertain and varies in the literature. In 1942, Stewart and Copeland,[71] reporting their experience from Memorial Hospital in New York,

maintained that "neurogenic sarcomas" comprised the majority of fibrosarcomas of soft tissue and that most occurred in patients without neurofibromatosis. Likewise, Geschickter,[27] in his review of cases from the Johns Hopkins Hospital, concluded that the tumor was among the most common of all soft tissue sarcomas. Both studies reflect a liberal diagnostic approach and willingness to accept many spindled collagen-producing sarcomas as neural, especially if they occur in certain locations or produce characteristic symptoms. On the other hand, Stout[73] proposed a stricter definition of the tumor. In his opinion, these tumors could not be separated from fibrosarcomas on histological grounds, and their diagnosis rested on documented origin from nerve or neurofibroma or association with von Recklinghausen's disease. The rarity of the tumor in his experience and its high association with neurofibromatosis reflect in large part his stringent criteria.

Our approach has generally been an intermediate one. We maintain that some, but certainly not all, MPNSTs can be recognized on histological grounds alone. Based on a review of a large number of typical cases of MPNST arising from nerve or in neurofibromatosis 1, we believe that certain histological features can help in the diagnosis of these tumors when they occur in less typical settings. Usually no one feature secures the diagnosis but, rather, several features in concert help distinguish MPNST from fibrosarcoma. These features, which are discussed in detail below, include peculiarities of nuclear shape, nuclear palisading, tactoid differentiation, perivascular changes, and occasionally the presence of heterologous elements (e.g., cartilage, bone, muscle). The ancillary techniques of electron microscopy and immunohistochemistry provide additional information that may aid in the distinction of MPNSTs from fibrosarcoma, monophasic synovial sarcoma, or other spindle cell sarcomas. Our approach implies that only the more typical MPNSTs will be diagnosed and that poorly differentiated ones not arising in a nerve or neurofibroma or in neurofibromatosis 1 will go undiagnosed.

---

*Rarely malignant tumors of nerve show differentiation along a purely nonschwannian line. Such tumors are classified by the respective line of differentiation (e.g., angiosarcoma of nerve[4]).

This approach offers an acceptable degree of diagnostic reproducibility and eliminates the potpourri of spindle cell tumors that have been diagnosed as MPNSTs in the past.

Clinical findings

In our consultation experience, MPNSTs account for approximately 10% of all soft tissue sarcomas; about half occur with neurofibromatosis 1.[23,40,68] Obviously the diagnostic criteria and type of pathological material affect these figures, as illustrated by the fact that the association with neurofibromatosis 1 varies from about one fourth[28] to over two thirds[83] in the literature. In large recent series in which there has been more consistency in histological diagnoses, the percentage of patients with MPNSTs having and not having neurofibromatosis 1 is roughly equal.[40,56] Patients with neurofibromatosis 1 are clearly at increased risk to develop these tumors. However, earlier estimates that patients with neurofibromatosis 1 had a risk as high as 13% of developing an MPNST are gross overestimates by current studies. About 4% of patients with neurofibromatosis 1 develop MPNSTs[69] (Chapter 31). Patients with neurofibromatosis 1 develop sarcomas usually after a relatively long latent period of 10 to 20 years,[35] and in some cases the MPNSTs are multiple.[68]

Although it might be expected that sarcomas arising in neurofibromatosis 1 would exhibit deletions of the neurofibromatosis 1 locus, this has not proved to be the case. Both Menon et al.[58] and Reynolds et al.[65] documented various abnormalities on chromosome 17 but outside the region of the neurofibromatosis 1 gene, possibly involving the p53 gene. The exact mechanism of malignant transformation or tumor progression in neurofibromatosis 1 is not fully understood, but it may involve a multistep process in which genes apart from the neurofibromatosis 1 gene also participate. Aside from the foregoing genetic predilection to develop MPNSTs, little is known concerning the pathogenesis of these tumors in humans. About 10% of cases occur as a result of therapeutic or occupational irradiation after a latent period of over 15 years.[22,23] The tumors do not differ significantly from other MPNSTs.

Experimentally these tumors can be induced in laboratory animals by transplacental injection of ethylnitrosourea[44] or administration of methylcholanthrene.[66] As a result of these studies, it has been suggested that a search for chemical carcinogens in the environment might prove fruitful.

MPNST is typically a disease of adult life; most tumors occur in patients between 20 and 50 years of age.[3,13-15,23,35,69] Patients with neurofibromatosis 1 develop these tumors at an earlier age, however. The average age at the time of diagnosis for patients with neurofibromatosis 1 was 29 and 36 years in the Mayo Clinic[23] and Memorial Sloan Kettering[40] studies, respectively, compared with

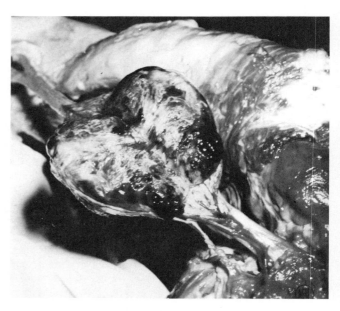

FIG. 32-1. Malignant peripheral nerve sheath tumor arising as a large fusiform mass from the sciatic nerve. Cut section of tumor shows prominent hemorrhage and necrosis.

40 and 44 years, respectively, for patients without the disease. Our experience indicates an average age of 32 years for both groups but a wider age range among patients without neurofibromatosis 1.[35] The sex ratio of patients with MPNSTs varies, depending on patient selection. Men predominate in studies having a high percentage of patients with neurofibromatosis 1 as a result of the bias toward men in this disease.[14,35] In studies of sporadic cases of MPNST, the sex ratio is roughly equal or slightly biased toward women.[13,28] These observations parallel our experience. Eighty percent of patients with neurofibromatosis 1 and MPNST are men,[35] whereas only 56% of patients with sporadic MPNST are men.[35]

Like other sarcomas, these lesions present as enlarging masses that are usually noted several months before diagnosis. Pain is variable but seems to be more prevalent in patients with neurofibromatosis 1. In fact, pain or sudden enlargement of a preexisting mass in this setting should lead to immediate biopsy in order to exclude the possibility of malignant transformation of a neurofibroma. MPNSTs that arise from major nerves typically give rise to a striking constellation of sensory and motor symptoms, including projected pain, paresthesias, and weakness. The symptoms rarely antedate the detection of a mass.

Most MPNSTs arise in association with major nerve trunks, including the sciatic nerve, brachial plexus, and sacral plexus. Consequently, the most common anatomical sites include the proximal portions of the upper and lower extremities and trunk. Comparatively few arise in the head

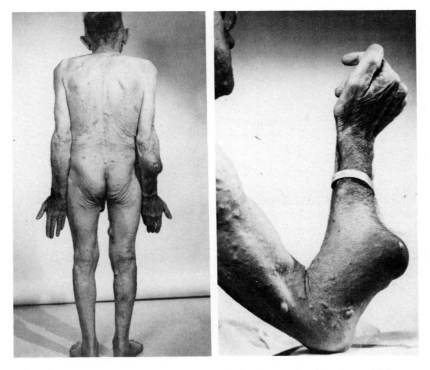

FIG. 32-2. Malignant peripheral nerve sheath tumor of arm occurring in patient with long-standing neurofibromatosis.

and neck, a feature that contrasts with the distribution of the neurilemoma.

Gross findings

In its classic form, an MPNST arises as a large fusiform or eccentric mass within a major nerve (Fig. 32-1). Thickening of the nerve proximally and distally to the main mass usually indicates spread of the neoplasm along the epineurium and perineurium. In neurofibromatosis 1, MPNSTs may develop within a preexisting neurofibroma (Fig. 32-2). The vast majority of these lesions are deeply situated, whereas only rare ones arise from superficial neurofibromas. Regardless of the clinical setting, the gross appearance of MPNSTs is essentially similar to that of other soft tissue sarcomas. It is usually large, averaging more than 5 cm in diameter, and has a fleshy, white-tan surface marked by areas of secondary hemorrhage and necrosis.

Microscopic findings

The majority of MPNSTs resemble fibrosarcomas in their overall organization (Fig. 32-3) but manifest certain modifying features. Classically, the cells recapitulate the features of the normal Schwann cell. Unlike the symmetrical spindled cells of fibrosarcoma, they have markedly irregular contours. In profile the nuclei are wavy, buckled, or comma-shaped, whereas when viewed en face they are asymmetrically oval (Fig. 32-3, *B*). The cytoplasm is lightly stained and usually indistinct (Fig. 32-4).

The cells are arranged in sweeping fascicles, but there is greater variation in organization than in the fibrosarcoma. Densely cellular fascicles alternate with hypocellular, myxoid zones (Fig. 32-5, *A*) where the parallel orientation of the cells is lacking (Fig. 32-5, *B*). Some lesions possess, in addition, rounded or short fusiform (Fig. 32-6) cells. Others display a peculiar nodular, curlicue, or whorled arrangement of spindled cells (Figs. 32-7 to 32-9). The last feature suggests rudimentary tactoid differentiation, but it is never as well developed as in the Wagner-Meissner or pacinian bodies of benign neurofibromas. Nuclear palisading may be present, but in our cases it occurs in fewer than 10% of all malignant schwannomas and, when present, is usually of a focal nature (Fig. 32-10).

There are several other subtle features that are also quite characteristic of MPNST. Because they are not completely specific, they must be evaluated in the context of the foregoing discussion before a given tumor is termed MPNST. These features include hyaline bands (Fig. 32-11, *A*) and nodules, which in cross-section can be likened to giant rosettes (Fig. 32-11, *B*), extensive perineural and intraneural spread of tumor (Fig. 32-12), and a peculiar proliferation of tumor in the subendothelial zones of vessels so that the neoplastic cells appear to herniate into the lumen (Fig. 32-

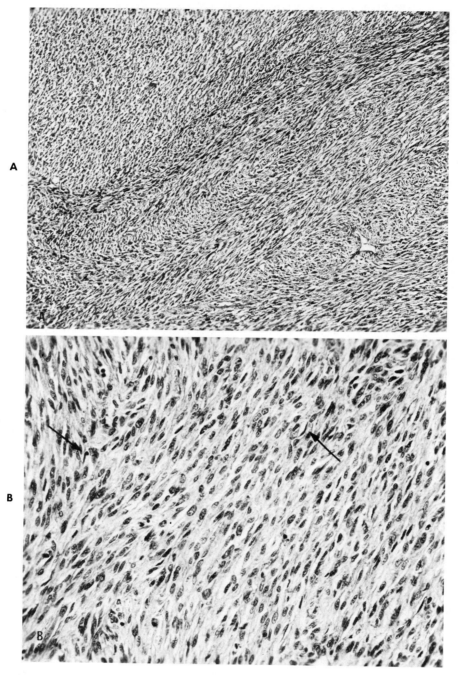

FIG. 32-3. Typical appearance of malignant peripheral nerve sheath tumor. **A,** Long sweeping fascicles similar to a fibrosarcoma compose majority of these tumors. (×100.) **B,** Unlike a fibrosarcoma, nuclei are twisted, buckled, and more irregular in shape. Note occasional comma-shaped cells similar to those seen in benign nerve sheath tumors *(arrows).* (×250.)

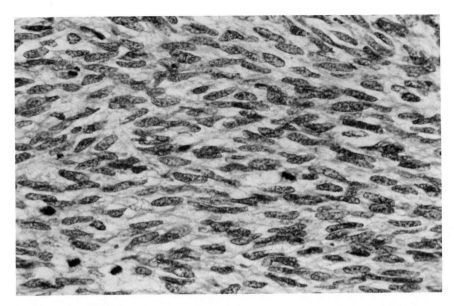

FIG. 32-4. Cells of malignant peripheral nerve sheath tumor showing wavy or buckled shape of nuclei and indistinct cytoplasmic borders. (×400.)

13). Likewise, heterotopic elements present in about 10% to 15% of MPNSTs[40] seem to be more common in MPNSTs than in other sarcomas,[21] and their presence may initially suggest the diagnosis in a tumor that otherwise resembles fibrosarcoma.

Mature islands of cartilage and bone are the most common elements (Fig. 32-14), whereas skeletal muscle and mucin-secreting glands are quite rare. In addition, we have seen one malignant schwannoma with squamous differentiation (Fig. 32-15), and one malignant schwannoma reported in the literature arising in von Recklinghausen's disease showed foci of liposarcoma, although the illustrations are not entirely convincing.[14] These unusual MPNSTs seem to occur more often in neurofibromatosis 1 and have been referred to in the past as *malignant mesenchymomas of nerve sheath*.[36] Because they are composed predominantly of recognizable schwannian elements, we still consider them variants of MPNST.

Although most MPNSTs conform to this description, a small percentage appear quite different. Some of these tumors closely resemble neurofibromas except that they manifest a greater degree of cellularity, pleomorphism, and, most importantly, mitotic activity (Fig. 32-16). These MPNSTs are typically found in the setting of von Recklinghausen's disease and have sometimes been termed *malignant neurofibromas*. At the opposite end of the spectrum are anaplastic MPNSTs, which may be difficult to distinguish from other pleomorphic sarcomas such as malignant fibrous histiocytoma (Fig. 32-17, *B*). They contain sheets of plump, spindled and giant cells intermixed with areas of

hemorrhage and necrosis. These pleomorphic tumors have been documented more often in the setting of von Recklinghausen's disease. To some extent this may indicate the general reluctance to make the diagnosis of anaplastic MPNST outside the setting of neurofibromatosis 1. Diagnosis of these tumors depends on identification of areas of typical MPNST (Fig. 32-17, *A*). Infrequently, MPNSTs contain areas of primitive neuroepithelial differentiation consisting of cords or nests of small round cells and, in extraordinary cases, even rosettes. Primitive neuroepithelial differentiation appears to be a more common feature of MPNSTs occurring in children.[56]

Immunohistochemical findings

There are a number of antigens that are useful in identifying nerve sheath differentiation. These include S-100 protein, Leu-7, and myelin basic protein. S-100 protein, the most widely used antigen for neural differentiation, can be identified in 50% to 90% of MPNSTs, although typically the staining is focal and limited to small numbers of cells.[53,61,82,85] Since it is rare to encounter an MPNST with strong, diffuse immunoreactivity for S-100 protein, such a staining pattern should always suggest reconsideration of various benign diagnoses such as cellular schwannoma. Leu-7 and myelin basic protein are found in about 50% and 40% of MPNSTs, respectively.[84] Since none of these markers are specific for neural differentiation, it is prudent to assess a panel of antigens to determine whether a given tumor is displaying neural differentiation.

Text continued on p. 901.

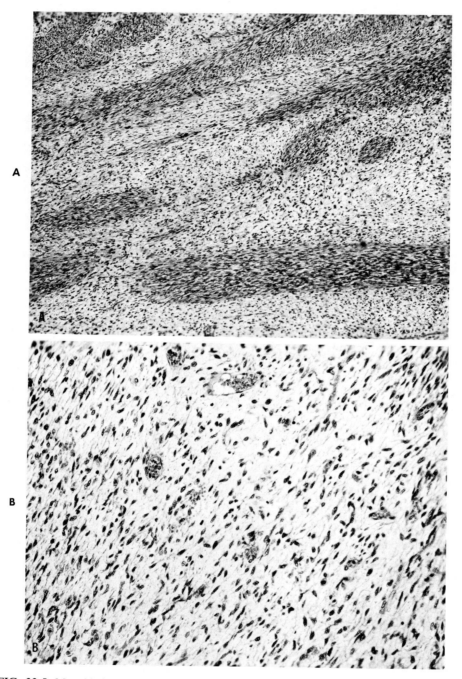

FIG. 32-5. Myxoid change is commonly seen in malignant peripheral nerve sheath tumor. Fascicles become widely separated (**A**), and in myxoid zones cells often lose their parallel orientation (**B**). (**A** ×60; **B** ×160.)

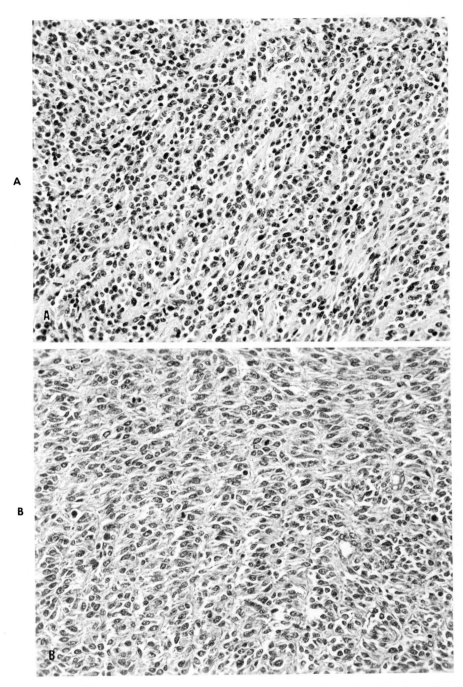

FIG. 32-6. Malignant peripheral nerve sheath tumor showing areas composed of rounded (**A**) or short fusiform (**B**) cells. In **B**, vague alignment of nuclei (early nuclear palisading) can be seen. (**A** and **B**, ×250)

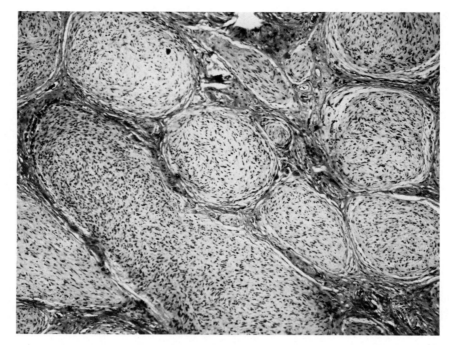

FIG. 32-7. Nodular or plexiform pattern within a malignant peripheral nerve sheath tumor. (×60.)

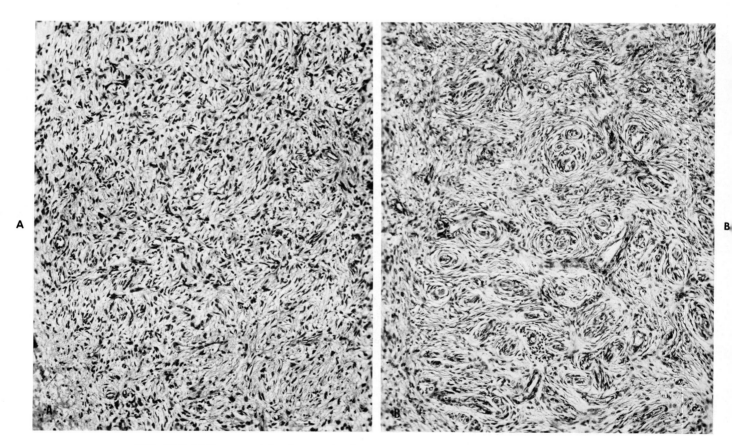

FIG. 32-8. Malignant peripheral nerve sheath tumor showing curlicue arrangement (A) and whorling of tumor cells (B). The latter is reminiscent of rudimentary tactoid differentiation. (A and B, ×100.)

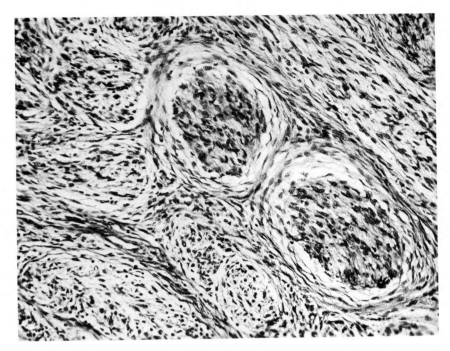

FIG. 32-9. Whorled structures within a malignant peripheral nerve sheath tumor. (×160.)

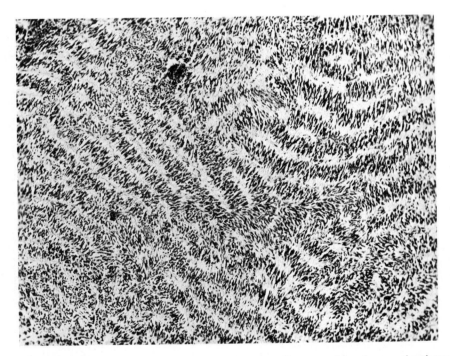

FIG. 32-10. Well-developed nuclear palisading within a malignant peripheral nerve sheath tumor. This feature is rather uncommon and is rarely as striking as is portrayed in this tumor. (×75.)

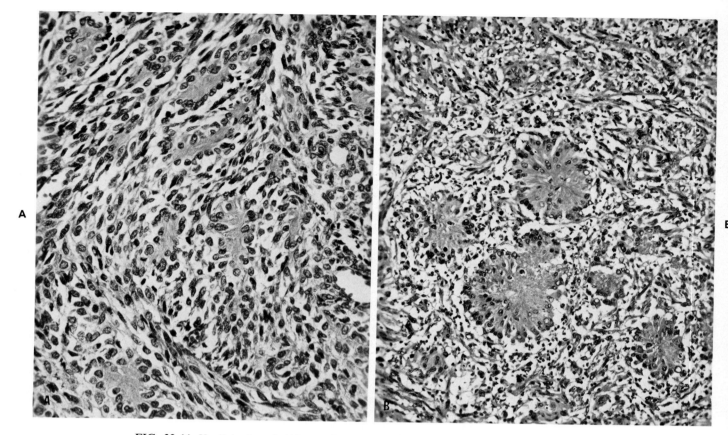

FIG. 32-11. Hyalinized cords **(A)** or nodules **(B)** are uncommon but distinctive features of malignant peripheral nerve sheath tumor. Similar structures may also be seen in neurilemomas. (**A**, ×250; **B**, ×160.)

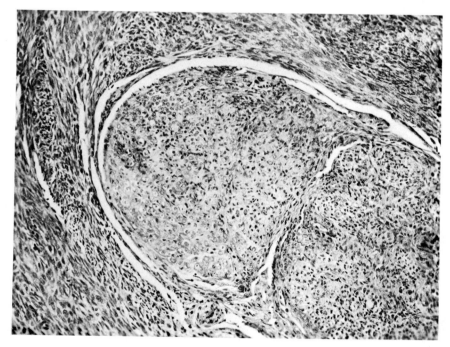

FIG. 32-12. Replacement of peripheral nerve by malignant peripheral nerve sheath tumor. Perineural extension is a common mode of spread. (×160.)

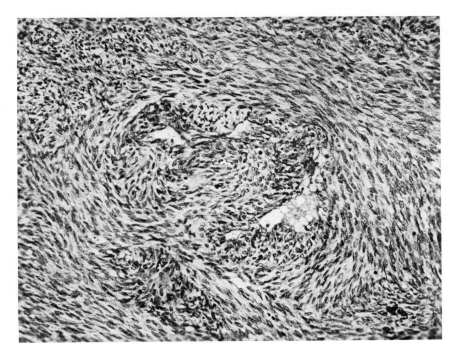

FIG. 32-13. Peculiar "proliferative" change occurring around small vessel in malignant peripheral nerve sheath tumor. (×160.)

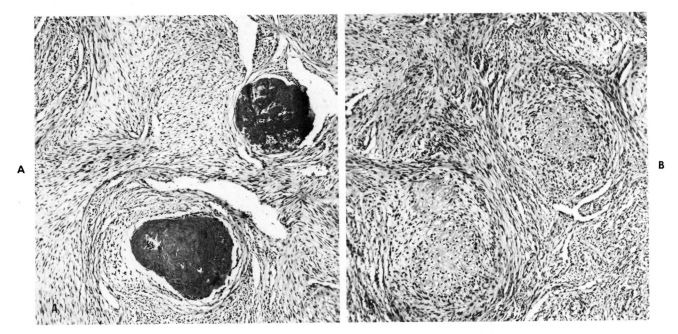

FIG. 32-14. Heterologous elements with a malignant peripheral nerve sheath tumor are most often bone (**A**) and cartilage (**B**). (**A** and **B**, ×60.)

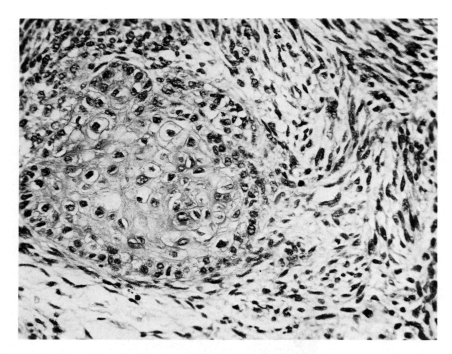

FIG. 32-15. Unique example of squamous elements as a form of heterologous differentiation within a malignant peripheral nerve sheath tumor. (×250.)

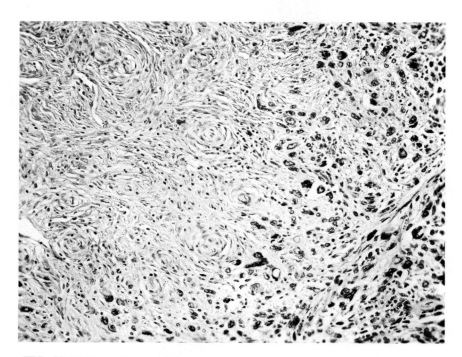

FIG. 32-16. Neurofibroma *(left)* showing focus of malignant change *(right)*. (×160.)

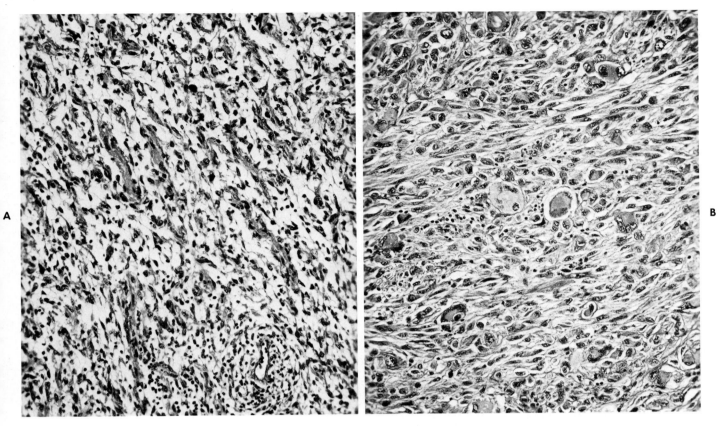

FIG. 32-17. Malignant peripheral nerve sheath tumor (**A**) with pleomorphic areas resembling a malignant fibrous histiocytoma (**B**). (**A** and **B**, ×160.)

Electron microscopic findings

MPNSTs are characterized by many of the same features as benign nerve sheath tumors. Most significantly, the spindled or polygonal cells give off nontapered branching cytoplasmic processes that extend for appreciable distances from the cell body and contain microtubules and neurofilaments (Fig. 32-18). The processes usually lie close to one another and form junctional complexes.[55] In well-differentiated MPNSTs, the cells and processes are coated with basal lamina,[7,24,39,54] and occasional wisps of cytoplasm curl around themselves in the manner of mesaxon formation.[54] In less well-differentiated MPNSTs, the cell processes are broader[24] and the basal laminae are poorly developed or incomplete.[24,54] The matrix contains collagen in various forms (e.g., typical, long spacing, and broad amianthoid fibers)[61] as well as wisps and scrolls of basal lamina. One unique example of MPNST contained annulate lamellae.[31] These ultrastructural features are most compatible with schwannian differentiation. However, there is some evidence that fibroblast-like cells may participate in MPNST associated with von Recklinghausen's disease,[7] just as they participate in benign neurofibromas. Nonethe-

less, it should be recalled that the perineural fibroblast and Schwann cell are closely related and may represent structural modulations of the same cell determined by their locations within the nerve sheath.[11]

Differential diagnosis

Most MPNSTs are easily diagnosed as malignant tumors, and the major challenge resides in distinguishing them from other sarcomas such as fibrosarcoma, monophasic synovial sarcoma, and leiomyosarcoma. As implied previously, both fibrosarcoma and synovial sarcoma have a more uniform fascicular pattern, contain symmetrical fusiform cells resembling fibroblasts, and obviously lack features of neural differentiation. Monophasic synovial sarcoma often contains densely hyalinized or calcified areas, or both, in combination with areas suggesting rudimentary epithelial differentiation in the form of clusters of rounded cells with clear cytoplasm.

Immunostaining for cytokeratin and S-100 protein also aids in the differential diagnosis. Immunoreactive cytokeratin can be detected within a significant number of monophasic synovial sarcomas but is absent except within

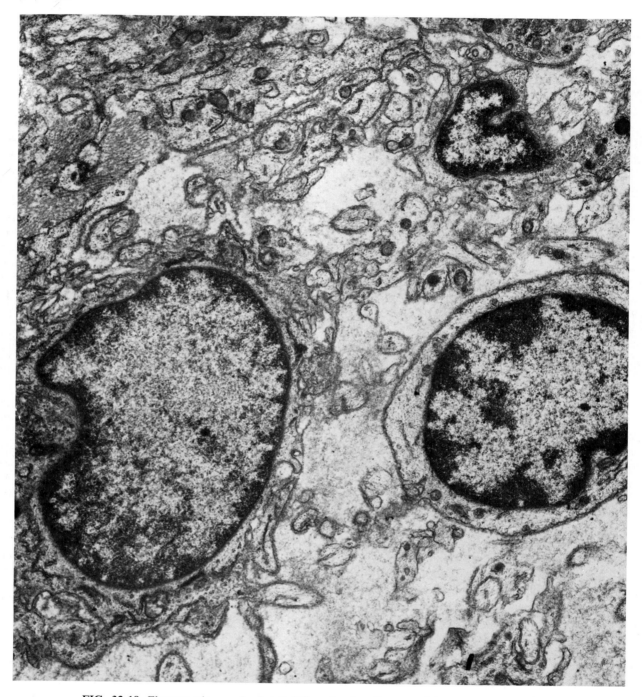

FIG. 32-18. Electron micrograph of well-differentiated malignant peripheral nerve sheath tumor (epithelioid type). Elaborate branched cytoplasmic processes covered by basal lamina characterize the tumor. (×4600.) (Courtesy Dr. Michael D. Lagios.)

the glands of glandular malignant schwannoma (see p. 904). On the other hand, S-100 protein is only occasionally identified within synovial sarcomas, but is present in 50% to 90% of MPNSTs.[16,52,60,81,84] Typically the staining is rather focal and the number of immunoreactive cells is small compared with neurofibroma and neurilemoma, reflecting either a loss of differentiation or a shift from a Schwann cell (S-100 protein positive) to a perineural cell (S-100 protein negative) population. Myelin basic protein has been identified in about half of MPNSTs,[84] but there are far fewer data concerning the specificity of immunostaining for this antigen in mesenchymal tumors. Neuron-specific enolase and neurofilament proteins have also been identified in malignant schwannoma, where their presence has been interpreted as evidence that these tumors occasionally display neuronal differentiation.[52]

Leiomyosarcoma can usually be separated from malignant schwannoma without undue difficulty. Its cells have distinct eosinophilic cytoplasm, centrally placed, blunt-ended nuclei, and occasional juxtanuclear vacuoles. In ambiguous situations special stains are helpful, as the cytoplasm of leiomyosarcoma is fuchsinophilic with longitudinal striations (Masson trichrome stain) and contains at least moderate amounts of glycogen (PAS preparation). The cytoplasm of MPNSTs is usually less fuchsinophilic (with no longitudinal striations) and contains little or no glycogen.

Only occasionally must a benign nerve sheath tumor be distinguished from an MPNST. This occurs typically with "borderline" neurofibromatous lesions of von Recklinghausen's disease. These neurofibromas may be quite cellular and even contain pleomorphic cells. However, it is the presence of mitotic activity that should be used as the principal criterion in establishing the diagnosis of malignancy. In rare instances, one may encounter a typical neurofibroma in which small foci may appear malignant by virtue of the pleomorphism and mitotic activity. We have interpreted such lesions as "neurofibroma with focal malignant change" and recommended conservative excision if the focus constitutes a small portion of the entire neurofibroma and the focus appeared totally removed by the excision. Preliminary follow-up in these cases supports this conservative approach to management.

The criterion of mitotic activity, paradoxically, does not apply to neurilemomas. Neurilemoma displaying mitotic activity pursues a benign course, and rarely has this tumor been known to undergo malignant degeneration. Thus when material from a small biopsy specimen is evaluated, it is hazardous to attempt to distinguish a cellular neurilemoma from a malignant schwannoma solely on the basis of mitotic activity. In this situation, a larger sample of the mass is necessary to determine if the tumor in question has an Antoni A and B pattern, perivascular hyalinization, encapsulation, or other typical features of a neurilemoma.

Discussion

The majority of MPNSTs are high-grade sarcomas, with a high likelihood of producing local recurrence and distant metastasis. There has been a growing body of literature indicating that those tumors associated with neurofibromatosis 1 have a particularly poor prognosis when compared with those occurring on a sporadic basis.* This has not been a surprising observation because of the presumed tendency of tumors in neurofibromatosis 1 to be large, central, and deep. In two recent large studies this has not been confirmed, however.[40,79] In a large series from Memorial Hospital in which the authors compared tumors of roughly comparable size and location (buttock and leg) in patients with and without neurofibromatosis 1, there was no significant difference in behavior. Approximately 40% of patients in both groups developed local recurrence, and this could be correlated with the type of surgery and the presence of positive margins.[40,79] Sixty-five percent of patients in both groups developed distant metastasis with a comparable interval between surgery and metastasis (14 to 18 months).[40] The overall 5-year survival rate in the experience of Wanebo et al. was 43.7%, with factors such as age of patient, size and location of tumor, and margins most influential on outcome.[79] The most common metastatic site in this tumor is the lung (22 cases), followed by bone (9 cases), the pleura (6 cases), and the retroperitoneum (4 cases). Only 2 of 22 patients with metastatic disease developed regional node metastasis, indicating that routine lymph node dissections do not play an important role in the treatment of this disease. This also emphasizes the fact that metastatic spindle cell lesions with Schwann cell–like features are apt to be metastatic desmoplastic or neurotropic melanoma or some other spindle cell tumor mimicking MPNST. One should also be aware of the propensity of this tumor to spread for considerable distances along the nerve sheath, and there are reports of tumors entering the subarachnoid space of the spinal cord via this route.[71] Therefore it is wise to obtain a frozen section of the nerve margins in order to assess the adequacy of the excision. In the experience of most, regional lymph node metastasis is uncommon[28,71]; consequently, lymph node dissections do not play a role in the primary surgical therapy of this disease. However, in our experience, lymph node metastasis may be seen in the face of widely metastatic disease.

Although MPNST does not occur very often in the pediatric age group, a recent large study by Meis et al. of 78 children under 14 years of age indicates that the long-term prognosis is no different in children.[56] In this study, 50% of patients developed metastasis within 2 years. Independent variables that influenced the prognosis adversely included large tumor size, age under 7 years, tumor

---

*References 13, 14, 23, 56, 68, 71.

necrosis of more than 25%, and the presence of neurofibromatosis 1.

Malignant peripheral nerve sheath tumor with rhabdomyoblastic differentiation (malignant Triton tumor)

In the broadest sense, a Triton tumor is any neoplasm showing both neural and skeletal muscle differentiation and includes neuromuscular hamartoma (benign Triton tumor),[33,62] medulloblastoma with rhabdomyosarcoma,[89] rhabdomyosarcoma with ganglion cells (ectomesenchymoma),[42] and MPNST with rhabdomyosarcoma.[5,16,35,87] By convention the term *malignant Triton tumor* is usually applied only to MPNST with rhabdomyosarcoma because it is the most widely recognized of the foregoing entities. This composite neoplasm was first described in 1932 by Masson and Martin,[51] who suggested the neural elements in the tumor induced the differentiation of skeletal muscle in much the same fashion as normal nerve was believed to induce the regeneration of skeletal muscle in the Triton salamander. As a result, these tumors were eventually accorded the name of the amphibian.

A review of all reported cases of Triton tumors in the literature attests to their relative rarity and their tendency to occur in neurofibromatosis 1.[87] About two thirds of the reported cases in the literature have occurred in patients with von Recklinghausen's disease.[5,21] However, our experience suggests the tumor may occur outside the setting of neurofibromatosis 1 more often than is generally appreciated. Low estimates of sporadic cases seem to result from errors in diagnosis, as evidenced by the fact that most cases are referred to us with a diagnosis of fibrosarcoma or rhabdomyosarcoma, depending on the prominence of the muscle component. Because most reported cases occur in patients with von Recklinghausen's disease, affected individuals are usually young (average age 35 years). The tumors are widely distributed, but most occur on the head, neck, and trunk. Like other MPNSTs, symptoms are related to a progressively enlarging mass that may give rise to neurological symptoms. Of the cases reviewed in the literature by Brooks et al., the 5-year survival rate was 12%.[5]

The hallmark of this tumor is the presence of rhabdomyoblasts scattered throughout a stroma indistinguishable from an ordinary MPNST (Fig. 32-19). The number of rhabdomyoblasts varies greatly from tumor to tumor and even from area to area within the same tumor. They are usually relatively mature, and their abundant eosinophilic cytoplasm contrasts sharply with the pale-staining cytoplasm of the Schwann cells. Cross-striations can be identified but, as in rhabdomyosarcomas, are more readily identified in cells possessing elongated tapered cytoplasm (Fig. 32-19, *B*). Both desmin and myoglobin can be demonstrated within the

rhabdomyoblasts, although the latter tends to be present in only the most mature elements (Chapter 22).

The histogenesis of these unusual tumors has occasioned much discussion. Although Masson believed that one cell line induced the other, it seems just as likely that both cell lines originate from less well-differentiated neural crest cells. Normally the neural crest contributes to the formation of mesenchyme in certain vertebrates and ultimately forms portions of branchial cartilage, connective tissue, and muscle in the facial region.[82] Thus, these tumors recapitulate both the schwannian and the mesenchymal potentiality of the neural crest.

Malignant peripheral nerve sheath tumor with glands (glandular malignant schwannoma)

In 1892, Garre[26] published a report of a patient with von Recklinghausen's disease and an MPNST of the sciatic nerve. Scattered throughout the schwannian background of the tumor were numerous well-differentiated glands. Since that time, fewer than 10 additional cases of these tumors have been published, probably making it the rarest form of MPNST. Almost all of these tumors have occurred in patients with von Recklinghausen's disease, a fact that easily accounts for the young median age (about 30 years)[86] of affected patients. The tumors usually arise from major nerves, including the sciatic,[26,59] median,[10] brachial plexus, and spinal nerves.[86] Characteristically, they have a spindle cell background indistinguishable from ordinary MPNST and may contain other heterotopic elements such as muscle, cartilage, and osteoid. The glands are usually few in number and are made up of well-differentiated, nonciliated cuboidal or columnar cells with clear cytoplasm and occasional goblet cells (Fig. 32-20). Intracellular and extracellular mucin, which are histochemically identical to conventional epithelial mucins, can be demonstrated within the glands. By electron microscopy, the glands have features of intestinal epithelium and possess numerous well-oriented microvilli with core rootlets.[77] Some of the cells within the glands are argyrophilic and contain dense core granules.[80] Somatostatin immunoreactivity has been noted in the glands of one glandular schwannoma.[80] On rare occasion, the glands may appear histologically malignant. There may be some difficulty in separating these tumors from biphasic synovial sarcomas because the glandular elements may be virtually identical. It is the nature of the spindled element that distinguishes them. In synovial sarcomas the spindled element resembles a conventional fibrosarcoma and may be secondarily modified by dense hyalinization or calcification. Subtle degrees of epithelial differentiation may also be evident in the spindled stroma of the synovial sarcoma. This feature is not present in glandular MPNST, because the epithelial elements invariably arise rather abruptly from the stroma. The immunological phe-

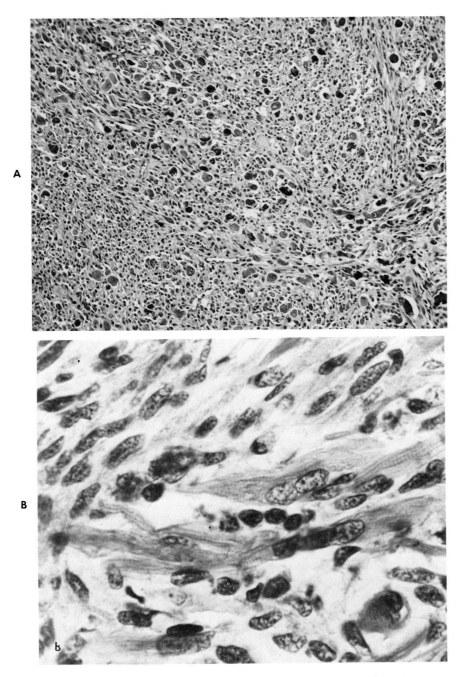

FIG. 32-19. Malignant peripheral nerve sheath tumor with rhabdomyoblastic differentiation (malignant Triton tumor). **A,** Large, rounded or elongated rhabdomyoblasts are scattered throughout the tumor. (×100.) **B,** Distinct cross-striations can be identified within the rhabdomyoblasts. (×750.)

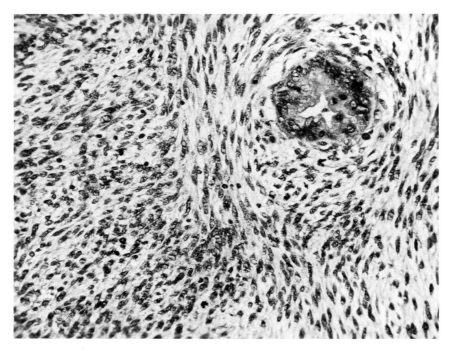

FIG. 32-20. Malignant peripheral nerve sheath tumor with glandular differentiation (glandular malignant schwannoma). (×250.)

notype of synovial sarcoma and glandular MPNST differs. The former often contains keratin-positive cells in the spindled zones (and very rarely S-100 protein-positive ones), whereas the latter displays only focal S-100 protein positivity.

Although the glandular elements set this tumor apart as a peculiar histological variant, they serve essentially no role in grading the tumor or in predicting its biological behavior. Tumors having a highly malignant schwannian component may be expected to do poorly regardless of the degree of differentiation of the glands. Most tumors reported in the literature seem to fall into this category. On the other hand, tumors having a low-grade schwannian element may do extremely well, as illustrated by the fact that the two patients with tumors of this type reported by Woodruff[86] are alive and well.

The source of the epithelial elements within these tumors has remained controversial. Some authors have suggested that they arise from heterotopic ependymal cells located within the peripheral nerve,[16,27] and some authors claim to have documented ependymal features. The presence of goblet cells within these glands, the degree of mucin production, and the consistent absence of blepharoplasts argue against this interpretation. A more tenable suggestion is that the Schwann cell or a less committed precursor differentiates along epithelial and schwannian lines.

Epithelioid malignant peripheral nerve sheath tumor (epithelioid malignant schwannoma)

Epithelioid MPNST is an unusual form of MPNST that closely resembles carcinoma or melanoma.* Although we estimated that 5% or less of MPNSTs belong to this group, this estimate may be far too generous. In fact, for many years the exact nature of this unusual group of tumors was questioned, as indicated by Stewart and Copeland: "We have observed tumors of deeper nerve trunks which looked like certain nonpigmented melanomas yet did not run the clinical course of melanoma. Are these melanomas or neurosarcomas?"[71]

There is convincing evidence that these tumors do represent nerve sheath tumors rather than melanomas or metastatic carcinomas. First, the tumors follow a similar distribution to ordinary MPNST, with most occurring in patients 20 to 50 years of age. In our recently published experience of 26 cases, the median age was 36 years; men were slightly more often affected than women. The majority of those tumors reported in the literature originated in major nerves, including the sciatic,[10,32,48] tibial,[59] peroneal,[53] facial,[74] antebrachial cutaneous,[32] and digital nerves.[32] In our experience, 8 of 10 deeply situated epithelioid MPNSTs originated from a major nerve, including the

*References 1, 20, 27, 32, 48, 49, 53, 71, 74.

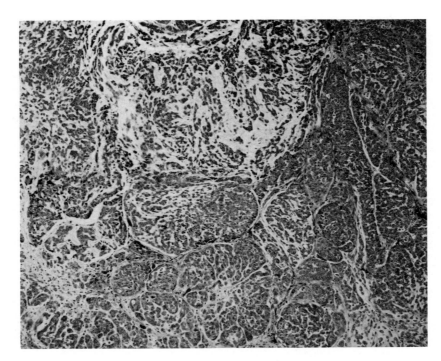

FIG. 32-21. Epithelioid malignant peripheral nerve sheath tumor showing vague nodular growth. Tumor varies from slightly myxoid to cellular. (×60.)

sciatic (3 cases), brachial plexus, femoral, radial, and median nerves (1 case each). It is those cases in which origin from a nerve or neurofibroma cannot be documented that pose the most challenging and sometimes unresolvable problems in diagnosis. Although this form of MPNST may occur in neurofibromatosis 1,[32,71,73,83] this seems to occur less frequently than in ordinary MPNST. Lodding et al.[48] encountered one case in their series of 16, whereas none of our 26 patients had the disease.

Histologically, the tumor is quite variable. In our cases the most characteristic appearance is that of short cords of large epithelioid cells arranged in a vague nodular pattern (Figs. 32-21 and 32-22). The cells within these tumors usually have large round nuclei with prominent melanoma-like nucleoli (Fig. 32-23). The tumors may appear densely cellular or myxoid (Fig. 32-24), depending on the accumulation of acid mucin between the cords, and there is often a subtle blending of the epithelial areas with spindled areas resembling conventional MPNST (Fig. 32-25). However, it is our belief that the term *epithelioid MPNST* should be reserved for those tumors in which the predominant pattern is epithelioid. Although the combination of all of these features is usually sufficient to make the correct diagnosis, many tumors lack this distinctive appearance. In fact, most tumors reported in the literature have resembled melanomas or carcinomas and have consisted

simply of small nests of epithelial cells admixed with a spindled component.

There are a number of rather unusual forms of epithelioid MPNST that deserve comment in passing. Some contain a predominance of clear cells (Fig. 32-26); others may be made up of rhabdoid cells with a prominent glassy eosinophilic perinuclear zone corresponding ultrastructurally to the presence of whorls of intermediate filaments (Fig. 32-27). Still other tumors consist of sheets of rounded pleomorphic cells suggestive of a pleomorphic carcinoma.

Consequently, the diagnosis has largely depended on established origin from a nerve. In the absence of this feature, the diagnosis can sometimes be suspected by a delicate "mesenchymal" pattern of collagenization and a transition to spindled "schwannian" areas (Fig. 32-25). Unlike many melanomas, neither melanin pigment nor glycogen can be demonstrated within the cytoplasm of these tumors. In one unique case we reviewed, the diagnosis of "malignant epithelioid schwannoma" was established by virtue of the presence of true rosettes in a tumor that otherwise resembled melanoma (Fig. 32-28). It should be emphasized that a clear-cut distinction from melanoma or carcinoma is not always possible on routine sections, a dilemma compounded by the fact that occasionally metastatic spindled melanomas are virtually indistinguishable from malignant schwannoma (Fig. 32-29).

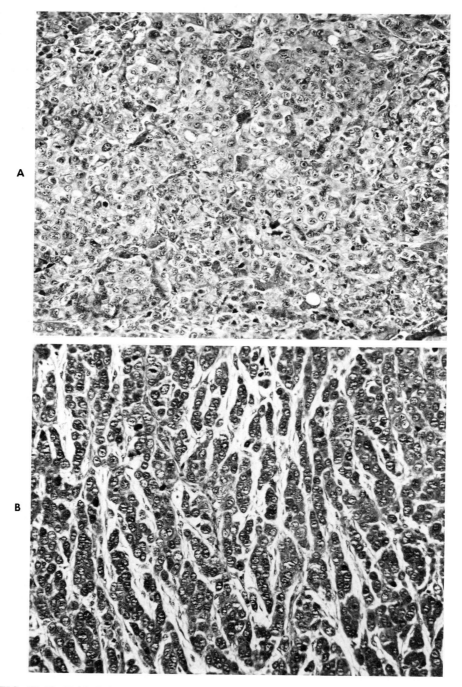

FIG. 32-22. Epithelioid malignant peripheral nerve sheath tumor. Tumor arose from buttock of 9-year-old child. **A,** Original tumor was initially considered a carcinoma because of sheetlike epithelioid pattern. **B,** Recurrence demonstrated more typical cordlike pattern. No tumor was identified elsewhere in patient. (**A** and **B,** ×160.)

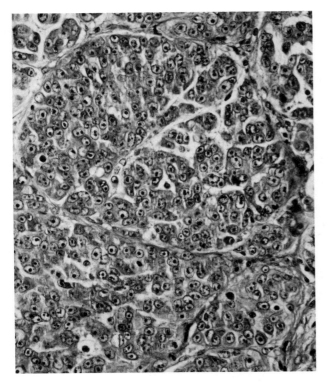

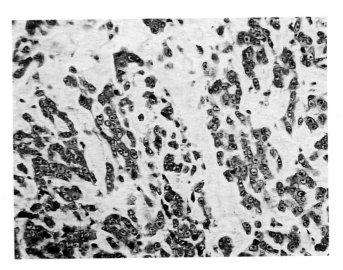

FIG. 32-24. Myxoid change within an epithelioid malignant peripheral nerve sheath tumor. (×250.)

FIG. 32-23. Epithelioid malignant peripheral nerve sheath tumor showing polygonal shape of cells and prominent nucleoli. (×250.)

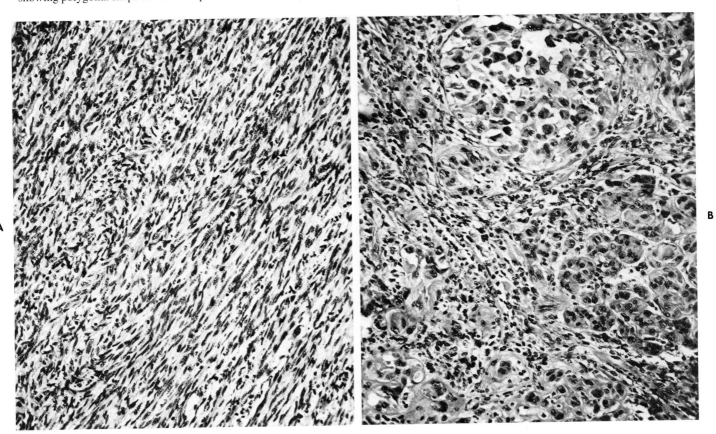

A

B

FIG. 32-25. Epithelioid malignant peripheral nerve sheath tumor. Tumor can be recognized by virtue of its spindled areas (A), which are typical of conventional forms of malignant peripheral nerve sheath tumor. Areas of epithelial differentiation (B) are indistinguishable from a carcinoma or melanoma. (A and B, ×160.)

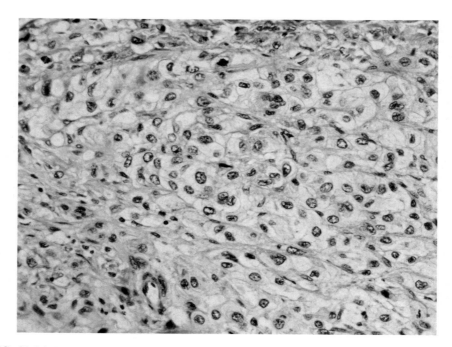

FIG. 32-26. Rare example of an epithelioid malignant peripheral nerve sheath tumor having clear cell features. (×250.)

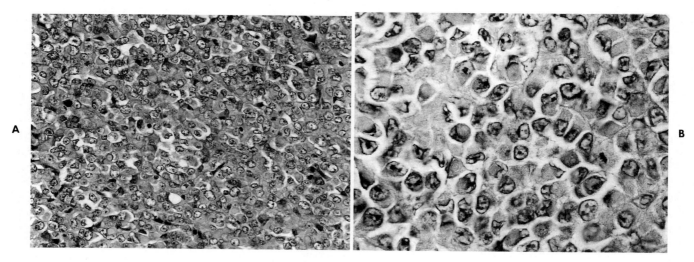

FIG. 32-27. A, Epithelioid malignant peripheral nerve sheath tumor with rhabdoid cells. **B,** High power of rhabdoid cells showing glassy perinuclear zone. (**A,** ×250; **B,** ×400.)

In our experience, about 80% of these tumors are strongly and diffusely positive for S-100 protein, a pattern of immunoreactivity that contrasts with conventional MPNST.[46] They do not express a melanoma-associated antigen or keratin in the limited cases we have studied. Thus, these two antigens could help distinguish this tumor from melanoma or carcinoma in some instances. Care must be

employed in interpreting the results of immunostaining, however, since aberrant expression of keratin has come to be accepted as part of the repertoire of a variety of sarcomas. Type IV collagen can be identified readily between individual cells as well as groups of cells with immunohistochemical procedures, but regrettably the pattern of basal lamina deposition does not help in distinguishing this tu-

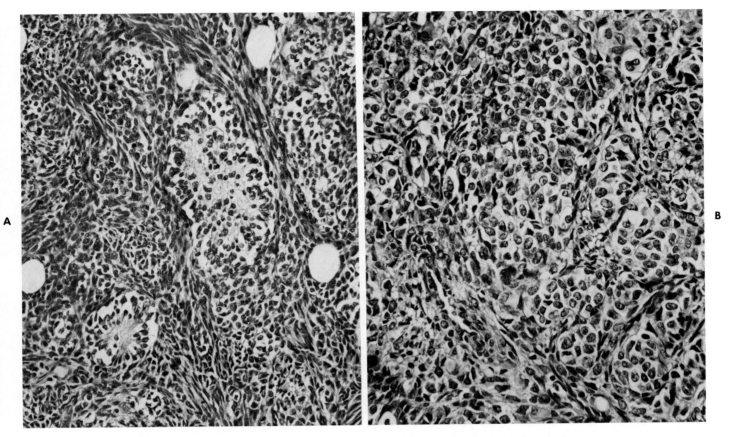

FIG. 32-28. Unique example of malignant peripheral nerve sheath tumor showing focal rosette differentiation in the original tumor **(A)** and purely epithelial differentiation in the recurrence **(B)** and metastasis. **(A, ×160; B, ×250.)**

mor from melanoma, which also shares considerable overlap.[46]

The ultrastructural features of epithelioid MPNST vary as a function of differentiation. Whereas it is possible to identify interlocking cell processes invested with basal lamina and displaying cell junctions, these features are not invariably present.

Despite the limited number of reported cases, there is no doubt that they are fully malignant tumors and should be treated accordingly. At least half of the patients reported in the literature developed distant metastases, usually in the lung. In our experience with 10 tumors occurring within deep soft tissue, 3 developed metastatic disease.[46] Because of the melanoma-like appearance of these tumors, the question has been raised as to whether they commonly spread to regional lymph nodes. Lodding et al. noted lymph node metastasis in three of their 14 cases,[48] while we had no instances of lymph node metastasis in 16 cases.[46] Until additional cases adequately address the question, it seems prudent to at least clinically evaluate these tumors before deciding on definitive therapy.

Superficial epithelioid malignant peripheral nerve sheath tumor

A significant number of epithelioid MPNSTs may occur in the superficial soft tissues. Until recently, such tumors were unrecognized probably because they were diagnosed as other forms of malignancy. In our recent study of epithelioid MPNSTs, over half of the tumors occurred in the dermis or subcutaneous tissue. Unlike deep lesions, these were not multinodular, but rather uninodular masses circumscribed by the capsule of a preexisting nerve or neurofibroma. Within the nodule, the cells are arranged in small groups or cohesive nests somewhat reminiscent of those in a nevus (Fig. 32-30). The cells typically mold to one another with little or no intervening stroma, although the nests are separated by a fibrous or myxoid stroma. The cells, however, display the same prominence of nucleoli and mitotic activity as those in soft tissue. Like their deep counterparts, S-100 protein can usually be identified. The behavior of this group of lesions is quite good, probably because of their superficial location, sharp circumscription, and smaller size. In this group only one of 16 patients in our review developed metastasis to the lung.

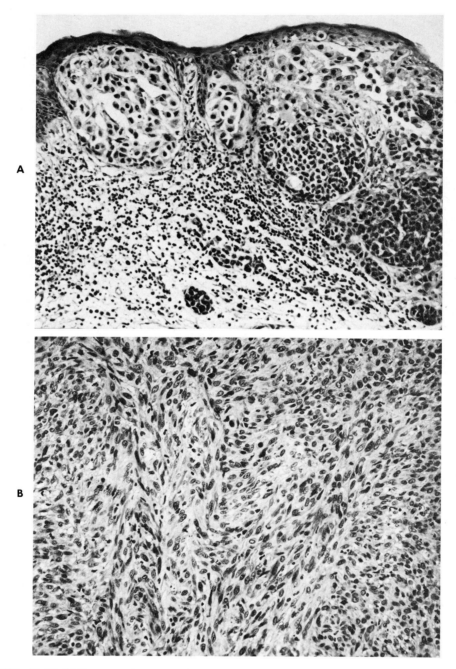

FIG. 32-29. Malignant melanoma of back **(A)** with axillary metastasis **(B)** that resembled malignant peripheral nerve sheath tumor. Spindled malignant melanoma and malignant peripheral nerve sheath tumor may occasionally be indistinguishable from each other. **(A** and **B,** ×160.)

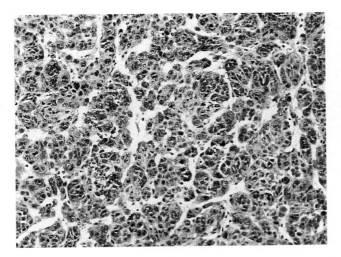

FIG. 32-30. Superficial form of epithelioid malignant peripheral nerve sheath tumor consisting of nests of epithelioid cells. (×160.)

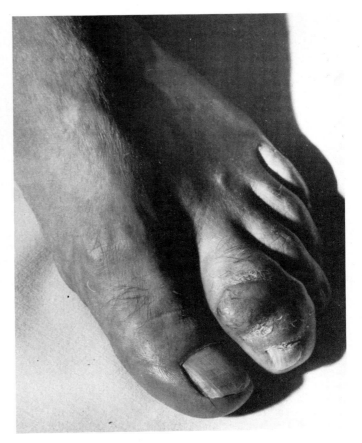

FIG. 32-31. Clear cell sarcoma of the second toe.

CLEAR CELL SARCOMA (MALIGNANT MELANOMA OF SOFT PARTS)

Described in 1968 by Enzinger,[101] clear cell sarcoma has become a well-accepted clinicopathological entity. Although it possesses the ability to produce melanin,[91,93,100,123,131] it has a clinical presentation quite different from conventional melanoma in that it is more deeply located, is nearly always intimately associated with tendons or aponeuroses, lacks epidermal involvement and junctional changes, and displays a more uniform growth pattern characterized by pale-staining fusiform tumor cells that are arranged in nestlike aggregates. Moreover, recent cytogenetic analysis of a small number of clear cell sarcomas indicates that in most there is a translocation of chromosomes 12 and 22, an alteration not encountered in malignant melanoma.* Although the term *malignant melanoma of soft parts* is used as a synonym for this tumor, it is important that this lesion not be loosely considered a malignant melanoma, but rather segregated as a unique tumor of soft tissue.

Clinical findings

Clear cell sarcoma mainly afflicts young adults between the ages of 20 and 40 years, but in rare instances it may occur in the very young and the very old. The age range in our series of 141 patients[97] was 7 to 83 years; the median age was 27 years. Women were affected more commonly than men. The principal sites of the neoplasm are the extremities, especially the region of the foot and ankle; 63 (43%) of our 141 cases originated in this general region. Next in frequency are the knee, thigh, and hand, where another 51 (36%) of the cases occurred (Fig. 32-31). The head

*References 94, 95, 118, 127, 129, 132.

Table 32-1. Anatomical distribution of 141 cases of clear cell sarcoma (malignant melanoma of soft parts)[97]

Location	No. patients	Percent
Head and neck	1	0.8
Trunk	3	2.1
Upper extremity	31	22.0
Lower extremity (foot 28; knee 21; heel 15; ankle 11)	106	75.1
TOTAL	141	100.0

and neck region and the trunk are only rarely involved (Table 32-1). Clear cell sarcoma is usually deep seated and, like epithelioid sarcoma, is often intimately bound to tendons or aponeuroses. The overlying skin tends to be uninvolved, although many of the larger tumors extend into the subcutis and lower dermis.

At the time of diagnosis, the tumor presents as a slowly enlarging mass causing tenderness or pain in about half of the cases. At the time of operation the duration of symp-

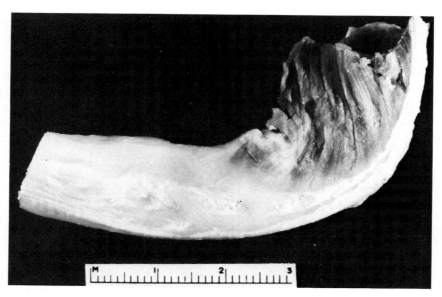

FIG. 32-32. Clear cell sarcoma of the Achilles tendon in a 50-year-old man. Note diffuse infiltration into tendon and muscle tissue. (From Enzinger FM: *Cancer* 18:1163, 1965.)

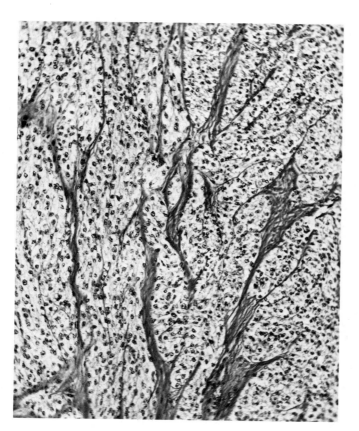

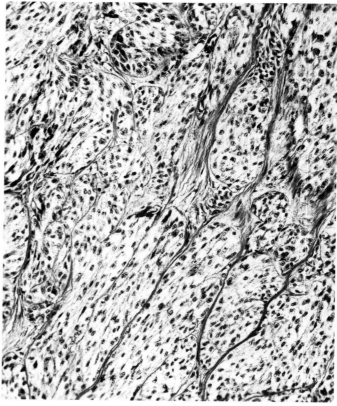

FIG. 32-33. Clear cell sarcoma showing arrangement of the pale-staining tumor cells in short fascicles separated by dense fibrous septa. (×130.)

FIG. 32-34. Clear cell sarcoma. Fibrous tissue septa divide the tumor into well-defined nests and groups of pale-staining tumor cells. (×160.)

toms varies substantially, averaging 2 years but ranging from a few weeks to 20 years. In fact, clear cell sarcomas that have been present for 5 or more years are not uncommon. A history of trauma or injury to the site of the tumor is given in slightly less than half of the patients.

Roentgenograms are of little help in diagnosis. Nearly always they merely reveal a soft tissue mass without calcification and without any changes in the underlying bone. Raynor et al.[123] noted destruction of the phalanx in a patient with clear cell sarcoma of the left thumb. Angiograms vary in appearance, and both richly vascular and poorly vascular clear cell sarcomas have been observed.[90]

Pathological findings

Macroscopically the tumor consists of a circumscribed, but rarely encapsulated, lobulated or multinodular mass that displays a gray-white surface on sectioning. Frequently the mass is attached to tendons or aponeuroses and there is no connection with the overlying skin (Fig. 32-32). The tumor ranges in size from 1 cm to more than 10 cm, but in the majority of cases it measures 2 to 6 cm in diameter. The cut surface may be distorted by focal hemorrhage, ne-

crosis, or cystic change. Foci of dark brown or black pigmentation occur in about 2 out of 10 cases.[97]

Microscopic examination discloses a rather uniform pattern composed of compact nests or fascicles of rounded or fusiform cells with a clear cytoplasm bordered and defined by a delicate framework of fibrocollagenous tissue, which is often contiguous with adjacent tendons or aponeuroses. The individual cells have a fairly regular appearance, but they vary somewhat from tumor to tumor. In most instances they possess round to ovoid vesicular nuclei with prominent basophilic nucleoli and clear or pale-staining cytoplasm. They are associated with occasional multinucleated giant cells having 10 to 15 peripherally placed nuclei that are similar to those of the surrounding mononuclear tumor cells (Figs. 32-33 to 32-36). Less commonly the cells have a finely stippled eosinophilic cytoplasm and resemble those of a fibrosarcoma. Sometimes clear cells and eosinophilic cells coexist in different portions of the same neoplasm with focal transitions (Fig. 32-37). Rarely, especially in recurrent and metastatic neoplasms, the cells may become more pleomorphic with features suggesting diagnoses such as carcinoma or melanoma (Fig. 32-38). Mitotic figures

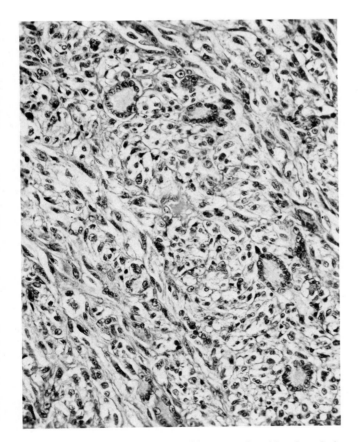

FIG. 32-35. Clear cell sarcoma with scattered multinucleated giant cells. The giant cells possess a wreath of peripherally placed nuclei of uniform size and shape. (×250.)

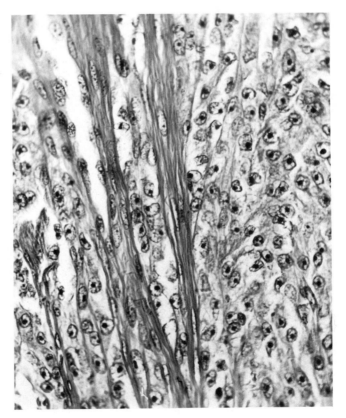

FIG. 32-36. Clear cell sarcoma exhibiting prominent vesicular nuclei with a large single nucleolus. Mitotic figures are rare. (×395.)

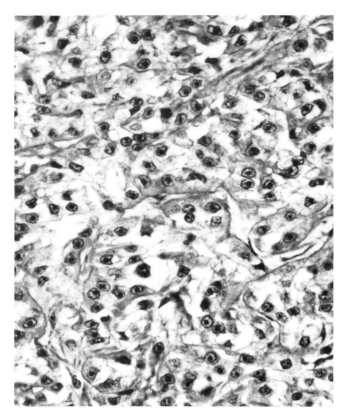

FIG. 32-37. Clear cell sarcoma showing a transition between clear cells and cells with a finely stippled eosinophilic cytoplasm. (×395.)

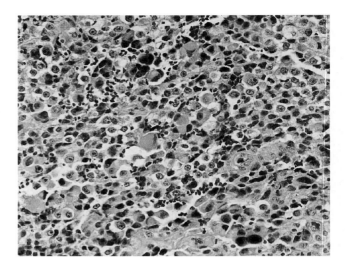

FIG. 32-38. Metastatic clear cell sarcoma displaying marked pleomorphism and essentially no spindling. Metastatic deposits of this type resemble melanoma or carcinoma. (×250.)

tend to be rare and usually amount to fewer than 2 or 3 mitotic figures/10 HPF. In contrast to synovial sarcoma, intracellular mucin is absent, but alcian blue-positive, hyaluronidase-sensitive mucoid material is sometimes deposited outside the tumor cells. It may lead to loss of cellular cohesion and may mimic a richly myxoid sarcoma. In general, however, there is little or no mucoid material, and the clear cell appearance is a result of the presence of large amounts of intracellular glycogen. Reticulin preparations accentuate the nestlike pattern and clearly outline the collagenous framework that separates the cellular aggregates (Fig. 32-39). In some tumors, the nestlike pattern is absent or inconspicuous. Intracellular melanin is rarely seen with hematoxylin-eosin stain, but it is detected with Fontana's stain in almost 50% of cases (Fig. 32-40), and with the more sensitive Warthin-Starry preparation (at pH 3.2) in 60% to 75% of cases. It is also noteworthy that in some instances melanin is absent in the primary tumor but is abundant in the metastasis, and that many clear cell sarcomas contain hemosiderin that may stain positively with Fontana's stain or Warthin-Starry preparation. In cases of

doubt, an iron preparation is necessary to clearly distinguish melanin from hemosiderin.

Immunohistochemically, the cells of nearly all cases express antigens for S-100 protein and many a melanoma-associated antigen (as defined by HMB45),[129] reflective of melanin synthesis. Neuron-specific enolase, Leu-7, and LN3 have also been noted within these lesions.[130] Under the electron microscope, the tumor consists of oval or fusiform cells with rounded nuclei, evenly dispersed chromatin at the nuclear membrane, and a large, centrally placed, single nucleolus. The cytoplasm contains multiple, rounded and swollen mitochondria, membrane-bound vesicles, and ribosomes and polyribosomes in varying numbers.[91,123] There are also aggregates of rough endoplasmic reticulum, scanty amounts of glycogen, and occasional lipid droplets. Mononuclear and multinuclear cells display similar ultrastructural characteristics. Melanosomes in varying stages of development are present in most cases. Some of them show dense pigmentation; others exhibit the typical lamellar, striated, or "barrel-stave" internal structure of premelanosomes (Fig. 32-41). Basal laminae surround groups of closely apposed neoplastic cells. Collagen fibers are abundant in the extracellular spaces.[91,92,123] Benson et al.[92] also described occasional cells with stubby or fingerlike dendritic processes, a few of which contained longitudinally aligned filaments.

Differential diagnosis

Although several of the tumors in our series and the literature were initially diagnosed as synovial sarcoma[90,101,112] and a relationship between both tumors was

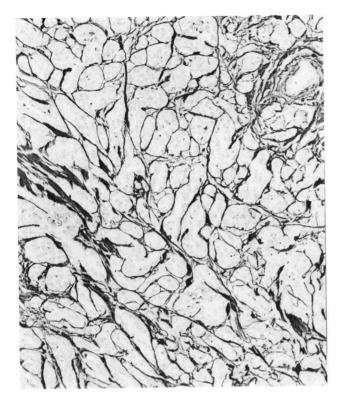

FIG. 32-39. Clear cell sarcoma. Reticulin preparation outlines loose meshwork of reticulin fibers, which surround the individual nests of tumor cells. (Reticulin preparation; ×410.)

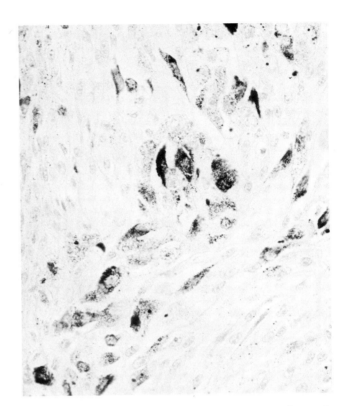

FIG. 32-40. Clear cell sarcoma. Fontana's stain revealing melanin pigment within some of the tumor cells. (Fontana's stain; ×400.)

claimed in the literature (tendosynovial sarcoma),[103] a reliable microscopic distinction of both tumors is feasible if attention is paid to the absence of a biphasic cellular pattern and intracellular mucin and, in more than half of cases, to the presence of intracellular melanin. Tsuneyoshi et al.[133] distinguished between "synovial" and "melanotic" types of clear cell sarcoma, a rather arbitrary and subjective division that is not possible in our opinion.

Differentiation from fibrosarcoma may be more problematic, particularly in those cases which lack the clear cell appearance of the tumor cells and consist of spindle-shaped cells with eosinophilic cytoplasm and smaller, less prominent nucleoli. In these cases, special stains may help in arriving at a reliable diagnosis, since the cells of fibrosarcoma are not arranged in distinct cellular aggregates, lack immunoreactivity for S-100 protein, and are devoid of glycogen. Separation from an epithelioid form of MPNST and a spindle cell melanoma may be much more difficult. In fact, it may be impossible in rare cases. MPNST, however, is often associated with a large peripheral nerve or with manifestations of neurofibromatosis; moreover, its cells rarely contain glycogen, have dense hyperchromatic nuclei, and

display more prominent mitotic activity. MPNSTs with melanin formation do exist, but they are exceedingly rare in our experience. As a rule, desmoplastic or spindle cell malignant melanoma,[125] a much more common condition, involves the dermis and is associated with pigmentation or junctional changes in the overlying or adjacent skin. Its cells also possess prominent nucleoli, infrequent mitotic figures, and intracellular glycogen, and show positive immunostaining for S-100 proteins, but they are rarely as pale-staining or as uniform as those of clear cell sarcoma. The prominent nucleoli and the more fusiform appearance of the tumor cells also assist in the differentiation from metastatic renal cell carcinoma.

Clinical course and behavior

Even in those cases which have been treated by seemingly adequate therapy, the prognosis is poor, and many patients develop recurrences and metastases. Among the 115 patients with follow-up information in our series,[97] 62 (54%) were alive and 53 (46%) had died, 50 of metastatic disease and three from some other unrelated cause. In 24 of the 50 cases the tumor recurred locally before metasta-

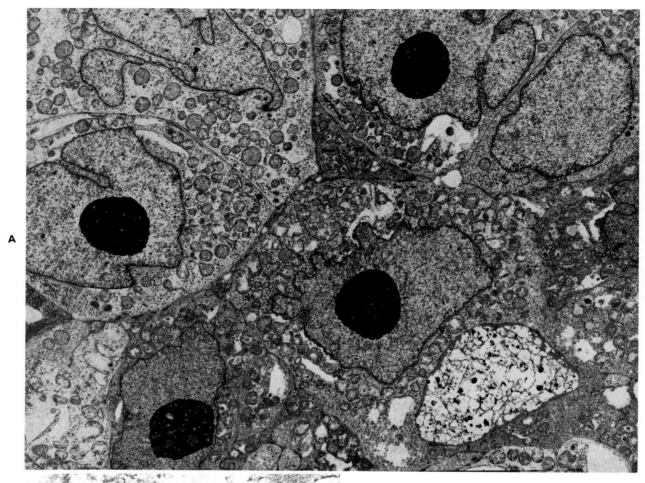

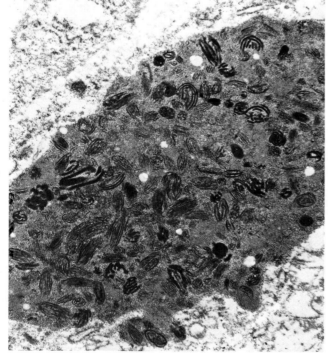

FIG. 32-41. A, Clear cell sarcoma (malignant melanoma of soft parts) showing tumor cells with irregular nuclear profiles, strikingly prominent nucleoli, and numerous mitochondria. (×4600.) (From Benson JD, Kraemer B, Mackay B: *Ultrastruct Pathol* 8:57, 1985.) B, Melanosomes with typical lamellar or "barrel-stave" internal structure in clear cell sarcoma. (×40,500.)

sis. Of the living patients, 34 were well without recurrence or metastasis, 21 with one or more recurrences, and seven with metastatic disease. Cases with four or more recurrences are common.[109,111] In our material the average time between diagnosis and recurrence was 2.6 years, between diagnosis and metastasis 3.5 years. It may be much longer, however. One of Mackenzie's patients[111] was alive after 26 years and four recurrences; similarly, one of our patients developed pulmonary metastasis 30 years after diagnosis. Prognostic factors in this disease include tumor size[116,128] and necrosis.[128] Other factors such as age, location, depth, or proliferation index have been found to be independent prognostic factors. The most common sites of metastasis are the lung, lymph nodes, and bone.[116,128]

The treatment that has been employed varies greatly. From our follow-up data it is obvious, however, that clear cell sarcoma is a highly malignant tumor that requires radical excision—or amputation if radical excision is not feasible—combined with radiotherapy and multiagent chemotherapy. Regional lymph node excision should be part of the therapy, especially if there is evidence of regional lymphadenopathy. Although our follow-up data are not particularly encouraging, apparent cures have been described with radiotherapy and chemotherapy (vincristine and bleomycin sulfate)[121] and with arterial limb perfusion (actinomycin D and L-phenylalanine mustard) and subsequent resection.[92] The fact that some tumors have recurred or metastasized 10 or more years after the initial tumor indicates that long-term follow-up is necessary before one can safely assume that the patient has been cured.

Discussion

There seems to be no doubt that clear cell sarcoma is a neuroectodermal tumor, although it is more difficult to place it clearly within the family of melanotic neuroectodermal tumors. In some cases the lesion seems akin to a pigmented MPNST, in others a deep and unusual form of malignant melanoma, or malignant cellular blue nevus possibly arising from melanocytes that have migrated to tendinous or aponeurotic structures during embryonic development. Schwann cell origin appears less likely for a number of reasons; among almost 200 examples of this tumor that we have seen in consultation, we have never observed the association of clear cell sarcoma and neurofibromatosis, nor have we ever encountered the tumor in a large peripheral nerve. Parker et al.[120] observed a "clear cell sarcoma" in the thoracic spinal cord, but from their illustrations it seems more likely that their tumor is an MPNST than a "bona fide" clear cell sarcoma. The frequency of lymph node metastasis in clear cell sarcoma and the presence of intracellular glycogen are also much more in keeping with a variant of malignant melanoma than an MPNST, in which both of these features are quite rare in our experience. In addition, positive immunostaining for S-100 protein and the ultra-

structural features support a melanoma-like neoplasm. It must be pointed out, however, that clear cell sarcoma, on the average, occurs in younger patients and displays a rather specific and less variable histological picture than malignant melanoma. Although Epstein et al.[102] concluded the tumor was closely related to melanoma on the basis of transplantation into nude mice, recent cytogenetic evidence indicates relative separateness of the two lesions.* In over three quarters of cases studied, there has been a translocation of chromosomes 12 and 22; in those lacking the translocation, various structural abnormalities in chromosome 22 have been observed. Melanomas, on the other hand, demonstrate primarily abnormalities on chromosomes 1, 6, 7, and 9.

NEUROTROPIC (DESMOPLASTIC) MELANOMA

In the first edition of this textbook we alluded to a form of epithelioid malignant schwannoma which, in our experience, appeared to arise from the dermal connective tissue and combine features of a conventional MPNST and malignant melanoma (malignant epithelioid schwannoma of superficial soft tissue). These are histologically identical to lesions described by Reed and Leonard[143] as "neurotropic melanoma" and by Conley et al.[137] as "desmoplastic melanoma." The choice of names in the former emphasizes the tendency for these tumors to migrate toward and spread along nerves, whereas the latter term highlights the remarkable desmoplastic properties of the tumor. In fact, both features may be seen to a varying degree within a given case. The term neurotropic melanoma is not used for conventional melanomas that simply display focal neurotropism. Most of these lesions probably originate from melanocytes of the epidermis, whereas only a small fraction arise de novo from the dermal structures. The size, appearance, and degree of melanocytic atypia within the precursor lesion are variable. It is not uncommon, in our experience, that a precursor lesion is overlooked entirely and that progression or recurrence of the lesion is assumed to be a primary soft tissue neoplasm.

About three quarters of neurotropic melanomas occur on the head and neck, usually in adult patients (Fig. 32-42). Cases in children have been recognized, and unusual sites such as the vulva may be affected.[145] The most common precursor lesion is lentigo maligna melanoma, but these tumors may also arise in superficial spreading and acral lentiginous melanomas.[143] Apart from the precursor lesion, the main tumor mass is firm and scarlike in consistency (Fig. 32-43) and is made up of spindled or slightly oval cells that form short packetlike fascicles, vaguely reminiscent of carcinoma, which infiltrate the connective tissue (Figs. 32-44 to 32-46). In some cases, collections of tumor cells with Schwann cell features may, in a rudimentary fashion, reca-

*References 94, 95, 118, 127, 129, 132.

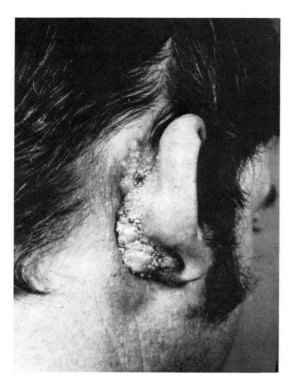

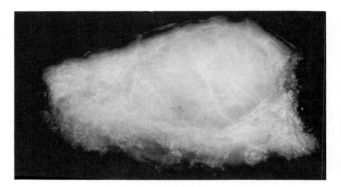

FIG. 32-42. Neurotropic melanoma. Tumor arose in posterior auricular region and produced a wartlike nonpigmented mass. Lesion recurred several times in the same region before metastasizing to the paraspinal area.

FIG. 32-43. Neurotropic melanoma. Note the ill-defined scarlike quality of this dermal tumor.

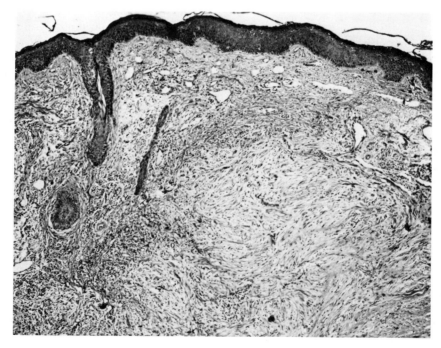

FIG. 32-44. Neurotropic melanoma. Highly desmoplastic tumor present in mid- and deep dermis. No epidermal lesion was present in sections studied. (×160.)

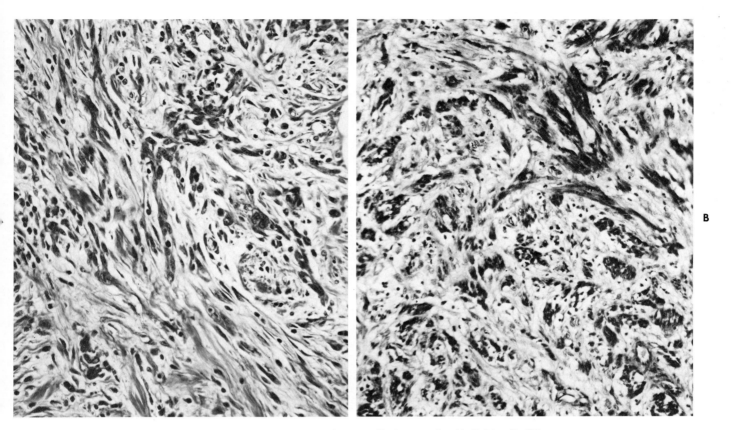

FIG. 32-45. Neurotropic melanoma varies from small clusters of epithelioid cells (**B**) to attenuated spindled elements surrounded by reactive fibroblasts (**A**). (**A**, ×160; **B**, ×250.)

pitulate the appearance of small nerves. Fine or dense collagen fibrils surround the cells. In other areas the cells lose their cohesion with one another and infiltrate singly. These areas are often collections of tumor cells that can be identified within both the endoneurium and perineurium of normal nerves (Fig. 32-47) and are believed to be one of the reasons for the high rate of local recurrence of this lesion following conservative excision. In recurrent tumors the cells acquire a more epithelial appearance and usually have more pleomorphism so that they look distinctly carcinomatous (Fig. 32-48). Although axons can be demonstrated within the tumor, melanin pigment is absent within the tumor, but it can be identified within the precursor lesion.

Ultrastructurally, the cells within neurotropic melanoma do not contain melanosomes or premelanosomes, but express Schwann cell features to a variable degree.[139,144] Most tumors exhibit positive immunostaining for S-100 protein. In these preparations the long attenuated shape of these schwannian cells is easily appreciated (Fig. 32-49). S-100 protein immunostaining is extremely helpful in distinguishing a bland neurotropic melanoma from a reactive fibroblastic proliferation of the skin. Likewise, immuno-

staining for cytokeratin clearly separates this tumor from most squamous carcinomas. Occasionally, spindled and epithelioid cell nevi (Spitz nevus) in children are quite desmoplastic,[136] but they are rarely, if ever, as infiltrative or as spindled as neurotropic melanoma.

These lesions are fully malignant tumors. Of the collected cases in the literature, about one third of patients died of their tumors. Local recurrence occurs in about half of patients and can be predicted by excision with margins of less than 1 cm, head and neck location, level V invasion, and tumor thickness of more than 4 mm. Common metastatic sites are the regional lymph nodes and the lung. It should be noted that occasionally conventional melanomas will display neurotropic or Schwann cell features in a metastatic site.[138,139] Thus, a lymph node with metastatic tumor reminiscent of a malignant schwannoma could be either a conventional or neurotropic melanoma but rarely an MPNST (see Fig. 32-29).

EXTRASPINAL (SOFT TISSUE) EPENDYMOMA

Soft tissue ependymomas are rare tumors that occur in subcutaneous locations dorsal to the sacrum and coccyx or

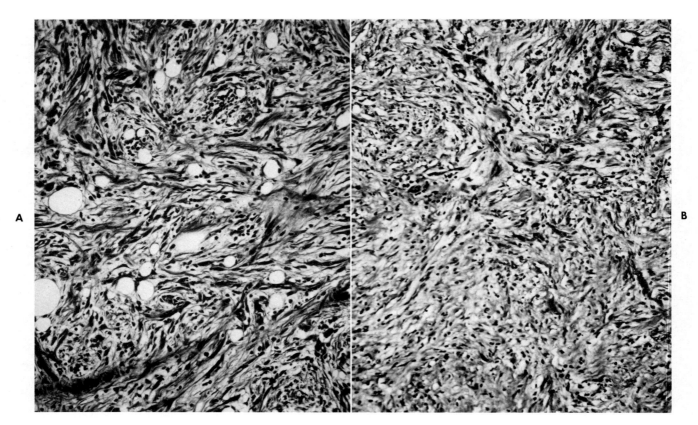

FIG. 32-46. Neurotropic melanoma showing areas that are composed of loosely cohesive spindled cells. These areas may be confused with neurofibroma. (**A** and **B**, ×160.)

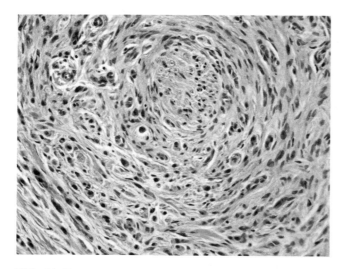

FIG. 32-47. Neurotropic melanoma showing targeting of tumor cells around nerve (neurotropism). (×250.)

in deep soft tissue anterior to the sacrum and posterior to the rectum. Many that occur in the latter location represent ependymomas of the cauda equina that have extended through the sacral foramina to present as presacral masses.[160] Thus, those situated dorsally to the sacrum represent the more significant group in terms of soft tissue tumors; consequently, this discussion is restricted to this group. Pathogenetically, the dorsal coccygeal ependymoma may arise from normal remnants of the neural tube (coccygeal medullary vestige) or from abnormal remnants resulting from embryological malformations. The latter contention is supported by the fact that a significant proportion of patients with this tumor[150,160] have developmental abnormalities such as spina bifida. Characteristically these tumors present as long-standing masses that are often diagnosed preoperatively as pilonidal cysts, teratomas, or sweat gland tumors. Although a few cases have proved to be quite extensive at the time of initial surgery,[150] most are encapsulated and easily separated from the fascia overlying the sacrum and coccyx. Grossly, they are myxoid multilobulated masses with focal areas of hemorrhage and necrosis (Fig. 32-50). The majority resemble the ependymomas arising

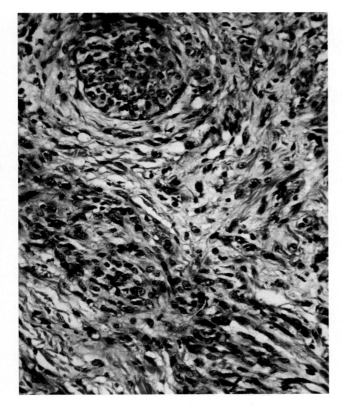

FIG. 32-48. Metastatic neurotropic melanoma showing increased pleomorphism with solid epithelioid areas. (×250.)

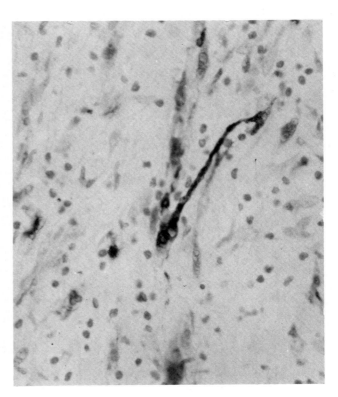

FIG. 32-49. Immunostaining of neurotropic melanoma for S-100 protein illustrating elongated schwannian cells. (Anti-S-100 protein, peroxidase-antiperoxidase; ×400.)

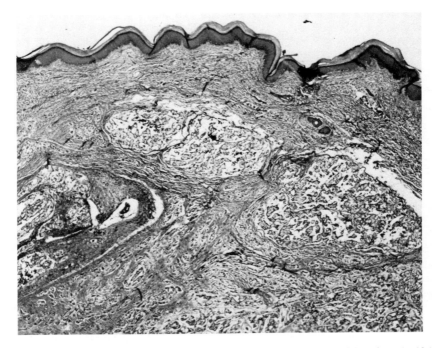

FIG. 32-50. Extraspinal ependymoma presenting in a dorsococcygeal location. (×40.)

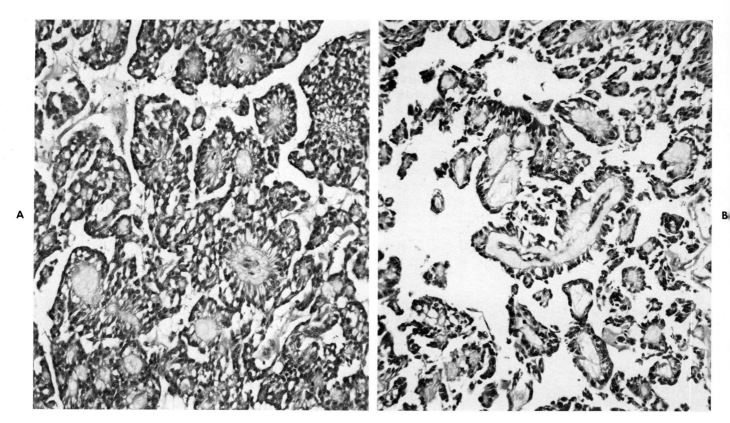

FIG. 32-51. Extraspinal ependymoma. Tumor resembles myxopapillary ependymoma of cauda equina and contains perivascular pseudorosettes (**A**) and papillary structures (**B**). (**A** and **B**, ×250.)

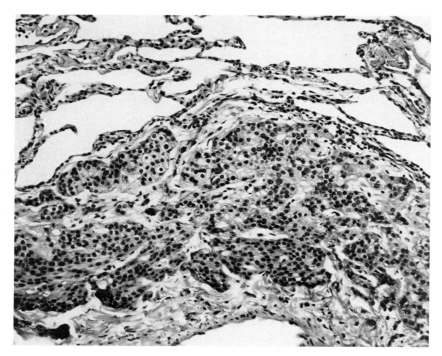

FIG. 32-52. Extraspinal ependymoma metastatic to lung. Nests of epithelioid tumor cells may mimic the pattern of carcinoma or carcinoid tumor. (×250.)

from the cauda equina and are of the "myxopapillary type." Cuboidal or columnar cells are arranged on fibrovascular stalks in a papillary configuration (Fig. 32-51). Secondary perivascular degenerative changes result in the peculiar myxoid and hyalinized appearance that characterizes the myxopapillary ependymoma. In cases where the degeneration is not marked, the tumor may resemble the more cellular papillary ependymoma of the brain. The cells are usually well differentiated with apically polarized nuclei. Occasionally blepharoplasts may be demonstrated by means of special stains (phosphotungstic acid-hematoxylin stain). Carminophilic intracytoplasmic mucin is not present in these cells despite its presence in the closely related "choroid plexus papilloma."[160] Ultrastructurally these cells have many of the features of normal ependymal cells. They contain microvilli and lateral desmosomes at their apical surfaces, whereas elaborate interdigitations of the plasma membrane and underlying basement membrane material characterize the basal surfaces. Parallel arrays of fine filaments and occasional microtubules are found within the cytoplasm.[160]

Although ependymomas are, in general, low-grade neoplasms and usually pose only problems in control of local disease, dorsal coccygeal ependymomas have a distantly greater propensity to metastasize than their intraspinal counterparts. This has been ascribed to their easier accessibility to lymphatic channels as well as to the longer survival time associated with these tumors. Thus of 11 primary dorsal coccygeal ependymomas, three metastasized either to regional (inguinal) nodes or the lung. Metastasis to the lung may be mistaken for a carcinoid tumor (Fig. 32-52). Distant metastasis is a late event, usually occurring 10 years or more after diagnosis of the primary tumor. Adequate treatment of these tumors should consist of wide local excision with radiation employed for residual or inoperable disease. The protracted course of this disease underscores the need for extended follow-up care and even resection of isolated metastases, if and when they appear.

REFERENCES
Malignant peripheral nerve sheath tumor

1. Alvira MM, Mandybur TI, Menefee MG: Light microscopic and ultrastructural observations of a metastasizing malignant epithelioid schwannoma. *Cancer* 38:1977, 1976.
2. Biggs FJ: Neurosarcoma of the median nerve. *Med J Aust* 1:687, 1935.
3. Bojsen-Moller M, Myrhe-Jensen O: A consecutive series of 30 malignant schwannomas: survival in relation to clinicopathological parameters and treatment. *Acta Pathol Microbiol Scand* 92A:147, 1984.
4. Bricklin AS, Rushton HW: Angiosarcoma of venous origin arising in radial nerve. *Cancer* 39:1556, 1977.
5. Brooks JS, Freeman M, Enterline HT: Malignant "Triton" tumors: natural history and immunohistochemistry of nine new cases with literature review. *Cancer* 55:2543, 1985.
6. Brown RW, Tornos C, Evans HL: Angiosarcoma arising from malignant schwannoma in a patient with neurofibromatosis. *Cancer* 70:1141, 1992.
7. Chitale AR, Dickerson GR: Electron microscopy in the diagnosis of malignant schwannomas: a report of six cases. *Cancer* 51:1448, 1983.
8. Chiu HF, Troster M: Ultrastructure of malignant schwannomas. *Lab Invest* 40A:246, 1979.
9. Coffin CM, Dehner LP: Peripheral neurogenic tumors of the soft tissues of children and adolescents: a clinicopathologic study of 139 cases. *Pediatr Pathol* 9:387, 1989.
10. Cohn I: Epithelial neoplasms of peripheral and cranial nerves: Report of three cases: review of the literature. *Arch Surg* 17:117, 1928.
11. Conley K, Rubinstein LJ, Spence AM: Studies on experimental malignant nerve sheath tumors maintained in tissue and organ culture systems. II. Electron microscopy observations. *Acta Neuropathol (Berl)* 34:293, 1976.
12. Cross PA, Clarke NW: Malignant nerve sheath tumor with epithelial elements. *Histopathology* 12:547, 1988.
13. D'Agostino AN, Soule EH, Miller RH: Primary malignant neoplasm of nerves (malignant neurilemomas) in patients without manifestations of multiple neurofibromatosis (von Recklinghausen's disease). *Cancer* 16:1003, 1963.
14. D'Agostino AN, Soule EH, Miller RH: Sarcomas of the peripheral nerves and somatic soft tissues associated with multiple neurofibromatosis (von Recklinghausen's disease). *Cancer* 16:1015, 1963.
15. Daimaru Y, Hashimoto H, Enjoji M: Malignant peripheral nerve-sheath tumors (malignant schwannomas): an immunohistochemical study of 29 cases. *Am J Surg Pathol* 9:434, 1985.
16. Daimaru Y, Hashimoto H, Enjoji M: Malignant "Triton" tumors: a clinicopathologic and immunohistochemical study of nine cases. *Hum Pathol* 15:768, 1984.
17. Das Gupta TK, Brasfield RD: Solitary malignant schwannoma. *Ann Surg* 171:419, 1970.
18. Denlinger RH, Koestner A, Wechsler W: Indication of neurogenic tumors in C3HeB/FEJ mice by nitrosourea derivatives. *Int J Cancer* 13:559, 1974.
19. DeSchryver K, Santa Cruz DJ: So-called glandular schwannoma: ependymal differentiation in a case. *Ultrastruct Pathol* 6:167, 1984.
20. DiCarlo EF, Woodruff JM, Bansal M, et al: The purely epithelioid peripheral nerve sheath tumor. *Am J Surg Pathol* 10:478, 1986.
21. Ducatman BS, Scheithauer BW: Malignant peripheral nerve sheath tumor with divergent differentiation. *Cancer* 54:1049, 1984.
22. Ducatman BS, Scheithauer BW: Port-irradiation neurofibrosarcoma. *Cancer* 51:1028, 1983.
23. Ducatman BS, Scheithauer BW, Piepgras DG: Malignant peripheral nerve sheath tumors: a clinicopathologic study of 120 cases. *Cancer* 57:2006, 1986.
24. Erlandson RA, Woodruff JM: Peripheral nerve sheath tumors: an electron microscopic study of 43 cases. *Cancer* 49:273, 1982.
25. Foraker AG: Glandlike elements in a peripheral neurosarcoma. *Cancer* 1:286, 1948.
26. Garre C: Uber sekundare Maligne Neurome. *Beitr Z Chir Z* 9:465, 1892.
27. Geschickter CF: Tumors of the peripheral nerves. *Am J Cancer* 25:377, 1935.
28. Ghosh BC, Ghosh L, Huvos AG, et al: Malignant schwannoma: a clinicopathologic study. *Cancer* 31:184, 1973.

29. Giannestras NJ, Bronson JL: Malignant schwannoma of the medial plantar branch of the posterior tibial nerve (unassociated with von Recklinghausen's disease). *J Bone Joint Surg* 57A:701, 1975.

30. Goldman RL, Jones SE, Heusinkveld RS: Combination chemotherapy of metastatic malignant schwannoma with vincristine, Adriamycin, cyclophosphamide, and imidazole carboxamide: a case report. *Cancer* 39:1955, 1977.

31. Goodlad JR, Fletcher CDM: Malignant peripheral nerve sheath tumour with annulate lamellae mimicking pleomorphic malignant fibrous histiocytoma. *J Pathol* 164:23, 1991.

32. Gore I: Primary malignant tumors of nerves: a report of eight cases. *Cancer* 2:278, 1951.

33. Gratia: Une curieuse anomalie anatomique constituee par la presence de tissu musculaire strie dans la substance du nerf pneumogastrique. *Ann Med Vet* 33:649, 1884.

34. Gray MH, Rosenberg AE, Dickersin GR, et al: Glial fibrillary acidic protein and keratin expression by benign and malignant nerve sheath tumors. *Hum Pathol* 20:1089, 1989.

35. Guccion JG, Enzinger FM: Malignant schwannoma associated with von Recklinghausen's neurofibromatosis. *Virchows Arch (Pathol Anat)* 383:43, 1979.

36. Harkin JC, Reed RJ: Tumors of the peripheral nervous system. In *Atlas of tumor pathology,* Armed Forces Institute of Pathology, 1969, second series, fascicle 3, Washington, DC.

37. Hedeman LA, Lewinsky BS, Lochridge GK, et al: Primary malignant schwannoma of the gasserian ganglion: report of two cases. *J Neurosurg* 48:279, 1978.

38. Heffner DK, Gnepp DR: Sinonasal fibrosarcomas, malignant schwannomas, and "Triton" tumors: a clinicopathologic study of 67 cases. *Cancer* 70:1089, 1992.

39. Herrera GA, deMoraes HP: Neurogenic sarcomas in patients with neurofibromatosis (von Recklinghausen's disease): light, electron microscopy and immunohistochemistry study. *Virchows Arch (Pathol Anat)* 403:361, 1984.

40. Hruban RH, Shiu MH, Senie RT, et al: Malignant peripheral nerve sheath tumors of the buttock and lower extremity. *Cancer* 66:1253, 1990.

41. Johnson K, Glick AD, Davis BW: Immunohistochemical evaluation of Leu-7, myelin basic protein, S-100 protein, glial fibrillary acidic protein, and LN3 immunoreactivity in nerve sheath tumors and sarcomas. *Arch Pathol Lab Med* 112:155, 1988.

42. Karcioglu Z, Somren A, Mathes SJ: Ectomesenchymoma: a malignant tumor of migratory neural crest (ectomesenchyme) remnants showing ganglionic, schwannian, melanocytic, and rhabdomyoblastic differentiation. *Cancer* 39:2486, 1977.

43. Katz LD, Creech JL, Makk L: Giant retroperitoneal sarcoma of nerve sheath origin. *South Med J* 67:349, 1974.

44. Koestner A, Swenberg JA, Wechsler W: Transplacental production of ethylnitrosourea of neoplasms of the nervous system in Sprague-Dawley rats. *Am J Pathol* 63:37, 1971.

45. Krumerman MS, Stingle W: Synchronous malignant glandular schwannomas in congenital neurofibromatosis. *Cancer* 41:2444, 1978.

46. Laskin WB, Weiss SW, Bratthauer GL: Epithelioid variant of malignant peripheral nerve sheath tumor (malignant epithelioid schwannoma). *Am J Surg Pathol* 15:1136, 1991.

47. Laurian N, Zohar Y: Malignant neurilemoma of parotid gland. *J Laryngol Otol* 84:1267, 1970.

48. Lodding P, Kindblom LG, Angervall L: Epithelioid malignant schwannoma: a study of 14 cases. *Virchows Arch (Pathol Anat)* 409:433, 1986.

49. Mannarino E, Watts JW: Malignant tumors arising from peripheral nerves. *J Int Coll Surg* 37:550, 1962.

50. Maseritz IH: Neurogenic sarcoma. *J Bone Joint Surg* 24:586, 1942.

51. Masson P, Martin JF: Rhabdomyomes des nerfs. *Bull Assoc Franc Etude Cancer* 27:751, 1938.

52. Matsunou H, Shimoda T, Kakimoto S, et al: Histopathologic and immunohistochemical study of malignant tumors of peripheral nerve sheath (malignant schwannoma). *Cancer* 56:2269, 1985.

53. McCormick LJ, Hazard JB, Dickson JA: Malignant epithelioid neurilemoma (schwannoma). *Cancer* 7:725, 1954.

54. McKay B, Osborne BM: The contribution of electron microscopy to the diagnosis of tumors. *Pathol Ann* 8:359, 1978.

55. McKeen EA, Bodurtha J, Meadows AT, et al: Rhabdomyosarcoma complicating multiple neurofibromatosis. *J Pediatr* 93:992, 1978.

56. Meis JM, Enzinger FM, Martz KL, et al: Malignant peripheral nerve sheath tumors (malignant schwannoma) in children. *Am J Surg Pathol* 16:694, 1992.

57. Mennemeyer RP, Hallman KO, Hammar SP, et al: Melanotic schwannoma: clinical and ultrastructural studies of three cases with evidence of intracellular melanin synthesis. *Am J Surg Pathol* 3:3, 1979.

58. Menon AG, Anderson KM, Riccardi VM, et al: Chromosome 17p deletions and p53 gene mutations associated with the formation of malignant neurofibrosarcomas in von Recklinghausen's neurofibromatosis. *Proc Natl Acad Sci U S A* 87:5435, 1990.

59. Michel SL: Epithelial elements in a malignant neurogenic tumor of the tibial nerve. *Am J Surg* 113:404, 1967.

60. Nakajima T, Watanaba S, Soto Y, et al: An immunoperoxidase study of S-100 protein distribution in normal and neoplastic tissues. *Am J Surg Pathol* 6:715, 1982.

61. Orenstein JM: Amianthoid fibers in synovial sarcoma and a malignant schwannoma. *Ultrastruct Pathol* 4:163, 1983.

62. Orlandi E: Rhabdomyoma del nervo ischiatico. *Arch Sci Med (Torino)* 19:113, 1895.

63. Payne RA: Metaplasia in a nerve sheath sarcoma in von Recklinghausen's disease. *Br J Surg* 47:688, 1960.

64. Rao SB, Dinakar I: Neurofibroma of sciatic nerve. *Indian J Cancer* 7:226, 1970.

65. Reynolds JE, Fletcher JA, Lytle CH, et al: Molecular characterization of a 17q11.2 translocation in a malignant schwannoma cell line. *Hum Genet* 90:450, 1992.

66. Rigdon RH: Neurogenic tumors produced by methylcholanthrene in the white Pekin duck. *Cancer* 8:906, 1955.

67. Rubinstein LJ, Conley FK, Herman MM: Studies on experimental malignant nerve sheath tumors maintained in tissue and organ culture systems. I. Light microscopy observations. *Acta Neuropathol (Berl)* 34:277, 1976.

68. Sordillo PP, Helson L, Hajdu SI, et al: Malignant schwannoma: clinical characteristics, surgery, and response to therapy. *Cancer* 47:2503, 1981.

69. Sorensen SA, Mulvihill JJ, Nielsen A: Long-term follow-up of von Recklinghausen neurofibromatosis. *N Engl J Med* 305:1617, 1981.

70. Spence AM, Rubenstein LJ, Conley FK, et al: Studies on experimental malignant nerve sheath tumors maintained in tissue and organ culture systems. III. Melanin pigment and melanogenesis in experimental neurogenic tumors, a reappraisal of the histogenesis of pigmented nerve sheath tumors. *Acta Neuropathol (Berl)* 35:27, 1976.

71. Stewart FW, Copeland MM: Neurogenic sarcoma. *Am J Cancer* 15:1235, 1931.

72. Storm FK, Eilber FR, Mirra J, et al: Neurofibrosarcoma. *Cancer* 45:126, 1980.

73. Stout AP: The malignant tumors of the peripheral nerves. *Am J Cancer* 25:1, 1935.

74. Taxy JB, Battifora HB: Epithelioid schwannoma: diagnosis by electron microscopy. *Ultrastruct Pathol* 2:19, 1981.

75. Trojanowski JQ, Kleinman GM, Proppe KH: Malignant tumors of nerve sheath origin. *Cancer* 46:1202, 1980.

76. Tsuneyoshi M, Enjoji M: Primary malignant peripheral nerve tumors (malignant schwannomas): a clinicopathologic and electron microscopic study. *Acta Pathol Jpn* 29:363, 1979.

77. Uri AK, Witzleben CL, Raney RB: Electron microscopy of glandular schwannoma. *Cancer* 53:493, 1984.

78. Vieta JO, Pack GT: Malignant neurilemomas of peripheral nerves. *Am J Surg* 82:416, 1951.

79. Wanebo JE, Malik JM, Vandenberg SR, et al: Malignant peripheral nerve sheath tumors: a clinicopathologic study of 28 cases. *Cancer* 71:1247, 1993.

80. Warner TFCS, Louie R, Hafez GR, et al: Malignant nerve sheath tumor containing endocrine cells. *Am J Surg Pathol* 7:583, 1983.

81. Weiss SW, Langloss JM, Enzinger FM: The role of S-100 protein in the diagnosis of soft tissue tumors with particular reference to benign and malignant Schwann cell tumors. *Lab Invest* 49:299, 1983.

82. Weston JA: The migration and differentiation of neural crest cells. *Adv Morphogen* 8:41, 1970.

83. White HR: Survival in malignant schwannoma: an 18-year study. *Cancer* 27:720, 1971.

84. Wick MR, Swanson PE, Scheithauer BW, et al: Malignant peripheral nerve sheath tumor: an immunohistochemical study of 62 cases. *Am J Clin Pathol* 87:425, 1987.

85. Wong SY, Teh M, Tan YO, et al: Malignant glandular Triton tumor. *Cancer* 67:1076, 1991.

86. Woodruff JM: Peripheral nerve tumors showing glandular differentiation (glandular schwannoma). *Cancer* 37:2399, 1976.

87. Woodruff JM, Chernik NL, Smith MC, et al: Peripheral nerve tumors with rhabdomyosarcomatous differentiation (malignant "Triton" tumors). *Cancer* 32:426, 1973.

88. Wuerker RB, Kirkpatrick JB: Neuronal microtubules, neurofilaments, and microfilaments. *Int Rev Cytol* 33:45, 1972.

89. Zimmerman LE, Font RL, Andersen SR: Rhabdomyosarcomatous differentiation in malignant intraocular medulloepitheliomas. *Cancer* 30:817, 1972.

Clear cell sarcoma (malignant melanoma of soft parts)

90. Angervall L, Stener B: Clear cell sarcoma of tendons: a study of four cases. *Acta Pathol Microbiol Scand* 77:589, 1969.

91. Bearman RM, Noe J, Kempson R: Clear cell sarcoma with melanin pigment. *Cancer* 36:977, 1975.

92. Benson JD, Kraemer BB, Mackay B: Malignant melanoma of soft parts: an ultrastructural study of four cases. *Ultrastruct Pathol* 8:57, 1985.

93. Boudreaux D, Waisman J: Clear cell sarcoma with melanogenesis. *Cancer* 41:1387, 1978.

94. Bridge JA, Borek DA, Neff JR, et al: Chromosomal abnormalities in clear cell sarcoma: implication for histogenesis. *Am J Clin Pathol* 93:26, 1990.

95. Bridge JA, Sreekantaiah C, Neff JR, et al: Cytogenetic findings in clear cell sarcoma of tendons and aponeuroses: malignant melanoma of soft parts. *Cancer Genet Cytogenet* 52:101, 1991.

96. Carpenter WM, Tsaknis PJ, Konzelman JL, et al: Clear cell sarcoma of tendons and aponeuroses. *Oral Surg Oral Med Oral Pathol* 45:580, 1978.

97. Chung EB, Enzinger FM: Malignant melanoma of soft parts: a reassessment of clear cell sarcoma. *Am J Surg Pathol* 7:405, 1983.

98. Dutra FR: Clear cell sarcoma of tendons and aponeuroses: three additional cases. *Cancer* 25:942, 1970.

99. Eckhardt JJ, Pritchard DL, Soule EH: Clear cell sarcoma: a clinicopathologic study of 27 cases. *Cancer* 52:1482, 1983.

100. Ekfors TO, Rantakokko V: Clear cell sarcoma of tendons and aponeuroses: Malignant melanoma of soft tissue: report of four cases. *Pathol Res Pract* 165:422, 1979.

101. Enzinger FM: Clear cell sarcoma of tendons and aponeuroses: an analysis of 21 cases. *Cancer* 18:1163, 1968.

102. Epstein AL, Martin AO, Kempson R: Use of a newly established human cell line (SU-CCS-1) to demonstrate the relationship of clear cell sarcoma to malignant melanoma. *Cancer Res* 44:1265, 1984.

103. Hajdu SI, Shiu MH, Fortner JG: Tendosynovial sarcoma: a clinicopathologic study of 136 cases. *Cancer* 39:1201, 1977.

104. Hernandez EJ: Malignant blue nevus: a light and electron microscopic study. *Arch Dermatol* 107:741, 1973.

105. Hirata K: Clear cell sarcoma arising from the right plantar aponeurosis. *Orthop Surg (Tokyo)* 20:1326, 1969.

106. Hoffman GJ, Carter D: Clear cell sarcoma of tendons and aponeuroses with melanin. *Arch Pathol* 95:22, 1973.

107. Katenkamp D, Perevoshikov AG, Raikhlin NT: Das Klarzellsarkom des Weichgewebes: Morphologie, Differentialdiagnose und Tumoreinordnung. *Zentralbl Allg Pathol* 129:521, 1984.

108. Kindblom LG, Lodding P, Angervall L: Clear cell sarcoma of tendons and aponeuroses: an immunohistochemical and electron microscopic analysis indicating neural crest origin. *Virchows Arch (Pathol Anat)* 401:109, 1983.

109. Kubo T: Clear cell sarcoma of patellar tendon studied by electron microscopy. *Cancer* 24:948, 1969.

110. Lucas DR, Nascimento AG, Sim FH: Clear cell sarcoma of soft tissues: Mayo Clinic experience with 35 cases. *Am J Surg Pathol* 16:1197, 1992.

111. Mackenzie DH: Clear cell sarcoma of tendon and aponeuroses with melanin production. *J Pathol* 114:231, 1974.

112. Mackenzie DH: Two types of soft tissue sarcoma of uncertain histogenesis. *Br J Cancer* 25:458, 1971.

113. McKlatshie S: An example of clear cell sarcoma of tendon. *E Afr Med J* 46:524, 1969.

114. Mechtersheimer G, Tilgen W, Klar E, et al: Clear cell sarcoma of tendons and aponeuroses: case presentation with special reference to immunohistochemical findings. *Hum Pathol* 20:914, 1989.

115. Merkow LP, Burt RC, Hayeslip DW, et al: A cellular and malignant blue nevus: a light and electron microscopic study. *Cancer* 24:888, 1969.

116. Montgomery EA, Meis JM, Ramos AG, et al: Clear cell sarcoma of tendons and aponeurosis: a clinicopathologic study of 58 cases with analysis of prognostic factors. *Int J Surg Pathol* 1:59, 1993.

117. Morimoto N: Clear cell sarcoma of the heel. *Jpn J Clin Pathol* 17:60, 1969.

118. Mrozek K, Karakousis CP, Perez-Mesa C, et al: Translocation t(12;22)(q13;q12.2-12.3) in a clear cell sarcoma of tendons and aponeuroses. *Genes Chromosom Cancer* 6:249, 1993.

119. Mukherjee AK, Gupta S: Clear cell sarcoma of tendons and aponeuroses: a case report. *Indian J Cancer* 15:69, 1978.

120. Parker JB, Marcus PB, Martin JH: Spinal melanotic clear cell sarcoma: a light and electron microscopic study. *Cancer* 46:718, 1980.

121. Radstone DJ, Revell PA, Mantell BS: Clear cell sarcoma of tendons and aponeuroses treated with bleomycin and vincristine. *Br J Radiol* 52:238, 1979.

122. Ramdhane BK, Lacombe MJ, Sevin D, et al: Les sarcomes a cellulaires claires des tissue mous: Reevalation des sarcomes a cellular claires des tendons et de gaines: A propos de 14 cas. *Ann Pathol* 4:349, 1984.

123. Raynor AC, Vargas-Crotes F, Alexander RW, et al: Clear cell sarcoma with melanin pigment: a possible soft tissue variant of malignant melanoma: Case report. *J Bone Joint Surg* 61A:276, 1979.

124. Reeves BR, Fletcher CD, Gusterson BA: Translocation t(12;22)(q12;q13) is a nonrandom rearrangement in clear cell sarcoma. *Cancer Genet Cytogenet* 64:101, 1992.

125. Reiman HM, Goellner JR, Woods JE, et al: Desmoplastic melanoma of the head and neck. *Cancer* 60:2269, 1987.

126. Rodriguez HA, Ackerman LV: Cellular blue nevus: clinicopathological study of 45 cases. *Cancer* 21:393, 1968.

127. Rodriquez E, Sreekantaiah C, Reuter VE, et al: t(12;22)(q13;q13) and trisomy 8 are nonrandom aberrations in clear cell sarcoma. *Cancer Genet Cytogenet* 64:107, 1992.

128. Sara AS, Evans HL, Benjamin RS: Malignant melanoma of soft parts

(clear cell sarcoma): a study of 17 cases with emphasis on prognostic factors. *Cancer* 15:367, 1990.

129. Stenman G, Kindblom LG, Angervall L: Reciprocal translocation t(12;22)(q13;q13) in clear cell sarcoma of tendons and aponeuroses. *Genes Chromsom Cancer* 4:122, 1992.

130. Swanson PE, Wick MR: Clear cell sarcoma: an immunohistochemical analysis of six cases and comparison with other epithelioid neoplasms of soft tissue. *Arch Pathol Lab Med* 113:55, 1989.

131. Toe TK, Saw D: Clear cell sarcoma with melanin: report of two cases. *Cancer* 41:235, 1978.

132. Travis JA, Bridge JA: Significance of both numerical and structural chromosomal abnormalities in clear cell sarcoma. *Cancer Genet Cytogenet* 64:104, 1992.

133. Tsuneyoshi M, Enjoji M, Kubo T: Clear cell sarcoma of tendons and aponeuroses: a comparative study of 13 cases with provisional subgrouping into the melanotic and synovial types. *Cancer* 42:243, 1978.

Neurotropic (desmoplastic) melanoma

134. Ackerman AB, Godomski J: Neurotropic malignant melanoma and other neurotropic neoplasms in the skin. *Am J Dermatopathol* 6 (suppl):63, 1984.

135. Barr RJ, Morales RV, Graham JH: Desmoplastic nevus: a distinct histologic variant of mixed spindle cell and epithelioid cell nevus. *Cancer* 46:557, 1980.

136. Bruijm JA, Mihm MC, Barnhill RL: Desmoplastic melanoma. *Histopathology* 20:197, 1992.

137. Conley J, Lattes R, Orr W: Desmoplastic malignant melanoma: a rare variant of spindle cell melanoma. *Cancer* 28:914, 1971.

138. Dabbs DJ, Bolen JW: Superficial spreading malignant melanoma with neurosarcomatous metastasis. *Am J Clin Pathol* 82:109, 1984.

139. DiMaio SM, Mackay B, Smith JL, et al: Neurosarcomatous transformation in malignant melanoma: an ultrastructural study. *Cancer* 50:2345, 1982.

140. Egbert B, Kempson R, Sagebiel R: Desmoplastic malignant melanoma: a clinicopathologic study of 25 cases. *Cancer* 62:2033, 1988.

141. Jain S, Allen PW: Desmoplastic malignant melanoma and its variants. *Am J Surg Pathol* 13:358, 1989.

142. Labrecque P, Hu C, Winkelman RK: On the nature of desmoplastic melanoma. *Cancer* 38:1025, 1976.

143. Reed PJ, Leonard DD: Neurotropic melanoma: a variant of desmoplastic melanoma. *Am J Surg Pathol* 3:301, 1979.

144. Smithers BM, McLeod GR, Little JH: Desmoplastic neural transforming and neurotropic melanoma: a review of 45 cases. *Aust N Z J Surg* 60:967, 1990.

145. Valensi Q: Desmoplastic malignant melanoma: a light and electron microscopic study of two cases. *Cancer* 43:1148, 1979.

146. Warner TFCS, Hafez GR, Buchler DA: Neurotropic melanoma of the vulva. *Cancer* 49:999, 1982.

147. Warner TFCS, Hafez GR, Finch RE, et al: Schwann cell features in neurotropic melanoma. *J Cutan Pathol* 8:177, 1981.

148. Warner TFCS, Lloyd RV, Hafez GR, et al: Immunocytochemistry of neurotropic melanoma. *Cancer* 53:254, 1984.

Extraspinal (soft tissue) ependymoma

149. Adson AW, Moersch FP, Kernohan JW: Neurogenic tumors arising from the sacrum. *Arch Neurol Psychiatr* 41:535, 1939.

150. Anderson MS: Myxopapillary ependymomas presenting in the soft tissues over the sacrococcygeal region. *Cancer* 19:585, 1966.

151. Brindley GV: Sacral and presacral tumors. *Ann Surg* 121:721, 1945.

152. Heath MH: Presacral ependymoma: case report and review of the literature. *Am J Clin Pathol* 39:161, 1963.

153. Hendren TH, Hardin CA: Extradural metastatic ependymoma. *Surgery* 54:880, 1963.

154. Jackman RJ, Clark PL, Smith ND: Retrorectal tumors. *JAMA* 145:956, 1951.

155. Kernohan JW, Fletcher-Kernohan HA: Ependymomas: a study of 109 cases. *Assoc Res Nerv Dis* 16:182, 1937.

156. Lovelady SB, Dockerty MB: Extragenital pelvic tumors in women. *Am J Obstet Gynecol* 58:215, 1949.

157. Mallory FB: Three gliomata of ependymal origin: two in the fourth ventricle, one subcutaneous over the coccyx. *J Med Res* 8:1, 1902.

158. Ross ST: Sacral and presacral tumors. *Am J Surg* 76:687, 1948.

159. Vagaiwala MR, Robinson JS, Galicich JH, et al: Metastasizing extradural ependymoma of the sacrococcygeal area: case report and review of the literature. *Cancer* 44:326, 1979.

160. Wolff M, Santiago H, Duby MM: Delayed distant metastasis from a subcutaneous sacrococcygeal ependymoma: case report with tissue culture, ultrastructural observations, and review of the literature. *Cancer* 30:1046, 1972.

CHAPTER 33

PRIMITIVE NEUROECTODERMAL TUMORS AND RELATED LESIONS

In previous editions of this textbook, neuroblastoma, peripheral neuroepithelioma, and extraskeletal Ewing's sarcoma were described in separate chapters to reflect their diverse sites of origin. Neuroblastoma, arising from the adrenal and autonomic nervous system, was described in conjunction with melanotic schwannoma, a tumor that also occurs along the parasympathetic axis of the body, whereas peripheral neuroepithelioma was described in the context of malignant tumors of peripheral nerve. Extraskeletal Ewing's sarcoma was, until recently, considered a malignant tumor of uncertain type. A number of lines of evidence suggest that Ewing's sarcoma and peripheral neuroepithelioma are closely related, the former perhaps representing a less-differentiated form of the latter. The evidence includes the fact that both share a common 11/22 chromosomal translocation and cell surface protein (p30/32^{mic-2}). In addition, Ewing's cells can be induced to differentiate along neural lines in tissue culture. It seems reasonable to consider these three lesions as a common family. Distinctions among the three should also be clearly made whenever possible. The difference in presentation, behavior, and therapy between neuroblastoma and the other two tumors requires clear-cut separation. Whereas it may be less important to make the distinction between Ewing's sarcoma and primitive neuroepithelioma, it will never be possible to learn important biological or therapeutic differences between the two unless an earnest attempt is made to classify these lesions accurately. Classification, in turn, will become increasingly more dependent on incorporating diverse observations gleaned from light microscopic, immunohistochemical, and molecular diagnostic techniques.

NEUROBLASTOMA AND GANGLIONEUROBLASTOMA

Neuroblastoma and the related tumors ganglioneuroblastoma and ganglioneuroma are derived from primordial neural crest cells that migrate from the mantle layer of the developing spinal cord and populate the primordia of the sympathetic ganglia and adrenal medulla. These tumors can be conceptualized as three different maturational manifestations of a common neoplasm. Neuroblastoma, the least differentiated, resembles the fetal adrenal medulla and is made up of primitive neuroblasts. Ganglioneuroblastoma (differentiating neuroblastoma) possesses primitive neuroblasts along with maturing ganglion cells; the number and arrangement of the cells vary so that the tumor may assume a wide range of appearances and is associated with a wide range in biological behavior. Ganglioneuroma, a fully differentiated tumor, is characterized by a mixture of mature Schwann cells and ganglion cells. Neuroblastoma and ganglioneuroblastoma are discussed together because both are considered malignant. In contrast, pure ganglioneuromas are benign tumors requiring only conservative therapy and are considered separately.

Etiological and genetic factors

The majority of neuroblastomas occur on a sporadic basis, with a small number occurring in a familial setting.[17,51,86] The tumor tends to be less common in blacks than whites, and in certain parts of the world, notably the Burkitt's lymphoma belt in Africa, it is practically nonexistent.[70] In situ neuroblastomas, small microscopic foci of neuroblastoma confined to the adrenal and discovered incidentally at autopsy, are rather common (1 out of 200 infants dying of other causes), in dramatic contrast with the low incidence of clinical neuroblastoma. Beckwith and Perrin[8] have suggested that host factors probably assume an important role in the resolution or maturation of these microscopic tumors.

A number of cytogenetic abnormalities have been identified in neuroblastomas, although the exact manner in which they are etiologically linked to the tumor is not fully understood.[13] The most common abnormality, deletion or rearrangement of the short arm of chromosome 1 between 1p32 and 1pter, occurs in about 80% of neuroblastomas. Alterations in this region probably represent a primary critical event in the development of neuroblastoma, suggesting this is the locus of a neuroblastoma suppressor gene. Extrachromosomal double-minute chromatin bodies as well as homogeneously staining regions, representing sites of N-myc amplified sequences, are additional common findings. N-myc amplification occurs in approximately 25% to 30% of patients with neuroblastoma and is strongly predictive of poor outcome, independent of stage. Since N-myc copy number in a given tumor is relatively constant with respect to time, N-myc amplification appears to be an intrinsic property of a given tumor and probably occurs as an early event following alterations of 1p.

Most recently attention has focused on abnormalities in the nerve growth factor/nerve growth factor receptor pathway. Nerve growth factor binds to a cell surface receptor protein and induces differentiation in sympathetic neurons. Nearly all neuroblastoma cell lines tested have displayed abnormalities in this pathway.[13] In addition, expression of the TRK gene (encoding the growth factor receptor protein) has been correlated with favorable clinical stage and outcome and is inversely related to N-myc amplification.[99] Brodeur et al.[13] have postulated that failure to maintain an intact growth factor/receptor pathway results in neuroblasts that remain in a relatively undifferentiated state, making them vulnerable to subsequent mutation events such as 1p loss and N-myc amplification.

Clinical findings

Neuroblastoma is the third most common malignant tumor in children; it occurs at a rate of about 1 out of 10,000 live births.[8] At most large children's centers it accounts for about 10% to 12% of all malignant tumors, preceded in frequency by leukemias and brain tumors.[25] It develops at a relatively younger patient age than rhabdomyosarcomas and extraskeletal Ewing's sarcomas. About one fourth of neuroblastomas are congenital. Half are diagnosed by the age of 2 years, 90% by the age of 5 years, and only sporadic cases during adolescence or adult life.[90] The peak age at the time of presentation is about 18 months. In most large series there is a slight male predominance documented as 1.22:1 by Kinnear-Wilson and Draper[62] and 1.26:1 by De-Lorimier et al.[25] The distribution of neuroblastomas and ganglioneuroblastomas generally follows the distribution of the sympathetic ganglia; hence they are found in a paramidline position at any point between the base of the skull and pelvis, in addition to the adrenal medulla and organ of Zuckerkandl. Some cases possibly also arise from the dorsal root ganglia. This location would explain those cases of dumbbell-shaped neuroblastomas in which significant enlargement of the intervertebral foramen occurs. Whether these neuroblastomas possess the same synthetic and functional attributes as neuroblastomas in more conventional locations is not certain. In the experience reported by De-Lorimier et al.,[25] based on the California Tumor Registry, 134 cases out of 212 occurred within the retroperitoneum,

33 in the mediastinum, five in the cervical region, and six in the sacral region. About half of all retroperitoneal tumors arise in the adrenal, although the difficulty in determining the origin of large tumors must be acknowledged.

The constellation of symptoms varies, depending on the age of the patient, location of the mass, and presence or absence of associated clinical syndromes.[92,95] Usually patients with neuroblastomas appear wasted and chronically ill and manifest a variety of nonspecific signs and symptoms, including fever, weight loss, gastrointestinal tract disturbances including watery diarrhea,[95] and anemia. Recently, watery diarrhea leading to hypokalemia and achlorhydria has been linked to multiple hormone gene expression in ganglioneuroblastoma. In half of the patients a nodular fixed mass extending across the midline can be palpated on physical examination. So protean are the manifestations that half of neuroblastomas are misdiagnosed initially[86] and a significant number of patients may be diagnosed as having rheumatic fever because of the frequent occurrence of fever and joint pain.[24] About one third of neonates with neuroblastoma present with blue-red cutaneous metastases, which have been likened to blueberries (blueberry muffin baby).[123] Although hypertension is neither as common nor as severe as in pheochromocytomas, about one fifth will have this symptom, which remits with tumor removal.[117] A relatively rare presentation of neuroblastoma usually associated with a good prognosis is the "myoclonus-opsoclonus" syndrome.[120] Characterized by rapid alternating eye movements and myoclonic movements of the extremities, this symptom complex also disappears following tumor eradication, suggesting it is due to a circulating antitumor factor that cross-reacts with cerebellar cells.[101] Other cases of neuroblastoma have been associated with myasthenia gravis,[92] Cushing's syndrome,[24] von Recklinghausen's disease,[9] and fetal hydantoin syndrome.[108]

Roentgenographic findings

Retroperitoneal neuroblastomas cause anterior, lateral, and downward displacement of the kidney, usually without hydronephrosis or calyceal distortion. Calcification, a characteristic finding, occurs in about half of the tumors.[27] Typically the calcification consists of finely stippled densities in the central portion of the tumor, although peripheral linear densities may also be seen. Metastatic lesions commonly occur in bone; therefore roentgenographic studies are a mandatory part of clinical staging. Bone metastases are osteolytic lesions that display a peculiar predilection for the skull, femur, and humerus and occasionally are bilaterally symmetrical in their distribution.

Laboratory findings

About 80% to 90% of patients with neuroblastoma have elevated levels of catecholamines (norepinephrine, epinephrine) and their metabolites (vanillylmandelic acid

[VMA], homovanillic acid [HVA], and 3-methoxy-4-hydroxyphenylglycol [MHPG]) in their urine (Fig. 33-1).[70] This may reflect either increased production or diminished storage of these substances by the tumor. Measurement of these substances has proved to be useful both for diagnosis and for monitoring the course of the disease during therapy. Persistent elevation following surgery suggests significant residual disease, and elevations of the metabolites sometimes occur before a recurrence is clinically evident. Recently the ratio of VMA to HVA has become an important prognostic factor. Ratios of 1.5 or more are associated with an improved prognosis.[29] Neuropeptide Y, a biologically active polypeptide that colocalizes with catecholamines, is found in high levels in the serum of patients with neuroblastomas compared with levels in those with ganglioneuroblastoma or ganglioneuroma. It is released during surgical manipulation of tumors, decreases following tumor removal, and reappears with recrudescence of disease, suggesting that it, too, may prove useful in monitoring disease.[83]

Serum ferritin can be detected in the serum of patients with active disease and is also used as a prognostic indicator. This iron-binding protein, presumably synthesized by the tumor, is capable of coating the surface of T lymphocytes and is responsible for E rosette inhibition, a phenomenon observed in patients with advanced neuroblastoma.[48,50] The presence of serum neuron-specific enolase has also been correlated with survival rates in neuroblastoma.[41]

Gross findings

Neuroblastomas are lobulated masses averaging 6 to 8 cm in diameter; they are intimately related to the adrenal gland or sympathetic chain. At surgery they often appear to have delicate membranous capsules, which are easily ruptured to yield the soft, fleshy, gray, partially hemorrhagic tumor. Tumors composed of large expanses of differentiated ganglioneuroma associated with neuroblastomatous foci (nodular ganglioneuroblastoma) have gray hemorrhagic nodules set within a firm white-gray tumor mass.

Microscopic findings

The nomenclature of neuroblastomas has undergone revision in the past decade. Old classification schemes utilizing terms such as "ganglioneuroblastoma" without further modification obviously ignore the vast range of behavior that can be encountered in tumors having both neuroblastic and ganglionic elements. The following discussion follows the Joshi modification[72,74] of the commonly employed Shimada system of classification.[101] Equivalent terms in old classification systems are indicated in Table 33-1 and depicted diagramatically in Fig. 33-2.

Table 33-1. Nomenclature of neuroblastoma

Joshi system	Shimada system	Conventional system
Neuroblastoma		
Undifferentiated type	Stromal-poor, undifferentiated histology	Neuroblastoma
Poorly differentiated type	Stromal-poor, undifferentiated histology	Neuroblastoma
Differentiating type	Stromal-poor, differentiated histology	Ganglioneuroblastoma
Ganglioneuroblastoma		
Nodular type	Stromal-rich, nodular type	Composite ganglioneuroblastoma
Intermixed type	Stromal-rich, intermixed type	Composite ganglioneuroblastoma
Borderline type	Stromal-rich, well-differentiated type	Ganglioneuroblastoma

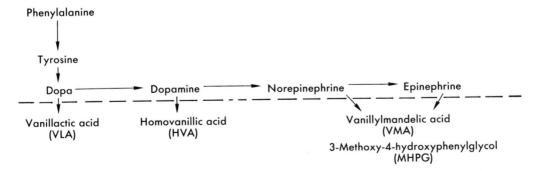

FIG. 33-1. Metabolic pathway showing enzymatic conversion of phenylalanine to epinephrine. Catabolites below dotted line are those that may be present in the urine of patients with neuroblastoma.

Components of neuroblastic tumors

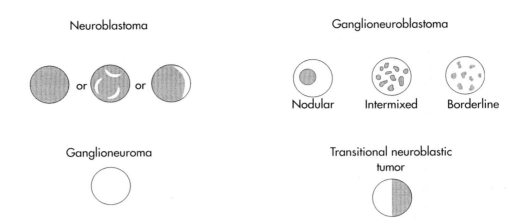

FIG. 33-2. Diagrammatic representation of terminology of neuroblastic tumors. Shaded areas represent neuroblastomatous component. Unshaded areas are ganglioneuromatous component. (Modified from Joshi et al: *Cancer* 69:2199, 1992.)

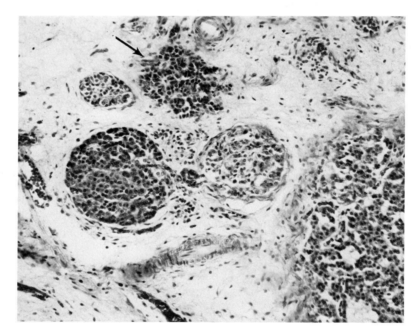

FIG. 33-3. Clusters of primitive neuroblasts *(arrow)* from the periadrenal area in developing fetus. (×160.)

Neuroblastoma. The term "neuroblastoma" refers to a tumor that is composed mostly of neuroblasts, which may display a variable degree of ganglionic differentiation (see below). These tumors are further subdivided into undifferentiated, poorly differentiated, and differentiating forms, depending on the percentage of cells showing ganglionic differentiation. Undifferentiated forms display no ganglionic differentiation, whereas the other two forms display less than or more than 5% differentiating cells, respec-

tively. However, unlike in ganglioneuroblastoma, mats of mature stroma composed of Schwann cells are not present.

The most primitive neuroblastomas resemble the anlage of the developing sympathetic nervous system and adrenal medulla (Fig. 33-3). They are composed of sheets of small rounded cells, which are divided into small lobules by delicate fibrovascular stroma (Fig. 33-4, *A*). The cells, which are almost devoid of cytoplasm, have round to polygonal deeply staining nuclei (Figs. 33-4, *B,* and 33-5) similar to

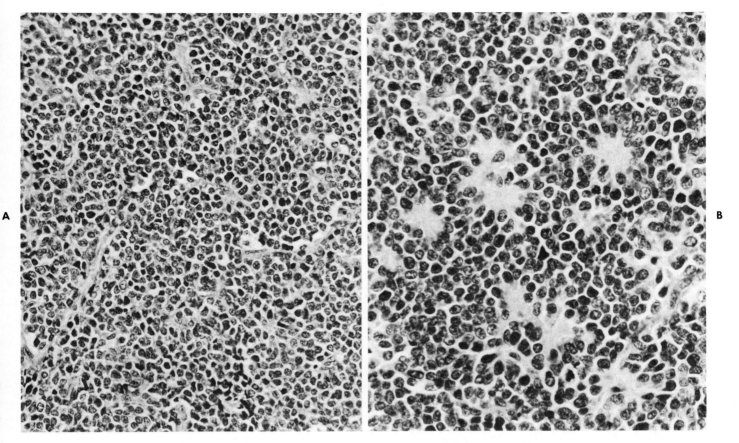

FIG. 33-4. A, Poorly differentiated neuroblastoma composed of monotonous sheets of cells with little cytoplasm. **B,** Some areas of the tumor contained rosettes. (**A,** ×160; **B,** ×400.)

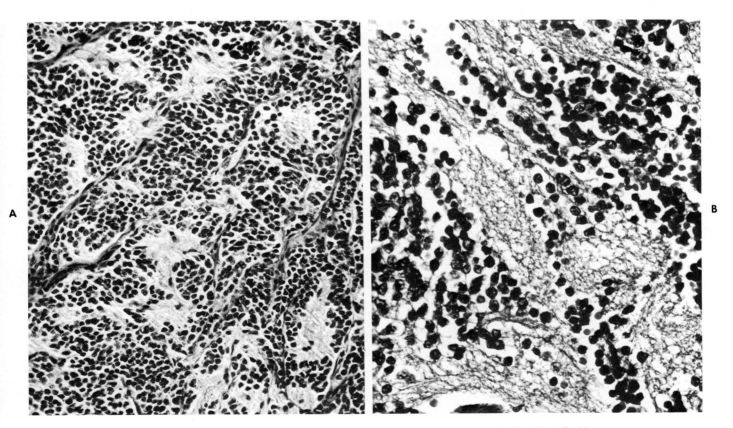

FIG. 33-5. A, Neuroblastoma showing greater degree of differentiation than in Fig. 33-4. **B,** Mats of neuropil were present throughout tumor. (×400.)

those of lymphocytes. Out of context, poorly differentiated neuroblastomas may be mistaken for round cell sarcomas such as Ewing's sarcoma, lymphoma, or nucleated erythrocytes of erythroblastosis fetalis, especially if cellular preservation is poor and the cells are artifactually crushed (Figs. 33-6 and 33-7). In contrast to Ewing's sarcoma there is usually a greater degree of nuclear irregularity and hyperchromatism. Diagnosis of poorly differentiated neuroblastoma is sometimes suggested by the presence of calcification or morula-like clusters of cells that represent the earliest form of rosette formation or, alternatively, by ancillary immunohistochemical or ultrastructural studies documenting neuroblastic features. With progressive differentiation, the neuroblasts acquire attenuated cytoplasmic processes (neurites), which are polarized toward a central point to form a rosette (Fig. 33-4, *B*) with a solid central core (Homer-Wright rosette). In addition, the stroma contains mats of neuropil, which are tangled networks of cell processes (Fig. 33-5). In the most-differentiated neuroblastomas, some of the cells show partial or even complete ganglionic differentiation (Figs. 33-8 to 33-10). Ganglionic differentiation is heralded by enlargement of the cells with acquisition of a discernible rim of eosinophilic cytoplasm. Binucleation occurs, and the nuclear chromatin pattern is distinctly vesicular.

Ganglioneuroblastoma. Ganglioneuroblastomas are tumors in which a portion of the tumor has the appearance of a neuroblastoma as described above and contains, in addition, a partial ganglioneuromatous stroma (see ganglioneuroma). The exact amount and arrangement of this stroma further determines the subclassification of the ganglioneuroblastoma. Nodular ganglioneuroblastoma contains gross nodules of neuroblastoma abutting large expanses of ganglioneuroma (Figs. 33-11 and 33-12). This form of ganglioneuroblastoma was previously referred to as "ganglioneuroblastoma with focal complete differentiation" by Beckwith and Martin[7] and as "composite neuroblastoma" by Stout. The second or intermixed form of ganglioneuroblastoma consists of microscopic nests of neuroblastoma situated within a ganglioneuromatous stroma (Fig. 33-13). The nests of neuroblasts appear discrete but unencapsulated. In the borderline form of ganglioneuroblastoma the tumor is composed of a few scattered foci of moderately differentiated neuroblasts and neuropil amidst a predominantly ganglioneuromatous stroma.

In the Joshi system two additional categories have been added. Transitional neuroblastoma contains equal proportions of ganglioneuroma and neuroblastoma, and unclassifiable neuroblastoma refers to tumors that defy classification because of extensive necrosis, hemorrhage, calcification, crush artifact, or problems related to tissue processing.

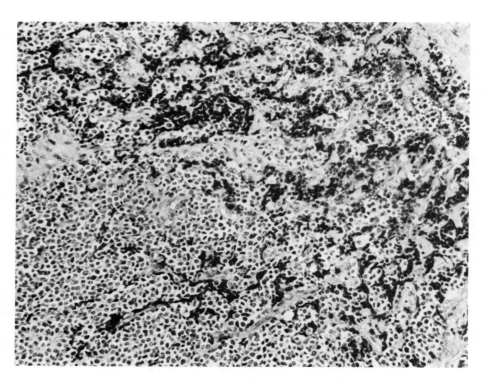

FIG. 33-6. Neuroblastoma with "crush artifact" of cells similar to that seen in oat cell carcinoma of the lung. (×160.)

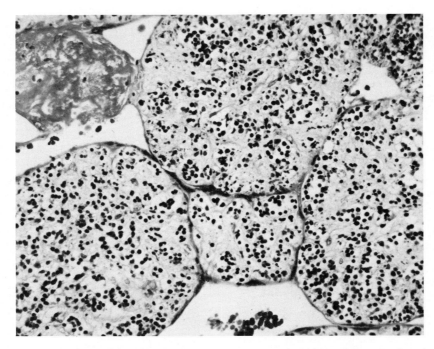

FIG. 33-7. Congenital neuroblastoma involving placenta. Tumor cells resemble nucleated erythrocytes and may be misinterpreted as evidence of erythroblastosis fetalis. (×160.)

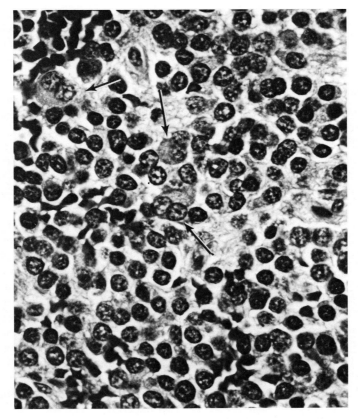

FIG. 33-8. Neuroblastoma showing early ganglionic differentiation. Primitive ganglion cells *(arrows)* have discernible cytoplasm and vesicular nuclei. Occasional binucleated forms are present. (×650.)

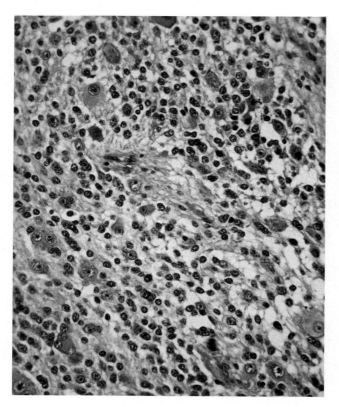

FIG. 33-9. Differentiating neuroblastoma. Neuroblasts and ganglion cells are intimately intermixed with one another. (×250.)

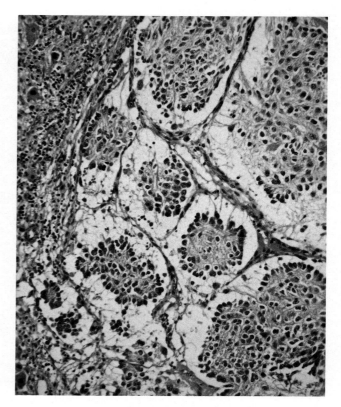

FIG. 33-10. Neuroblastoma with diffuse admixture of mature and immature cells. Note fibrovascular stroma, which is accentuated by retraction of tumor nodules. (×100.)

Immunohistochemical findings

A number of neuroectodermal antigens can be identified within neuroblastomas, although generally the extent and intensity are functions of the level of differentiation.[6] Neuron-specific enolase is probably the most sensitive but also least specific marker for neuroblastomas. It can be identified at least focally within even poorly differentiated tumors and is identified with increasing intensity in differentiating tumors and in ganglioneuroblastomas and ganglioneuromas. Because it is present in a variety of other small round cell tumors such as Ewing's sarcoma and rhabdomyosarcoma, it cannot be used alone in differential diagnosis. Neurofilament protein, the intermediate filament characteristic of neuronal cells, can be identified in many neuroblastomas, although the immunoreactivity appears to depend greatly on the degree of differentiation, type of antisera, and method of fixation.[4,6,78,84,121] Utilizing fresh tissue, Osborn et al.[84] were able to identify neurofilament protein in most neuroblastomas, where it is localized preferentially to cells showing evidence of ganglionic differentiation. Mukai et al.[78] were also able to demonstrate it within neuroblastomas but found monospecific antisera to the 68

kd subunit to be most sensitive. S-100 protein is only detected within ganglioneuromatous portions of these tumors and occasionally within the thin stromal network that separates the nodules of neuroblastic cells from cells that stain positively for S-100 protein in this location and has recently been used as one criterion to separate undifferentiated neuroblastomas into favorable and unfavorable histological types.[100] Presumably these cells represent precursor cells capable of producing a differentiated neuromatous stroma. Other markers that have proved useful in the diagnosis of neuroblastoma include protein gene product 9.5, chromogranin, vasoactive intestinal peptide, and synaptophysin.[76,121] All are best demonstrated in more differentiated tumors. Glial fibrillary acidic protein and myelin basic protein are usually not identified within neuroblastomas unless they contain more differentiated foci.[76] Although immunoreactivity for enzymes of catecholamine synthesis (tyrosine hydroxylase, dopamine decarboxylase) can be detected in neuroblastomas, it tends to be weak. Preliminary reports have described immunolocalization of β-integrins,[34] TGF-β,[73] N-CAM,[76] opiate receptors,[52,60] and microtubule-associated protein within these tumors.

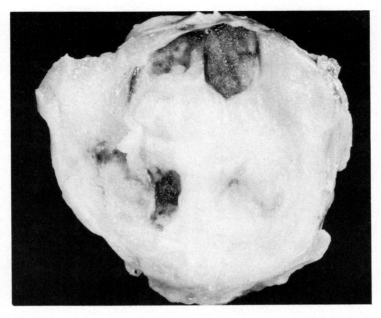

FIG. 33-11. Ganglioneuroblastoma. Hemorrhagic areas corresponded to neuroblastoma, whereas the remainder of the tumor was ganglioneuroma.

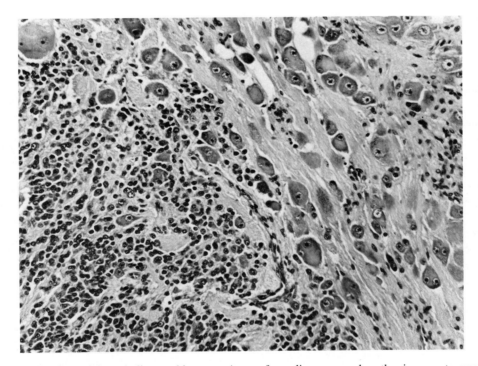

FIG. 33-12. Nodular ganglioneuroblastoma. Areas of ganglioneuroma abruptly give way to areas of neuroblastoma. (×160.)

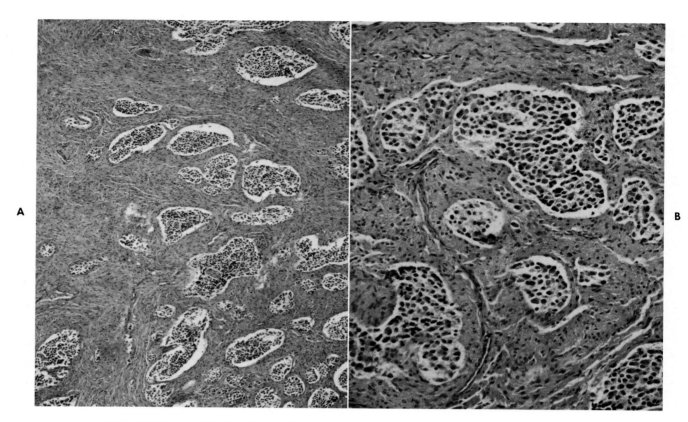

FIG. 33-13. A and B, Ganglioneuroblastoma showing patchy nodules of immature neuroblasts set within a mature ganglioneuromatous stroma. (**A**, ×60; **B**, ×160.)

Ultrastructural findings

Ultrastructurally neuroblastoma shows a wide range of cytological differentiation.[71,75,93,111,112] The least differentiated cells may be difficult to distinguish from primitive cells in other types of tumors because they have scant rims of cytoplasm, few organelles apart from free ribosomes, and small numbers of heterogeneous granules measuring about 50 nm.[75] More differentiated cells can be clearly recognized as neural by virtue of attenuated cytoplasmic processes containing fine neurofilaments (8 to 12 nm) and microtubules (24 to 26 nm).[111] Dense core neurosecretory granules, presumably representing the site of conversion of dopamine to norepinephrine, vary in numbers. Although they typically occur in small clusters in the elongated cell processes, they may also be found in the cell body. The granules, measuring approximately 100 nm in diameter, contain central dense cores surrounded by clear halos and delicate outer membranes. Occasionally clear vesicles are also noted. The significance of the latter structures is not clear, although they may contain acetylcholine or may be exhausted sites of catecholamine stores. Ganglionic differentiation within these tumors is accompanied by an increase in the cytoplasm, with concomitant increase in mitochon-

dria, ribosomes, polysomes, and perinuclear Golgi apparatus. Small dense core granules are found randomly throughout the cytoplasm (Fig. 33-14). In addition, larger heterogeneous granules containing myelin figures are present in significant numbers and are believed to represent sites for storage of degraded catecholamines. Ganglioneuromatous areas contain, in addition to mature ganglion cells, a proliferation of Schwann cells characterized by long tapered cytoplasmic processes invested with basal lamina.

Differential diagnosis

The young age of the patient, location along the sympathetic chain, and elevated urinary catecholamines establish the diagnosis of neuroblastoma in the majority of cases. Evaluation of needle biopsy specimens of poorly differentiated nonfunctioning tumors, however, may present diagnostic problems. The usual problem is the distinction of neuroblastoma from embryonal rhabdomyosarcoma or extraskeletal Ewing's sarcoma, but fortunately both immunohistochemical and electron microscopic studies have greatly improved the accuracy of light microscopic diagnosis.

The clinical presentations of neuroblastoma and rhabdomyosarcoma may be quite similar. Both occur in young

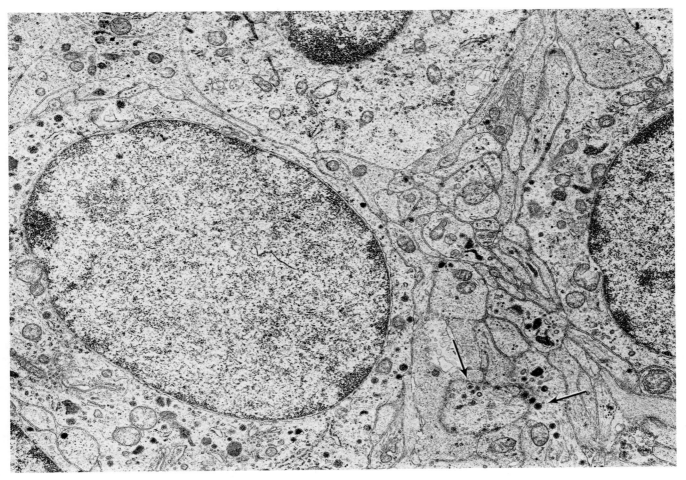

FIG. 33-14. Electron micrograph of neuroblastoma. Cells have numerous intertwining processes containing dense core granules *(arrows).* Occasional dense core granules are also present in cell body. (×17,000.) (Courtesy Dr. Tim Triche, National Cancer Institute, Bethesda, Maryland.)

persons, often in intraabdominal locations. Rhabdomyosarcomas usually show a greater degree of variability in the size and shape of cells and nuclei. The cytoplasm is usually more abundant, more sharply outlined, and endowed with an eosinophilic hue. Careful search for differentiated areas reveals typical strap cells and tadpole cells. Differentiated rhabdomyoblasts have both thin (8-nm) and thick (12-nm) myofilaments and occasionally Z-band material ultrastructurally. Moreover, the majority of rhabdomyosarcomas possess moderate amounts of cytoplasmic glycogen in contrast to neuroblastoma. Desmin is present in most rhabdomyosarcomas. Myoglobin, in our experience, is usually not present in rhabdomyosarcomas except, in the most-differentiated cells.

Although patients with Ewing's (extraskeletal) sarcoma usually are relatively older than those with neuroblastomas, we have found that histologically the two tumors can be quite difficult to separate, particularly when cellular preservation is not optimal. In well-preserved specimens Ewing's sarcomas have more regular nuclei, more finely stippled chromatin patterns, and cytoplasm filled with glycogen. Usually the cells are arranged in sheets and lobules. We have, however, seen several cases of Ewing's sarcoma in which rosettelike structures were plentiful. On electron microscopic studies these "pseudorosettes" consist of clusters of Ewing's cells having blebs of glycogen-filled cytoplasm polarized toward a central point in the same fashion as the neurofibrillary tangle of the neural rosette. The presence of p30/32, the product of the mic-2 gene, as detected by HBA71, has recently been identified as a relatively specific cell surface marker of Ewing's sarcoma and primitive neuroepitheliomas, but not of classic neuroblastoma. This provides an important diagnostic discriminant for the two tumors. As indicated above, the presence of neuron-specific enolase in occasional examples of Ewing's sarcoma and rhabdomyosarcoma render this a less-specific marker.

Behavior and treatment

Despite recent therapeutic advances, the survival rates of patients with neuroblastoma have remained relatively unchanged over the past 2 decades, a finding that contrasts with the prognosis of other childhood sarcomas. Survival rates depend on a number of partially interrelated factors (Tables 33-2 and 33-3; box, below), including age at diagnosis, clinical stage, location, histological type, presence of N-myc amplification and DNA ploidy, and certain laboratory findings (e.g., serum ferritin, neuron-specific enolase) (Tables 33-1 and 33-2).

Age and clinical stage, two independent variables, are the two most important prognostic factors. Children less than 2 years of age have statistically better survival rates (77%) than those older than 2 years (38%).[19] Likewise, patients with stage I or II disease (see box, p. 941) have an 88% 2-year survival rate compared with a 33% rate for patients with stage III or IV disease.[29] Location of the tumor, although important, is closely related to the stage of the disease. For instance, cervical, thoracic, and pelvic tumors have better prognoses than retroperitoneal and adrenal tumors (Table 33-3), but usually are detected at an earlier clinical stage. A notable exception to the trend of decreasing survival rates with increasing clinical disease is a special group of stage IV patients designated as stage IV-S.[30] These patients have small primary tumors, and metastases are limited to skin, liver, and bone marrow without involvement of bone. The survival rate of stage IV-S patients is between 75% and 100%, very similar to that of patients with stage I and II disease. The reason for the excellent prognosis in this group with heavy tumor burden is not completely understood, but it is probably related in part to the young age (usually less than 1 year) of the patients. Some have conceptualized stage IV-S as multiple primary tumors rather than metastases;[23] others have hypothesized that stage IV-S is a premalignant condition in which the final mutagenic event has not occurred.[63] In this respect stage IV-S could be considered comparable with in situ adrenal neuroblastoma, which regresses in most instances.

In the last several years numerous studies have attested to the importance of N-myc amplification in the prognosis of neuroblastoma. Consequently it is mandatory that from every suspected neuroblastoma a small aliquot of tissue

Table 33-2. Two-year survival rates in neuroblastoma by prognostic factors

	Number of patients	Survival (%)
Overall	124	60
Age in years		
<2	73	77
2+	51	38
Neuron specific enolase		
Normal (1-100 ng/ml)	60	76
Abnormal (>100 ng/ml)	23	17
Ferritin		
Normal (0-150 ng/ml)	64	83
Abnormal (>150 ng/ml)	39	19
E rosette inhibition		
Normal (0-15%)	56	60
Abnormal (>15%)	27	54
VMA/HVA ratio		
High (>1)	28	84
Low (<1)	22	44
Stage		
I	15	100
II	27	82
III	18	42
IV	51	30
IV-S	13	100
Pathology (Shimada system)		
Favorable type	52	94
Unfavorable type	36	39

From Evans AE et al: *Cancer* 59:1853, 1987.

Favorable prognostic factors in neuroblastoma

Young age (<2yrs)
Favorable histological type
Low stage (I, II, IV-S)
No N-myc amplification
Low serum ferritin
Hyperdiploidy
High expression of TRK gene

Table 33-3. Effect of location on survival rates (%) in neuroblastoma

	Location			
	Cervical	Thoracic	Adrenal	Retroperitoneal
Evans (1971) (100 cases)		47	26	
Duckett and Koop (1977) (81 cases)	33	56	24	34

should be obtained and frozen at the time of surgery so these studies can be carried out is the diagnosis must be confirmed on permanent sections. Approximately 25% to 30% of patients with neuroblastoma have N-myc amplification, corresponding to about 30% of patients with advanced-stage disease but less than 5% of patients with low-stage disease. The presence of amplification identifies patients with a rapid clinical course independent of stage, however. Tumor cell ploidy seems to provide data complementary to N-myc amplification, and together these data identify three clinicogenetic types of neuroblastoma (Table 33-4). Near diploid or tetraploid levels of DNA correspond to patients with advanced-stage disease, whereas hyperdiploidy is associated with a good prognosis.

Other factors that predict survival rates in this disease include serum levels of ferritin and neuron-specific enolase as well as histological grade. Serum ferritin levels greater than 150 ng/ml are found in patients with statistically poorer survival rates. Other factors such as the urinary ratio of VMA to HVA and E rosette inhibition also correlate with survival rates but not with the same level of statistical significance as the preceding factors.[29]

In the past it has been difficult to correlate the degree of differentiation with the outcome because, as indicated previously, terms such as "ganglioneuroblastoma" encompassed a broad range of tumors.[19,72,101] In 1984 Shimada and associates proposed a new system, which has generally replaced earlier systems for purposes of predicting the clinical course (Table 33-5). It divides neuroblastomas into those that have a differentiated stroma (stromal rich) and those that do not (stromal poor). The latter group, composed of pure neuroblastomas and some ganglioneuroblastomas, is further subdivided by age of patient, degree of cellular maturation, and nuclear pathologic characteristics (mitosis-karyorrhexis index) into favorable and unfavorable subtypes.

Table 33-4. Clinical and genetic types of neuroblastoma

Feature	Type 1	Type 2	Type 3
Age	<12 months	Any age	Any age
Stage	I, II, IV-S	III, IV	Any stage
Ploidy	Hyperdiploid	Near diploid	Near diploid
	Near triploid	Near tetraploid	Near tetraploid
Chromosome 1p	Normal	Normal	Deleted
dmins, HSR	Absent	Absent	Present
N-myc copy	Normal	Normal	Amplified
Outcome	Good	Intermediate	Bad

From Brodeur GM et al: Neuroblastoma: effect of genetic factors on prognosis and treatment. *Cancer* 70:1685, 1992.
dmins, Double-minute chromatin bodies; *HSR*, homogeneously staining region.

Table 33-5. Histological type of neuroblastoma and its effect on 2-year survival rates

Stromal character	Survival (%)
Stromal rich	
Well-differentiated type*	100
Intermixed type*	92
Nodular type†	18
Stromal poor	
Favorable type*	84
Unfavorable type†	4.5

From Shimada H et al.: *J Natl Cancer Inst* 73:405, 1984.
*Favorable histological type.
†Unfavorable histological type.

Clinical staging of neuroblastoma

Stage I: Tumor confined to the organ or structure of origin.

Stage II: Tumors extending in continuity beyond the organ or structure of origin, but not crossing the midline*; regional lymph nodes in the ipsilateral side may be involved.

Stage III: Tumors extending in continuity beyond the midline; regional lymph nodes may be involved bilaterally.

Stage IV: Remote disease involving the skeleton, organs, soft tissues, distant lymph node groups, or other structures.

Stage IV-S: Patients who would otherwise be stage I or II but who have remote disease confined to one or more of the following sites: liver, skin, or bone marrow (without radiographic evidence of bone metastases on complete skeletal survey).

From Evans AE et al.: *Cancer* 27:374, 1971.
*For tumors arising in midline structures (e.g., organ of Zuckerkandl), penetration beyond the capsule with involvement of lymph nodes on the same side is considered stage II disease. Extradural extension of paravertebral lesions is also considered stage II disease unless tumors cross the midline.

Table 33-6. Age and anatomical distributions of ganglioneuroma (AFIP, 1970-1980) (88 cases)

Age (years)	No. cases	Location	No. cases
0-4	5	Mediastinal	34
5-9	9	Retroperitoneal	27
10-19	23	Adrenal	19
20-29	22	Pelvic	5
30-39	12	Cervical	2
40-49	4	Parapharyngeal	1
50-59	6		
60-69	4		
Over 69	3		

The Shimada system appears to accurately identify two groups of patients (unfavorable stromal-poor, nodular stromal-rich) with a notably poor prognosis (Table 33-6). This is a more complex system than earlier ones and introduces an entirely new nomenclature, with which pathologists were less familiar. The recently proposed Joshi system, detailed above, blends the basic observations of the Shimada system with more traditional terms.

At the time of diagnosis about two thirds of patients will harbor metastatic disease, a finding that emphasizes the need for thorough clinical evaluation before institution of therapy. Metastatic disease is most common in bone, lymph nodes, liver, and skin. Although the presence of metastasis does not necessarily portend death from disease, bone metastasis accompanied by overt radiological changes is a notable exception. This pattern of metastasis almost always signifies a fatal outcome.

As indicated previously, a small percentage of tumors (1% to 2%) may undergo spontaneous regression or maturation. This occurs most often in children under 1 year of age. It is generally believed that most clinical cures of neuroblastomas, particularly in patients with stage IV-S disease, represent tumor regression rather than maturation.[30] Maturation is well documented in the literature.[20,28,37,44] In many recent cases the question has been raised as to whether therapy induced the maturation. Early cases, such as the one described by Cushing and Wolback,[20] leave little doubt that this represents a natural sequence of events in some cases. In this instance the patient received no therapy apart from administration of Coley's toxin and only a biopsy was done.

Therapy is usually based on the age of the patient and the stage of the disease. Complete extirpation of the tumor without radiotherapy has been recommended for stage I and II cases.[31,66] Surgery with postoperative radiation therapy for residual disease is advocated in stage III disease.[49] Unfortunately stage IV patients do not seem to benefit greatly from attempted removal of the primary tumor. Consequently, only when the operative risk is small and the patient is not debilitated from metastatic disease is this at-

tempted.[67] Radiotherapy, however, is used in these patients to reduce the size of the primary tumor and to minimize pain from metastatic disease. A notable exception to this approach is the treatment of patients with stage IV-S disease, who require removal of the primary tumor and, at most, conservative adjunctive therapy.

As a relatively new approach, some patients with disseminated neuroblastoma have been given total body irradiation and high-dose chemotherapy followed by bone marrow transplantation.[70] In order to remove tumor from autologous marrow intended for transplantation, magnetic microspheres, targeted with monoclonal antibodies against the tumor, have been employed.[90]

GANGLIONEUROMA

Ganglioneuroma is a fully differentiated tumor that contains no immature elements. They are quite rare compared with other benign neural tumors such as neurilemoma and neurofibroma, but they outnumber neuroblastomas occurring along the sympathetic axis by about 3:1 according to Stout's estimate.[109] In our experience at the AFIP, ganglioneuromas differ significantly in age distribution and location compared with neuroblastomas. The majority of ganglioneuromas are diagnosed in patients older than 10 years and are most often located in the posterior mediastinum, followed by the retroperitoneum (Table 33-6). Only a minor proportion occur in the adrenal proper. The differences in distribution of neuroblastomas and ganglioneuromas support the idea that all ganglioneuromas do not necessarily arise by way of maturation in a preexisting neuroblastoma; most, in our opinion, probably arise de novo.

Clinically, ganglioneuromas present as large masses in the retroperitoneum or mediastinum; they are usually of longer duration than neuroblastomas. We have reviewed one case in which the mass was allegedly present 20 years before the time of surgery. About one third have intralesional calcification. On ultrasonographic studies they are hypoechoic lesions that are typically hypovascular. We have seen a few cases in patients with neurofibromatosis. Occasional tumors may be associated with diarrhea,[74,95,114] sweating, hypertension, and rarely virilization[1] and myasthenia gravis.[74,80,114] Diarrheal symptoms in patients with these tumors have been related to the presence of vasoactive intestinal peptide, which can be localized to the cytoplasm of the ganglion cell by means of immunoperoxidase techniques.[74]

Grossly, ganglioneuroma is a well-circumscribed tumor having a fibrous capsule. On cut section it is gray to yellow and sometimes displays a trabecular or whorled pattern similar to that of leiomyoma (Fig. 33-15). Histologically, it has a uniform appearance throughout. The background consists of bundles of longitudinal and transversely oriented Schwann cells that crisscross each other in an irregular fashion (Figs. 33-16 and 33-17). Rarely, fat may

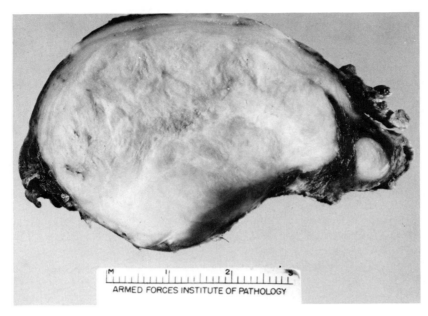

FIG. 33-15. White whorled gross appearance of ganglioneuroma.

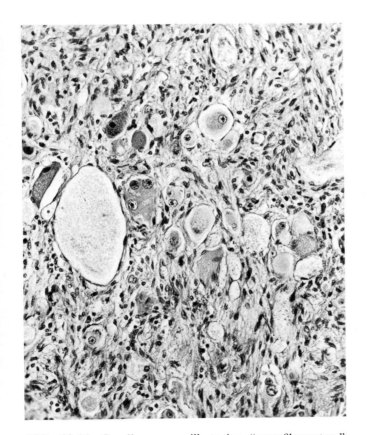

FIG. 33-16. Ganglioneuroma illustrating "neurofibromatous" stroma with atypical ganglion cells. (×160.)

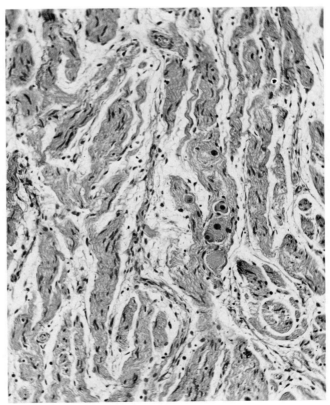

FIG. 33-17. Ganglioneuroma with slightly more mature stroma than that shown in Fig. 33-13.

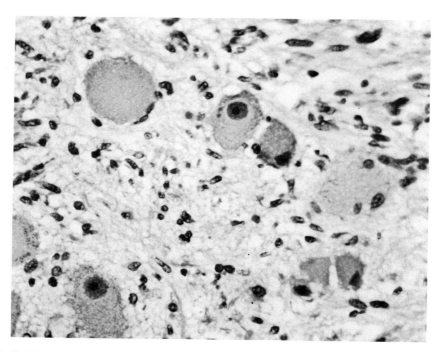

FIG. 33-18. Ganglion cells from ganglioneuroma having less Nissl substance and fewer satellite cells compared with their normal counterparts. (×400.)

be present within the stroma. Scattered throughout the schwannian backdrop are relatively mature ganglion cells. Although they may occur in an isolated fashion, usually they are found in small clusters or nests. In general, they are not fully mature and lack satellite cells and Nissl bodies (Fig. 33-18). Typically their voluminous cytoplasm is bright pink and contains one to three nuclei, which may show a mild to moderate degree of atypia. Pigment is sometimes present within the ganglion cells and is believed to represent catecholamine products that undergo autooxidation to a melanin-like substance (neuromelanin).[42,47,79] Although the pigment has tinctorial properties of dermal melanin (Fontana-positive), ultrastructurally it does not have the regular subunit structure but consists instead of large lysosomal structures with myelin figures.[79] There are now a number of reports in the literature of composite tumors composed of ganglioneuroma and pheochromocytoma. Such tumors have been associated with the symptom of watery diarrhea (Fig. 33-19).[74,114]

Biologically, ganglioneuromas are benign tumors. Of the 146 tumors studied by Stout,[109] none metastasized. However, it should be pointed out that rarely an apparent "metastatic" focus of ganglioneuroma may be encountered within a lymph node adjacent to the main tumor mass (Fig. 33-20) or in a more distant site.[38] It is assumed that these cases represent neuroblastomas in which the metastasis as well as the primary tumor matured. We have reviewed three examples of ganglioneuroma that underwent malignant transformation (Fig. 33-21). One case was that of a young woman with a neuroblastoma that matured to ganglioneuroma. It remained stable for 20 years, after which time it underwent transformation to malignant schwannoma. The second case was a de novo ganglioneuroma that had been present for several decades. The patient died of other causes and at autopsy had malignant foci resembling a malignant schwannoma within the ganglioneuroma. Other cases of malignant transformation of ganglioneuroma have also been reported,* some occurring in de novo ganglioneuromas and others in ganglioneuromas arising as a result of maturation in neuroblastoma. One case of malignant transformation of a ganglioneuroma in an HIV-positive patient has been reported.[16]

GANGLION CELL CHORISTOMA

Collections of mature ganglion cells occurring in the skin as an isolated and incidental finding have been termed "ganglion cell choristoma."[126-128] Rios et al.[128] reported a case in a 14-year-old child, consisting of a poorly circumscribed collection of mature ganglion cells within the dermis. The tumor was not associated with elevated levels of urinary VMA secretion nor was the patient known to have a neu-

---

*References 5, 16, 21, 35, 39, 61, 91.

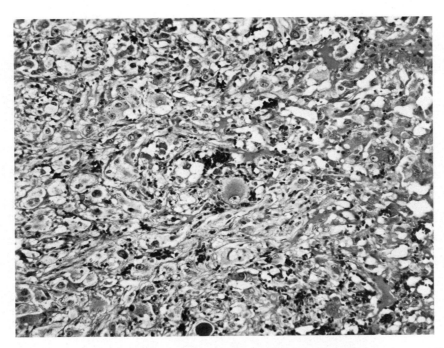

FIG. 33-19. Ganglioneuroma with focal areas of pheochromocytoma *(upper right).* (×160.)

roblastoma. Lee et al.[126] described a slightly different dermal lesion containing a superficial ganglionic component associated with a deep dermal neuromatous component. Traumatic pharyngeal neuromas arising adjacent to autonomic ganglia may contain ganglion cells and thus may superficially resemble a ganglioneuroma.[125]

PERIPHERAL NEUROEPITHELIOMA (PERIPHERAL NEUROBLASTOMA OR PRIMITIVE NEUROECTODERMAL TUMOR)

Peripheral neuroepithelioma is a primitive neuroblastic tumor arising outside the autonomic nervous system. An early description of this tumor was published by Stout. He reported a round cell tumor of the ulnar nerve that formed rosettes[187] and in tissue culture grew axons,[183] suggesting a close histogenetic relationship with neuroblastoma. Stout later reported a similar tumor that lacked rosettes and neurites and in tissue culture gave rise to "epithelium" similar to primitive neuroepithelium. Tumors of the latter type are comparable to poorly differentiated neuroepitheliomas of the central nervous system (i.e., medulloblastoma).[170] Most tumors described as small cell tumor of the thoracopulmonary wall of children, reported by Askin et al.,[160] are peripheral neuroepitheliomas. Thus, it is clear that many stages of developing neuroepithelium may be recapitulated in this group of tumors.

In the past, most examples of peripheral neuroepithelioma have been diagnosed by virtue of their origin from a peripheral nerve. The ability to identify neuroblastic differentiation by immunohistochemical and ultrastructural analysis has expanded our concept of this entity. Yet this approach has also created certain problems. Although it is relatively easy to recognize those neuroepitheliomas that arise from nerve and form rosettes, there is less agreement as to the minimum criteria for making this diagnosis when the tumor does not arise in a peripheral nerve and rosettes are absent or poorly formed. Such cases overlap with Ewing's sarcoma. One has only to peruse the various large studies in the literature to realize that the diagnostic criteria vary from institution to institution, making it difficult to compare and contrast data. For example, in the study from Memorial Sloan Kettering Cancer Center,[151] tumors with ganglionic differentiation were excluded from consideration, whereas the opposite was the case in the study of the German Society of Pediatric Oncology.[154] Some authors maintain that the presence of neuron-specific enolase identifies a lesion as a peripheral neuroepithelioma, whereas we believe that this enzyme, which also occurs in classic Ewing's sarcoma, should not by itself be used to discriminate Ewing's sarcoma from peripheral neuroepithelioma.

Despite the fact that peripheral neuroepitheliomas share certain common histological features with neuroblastoma, there are several significant differences: (1) They rarely display the capacity for differentiation and functional activity encountered in neuroblastoma. (2) Peripheral neuroepitheliomas do not possess the characteristic 1p deletions that characterize most neuroblastomas. Instead, they share the same cytogenetic abnormality (t(11;22)) as Ewing's sar-

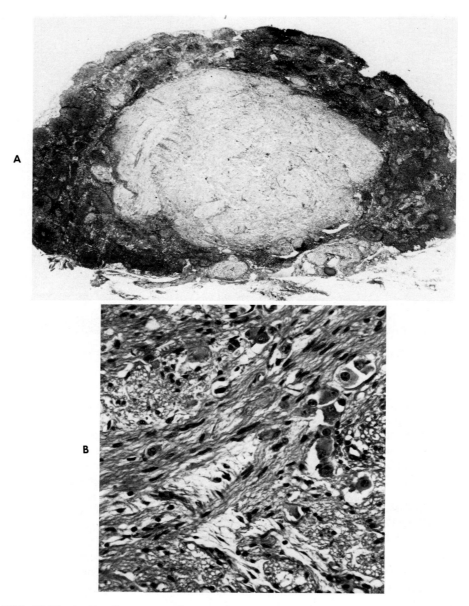

FIG. 33-20. A, Ganglioneuroma of retroperitoneum in which "metastatic" deposit was present within a regional lymph node. (×15.) **B,** Both primary and "metastatic" deposits had typical appearance and presumably occurred as a result of maturation of a preexisting neuroblastoma. (×160.)

coma,[162,169,188] a similar pattern of protooncogene expression (N-myc, c-myb, c-ets-1),[166] and the same surface protein (p30/32) encoded by the mic-2 gene.[129,131,175]

Clinical features

Despite increasing reports of this tumor, the incidence of this lesion, by all accounts, is still rare. In the experience cited by Hashimoto et al.,[149] it comprised 1% of all sarcomas. Kushner et al.[157] reported 54 cases treated at Memorial Sloan Kettering Cancer Hospital over a 20-year period, and Marina et al.[165] only 26 cases at St. Jude's Hos-

pital during a 25-year period. Unlike neuroblastoma, which usually occurs in patients younger than age 5 years, this tumor may occur at almost any age. In our experience with 52 cases studied at the AFIP, as well as that of others,[141,157] about three quarters of cases occur before age 35 years and the median age is approximately 20 years, a distribution corresponding roughly to that of extraskeletal Ewing's sarcoma. By definition, peripheral neuroepitheliomas do not arise from the sympathetic nervous system, and, thus, acceptable cases of neuroepitheliomas occur for the most part outside the vertebral axis of the body, usually in the ex-

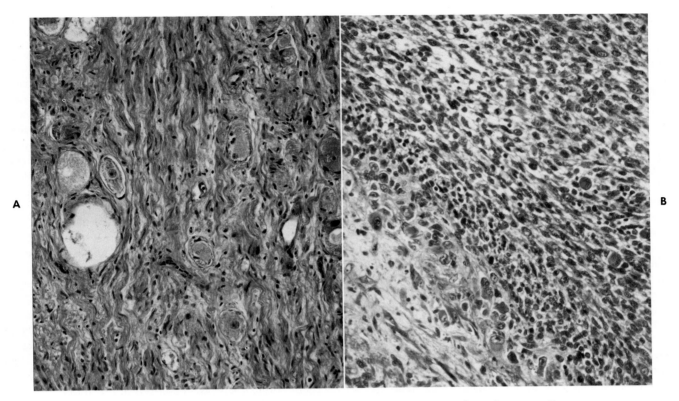

FIG. 33-21. Ganglioneuroma (A) which underwent malignant transformation to malignant schwannoma (B). Note that residual mature ganglion cells are present in lower left corner of B. (A and B, ×250.)

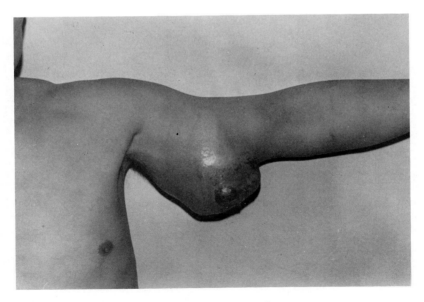

FIG. 33-22. Neuroepithelioma of upper arm.

tremities (Fig. 33-22). Studies reporting a high incidence of lesions in the paravertebral areas, especially in close relationship to the vertebral foramina, possibly have included examples of neuroblastoma. In our material, the most common anatomical sites are the buttock and upper thigh (32%) where the tumors were often intimately associated with the sciatic nerve.[141] The shoulder and upper arm accounted for an additional 25% of cases. Fully one third of our cases were intimately attached to a major nerve and gave rise to signs and symptoms related to diminished neurological function. There is no increased tendency for these tumors to occur in patients with von Recklinghausen's disease. With rare exceptions,[188] peripheral neuroepitheliomas have not been associated with elevated catecholamine levels.

Microscopic features

Generally these tumors resemble neuroblastomas. They are composed of sheets or lobules of small rounded cells containing darkly staining, round or oval nuclei (Figs. 33-23 and 33-24). The cytoplasm is indistinct except in areas where the cells are more mature, and the elongated hairlike cytoplasmic extensions coalesce to form rosettes. Most of the rosettes are similar to those seen in neuroblastoma and contain a central solid core of neurofibrillary material (Figs. 33-24 and 33-27) (Homer-Wright rosette). Rarely, the rosettes resemble those of retinoblastoma and contain a central lumen or vesicle (Flexner-Wintersteiner rosette). In some peripheral neuroepitheliomas, rosettes may be few in number and closely resemble Ewing's sarcoma (Fig. 33-25). In others, the tumor possesses cords or trabeculae of small round cells. These areas bear a resemblance to a carcinoid tumor or small cell undifferentiated carcinoma, although histogenetically they are properly compared with primitive neuroepithelium. Between 10% and 20% of neuroepitheliomas will display spindled areas that resemble a primitive fibrosarcoma or malignant schwannoma (Fig. 33-26). There are also examples of peripheral neuroepithelioma containing a variety of lines of differentia-

tion including glial, ependymal, cartilaginous, and epithelial.[146,179]

Immunohistochemical and ultrastructural features

The most characteristic ultrastructural feature is the presence of elongated cell processes that interdigitate with each other and contain small dense core granules (neurosecretory granules), which measure 50 to 100 nm, and occasionally contain microtubules.[130,163,181] The processes are most highly developed in the center of the rosettes and in the neurofibrillary areas, where they form a tangled mass. However, they are also noted in areas that display little neurofibrillary differentiation by light microscopy.

The immunohistochemical profile of this tumor varies depending on the study.[129,131,136,144,154] Most agree that the tumors strongly express neuron-specific enolase and the cell surface antigen (p30/32) encoded by the mic-2 gene and detected by the antibody HBA71. The latter is highly characteristic but not totally specific for neuroepithelioma and Ewing's sarcoma, since it may also be identified in some lymphomas and rhabdomyosarcomas.[129] Leu-7, synaptophysin, S-100 protein, neurofilament protein, and chromogranin are variably positive within these tumors, but glial fibrillary acidic protein is consistently negative. Recently, desmin has been described in two primitive neuroectodermal tumors that possessed rosettes on light microscopic studies and neural features on electron microscopic studies, but had no structural evidence of muscle differen-

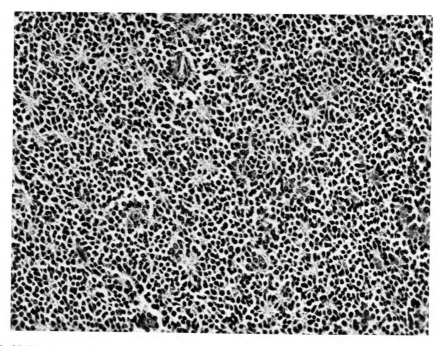

FIG. 33-23. Neuroepithelioma of thigh. Tumor is very similar to neuroblastoma but lacks mats of neuropil and ganglion cells. (×250.)

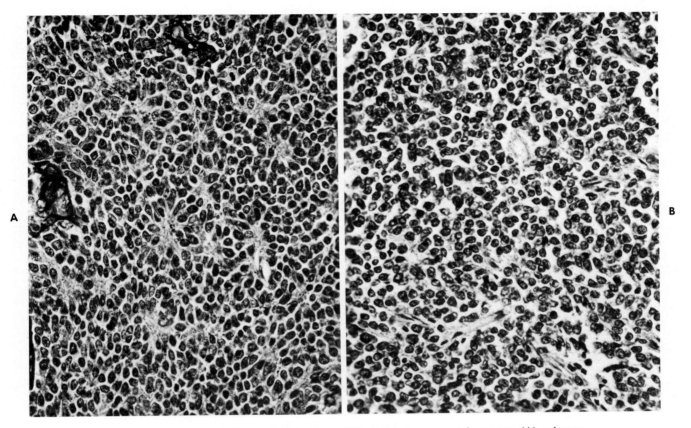

FIG. 33-24. Neuroepithelioma of thigh. Better differentiated areas contain rosettes **(A)**, whereas less-differentiated areas consist simply of primitive round cells **(B)**. (**A** and **B**, ×400.)

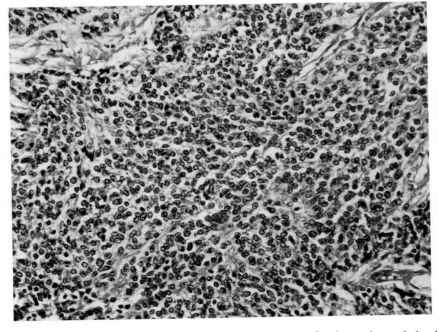

FIG. 33-25. Peripheral neuroepithelioma showing rosettes that are few in number and closely resemble Ewing's sarcoma.

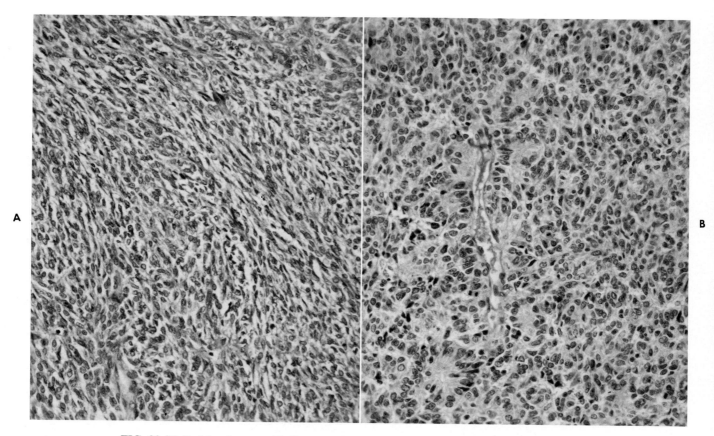

FIG. 33-26. Peripheral neuroepithelioma showing round cell areas containing rosettes **(A)** and spindled areas **(B)**, which coexisted in same tumor. (**A** and **B**, ×160.)

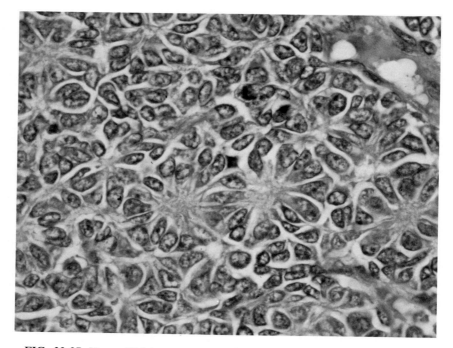

FIG. 33-27. Homer-Wright rosette within a peripheral neuroepithelioma. (×400.)

tiation.[176] This finding, supported by Western blot analysis, indicates that aberrant expression or lineage infidelity occurs in this group of lesions.

Differential diagnosis

These tumors present one of the most difficult diagnostic challenges to the pathologist. Since this tumor is either a close relative of extraosseous Ewing's sarcoma or part of the same morphological spectrum, it is not surprising that the differential diagnosis of these two lesions is the most problematic. Unfortunately, there are no uniformly accepted criteria as to where one should draw the line between the two. In our practice we have regarded a lesion as neuroepithelioma rather than extraosseous Ewing's sarcoma if it possessed well-defined rosettes of the Homer-Wright or Flexner-Wintersteiner type, if there was evidence of neural differentiation on electron microscopic studies (neurites or dense core granules), or if two or more neural markers were present (e.g., neuron specific enolase, Leu-7, synaptophysin, chromogranin). Since extraosseous Ewing's sarcoma may express neuron specific-enolase, we have not regarded the presence of this antigen alone as sufficient evidence to establish the diagnosis of neuroepithelioma. During childhood this tumor must be distinguished from metastasis of neuroblastoma. The presence of mats of neuropil, ganglionic differentiation, and calcification are usually features of either primary or metastatic neuroblastoma. Expression of mic-2 gene product and β-2-microglobulin is also strong presumptive evidence that one is dealing with either neuroepithelioma or Ewing's sarcoma rather than neuroblastoma.[175] In adults the possibility of metastatic neuroblastoma is remote, and the usual question is that of small cell carcinoma (either primary or metastatic). These tumors, which show distinct rosettes or neurofibrils or clearly arise in a nerve, present no problem in diagnosis. Less-differentiated tumors consisting of cords or ribbons of cells sometimes cannot be reliably distinguished from carcinoma by light microscopy. In these cases electron microscopic or immunohistochemical studies have proved valuable.[40] Although some small cell carcinomas possess dense core granules, they have less-elaborate processes than neuroepithelioma and possess more highly developed desmosomes and occasional tonofibrils.

Clinical course

These lesions are highly aggressive neoplasms that rapidly give rise to metastatic disease and death. Jurgens et al.[154] cited a survival rate of approximately 50% at 3 years, whereas Kushner et al.[157] indicated that only 25% of patients with tumors greater than 5 cm were alive at 24 months. Marina et al. reported a 10.8-month disease control interval, a period significantly shorter than that of classic osseous Ewing's sarcoma. Metastatic disease occurs most commonly to lung, bone, and liver. Most authors agree that the best outlook for cure resides with a combination of surgery, irradiation, and chemotherapy.

OLFACTORY NEUROBLASTOMA (ESTHESIONEUROBLASTOMA)

Described in 1924 by Berger, this lesion is a specialized form of neuroectodermal tumor arising from the nasal cavity.* Its origin has been debated and has been variously attributed to the neuroectodermal cells of the olfactory placode, the sympathetic fibers (ganglion of loci of the nervus terminalis) in the anterior portion of the nasal cavity, the sphenopalatine ganglion, and the organ of Jacobson. The identification of norepinephrine and dopamine β-hydroxylase (the enzyme that catalyzes the conversion of dopamine to norepinephrine) in a recent case indicates a functional similarity to neuroblastoma,[167] although currently some have suggested its close kinship with peripheral neuroepithelioma.[187] Its location high in the nasal vault, however, and the fact that some tumors have ultrastructural features of olfactory nerve cells[163] favor origin from the olfactory placode. Unlike neuroblastomas, these tumors rarely arise during early childhood. Approximately 90% occur in patients over the age of 10 years.[163] In localized lesions the most common presentation is unilateral nasal obstruction and epistaxis, followed less frequently by lacrimation, rhinorrhea, and anosmia. Extensive lesions involving the sinuses are accompanied by frontal headache and diplopia. One unique case has been associated with vasopressin secretion.[180] Radiographically, spotty calcification may be detected within the tumor, although the specific bone changes depend on the extent of the tumor. The lesions are fleshy gray polypoid masses that histologically consist of sheets of small dark cells similar to those of neuroblastoma. Both true rosettes with a central lumen and pseudorosettes containing a core of neurofibrillary material can be found within the tumor. In more mature lesions the stroma contains mats of neuropil. Ultrastructurally, the cells have features of primitive neuroblasts including dense core (neurosecretory) granules within neuritic processes.[133,156,163,186] Neurotubules and cilia are sometimes present. In one case, specific features of olfactory differentiation were present. The columnar cells possessed numerous apical microvilli and bulbous extensions similar to those of the neurogenous cell of the olfactory apparatus.[163] Both neurofilament protein[185] and neuron-specific enolase can be identified within the primitive neuroblastic cells. A fine network of cells that are positive for S-100 protein and vimentin surrounds the neuroblasts in a diagnostically distinctive fashion[134,178] and brings to mind the sustentacular network that is positive for S-100 protein within paragangliomas. These staining procedures, in conjunction with staining for

---

*References 133, 140, 142, 150, 156, 168, 173, 174, 180, 181.

cytokeratin and leukocyte common antigen to rule out carcinoma and lymphoma, respectively, have simplified the diagnosis of this previously elusive tumor.

A histological classification of these tumors into three subtypes has been suggested: (1) olfactory neuroepithelioma containing true rosettes, (2) olfactory neuroblastoma containing pseudorosettes, and (3) olfactory neurocytoma, which lacks rosettes altogether and is composed of more mature cells. Unfortunately this classification bears little relationship to the behavior of these tumors and has been abandoned by most authors in favor of staging as proposed by Kadish et al.[155] Stage A patients, with tumors limited to the nasal cavity, have a crude 5-year survival rate of 90%.[140] Stage B patients, with tumors involving the nasal cavity and one or more paranasal sinuses, have a 70.8% survival rate.[140] Stage C patients, with disease extending beyond the nasal cavity and sinuses, have a 46.7% survival rate.[140] Retrospective analysis of reported cases indicates that radiotherapy alone, surgery alone, or combined irradiation and surgery are all equally effective in controlling stage A and B disease, whereas combined therapy may be more valuable for patients with stage C disease.[140] Mills and Frierson[168] and others have pointed out that even the Kadish staging system is not fully predictive of survival rates. In their experience with 21 olfactory neuroblastomas, the only clinical feature that correlated with prognosis was completeness of surgical excision. Furthermore, no histological features could be correlated significantly with survival rates. Seven patients (33%) died of their disease, with an average survival time of 27 months. A recent study from the University of Michigan Hospitals with 21 patients suggested that the recent use of aggressive craniofacial resection as well as irradiation and chemotherapy for advanced disease has improved survival rates in recent years.[190]

EXTRASKELETAL EWING'S SARCOMA

Although Ewing's sarcoma of bone not infrequently breaks through the cortex and extends into the surrounding tissues, this tumor also occurs as a primary soft tissue neoplasm without involvement of bone. According to our experience with approximately 150 cases of this tumor, it is slightly more common in males than in females and affects predominantly adolescents and young adults between 15 and 30 years of age. It chiefly involves the soft tissues of the paravertebral region as well as the retroperitoneum and the lower extremities.[190,254,256]

Clinical findings

Clinical data regarding this tumor are still rather limited. In our series of 39 cases of extraskeletal Ewing's sarcoma,[190] the youngest patient was a 20-month-old boy and the oldest a 63-year-old woman. Seventy-seven percent of the patients were between 10 and 30 years of age, and the median age was 20 years. Males slightly predominated over

females.[190,249] These observations correspond closely with those given for Ewing's sarcoma of bone; in the series of Pritchard et al.,[240] for example, the patients ranged in age from 14 months to 59 years, with 70% being younger than 20 years. Blacks seem to be rarely affected by skeletal or extraskeletal Ewing's sarcoma.[205]

In general, the tumor presents as a rapidly growing, deeply located mass measuring 5 to 10 cm in greatest diameter. Superficially located cases do occur but are rare.[237] The tumor is painful in about one third of cases. If peripheral nerves or the spinal cord is involved, there may be progressive sensory or motor disturbances. As with other round cell sarcomas, the preoperative duration of symptoms is usually less than 1 year. Unlike in neuroblastoma, catecholamine determinations are within normal limits.[194,225,229,255]

The principal sites are the paravertebral region and chest wall, generally in close association with the vertebrae or the ribs. The tumor may also arise in the soft tissues of the lower extremities and, very rarely, in the pelvic and hip regions, the retroperitoneum, and the upper extremities (Table 33-7).[190,206,251] The most common sites in the study of Shimada et al.[249] were the trunk (especially the paravertebral region and chest wall), the extremities, and the retroperitoneum. Radiographs, CT scan, or magnetic resonance imaging is essential for establishing the extraskeletal site of the tumor.

Pathological findings

The gross appearance varies. In general, the tumor is multilobulated, soft, and friable and rarely exceeds 10 cm in greatest diameter. Its cut surface has a gray-yellow or gray-tan appearance, often with large areas of necrosis, cyst formation, or hemorrhage. Despite the extensive necrosis, calcification is rare.

Microscopically, typical examples of this tumor are marked by a solidly packed, lobular round cell pattern of striking uniformity. The individual cells possess a rounded or ovoid vesicular nucleus measuring 10 to 15 μm in diameter, with a distinct nuclear membrane, finely divided powdery chromatin, and a single minute nucleolus. There are no multinucleated giant cells. The cytoplasm is ill de-

Table 33-7. Anatomical distribution of 72 cases of extraskeletal Ewing's sarcoma

Location	No. patients	%
Chest wall	20	28
Lower extremity	18	25
Paravertebral region	16	22
Pelvic and hip region	10	14
Retroperitoneum	6	8
Upper extremity	2	3
TOTAL	72	100

fined, scanty, and pale staining and in many cases is irregularly vacuolated as a result of intracellular deposits of glycogen (Figs. 33-28 to 33-31). Intracellular glycogen is present in the majority of cases, but the amount varies from tumor to tumor and sometimes in different portions of the same neoplasm.[190,244] Complete absence of glycogen, however, is rare in Ewing's sarcoma (Figs. 33-32 and 33-33). The number of mitotic figures varies, and in many cases the paucity of mitotic figures contrasts with the immature appearance of the tumor cells[190] (Figs. 33-28 to 33-31).

Although the tumor is richly vascular, the thin-walled vessels are compressed and obscured by the closely packed tumor cells, and the rich vascularity is often discernible only in areas of degeneration and necrosis. In fact, the association of distinct vascular structures with degenerated or necrotic "ghost" cells is a common striking feature that has been described as the "filigree pattern" of Ewing's sarcoma[215] (Fig. 33-34). Aside from the prominent vascularity, there is occasionally a pseudovascular or pseudoalveolar pattern caused by small fluid-filled pools or spaces amidst the solidly arranged tumor cells; this feature should not be mistaken for evidence of angiosarcoma or alveolar rhabdomyosarcoma. Presumably, this pattern is responsible for Ewing's initial designation of the tumor as "diffuse endothelioma"[203] (Fig. 33-35).

Reticulin preparations outline the tumor lobules, but there are hardly any reticulin fibrils between the densely packed tumor cells, and tissue culture studies reveal complete lack of collagen production, a feature that aids in distinguishing the tumor from poorly differentiated fibrosarcoma, chondrosarcoma, and small cell osteosarcoma.

Round cell tumors that deviate from the typical pattern by cell size or cellular atypism have been described in the literature as "small cell" (lymphocytoid), "large cell," or "atypical" Ewing's sarcoma.[233,234]

Immunohistochemical findings

Although the results (and criteria for diagnosis) of the various immunohistochemical studies vary greatly, there is general agreement that in one half to two thirds of cases the cells stain positively for vimentin[138,200,204] and that in nearly all cases the tumor cells, like those of peripheral neuroepithelioma, diffusely express the mic-2 gene, a glycoprotein located in the pseudoautosomal region of both the X and Y chromosomes.[129,204,236] Less frequently the cells stain with antibodies to neuron-specific enolase, Leu-7 (HNK-1), and synaptophysin, but the reported results vary greatly among different reviewers.* Immunostaining for neurofilaments, S-100 protein, and chromogranin is usually but not always negative.[195,249] There are also a few reports of Ewing's sarcoma of bone that stains focally for low-

---

*References 151, 213, 219, 239, 246, 258.

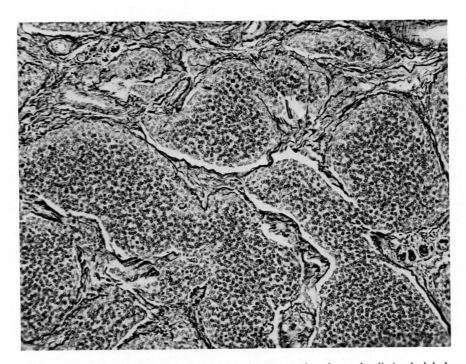

FIG. 33-28. Extraskeletal Ewing's sarcoma. Reticulin preparation shows the distinctly lobular arrangement of the tumor and the absence of reticulin fibers between the tumor cells. (Reticulin preparation, ×120.) (From Angervall L, Enzinger FM: *Cancer* 36:240, 1975.)

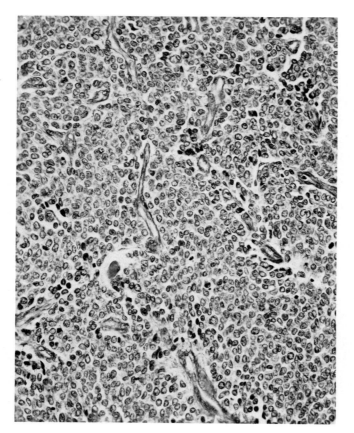

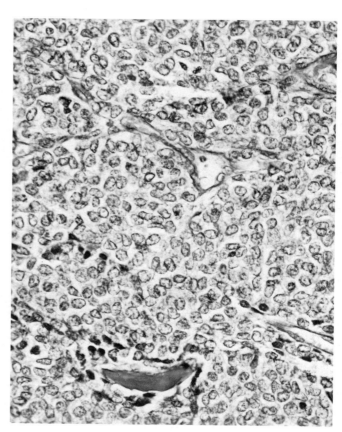

FIG. 33-29. Extraskeletal Ewing's sarcoma. Solidly packed tumor cells of striking uniformity with interspersed thin-walled vascular structures. (×160.)

FIG. 33-30. Extraskeletal Ewing's sarcoma. The cellular elements possess rounded or ovoid vesicular nuclei and an indistinct, pale-staining cytoplasm. (×390.)

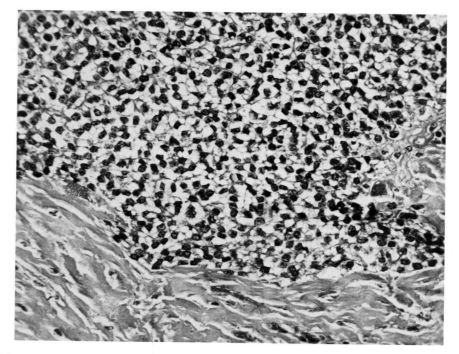

FIG. 33-31. Extraskeletal Ewing's sarcoma. Vacuolated appearance of the tumor is the result of deposition of abundant intracellular glycogen. (×295.)

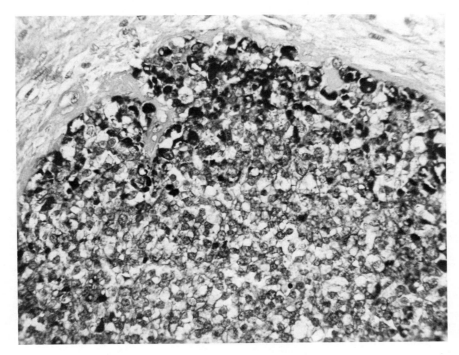

FIG. 33-32. Extraskeletal Ewing's sarcoma. PAS preparation reveals intracellular glycogen, especially in the peripheral portion of the tumor. (×295.)

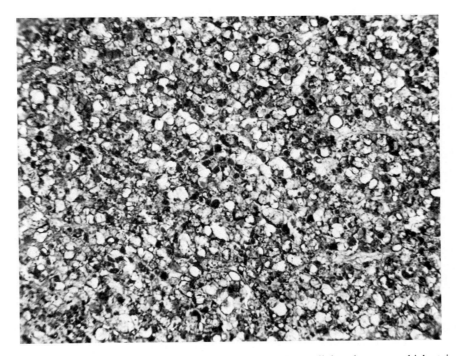

FIG. 33-33. Extraskeletal Ewing's sarcoma with abundant intracellular glycogen, which stains a deep purple with PAS preparation. (×350.)

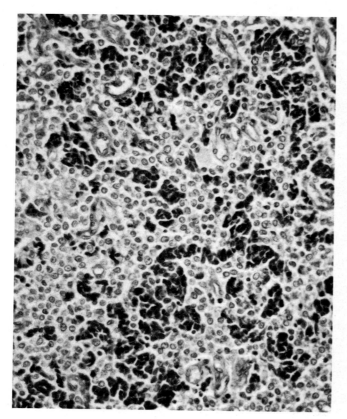

FIG. 33-34. Ewing's sarcoma showing a biphasic pattern caused by partial degeneration and necrosis of tumor cells (filigree pattern). (×250.)

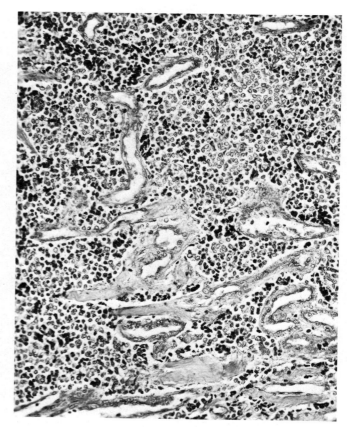

FIG. 33-35. Extraskeletal Ewing's sarcoma. Prominent hemangioma-like vascular pattern in area of cellular degeneration.

weight cytokeratin.[220,223] There is general agreement that the tumor cells do not express glial fibrillary acidic protein, desmin, muscle-specific actin, myoglobin, factor VIII, or leukocyte common antigen.[231,234]

Ultrastructural findings

Examination of skeletal and extraskeletal Ewing's sarcoma with the electron microscope reveals primitive undifferentiated cells with uniform rounded or ovoid nuclei, a smooth nuclear envelope, and finely granular chromatin with one or two small nucleoli.[206,217,234] Characteristically, the cytoplasm contains few organelles, including a small number of mitochondria, a poorly developed Golgi complex, and abundant glycogen sometimes containing small lipid droplets (Fig. 33-36). There are also free ribosomes, inconspicuous rough endoplasmic reticulum, occasional membrane-bound dense bodies (presumably lysosomes), and bundles of intermediate nonspecific filaments. The cells are closely apposed and are joined by infrequent and rudimentary cell junctions. There is hardly any collagen in the extracellular spaces. Bundles of myofilaments, Weibel-Palade bodies, and distinct basal laminae are absent in the

tumor.[163,202,262] Evidence of neural differentiation (cytoplasmic processes, microtubules, or neurosecretory granules) has been reported in a small number of tumors.[151,202,222,228,240]

Cytogenetic findings

Cytogenetic analysis of osseous and extraosseous Ewing's sarcoma reveals in 80% to 90% of tumors reciprocal translocation of the long arm of chromosomes 11 and 22 (t(11;22)(q24;q12)). This feature was first demonstrated by Aurias et al.[192] in 1983 and has been confirmed since by several other investigators, sometimes together with additional but less-specific chromosomal changes.* Besides skeletal and extraskeletal Ewing's sarcoma, this characteristic genetic abnormality of chromosomes 11 and 22 has also been demonstrated in peripheral neuroepithelioma,[187] Askin tumor,[248] and esthesioneuroblastoma.[189] A similar translocation, t(11;22)(q13;q12), has also been demonstrated in the intraabdominal desmoplastic small cell tumor of childhood.[243] This abnormality is absent in other round

*References 189, 193, 201, 219, 226, 260, 261.

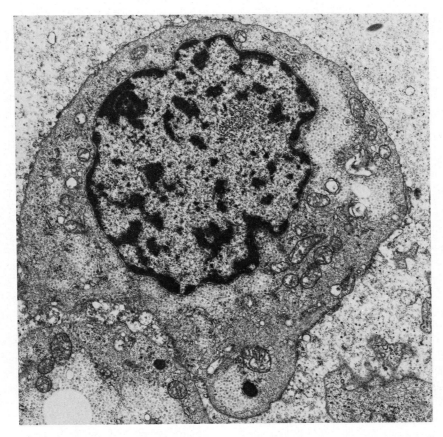

FIG. 33-36. Electron microscopic picture of extraskeletal Ewing's sarcoma. The individual tumor cell has a prominent nucleus with marginated chromatin, few organelles, and abundant glycogen. (×10,500.)

cell sarcomas, especially rhabdomyosarcoma and neuroblastoma. A similar translocation, t(11;22)(q23;q11), has been reported in numerous families as a constitutional rearrangement without increased tumor incidence.[265] Stephenson et al.[252] give a detailed account of the molecular genetics in Ewing's sarcoma.

Differential diagnosis

Distinction from other round cell sarcomas may cause considerable difficulties. Ewing's sarcoma and peripheral neuroepithelioma may show similar morphological features under the light microscope, but separation of these two tumors is important because of the better prognosis of Ewing's sarcoma. As previously pointed out, a diagnosis of neuroepithelioma rather than Ewing's sarcoma should be rendered if the tumor shows well-defined rosettes of the Homer-Wright or Flexner-Wintersteiner type, if there are two or more positive neural markers, or if there is ultrastructural evidence of neural differentiation such as multiple cellular processes and dense core granules. Neuron-specific enolase is frequently demonstrable in the cells of both tumors and does not seem to constitute a useful differential diagnostic criterion. Also helpful in differential diagnosis are the more uniform nuclei, the lesser amount of nuclear chromatin, and the presence of intracellular glycogen and immunoreactive vimentin in most cases of Ewing's sarcoma. Age of patient and tumor location are of little help in differential diagnosis. Occurrence of the tumor in a large nerve trunk such as the brachial plexus or the sciatic nerve is unknown in Ewing's sarcoma and strongly favors a diagnosis of neuroepithelioma.

"Malignant small cell tumor of the thoracopulmonary region in childhood," or "Askin tumor,"[136,191] is a tumor that affects mostly the chest wall and ribs, with frequent involvement of intercostal nerves. It seems to be more closely related to neuroepithelioma than Ewing's sarcoma, mainly because this tumor expresses neural markers more frequently than Ewing's sarcoma.[248] Glycogen may or may not be present in this tumor.[221]

Neuroblastoma enters into the differential diagnosis because of the young age of some patients, the frequent paravertebral location of the tumor, and the presence of rosettelike structures of the Homer-Wright type in about 20% to 30% of cases. The average patient with extraskeletal Ewing's sarcoma is older than the average patient with neuroblastoma and the cells are more rounded and contain glycogen, lack catecholamine fluorescence, and express the mic-2 gene. Intracellular glycogen is rare in neuroblastoma and may be discernible only with the electron microscope. Also, in contrast to neuroblastoma, the necrotic areas in Ewing's sarcoma rarely undergo calcification.[257] Another important distinguishing feature is the deletion of chromosome 1, del(1)(p32;p36), in most cases of neuroblastoma.

Alveolar rhabdomyosarcoma may display similar densely packed cellular areas, especially at its periphery, but in general its nuclei contain a greater amount of chromatin and tend to be more irregular in outline. When multiple sections are examined, the solid round cell areas are nearly always associated with areas showing loss of cellular cohesion and a distinct alveolar pattern, multinucleated giant cells with marginally placed nuclei, and, in about 20% to 30% of cases, eosinophilic cells characteristic of rhabdomyoblasts with or without cross-striations. Furthermore, the majority of these tumors show positive immunostaining for muscle-specific actin (with HHF35 antibodies) and desmin as well as a characteristic genetic abnormality, t(2;13)(q37;q14), different from that in Ewing's sarcoma and peripheral neuroepithelioma.[199]

Malignant (non-Hodgkin's) lymphoma is often suspected because of the undifferentiated appearance of the tumor cells. This diagnosis can be ruled out in most cases if attention is paid to the lobular arrangement and monotonous uniformity of the nuclei in extraskeletal Ewing's sarcoma, the presence of stainable intracellular glycogen, and the lack of reticulin fibrils within the tumor lobules. The presence or absence of lymph node involvement may be significant, since lymph node metastasis of extraskeletal Ewing's sarcoma is rare. Furthermore, malignant lymphomas, unlike Ewing's sarcoma and some acute nonlymphoid leukemias, express leukocyte common antigen.

Metastatic pulmonary small cell carcinoma and trabecular carcinoma of the skin (Merkel cell tumor) must be considered in the differential diagnosis, particularly when the tumor occurs in patients older than 45 years and is superficially located. In general, metastatic pulmonary small cell carcinoma can be ruled out if a thorough clinical history and x-ray study fail to reveal any pulmonary involvement. The cells of Merkel cell tumor have large, closely packed nuclei and little cytoplasm and are frequently arranged in a trabecular pattern. The cytoplasm contains perinuclear immunocytokeratin in a characteristic globular or punctate pattern and, ultrastructurally, neurosecretory granules. Trabecular carcinoma is chiefly located in the dermis or subcutis, and two thirds of cases occur in patients older than 60 years. The absence of atypical osteoid or cartilage production by the cells of extraskeletal Ewing's sarcoma permits separation from mesenchymal chondrosarcoma and small cell osteosarcoma.[227,250]

Clinical behavior and therapy

Until the introduction of modern therapy the outlook for patients with extraskeletal Ewing's sarcoma was bleak and only a small percentage of patients with this tumor survived. For instance, in our series of 35 cases of extraskeletal Ewing's sarcoma with follow-up information, 22 died of metastatic disease and only 13 were alive, two with metastasis and one with recurrence. The most common metastatic sites were the lung and the skeleton. Lymph node metastasis was rare.

More recently, however, prolonged disease-free survival times and cure have been achieved in a significant percentage of patients: Schmidt et al.,[246] for instance, reported a 66% 5-year survival rate in extraskeletal Ewing's sarcoma. Similar or even better 5-year survival rates have been observed in Ewing's sarcoma of bone.[209,263] Therapy chiefly consists of intensive sequential chemotherapy (doxorubicin hydrochloride, cyclophosphamide, dactinomycin, and vincristine) and limited radical excision following histological diagnosis by biopsy or excision. Radiation therapy may be added as adjunctive therapy.[209,212,214,238] There are sporadic reports of a second malignant neoplasm after radiotherapy[253] and of late recurrence and central nervous system involvement after chemotherapy.[207,224,241]

Key prognostic factors that adversely influence the outcome of the disease are large size of the tumor and extensive necrosis (filigree pattern).[198,226,247] Most Ewing's sarcomas are diploid, but there seems to be no reliable correlation between DNA ploidy and survival rates.[218]

Discussion

While most reviewers agree that the skeletal and extraskeletal forms of Ewing's sarcoma represent a morphologically distinct entity, opinions as to the differentiation of this neoplasm are divided; some believe that it is a tumor of primitive or uncommitted mesenchymal cells, but most favor neural origin and believe that the tumor is closely related to peripheral malignant neuroepithelioma.[151,196,230,249] In fact, it has been suggested that Ewing's sarcoma and peripheral neuroepithelioma occupy opposite ends of a spectrum of primitive neural tumors.[138] The concept of neuroectodermal origin is supported by the described immunochemical findings, the in vitro neural differentiation of Ewing's sarcoma cell lines, and especially the presence of distinct identical cytogenetic anomalies shared by Ewing's sarcoma and peripheral neuroepithelioma.

A genetic basis in the oncogenesis of the tumor is also suggested by the occurrence of multiple tumors in some families and in some patients affected by the tumor.[207] For example, in one of our cases of extraskeletal Ewing's sarcoma, a sibling died of Ewing's sarcoma of bone; in another the mother of the patient was treated for myxoid liposarcoma of the retroperitoneum and osteosarcoma of the tibia. There also are several reports in the literature of Ewing's sarcoma of bone occurring in siblings[210,211,228,266] and in patients following treatment of retinoblastoma,[245]

and the tumor has also been seen in association with multiple birth anomalies, particularly of the urogenital tract and skeleton.[228]

REFERENCES

Neuroblastoma, ganglioneuroblastoma, and ganglioneuroma

1. Adam A, Hochholzer L: Ganglioneuroblastoma of the posterior mediastinum: a clinicopathologic review of 80 cases. *Cancer* 47:373, 1981.
2. Aoyama C, Qualman SJ, Regan M, et al: Histopathologic features of composite ganglioneuroblastoma: immunohistochemical distinction of the stromal component is related to prognosis. *Cancer* 65:255, 1990.
3. Aquire P, Scully RE: Testosterone-secreting adrenal ganglioneuroma containing Leydig cells. *Am J Surg Pathol* 7:699, 1983.
4. Artlieb U, Krepler R, Wiche G: Expression of microtubule-associated proteins Map-1 and Map-2 in human neuroblastoma and differential diagnosis of immature neuroblasts. *Lab Invest* 53:684, 1985.
5. Banks E, Yum M, Brodhecker C, et al: A malignant peripheral nerve sheath tumor in association with paratesticular ganglioneuroma. *Cancer* 64:1738, 1989.
6. Becker H, Wirnsberger G, Ziervogel K, et al: Immunohistochemical markers in (ganglio)neuroblastomas. *Acta Histochem Suppl* 38:107, 1990.
7. Beckwith JB, Martin RF: Observations on the histopathology of neuroblastoma. *J Pediatr Surg* 3:106, 1968.
8. Beckwith JB, Perrin EV: In situ neuroblastomas: a contribution to the natural history of neural crest tumors. *Am J Pathol* 43:1089, 1963.
9. Berry CL, Keeling J, Hilton C: Coincidence of congenital malformation and embryonic tumours of childhood. *Arch Dis Child* 45:229, 1970.
10. Bertolone S: Neuroblastoma. *Pediatr Clin North Am* 24:589, 1977.
11. Bolande RP, Towler WF: A possible relationship of neuroblastoma to von Recklinghausen's disease. *Cancer* 26:162, 1970.
12. Breslow N, McCann B: Statistical estimation of prognosis for children with neuroblastoma. *Cancer Res* 31:2098, 1971.
13. Brodeur GM, Azar C, Brother M, et al: Neuroblastoma: effect of genetic factors on prognosis and treatment. *Cancer* 70:1685, 1992.
14. Brodeur GM, Green AA, Hayes FA: Cytogenetic studies of primary human neuroblastoma. In Evans AE, editor: *Advances in neuroblastoma research,* New York, 1980, Raven Press.
15. Brodeur GM, Seeger RC, Barrett A, et al: International criteria for diagnosis, staging, and response to treatment in patients with neuroblastoma. *J Clin Oncol* 6:1874, 1988.
16. Chandrasoma P, Shibata D, Radin R, et al: Malignant peripheral nerve sheath tumor arising in an adrenal ganglioneuroma in an adult male homosexual. *Cancer* 57:2022, 1986.
17. Chatten J, Voorhess M: Familial neuroblastoma. *N Engl J Med* 277:1230, 1967.
18. Chetty R, Duhig JD: Bilateral pheochromocytoma-ganglioneuroma of the adrenal in type 1 neurofibromatosis. *Am J Surg Pathol* 17:837, 1993.
19. Coldman AJ, Fryer CJH, Elwood JM, et al: Neuroblastoma: influence of age at diagnosis, stage, tumor site, and sex on prognosis. *Cancer* 46:1896, 1980.
20. Cushing H, Wolback SB: Transformation of malignant paravertebral sympathoblastoma into benign ganglioneuroma. *Am J Pathol* 3:203, 1927.
21. Damiani S, Manetto V, Carrillo G, et al: Malignant peripheral nerve sheath tumor arising in a "de novo" ganglioneuroma: a case report. *Tumori* 77:90, 1991.
22. D'Amore ES, Manivel JC, Pettinato G, et al: Intestinal ganglioneuromatosis: mucosal and transmural types: a clinicopathologic and immunohistochemical study of six cases. *Hum Pathol* 22:276, 1991.
23. D'Angio GJ, Lyster KM, Urunay G: Neuroblastoma: stage IV-S: a special entity? *Memorial Sloan-Kettering Cancer Center Bull* 2:61, 1971.
24. Dehner LP: *Pediatric surgical pathology.* St Louis, 1975, Mosby.
25. DeLorimier AA, Bragg KU, Linden G: Neuroblastoma in childhood. *Am J Dis Child* 118:441, 1969.
26. Donner L, Triche TJ, Israel MA, et al: A panel of monoclonal antibodies which discriminate neuroblastoma from Ewing's sarcoma, rhabdomyosarcoma, neuroepithelioma, and hematopoietic malignancies. In Evans A, editor: *Advances in neuroblastoma research,* New York 1988, Alan R. Liss.
27. Duckett JW, Koop CE: Neuroblastoma. *Urol Clin North Am* 4:285, 1977.
28. Dyke PC, Mulkey DA: Maturation of ganglioneuroblastoma to ganglioneuroma. *Cancer* 20:1343, 1967.
29. Evans AE, Angio GJ, Propert K, et al: Prognostic factors in neuroblastoma. *Cancer* 59:1853, 1987.
30. Evans AE, Chatten J, D'Angio GJ, et al: A review of 17 IV-S neuroblastoma patients at the Children's Hospital of Philadelphia. *Cancer* 45:833, 1980.
31. Evans AE, D'Angio GJ, Koop CE: Diagnosis and treatment of neuroblastoma. *Pediatr Clin North Am* 23:161, 1976.
32. Evans AE, D'Angio GJ, Randolph J: A proposed staging for children with neuroblastoma. *Cancer* 27:374, 1971.
33. Fabbretti G, Valenti C, Loda M, et al: N-myc gene amplification/expression in localized stroma-rich neuroblastoma (ganglioneuroblastoma). *Hum Pathol* 24:294, 1993.
34. Favrot MC, Combaret V, Goillot E, et al: Expression of integrin receptors on 45 clinical neuroblastoma specimens. *Int J Cancer* 49:347, 1991.
35. Fletcher CDM, Fernando IN, Braimbridge MV, et al: Malignant nerve sheath tumor arising in a ganglioneuroma. *Histopathology* 12:445, 1988.
36. Fortner J, Nicashi A, Murphy ML: Neuroblastoma: natural history and results of treating 133 cases. *Ann Surg* 167:132, 1968.
37. Fox F, Davidson J, Thomas LB: Maturation of sympathicoblastoma into ganglioneuroma: report of two patients with 20 and 46 years survival respectively. *Cancer* 12:108, 1959.
38. Gargin JH, Lack EE, Berenberg W, et al: Ganglioneuroma presenting with differentiated skeletal metastases: report of a case. *Cancer* 54:357, 1984.
39. Ghali VS, Gold JE, Vincent RA, et al: Malignant peripheral nerve sheath tumor arising spontaneously from retroperitoneal ganglioneuroma: a case report, review of the literature, and immunohistochemical study. *Hum Pathol* 23:72, 1992.
40. Gitlow SE, Dziedzic LB, Strauss L, et al: Biochemical and histologic determinants in the prognosis of neuroblastoma. *Cancer* 32:898, 1973.
41. Gonzalez-Angula A, Reyes HA, Reyna AN: The ultrastructure of ganglioneuroblastoma: observation on neoplastic ganglion cells. *Neurology* 15:242, 1965.
42. Graham DG: On the origin and significance of neuromelanin. *Arch Pathol Lab Med* 103:359, 1979.
43. Greenfield LJ, Shelley WM: The spectrum of neurogenic tumors of

the sympathetic nervous system: maturation and adrenergic function. *J Natl Cancer Inst* 35:215, 1965.

44. Griffin ME, Bolande RP: Familial neuroblastoma with regression and maturation to ganglioneurofibroma. *Pediatrics* 43:377, 1969.

45. Gross RE, Farber S, Martin LW: Neuroblastoma sympatheticum: a study and report of 217 cases. *Pediatrics* 23:1179, 1959.

46. Guin GH, Gilbert EF, Jones B: Incidental neuroblastoma in infants. *Am J Clin Pathol* 51:126, 1969.

47. Hahn JF, Netsky MG, Butler AB, et al: Pigmented ganglioneuroblastoma: relation of melanin and lipofuscin to schwannomas and other tumors of neural crest origin. *J Neuropathol Exp Neurol* 35:393, 1976.

48. Hann HWL, Evans AE, Cohen IJ, et al: Biologic differences between neuroblastoma stages IV-S and IV: measurement of serum ferritin and E-rosette inhibition in 30 children. *N Engl J Med* 305:425, 1981.

49. Hann HW, Levy HM, Evans AE: Serum ferritin as a guide to therapy of neuroblastoma. *Cancer Res* 40:1411, 1980.

50. Hann HW, Stahlhut MW, Evans AE: Serum ferritin as a prognostic indicator in neuroblastoma: biological effects of isoferritins. *Advances in neuroblastoma research,* New York, 1985, Alan R. Liss.

51. Hardy PC, Nesbit ME: Familial neuroblastoma: report of a kindred with a high incidence of infantile tumors. *J Pediatrics* 80:74, 1972.

52. Hochhaus G, Yu VC, Sadee W: Delta opioid receptors in human neuroblastoma cell lines. *Brain Res* 382:327, 1987.

53. Horn RC, Koop CE, Kiesewetter WB: Neuroblastoma in childhood: clinicopathologic study of 44 cases. *Lab Invest* 5:106, 1956.

54. Hortnagel H, Hortnagel H, Winkler H, et al: Storage of catecholamines in neuroblastoma and ganglioneuroma. *Lab Invest* 27:613, 1972.

55. Hughes M, Marsden HB, Palmer HK: Histologic patterns of neuroblastoma related to prognosis and clinical staging. *Cancer* 34:1706, 1974.

56. Joshi VV, Cantor AB, Altshuler G, et al: Age-linked prognostic categorization based on a new histologic grading system of neuroblastomas: a clinicopathologic study of 211 cases from the Pediatric Oncology Group. *Cancer* 69:2197, 1992.

57. Joshi VV, Cantor AB, Altshuler G, et al: Recommendations for modification of terminology of neuroblastic tumors and prognostic significance of Shimada classification: a clinicopathologic study of 213 cases from the Pediatric Oncology Group. *Cancer* 69:2183, 1992.

58. Joshi VV, Silverman JF, Altshuler G, et al: Systematization of primary histopathologic and fine-needle aspiration cytology feature and description of unusual histopathologic features of neuroblastic tumors: a report from the Pediatric Oncology Group. *Hum Pathol* 24:493, 1993.

59. Kabisch H, Heinshohn S, Milde K, et al: Detection of neuroblastoma cells in bone marrow by in situ hybridization. *Eur J Pediatr* 145:323, 1986.

60. Kazmi SMI, Mishra RK: Opioid receptors in human neuroblastoma SH-SY5Y cells: evidence for distinct morphine (mu) and enkephalin (delta) binding sites. *Biochem Biophys Res Comm* 137:813, 1986.

61. Keller SM, Papazoglou S, McKeever P, et al: Late occurrence of malignancy in a ganglioneuroma 19 years following radiation therapy to a neuroblastoma. *J Surg Oncol* 25:227, 1984.

62. Kinnear-Wilson LM, Draper GJ: Neuroblastoma, its natural history and prognosis: a study of 487 cases. *Br Med J* 3:301, 1974.

63. Knudson AG Jr, Meadows AT: Regression of neuroblastoma IV-S: a genetic hypothesis. *N Engl J Med* 302:1254, 1980.

64. Knudson AG, Strong LC: Mutation and cancer: neuroblastoma and pheochromocytoma. *Am J Hum Genet* 24:514, 1972.

65. Kogner P, Bjork O, Theodorsson E: Neuropeptide Y in neuroblastoma: increased concentration in metastasis, release during surgery,

66. Koop CE, Hernandez JR: Neuroblastoma: experience with 100 cases in children. *Surgery* 56:726, 1964.

67. Koop CE, Schnaufer L: The management of abdominal neuroblastomas. *Cancer* 35:905, 1975.

68. Kramer SA, Bradford WD, Anderson EE: Bilateral adrenal neuroblastoma. *Cancer* 45:2208, 1980.

69. Lopez R, Karakousis C, Rao U: Treatment of adult neuroblastoma. *Cancer* 45:840, 1980.

70. Lopez-Ibor B, Schwartz AD: Neuroblastoma. *Pediatr Clin North Am* 32:755, 1985.

71. Luse SA: Synaptic structure occurring in a neuroblastoma. *Arch Neurol* 11:185, 1964.

72. Mauakinen J: Microscopic patterns as a guide to prognosis of neuroblastomas in childhood. *Cancer* 29:1637, 1972.

73. McCune BK, Patterson K, Chandra RS, et al: Expression of transforming growth factor-beta isoforms in small round cell tumors of childhood: an immunohistochemical study. *Am J Pathol* 142:49, 1993.

74. Mendelsohn G, Eggleston JC, Olson JL, et al: Vasoactive intestinal peptide and its relationship to ganglion cell differentiation in neuroblastic tumors. *Lab Invest* 41:144, 1979.

75. Misugi K, Misugi N, Newton WAS: Fine structural study of neuroblastoma, ganglioneuroblastoma, and pheochromocytoma. *Arch Pathol* 86:160, 1968.

76. Molenaar WM, deLeiji L, Trojanowski JQ: Neuroectodermal tumors of the peripheral and central nervous system share neuroendocrine N-CAM-related antigens with small cell lung carcinoma. *Acta Neuropathol (Berl)* 83:46, 1991.

77. Moriwaki Y, Miyake M, Yamamoto T, et al: Retroperitoneal ganglioneuroma: a case report and review of the Japanese literature. *Int Med* 31:82, 1992.

78. Mukai M, Torikata C, Iri H, et al: Expression of neurofilament triplet proteins in human neural tumors: an immunohistochemical study of paraganglioma, ganglioneuroma, ganglioneuroblastoma, and neuroblastoma. *Am J Pathol* 122:28, 1986.

79. Mullins JD: A pigmented differentiating neuroblastoma: a light and ultrastructural study. *Cancer* 46:522, 1980.

80. Nagashima F, Hayashi J, Araki Y, et al: Silent mixed ganglioneuroma/pheochromocytoma which produces a vasoactive intestinal polypeptide. *Int Med* 32:63, 1993.

81. Nakagawara A, Arima-Nakagawara M, Scavarda NJ, et al: Association between high levels of expression of the TRK gene and favorable outcome in human neuroblastoma. *N Engl J Med* 328:847, 1993.

82. Nickerson BG, Hutter JJ: Opsomyoclonus and neuroblastoma. *J Clin Pediatrics* 18:446, 1979.

83. Orr JD: Cervical neuroblastoma in childhood: a better prognosis? *Clin Oncol* 4:353, 1978.

84. Osborn M, Dirk T, Kaser H, et al: Immunohistochemical localization of neurofilaments and neuron specific enolase in 29 cases of neuroblastoma. *Am J Pathol* 122:433, 1986.

85. Page LB, Jacoby GA: Catecholamine metabolism and storage granules in pheochromocytoma and neuroblastoma. *Medicine* 43:379, 1964.

86. Pegelow C, Ebbin AJ, Powars D, et al: Familial neuroblastoma. *J Pediatrics* 87:763, 1975.

87. Pendergrass TW, Hanson JW: Fetal hydantoin syndrome and neuroblastoma. *Lancet* 2:150, 1976.

88. Potter EL, Parrish JM: Neuroblastoma, ganglioneuroblastoma, and fibroneuroma in a stillborn fetus. *Am J Pathol* 18:181, 1942.

89. Qualman SJ, Dorisio MS, Fleshman DJ, et al: Neuroblastoma: correlation of neuropeptide expression in tumor tissue with other prognostic factors. *Cancer* 70:2005, 1992.

and characterization of plasma and tumor extracts. *Med Pediatr Oncol* 21:317, 1993.

90. Reynolds CP, Seeger RC, Vo DD, et al: Model system for removing neuroblastoma cells from bone marrow monoclonal antibodies and magnetic immunobeads. *Cancer Res* 46:5882, 1986.

91. Ricci A, Parham DM, Woodruff JM, et al: Malignant peripheral nerve sheath tumors arising from ganglioneuromas. *Am J Surg Pathol* 8:19, 1984.

92. Robinson MJ, Howard RN: Neuroblastoma, presenting as myasthenia gravis in a child aged 3 years. *Pediatrics* 43:111, 1969.

93. Romansky SG, Crocker DW, Shaw KNF: Ultrastructural studies on neuroblastoma. *Cancer* 42:2392, 1978.

94. Rosen N, Reynolds CP, Thiele CJ, et al: Increased N-myc expression following progressive growth of human neuroblastoma. *Cancer Res* 46:4139, 1986.

95. Rosenstein BJ, Engelman K: Diarrhea in a child with a catecholamine-secreting ganglioneuroma: case report and review of the literature. *J Pediatrics* 63:217, 1963.

96. Sandstedt B, Jereb B, Eklund G: Prognostic factors in neuroblastomas. *Acta Pathol Microbiol Immunol Scand (Sect A)* 91:365, 1983.

97. Sasaki A, Ogawa A, Nakazato Y, et al: Distribution of neurofilament protein and neuron-specific enolase in peripheral neuronal tumors. *Virchows Arch (Pathol Anat)* 407:33, 1985.

98. Schwarz A, Dadash-Fadeh M, Lee H, et al: Spontaneous regression of disseminated neuroblastoma. *J Pediatrics* 85:760, 1974.

99. Seeger RC, Brodeur GM, Sather H: Association of multiple copies of the N-myc oncogene with rapid progression of neuroblastoma. *N Engl J Med* 313:111, 1985.

100. Shimada H, Aoyama C, Chiba T, et al: Prognostic subgroups for undifferentiated neuroblastoma: immunohistochemical study with anti-S-100 protein antibody. *Hum Pathol* 16:471, 1985.

101. Shimada H, Chatten J, Newton WA Jr, et al: Histopathologic prognostic factors in neuroblastic tumors: definition of subtypes of ganglioneuroblastoma and an age-linked classification of neuroblastoma. *J Natl Cancer Inst* 73:405, 1984.

102. Shown TE, Durfee MF: Blueberry muffin baby: neonatal neuroblastoma with subcutaneous metastasis. *J Urol* 104:193, 1970.

103. Silverman L, et al: Ganglioneuroblastoma: studies of pathologic changes and content of catecholamine. *Am J Clin Pathol* 42:145, 1964.

104. Slamon DJ, Boone TC, Seeger RC, et al: Identification and characterization of the protein encoded by the human N-myc oncogene. *Science* 232:768, 1986.

105. Smith RA, et al: Functionally active intrathoracic neuroblastoma. *Arch Dis Child* 36:82, 1961.

106. Snyder WH, Hastings TN, Pollock WF: Neurogenic tissue tumors: neuroblastomas. In Mustard WT, et al: *Pediatric surgery*, ed 2, Chicago, 1969, Year Book Medical Publishers.

107. Spandisos DA, Arvanitis D, Field JK: Ras p21 expression in neuroblastomas and ganglioneuroblastoma: correlation with patients' progress. *Int J Oncol* 1:53, 1992.

108. Stella JG, Schweisguth O, Schlienger M: Neuroblastoma: a study of 144 cases treated in the Institut Gustave-Roussy over a period of 7 years. *Am J Roentgenol* 108:325, 1970.

109. Stout AP: Ganglioneuroma of the sympathetic nervous system. *Surg Gynecol Obstet* 84:101, 1947.

110. Swank RL, Fetterman GH, Sieber WR, et al: Prognostic factors in neuroblastoma. *Ann Surg* 174:428, 1971.

111. Tannenbaum M: Ultrastructural pathology of adrenal medullary tumors. *Pathol Ann* 5:145, 1970.

112. Taxy JB: Electron microscopy in the diagnosis of neuroblastoma. *Arch Pathol Lab Med* 104:355, 1980.

113. Triche TJ, Ross WE: Glycogen-containing neuroblastoma with clinical and histopathologic features of Ewing's sarcoma. *Cancer* 41:1425, 1978.

114. Trump DL, Livingston JN, Baylin SB: Watery diarrhea syndrome in an adult with ganglioneuroma-pheochromocytoma. *Cancer* 40:1526, 1977.

115. Tsokos M, Linnoila RI, Chandra RS, et al: Neuron specific enolase in the diagnosis of neuroblastoma and other small round-cell tumors in children. *Hum Pathol* 15:575, 1984.

116. Turkel SB, Itabashi HH: The natural history of neuroblastic cells in the fetal adrenal gland. *Am J Pathol* 76:225, 1974.

117. Weinblatt ME, Heisel MA, Siegel SE: Hypertension in children with neurogenic tumors. *Pediatrics* 71:947, 1983.

118. Whang-Peng J, Triche TJ, Knutsen T, et al: Cytogenetic characterization of selected small round cell tumors of childhood. *Cancer Genet Cytogenet* 21:185, 1986.

119. Wilkerson JA, Van deWater JM, Goepfert H: Role of embryonic induction in benign transformation of neuroblastoma. *Cancer* 20:1335, 1967.

120. Williams TH, House RF, Burgert EO, et al: Unusual manifestations of neuroblastoma, chronic diarrhea, polymyoclonia-opsoclonus, and erythrocyte abnormalities. *Cancer* 24:475, 1972.

121. Wirnsberger GH, Becker H, Ziervogel K, et al: Diagnostic immunohistochemistry of neuroblastic tumors. *Am J Surg Pathol* 16:49, 1992.

122. Wright JH: Neurocytoma or neuroblastoma, a kind of tumor not generally recognized. *J Exp Med* 12:556, 1910.

123. Yunis E, Walpusk JA, Agostini RM, et al: Glycogen in neuroblastomas: a light and electron microscopic study of 40 cases. *Am J Surg Pathol* 3:313, 1979.

124. Zeltzer PM, Parma AM, Dalton A, et al: Raised neuron-specific enolase in serum of children with metastatic neuroblastoma: a report from the Children's Cancer Study Group. *Lancet* 1:361, 1983.

Ganglion cell tumors

125. Daneshvar A: Pharyngeal traumatic neuromas and traumatic neuromas with mature ganglion cells (pseudoganglioneuromas). *Am J Surg Pathol* 14:565, 1990.

126. Lee JY, Martinez AJ, Abell E: Ganglioneuromatous tumor of the skin: a combined heterotopia of ganglion cells and hamartomatous neuroma: report of a case. *J Cutan Pathol* 15:58, 1988.

127. Radice F, Gianotti R: Cutaneous ganglion cell tumor of the skin: case report and review of the literature. *Am J Dermatopathol* 15:488, 1993.

128. Rios JJ, Diaz-Cano SJ, Rivera-Hueto F, et al: Cutaneous ganglion cell choristoma: report of a case. *J Cutan Pathol* 18:469, 1991.

Peripheral neuroepithelioma and olfactory neuroblastoma

129. Ambros IM, Ambros PF, Strehl S, et al: MIC2 is a specific marker for Ewing's sarcoma and peripheral primitive neuroectodermal tumors: evidence for a common histogenesis of Ewing's sarcoma and peripheral primitive neuroectodermal tumors from MIC2 expression and specific chromosomal aberration. *Cancer* 67:1886, 1991.

130. Bolen JW, Thorning D: Peripheral neuroepithelioma: a light and electron microscopic study. *Cancer* 46:2456, 1980.

131. Cavazzana AO, Ninfo V, Roberts J, et al: Peripheral neuroepithelioma: a light microscopic, immunocytochemical, and ultrastructural study. *Mod Pathol* 5:71, 1992.

132. Cavazzana AO, Santopietro R, Sforza V, et al: Morphometry and the differential diagnosis between peripheral neuroepithelioma and neuroblastoma. *Mod Pathol* 4:615, 1991.

133. Chaudhry AP, Haar JG, Koul A, et al: Olfactory neuroblastoma (esthesioneuroblastoma): a light and ultrastructural study of two cases. *Cancer* 44:564, 1979.

134. Choi HS, Anderson PJ: Immunohistochemical diagnosis of olfactory neuroblastoma. *J Neuropathol Exp Neurol* 44:18, 1985.

135. Christiansen H, Altmannsberger M, Lampert F: Translocation (5;22) in an Askin's tumor. *Cancer Genet Cytogenet* 62:203, 1992.

136. Contesso G, Llombart-Bosch A, Terrier P, et al: Does malignant small round cell tumor of the thoracopulmonary region (Askin tumor) constitute a clinicopathologic entity? An analysis of 30 cases with immunohistochemical and electron microscopic support treated at the Institute Gustave Roussy. *Cancer* 69:1012, 1992.

137. Dehner LP: Peripheral and central primitive neuroectodermal tumors: a nosologic concept seek a consensus. *Arch Pathol Lab Med* 110:997, 1986.

138. Dehner LP: Primitive neuroectodermal tumor and Ewing's sarcoma. *Am J Surg Pathol* 17:1, 1993.

139. Dehner LP: Whence the primitive neuroectodermal tumor? *Arch Pathol Lab Med* 114:16, 1990.

140. Elkon D, Hightower SI, Lim ML, et al: Esthesioneuroblastoma. *Cancer* 44:1087, 1979.

141. Enzinger FM: *Case 12 in proceedings of the forty-ninth annual anatomic pathology slide seminar.* Chicago, 1983, American Society of Clinical Pathology Press.

142. Frierson HF, Ross GW, Mills SE, et al: Olfactory neuroblastoma: additional immunohistochemical characterization. *Am J Clin Pathol* 94:547, 1990.

143. Fuzesi L, Heller R, Schreiber H, et al: Cytogenetics of Askin's tumor: case report and review of the literature. *Pathol Res Pract* 189:235, 1993.

144. Gariepy G, Drouin R, Lemieux N, et al: Ultrastructural, immunohistochemical, and cytogenetic study of a malignant peripheral neuroectodermal tumor in a patient seropositive for human immunodeficiency virus. *Am J Clin Pathol* 93:818, 1990.

145. Gerard-Marchant R, Micheau C: Microscopical diagnosis of olfactory esthesioneuromas: general review and report of five cases. *J Natl Cancer Inst* 35:75, 1965.

146. Hachitanda Y, Tsuneyoshi M, Enjoji M, et al: Congenital primitive neuroectodermal tumor with epithelial and glial differentiation: an ultrastructural and immunohistochemical study. *Arch Pathol Lab Med* 114:101, 1990.

147. Harper PG, Pringle J, Souhami RL: Neuroepithelioma: a rare malignant peripheral nerve tumor of primitive origin: report of two new cases. *Cancer* 48:2282, 1981.

148. Hasegawa T, Hirose T, Kudo E, et al: Atypical primitive neuroectodermal tumors: comparative light and electron microscopic and immunohistochemical studies on peripheral neuroepitheliomas and Ewing's sarcoma. *Acta Pathol Jpn* 41:444, 1991.

149. Hashimoto H, Enjoji M, Nakajima T, et al: Malignant neuroepithelioma (peripheral neuroblastoma): a clinicopathologic study of 15 cases. *Am J Surg Pathol* 7:309, 1983.

150. Hutter RVP, Lewis JS, Foote FW, et al: Esthesioneuroblastoma: a clinical and pathological study. *Am J Surg* 106:748, 1963.

151. Jaffe R, Santamaria M, Yunis EJ, et al: The neuroectodermal tumor of bone. *Am J Surg Pathol* 8:885, 1984.

152. Jensen KJ, Elbrond O, Lund C: Olfactory esthesioneuroblastoma. *J Laryngol Otol* 90:1007, 1976.

153. Joachim HZ, Altman MM, Mayer SW: Olfactory neuroblastoma. *J Laryngol Otol* 89:335, 1975.

154. Jurgens H, Bier V, Harms D, et al: Malignant peripheral neuroectodermal tumors: a retrospective analysis of 42 patients. *Cancer* 61:349, 1988.

155. Kadish S, Goodman M, Wang CC: Olfactory neuroblastoma: a clinical analysis of 17 cases. *Cancer* 37:1571, 1976.

156. Kahn LB: Esthesioneuroblastoma: a light and electron microscopic study. *Hum Pathol* 5:364, 1974.

157. Kushner BH, Hajdu SI, Gulati SC, et al: Extracranial primitive neuroectodermal tumors: the Memorial Sloan-Kettering Cancer Center experience. *Cancer* 67:1825, 1991.

158. Lagerkvist B, Ivermark B, Sylven B: Malignant neuroepithelioma in childhood: a report of three cases. *Acta Chir Scand* 135:641, 1969.

159. Lattes R, Enzinger FM: Proceedings of the Thirty-ninth Annual An-

160. Linnoila RI, Tsokos M, Triche TJ, et al: Evidence for neural origin and periodic acid-Schiff positive variants of the malignant small cell tumor of thoracopulmonary region ("Askin tumor"). *Lab Invest* 48:51A, 1983.

161. Llombart-Bosch A, Terrier-Lacombe MJ, Reydro-Olaya A, et al: Peripheral neuroectodermal sarcoma of soft tissue (peripheral neuroepithelioma): a pathologic study of ten cases with differential diagnosis regarding other small, round-cell sarcomas. *Hum Pathol* 20:273, 1989.

162. Lopez-Gines C, Pellin A, Llombart-Bosch A: Two new cases of primary peripheral neuroepithelioma of soft tissue with translocation t(11;22)(q24;q12). *Cancer Genet Cytogenet* 33:291, 1988.

163. Mackay B, Luna MA, Butler JJ: Adult neuroblastoma: electron microscopic observations in nine cases. *Cancer* 37:1334, 1976.

164. Mancer K, Gillespie R, Thulbourne T: Neuroepithelioma of peripheral nerve. *Lab Invest* 32:451, 1975.

165. Marina NM, Etcubanas E, Parham DM, et al: Peripheral primitive neuroectodermal tumor (peripheral neuroepithelioma) in children: a review of the St. Jude experience and controversies in diagnosis and management. *Cancer* 64:1952, 1989.

166. McKeon C, Thiele CJ, Ross RA, et al: Indistinguishable patterns of protooncogene expression in two distinct but closely related tumors: Ewing's sarcoma and neuroepithelioma. *Cancer Res* 48:4307, 1988.

167. Micheau C, Guerinot F, Bohuon C, et al: Dopamine-hydroxylase and catecholamines in an olfactory esthesioneuroma. *Cancer* 35:1309, 1975.

168. Mills SE, Frierson HF: Olfactory neuroblastoma: a clinicopathologic study of 21 cases. *Am J Surg Pathol* 9:317, 1985.

169. Miozzo M, Sozzi G, Calderone C, et al: t(11;22) in three cases of peripheral neuroepithelioma. *Genes Chromosom Cancer* 2:163, 1990.

170. Nakamura Y, Becker LE, Mancer K, et al: Peripheral medulloepithelioma. *Acta Neuropathol (Berl)* 57:137, 1982.

171. Nesbitt KA, Vidone RA: Primitive neuroectodermal tumor (neuroblastoma) arising in sciatic nerve of a child. *Cancer* 37:1562, 1976.

172. Ninfo V, Ziliotto GR: Il neuroepithelioma maligno dei nervi periferici (considdetto medulloblastoma dei nervi periferici). *Patholgica* 65:393, 1973.

173. Oberman HA, Rice DH: Olfactory neuroblastoma: a clinicopathologic study. *Cancer* 38:2494, 1976.

174. Osamura RY, Fine G: Ultrastructure of esthesioneuroblastoma. *Cancer* 38:173, 1976.

175. Pappo AS, Douglass EC, Meyer WH, et al: Use of HBA71 and anti-beta-microglobulin to distinguish peripheral neuroepithelioma from neuroblastoma. *Hum Pathol* 24:880, 1993.

176. Parham DM, Dias P, Kelly DR, et al: Desmin positivity in primitive neuroectodermal tumors of childhood. *Am J Surg Pathol* 16:483, 1992.

177. Schmidt D, Harms D, Burdach S: Malignant peripheral neuroectodermal tumours of childhood and adolescence. *Virchows Arch (Pathol Anat)* 406:351, 1985.

178. Schmidt JL, Zarbo RJ, Clark JL: Olfactory neuroblastoma: clinicopathologic and immunohistochemical characterization of four representative cases. *Laryngoscope* 100:1052, 1990.

179. Seemayer TA, Thelmo WL, Boland R, et al: Peripheral neuroectodermal tumors. *Perspect Pediatr Pathol* 2:151, 1975.

180. Singh W, Ramage C, Best P, et al: Nasal neuroblastoma secreting vasopressin: a case report. *Cancer* 45:961, 1980.

181. Skolnick EM, Massari FS, Tenta LT: Olfactory neuroepithelioma: review of the world literature and presentation of two cases. *Arch Otolaryngol* 84:644, 1966.

182. Stout AP: Tumor of the ulnar nerve. *Proc NY Pathol Soc* 18:2, 1918.

183. Stout AP, Murray MD: Neuroepithelioma of the radial nerve with a study of its behavior in vitro. *Rev Can Biol* 1:651, 1942.

184. Taxy JB, et al: The spectrum of olfactory neural tumors: a light-microscopic immunohistochemical and ultrastructural analysis. *Am J Surg Pathol* 10:687, 1986.

185. Trojanowski JQ, Lee V, Pillsbury N, et al: Neuronal origin of human esthesioneuroblastoma demonstrated with antineurofilament monoclonal antibodies. *N Engl J Med* 307:159, 1982.

186. Voss BL, Pysher TJ, Humphrey GB: Peripheral neuroepithelioma in childhood. *Cancer* 54:3059, 1984.

187. Whang-Peng J, Freter CE, Knutsen T, et al: Translocation t(11;22) in esthesioneuroblastoma. *Cancer Genet Cytogenet* 29:155, 1987.

188. Whang-Peng J, Triche TJ, Knutsen T, et al: Chromosome translocation in peripheral neuroepithelioma. *N Engl J Med* 311:584, 1984.

189. Zappia JJ, Carroll WR, Wolf GT, et al: Olfactory neuroblastoma: the results of modern treatment approaches at the University of Michigan. *Head Neck* 15:190, 1993.

Extraskeletal Ewing's sarcoma

190. Angervall L, Enzinger FM: Extraskeletal neoplasm resembling Ewing's sarcoma. *Cancer* 36:240, 1975.

191. Askin FB, Rosai J, Sibley RK, et al: Malignant small cell tumor of the thoracopulmonary region in childhood. *Cancer* 43:2438, 1979.

192. Aurias A, Rimbaut C, Buffe D, et al: Chromosomal translocation in Ewing's sarcoma. *N Engl J Med* 309:496, 1983.

193. Aurias A, Rimbaut C, Buffe D, et al: Translocation involving chromosome 22 in Ewing's sarcoma: a cytogenetic study of four fresh tumors. *Cancer Genet Cytogenet* 12:1, 1984.

194. Berthold F, Kracht J, Lampert F, et al: Ultrastructural, biochemical, and cell culture studies of a presumed extraskeletal Ewing's sarcoma with special reference to differential diagnosis from neuroblastoma. *J Cancer Res Clin Oncol* 103:293, 1982.

195. Carter RL, Al-Sam SZ, Corbett RP, et al: A comparative study of immunohistochemical staining for neuron-specific enolase, protein gene product 9.5, and S-100 protein in neuroblastoma, Ewing's sarcoma, and other round cell tumours in children. *Histopathology* 16:461, 1990.

196. Cavazzana AO, Miser JS, Jefferson J, et al: Experimental evidence for a neural origin of Ewing's sarcoma of bone. *Am J Pathol* 127:507, 1987.

197. Dahlin DC, Coventry MB, Scanlon PW: Ewing's sarcoma: a critical analysis of 165 cases. *J Bone Joint Surg* 43A:185, 1961.

198. de Stefani E, Carziglio J, Deneo Pellegrini H, et al: Ewing's sarcoma: value of tumor necrosis as a predictive factor. *Bull Cancer (Paris)* 71:16, 1984.

199. Dickman PS, Triche TJ: Extraosseous Ewing's sarcoma versus primitive rhabdomyosarcoma: diagnostic criteria and clinical correlation. *Hum Pathol* 17:881, 1986.

200. Dierick AM, Roels H, Langlois M: The immunophenotype of Ewing's sarcoma: an immunohistochemical analysis. *Pathol Res Pract* 189:26, 1993.

201. Douglass EC, Rowe ST, Valentine M, et al: A second nonrandom translocation, der(16)t(1;16)(q21;q13), in Ewing's sarcoma and peripheral neuroectodermal tumor. *Cytogenet Cell Genet* 53:87, 1990.

202. Erlandson A: Ultrastructural distinction between rhabdomyosarcoma and other undifferentiated "sarcomas." *Ultrastruct Pathol* 11:83, 1987.

203. Ewing J: Diffuse endothelioma of bone. *Proc NY Pathol Soc* 21:17, 1921.

204. Fellinger EJ, Garin-Chesa P, Glasser DB, et al: Comparison of cell surface antigen HBA71 (p30/32MIC2), neuron specific enolase, and vimentin in the immunohistochemical analysis of Ewing's sarcoma of bone. *Am J Surg Pathol* 16:746, 1992.

205. Fraumeni JF Jr, Glass AG: Rarity of Ewing's sarcoma among U.S. Negro children. *Lancet* 1:366, 1979.

206. Gillespie JJ, Roth LM, Wills ER, et al: Extraskeletal Ewing's sarcoma: histologic and ultrastructural observations in three cases. *Am J Surg Pathol* 3:99, 1979.

207. Greene MH, Glaubiger DL, Mead GD, et al: Subsequent cancer in patients with Ewing's sarcoma. *Cancer Treat Rep* 63:2043, 1979.

208. Hashimoto H, Tsuneyoshi M, Daimaru Y, et al: Extraskeletal Ewing's sarcoma: a clinicopathologic and electron microscopic analysis of 8 cases. *Acta Pathol Jpn* 35:1087, 1985.

209. Hayes FA, Thompson EI, Hustu HO, et al: The response of Ewing's sarcoma to sequential cyclophosphamide and adriamycin induction therapy. *J Clin Oncol* 1:45, 1983.

210. Huntington RW, Sheffel DJ, Iger M, et al: Malignant bone tumors in siblings: Ewing's tumor and an unusual tumor perhaps a variant of Ewing's tumor: a case report. *J Bone Joint Surg* 42A:1065, 1960.

211. Joyce MJ, Harmon DC, Mankin JH, et al: Ewing's sarcoma in female siblings: a clinical report and review of the literature. *Cancer* 53:1959, 1984.

212. Jürgens H, Exner U, Gadner H, et al: Multidisciplinary treatment of primary Ewing's sarcoma of bone: a 6-year experience of a European cooperative trial. *Cancer* 61:23, 1988.

213. Kawaguchi K, Koike M: Neuron-specific enolase and Leu-7 immunoreactive small round-cell neoplasm: the relationship to Ewing's sarcoma in bone and soft tissue. *Am J Clin Pathol* 86:79, 1986.

214. Kinsella TJ, Triche TJ, Dickman PS, et al: Extraskeletal Ewing's sarcoma: results of combined modality treatment. *J Clin Oncol* 1:489, 1983.

215. Kissane JM, Askin FV, Foukes M, et al: Ewing's sarcoma of bone: clinicopathologic aspects of 303 cases from the Intergroup Ewing's sarcoma study. *Hum Pathol* 14:773, 1983.

216. Kodama K, Doi O, Higashiyama M, et al: Establishment and characterization of a new Ewing's sarcoma cell line. *Cancer Genet Cytogenet* 57:19, 1991.

217. Komiya S, Irie K, Sasaguri Y, et al: An ultrastructural study of extraskeletal Ewing's sarcoma. *Acta Pathol Jpn* 34:445, 1984.

218. Kowal-Vern A, Walloch J, Chou P, et al: Flow and image cytometric DNA analysis in Ewing's sarcoma. *Mod Pathol* 5:56, 1992.

219. Ladanyi M, Heinemann FS, Huvos AG, et al: Neural differentiation in small round cell tumors of bone and soft tissue with the translocation t(11;22)(q24;q12): an immunohistochemical study of 11 cases. *Hum Pathol* 21:1245, 1990.

220. Ladanyi M, Lewis R, Gari-Chesa P, et al: EWS rearrangement in Ewing's sarcoma and peripheral neuroectodermal tumor: molecular detection and correlation with cytogenetic analysis and MIC2 expression. *Diagn Mol Pathol* 2:141, 1993.

221. Linnoila RI, Tsokos M, Triche TJ, et al: Evidence for neural origin and PAS-positive variants of the malignant small cell tumor of thoracopulmonary origin ("Askin tumor"). *Am J Surg Pathol* 10:124, 1986.

222. Llombart-Bosch A, Blache R, Peydro-Olaya A: Ultrastructural study of 28 cases of Ewing's sarcoma: typical and atypical forms. *Cancer* 41:1362, 1978.

223. Llombart-Bosch A, Carda C, Peydro-Olaya A, et al: Soft tissue Ewing's sarcoma: characterization in established cultures and xenografts with evidence of a neuroectodermic phenotype. *Cancer* 66:2589, 1990.

224. Macintosh DJ, Price CHG, Jeffree GM: Ewing's tumor: a study of behavior and treatment in 47 cases. *J Bone Joint Surg* 57B:331, 1975.

225. Mahoney JP, Ballinger WE Jr, Alexander RW: So-called extraskeletal Ewing's sarcoma: report of a case with ultrastructural analysis. *Am J Clin Pathol* 79:926, 1978.

226. Maletz N, McMorrow LE, Greco MA, et al: Ewing's sarcoma: pathology, tissue culture, and cytogenetics. *Cancer* 58:252, 1986.

227. Martin SE, Dwyer A, Kissane JM, et al: Small cell osteosarcoma. *Cancer* 50:990, 1982.

228. McKeen EA, Hanson MR, Mulhivill J, et al: Birth defects in Ewing's sarcoma. *N Engl J Med* 309:1522, 1983.

229. Meister P, Gokel JM: Extraskeletal Ewing's sarcoma. *Virchows Arch (Pathol Anat)* 378:173, 1978.

230. Mieran H, et al: Extraskeletal Ewing's sarcoma (peripheral neuroepithelioma). *Ultrastruct Pathol* 9:91, 1985.

231. Miettinen M, Lehto VP, Virtanen J: Histogenesis of Ewing's sarcoma: an evaluation of intermediate filaments and endothelial cell markers. *Virchows Arch (Cell Pathol)* 41:277, 1982.

232. Mugneret F, Lizard S, Aurias A, et al: Chromosomes in Ewing's sarcoma. II. Nonrandom additional changes, trisomy 8, and der (16)t(1;16). *Cancer Genet Cytogenet* 32:239, 1988.

233. Nascimento AG, Unni KK, Pritchard DJ, et al: A clinicopathologic study of 20 cases of large-cell (atypical) Ewing's sarcoma of bone. *Am J Surg Pathol* 4:29, 1980.

234. Navas-Palacios JJ, Aparicio-Duque R, Valdes MD: On the histogenesis of Ewing's sarcoma: an ultrastructural, immunohistochemical, and cytochemical study. *Cancer* 53:1882, 1984.

235. Noguera R, Navarro S, Triche TJ: Translocation t(11;22) in small cell osteosarcoma. *Cancer Genet Cytogenet* 45:121, 1990.

236. Perlman EJ, Dickman BS, Askin FB, et al: Ewing sarcoma: routine diagnostic utilization of MIC 2 analysis: a Pediatric Oncology Group/Children's Cancer Group Intergroup study. *Hum Pathol* 25:304, 1994.

237. Peters MS, Reiman HM, Muller SA: Cutaneous extraskeletal Ewing's sarcoma. *J Cutan Pathol* 12:476, 1985.

238. Pilepich MV, Vietti TJ, Nesbit ME, et al: Radiotherapy and combination chemotherapy in advanced Ewing's sarcoma: intergroup study. *Cancer* 47:1930, 1981.

239. Pinto A, Grant LH, Hayes FA, et al: Immunohistochemical expression of neuron specific enolase and Leu-7 in Ewing's sarcoma of bone. *Cancer* 64:1266, 1989.

240. Pritchard DJ, Dahlin DC, Dauphine RT: Ewing's sarcoma. *J Bone Joint Surg* 57A:10, 1974.

241. Rud NP, Reiman HM, Pritchard DJ, et al: Extraosseous Ewing's sarcoma: a study of 42 cases. *Cancer* 64:1548, 1989.

242. Salzer-Kuntschik M, Wunderlich M: Das Ewing-Sarkom in der Literatur. *Arch Orthop Unfall-Chir* 71:297, 1971.

243. Sawyer JR, Tryka AF, Lewis JM: A novel reciprocal chromosome translocation t(11;22)(p13;q12) in an intraabdominal desmoplastic small round-cell tumor. *Am J Surg Pathol* 16:411, 1992.

244. Schajowicz F: Ewing's sarcoma and reticulum cell sarcoma of bone: with special reference to the histological demonstration of glycogen as an aid to differential diagnosis. *J Bone Joint Surg* 41A:349, 1954.

245. Schifter S, Vendelbo L, Myhre O, et al: Ewing's tumor following bilateral retinoblastoma. *Cancer* 51:1746, 1983.

246. Schmidt D, Herrmann C, Jurgens H, et al: Malignant peripheral neuroectodermal tumor and its necessary distinction from Ewing's sarcoma: a report from the Kiel Pediatric Tumor Registry. *Cancer* 68:2251, 1991.

247. Schmidt D, Mackay B, Ayala AG: Ewing sarcoma with neuroblastoma-like features. *Ultrastruct Pathol* 3:143, 1982.

248. Seemayer TA, Vekemans M, de Chadarevian JP: Histological and cytogenetic findings in a malignant tumor of the chest wall and lung (Askin tumor). *Virchows Arch (Pathol Anat)* 408:289, 1985.

249. Shimada H, Newton WA Jr, Soule EH, et al: Pathologic features of extraosseous Ewing's sarcoma: a report from the Intergroup Rhabdomyosarcoma Study. *Hum Pathol* 19:442, 1988.

250. Sim FH, Unni KK, Beabout JW, et al: Osteosarcoma with small cells simulating Ewing's sarcoma. *J Bone Joint Surg* 61A:207, 1979.

251. Soule EH, Newton W Jr, Moon TE, et al: Extraskeletal Ewing's sarcoma: a preliminary review of 26 cases encountered in the Intergroup Rhabdomyosarcoma Study. *Cancer* 42:259, 1978.

252. Stephenson CF, Bridge JA, Sandberg AA: Cytogenetic and pathologic aspects of Ewing's sarcoma and neuroectodermal tumors. *Hum Pathol* 23:1270, 1993.

253. Strong LC, Herson J, Osborne BM, et al: Risk of radiation-related subsequent malignant tumors in survivors of Ewing's sarcoma. *J Natl Cancer Inst* 52:1401, 1979.

254. Stuart-Harris R, et al: Extraskeletal Ewing's sarcoma: a clinical morphological and ultrastructural analysis of five cases. *Eur J Cancer Clin Oncol* 22:393, 1986.

255. Szakacs JE, Carta M, Szakacs MR: Ewing's sarcoma, extraskeletal and of bone. *Ann Clin Lab Sci* 4:306, 1974.

256. Tefft M, Vauter GF, Mitus A: Paravertebral "round cell" tumors in children. *Radiology* 92:1501, 1969.

257. Triche TJ, Ross WE: Glycogen-containing neuroblastoma with clinical and histopathological features of Ewing's sarcoma. *Cancer* 41:1425, 1978.

258. Tsokos M, Linnoila RI, Triche TJ, et al: Neuron-specific enolase in the diagnosis of neuroblastoma and other small-, round-cell tumors in children. *Hum Pathol* 15:575, 1984.

259. Tsuneyoshi M, Yokoyama R, Hashiomoto H, et al: Comparative study of neuroectodermal tumor and Ewing's sarcoma of the bone: histopathologic, immunohistochemical, and ultrastructural features. *Acta Pathol Jpn* 39:573, 1989.

260. Turc-Carel C, Aurias A, Mugneret F, et al: Chromosomes in Ewing's sarcoma. I. An evaluation of 85 cases and remarkable consistency of t(11;22)(q24;q12). *Cancer Genet Cytogenet* 32:229, 1988.

261. Turc-Carel C, Philip I, Berger MP, et al: Chromosome study of Ewing's sarcoma (ES) cell lines, consistently of a reciprocal translocation T(11,22)(q24;q12). *Cancer Genet Cytogenet* 12:1, 1984.

262. Wigger HJ, Salazar GH, Blane WA: Extraskeletal Ewing's sarcoma: an ultrastructural study. *Arch Pathol* 101:446, 1977.

263. Wilkins RM, Pritchard DJ, Burgert EO, et al: Ewing's sarcoma of bone: experience with 140 patients. *Cancer* 58:2551, 1986.

264. Yunis EJ: Ewing's sarcoma and related small round cell neoplasms in children. *Am J Surg Pathol* 10(Suppl):54, 1986.

265. Zachai EH, Emanuel BS: Site specific reciprocal translocation t(11;22)(q23;q11) in several unrelated families with 3 : 1 meiotic disjunction. *Am J Med Genet* 7:507, 1980.

266. Zamora P, et al: Ewing's tumor in brothers: an unusual observation. *Am J Clin Oncol* 9:358, 1986.

CHAPTER 34

PARAGANGLIOMA

The paraganglia are widely dispersed collections of specialized neural crest cells that arise in association with the segmental or collateral autonomic ganglia throughout the body. This system includes the adrenal medulla, the chemoreceptors (i.e., carotid and aortic bodies), vagal body, and small groups of cells associated with the thoracic, intraabdominal, and retroperitoneal ganglia. Although the paraganglia are closely related structures, the present trend is to regard them as a large group of embryologically similar structures that manifest certain anatomical differences and functional specializations. For example, the adrenal medulla is a neuroendocrine organ that secretes large amounts of epinephrine and norepinephrine; its cells are chromaffin positive, and tumors arising from this organ are often functionally active. On the other hand, the carotid and aortic bodies are chemoreceptors, which are specialized to detect changes in the blood pH and oxygen tension. Although catecholamine storage can be documented within their chief cells by sensitive fluorometric techniques, their cells are usually chromaffin negative, and tumors arising from these structures are usually nonfunctional.

According to Glenner and Grimley,[4] the extraadrenal paraganglion system can be divided into several anatomical groups (Figs. 34-1 and 34-2).

The *branchiomeric paraganglia* arise in association with arterial vessels and cranial nerves of the head and neck region and include the jugulotympanic, intercarotid (carotid body), subclavian, laryngeal, coronary, aorticopulmonary, and orbital paraganglia. Their cells are generally chromaffin negative and are arranged in small cohesive nests (zellballen). The carotid body tumor and glomus jugulare tumor epitomize the neoplasms arising from branchiomeric paraganglia.

The *intravagal paraganglia* are located within the perineurium of the vagus nerve, usually at the level of the jugular or nodose ganglion. The tumors arising from these structures are histologically and cytochemically indistinguishable from those arising in the branchiomeric paraganglia. In fact, those arising from the jugular ganglion and

invading the temporal bone may be quite difficult to distinguish from glomus jugulare tumors.

Aorticosympathetic paraganglia arise in association with the sympathetic nervous system, particularly at the bifurcation of the aorta (Figs. 34-2 to 34-4). They may also be found along the courses of the iliac and femoral vessels and in the thorax. Tumors arising from these structures vary in chromaffinicity, functional activity, and histological appearance. Some may resemble branchiomeric paragangliomas, whereas others may be virtually indistinguishable from adrenal pheochromocytomas.

The nomenclature of paragangliomas is confusing and before the work of Glenner and Grimley,[4] was poorly standardized. Early authors classified paragangliomas according to the chromaffin reaction (i.e., chromaffin and nonchromaffin paragangliomas) on the assumption that catecholamine-secreting tumors such as pheochromocytomas would be chromaffin positive and nonfunctional tumors chromaffin negative. The chromaffin reaction is an unreliable procedure that does not always correspond to functional activity and is not specific for catecholamines. Moreover, nonfunctional tumors such as carotid body paragangliomas synthesize and store small amounts of catecholamine, further underscoring the fact that the chromaffin reaction is at best only a crude means of classifying this group of tumors. The most rational approach is that paragangliomas be named according to their anatomical sites and further modified depending on whether functional activity is documented clinically. Thus the common nonfunctioning carotid body tumor would be designated "carotid body paraganglioma, nonfunctional." This is the nomenclature used in this chapter.

CAROTID BODY PARAGANGLIOMA (CHEMODECTOMA, NONCHROMAFFIN PARAGANGLIOMA)

The normal carotid body lies on the posterior aspect of the bifurcation of the common carotid artery, usually buried in the adventitia of the vessel.[2] It is a specialized chemoreceptor that monitors changes in the arterial oxygen ten-

965

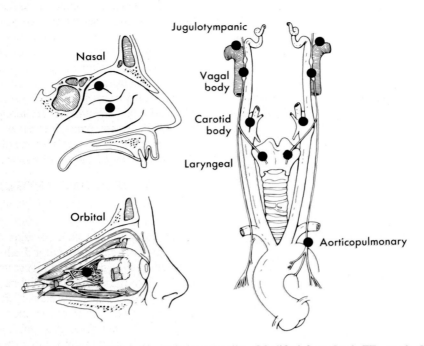

FIG. 34-1. Distribution of branchiomeric paraganglia. (Modified from Lack EE, et al: *Cancer* 39:397, 1977.)

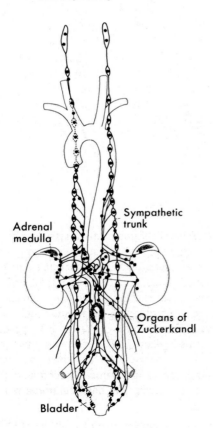

FIG. 34-2. Distribution of aorticosympathetic paraganglia. (Modified from Glenner CG, Grimley PM: Tumors of the extraadrenal paraganglion system (including chemoreceptors). In *Atlas of tumor pathology*, Fascicle 9, Second Series, Washington, D.C., 1974, Armed Forces Institute of Pathology.)

sion and pH of the blood and in turn influences in a reflex fashion the rate and depth of respiration and to a lesser extent the heart rate. It is among the largest of the paraganglia and can usually be identified during routine autopsy as a small red body approximately the size of a rice grain. It may assume a size of several millimeters in persons with chronic lung disease or those subjected to the chronic hypoxemia of high altitudes as a result of compensatory hyperplasia. The body receives its blood supply from the common or external carotid and receives its innervation primarily from sensory (afferent) fibers of the glossopharyngeal (IX) nerve, with lesser contributions from the vagus (X) nerve and superior cervical ganglion of the sympathetic nervous system. The organ is made up of round or polygonal cells (chief cells) surrounded by delicate sustentacular cells, an arrangement that creates the nestlike or zellballen appearance. The chief cells possess small dense core granules measuring 100 to 200 nm, which are the sites of norepinephrine storage as confirmed by the formalin vapor–induced fluorescence of the cells (see Special Staining Procedures). The exact function of the chief cells is unclear, although it seems likely they influence the level of activity of the autonomic nerves within the organ. The sustentacular cells are modified Schwann cells that appear to conduct nerves to their synaptic terminations on the chief cells. Although the chief cells and sustentacular cells are believed to be of neural crest origin, the supporting structures of the body are presumably of mesenchymal origin.

The carotid body tumor is the most common of the extraadrenal paragangliomas. In the review by Saldana et al.[41] of the literature and in the experience of the Memorial Hos-

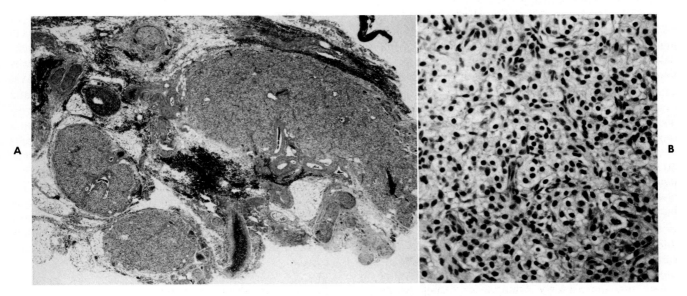

FIG. 34-3. A and **B**, Organ of Zuckerkandl removed at autopsy from a child. (**A**, ×15; **B**, ×100.)

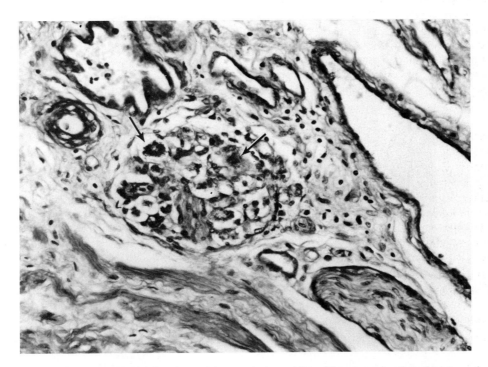

FIG. 34-4. Normal paraganglion located in association with small autonomic nerve in retroperitoneum. Pigment, probably lipochrome, is present with some of the paraganglion cells *(arrows)*. (×400.)

pital reported by Lack et al.,[29] about 60% of all head and neck paragangliomas arise from the carotid body. The overall incidence of these tumors, however, is low, calculated at 0.012% of the surgical specimens at Memorial Hospital.[29] The tumor is considerably more common in areas of high altitude such as Peru, Mexico, and Colorado. In fact, Saldana et al.[41] observed that it is nearly 10 times more frequent in high-altitude areas in Peru than in sea level locales, and this suggests that prolonged hyperplasia of the organ may eventually cause neoplasia. Males are affected about as often as females in most series, except for those reported at high altitudes, where females predominate.[41] Usually the tumor occurs in patients between the ages of 40 and 60 years, although occasional cases in children have been reported.[43] The most common sign is that of a painless, slowly enlarging mass located in the upper portion of the neck below the angle of the jaw (Fig. 34-5). The tumor is usually movable from side to side but not in a vertical direction. A bruit may be audible over the tumor, and pressure on the tumor may cause an increase in the heart rate (carotid sinus syndrome). Large tumors encroaching on nearby structures cause a variety of associated symptoms. Lesions impinging on the hypopharynx cause hoarseness, whereas involvement of the vagus or sympathetic nerve results in vocal cord paralysis or Horner's syndrome. Rarely, carotid body tumors are functional. Two cases in elderly men were associated with elevated urinary catecholamines.[16,25] In one case the patient suffered clinical hypertension; in the other, surgical manipulation of the tumor produced elevation of the systolic blood pressure. In one

of the cases the tumor had combined features of pheochromocytoma and carotid body tumor. Other functional tumors in the vicinity of the carotid body were reported by Fries and Chamberlin,[20] Glenner et al.,[22] and Cone.[18] In each instance, however, the tumor seemed to arise from the cervical sympathetic chain rather than the carotid bifurcation. In the past the level of accurate preoperative diagnosis was extremely low, and these tumors were often confused with tuberculous lymphadenitis, branchial cleft cyst, metastatic carcinoma, carotid artery aneurysm, schwannoma, or lymphoma. Selective arteriography in recent years has led to a higher level of preoperative diagnosis. Typically these studies indicate enlarged tortuous carotid vessels with widening and lateral displacement of the bifurcation point (Fig. 34-6). These studies are also useful in documenting the extent of the lesion. Contralateral carotid angiography may be necessary in some patients to exclude bilateral tumors or to document the amount of collateral cerebral blood flow should ligation of the carotid vessels be necessary during surgery.

Familial and multifocal tumors

Paragangliomas have a tendency to occur multifocally. Approximately 2% to 5% of carotid body tumors are bilateral, although seldom do both tumors come to clinical attention simultaneously.[29,30,40] Carotid body tumors may also occur within certain families.[17,27,40,45,47] Analysis of one family with hereditary paraganglioma has localized the putative gene to the proximal region of chromosome 11q.[9] In such cases the high incidence of bilaterality, estimated

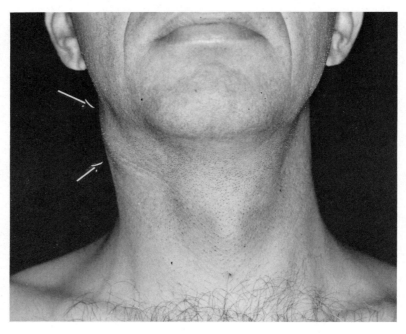

FIG. 34-5. Patient with carotid body paraganglioma of right cervical region *(arrows)*. (Courtesy Dr. Thomas J. Whelan, Honolulu, Hawaii.)

at about one third,[47] underscores the need to perform bilateral carotid angiography. One particularly striking case was reported by Sprong and Kirby,[45] in which carotid body tumors developed in nine of 11 siblings and one parent. In addition, various combinations of paragangliomas have been noted and have included carotid body tumors with tumors of the glomus jugulare,[28,33] organ of Zuckerkandl,[19] vagal body,[84] aortic body,[84] and adrenal medulla.[18] A case of carotid body paraganglioma was reported in association with nonmedullary thyroid carcinoma,[14] although this association may be fortuitous.

Gross and microscopic findings

Carotid body tumors typically lie in the bifurcation of the common carotid artery (Fig. 34-7, *A*) and may be only partially attached to the vessel or may completely encase it. The intimacy of this relationship is a major factor in determining the surgical resectability of a given tumor. Most carotid body tumors have a lobular, beefy red to brown appearance and measure a few centimeters in diameter (Fig. 34-7, *B*). Hemorrhage and fibrosis are seen in some cases. The tumor is surrounded by a thin or incomplete capsule of connective tissue that is periodically penetrated by fine nerve branches. Within the capsule the round or polygonal epithelioid cells are arranged in small nests or zellballen

around an elaborate vasculature that can be clearly outlined with a reticulin preparation (Fig. 34-8). In contrast to the normal gland, the zellballen of the carotid body tumor are larger and more irregular in shape, and the cells comprising the tumor are usually larger and more atypical than normal chief cells (Fig. 34-9). Their centrally located nuclei have finely clumped chromatin, and the cytoplasm has either an amphophilic or granular eosinophilic appearance. The cytoplasm of one cell occasionally envelops that of an adjacent cell, a phenomenon termed "cell embracing" (see Fig. 34-22). Frequently, shrinkage or retraction of the cells away from the tiny vessels results in loss of the classic zellballen pattern. In these regions the cells seem to be arranged in short ribbons or cords similar to those in a carcinoid tumor (Fig. 34-10), in pseudoglands in an adenocarcinoma, or in pseudorosettes as in a neuroblastic tumor. Paragangliomas with these patterns are often misdiagnosed, a fact that emphasizes the need for special staining procedures. In addition to the specific staining procedures for paragangliomas discussed below, staining for glycogen and mucin is occasionally useful because they are negative in paragangliomas and often positive in carcinomas. Another peculiar but frequent artifact of the carotid body tumor is the foamy or vacuolar cytoplasmic change of the chief cell. The cytoplasm contains one or more clear vacuoles, which indent

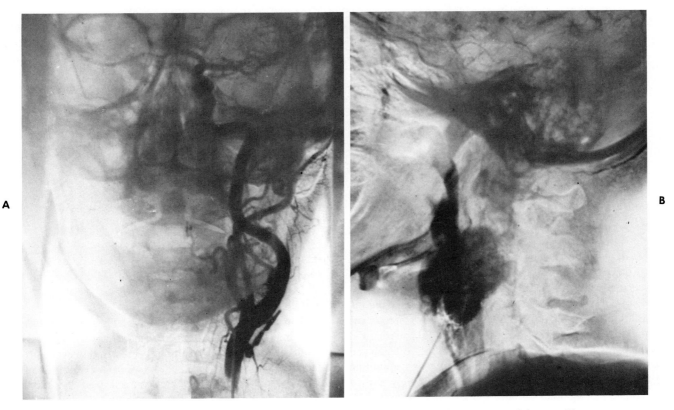

FIG. 34-6. A, Carotid angiography demonstrated widening and lateral displacement of the carotid bifurcation point caused by carotid body tumor. **B,** Tumor blush is evident in later phase of study.

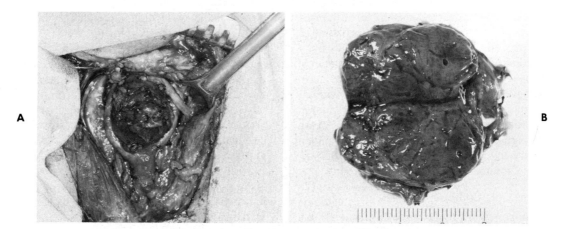

FIG. 34-7. A, Carotid body tumor located at bifurcation of internal and external carotid arteries. **B,** Cut section of carotid body tumor. (Courtesy Dr. Thomas J. Whelan, Honolulu, Hawaii.)

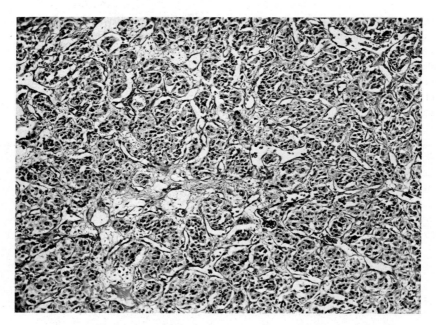

FIG. 34-8. Low-power view of carotid body paraganglioma illustrating nestlike or zellballen pattern. (×100.)

the small pyknotic nucleus in the same fashion that fat droplets displace or indent the nucleus of the lipoblast (Fig. 34-11). It is possible to distinguish these cells from true lipoblasts by their close associations with other cells having the conventional features of chief cells. Markedly sclerotic carotid body tumors have little or no nesting pattern, and small aggregates of cells lie isolated within the collagenized matrix (Fig. 34-12). In a small number of cases, spindling of the chief cell occurs. This change, descriptively termed "sarcomatoid" by Lack et al.,[29] does not appear to adversely affect the prognosis. Occasionally carotid body tumors may be mistaken for vascular tumors, specifically he-

mangiopericytomas, if the vessels become ectatic and compress the intervening chief cells (Fig. 34-13).

Malignant carotid body tumors

It is usually difficult to recognize the potentially metastasizing carotid body tumor because many are virtually devoid of "malignant" features. A few, however, possess atypical features that we believe warrant a diagnosis of malignancy. These tumors are characterized by extremely large zellballen, which blend into broad sheets made up of pleomorphic cells with mitotic figures (Fig. 34-14). Focal necrosis is usually present within the zellballen, and vas-

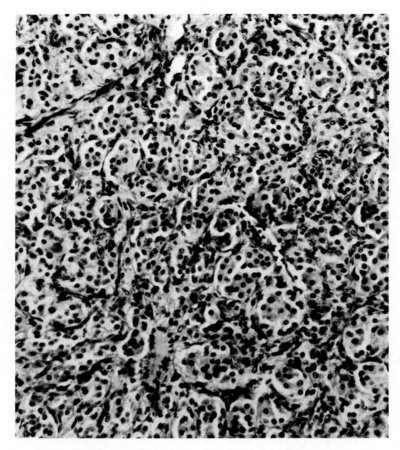

FIG. 34-9. Carotid body paraganglioma composed of nests of rounded regular cells surrounding a delicate vasculature. (×250.)

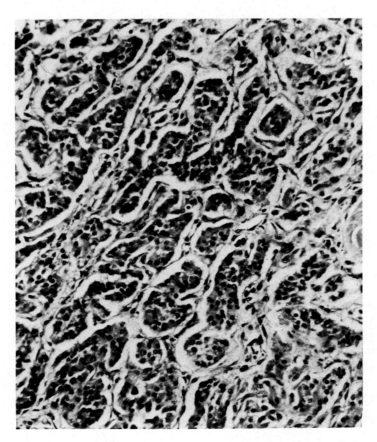

FIG. 34-10. Carcinoid-like pattern occurring within a carotid body paraganglioma. (×250.)

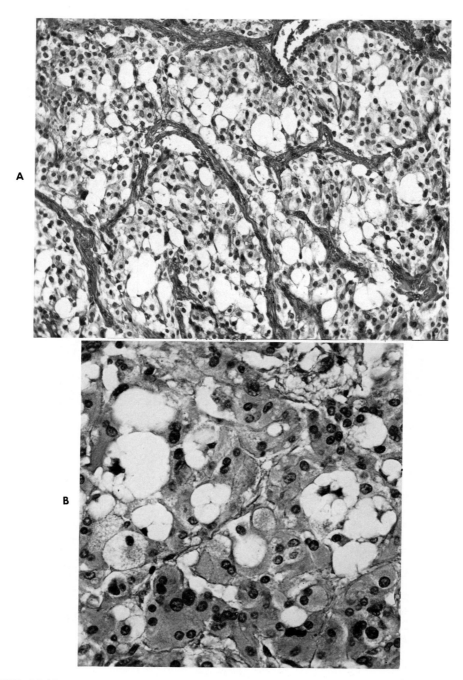

FIG. 34-11. Paraganglioma illustrating vacuolization of the cells **(A)**, some of which resemble lipoblasts **(B)**. **(A,** ×65; **B,** ×350.)

cular invasion may also be documented. Tumors having these features are quite uncommon, so that an outright diagnosis of malignancy is infrequently made by us in carotid body tumors. It should be emphasized that nuclear pleomorphism and giant cell formation may be seen in benign carotid body tumors and should not be regarded as sufficient evidence of malignancy.

Special staining procedures and other procedures

In the past the chromaffin reaction, based on the observation that chromic acid oxidizes catecholamines (i.e., norepinephrine, epinephrine) and indole amines (i.e., serotonin) to a brown polymer, was used to identify tissue containing catecholamines. As indicated recently by Glenner and Grimley,[4] this is an insensitive, nonspecific, and ca-

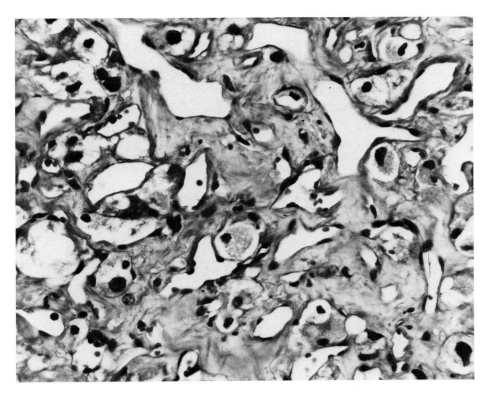

FIG. 34-12. Hyalinized carotid body tumor. (×300.)

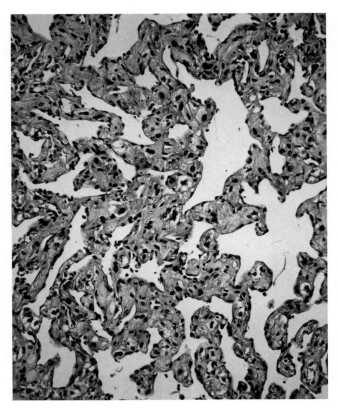

FIG. 34-13. Paraganglioma showing ectatic vasculature simulating the appearance of a hemangiopericytoma. (×160.)

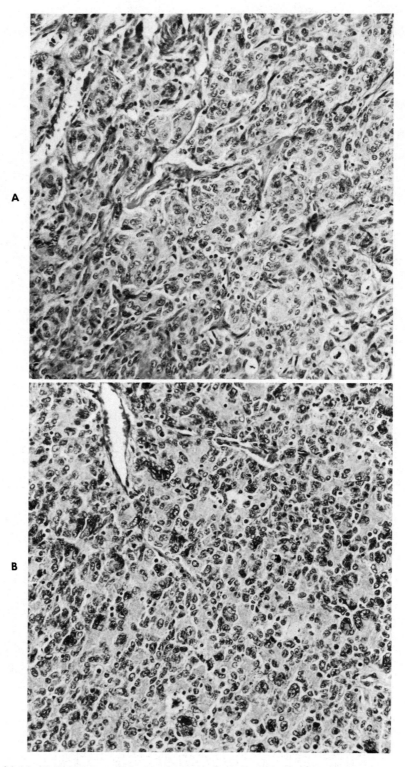

FIG. 34-14. Malignant carotid body tumor. **A,** Occasional areas have a zellballen arrangement. **B,** Others are composed of broad sheets of pleomorphic cells with mitotic figures. (**A** and **B,** ×250.)

pricious method for demonstrating catecholamines. It is usually invalidated by prior formalin fixation, excessive washing, or dehydration of the tissue, and it fails to detect small amounts of catecholamine. Moreover, it does not invariably identify tissues that presumably have large amounts of this substance, possibly because of anoxic loss of the biogenic amine, low concentration of the substance within a given cell, or differences in the protein envelope surrounding the compound. Although both the normal carotid body and carotid body paraganglioma contain small amounts of catecholamines, the chromaffin reaction is not sensitive enough to detect these quantities; consequently, with few exceptions, carotid body tumors are chromaffin negative. A more sensitive, reliable technique is formaldehyde-induced fluorescence of these compounds. When exposed to vaporous formaldehyde, catecholamines form a green fluorescent dicyclic compound, whereas serotonin forms a yellow compound. This method may be used with fresh or frozen tissue and is usually successful in identifying catecholamines within carotid body tumors. Because catecholamines can reduce silver salts, the modified Grimelius stain (2% silver nitrate) for argyrophil granules[5,6] can also be used in the diagnosis of carotid body tumors[28] (Fig. 34-15). This procedure is by no means as specific as the fluorescent technique described earlier, but it offers the advantage that it can be performed on paraffin-embedded

tissue. Caution must be exercised in interpreting these stains because degenerating cells are argyrophilic, as are other neural crest tumors. Fontana's stain for argentaffin granules is usually negative in carotid body tumors. False-positive reactions may occur as a result of lipochrome pigment in sustentacular cells.

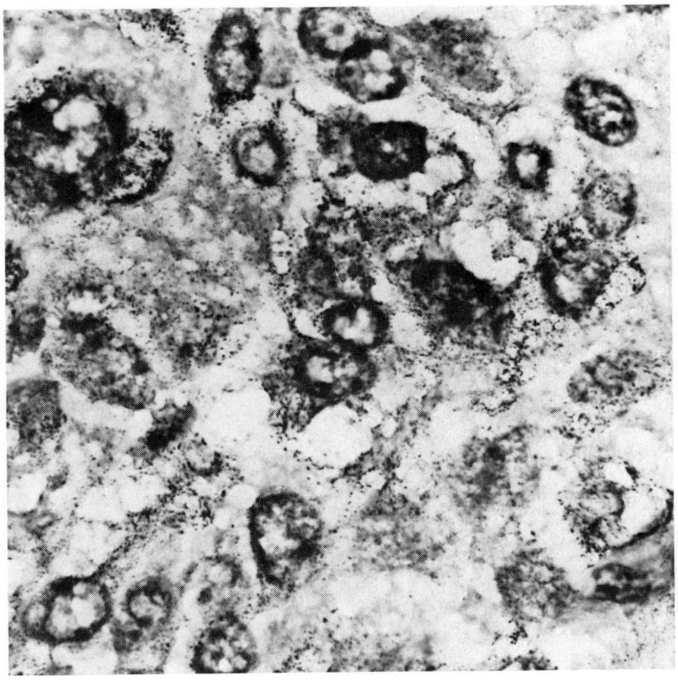

Immunohistochemical findings

With optimally fixed material, neuron-specific enolase and neurofilament protein can be demonstrated within the chief cells of most, if not all, branchiomeric paragangliomas. In addition, the delicate sustentacular network can be elegantly demonstrated using antisera to S-100 protein, and in a few instances these same cells may coexpress glial fibrillary acidic protein[9] (Fig. 34-16). A variety of other polypeptides can also be demonstrated within chief cells, but the actual immunological profile seems to vary slightly, depending on the type of paraganglioma. For example, 10 of 11 carotid body tumors expressed multiple peptide hormones in the experience reported by Warren et al.[10] These included various combinations of the following: serotonin, leu-enkephalin, gastrin, substance P, vasoactive intestinal

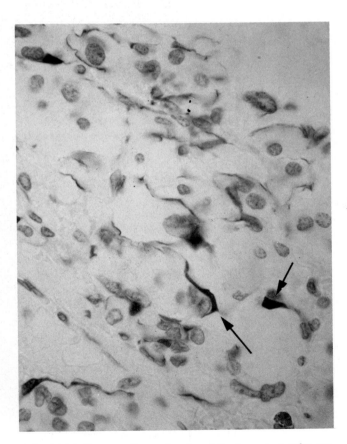

FIG. 34-15. Delicate intracytoplasmic argyrophyilic granules within a paraganglioma as documented by Grimelius stain. (×600.)

FIG. 34-16. Paraganglioma showing delicate sustentacular network *(arrows)* outlined by immunostaining for S-100 protein. (Anti–S-100 protein, peroxidase-antiperoxidase, ×400.)

peptide, somatostatin, bombesin, α-melanocyte-stimulating hormone, and adrenocorticotropic hormone. Only a few tumors of the glomus tympanicum expressed these hormones and none of the glomus jugulare did. A detailed listing of the incidence of neuropeptide hormones in paragangliomas collated from all sites is given in Table 34-1.

Ultrastructural findings

Electron microscopic studies have been performed by a number of investigators, and the results are quite similar.[15,23,29,48] The predominant cell, which resembles the normal chief cell, is round or polyhedral and closely interdigitates with other cells by means of intercellular junctions. The number of ribosomes and mitochondria varies from cell to cell so that the density of the cytoplasm ranges from "dark" to "light." The hallmark of the cell is the presence of small dense core granules measuring 100 to 200 nm in diameter (Fig. 34-17). These represent the sites of

Table 34-1. Immunohistochemical findings in paragangliomas

Substance	% Positive (n = 99)
Neuron-specific enolase	100
Leu-enkephalin	76
Met-enkephalin	75
Somatostatin	67
Pancreatic polypeptide	51
Vasoactive intestinal peptide	43
Substance P	31
Adrenocorticotropic hormone	28
Calcitonin	23
Bombesin	15
Neurotensin	12

From Linnoila RI et al: *Hum Pathol* 19:41, 1988.

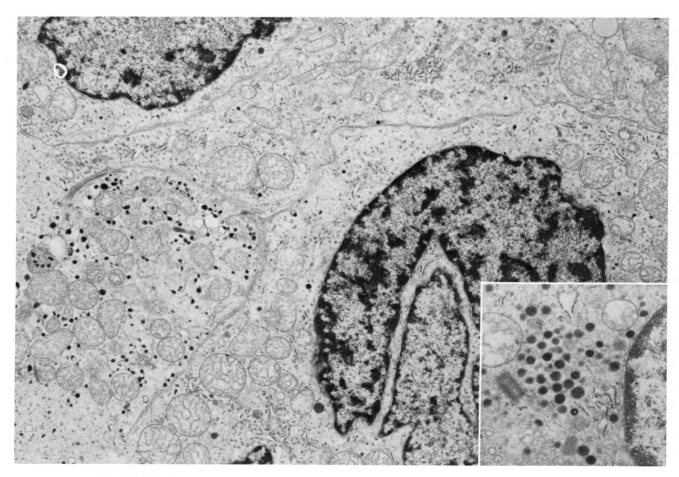

FIG. 34-17. Electron micrograph of a paraganglioma illustrating closely apposed cells characterized by small dense core granules *(insert)*. (From Taxy JB, Battifor H: The electron microscope in the diagnosis of soft tissue tumors. In Trump B, Jones RT, editors: *Diagnostic electron microscopy,* New York, 1980, John Wiley & Sons.)

catecholamine storage and in rare sections can be demonstrated to arise from the Golgi apparatus.[15] Sustentacular cells, which have elongated cell processes, are usually not demonstrable in carotid body tumors.[15,29,48] In the few cases where they were present, they were markedly reduced in number.[23] Their relative rarity provides additional support for the contention that these carotid body lesions are true neoplasms and not hyperplasias. Nerve fibers are markedly reduced in number and if present do not bear the normal relationship to chief cells.

Behavior and treatment

Most carotid body tumors are benign and are cured if total excision can be accomplished at the time of initial surgery. A small number of patients will develop metastases. Patients who develop local tumor recurrence[47] or who have untreated tumors of long duration seem to be at greatest risk for this complication. The incidence of metastasis is estimated at 6% to 9%.[29,30,49] In the study by Gaylis and Mieny[21] an incidence of 30% is reported and is claimed to be the result of extended follow-up information. The incidence of malignancy, reported as 50% from an early study at the Mayo Clinic, was based on evaluation of histological features alone and was not borne out by subsequent follow-up information.[26] About half of metastases appear within regional lymph nodes, while the remainder occur in distant sites, particularly lung and bone.[44] Typically the interval between the time of diagnosis and metastasis is quite long. The patient reported by Gustilo et al.[24] developed a metastasis in the pelvis 35 years after resection of the primary tumor. Thus extended follow-up care is advisable.

Technological advances in vascular surgery and anesthesia now make it possible to resect a greater number of carotid body tumors with fewer complications than before. Before surgery bilateral carotid arteriography is advisable to document the extent of the lesion, determine the presence of a contralateral lesion, and assess the degree of collateral cerebral blood flow should ligation of the carotid become necessary. Functional activity should be excluded by means of preoperative catecholamine levels. Patients with functional tumors should be premedicated in the same fashion as patients with adrenal pheochromocytomas.[33]

Localized lesions are easily removed by a subadventitial dissection of the carotid artery with preservation of the entire system. More extensive lesions, which wrap themselves around the entire vessel, may require resection of the vessel with grafting.[33] Selection of patients for the latter procedure is usually based on several factors including patient age, degree of histological aggressiveness, and whether basic functions such as swallowing or breathing are compromised. Radiotherapy has been advocated for unresectable lesions[34] as well as for metastasis. High response rates have been noted in these tumors with irradiation in dosages of 3400 to 6000 rads.[33]

JUGULOTYMPANIC PARAGANGLIOMA (GLOMUS JUGULARE TUMOR)

Paragangliomas involving the temporal bone and specifically the middle ear take their origin from the paraganglia that follow the auricular branch of the vagus nerve or the tympanic branch of the glossopharyngeal nerve or those related to the bulb of the jugular vein. Although it is conventional to refer to these tumors collectively as glomus jugulare tumors, some prefer to separately designate the tumors involving the middle ear as glomus tympanicum and to reserve glomus jugulare for those that grow upward from the jugular bulb.[58] In some cases, particularly those of long duration, it may be difficult to clearly define the origin of the tumor.

Paraganglioma is the most common neoplasm of the middle ear, and it represents the second most common type of extraadrenal paraganglioma. Most occur in women, and the peak incidence is in the fifth decade. The manner of presentation depends on the rate of growth and the location. Those that arise within the temporal bone usually extend laterally, eventually to present as masses in the middle ear or the external auditory canal. In such patients the initial symptoms develop early and include dizziness, pulsating tinnitus, and conductive hearing loss. Usually after several years, discoloration of the tympanic membrane or a friable hemorrhagic mass in the auditory canal appears. Often the diagnosis of aural polyp, cholesteatoma, or vascular tumor is erroneously made. Tumors of the jugular bulb, in contrast, grow upward, enlarging the jugular foramen and producing characteristic crescentic erosions of the bone crest between the jugular vein and carotid artery radiographically.[69] Although these tumors also involve the middle ear, they often, in addition, extend to the base of the brain, causing palsies of the cranial nerves in almost 40% of patients.[68] It has been suggested that retrograde venography is helpful in documenting the superior extent of these lesions. As in other branchiomeric paragangliomas, arteriography has been recommended to rule out ipsilateral or contralateral carotid body tumors, which may occur in about 10% of patients. The incidence of overt functional activity is estimated at 1% in jugulotympanic paragangliomas. One particularly striking case was reported in which the patient experienced cyclic changes in blood pressure at 10- to 17-minute intervals associated with increased norepinephrine levels.[68] Several other jugulotympanic paragangliomas have given rise to hypertensive crises during intraoperative manipulation.[54,69]

Histologically, these tumors are virtually identical to carotid body tumors. They are usually arranged in a zellballen configuration, although the zellballen are smaller and less uniform than those of the carotid body tumor. They are usually highly vascular tumors, a feature that has often led to the mistaken diagnosis of hemangioma when biopsy specimens of these tumors are taken from the external auditory canal. Typically the tumors are chromaffin negative, although argyrophilic granules can be demonstrated by means of Grimelius stain and catecholamine storage can be documented by using formalin-induced fluorescence. Ultrastructurally, the tumors are composed of chief cells with small dense core granules, occasional microtubules, and cilia. One recent report has described rhomboid crystals with a periodicity of 6 to 9 nm and delimited by a single membrane. Sustentacular cells are scarce.[63] The immunohistochemical findings are similar to those of carotid body tumors with minor differences.

The behavior and treatment of jugulotympanic paragangliomas can be most accurately assessed by clinical stage.[58] Stage 0 lesions are confined to the middle ear and present with symptoms of deafness and tinnitus. Stage 1 lesions are those which, in addition, penetrate the tympanic membrane and produce discharge. Stage 2 lesions are associated with facial nerve paralysis and, occasionally, radiographic changes in the mastoid bone. Hoarseness and vertigo, indicative of extension beyond the middle ear, characterize stage 3 lesions, whereas stage 4 tumors have multiple otological and neurological symptoms. Most stage 0, 1, and 2 lesions are adequately treated by surgery, either radical mastoidectomy or a lesser procedure, if the lesion is small and localized. Of the 150 patients in these three stages reported by Brown,[53] 138 were alive and without disease at 10 years. Stage 3 and 4 lesions usually require a combination of surgery and radiotherapy.[53,62] Fourteen of the 81 patients in these two groups died as a direct result of their tumor. However, in only two of 231 patients did metastasis actually develop, one to the lung and one to the liver. This rate is slightly lower than the 4% rate reported by Borsanyi,[52] derived from 200 cases reported in the literature. Fuller et al.,[56] in an analysis of 73 cases from the Mayo Clinic, found no metastasis, and a similar experience was reported by Cole[54] with 20 glomus jugulare tumors. Johnstone et al.[64] reviewed 20 cases of jugulotympanic paragangliomas that produced metastasis and found the common metastic sites were lung (nine cases), vertebra or bone (six cases), and liver (four cases). Only three of the 20 cases produced metastasis in regional lymph nodes.

VAGAL PARAGANGLIOMA (VAGAL BODY TUMOR)

The first vagal body tumor was described by Stout in 1935; since that time approximately 70 additional cases have been reported in the English literature, making it the third most common paraganglioma of the head and neck after the carotid body and glomus jugulare tumors. These tumors arise from small dispersed collections of paraganglia that follow the cervical course of the vagus nerve, particularly at the level of the jugular and nodose ganglia. These paraganglia usually lie just beneath the perineurium, but occasionally they are embedded in the substance of the nerve. Consequently, vagal body tumors develop as high cervical masses between the mastoid process and the angle of the jaw in the parapharyngeal space. The close relationship with the nerves at the base of the brain results in neurological symptoms including weakness of the tongue, vocal cord paralysis, hoarseness, and Horner's syndrome. Rare cases have been functional.[74,78] Like glomus jugulare tumors, these lesions are more frequent in women than in men, and in about 10% to 15% of cases multiple tumors have been noted.[73] They can be clearly distinguished from carotid body tumors arteriographically because they usually lie above the carotid bifurcation, causing anterior displacement of the vessels without widening of the bifurcation point. At surgery the tumor is usually wrapped around the nerve, although occasionally the nerve fibers may be splayed over the tumor, presumably in cases where the lesion arises from intravagal paraganglia. They are histologically similar to carotid body tumors, except they are often traversed by dense fibrous bands representing the residual vagal perineurium. The cells are chromaffin negative, but staining for argyrophilic granules is positive.[83] Ultrastructurally, the tumors contain chief cells that show a gradation in cytoplasmic density similar to the light and dark cells of the carotid body. They contain dense core neurosecretory granules, some of which have a more elongated or "pleomorphic" appearance than those of the carotid body tumor.[29,73] Sustentacular cells and synaptic endings on chief cells were described in one vagal paraganglioma[70] but not in others.[71,73]

Vagal body tumors occasionally metastasize. Local infiltration and extension into the cranial vault represent significant problems in disease control, however. The rate of metastasis has been estimated at 16%.[73] The vast majority of these cases represent regional lymph node metastasis. Only rare cases have metastasized distantly to lung and bone. Surgical resection is the treatment of choice, although it is usually not possible to excise these lesions without sacrifice of the vagus nerve.

MEDIASTINAL PARAGANGLIOMA (AORTIC BODY TUMOR, MEDIASTINAL AORTICOSYMPATHETIC PARAGANGLIOMA)

Mediastinal paragangliomas arise from paraganglia associated with the pulmonary artery and aortic arch or from the segmental paraganglia associated with the sympathetic chain. The former tumors are located in the anterior mediastinum and are termed "aortic body tumors," whereas the latter are located in the posterior mediastinum and are the mediastinal equivalent of the retroperitoneal (extraadrenal) paragangliomas.

Aortic body paragangliomas can originate at any site where the aortic body chemoreceptor has been identified. These include the areas (1) anterolateral to the aortic arch, (2) lateral to the innominate artery, (3) at the angle of the ductus arteriosus and descending aorta, and (4) to the upper right of the main pulmonary artery.[4] Clinically, these tumors usually present as asymptomatic masses that are noted at the time of chest radiography for other causes. The majority of reported cases have occurred in persons over age 40 years, and they affect the sexes equally. They may be associated with paragangliomas at other sites, as illustrated by the original case described by Lattes,[83] in which the patient had tumors of the aortic, vagal, and carotid bodies. Radiographically, they are highly vascular masses of the anterior or superior mediastinum, which are fed by vessels from the subclavian, internal mammary, or intercostal arteries, with early drainage into the superior vena cava.[81] Histologically, they are identical to the tumors of the carotid body. Although formerly regarded as relatively benign lesions, Olson and Salyer[85] recently emphasized the rather aggressive course of the anterior mediastinal paraganglioma. Although only about 10% of patients develop metastasis, most patients eventually die of the disease. Of the 41 cases reported in the literature and reviewed by Olson and Salyer,[85] only 19 patients were alive and well without evidence of disease. Of the remainder, 14 had either inoperable disease or died as a result of the tumor. Three were alive with residual mediastinal tumor; four had tumor documented incidentally at autopsy; one was lost to follow-up, and one had multiple tumors. Optimum therapy is complete surgical excision. When complete excision cannot be accomplished, the prognosis is guarded, as slow progression and death from tumor may ensue.

Posterior mediastinal paragangliomas are far less common than the foregoing type.[82] In contrast to the preceding group, they occur in younger persons (average age, 29 years) and in about half of cases are associated with symptoms referable to functional activity by the tumor. In the remainder of patients the mass, which is usually located in the costovertebral sulcus at the level of the fifth to seventh ribs, is discovered incidentally at the time of a chest radiograph. The tumors are related to the sympathetic chain, and for this reason they can be considered histogenetically and embryologically similar to the extraadrenal paragangliomas of the retroperitoneum. They may combine features of classic carotid body tumor or adrenal pheochromocytoma. The histological features of retroperitoneal paraganglioma, as discussed in the following section, are equally applicable to this tumor. Although only two out of 31 cases (7%) reported in the English literature metastasized, five displayed locally aggressive features.[82] Complete surgical excision is the preferred treatment and is usually accomplished more readily than with paragangliomas in the anterior mediastinum.

RETROPERITONEAL PARAGANGLIOMA

Approximately 10% to 20% of paragangliomas of the retroperitoneum arise outside the adrenal from paraganglia that lie along the aortic axis in close association with the sympathetic chain. The largest collection of paraganglia includes the organs of Zuckerlandl (see Figs. 34-3 and 34-4), paired structures overlying the aorta at the level of the inferior mesenteric artery. These structures are prominent during early infancy but gradually regress after the age of 12 to 18 months, leaving behind only small microscopic residua. Although they are believed to serve chemoreceptor functions in animals, their physiological role in humans is not understood. Most extraadrenal paragangliomas arise from this organ, whereas a smaller number are derived from the paraganglia lying at other points along the aortic or iliac vessels.

Retroperitoneal paragangliomas occur at a relatively earlier patient age than those of the head and neck. Most occur in persons between 30 and 45 years of age; the malignant forms may have an even younger median age.[105] Men and women are affected in approximately equal numbers in most series, although in our cases women predominate. Occasionally these tumors may be multiple, or they may be associated with paragangliomas of other sites[19] or with other tumors such as gastric leiomyoblastoma and pulmonary chondroma[93,94] (Chapter 20). Back pain and a palpable mass are the two most common presenting symptoms. About 10% of patients will present initially with metastatic disease, and about 20% of these tumors are discovered incidentally at the time of autopsy. Symptoms related to production of norepinephrine occur in 25% to 60% of patients with these tumors. Such patients develop chronic or intermittent hypertension, headaches, and palpitations. In contrast, functional adrenal paragangliomas (pheochromocytomas) may be associated with increased serum levels of both epinephrine and norepinephrine, and the exact constellation of symptoms depends on the relative amounts of each. Hypertension predominates in norepinephrine-secreting tumors, whereas hypotension, hypovolemia, palpitations, and tachyarrhythmias are hallmarks of those producing large amounts of epinephrine.[108] The difference in the secretory pattern is believed to be related to the presence of methyltransferase in some adrenal pheochromocytomas (which converts norepinephrine to epinephrine) and its absence in extraadrenal paragangliomas.

Diagnosis of extraadrenal paraganglioma is rarely made preoperatively unless the lesion is functional. In the latter instance, the diagnosis can be made by measurement of total urinary catecholamines, and the lesions can be localized by means of angiography. More recently, scintigraphic localization of both adrenal and extraadrenal lesions has been accomplished by means of I-131 meta-iodobenzylguanidine, a structural analog of norepinephrine. It is concentrated in adrenergic tissue by the same mechanism as that of a neurotransmitter and has allowed visualization of paragangliomas as small as 0.2 g.[109]

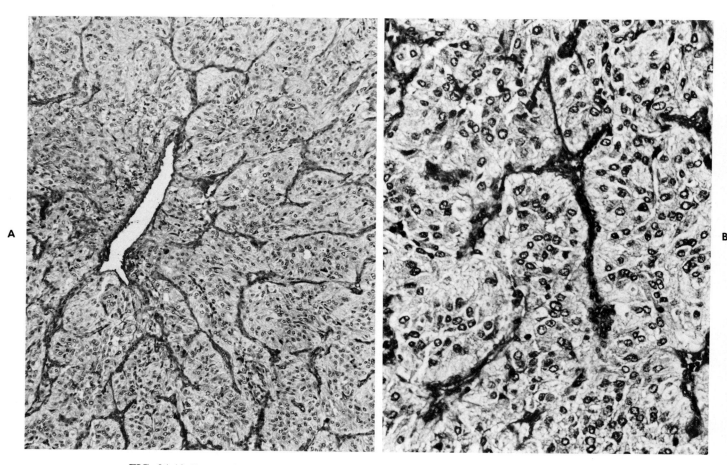

FIG. 34-18. Retroperitoneal paraganglioma depicting irregular anastomotic sheets of cells **(A)** that surround an intricate vasculature **(B)**. Cytoplasmic borders are often indistinct. **(A,** ×160; **B,** ×400.)

Gross and microscopic findings

These tumors are partially encapsulated brown masses that usually measure several centimeters in diameter. Hemorrhage is a common finding. Histologically, retroperitoneal paragangliomas may resemble a branchiomeric paraganglioma or adrenal pheochromocytoma, or they may combine features of both. Most, however, are similar to the adrenal pheochromocytoma. They are composed of small polygonal or slightly spindled cells with an amphophilic or eosinophilic cytoplasm. The cells are arranged in short, irregular anastomosing sheets around a delicate vasculature (Figs. 34-18 and 34-19). The cell outlines are often indistinct so that the sheets have a syncytial quality. Eosinophilic globules may be identified within the cytoplasm of the cells and vary in size from a few micra to the size of a nucleus. These structures seem to represent remnants of dense core granules and their presence has been correlated with benignancy (see below). Hemorrhage within these nests of cells is not infrequent (Fig. 34-20). Although few retroperitoneal paragangliomas resemble carotid body tumors in their entirety, it is often possible to find occasional areas within these lesions where the cells are rounded and grow in small nests (Fig. 34-21). A few retroperitoneal paragangliomas are highly pleomorphic lesions made up of spindled or angular cells with deeply eosinophilic cytoplasm and large hyperchromatic nuclei. Such tumors grow in extremely large sheets and often lack the organization of the usual paraganglioma (Fig. 34-22). On initial inspection these pleomorphic tumors are very worrisome and may be mistaken for carcinomas, except that little mitotic activity accompanies the pleomorphic changes. In rare instances, areas of ganglioneuroma may be encountered within retroperitoneal paragangliomas (Chapter 33). Chromaffin reactions are positive in about two thirds of retroperitoneal paragangliomas in the experience of Brantigan and Katase,[89] although not all such tumors are functional (Fig. 34-23). Argyrophilic granules were demonstrated in all the retroperitoneal paragangliomas reported by Lack et al.[100]

Criteria of malignancy

The criteria of malignancy in paragangliomas has been a controversial subject. In the opinion of some, the only def-

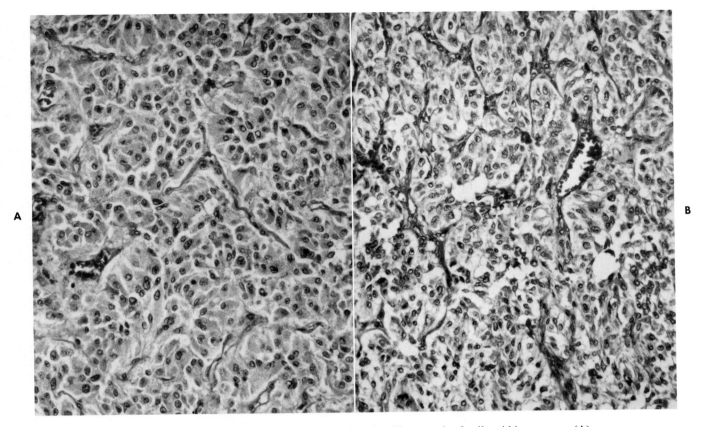

FIG. 34-19. Extraadrenal paraganglioma showing sheetlike growth of cells within one area (**A**). In other areas cells have lost cohesion with formation of clear spaces (**B**). (**A** and **B**, ×250.)

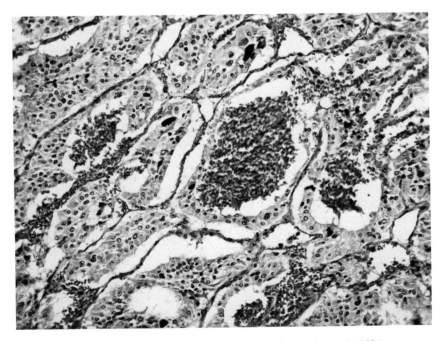

FIG. 34-20. Paraganglioma showing cystic hemorrhage. (×160.)

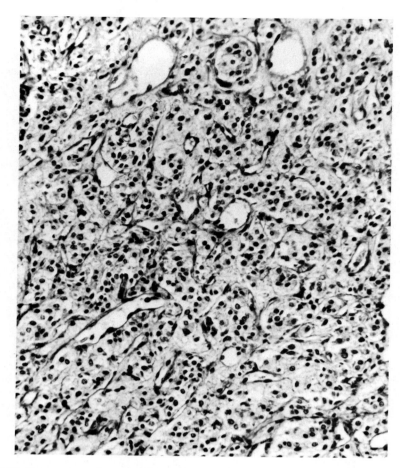

FIG. 34-21. Retroperitoneal paraganglioma showing areas resembling carotid body tumor. (×250.)

inite criterion of malignancy is metastatic disease. Recently, Linnoila et al.[102] have analyzed various features in clinically benign and malignant paragangliomas and have concluded that extraadrenal location, coarse nodularity, confluent necrosis, and absence of hyaline globules may be predictive of malignancy. Seventy-one percent of malignant tumors had two or three of these features, whereas 89% of benign tumors had one or none of the features. The same authors have suggested that decreased expression of a variety of neuropeptides may also correlate with malignancy and may, therefore, serve as an adjunctive means of identifying aggressive behavior. Benign lesions typically express five or more neuropeptides and malignant lesions only two.[103] The relative value of flow cytometry has recently been studied in the evaluation of malignancy in these tumors.[106] Although aneuploid and tetraploid DNA histograms have been identified within tumors that metastasized, similar histograms are seen within the benign group as well. Whereas a normal histogram is usually indicative of a benign lesion, abnormal histograms cannot be equated with malignancy.

Immunohistochemical findings

The immunological profile of this form of paraganglioma is similar to the branchiomeric forms in that neuron-specific enolase and neurofilament protein can be identified in chief cells, which, in turn, are surrounded by a sustentacular network of cells that stains positively for S-100 protein.[9] Leu-enkephalin, an opiate-like pentapeptide that comprises part of the β-endorphin molecule, can be identified within many adrenal and extraadrenal paragangliomas.[3] This finding is to be expected in view of the fact that this pentapeptide is normally produced by normal and hyperplastic adrenal medullary cells. Chromagranin, one of the matrix proteins of the dense core granule, can also be localized immunologically to these tumors, although the amount appears to be less than in normal medullary tissue.[8] Insulin-like growth factor II, a polypeptide of 67 amino acids that is homologous to the beta chain of proinsulin, has recently been identified within adrenal tissues, carotid body, and paraganglia and can also be localized to most chief cells within adrenal and extraadrenal paragangliomas.[110] Its exact significance is unclear, but it is known to

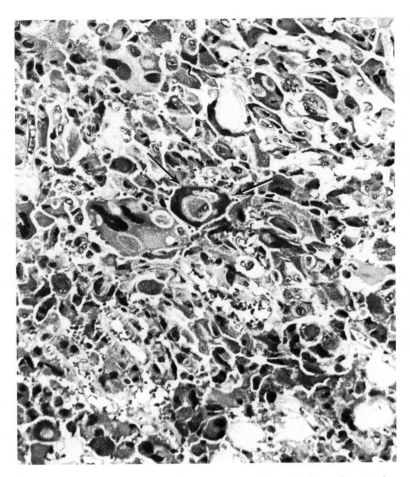

FIG. 34-22. Pleomorphic form of retroperitoneal paraganglioma. Cells are large and angular and have a deeply staining cytoplasm. Cell embracing, a general feature of paragangliomas, is evident in this tumor *(arrows)*. (×250.)

have a mitogenic influence on fibroblasts and can enhance differentiation in myoblasts and neuroblastoma cell lines. A variety of neuropeptides can be localized to the chief cells and are detailed in Table 34-1.[103] There also appears to be a correlation between the number of peptides expressed and the level of malignancy (see above).

Behavior and treatment

Earlier reports in the literature consistently indicated that extraadrenal paragangliomas had a more aggressive course than those within the adrenal.[95,100,104,105,108] A recent study based on experience from the Memorial Hospital offers evidence to the contrary.[107] Approximately 50% of both adrenal and extraadrenal tumors were malignant as evidenced by either metastatic disease or locally aggressive disease. The 5-year survival rate was 77% for patients with adrenal tumors compared with 82% for those with extraadrenal tumors, figures that are not significantly different. When patients with malignant tumors were compared by

site, there was still no statistical difference in disease-free survival rates. Treatment of these tumors consists of total excision. There is little correlation between the functional activity of the tumor and the degree of malignancy. Dissemination of this tumor occurs both lymphatically and hematogenously, and the most common sites of metastasis are the regional lymph nodes, bone, liver, and lung.

If the diagnosis of retroperitoneal paraganglioma is suspected clinically, appropriate steps to document functional activity should be undertaken before surgery. Premedication of patients with β-adrenergic blocking agents is mandatory so as to avert intraoperative hypertensive crises or tachyarrythmias during surgical manipulation of the tumor. Surgery should be aimed at complete removal, since adjunctive radiotherapy and chemotherapy can only be considered palliative measures. It has recently been suggested that serum neuropeptide Y levels may be a reliable and sensitive means of following patients, since levels of this substance can be correlated with tumor recurrence.[99]

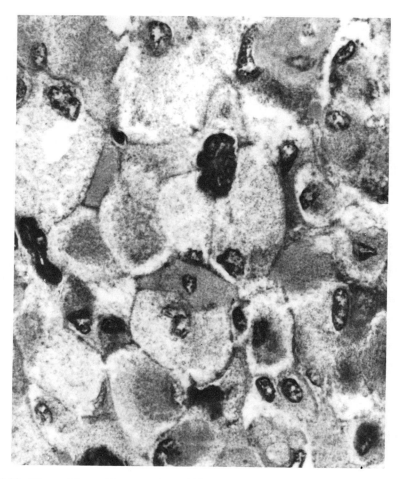

FIG. 34-23. Chromaffin-positive granules within the cells of a retroperitoneal paraganglioma. (Chromaffin fixation, ×600.)

MISCELLANEOUS PARAGANGLIOMAS

Paragangliomas may arise in numerous locations besides those already mentioned, including the nasopharynx,[119,120,132] larynx,[111,112,117] orbit,[144,145] gallbladder,[131] duodenum,* kidney,[127] bladder,[126,138,146] and heart.[122] Although it has been claimed that they may also arise in the extremities from paraganglia that follow the arterial vessels, systematic microscopic search by Karnauchow[123] of 38 autopsy cases failed to reveal acceptable structures. Moreover, some cases reported as paragangliomas of the extremity seem in reality to be alveolar soft part sarcomas. In our opinion the diagnosis of paraganglioma of the extremity should be made with great reserve and only after alternative diagnoses such as carcinoma, melanoma, and alveolar soft part sarcoma have been excluded by appropriate staining procedures, clinical history taking, and electron microscopic studies.

*References 116, 118, 124, 125, 128, 129, 133, 134-137, 143.

Nasopharyngeal paraganglioma

Most paragangliomas involving the nasopharynx arise from adjacent structures such as the glomus jugulare and vagal body and extend secondarily into this region.[1] Primary nasopharyngeal tumors arising from submucosal paraganglia are rare, and this diagnosis is an exclusionary one. These tumors are pulsatile blue masses arising high in the nasopharynx. They produce symptoms of dysphonia, dysphagia, nasal obstruction, and epistaxis. Their appearance is similar to that of carotid body tumor.

Laryngeal paraganglioma

Laryngeal paragangliomas arise from the paired paraganglia that are situated in the soft tissue of the larynx. The superior pair is located at the level of the superior margin of the thyroid cartilage, whereas the inferior pair is located at the border of the thyroid and cricoid cartilage. Aberrant locations near the upper tracheal rings have also been identified. Most laryngeal paragangliomas occur in men, and

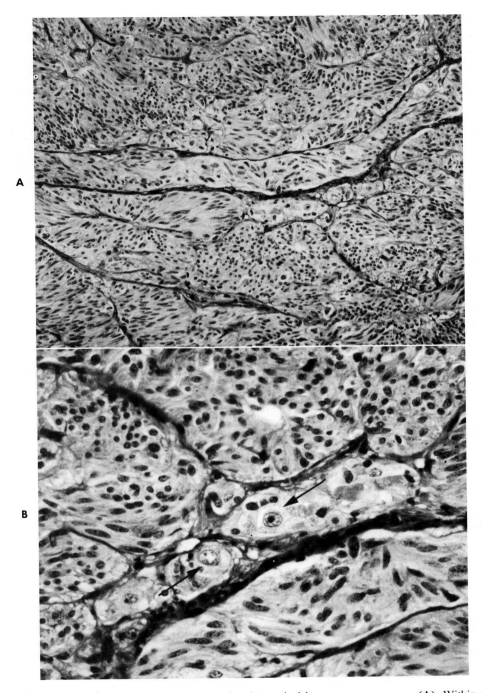

FIG. 34-24. Gangliocytic paraganglioma showing typical low-power appearance **(A)**. Within epithelioid areas, focal differentiating ganglion cells are seen *(arrow)* **(B)**. (A, ×100; B, ×250.)

the average patient age is 47 years.[117] Almost all arise above the level of the vocal cords and involve the ipsilateral aryepiglottic fold. Affected patients usually develop hoarseness, dysphagia, and dyspnea. These tumors are histologically similar to other branchiomeric paragangliomas. The relative malignancy of these tumors has been disputed.[117] Batsakis[1] maintains that most are benign and that the high incidence of metastasis reported as 25% in a review of the literature by Gallivan et al.[117] is most likely the result of misdiagnosis of laryngeal carcinomas. Laryngeal paragangliomas that have metastasized have a peculiar predilection to involve the subcutis of the neck.[117]

Orbital paraganglioma

Orbital paragangliomas are exceedingly rare tumors that are presumed to arise from the paraganglia associated with the ciliary ganglion. They produce symptoms of visual loss and throbbing pain and deficits of one or more cranial nerves. Unfortunately, many cases of orbital paragangliomas reported in the past are, in fact, alveolar soft part sarcomas that have been misdiagnosed. Excluding 13 of the 29 reported cases, Archer et al.[113] found that the 16 acceptable examples of orbital paraganglioma occurred at a wide range of ages (3 to 68 years) with an equal sex distribution. Nearly 40% of those treated with exenteration recurred. However, no case to date has produced metastatic disease.

Gangliocytic paraganglioma

Described in 1962 by Taylor and Helwig,[143] gangliocytic paraganglioma is an unusual tumor that combines features of paraganglioma, carcinoid, and ganglioneuroma and that almost always occurs in the second portion of the duodenum. Rarely, the third portion of the duodenum is involved. The tumor predominantly affects men and makes its appearance during adult life with the onset of gastrointestinal tract bleeding. The majority can be demonstrated on upper gastrointestinal tract series as pedunculated or sessile lesions that arise in the submucosa and deform the overlying mucosa. Histologically the tumors are quite distinctive. They are composed of epithelioid areas that may appear indistinguishable from conventional paraganglioma (Fig. 34-24, A) or may have a ribbonlike or trabecular arrangement similar to that of carcinoid. These cells are argyrophilic and only rarely contain argentaffin granules.[134] The epithelioid areas are surrounded by a delicate network of Schwann cells and nerve axons. Scattered among the epithelioid areas are variably differentiated ganglion cells (Fig. 34-24, B). Although most do not appear fully differentiated, they can be easily recognized by their abundant cytoplasm, vesicular nuclei, and faint cytoplasmic basophilia. In some gangliocytic paragangliomas, a very prominent neuromatous stroma may be seen so that portions of the tumor out of context resemble ganglioneuroma.

A variety of antigens can be identified within the epithelioid cells of these tumors, including neuron-specific enolase,[118,137] insulin,[134] glucagon,[134] leu-enkephalin,[134] pancreatic polypeptide,[118,134,137] somatostatin,[134,137] vasoactive intestinal peptide,[134] molluskan cardioexcitatory peptide,[134] and serotonin.[134] Chromagranin has been identified within carcinoid-like areas of these tumors.[118] The ganglion cells express neuron-specific enolase and neurofilament protein, whereas S-100 protein is easily demonstrable within the sustentacular network surrounding the epithelioid cells (Fig. 34-25). It has been postulated that this tumor arises from the primordium of the pancreas, which undergoes hyperplasia and recapitulates, in an exaggerated fashion, the

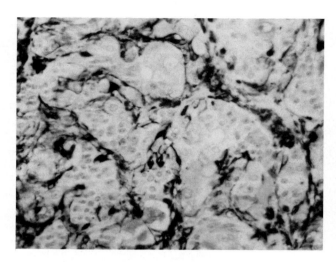

FIG. 34-25. S-100–positive sustentacular network surrounding epithelioid nests within a gangliocytic paraganglioma. (Anti–S-100 protein, peroxidase-antiperoxidase, ×250.)

endodermal-neuroectodermal complexes of van Campenout, which normally occur in the duodenum. However, as pointed out by Scheithauer et al.,[137] about half of paragangliomas of the cauda equina also show ganglionic differentiation, so that it does not seem necessary to specifically impute van Campenout complexes in the pathogenesis of this type of paraganglioma.

All tumors reported have proved to be benign. Hence simple excision to prevent recurrent gastrointestinal hemorrhage is adequate therapy.

Paraganglioma of the cauda equina

Paraganglioma of the cauda equina has been recognized only recently as a distinct entity.[115,121,140-142] Earlier cases were probably misdiagnosed as ependymomas or carcinomas. Approximately 50 cases have been reported in the literature.[141] Males are affected slightly more often, and the median age is approximately 50 years. All patients present with "cauda equina syndrome," which includes back pain, weakness of the extremity, or urinary or fecal incontinence. Extreme elevations in cerebrospinal fluid protein can be documented in a significant proportion of cases. The tumors are extramedullary, intradural masses, which may or may not be attached to the cauda equina. The tumors resemble other paragangliomas in all respects, although in about half, ganglionic differentiation is noted.[131] The chief cells contain neuron-specific enolase, neurofilament protein, and somatostatin. Electron microscopic studies document typical dense core granules in addition to paranuclear intermediate filaments and, rarely, cilia.[115] Although these are benign tumors, their location may complicate complete surgical excision, thereby leading to local recurrences in about 10% of patients. Radiotherapy has been recommended for unencapsulated or incompletely excised tumors.

Cardiac paraganglioma

This is one of the rarest forms of paraganglioma, with only 15 cases reported in the literature.[117] Most cases have occurred in women, with an average age of 45 years. The tumor occurs primarily on the left atrium or in the interventricular groove at the aortic root and commonly gives rise to hypertensive symptoms. The lesions are histologically and immunohistochemically quite similar to other forms of paraganglioma. Treatment of these inaccessible tumors usually requires resection of the posterior atrial wall with coronary artery bypass. Two of the 15 cases reported in the literature have developed metastasis.

REFERENCES
General

1. Batsakis JG: Paragangliomas of the head and neck. In *Tumors of the head and neck*. Baltimore, 1979, Williams & Wilkins.
2. Biscoe TJ: Carotid body: structure and function. *Physiol Rev* 51:437, 1971.
3. DeLellis RA, Tischler AS, Lee AK, et al: Leu-enkephalin-like immunoreactivity in proliferative lesions of the human adrenal medulla and extraadrenal paraganglia. *Am J Surg Pathol* 7:29, 1983.
4. Glenner GG, Grimley PM: Tumors of the extraadrenal paraganglion system (including chemoreceptors). *Atlas of tumor pathology*, Armed Forces Institute of Pathology, 1974, fascicle 9, second series.
5. Gomori G: Staining of chromaffin tissue. *Am J Clin Pathol* 16:115, 1946.
6. Kliewer CE, Cochran AJ: A review of the histology, ultrastructure, immunohistology, and molecular biology of extraadrenal paragangliomas. *Arch Pathol Lab Med* 113:1209, 1989.
7. Lack EE, Mercer L: A modified Grimelius argyrtophil technique for neurosecretory granules. *Am J Surg Pathol* 1:275, 1977.
8. Lloyd RV, Blaivas M, Wilson BS: Distribution of chromagranin and S-100 protein in normal and abnormal adrenal medullary tissues. *Arch Pathol Lab Med* 109:633, 1985.
9. Mariman EC, van Beersum SE, Cremers CW, et al: Analysis of a second family with hereditary nonchromaffin paragangliomas locates the underlying gene at the proximal region of chromosome 11q. *Hum Genet* 91:357, 1993.
10. Pearse AGE, Polak JM, Rost FWD, et al: Demonstration of the neural crest origin of type I (APUD) cells in the avian carotid body using a cytochemical marker system. *Histochemie* 34:191, 1973.
11. Schroder HD, Johannsen L: Demonstration of S-100 protein in sustentacular cells of pheochromocytomas and paragangliomas. *Histopathology* 10:1023, 1986.
12. Warren WH, Lee I, Gould VE, et al: Paragangliomas of the head and neck: ultrastructural and immunohistochemical analysis. *Ultrastruct Pathol* 8:333, 1985.
13. Willis AG, Birrell JW: The structure of a carotid body tumor. *Acta Anat (Basel)* 25:220, 1955.

Carotid body paraganglioma

14. Albores-Saavedra J, Duncan ME: Association of thyroid cancer and chemodectomas. *Am J Surg* 116:887, 1968.
15. Alpert LI, Bochetto JF Jr: Carotid body tumor: ultrastructural observations. *Cancer* 34:564, 1974.
16. Berdal P, Braaten M, Cappelen C Jr, et al: Noradrenaline-adrenaline producing nonchromaffin paraganglioma. *Acta Med Scand* 172:249, 1962.
17. Chase WH: Familial and bilateral tumors of the carotid body. *J Pathol Bacteriol* 36:1, 1933.
18. Cone TE Jr: Recurrent pheochromocytoma: report of a case in a previously treated child. *Pediatrics* 21:994, 1958.
19. Cragg RW: Concurrent tumors of the left carotid body and Zuckerkandl bodies. *Arch Pathol* 18:635, 1934.
20. Fries JG, Chamberlin JA: Extraadrenal pheochromocytoma: litera-

ture review and report of a cervical pheochromocytoma. *Surgery* 63:268, 1968.
21. Gaylis H, Mieny CJ: The incidence of malignancy in carotid body tumors. *Br J Surg* 64:885, 1977.
22. Glenner GG, Crout JR, Roberts WC: A functional carotid-body-like tumor secreting levarterenol. *Arch Pathol* 73:230, 1962.
23. Grimley PM, Glenner GC: Histology and ultrastructure of carotid body paragangliomas: comparison with the normal gland. *Cancer* 20:1473, 1967.
24. Gustilo RB, Lober PH, Salovich EL: Chemodectoma metastasizing to bone: case report. *J Bone Joint Surg* 47A:155, 1965.
25. Hamberger CA, Hamberger CB, Wersall J, et al: Malignant catecholamine-producing tumor of the carotid body. *Acta Pathol Microbiol Scand* 69(A):489, 1967.
26. Harrington SW, Claggett OT, Dockerty MB: Tumors of the carotid body: clinical and pathologic considerations of 20 tumours affecting 19 patients (1 bilateral). *Ann Surg* 114:820, 1941.
27. Katz AD: Carotid body tumors in a large family group. *Am J Surg* 108:570, 1964.
28. Kipkie GF: Simultaneous chromaffin tumors of the carotid body and glomus jugular. *Arch Pathol* 4:113, 1947.
29. Lack EE, Cubilla AL, Woodruff JM: Paragangliomas of the head and neck region: a pathologic study of tumors from 70 patients. *Hum Pathol* 10:199, 1979.
30. Lack EE, Cubilla AL, Woodruff JM, et al: Paragangliomas of the head and neck region: a clinical study of 69 patients. *Cancer* 39:397, 1977.
31. Malinatti GM, Camanni F, Pizzini A: Malignant hypertension in a case of nonchromaffin paraganglioma with a high concentration of catecholamine. *Cancer* 12:878, 1959.
32. Martin CE, Rosenfeld L, McSwain B: Carotid body tumors: A 16-year follow-up of seven malignant cases. *South Med J* 66:1236, 1973.
33. McGuirt WF, Harker LA: Carotid body tumors. *Arch Otolaryngol* 101:58, 1975.
34. Mitchell DC, Clyne CAC: Chemodectoma of the neck: the response to radiotherapy. *Br J Surg* 72:903, 1985.
35. Nabarra B, Sonsino E, Andrianarison I: Ultrastructure of a polysome-lamellae complex in a human paraganglioma. *Am J Pathol* 86:523, 1977.
36. Pryse-Davies J, Dawson IMP, Westbury G: Some morphologic, histochemical, and chemical observations on chemodectomas and the normal carotid body, including a study of the chromaffin reaction and possible ganglion cell elements. *Cancer* 17:185, 1964.
37. Rangwala AF, Sylvia LC, Becker SM: Soft tissue metastasis of a chemodectoma: a case report and a review of the literature. *Cancer* 42:2865, 1978.
38. ReMine WH, Weiland LH, ReMine SG: Carotid body tumors: chemodectomas. *Curr Probl Cancer* 2:1, 1978.
39. Robertson DI, Cooney TP: Malignant carotid body paraganglioma: light and electron microscopic study of the tumor and its metastases. *Cancer* 46:2623, 1980.

40. Rush BF Jr: Familial bilateral carotid body tumors. *Ann Surg* 157:633, 1963.

41. Saldana MJ, Salem LE, Travezan R: High altitude hypoxia and chemodectomas. *Hum Pathol* 4:251, 1973.

42. Sclafani LM, Woodruff JM, Brennan MF: Extraadrenal retroperitoneal paragangliomas: natural history and response to treatment. *Surgery* 108:1124, 1990.

43. Shamblin WR, ReMine WH, Sheps SG, et al: Carotid body tumor (chemodectoma): clinicopathologic analysis of 90 cases. *Am J Pathol* 122:732, 1971.

44. Smith SA, Kuhns J, McMurry GT: Metastasizing carotid paragangliomas. *J Ky Med Assoc* 76:65, 1978.

45. Sprong DH, Kirby FG: Familial carotid body tumors: report of nine cases in eleven siblings. *Ann West Med Surg* 3:241, 1949.

46. Staats EF, Brown RI, Smith RR: Carotid body tumors, benign and malignant. *Laryngoscope* 76:907, 1966.

47. Sugarbaker EV, Chretien PB, Jacobs JB: Bilateral familial carotid body tumors: report of a patient with occult contralateral tumor and postoperative hypertension. *Ann Surg* 174:242, 1971.

48. Toker C: Ultrastructure of a chemodectoma. *Cancer* 20:271, 1967.

49. Tu H, Bottomley RH: Malignant chemodectoma presenting as miliary pulmonary infiltrate. *Cancer* 33:244, 1974.

50. Whimster WF, Masson AF: Malignant carotid body tumor with extradural metastases. *Cancer* 26:239, 1970.

Jugulotympanic paraganglioma

51. Azzarelli B, Felten S, Muller J, et al: Dopamine in paragangliomas of the glomus jugulare. *Laryngoscope* 98:573, 1988.

52. Borsanyi SJ: Glomus jugulare tumors. *Laryngoscope* 72:1336, 1962.

53. Brown JS: Glomus jugulare tumors revisited: a ten-year statistical follow-up of 231 cases. *Laryngoscope* 95:284, 1985.

54. Cole JM: Glomus jugulare tumors of the temporal bone: radiation of glomus tumor of the temporal bone. *Laryngoscope* 89:1623, 1979.

55. Duke WW, Boshell BR, Soteres P, et al: A norepinephrine-secreting glomus jugulare tumor presenting as pheochromocytoma. *Ann Intern Med* 60:1040, 1964.

56. Fuller AM, Brown HA, Harrison EG Jr, et al: Chemodectomas of the glomus jugulare. *Laryngoscope* 77:218, 1967.

57. Gaffney JC: Carotid-body-like tumours of jugular bulb and middle ear. *J Pathol Bacteriol* 66:157, 1953.

58. Glascock ME, Harris PF, Newsome G: Glomus tumors: diagnosis and treatment. *Laryngoscope* 84:2006, 1974.

59. Glascock ME, Jackson CG, Dickens JRE, et al: Glomus jugulare tumors of the temporal bone: surgical management of glomus tumors. *Laryngoscope* 89:1640, 1979.

60. Gulya AJ: The glomus tumor and its biology. *Laryngoscope* 103 (Pt 2 suppl):7, 1993.

61. Hatfield PM, James AE, Schulz MD: Chemodectomas of the glomus jugulare. *Cancer* 30:1164, 1972.

62. Hawthorne MR, Makek MS, Harris JP, et al: The histopathological and clinical features of irradiated and nonirradiated temporal paragangliomas. *Laryngoscope* 98:325, 1988.

63. Horvath KK, Ormos J, Ribari O: Crystals in a jugulotympanic paraganglioma. *Ultrastruct Pathol* 10:257, 1986.

64. Johnstone PA, Foss RD, Desilets DJ: Malignant jugulotympanic paraganglioma. *Arch Pathol Lab Med* 114:976, 1990.

65. Lattes R, Waltner JG: Nonchromaffin paraganglioma of middle ear (carotid-body-like tumor; glomus-jugular tumor). *Cancer* 2:447, 1949.

66. Matsuguchi H, Tsuneyoshi M, Takeshita A, et al: Noradrenaline secreting glomus jugulare tumor with cyclic change of blood pressure. *Arch Intern Med* 135:1110, 1975.

67. Ogura JII, Spector GJ, Gado M: Glomus jugulare and vagale. *Ann Otol* 87:622, 1978.

68. Spector GJ, Sobel S, Thawley SE, et al: Glomus jugulare tumors of the temporal bone: patterns of invasion in the temporal bone. *Laryngoscope* 89:1628, 1979.

69. Wright JW Jr, Wright JW III, Hicks GW: Glomus jugulare tumors of the temporal bone: radiologic appearance of glomus tumors. *Laryngoscope* 89:1620, 1975.

Intravagal paraganglioma

70. Chaudhry AP, Haar JG, Kous A, et al: A nonfunctioning paraganglioma of vagus nerve. *Cancer* 43:1689, 1979.

71. Fernandez BB, Hernandez FJ, Staley CJ: Chemodectoma of the vagus nerve: report of a case with ultrastructural study. *Cancer* 35:263, 1975.

72. Heinrich MC, Harris AE, Bell WR: Metastatic intravagal paraganglioma: case report and review of the literature. *Am J Med* 78:1017, 1985.

73. Kahn LB: Vagal body tumor (nonchromaffin paraganglioma, chemodectoma, and carotid-body-like tumor) with cervical node metastasis and familial association: ultrastructural study and review. *Cancer* 38:2367, 1976.

74. Levit SA: Catechol secreting paraganglioma of the glomus jugular region resembling pheochromocytoma. *N Engl J Med* 281:805, 1969.

75. Moore G, Yarington CT, Mangham CA: Vagal body tumors: diagnosis and treatment. *Laryngoscope* 96:533, 1986.

76. Someren A, Karcioglu Z: Malignant vagal paraganglioma. report of a case and review of the literature. *Am J Clin Pathol* 68:400, 1977.

77. Tannir NM, Cortas, Allam C: A functioning catecholamine-secreting vagal body tumor: a case report and review of the literature. *Cancer* 52:932, 1983.

Mediastinal paraganglioma

78. Assaf HM, al-Momen AA, Martin JG: Aorticopulmonary paraganglioma: a case report with immunohistochemical studies and literature review. *Arch Pathol Lab Med* 116:1085, 1992.

79. Bird DJ, Seiler MW: Aorticopulmonary paraganglioma (aortic body tumor): report of a case. *Ultrastruct Pathol* 15:475, 1991.

80. D'Altoria RA, Rishi US, Bhagwanani DG: Arteriographic findings in mediastinal chemodectoma. *J Thorac Cardiovasc Surg* 67:963, 1974.

81. Gallivan MVE, Chun B, Rowden G, et al: Intrathoracic paravertebral malignant paraganglioma. *Arch Pathol Lab Med* 104:4, 1980.

82. Lack EE, Stillinger RA, Colvin DB, et al: Aortico-pulmonary paraganglioma: report of a case with ultrastructural study and review of the literature. *Cancer* 43:269, 1979.

83. Lattes R: Nonchromaffin paraganglioma of ganglion nodosum, carotid body, and aortic arch bodies. *Cancer* 3:667, 1950.

84. Mendelow II, Slobodkin M: Aortic body tumor of the mediastinum. *Cancer* 10:1008, 1957.

85. Olson JL, Salyer WR: Mediastinal paragangliomas (aortic body tumor): a report of four cases and a review of the literature. *Cancer* 41:2405, 1978.

86. Tama L, Ellis FH, Hidgson CH, et al: Chemodectoma of the mediastinum: report on patient with superior vena caval obstruction treated by shunt from right innominate vein to right atrium. *J Thorac Cardiovasc Surg* 43:585, 1962.

87. Wilkinson R, Forgan-Smith R: Chemodectoma in relation to the aortic arch (aortic body tumor): a clinical report. *Thorax* 24:28, 1969.

Retroperitoneal paraganglioma

88. Attia A, Golden RL, Ziffer H: Nonchromaffin staining functional tumor of the organ of Zuckekandl. *N Engl J Med* 264:1130, 1961.

89. Brantigan CO, Katase RY: Clinical and pathologic features of paraganglioma of the organ of Zuckerkandl. *Surgery* 65:898, 1969.

90. Brown WJ, Barajas L, Waisman J, et al: Ultrastructural and biochemical correlates of adrenal pheochromocytoma. *Cancer* 29:744, 1972.

91. Capella C, Riva C, Cornaggia M, et al: Histopathology, cytology, and cytochemistry of pheochromocytomas and paragangliomas including chemodectomas. *Pathol Res Pract* 183:176, 1988.

92. Carney JA: The triad of gastric epithelioid leiomyosarcoma, pulmonary chondroma, and functioning extraadrenal paraganglioma: a five year review. *Medicine (Balt)* 62:159, 1983.

93. Carney JA, Sheps SG, Go VLW, et al: The triad of gastric leiomyosarcoma, functioning extraadrenal paraganglioma, and pulmonary chondroma. *N Engl J Med* 296:1517, 1977.

94. Cross DA, Meyer JS: Postoperative deaths due to unsuspected pheochromocytoma. *South Med J* 70:1320, 1977.

95. Glenn F, Gray GF: Functional tumors of the organ of Zuckerkandl. *Ann Surg* 183:578, 1976.

96. Gullotta F, Helpap B: Tissue culture, electron microscopic, and enzyme histochemical investigations of extraadrenal paragangliomas. *Pathol Eur* 11:257, 1976.

97. Hellman LJ, Cohen PS, Averbuch SD, et al: Neuropeptide Y distinguishes benign from malignant pheochromocytoma. *J Clin Oncol* 7:720, 1989.

98. Kimura N, Miura Y, Nagatsu I, et al: Catecholamine synthesizing enzymes in 70 cases of functioning and non-functioning phaeochromocytoma and extra-adrenal paraganglioma. *Virchows Arch (Pathol Anat Histopathol)* 421:25, 1992.

99. Kuvshinoff BW, Nussbaum MS, Richards AI, et al: Neuropeptide Y secretion from a malignant extraadrenal retroperitoneal paraganglioma. *Cancer* 70:2350, 1992.

100. Lack EE, Cubilla AL, Woodruff JM, et al: Extraadrenal paragangliomas of the retroperitoneum. a clinicopathologic study of 12 tumors. *Am J Surg Pathol* 4:109, 1980.

101. Lee SP, Nicholson GI, Hitchcock G: Familial abdominal chemodectomas with associated angiolipomas. *Pathology* 9:1063, 1971.

102. Linnoila RI, Keiser HR, Steinberg SM, et al: Histopathology of benign versus malignant sympathoadrenal paragangliomas: clinicopathologic study of 120 cases including unusual histologic features. *Hum Pathol* 21:1168, 1990.

103. Linnoila RI, Lack EE, Steinberg SM, et al: Decreased expression of neuropeptides in malignant paragangliomas: an immunohistochemical study. *Hum Pathol* 19:47, 1988.

104. Melicow MM: One hundred cases of pheochromocytoma (107 tumors) at the Columbia-Presbyterian Medical Center 1926-1976. A clinicopathologic analysis. *Cancer* 40:1987, 1977.

105. Olson JR, Abell MR: Nonfunctional nonchromaffin paragangliomas of the retroperitoneum. *Cancer* 23:1358, 1969.

106. Pang LC, Tsao KC: Flow cytometric DNA analysis for the determination of malignant potential in adrenal and extraadrenal pheochromocytomas or paragangliomas. *Arch Pathol Lab Med* 117:1142, 1993.

107. Pommier RF, Vetto JT, Billingsly K, et al: Comparison of adrenal and extraadrenal pheochromocytomas. *Surgery* 114:1160, 1993.

108. Scott HW Jr, Oates JA, Nies AS, et al: Pheochromocytoma: recent diagnosis and management. *Ann Surg* 183:587, 1976.

109. Sisson JC, Frager MS, Valk TW, et al: Scintigraphic localization of pheochromocytoma. *N Engl J Med* 305:12, 1981.

110. Suzuki T, Watanabe K, Sugino T, et al: Immunocytochemical demonstration of IGF-II immunoreactivity in human phaeochromocytoma and extraadrenal paraganglioma. *J Pathol* 167:199, 1992.

Miscellaneous paragangliomas

111. Adlington P, Woodhouse MA: The ultrastructure of chemodectoma of the larynx. *J Laryngol Otol* 86:1219, 1972.

112. Andrews AH: Glomus tumors (nonchromaffin paragangliomas) of the larynx: case report. *Ann Otol Rhinol Laryngol* 64:1034, 1955.

113. Archer KF, Hurwitz JJ, Balogh JM, et al: Orbital nonchromaffin paraganglioma: a case report and review of the literature. *Ophthalmology* 96:1659, 1989.

114. Bilbao JM, Horvath E, Kovacs K, et al: Intrasellar paraganglioma associated with hypopituitarism. *Arch Pathol Lab Med* 102:95, 1978.

115. Cabello A, Ricoy JR: Paraganglioma of the caude equina. *Cancer* 52:751, 1983.

116. Cooney T, Sweeney EC: Paraganglioma of the duodenum: an evolutionary hybrid? *J Clin Pathol* 31:233, 1978.

117. Gallivan MVE, Chun B, Rowden G, et al: Laryngeal paraganglioma: a case report with ultrastructural analysis and literature review. *Am J Surg Pathol* 3:85, 1979.

118. Hamid QA, Bishop AE, Rode J, et al: Duodenal gangliocytic paraganglioma: a study of 10 cases with immunocytochemical neuroendocrine markers. *Hum Pathol* 17:1151, 1986.

119. Harkins WB: Nonchromaffin paraganglioma of the nasal sinuses. *Laryngoscope* 67:246, 1957.

120. House JM, Goodman ML, Gacek RR, et al: Chemodectomas of the nasopharynx. *Arch Otolaryngol* 96:138, 1972.

121. Ironside JW, Royds JA, Taylor CV, et al: Paraganglioma of the cauda equina: a histological, ultrastructural, and immunocytochemical study of two cases with a review of the literature. *J Pathol* 145:195, 1985.

122. Johnson TL, Shapiro B, Beierwaltes WH, et al: Cardiac paragangliomas: a clinicopathologic and immunohistochemical study of four cases. *Am J Surg Pathol* 9:827, 1985.

123. Karnauchow PN: Investigation into the occurrence of paraganglia in lower limbs. *Lab Invest* 6:368, 1957.

124. Kepes JJ, Zacharias DI: Gangliocytic paragangliomas of the duodenum: a report of two cases with light and electron microscopic examination. *Cancer* 27:61, 1971.

125. Kheir SM, Halpern NB: Paraganglioma of the duodenum in association with congenital neurofibromatosis. *Cancer* 53:2491, 1984.

126. Leestma JE, Price EB: Paraganglioma of the urinary bladder. *Cancer* 28:1063, 1971.

127. Legace R, Tremblany M: Nonchromaffin paraganglioma of kidney with distant metastasis. *Can Med Assoc J* 99:1095, 1968.

128. Lukash WM, Hyams VJ, Nilsson OF: Neurogenic neoplasms of small bowel: benign nonchromaffin paraganglioma of the duodenum: report of a case. *Am J Dig Dis* 11:575, 1966.

129. Matilla A, Rivera F, Fernandez-Sanz J, et al: Nonchromaffin paraganglioma of the duodenum. *Virchows Arch (Pathol Anat)* 383:217, 1979.

130. Mehta M, Nadel NS, Lonni Y, et al: Malignant paraganglioma of the prostate and retroperitoneum. *J Urol* 121:376, 1979.

131. Miller TA, Webber TR, Appleman HD: Paraganglioma of the gallbladder. *Arch Surg* 15:631, 1972.

132. Moran TE: Nonchromaffin paraganglioma of the nasal cavity. *Laryngoscope* 72:201, 1962.

133. Perrone T: Duodenal gangliocytic paraganglioma and carcinoid. *Am J Surg Pathol* 10:147, 1986.

134. Perrone T, Sibley RK, Rosai J: Duodenal gangliocytic paraganglioma: an immunohistochemical and ultrastructural study and a hypothesis concerning its origin. *Am J Surg Pathol* 9:31, 1985.

135. Qizelbash AH: Benign paraganglioma of the duodenum: a case report with light and electron microscopic examination and brief review of the literature. *Arch Pathol* 96:276, 1973.

136. Reed RJ, Daroca PJ, Harkin JC: Gangliocytic paraganglioma. *Am J Surg Pathol* 1:207, 1977.

137. Scheithauer BW, Nora FE, LeChago J, et al: Duodenal gangliocytic paraganglioma: clinicopathologic and immunocytochemical study of 11 cases. *Am J Clin Pathol* 86:559, 1986.

138. Scott WW, Eversole SL: Pheochromocytoma of the urinary bladder. *J Urol* 83:656, 1960.

139. Smith WT, Hughes B, Emocilla R: Chemodectoma of the pineal body and chemoreceptor tissue. *J Pathol* 92:69, 1966.
140. Soffer LD, Pittaluga S, Caine Y, et al: Paraganglioma of cauda equina: a report of a case and review of the literature. *Cancer* 51:1907, 1983.
141. Sonnenland PRL, Scheithauer BW, LeChago J, et al: Paragangli-oma of the caude equina region: clinicopathologic study of 31 cases with special reference to immunocytology and ultrastructure. *Cancer* 58:1720, 1986.
142. Taxy JB: Paraganglioma of the cauda equina: report of a rare tu-mor. *Cancer* 51:1904, 1983.

143. Taylor HB, Helwig EB: Benign nonchromaffin paragangliomas of the duodenum. *Virchows Arch (Pathol Anat)* 335:356, 1962.
144. Thacker WC, Duckworth JK: Chemodectoma of the orbit. *Cancer* 23:1233, 1969.
145. Tye AA: Nonchromaffin paraganglioma of the orbit. *Trans Ophthal-mol Soc Aust* 21:113, 1961.
146. Zimmerman IJ, Biron RE, MacMahon HE: Pheochromocytoma of the urinary bladder. *N Engl J Med* 249:25, 1953.

CHAPTER 35

CARTILAGINOUS SOFT TISSUE TUMORS

Benign extraosseous cartilaginous lesions are uncommon. They usually present as tumorlike masses, but it is still largely conjectural whether these lesions are neoplastic or metaplastic in origin or are inborn errors in tissue development. In the past we have employed rather arbitrarily the term *soft part or extraskeletal chondroma* for small well-defined solitary nodules of hyaline cartilage that are unattached to bone and occur primarily in the distal extremities, especially the fingers and the hand. We have used the same designation for the rare chondroma-like lesions occurring in the alimentary and respiratory tracts. These lesions, however, must be distinguished from the cartilaginous rests of branchial origin that are usually found in the soft tissues of the lateral neck in infants and small children[15] and from metaplastic cartilage that is encountered in some benign lipomatous (chondrolipoma) and fibromatous neoplasms (calcifying aponeurotic fibroma); they must also be separated from multiple cartilaginous nodules in the synovium (synovial chondromatosis) and from cartilage occurring within myositis ossificans and its variants.

Malignant cartilaginous tumors also occur as primary soft tissue neoplasms, but they are much less common than primary chondrosarcomas of bone. There are chiefly two distinctive types: *myxoid chondrosarcoma* and *mesenchymal chondrosarcoma*. There are sporadic reports of other morphological types of extraskeletal chondrosarcoma in the literature, but these are in need of further definition.[55]

Well-differentiated extraosseous chondrosarcomas are extremely rare. In fact, if such a tumor is encountered in soft tissue, it is more likely an extension or metastasis of a bone tumor than a primary soft tissue neoplasm. Well-differentiated chondrosarcomas, however, do arise from the synovium, sometimes secondary to synovial chondromatosis,[11,25,42,49,56] and from the periosteum (periosteal chondrosarcoma).[23] They also occur following radiation therapy[36] or injection of radioactive material, usually after a latent period of many years. For example, Ghalib et al.[46] recorded a chondrosarcoma of the larynx that appeared 40 years after a course of radiation for hyperthyroidism, and Schajowicz et al.[79] reported a chondrosarcoma of the ax-

illa secondary to injection of thorotrast for the diagnosis of hemangioma. Rare instances of chondrosarcoma also occur in the respiratory tract, especially the nasal passages, larynx,[35] trachea, and bronchi.[39] They also are found in the heart and great vessels, especially the pulmonary artery.[64]

Chondrosarcomas of the urinary bladder and uterus are most likely malignant mixed mesodermal tumors or carcinosarcomas that have differentiated along two or more cell lines but have been sampled inadequately. Equally rare are chondrosarcomas of the mammary gland. Most of them display an epithelial or fibroadenomatous component, and many show transitions toward liposarcoma or osteosarcoma.

EXTRASKELETAL CHONDROMA

There are two comprehensive reports of this entity. One of them was published by Dahlin and Salvador[7]; it gives the Mayo Clinic experience with 70 examples of this tumor. The other[5] reviews 104 cases from the files of the Armed Forces Institute of Pathology (AFIP). Both series agree as to the predominant location of this tumor in the hands and feet, its benign clinical course, and its variable histological appearance that not infrequently leads to a mistaken diagnosis of chondrosarcoma.

Clinical findings

The tumor occurs primarily in the soft tissues of the hands and feet, usually without any connection to the underlying bone. Its predominant single site is the fingers, where over 80% of extraskeletal chondromas are found. Less frequent sites are the hands, toes, feet, and trunk. Extraskeletal chondroma usually manifests as a slowly enlarging nodule or mass that seldom causes pain or tenderness; the tumor mainly affects adults between 30 and 60 years of age; it is often associated with tendon, tendon sheath, or the joint capsule, and, unlike periosteal chondroma, is located outside the periosteum.[10,21,26,29] A trigger finger secondary to soft part chondroma is a rare event.[27]

Nearly all of the tumors are solitary, but Dellon et al.[9] described bilateral chondromas in the right index and left

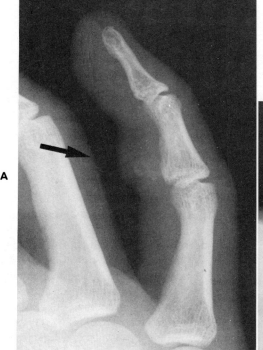

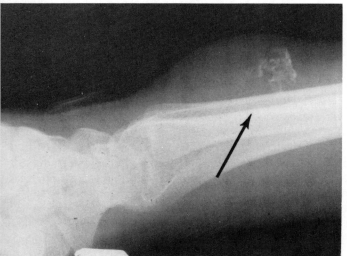

FIG. 35-1. Chondroma of soft parts. **A,** Roentgenograph of right fifth finger showing a small soft tissue mass with foci of calcification. **B,** X-ray film of similar lesion in the right distal forearm. Note the intact ulnar and radial bones. (**B,** From Chung EB, Enzinger FM: *Cancer* 41:1414, 1978.)

ring fingers in a patient with renal failure. In general, however, multiple lesions are more likely examples of synovial chondromatosis. The association of pulmonary chondroma, gastric epithelioid leiomyosarcoma, and extraadrenal paraganglioma is known as *Carney's triad.*

Roentgenographically, the lesion is well demarcated and does not involve bone, although some tumors cause com-

pression deformities or bone erosion. Discrete, irregular, ringlike or curvilinear calcifications are often demonstrable[30] (Fig. 35-1, *A* and *B*). CT scan and MRI are very useful in determining the exact localization of the tumor and its relationship to the adjacent bone.[29,58]

Pathological findings

The excised chondromas are usually well demarcated, have rounded or ovoid configurations, and are firm on palpation. Occasional chondromas are soft or friable with focal cystic change. Nearly all are small and seldom exceed 3 cm in greatest diameter. They may be attached to tendon or tendon sheath (Fig. 35-2). Microscopically, they vary considerably in appearance: About two thirds consist of mature or fairly mature hyaline cartilage arranged in a more or less distinct lobular pattern with sharp borders (Figs. 35-3 and 35-4). Some of these tumors are altered by focal fibrosis *(fibrochondroma)* or ossification *(osteochondroma);* others show myxoid change *(myxochondroma),* sometimes together with focal hemorrhage. About one third display focal or diffuse calcification, usually a late feature that may completely obscure the cartilaginous nature of the tumor and may mimic tumoral calcinosis. The calcified material is granular, floccular, or crystalline (Fig. 35-5) and often outlines the contours of the chondrocytes in a lacelike pattern (Fig. 35-6). Calcification tends to be more pronounced in the center than the periphery of the tumor lobule. It is often accompanied by cellular degeneration and necrosis,

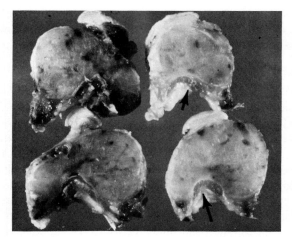

FIG. 35-2. Cross-sections of chondroma of soft parts removed from the second toe of a 62-year-old woman. The tumor is well circumscribed and is firmly attached to a tendon *(arrows).* (From Chung EB, Enzinger FM: *Cancer* 41:1414, 1978.)

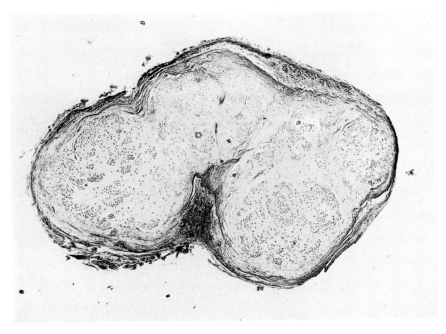

FIG. 35-3. Cross-section of chondroma of soft parts showng circumscription and multinodular growth pattern. (×45.) (From Chung EB, Enzinger FM: *Cancer* 41:1414, 1978.)

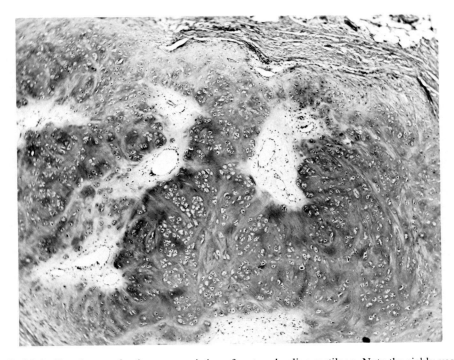

FIG. 35-4. Chondroma of soft parts consisting of mature hyaline cartilage. Note the richly vascular interlobular connective tissue. (×50.)

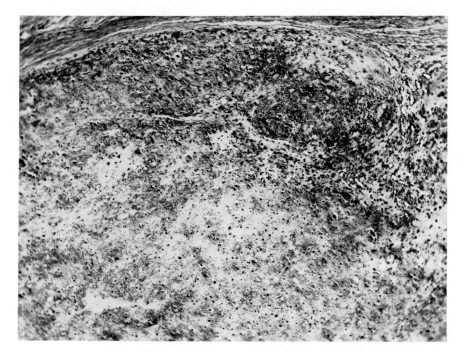

FIG. 35-5. Chondroma of soft parts distorted by marked calcification of the cartilaginous tissue. (×50.) (From Chung EB, Enzinger FM: *Cancer* 41:1414, 1978.)

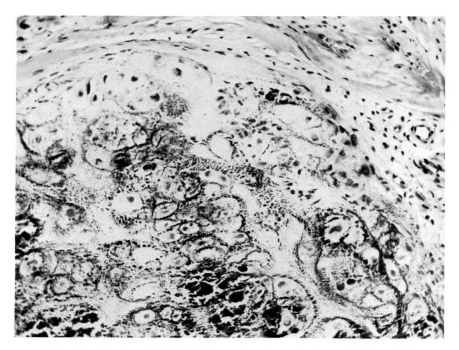

FIG. 35-6. Calcified chondroma of soft parts. Calcium deposits surround and partly replace the cartilage cells. (×165.) (From Chung EB, Enzinger FM: *Cancer* 41:1414, 1978.)

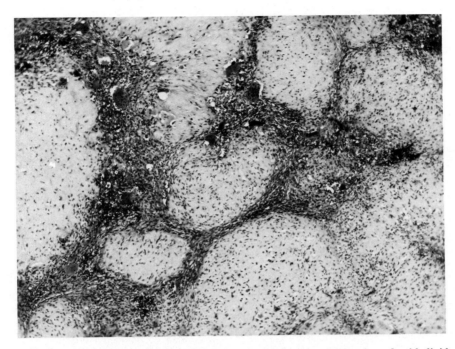

FIG. 35-7. Chondroma of soft parts altered by a granuloma-like proliferation of epithelioid and multinucleated giant cells. (×60.)

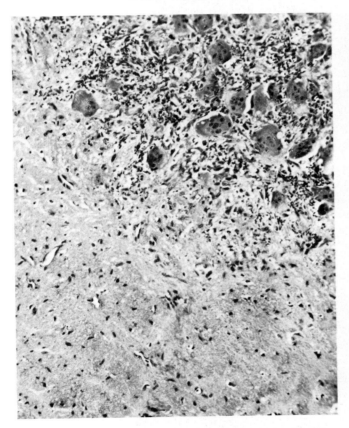

FIG. 35-8. Calcified chondroma of soft parts with proliferation of multinucleated giant cells at the periphery of the calcified nodule. (×130.)

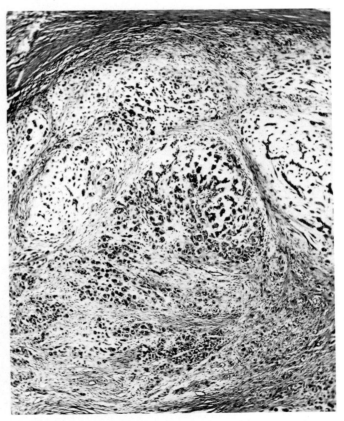

FIG. 35-9. Chondroma of soft parts consisting of immature-appearing cells within a myxoid matrix. (×50.) (From Chung EB, Enzinger FM: *Cancer* 41:1414, 1978.)

which accounts for the softened gross appearance of some of these tumors.

Another striking feature, which occurs in about 15% of the cases, is a focal granuloma-like proliferation of epithelioid and multinucleated giant cells somewhat reminiscent of a fibroxanthoma or a giant cell tumor. This proliferation is most conspicuous at the tumor margin and along the interlobular vascular channels (Figs. 35-7 and 35-8).

There are also rare examples of extraskeletal chondromas in which the presence of plump immature-appearing cells within a myxoid background simulates a chondrosarcoma (Fig. 35-9). In general, however, these tumors can

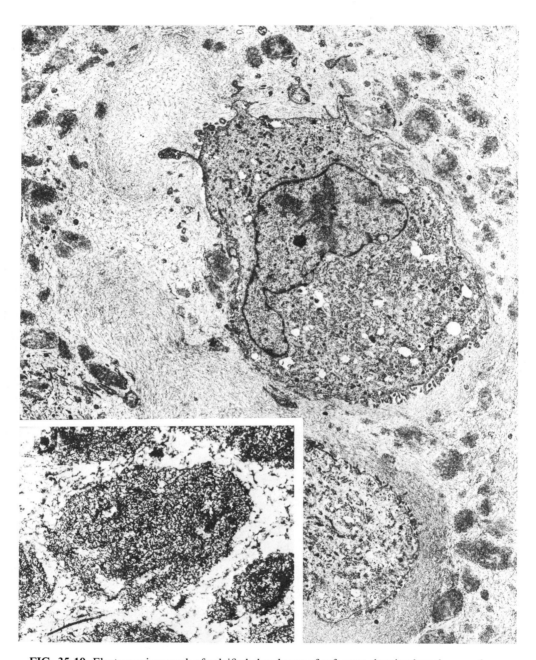

FIG. 35-10. Electron micrograph of calcified chondroma of soft parts showing loosely spaced cartilage cells having abundant rough endoplasmic reticulum, free ribosomes, and short irregular microvillous processes surrounded by aggregates of calcium crystals. (×2650.) Inset shows aggregates of hydroxyapatite crystals under higher magnification. (×10,800). (From Chung EB, Enzinger FM: *Cancer* 41:1414, 1978.)

be recognized as chondromas by the presence of more mature and less cellular cartilaginous areas at the periphery. There is also one report of an extraskeletal chondroma displaying chondroblastic features and multinucleated giant cells.[13]

Like normal chondrocytes, the cells of extraskeletal chondroma are positive for vimentin and S-100 protein. The electron microscopic picture reveals chondrocytes that have large indented nuclei, abundant rough endoplasmic reticulum, and occasional membrane-bound vacuoles. Short microvillous processes or filopodia extend from the cytoplasmic surfaces into the surrounding intercellular matrix. In the calcified cases the latter contains variously sized aggregates of hydroxyapatite crystals (Fig. 35-10).

Differential diagnosis

Distinction from other benign lesions should not be too difficult; calcifying aponeurotic fibroma is characterized by short barlike foci of cartilaginous metaplasia within a dense, poorly circumscribed fibromatous background. It occurs in the hand rather than in the distal portion of the digits and in patients younger than 25 years. Tumoral calcinosis may mimic a heavily calcified chondroma, but it lacks cartilage and usually shows a distinct histiocytic response to the calcified material. Giant cell tumors have more uniform cellular patterns and contain very rarely metaplastic cartilage or bone. Radiographs usually allow distinction from periosteal or juxtacortical chondroma, a small well-circumscribed tumor that is located beneath the periosteum and causes erosion of the underlying cortex with "ledges" or "buttresses" at the margin of the tumor,[3,12,14,17,23] and from subungual osteochondroma,[1,2] a lesion that shows cartilage overlying well-developed bone. A related calluslike lesion of the cortical surfaces of the hands and feet marked by a proliferation of bizarre chondrocytes was reported by Nora et al.[24] as "bizarre, parosteal osteochondromatous proliferation." "chondroid lipoma,"[19] and "extraskeletal chondroma with lipoblast-like cells"[4] refer to a peculiar extraskeletal chondroid lesion that consists of multivacuolated lipoblast-like cells and chondroid matrix (see Chapter 16). The "subcutaneous or skeletal chordomoid nodules in an infant" described by Tang et al.[28] may be another variant of this process.

Synovial chondromatosis[8,22] differs from extraskeletal chondroma by its occurrence in large joints, such as the knee, hip, elbow, or shoulder joint, and the formation of numerous, small, metaplastic cartilaginous or osteocartilaginous nodules of varying size attached to the synovial membrane of the joint, tendon sheath, or lining of the adjacent extraarticular bursa or popliteal cyst. Rarely it occurs in the surrounding soft tissues (extraarticular synovial chondromatosis) (Fig. 35-11). These synovial nodules often become detached and are found as loose bodies in the joint space. Some of them are hypercellular with clustering of tumor cells and increased mitotic activity. Most become calcified or ossified, and can be readily demonstrated by routine radiographs as multiple, discrete radiopaque bodies of small size (loose bodies or joint mice). Nonmineralized "loose bodies" are demonstrable on arthrograms or CT scans as multiple filling defects outlined by contrast material. Bone scintigraphy also shows intense radionuclide uptake within the nodules.[15,58] As in soft part chondroma, hypercellularity, binucleate cells, and nuclear atypia are compatible with a benign clinical course. Rare instances of chondrosarcoma arising in synovial chondromatosis have been reported.[25,34] Periosteal chondrosarcoma must also be included in the differential diagnosis.[23]

Drawing a sharp line between myxoid chondrosarcoma and the myxoid variant of chondroma may be difficult, especially in those rare examples that exhibit a moderate degree of cellular pleomorphism. Usually, however, the cartilage cells of these tumors are better differentiated, especially in the peripheral portion of the tumor. Moreover, myxoid chondromas tend to be less cellular, are smaller, and, as a rule, occur in the soft tissues of the hands and

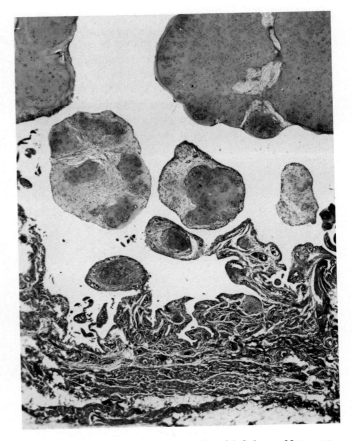

FIG. 35-11. Synovial chondromatosis of left knee. Note metaplastic cartilaginous nodules within synovial villi. (×25.)

feet, unusual locations for myxoid chondrosarcoma. A case of extraskeletal chondroblastoma has also been described.[57]

Discussion

Although some of the chondroblastic or myxoid forms of extraskeletal chondroma may cause concern because of their atypical cellular features, there is no evidence that these tumors behave differently from the well-differentiated forms composed of adult-type hyaline cartilage. We have observed a few tumors that recurred locally, but all of these were effectively treated by reexcision of the tumor. It is noteworthy that we have never encountered transformation of extraskeletal chondroma to chondrosarcoma, although this is by no means rare in chondroid lesions of bone. Local excision is the preferred mode of therapy.

EXTRASKELETAL MYXOID CHONDROSARCOMA (CHORDOID SARCOMA)

This tumor bears a superficial resemblance to myxoid liposarcoma, but its distinctive structure and staining characteristics identify it as a separate entity and establish its chondroblastic origin. Although a good number of these neoplasms have been recorded in the literature, including a series of 34 cases from the AFIP files,[44] the tumor is rare. Tsuneyoshi et al.[87] noted an incidence of 2.3% among 603 soft tissue sarcomas.

Examples of myxoid chondrosarcoma have also been described by Martin et al.[62] as chordoid sarcoma and by Hajdu et al.,[51] who coined the term *tendosynovial sarcoma* for a group of neoplasms composed of synovial sarcoma, epithelioid sarcoma, clear cell sarcoma, and myxoid chondrosarcoma. Parachordoma, a neoplasm reported by Dabska,[37] seems to be different from myxoid chondrosarcoma (see Chapter 37).

Myxoid chondrosarcoma occurs primarily in the deep tissues of the extremities, especially the musculature. Since a morphologically identical tumor also occurs in bone, x-ray examination, CT scan, or magnetic resonance imaging may be necessary to clearly establish its soft tissue origin. Usually, myxoid chondrosarcoma is a relatively slow-growing tumor, which, nonetheless, is capable of recurrence and metastasis, sometimes years after the initial diagnosis.

Clinical findings

The tumor most commonly afflicts patients older than 35 years, and only a few cases have been encountered in children and adolescents.[50] In our series[44] the median age was 48 years; others reported a mean age of 46 years,[40] 51 years,[67] and 57 years.[77] Males are affected about twice as often as females. The clinical signs and symptoms are nonspecific: The patient complains of a slowly growing, deep-seated mass that causes pain and tenderness in approximately one third of cases. Complications such as ulceration and hemorrhage may be encountered with large tumors. The duration of symptoms varies considerably and ranges from a few weeks to several years. In our series prior injury to the site of the tumor was reported in 8 of the 34 cases, but as with other sarcomas, the significance of this finding remains uncertain.

More than two thirds of the tumors occur in the extremities, especially the thigh and popliteal fossa, similar to myxoid liposarcoma.[40,44,67,77] Most are deep seated, but occasional tumors are confined to the subcutis. These tumors may cause difficulties in differential diagnosis from myxoid forms of benign chondroma. There are also accounts of synovial and pleural myxoid chondrosarcomas.[47,55]

Roentgenographs and CT scans show a soft tissue mass without any distinctive radiological features that would set the tumor apart from other types of soft tissue sarcoma.

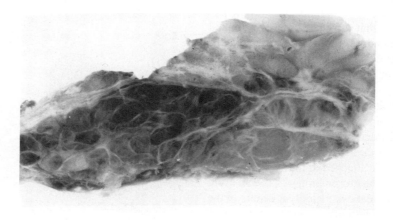

FIG. 35-12. Gross picture of myxoid chondrosarcoma displaying characteristic gelatinous appearance and multinodular growth pattern of this tumor. The dark appearance of some of the nodules is the result of hemorrhage. (From Enzinger FM, Siraki M: *Hum Pathol* 3:421, 1972.)

Pathological findings

Macroscopically, the neoplasm occurs as a soft to firm, ovoid, lobulated to nodular mass that is generally well circumscribed, often with a distinct fibrous capsule. On section it has a gelatinous, gray to tan-brown surface; its color largely depending on the amount of hemorrhage, a frequent feature of the tumor (Fig. 35-12). Occasionally hemorrhage may be so severe that the tumor is mistaken for a hematoma. Despite the distinct multinodular pattern, there is no evidence of multicentric origin.

The size of the tumor varies from a few centimeters to 15 cm or more; most, however, measure 4 to 7 cm in greatest diameter at the time of excision. Meis and Martz[67] reported a range from 1.1 to 24 cm and a median tumor size of 7 cm.

Under the microscope the characteristic multinodular pattern is clearly evident. The individual tumor nodules consist of rounded or slightly elongated cells of uniform shape and size separated by variable amounts of mucoid material (Fig. 35-13). The individual cells possess small hyperchromatic nuclei and a narrow rim of deeply eosinophilic cytoplasm, features characteristic of chondroblasts (Fig. 35-14, A and B). Occasional cells are vacuolated. Unlike chondrosarcoma of bone, differentiated cartilage cells with distinct lacunae are rare but on careful and prolonged search of multiple sections can be detected in about one third of the cases (Fig. 35-14, C). Mitotic figures are rare in typical cases but may be numerous in less well-differentiated and more cellular forms of the tumor.

Characteristically, the individual cells are arranged in short anastomosing cords and strands, often creating a lacelike appearance (Figs. 35-14, A and B, and 35-15). Less frequently the cellular elements are disposed in small loosely textured whorls or aggregates, reminiscent of an epithelial neoplasm (Fig. 35-16). There are also less well differentiated, hypercellular tumors that display no particular pattern and are largely devoid of a myxoid matrix. Indeed, if these features prevail throughout the tumor, a positive diagnosis of chondrosarcoma may be impossible. In the more typical tumors, however, the extracellular mucinous material is abundant and consists largely of chondroitin 4-sulfate, chondroitin 6-sulfate, and keratan sulfate.[45] It stains deeply with the colloidal iron stain, the alcian blue preparation, and, unlike other richly mucinous soft tissue tumors—with the exception of myxochondroma and chordoma—the staining reaction is not inhibited by prior treatment of the sections with hyaluronidase (Fig. 35-17). The mucinous matrix also stains with the mucicarmine stain, metachromatically with toluidine blue, and a deep purple with the aldehyde-fuchsin preparations at pH 1.7. The intensity of mucin staining depends on the pH level of the staining solution.[32,44,54] Kindblom and Angervall,[55] using the critical electrolyte method designed by Scott and Dorling,[80] demonstrated that alcian blue stained the matrix with

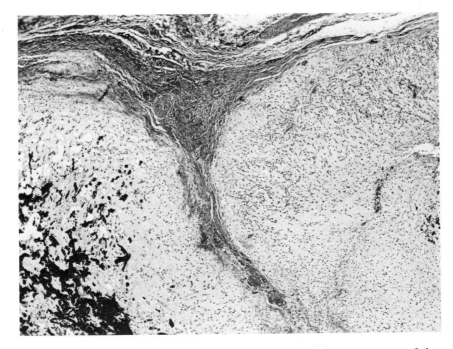

FIG. 35-13. Myxoid chondrosarcoma showing the distinctly nodular arrangement of the small chondroblasts and the associated myxoid matrix. Hemorrhage is present in one of the nodules. (×30.)

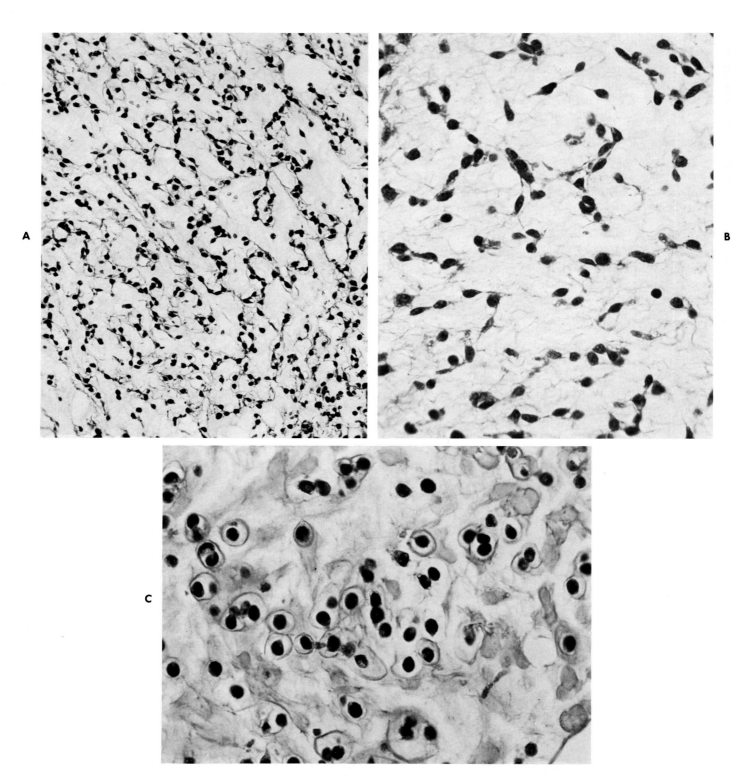

FIG. 35-14. Myxoid chondrosarcoma. **A,** Characteristic alignment of the tumor cells in strands and cords separated by large amounts of mucoid material. (×195.) **B,** Higher magnification showing typical chondroblasts with oval nuclei and a narrow rim of eosinophilic cytoplasm. (×440.) **C,** Focal cartilaginous differentiation. (×395.)

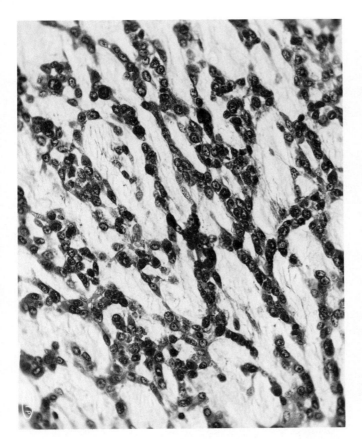

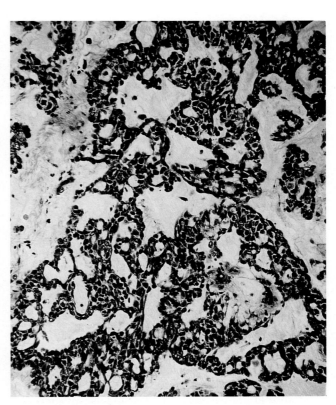

FIG. 35-15. Extraskeletal myxoid chondrosarcoma of the popliteal fossa in a 60-year-old man. The cells are large and poorly differentiated but also exhibit the characteristic lacelike growth pattern. (×300.) (From Enzinger FM, Shiraki M: *Hum Pathol* 3:421, 1972.)

FIG. 35-16. Extraskeletal myxoid chondrosarcoma displaying grouping and pseudopapillary arrangement of poorly differentiated, hyperchromatic tumor cells. (×160.)

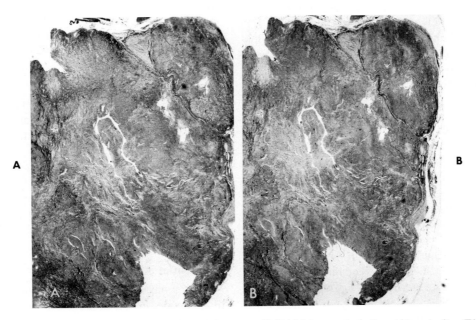

FIG. 35-17. Extraskeletal myxoid chondrosarcoma. Colloidal iron stain before (A) and after (B) treatment with testicular hyaluronidase revealing no change in staining characteristics, a feature typical of chondroid and chordoid tumors. (×7.) (From Enzinger FM, Shiraki M: *Hum Pathol* 3:421, 1972.)

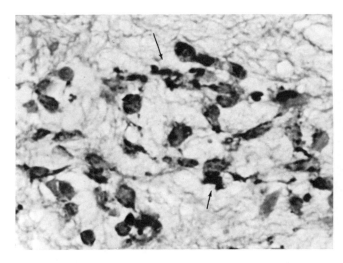

FIG. 35-18. Glycogen *(arrows)* within the chondroblasts of myxoid chondrosarcoma demonstrated with the periodic acid–Schiff preparation (PAS). (×300.)

a magnesium chloride concentration of up to 0.55 M compared with a magnesium chloride concentration of only 0.1 M for myxoid liposarcoma and intramuscular myxoma. As in normal cartilage cells, intracellular PAS-positive and diastase-sensitive material (glycogen) is another typical feature of the tumor (Fig. 35-18). Secondary changes such as fibrosis and hemorrhage are common, but calcification or bone formation is rare.

The cells of myxoid chondrosarcoma stain strongly for vimentin and less intensely for S-100 protein and Leu-7; they also display tubulin immunoreactivity.* Although most reviewers reported that immunostaining for cytokeratin and epithelial membrane antigen was negative, Meis and Martz[67] reported positive staining with these antibodies in several tumors.

Ultrastructural findings

The tumor is composed of fusiform spindle-shaped or ovoid cells with rounded nuclei, distinct nucleoli, and abundant cytoplasm with a well-developed Golgi complex, glycogen granules, microfilaments, and a prominent rough endoplasmic reticulum containing granular amorphous material.[40,63,72] Densely packed bundles or parallel arrays of microtubules may also be present, a feature that has also been observed in myxoid chondrosarcomas of bone and other neoplasms[41,61,85,92] (Fig. 35-19). The cellular surfaces are slightly scalloped and there are fingerlike cytoplasmic projections, but these features are less well pronounced than in normal developing chondroblasts.[90] There are also intracytoplasmic inclusions of matrix material and macular or

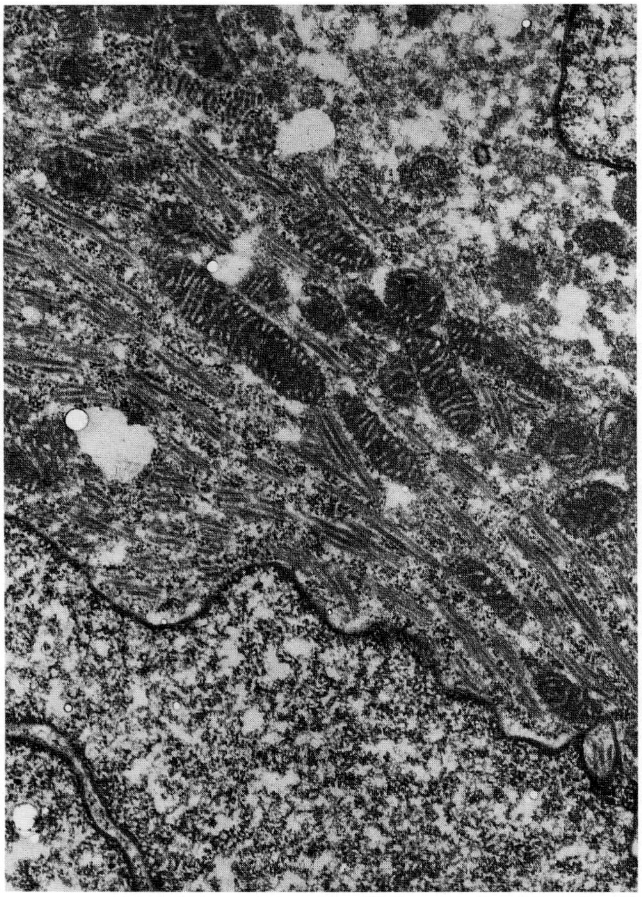

FIG. 35-19. Electon micrograph of extraskeletal myxoid chondrosarcoma showing multiple mitochondria and arrays of microtubules, a frequent finding in this tumor. (×34,500.) (Courtesy Dr. Kent Bottles, Department of Pathology, University of Iowa.)

desmosomal intercellular attachments without tonofilaments. The extracellular spaces contain copious amounts of an amorphous, granular or finely fibrillary matrix and a varying number of collagen fibers.[65,71,72,91]

Molecular analysis of myxoid chondrosarcoma may be helpful in diagnosis. There are only a few cytogenetic studies of this tumor but so far all of them show a characteristic pattern marked by a nonrandom reciprocal translocation between chromosomes 9 and 22, t(9;22)(q22-31;q11-12).[70,81,88]

Differential diagnosis

Among the various types of chondroid tumors, the "cartilage tumors in soft tissue" described by Lichtenstein and Goldman[16] bear some resemblance to myxoid chondrosarcoma. They differ, however, by their exclusive occurrence in the hand, their comparatively small size, and their benign behavior. They show a close similarity to the myxoid

*References 31, 50, 68, 70, 85, 93.

variant of soft part chondroma. *Chondromyxoid fibroma* very rarely occurs as a periosteal tumor or in soft tissue as secondary tissue implantations.[59,73] It can be recognized by its greater degree of cellular pleomorphism and condensation of the tumor cells beneath a narrow, richly vascularized fibrous band that borders the individual tumor nodules. In addition, there may be multinucleated giant cells and foci of calcification or ossification, features that are rarely seen in myxoid chondrosarcoma.

Juxtacortical (parosteal) chondrosarcomas lack the myxoid component and show a broad attachment to the perichondrium or periosteum of the involved bone, sometimes with invasion of the underlying cortex and cortical irregularities on roentgenographs.[78] *Chordoma,* especially its myxoid form, enters into the differential diagnosis, but this diagnosis is unlikely if the tumor occurs outside its usual location in the sacrococcygeal region, the base of the skull, or the cervical spine; shows no radiographic evidence of bone involvement; and lacks multivacuolated, physaliphorous tumor cells. Ultrastructurally, chordoma cells show peculiar multilayered structures composed of rough endoplasmic reticulum and mitochondria in close juxtaposition. More importantly, chordoma cells are positive with markers for cytokeratin and epithelial membrane antigen.[31,66,68]

Myxoma and *myxoid liposarcoma* must also be considered in differential diagnosis: *Myxoma* displays a similar paucity of vascular structures, but it is less cellular, and its cellular elements are less well defined than those of myxoid chondrosarcoma. *Myxoid liposarcoma,* on the other hand, almost always displays a striking plexiform vascular pattern and contains typical lipoblasts, especially at the margin of the tumor lobules. Both myxoma and liposarcoma can be clearly distinguished from myxoid chondrosarcoma by the absence of stainable mucin after treatment of the sections with hyaluronidase (Table 35-1). This is also true of *parachordoma*[37] (see Chapter 37).

Still another problem is the distinction of extraskeletal myxoid chondrosarcoma from benign and malignant *mixed tumor of salivary gland origin (pleomorphic adenoma)* and *sweat gland origin (chondroid syringoma)*. Obviously most of these tumors are more superficially located than chondrosarcoma, but they may show myxoid areas that are difficult to separate in the absence of epithelial structures. In fact, some of the deep-seated mixed tumors described in the literature may be myxoid chondrosarcomas[43] or perhaps parachordomas.[37] Immunohistochemical and electron microscopic studies will help in differential diagnosis. Most mixed tumors show, in addition to cells indistinguishable from chondrocytes, transitional forms between chondrocytes and myoepithelial or epithelial cells, with positive staining for vimentin, cytokeratin, and epithelial membrane antigen; ultrastructurally, there are also occasional actin microfilaments, desmosomes, and perinuclear tonofilaments.[69,74] *Myxopapillary ependymoma* can be distin-

guished by its perivascular growth, positivity for glial fibrillary acidic protein, and the presence of glial-type microfilaments[83] (see Table 37-1).

Discussion

Although the clinical behavior of myxoid chondrosarcoma varies considerably from case to case, it is in general a relatively slow-growing tumor that recurs and eventually metastasizes in the majority of cases. The rate of recurrence and metastasis is closely related to the degree of cellularity and the relative amounts of myxoid material. Therefore, the least cellular and most myxoid tumors carry the best prognoses. Of the 31 patients in our series,[44] 20 were alive at last follow up, but during the follow-up period, six of these patients developed recurrence and 2 developed metastasis. Four died of metastatic disease and seven of some unrelated cause. Meis and Martz[67] also report a protracted clinical course, with 73% of patients being alive at 10 years, including 53% with local recurrence and 44% with metastasis. Late recurrence and metastasis are common: One of our cases recurred 18 years after the initial excision; in another case pulmonary metastasis became evident 10 years after surgical removal of the tumor and 4 years after removal of a regional lymph node metastasis. Tanaka and Asao[86] observed recurrence 30 years after the clinical onset of the tumor. In the series of Saleh et al.[77] 3 of the 10 patients with metastasis were alive at 13, 14, and 16 years after the initial therapy. The most frequent metastatic sites are the lung, soft tissues, and lymph nodes. Radical local excision with or without adjunctive radiotherapy seems to be the treatment of choice. Good results with high-dose irradiation (6000 cGy) have been reported.[53] DNA analysis, reported in only a few cases, showed that the tumors were uniformly diploid.[70]

There seems to be little doubt as to the chondroblastic origin of myxoid chondrosarcoma; the close histological resemblance of the tumor cells to chondroblasts, the typical staining characteristics, and the presence of occasional foci of more mature and readily identifiable cartilage cells clearly support this concept. As mentioned, alterations of chromosomes 9 and 22 are a characteristic feature of myxoid chondrosarcoma.[52,81,88]

Table 35-1. Critical electrolyte concentration (CEC)* of myxoid soft tissue tumors†

Intramuscular myxoma	0.1
Myxoid liposarcoma	0.1
Myxoid malignant fibrous histiocytoma	0.2
Botryoid rhabdomyosarcoma	0.2
Myxoid chondrosarcoma	0.5

*Extinction of alcian blue stain at pH 5.6 with increasing mortality of magnesium chloride.
†From Kindblom LG, Angervall L: *Cancer* 36:985, 1975.

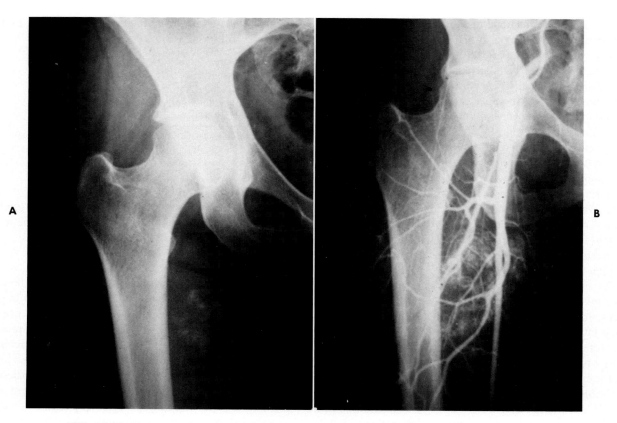

FIG. 35-20. Extraskeletal mesenchymal chondrosarcoma of right thigh. **A,** Roentgenogram illustrating soft tissue mass with focal calcification. **B,** Angiogram demonstrating the rich vascularity of the tumor.

EXTRASKELETAL MESENCHYMAL CHONDROSARCOMA

This neoplasm, first described as a distinct entity by Lichtenstein and Bernstein[60] in 1959, is a cartilaginous tumor of characteristic bimorphic appearance composed of sheets of primitive mesenchymal or precartilage cells and interspersed islands of well-differentiated cartilaginous tissue.[99,100,106,110] Because of its prominent vascular pattern, several cases reported in the earlier literature were initially interpreted as hemangiopericytoma with cartilaginous differentiation.[75,97] Mesenchymal chondrosarcoma is a rare tumor. It is two to three times as common in bone as in soft tissue.[100,107,110] Unlike myxoid chondrosarcoma it is a rapidly growing tumor with a high incidence of metastasis.

Clinical findings

This neoplasm differs from other forms of chondrosarcoma by its preponderance in young adults between 15 and 35 years of age and its slightly more frequent occurrence in females than in males. The tumor may also occur in young children.[99,114] Louvet et al.[105] pointed out a relationship between the age of the patient and the location of the tumor: patients with neural and muscular forms of the disease are considerably younger (mean age 23.5 years) than those with mesenchymal chondrosarcomas arising from the musculature (mean age 43.9 years). The principal anatomical sites of mesenchymal chondrosarcoma are the region of the head and neck, particularly the orbit, the cranial and spinal dura mater, and the occipital portion of the neck, followed by the lower extremities, especially the thigh.[103] In comparison, mesenchymal chondrosarcomas of bone arise chiefly in the jaws and ribs.[97,100,110]

Orbital lesions tend to produce exophthalmos, orbital pain, blurring of vision, and headaches;[98,113] intracranial and intraspinal tumors are accompanied by vomiting, headaches, and various motor and sensory defects.[109,111] Tumors in the extremities usually manifest as painless, slowly enlarging masses situated in the musculature. There are also cases in our files in which a metastasis from a primary mesenchymal chondrosarcoma of bone mimicked a soft tissue tumor. Therefore a bone survey is essential, particularly when the tumor occurs in an unusual location. In most cases roentgenograms reveal a well-defined soft tissue mass, often with irregular radiopaque stipplings, arcs, flecks, or

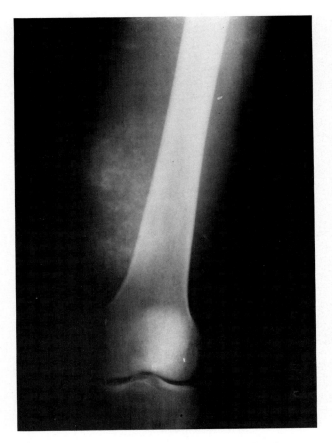

FIG. 35-21. Roentgenograph of mesenchymal chondrosarcoma showing soft tissue mass with calcification.

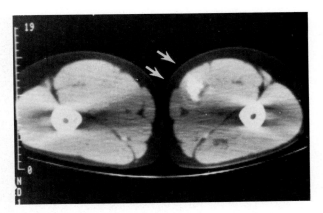

FIG. 35-22. CT scan of extraskeletal mesenchymal chondrosarcoma of the left thigh.

streaks as the result of focal calcification or bone formation within the cartilaginous areas (Figs. 35-20 and 35-21).[107,114] CT scans, magnetic resonance images, and angiograms are also helpful in outlining the tumor prior to surgical therapy (Fig. 35-22).

Pathological findings

Grossly, mesenchymal chondrosarcoma presents as a multilobulated circumscribed mass that shows considerable variations in size. In our series[103] the smallest tumor measured 2.5 cm in greatest diameter and the largest 37 cm. Cut sections show a mixture of fleshy soft gray-white tissue and scattered foci of irregularly sized cartilage and bone. At times there are also small areas of hemorrhage and necrosis, but hemorrhage is much less prominent than in myxoid chondrosarcoma.

Microscopically, the mesenchymal chondrosarcoma exhibits a characteristic bimorphic pattern composed of sheaths of undifferentiated round, oval, or spindle-shaped cells and small, usually well-defined islets or nodules of well-differentiated, benign-appearing cartilaginous tissue, frequently with central calcification and ossification (Fig.

35-23). The undifferentiated cells possess ovoid or elongated hyperchromatic nuclei and scanty, poorly outlined cytoplasm; they are arranged in small aggregates or in a hemangiopericytoma-like pattern about sinusoidal vascular channels lined by a single layer of endothelium (Fig. 35-24). PAS staining fails to demonstrate significant amounts of intracellular glycogen. Solid cellular and richly vascular patterns may be present in different portions of the same neoplasm. The cartilaginous foci are usually well defined (Figs. 35-23 and 35-25), but there are also poorly circumscribed cartilaginous areas that blend with the undifferentiated tumor cells (Fig. 35-26). Spindle cell areas, with or without collagen formation, are present in some cases but are rarely a prominent feature of the tumor (Fig. 35-27). The staining characteristics of the cartilaginous areas are indistinguishable from those of other forms of chondrosarcoma. Immunohistochemical preparations reveal S-100 protein positivity in the cartilaginous portion of the tumor and in isolated cells within the undifferentiated areas. Moreover, as in other round cell tumors, the undifferentiated cells may stain for neuron-specific enolase and Leu-7. None of the cells expresses desmin, actin, cytokeratin, or epithelial membrane antigen.[115,116]

Ultrastructural findings

The cells within the well-differentiated cartilaginous areas have irregular round to stellate or scalloped configurations with short cytoplasmic processes, large ovoid nuclei, abundant rough endoplasmic reticulum with focal saclike dilatations, a well-developed Golgi apparatus, and variable amounts of glycogen. The extracellular spaces contain filamentous, finely granular material. In contrast, the undifferentiated, round, ovoid, or polygonal cells possess prominent nuclei and nucleoli and inconspicuous cytoplasm with few organelles. The cells bear some resemblance to the cells of Ewing's sarcoma, but there is little intracytoplasmic gly-

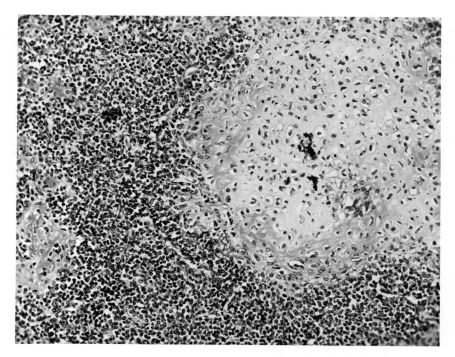

FIG. 35-23. Mesenchymal chondrosarcoma illustrating the characteristic bimorphic picture: islands of well-differentiated cartilage surrounded by sheets of small, undifferentiated tumor cells. (×145.)

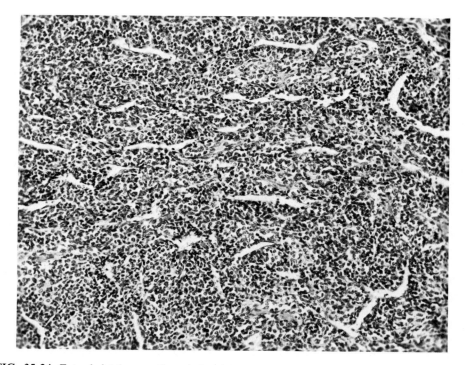

FIG. 35-24. Extraskeletal mesenchymal chondrosarcoma. Same neoplasm as in Fig. 35-23 illustrating the frequent hemangiopericytoma-like pattern of this tumor. (×145.)

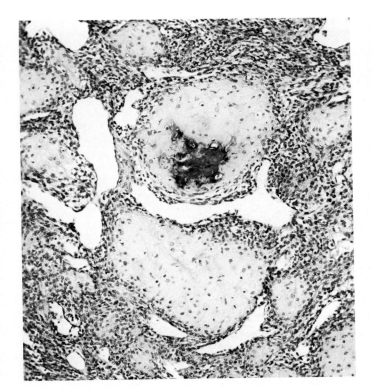

FIG. 35-25. Extraskeletal mesenchymal chondrosarcomoa showing calcification within the islands of cartilaginous tissue and dilatation of vascular spaces. (×115.) (From Guccion JG, Font RL, Enzinger FM, et al: *Arch Pathol* 95:336, 1973. Copyright 1973, American Medical Association.)

cogen. The cellular elements are closely packed with cohesive cell membranes and desmosomes but without cytoplasmic projections. Fibroblast-like cells with increased rough endoplasmic reticulum and occasional desmosome-like junctions may also be present in the tumor. Basal laminae are confined to the interspersed endothelial cell and pericytes.[63,72,101,109]

Differential diagnosis

Although typical examples of mesenchymal chondrosarcomas pose no particular problem in diagnosis, diagnosis may be extremely difficult, with small biopsies or needle biopsies showing only one of the two tissue elements. In particular, cases without the cartilaginous element may be mistaken for a malignant hemangiopericytoma[75,97] or a poorly differentiated synovial sarcoma with a prominent hemangiopericytoma-like pattern. Although we have observed well-differentiated cartilage in one case of benign hemangiopericytoma, this is an extremely rare finding, and as a rule, the presence of cartilage excludes a diagnosis of hemangiopericytoma. Metaplastic cartilage may also occur in poorly differentiated synovial sarcoma, but it is much less common in this tumor than foci of calcification or bone. Careful search for a biphasic pattern or epithelial differentiation with antibodies against cytokeratin or epithelial membrane antigen is indicated in doubtful cases. The presence of cartilaginous differentiation and negative staining for HBA71 antigen will assist in ruling out Ewing's sarcoma.

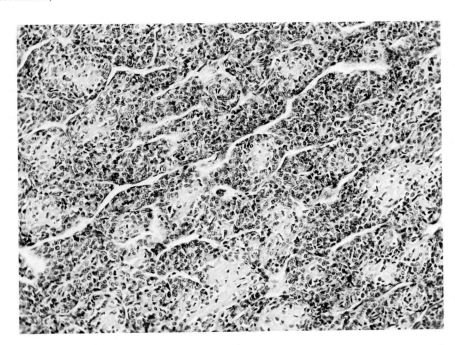

FIG. 35-26. Extraskeletal mesenchymal chondrosarcoma with prominent vascular pattern and early cartilaginous differentiation. (×165.) (From Guccion JG, Font RL, Enzinger FM, et al: *Arch Pathol* 95:336, 1973. Copyright 1973, American Medical Association.)

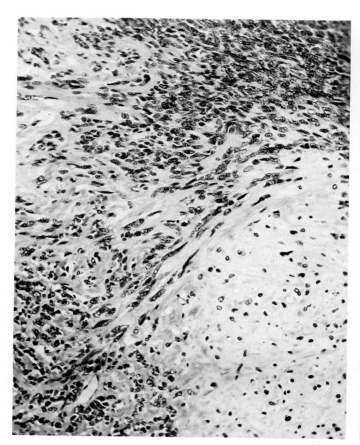

FIG. 35-27. Cartilaginous and spindle cell proliferation in mesenchymal chondrosarcoma. (×165.)

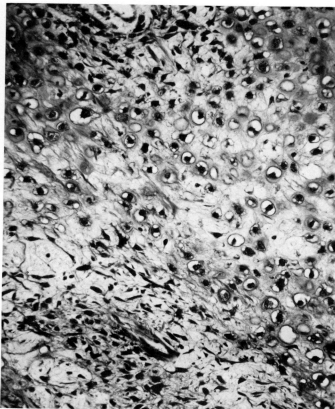

FIG. 35-28. Extraskeletal chondrosarcoma with focal well-differentiated and myxoid areas. (×250.)

Distinction from differentiated forms of extraskeletal chondrosarcoma may also cause some difficulties in diagnosis. These very rare tumors, however, always display a more uniform pattern and lack the contrasting differentiated and undifferentiated areas[89] (Fig. 35-28).

Discussion

Mesenchymal chondrosarcoma is a fully malignant tumor that pursues a rapid clinical course and metastasizes in a high percentage of cases.[103] Nakashima et al.[107] reported that in a group of 23 patients the 5-year survival rate was 54.6% and the 10-year survival rate was 27.3%. The principal metastatic site is the lung. Lymph node metastasis is less common than in myxoid chondrosarcoma. Several of our patients had a protracted clinical course and late metastases, but there seems to be no reliable prognostic relationship to the patient's age or degree of cellular differentiation. Combined radical surgery and chemotherapy or radiotherapy appears to be the treatment of choice.

The tumor is probably derived from primitive, precartilaginous mesenchymal cells with focal, nodular cartilaginous differentiation. There is no convincing evidence that trauma plays a significant etiological role, but an instance of this tumor has been observed in the lumbar spine 12 years after radiotherapy for Wilms' tumor.[112]

REFERENCES
Extraskeletal chondroma

1. Apfelberg DB, Druker D, Maser MR, et al: Subungual osteochondroma: differential diagnosis and treatment. *Arch Dermatol (Chicago)* 115:472, 1979.
2. Ayala F, Lembo G, Montesano M: A rare tumor: subungual chondroma: report of a case. *Dermatologica* 167:339, 1983.
3. Bauer TW, Dorfman HD, Latham JT: Periosteal chondroma. *Am J Surg Pathol* 6:631, 1982.
4. Chan JK, Lee KC, Saw D: Extraskeletal chondroma with lipoblast-like cells. *Hum Pathol* 17:1285, 1986.
5. Chung EB, Enzinger FM: Benign chondromas of soft parts. *Cancer* 41:1414, 1978.
6. Cocchia D, Lauriola L, Stolfi VM, et al: S-100 antigen labels neoplastic cells in liposarcoma and cartilaginous tumours. *Virchows Arch (Pathol Anat)* 402:139, 1983.
7. Dahlin C, Salvador H: Cartilaginous tumors of the soft tissues of the hands and feet. *Mayo Clin Proc* 49:721, 1974.

8. DeBenedetti MJ, Schwinn CP: Tenosynovial chondromatosis in the hand. *J Bone Joint Surg* 61A:898, 1979.

9. Dellon A, Weiss SW, Mitch WE: Bilateral extraosseous chondromas of the hand in a patient with chronic renal failure. *Am Soc Surg Hand* 3:139, 1978.

10. DelSignore JL, Torre BA, Miller RJ: Extraskeletal chondroma of the hand: case report and review of the literature. *Clin Orthop* 254:147, 1990.

11. Dunn EJ, McGavran M, Nelson P, et al: Synovial chondrosarcoma: report of a case. *J Bone Joint Surg* 56A:811, 1974.

12. Fornasier VL: Periosteal chondroma. *Clin Orthop* 124:233, 1977.

13. Isayama T, Iwasaki H, Kikuchi M: Chondroblastoma-like extraskeletal chondroma. *Clin Orthop* 268:214, 1991.

14. Jaffe HL: Juxtacortical chondroma. *Bull Hosp Joint Dis* 17:20, 1956.

15. Karlin CA, De Smet AA, Neff J, et al: The variable manifestations of extraarticular synovial chondromatosis. *Am J Roentgenol* 137:731, 1981.

16. Lichtenstein L, Goldman RL: Cartilage tumors in soft tissues, particularly in the hand and foot. *Cancer* 17:1203, 1964.

17. Lichtenstein L, Hall JE: Periosteal chondroma: a distinctive benign cartilage tumor. *J Bone Joint Surg* 34A:691, 1952.

18. Matthews WB: Congenital cartilaginous rests in the neck. *Arch Surg* 28:59, 1934.

19. Meis JM, Enzinger FM: Chondroid lipoma: a unique tumor simulating liposarcoma and myxoid chondrosarcoma. *Am J Surg Pathol* 17:1103, 1993.

20. Mullins F, Berard C, Eisenberg SH: Chondrosarcoma following synovial chondromatosis: a case study. *Cancer* 18:1180, 1965.

21. Murphy AF, Wilson JN: Tenosynovial osteochondroma in the hand. *J Bone Joint Surg* 40A:1236, 1958.

22. Murphy FP, Dahlin DC, Sullivan CR: Articular synovial chondromatosis. *J Bone Joint Surg* 44A:77, 1962.

23. Nojima T, Unni KK, McLeod RA, et al: Periosteal chondroma and periosteal chondrosarcoma. *Am J Surg Pathol* 9:661, 1985.

24. Nora FE, Dahlin DC, Beabout JW: Bizarre parosteal osteochondromatous proliferations of the hands and feet. *Am J Surg Pathol* 7:245, 1983.

25. Perry BE, McQueen Da, Lin JJ: Synovial chondromatosis with malignant degeneration to chondrosarcoma. *J Bone Joint Surg* 70A:1259, 1987.

26. Someren A, Merritt WH: Tenosynovial chondroma of the hand: a case report with a brief review of the literature. *Hum Pathol* 9:476, 1978.

27. Stockley I, Norris SH: Trigger finger secondary to soft tissue chondroma. *J Hand Surg* 15:468, 1990.

28. Tang TT, Dunn DK, Hodach AE, et al: Subcutaneous and skeletal chordomoid nodules in an infant. *Am J Dermatopathol* 3:303, 1981.

29. Wong L, Dellon AL: Soft tissue chondroma presenting as a painful finger: diagnosis by magnetic resonance imaging. *Ann Plast Surg* 28:304, 1992.

30. Zlatkin MB, Lander PH, Begin LR, et al: Soft tissue chondromas. *Am J Roentgenol* 144:1263, 1985.

Extraskeletal myxoid chondrosarcoma

31. Abenoza P, Sibley RK: Chordoma: an immunohistochemical study. *Hum Pathol* 17:744, 1986.

32. Angervall L, Enerbäck L, Knutson H: Chondrosarcoma of soft tissue origin. *Cancer* 32:507, 1973.

33. Ariel JM, Jakobs PA: Extraosseous chondrosarcoma arising from the tendon Achilles. *Bull Hosp Joint Dis* 22:129, 1961.

34. Bertoni F, Unni KK, Beabout JW, et al: Chondrosarcomas of the synovium. *Cancer* 67:155, 1991.

35. Brandenburg JH, Harris DD, Bennett M: Chondrosarcoma of the larynx. *Laryngoscope* 77:752, 1967.

36. Brenner RW, Garret R: Soft tissue chondrosarcoma-like tumor. *Arch Surg* 86:471, 1963.

37. Dabska M: Parachordoma: a new clinicopathologic entity. *Cancer* 40:1586, 1977.

38. D'Ambrosio FG, Shiu MH, Brennan MF: Intrapulmonary presentation of extraskeletal myxoid chondrosarcoma of the extremity: report of two cases. *Cancer* 58:1144, 1986.

39. Daniels AC, Conner GH, Straus FH: Primary chondrosarcoma of the tracheobronchial tree. *Arch Pathol* 84:615, 1967.

40. Dardick I, Lagacé R, Carlier MT, et al: Chordoid sarcoma (extraskeletal myxoid chondrosarcoma). A light and electron microscopic study. *Virchows Arch (Pathol Anat)* 399:61, 1983.

41. DeBlois G, Wang S, Kay S: Microtubular aggregates within rough endoplasmic reticulum: an unusual ultrastructural feature of extraskeletal myxoid chondrosarcoma. *Hum Pathol* 17:469, 1986.

42. Dunn EJ, McGavran MH, Nelson P, et al: Synovial chondrosarcoma: report of a case. *J Bone Joint Surg* 56A:811, 1974.

43. Dutra RR: Mixed tumor, salivary gland type, of deep fascial region of thigh. *Arch Pathol* 70:562, 1960.

44. Enzinger FM, Shiraki M: Extraskeletal myxoid chondrosarcoma: an analysis of 34 cases. *Hum Pathol* 3:421, 1972.

45. Fletcher CD, Powell G, McKee PH: Extraskeletal myxoid chondrosarcoma: a histochemical and immunohistochemical study. *Histopathology* 10:499, 1986.

46. Ghalib SH, Warner ED, DeGowin EL: Laryngeal chondrosarcoma after thyroid irradiation. *JAMA* 210:1762, 1969.

47. Goetz SP, Robinson RA, Landas SK: Extraskeletal myxoid chondrosarcoma of the pleura: report of a case clinically simulating mesothelioma. *Am J Clin Pathol* 97:498, 1992.

48. Goldenberg R, Cohen P, Steinlauf P: Chondrosarcoma of the extraskeletal soft tissues: a report of seven cases and review of the literature. *J Bone Joint Surg* 49A:1487, 1967.

49. Goldman RL, Lichtenstein L: Synovial chondrosarcoma. *Cancer* 17:1233, 1964.

50. Hachitanda Y, Tsuneyoshi M, Daimaru Y, et al: Extraskeletal myxoid chondrosarcoma in young children. *Cancer* 61:2521, 1988.

51. Hajdu SI, Shiu MH, Fortner JG: Tendosynovial sarcoma: a clinicopathologic study of 136 cases. *Cancer* 39:1201, 1977.

52. Hinrichs SH, Jaramillo MA, Gumerlock PH: Myxoid chondrosarcoma with a translocation involving chromosomes 9 and 22. *Cancer Genet Cytogenet* 14:219, 1985.

53. Hitchon H, Nobler MP, Wohl M, et al: The radiotherapeutic management of chordoid sarcoma. *Am J Clin Oncol* 13:208, 1990.

54. Kindblom LG, Angervall L: Histochemical characterization of mucosubstances in bone and soft tissue tumors. *Cancer* 36:985, 1975.

55. Kindblom LG, Angervall L: Myxoid chondrosarcoma of the synovial tissue. A clinicopathologic, histochemical, and ultrastructural analysis. *Cancer* 52:1886, 1983.

56. King JW, Spjut HJ, Fechner RE, et al: Synovial chondrosarcoma of the knee joint. *J Bone Joint Surg* 49A:1389, 1967.

57. Kingsley TC, Markel SF: Extraskeletal chondroblastoma: a report of the first recorded case. *Cancer* 27:203, 1971.

58. Kransdorf MJ, Meis JM: Extraskeletal osseous and cartilaginous tumors of the extremities. *RadioGraphics* 13:853, 1993.

59. Kyriakos M: Soft tissue implantation of chondromyxoid fibroma. *Am J Surg Pathol* 3:363, 1979.

60. Lichtenstein L, Bernstein D: Unusual benign and malignant chondroid tumors of bone: a survey of some mesenchymal cartilage tumors and malignant chondroblastic tumors including a few multicentric ones and chondromyxoid fibromas. *Cancer* 12:1142, 1959.

61. Mackay B, Ayala AG: Intracisternal tubules in human melanoma cells. *Ultrastruct Pathol* 1:1, 1980.

62. Martin RF, Melnick PJ, Warner NE, et al: Chordoid sarcoma. *Am J Clin Pathol* 59:623, 1973.

63. Martinez-Tello FJ, Navas-Palacios JJ: Ultrastructural study of conventional chondrosarcomas and myxoid and mesenchymal chondrosarcomas. *Virchows Arch (Pathol Anat)* 396:197, 1982.

64. McConnell TH: Bony and cartilaginous tumors of the heart and great vessels: report of an osteosarcoma of the pulmonary artery. *Cancer* 25:611, 1970.

65. Mehio AR, Ferenczy A: Extraskeletal myxoid chondrosarcoma with "chordoid" features (chordoid sarcoma). *Am J Clin Pathol* 70:700, 1978.

66. Meis JM, Giraldo AA: Chordoma: an immunohistochemical study of 20 cases. *Arch Pathol Lab Med* 112:553, 1988.

67. Meis JM, Martz KL: Extraskeletal myxoid chondrosarcoma: a clinicopathologic study of 120 cases. *Lab Invest* 66:9A, 1992.

68. Miettinen M, Lehto VP, Dahl D, et al: Differential diagnosis of chordoma, chondroid, and ependymal tumors as aided by antiintermediate filament antibodies. *Am J Pathol* 112:160, 1983.

69. Mills SE, Cooper PH: An ultrastructural study of cartilaginous zones and surrounding epithelium in mixed tumors of salivary glands and skin. *Lab Invest* 44:6, 1981.

70. Orndal C, Carlen B, Akerman M, et al: Chromosomal abnormality t(9;22)(q22;q12) in an extraskeletal myxoid chondrosarcoma characterized by fine needle aspiration cytology, electron microscopy, immunohistochemistry, and DNA flow cytometry. *Cytopathology* 2:261, 1991.

71. Pardo-Mindan FJ, Guillen FJ, Villas C, et al: A comparative ultrastructural study of chondrosarcoma, chordoid sarcoma, and chordoma. *Cancer* 47:2611, 1981.

72. Povysil C, Matejovsky Z: A comparative ultrastructural study of chondrosarcoma, chordoid sarcoma, chordoma, and chordoma periphericum. *Pathol Res Pract* 179:546, 1985.

73. Rahimi A, Beabout JW, Ivins JC, et al: Chondromyxoid fibroma: a clinicopathologic study of 76 cases. *Cancer* 30:726, 1972.

74. Redono C, Rocamura A, Vittoria F, et al: Malignant mixed tumor of the skin: malignant chondroid syringoma. *Cancer* 49:1690, 1982.

75. Reeh MJ: Hemangiopericytoma with cartilaginous differentiation involving orbit. *Arch Ophthalmol* 75:82, 1966.

76. Reiman HM, Dahlin DC: Cartilage- and bone-forming tumors of the soft tissues. *Semin Diagn Pathol* 3:288, 1986.

77. Saleh G, Evans HL, Ro JY, et al: Extraskeletal myxoid chondrosarcoma: a clinicopathologic study of ten patients with long-term follow-up. *Cancer* 70:2827, 1992.

78. Schajowicz F: Juxtacortical chondrosarcoma. *J Bone Joint Surg* 59B:473, 1977.

79. Schajowicz F, Defilippi-Novoa CA, Firpo CA: Thorotrast-induced chondrosarcoma of the axilla. *Am J Roentgenol* 100:931, 1967.

80. Scott JE, Dorling J: Differential staining of acid glucosaminoglycans (mucopolysaccharides) by alcian blue in salt solutions. *Histochemie* 5:221, 1965.

81. Shen WP, Young RF, Walter BN, et al: Molecular analysis of a myxoid chondrosarcoma with rearrangements of chromosomes 10 and 22. *Cancer Genet Cytogenet* 45:207, 1990.

82. Smith MT, Farinacci CJ, Carpenter HA, et al: Extraskeletal myxoid chondrosarcoma: a clinicopathologic study. *Cancer* 37:821, 1976.

83. Specht C, Smith TW, De Girolami U, et al: Myxopapillary ependymoma of the filum terminale. *Cancer* 58:310, 1986.

84. Stout AP, Verner EW: Chondrosarcoma of the extraskeletal soft tissues. *Cancer* 6:581, 1953.

85. Suzuki T, Kaneko H, Kojima K, et al: Extraskeletal myxoid chondrosarcoma characterized by microtubular aggregates in the rough endoplasmic reticulum and tubuline immunoreactivity. *J Pathol* 156:51, 1988.

86. Tanaka N, Asao T: Chordoid sarcoma of the soft tissue of the nape of the neck: a case with a 20-year follow-up. *Virchows Arch (Pathol Anat)* 379:261, 1978.

87. Tsuneyoshi M, Enjoji M, Iwasaki H, et al: Extraskeletal myxoid chondrosarcoma: a clinicopathologic and electron microscopic study. *Acta Pathol Jpn* 31:439, 1981.

88. Turc-Carel C, Dal Cin P, Rao U, et al: Recurrent breakpoints at 9q31 and 22q12.2 in extraskeletal myxoid chondrosarcoma. *Cancer Genet Cytogenet* 30:145, 1988.

89. Ujiki GT, Method HL, Putong PB, et al: Primary chondrosarcoma of the diaphragm. *Am J Surg* 122:132, 1971.

90. Weiss C, Rosenberg L, Helfet AJ: An ultrastructural study of normal young adult human articular cartilage. *J Bone Joint Surg* 50A:663, 1968.

91. Weiss SW: Ultrastructure of the so-called "chordoid sarcoma": evidence supporting cartilaginous differentiation. *Cancer* 37:300, 1976.

92. Wetzel WJ, Reuhl KR: Microtubular aggregates in the rough endoplasmic reticulum of a myxoid chondrosarcoma. *Ultrastruct Pathol* 1:519, 1980.

93. Wick MR, Burgess JH, Manivel JC: A reassessment of "chordoid sarcoma": ultrastructural and immunohistochemical comparison with chordom and skeletal myxoid chondrosarcoma. *Mod Pathol* 1:433, 1988

94. Wu KK, Collon DJ, Guise ER: Extraosseous chondrosarcoma: report of five cases and review of the literature. *J Bone Joint Surg* 62A:189, 1980.

Extraskeletal mesenchymal chondrosarcoma

95. Bagchi M, Husain N, Goel MM, et al: Extraskeletal mesenchymal chondrosarcoma of the orbit. *Cancer* 72:2224, 1993.

96. Bertoni F, Picci P, Bacchini P, et al: Mesenchymal chondrosarcoma of bone and soft tissues. *Cancer* 52:533, 1983.

97. Bloch DM, Bragolia J, Collins DN, et al: Mesenchymal chondrosarcoma of the head and neck. *J Laryngol Otol* 93:405, 1979.

98. Cardenas-Ramirez L, Albores-Saavedra J, DeBuen S: Mesenchymal chondrosarcoma of the orbit. *Arch Ophthalmol* 86:510, 1971.

99. Dabska M, Huvos AG: Mesenchymal chondrosarcoma in the young. *Virchows Arch (Pathol Anat)* 399:89, 1983.

100. Dahlin DC, Henderson ED: Mesenchymal chondrosarcoma: further observations on a new entity. *Cancer* 15:410, 1962.

101. Fu YS, Kay S: A comparative ultrastructural study of mesenchymal chondrosarcoma and myxoid chondrosarcoma. *Cancer* 33:1531, 1974.

102. Goldman RL: "Mesenchymal" chondrosarcoma, a rare malignant chondroid tumor usually primary in bone: report of a case arising in extraskeletal soft tissue. *Cancer* 20:1494, 1967.

103. Guccion JG, Font RL, Enzinger FM, et al: Extraskeletal mesenchymal chondrosarcoma. *Arch Pathol* 95:336, 1973.

104. Hedinger C: Mesenchymales Chondrosarkom der Weichteile. *Schweiz Med Wochenschr* 99:1142, 1969.

105. Louvet C, de Gramont A, Krulik M, et al: Extraskeletal mesenchymal chondrosarcoma: case report and review of the literature. *J Clin Oncol* 3:858, 1985.

106. Mazabraud A: Le chondrosarcome mésenchymateux: a propos des six observations. *Rev Chir Orthop* 60:197, 1974.

107. Nakashima Y, Unni KK, Shives TC, et al: Mesenchymal chondrosarcoma of bone and soft tissue: a review of 111 cases. *Cancer* 57:2444, 1986.

108. Nezelof C, Mazabraud A, Meary R: Le chondrosarcome mésenchymateux: a propos d'un cas de localization para-rachidienne. *Arch Anat Pathol* 13:26, 1965.

109. Rollo JL, Green WR, Kahan LB: Primary meningeal mesenchymal chondrosarcoma. *Arch Pathol Lab Med* 103:239, 1979.

110. Salvador AH, Beabout JW, Dahlin DC: Mesenchymal chondrosarcoma: observations on 30 new cases. *Cancer* 28:605, 1971.

111. Scheithauer BW, Rubinstein LJ: Meningeal mesenchymal chondrosarcoma: report of 8 cases with review of the literature. *Cancer* 42:2744, 1978.

112. Sears WP, Tefft M, Cohen J: Postirradiation mesenchymal chondrosarcoma: a case report. *Pediatrics* 40:254, 1967.

113. Sevel D: Mesenchymal chondrosarcoma of the orbit. *Br J Ophthalmol* 58:882, 1974.

114. Shapeero LG, Vanel D, Couanet D, et al: Extraskeletal mesenchymal chondrosarcoma. *Radiology* 186:819, 1993.
115. Swanson PE, Lillemoe TJ, Manivel JC, et al: Mesenchymal chondrosarcoma: an immunohistochemical study. *Arch Pathol Lab Med* 114:943, 1990.
116. Ushigome S, Takakuwa T, Shinagawa T, et al: Ultrastructure of cartilaginous tumors and S-100 protein in the tumors: with reference to the histogenesis of chondroblastoma, chondromyxoid fibroma, and mesenchymal chondrosarcoma. *Acta Pathol Jpn* 34:1285, 1984.

CHAPTER 36

OSSEOUS SOFT TISSUE TUMORS

We are principally concerned in this chapter with three extraskeletal bone-forming lesions: (1) myositis ossificans and related nonneoplastic, heterotopic ossifications, (2) fibroosseous pseudotumor of the digits, (3) fibrodysplasia (myositis) ossificans progressiva, and (4) extraskeletal osteosarcoma.

Myositis ossificans, by far the most common of the four lesions, is a localized, self-limiting ossifying process that follows mechanical trauma in the majority of cases. Identical lesions also occur in persons without an apparent history of preceding injury, and in some of these cases an infectious process has been claimed as a possible cause or initiating factor. While the majority of these lesions originate in muscle tissue, morphologically similar lesions also arise in the subcutis, tendons, fasciae, and periosteum. Depending on their location, these heterotopic ossifications have been variously classified as *panniculitis ossificans, fasciitis ossificans, florid reactive periostitis,* and *fibroosseous pseudotumor of digits.*

Not further discussed in this chapter are other rare heterotopic ossifications that occur after various kinds of soft tissue injury. Such lesions have been described in surgical scars, particularly those of the abdomen,[4,38,41] in burns,[28] and in association with dislocations of the elbow and other joints and total hip arthroplasty.[2] They have also been observed in patients with tetanus,[4,43] in hemophiliacs, in paraplegics secondary to traumatic spinal injury,[21,39,42,59] and in patients with spina bifida, myelomeningocele, syringomyelia, cerebral palsy, or poliomyelitis, probably induced by passive movement or forced exercise.[11,19,22] Repeated minor soft tissue trauma is also the cause of the "drill bone" or "shooter bone" in the deltoid and pectoralis muscles, the "rider bone" in the adductor muscles of the thigh, and the "shoemaker's bone" in the rectus muscle of the lower abdominal wall—all lesions that are rarely encountered today but have been repeatedly described in the earlier literature.

Besides these more deeply seated lesions, localized bone formations in the dermis and subcutis are not particularly rare. They may be solitary or multiple, and occur spontaneously or in connection with a variety of neoplastic (e.g., linear basal cell nevus, basal cell carcinoma, chondrosyringoma, calcifying epithelioma) and nonneoplastic processes (e.g., scars, acne, puncture wounds, injections, organizing hematomas, pseudohypoparathyroidism, dermatomyositis). Many of these lesions have been reported as *osteoma cutis,* but they too seem to be products of metaplasia rather than neoplasia.*

Fibroosseous pseudotumor of the digits is a rare heterotopic ossification related to myositis ossificans. It occurs chiefly in the fingers of young adults where it involves the subcutaneous tissue and adjacent fibrous structures. It shows a rather irregular growth pattern, without the typical zoning of myositis ossificans. Despite some cellular atypia and mitotic activity the lesion is benign and curable by local excision.

Fibrodysplasia ossificans progressiva (myositis ossificans progressiva) is a heritable disorder in which massive crippling ossification occurs following diffuse fibroblastic proliferation in muscle and associated soft tissues, especially those of the back, shoulder, and neck. The process has its onset in early childhood and follows a relentless clinical course with total disability in its later stages. Although microscopically the early phase of the lesion may be confused with fibromatosis, it can be positively identified radiographically in nearly all cases by the presence of microdactylia and other malformations of the hands and feet.

Extraskeletal osteosarcoma, the fourth category and the only true neoplasm discussed in this chapter, is a highly malignant tumor that afflicts a much older age group than osteosarcoma of bone. Occasionally it occurs in radiation-damaged tissues, but there is no convincing evidence that it ever occurs as a malignant transformation of myositis ossificans.

MYOSITIS OSSIFICANS

Myositis ossificans is a benign ossifying process that is generally solitary and well circumscribed. It is found most

---

*References 3, 6, 17, 18, 33, 52.

commonly in the musculature, but it may also occur in other tissues, especially in tendons[53] and subcutaneous fat.[42] The latter lesions are sometimes referred to as *panniculitis ossificans* or *fasciitis ossificans*. Distinguishing between traumatic and nontraumatic forms of myositis ossificans seems to serve little purpose, since both forms are morphologically identical and are most likely secondary to some kind of injury.

Despite countless reports of this lesion in the literature, myositis ossificans still causes considerable difficulties in diagnosis. This is particularly true of the early stage of the disease, in which the immature and highly cellular portions of the lesions are often confused with those of extraskeletal osteosarcoma. In fact, there are several reports of cases in which the lesion was initially incorrectly diagnosed, and the patient was treated by unnecessarily radical surgery. Late examples of myositis ossificans, consisting entirely of mature lamellar bone, are sometimes misinterpreted as osteomas.

As Ackerman[1] and others have pointed out, the term *myositis ossificans* is a misnomer because the lesion is not confined to the musculature, is devoid of bone in its early proliferative phase, and lacks a significant degree of inflammation. If inflammation occurs, it is usually minimal and is mostly evident in the tissues surrounding the lesion. For these reasons myositis ossificans and related processes have also been discussed under the designations "pseudomalignant osseous tumors of soft tissues"[9,62] and "extraosseous localized, nonneoplastic bone and cartilage formation."[1] Although undoubtedly these terms are more accurate and less confining, they are more cumbersome and so far have not been widely accepted in the literature. For this reason the conventional term *myositis ossificans* is retained for this chapter.

Clinical findings

The initial complaint, noted within hours or days after injury, is pain or tenderness, followed by a diffuse, doughy soft tissue swelling. Later, usually in the second or third week after onset, the swelling becomes more circumscribed and indurated and gradually changes into a mass that is distinctly outlined and firm to stony on palpation. The mass averages 3 to 6 cm in greatest diameter, but lesions measuring as large as 15 cm have been observed.

The condition chiefly affects young, vigorous, athletically active adolescents and adults, predominantly males, but it may also be found in older persons and females. Among our cases about half of the patients were younger than 30 years of age; the youngest was a 9-year-old boy and the oldest an 84-year-old man. For unknown reasons myositis ossificans is rare in small children, and most ossifying soft tissue lesions in this age-group are examples of fibrodysplasia ossificans progressiva. Nuovo et al.[46] observed three examples of myositis ossificans in children younger than 10 years of age. In about 80% of cases the lesion involves the limbs; the favored site in the lower extremity is the quadriceps muscle and the gluteus, and in the upper extremity the flexor muscles, especially the brachialis muscle. Deep-seated lesions may involve both muscle and underlying periosteum.

There are also myositis ossificans–like lesions that are confined to the subcutaneous fat (*panniculitis ossificans*). According to our material, these lesions prevail in the upper extremity, and, unlike the intramuscular lesions, predominate in women rather than men. The age incidence is the same as that of myositis ossificans.

Laboratory findings in myositis ossificans are largely normal. There are no significant changes in serum calcium or phosphorus levels, but sometimes the sedimentation rate, white blood count, and alkaline phosphatase levels are slightly elevated; these changes return to normal after removal of the lesion.

Roentgenographic findings

At the initial stage radiographs show merely a slight increase in soft tissue density. Calcification is rarely seen before the end of the third week after injury and initially presents as rather faint irregular, floccular radiopacities, sometimes described as the "dotted veil" pattern of myositis ossificans. As the lesion progresses and becomes increasingly calcified, it presents as a well-outlined soft tissue mass, which is most densely calcified at its periphery.[23] Calcification becomes clearly apparent radiographically 4 to 6 weeks after the onset of the lesion (Figs. 36-1 and 36-2); it proceeds from the periphery toward the center of the process, but even in late lesions the central core tends to remain uncalcified. The presence of a distinct radiolucent cleft between the lesion and the underlying bone helps to distinguish myositis ossificans from osteochondroma.[45] Angiograms reveal a diffuse blush and fine neovascularity in the early phase of the process.[60] The appearance of myositis ossificans on CT scan and MRI has been described in detail by Kransdorf et al.[31,32] and De Smet et al.[15,16]

Pathological findings

Grossly, most of the lesions measure 3 to 6 cm in greatest diameter. They tend to be well circumscribed and cut with a gritty sensation; they are white, soft, and rather gelatinous (or hemorrhagic) in the center and yellow-gray and firm with a rough granular surface at the periphery (Fig. 36-3).

Under the microscope, myositis ossificans is generally characterized by the presence of a distinct zonal pattern that reflects different degrees of cellular maturation, a pattern that is most conspicuous in lesions of 3 or more weeks' duration[29] (Figs. 36-4 to 36-6). In these cases the innermost portion of the lesion is composed of immature, loosely textured, often richly vascular fibroblastic tissue bearing a

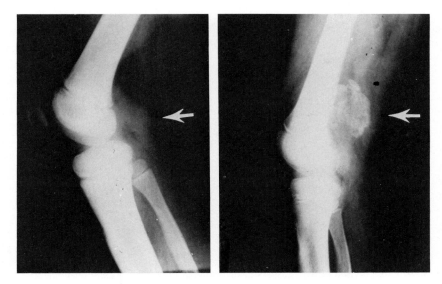

FIG. 36-1. Myositis ossificans of the popliteal fossa showing evidence of progressive ossification within a 22-day period.

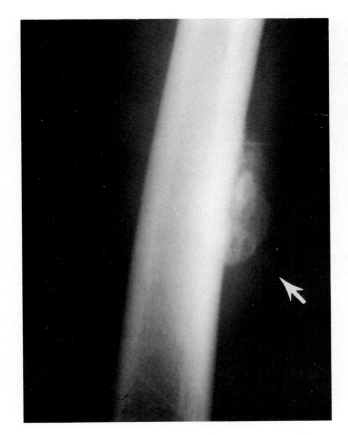

FIG. 36-2. Radiograph of myositis ossificans *(arrow)* of the upper thigh. The lesion had been present for 5 weeks.

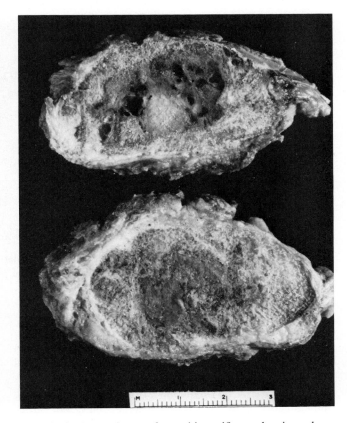

FIG. 36-3. Gross picture of myositis ossificans showing a hemorrhagic center surrounded by a broad zone of ossification and small amounts of residual muscle tissue.

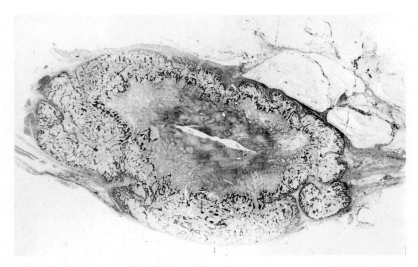

FIG. 36-4. Cross-section of myositis ossificans showing the typical zoning phenomenon: a fibroblastic center and a broad zone of ossification at the periphery. (×4.5.)

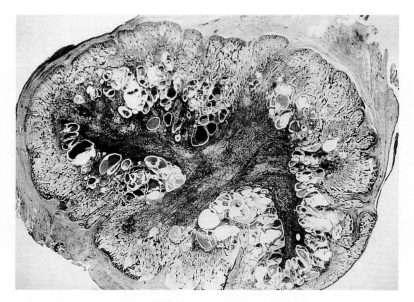

FIG. 36-5. Myositis ossificans showing similar features as Fig. 36-4, but in addition dilated vessels and focal hemorrhage in the more central portion of the lesion. (×45.)

close resemblance to nodular fasciitis or granulation tissue. The constituent fibroblasts and myofibroblasts display a mild to moderate degree of cellular pleomorphism and rather prominent mitotic activity (Fig. 36-7). They are intermingled with a varying number of macrophages, chronic inflammatory cells, fibrinous material, and, not infrequently, multinucleated giant cells. In addition, there may be prominent endothelial proliferation, focal hemorrhage, fibrin, and entrapped atrophic or necrotic muscle fibers.

Bordering these areas is an intermediate zone in which the cells become condensed into ill-defined trabeculae consisting of a mixture of fibroblasts, osteoblasts, and varying amounts of osteoid separated by thin-walled, ectatic vascular channels (Fig. 36-8). Further toward the periphery the osteoid increasingly undergoes calcification and evolves into mature lamellar bone. Not infrequently islets of immature or mature cartilage are present and precede bone formation. Characteristically, bone formation is most promi-

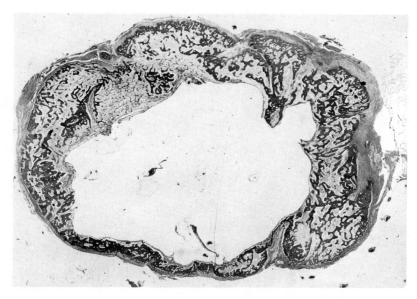

FIG. 36-6. Late form of myositis ossificans with a central fluid-filled space surrounded by mature bone and dense fibrous tissue. (×45.)

nent at the margin of the lesion, often with rimming of the osteoid by a monolayer of osteoblasts showing little variation in size and shape. The bone is separated from the surrounding muscle tissue by a zone of loose, myxoid, or compressed fibrous tissue (Fig. 36-9). The surrounding muscle often shows atrophic changes, sometimes together with a mild inflammatory infiltrate and focal sarcolemmal proliferation. In some tumors, particularly those arising in the subcutaneous fat *(panniculitis ossificans)* the zonal pattern is absent or inconspicuous. Older lesions consist only of mature lamellar bone together with interspersed fat cell, fibrous tissue, and thin-walled vascular spaces, indistinguishable from osteoma.

Special staining techniques are generally not helpful. As in other bone-forming lesions, the osteoblasts contain large amounts of alkaline phosphatase, and the osteoclast-like giant cells contain abundant acid phosphatase.[7]

Ultrastructurally, myositis ossificans consists of fibroblasts and myofibroblasts with focally condensed myofilaments and without basal laminae, macrophages, and preosteoblasts and osteoblasts with numerous mitochondria and prominent rough endoplasmic reticulum.[50] Caulet et al.[7] also reported the presence of coarsely banded collagen in the extracellular spaces.

Malignant transformation of myositis ossificans

There are no convincing cases of malignant transformation in our files or in Ackerman's series,[1] but there are several accounts in the literature in which transformation of myositis ossificans into extraskeletal osteosarcoma is claimed.* In most of these cases the presence of myositis ossificans is poorly documented, and in only a few is the diagnosis based on biopsy. In some of the reported cases, long duration and dedifferentiation of a well-differentiated osteosarcoma may have simulated origin in myositis ossificans. Eckardt et al.[118] described a patient with a history of dermatomyositis who developed an extraskeletal osteosarcoma of the thigh 29 years after a soft tissue ossification was noted in the same location.

Differential diagnosis

It is of paramount importance to clearly distinguish this lesion from extraskeletal osteosarcoma. This is best accomplished on the basis of the characteristic zoning phenomenon of myositis ossificans, that is, the presence of immature cellular areas in the center and more mature, ossifying areas with osteoblastic rimming at the periphery. In sharp contrast, osteosarcoma displays a more disorderly growth of hyperchromatic and often pleomorphic cells with lacelike rather than trabecular osteoid formation and sometimes a "reverse zoning effect," namely osteoid or bone formation in the interior and older portion of the lesion and immature spindle cell formation at its margin.[142] Moreover, unlike myositis ossificans, extraskeletal osteosarcoma shows a greater degree of cellular atypia, no subsidence of growth at the periphery, and infiltration of neighboring tissues in a destructive manner. Mitotic figures are present in both the immature portion of myositis ossificans and osteo-

*References 24, 26, 48, 55, 119, 126.

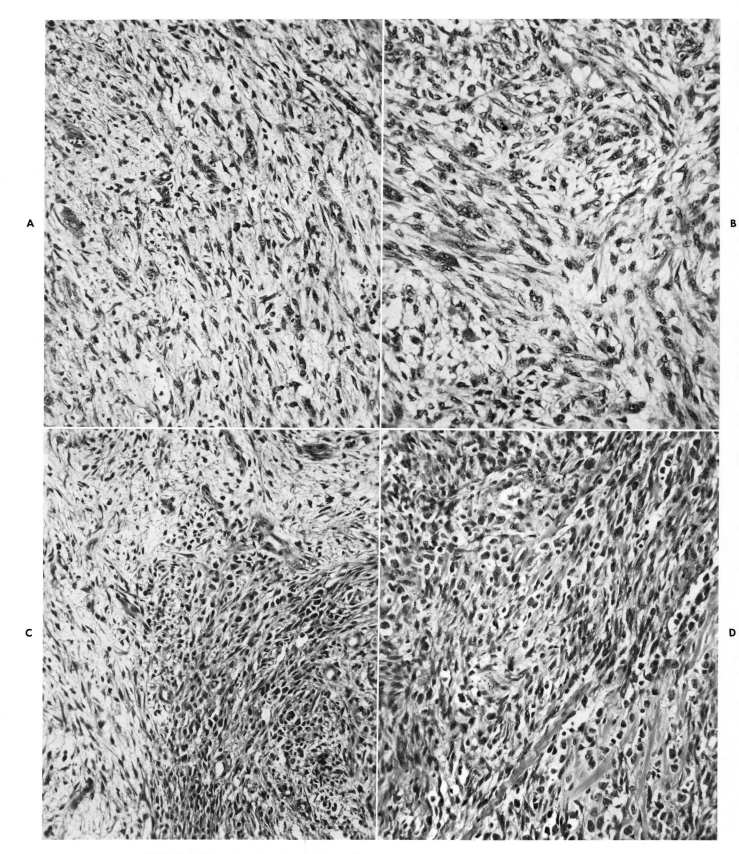

FIG. 36-7. Central portion of myositis ossificans showing fibroblastic proliferation varying in cellularity and number of mitotic figures. **A** and **B,** Loosely textured fibroblastic areas. **C** and **D,** Cellular areas showing some pleomorphism mimicking a sarcoma. (**A, C,** and **D,** ×160; **B,** ×250.)

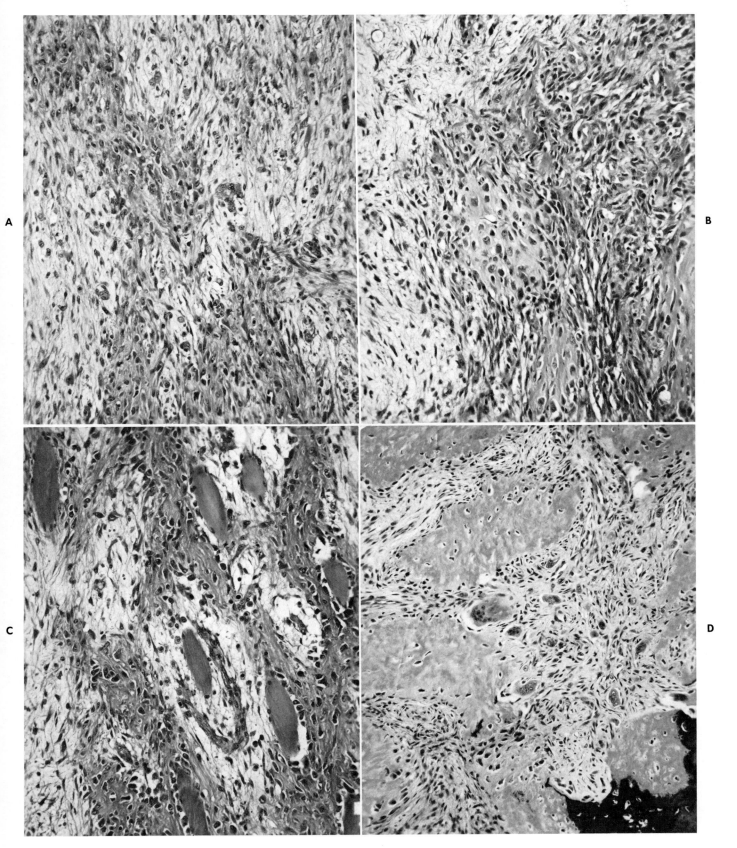

FIG. 36-8. Intermediate portion of myositis ossificans. **A** and **B,** Depositions of collagen and osteoid among proliferated spindle cells with early trabeculation of ossifying areas. **C,** Trabeculae of osteoid between atrophic residual muscle fibers (same case as **A**). **D,** Masses of osteoblasts and osteoid associated with osteoclast-like, multinucleated giant cells. (**A** to **D,** ×160.)

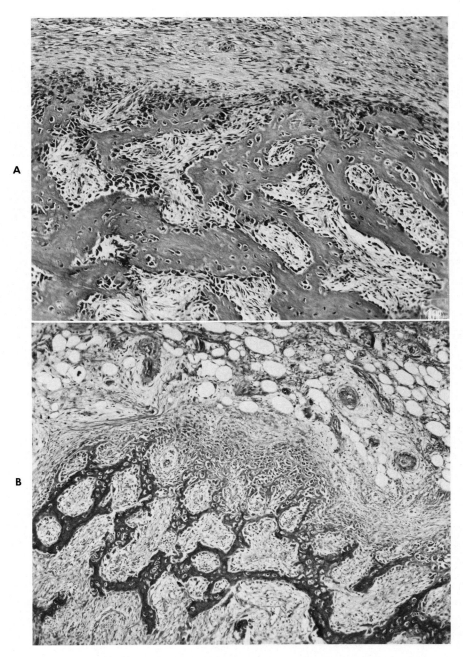

FIG. 36-9. Peripheral portion of myositis ossificans displaying a zone of osteoid trabeculae rimmed by osteoblasts and bone **(A)** surrounded by loose fibrous tissue and atropic fat **(B). (A,** ×100; **B,** ×60.)

sarcoma, but several clearly atypical or tripolar forms of mitotic figures point toward malignancy.

Confusion of myositis ossificans with osteosarcoma is most likely with small or minute biopsy specimens taken during the initial proliferative phase or obtained from the cellular center of an early lesion. Differential diagnosis may also be a problem in those cases in which the lesion lacks the characteristic zoning phenomenon and grows in an irregular multifocal or multilobulated fashion, as in most cases of fibroosseous pseudotumor involving the distal portions of the fingers or toes. Because extraskeletal osteosarcomas occur rarely in young persons, consideration of the age of the patient may help in reaching a correct diagnosis.[57] Very rarely, a soft tissue metastasis of a silent osteoblastic carcinoma may masquerade as myositis ossificans.

There are also benign lesions that may be confused with myositis ossificans; they include purely reactive lesions such as nodular fasciitis, proliferative myositis, posttraumatic periostitis, and exuberant fracture callus. Proliferative myositis rarely contains minute foci of osteoid or bone, but characteristically this feature is associated with a diffuse proliferation of plump fibroblasts resembling ganglion cells. Posttraumatic periostitis manifests as an ossified mass that is attached to bone with a broad base. Exuberant callus is usually associated with a discernible fracture line on standard x-rays.

Pathogenesis

Although there is general agreement that myositis ossificans is a nonprogressive benign process without neoplastic potential, its pathogenesis is still poorly understood. In cases with a definite history of traumatic injury it can be assumed that the process commences with tissue necrosis or hemorrhage, or both, followed by exuberant reparative fibroblastic and vascular proliferation, eventually leading to progressive ossification. The exact environmental or humoral conditions underlying the ossifying process are unclear. It seems unlikely, however, that detachment and intramuscular implantation of periosteal cells are necessary prerequisites for the ossification, especially since this ossifying process also takes place in the subcutis and in abdominal scars at considerable distance from bone. Similarly, the occurrence of ectopic ossifications in paraplegics and patients with tetanus may be explained by trauma resulting from passive exercise rather than disturbed neurotrophic factors. There are no reliable studies as to the source of the osteoblasts. They may be transformed fibroblasts, or they may be derived from primitive perivascular mesenchymal cells secondary to injury and necrosis of muscle and other tissues.[8]

A satisfactory explanation of the so-called nontraumatic cases of myositis ossificans is even more problematic. They amount to almost half of the total number of cases in our material and have been repeatedly reported by others.[1,13,27,47,54] It is likely that in most of these cases minor injury, such as a spontaneous muscle tear or a similar disruptive lesion, associated with heavy manual labor, weight lifting, or some other strenuous exercise or activities, has been overlooked or forgotten; yet it is difficult to exclude the possibility that some of these cases are caused or initiated by an infectious process. Lagier and Cox[36] have reported on a patient who had an antiinfluenza vaccination 15 days before the onset of the lesion. A similar infectious origin has been considered for the related "fibroosseous pseudotumors of the digits."[62]

Discussion

Because myositis ossificans is a benign self-limiting process, the prognosis is excellent, and there is no need for further therapy once the diagnosis of myositis ossificans has been established by biopsy or local excision. However, if only a biopsy was done or if the lesion was partly excised at an early phase of its growth, it may continue to grow for a limited period; in these cases repeated x-ray examinations should be made during the follow-up period to document the maturation of the lesion and the absence of destructive growth. Spontaneous regression of myositis ossificans has also been observed.[1]

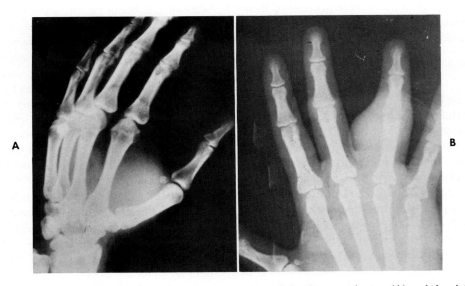

FIG. 36-10. Radiographs of fibroosseous pseudotumor of the thenar eminence **(A)** and the right ring finger **(B).**

FIBROOSSEOUS PSEUDOTUMOR OF THE DIGITS

This condition, which is a heterotopic ossification closely related to myositis ossificans, occurs in the subcutaneous tissue of the digits[65]; the terms *florid reactive periostitis of the tubular bones of hands and feet*[69] and *parosteal fascii-tis*[67] also refer to this lesion when it is attached to bone. Clinically, this process presents as a painful, localized, fusiform, often erythematous swelling in the soft tissues of the fingers, especially the region of the proximal phalanx, and less commonly of the toes. It is most common in young adults and, unlike myositis ossificans, predominates in women (Fig. 36-10).

When examined under the microscope, the lesion closely resembles myositis ossificans but lacks its orderly zonal pattern and consists merely of an irregular, often nodular mixture of loosely arranged fibroblasts, a prominent myxoid matrix, and deposits of osteoid rimmed by uniform osteoblasts.[65] Although some of these lesions have been confused with extraskeletal osteosarcoma because of their focal hypercellularity, the presence of immature and sometimes atypical fibroblasts, the increased mitotic rate, and the lack of a typical zonal arrangement, they can be recognized as a benign process if attention is paid to their characteristic location in the digits and the absence of pleomorphic or hyperchromatic cells and atypical mitotic figures[9,63,64,66,68] (Fig. 36-11).

As in the conventional form of myositis ossificans, the exact pathogenetic mechanism of this process is not clear. In our series a history of trauma was given in only 9 of 21 patients, and both a neglected minor injury and an infectious process have to be considered as a possible cause.[65] There was no history of an associated infection in our cases, but Angervall et al.,[62] who favored an infectious pathogenesis, were able to demonstrate elevated white blood counts as well as increased streptolysin O titers in some of their patients. There is no tendency toward recurrence, and complete excision is curative.

FIBRODYSPLASIA (MYOSITIS) OSSIFICANS PROGRESSIVA

This is a rare, slowly progressive hereditary disease that principally affects children under the age of 10 years. It is characterized by progressive fibroblastic proliferation and subsequent calcification and ossification of subcutaneous fat, muscles, tendons, aponeuroses, and ligaments. The disorder is often associated with symmetrical malformations of the digits, especially microdactyly or adactyly of the thumbs and great toes that precedes the onset of the fibroblastic proliferations and calcifications. Its prevalence in children, diffuse or multinodular soft tissue involvement, progressive clinical course, and increased familial incidence distinguish it from localized myositis ossificans. Sporadic examples of this condition have been described in the literature since the seventeenth century.

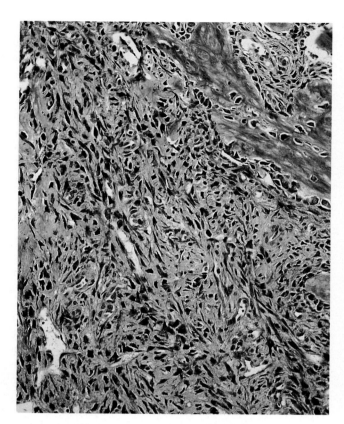

FIG. 36-11. Fibroosseous pseudotumor of the right index finger showing a mixture of proliferated, slightly pleomorphic fibroblasts and trabeculae of osteoid rimmed by small, uniform osteoblasts. (×160.)

Clinical findings

The disease has its onset primarily between birth and 6 years of age, but in rare instances it may also arise in older children and even in young adults.[72] Males and females are about equally affected and there is no predilection for any particular race. As in localized myositis ossificans, the lesion presents as a painful, doughy soft tissue swelling that is often but not always precipitated by injury or infectious disease. It is found most commonly in the musculature of the back, shoulder, paravertebral region, and upper arms and is often preceded by similar lesions in the occipital portion of the scalp and the region of the sternocleidomastoid muscle.[86] Early nonossified lesions of this disease have been confused with fibromatosis of the sternocleidomastoid muscle. The facial muscle may also be affected. In the case reported by Cramer et al.[76] the disorder commenced in the lip at age 3 months and subsequently involved the entire left side of the face with ankylosis of the temporomandibular joint (Figs. 36-12 and 36-13, *A*). Although increased familial incidence is rare, the disorder is probably inherited as an autosomal dominant trait.[84]

As the lesion progresses, other areas such as the proxi-

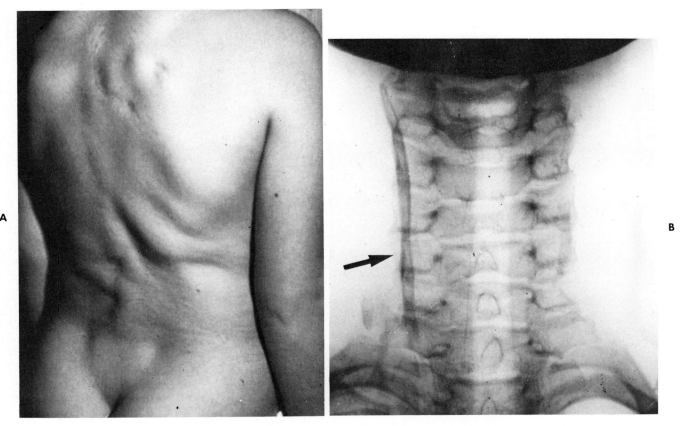

FIG. 36-12. A, Fibrodysplasia (myositis) ossificans progressiva involving the back of a child with ill-defined, indurated nodules caused by focal fibroblastic proliferation and ossification of the musculature. **B,** Radiograph of linear ossification of paraspinal muscles *(arrow).* (Courtesy Prof. Dr. Günther Möbius, Schwerin.)

mal portions of the upper extremities become involved, and there is increasing multifocal induration of muscle and subcutis with irregular and focal calcification and ossification. This causes progressive muscle stiffening, immobilization, and contraction deformities leading to severe changes in posture and gait as well as increasing difficulties in respiration. Involvement of the masseter muscle may impair normal mastication and may result in severe weight loss. Death may result from respiratory failure or pneumonia during early adult life.[84]

Malformation or absence of one or more digits is an almost constant finding that helps to distinguish this disease from infantile forms of fibromatosis. The malformations are usually present at birth or appear soon thereafter; in the earliest stage they are best identified roentgenographically; they consist mainly of bilateral shortening of the fingers (microdactyly), absence of both thumbs and great toes (adactyly), or digital deviations, particularly valgus position of the great toe (bilateral hallux valgus) (Fig. 36-13, *B* and *C*). Frequently other digits are also involved.[94] Con-

nor and Evans,[73] in a review of 34 affected patients, reported hallux valgus in 79%, short first metacarpals in 59%, and deviation (clinodactyly) of the fifth fingers in 42%. In 29 of the 34 cases the skeletal alterations were present at birth. Sometimes the significance of these osseous malformations is not immediately recognized, and surgical correction is attempted. Additional roentgenographic changes, which appear at a later stage of the disease, consist of bony bridges within muscles and tendons, contractures and ankylosis of the shoulder, elbow, and other joints, exostosis of the tibia and other bones, and osteoporosis. Deformity of the ears, absence of teeth, deafness, and sexual infantilism may also be part of the clinical picture.[91,94] Laboratory findings are generally unremarkable, except for elevated alkaline phosphatase levels and a markedly increased turnover rate of minerals.[84,95]

Roentgenographs show ectopic barlike and bridgelike soft tissue ossifications and various abnormalities of the short bones and vertebrae. Microdactyly of the thumb and great toe and bilateral shortening and deviation of the fifth

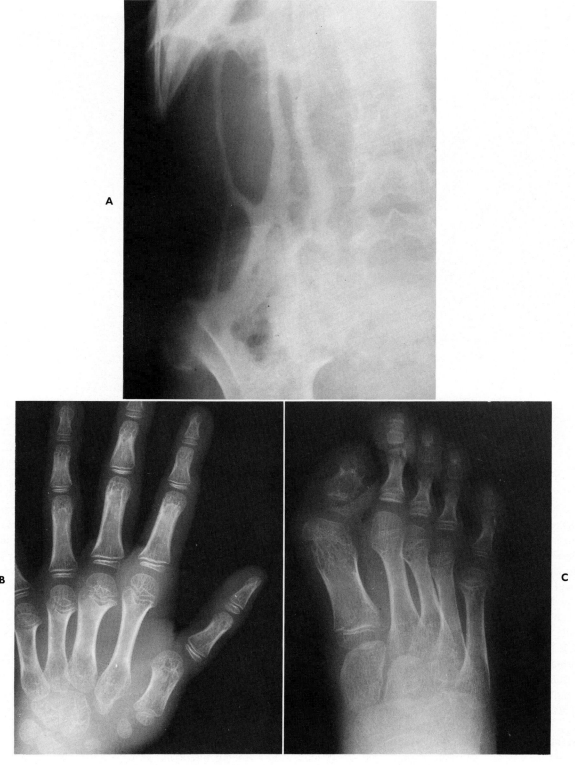

FIG. 36-13. Fibrodysplasia (myositis) ossificans progressiva with soft tissue ossification of the back (**A**), shortening and deviation of the thumb (**B**), and malformation of the great toe (**C**).

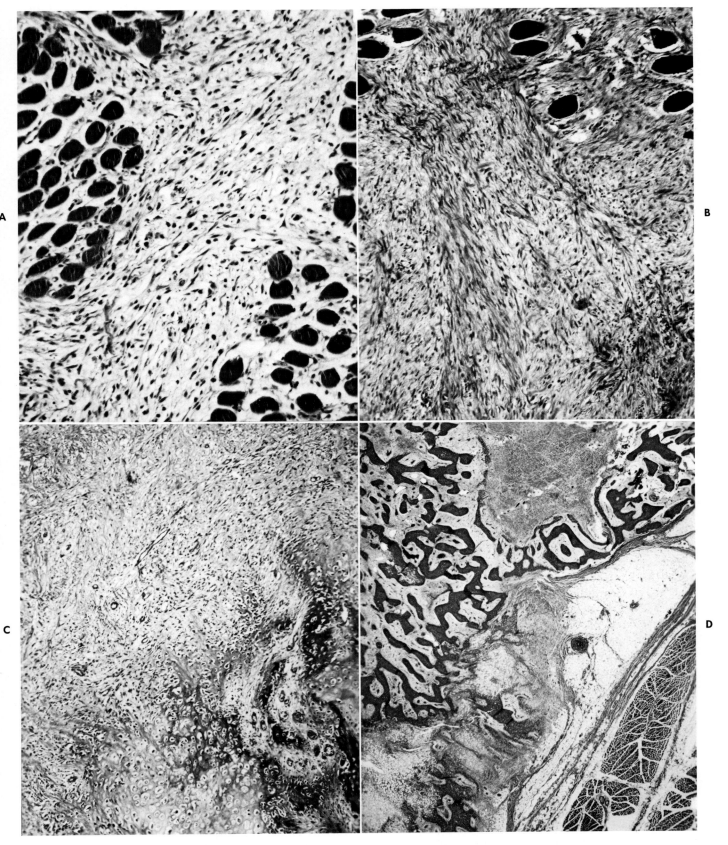

FIG. 36-14. Fibrodysplasia (myositis) ossificans progressiva of the scapular region in a 7-year-old girl. **A** and **B,** Edema and ill-defined, loosely textured fibroblastic proliferation of muscle superficially resembling infantile fibromatosis, proliferative myositis, or nodular fasciitis. **C** and **D,** Irregular ossification of the fibroblastic tissue lacking the zoning phenomenon of localized myositis ossificans. (**A,** ×100; **B,** ×160; **C,** ×60; **D,** ×15.)

finger are frequent findings. Less often there is a calcaneal spur, a short femoral neck, and medial cortical thickening of the proximal tibia. CT scan and MRI may help in demonstrating early changes of the disease. Bone scintigraphs reveal increased tracer uptake at the sites of ossification.[31,71,89,97]

Pathological findings

There are essentially two stages of the disease. The first consists of nodular swelling of muscle and subcutis caused by interstitial edema and loose proliferation of fibroblasts, usually in the endomysium and perimysium (Fig. 36-14, *A* and *B*). In the second stage, collagen is laid down between the fibroblasts, followed by variable muscular atrophy, calcification, ossification of the collagenized fibrous tissue, and formation of mature bone and cartilage. Unlike localized myositis ossificans, the ossification occurs in the center of the nodules. The nodules often interconnect, leading eventually to the formation of bony bridges that replace muscle, tendons, and ligaments (Fig. 36-14, *C* and *D*). Histochemical and ultrastructural studies, as described by Maxwell et al.,[85] show active fibroblasts with a prominent endoplasmic reticulum, collagen fibers of normal periodicity, and increased mucosubstances. Positive staining for S-100 protein was noted in sections of the earliest lesions.[81]

Prognosis and therapy

The outlook is poor, and usually the disease proves fatal within a period of 10 to 15 years, frequently as the result of severe respiratory insufficiency caused by progressive immobilization of the thorax. Biopsy and trauma may lead to the development of new lesions and should be avoided. Dietary measures, steroids,[77] and agents binding minerals or blocking calcification (EDTA and EHDP) have been tried with disappointing results. In fact, Rogers and Dorst[90] reported ricketlike osseous abnormalities following therapy with high doses of disodium etidronate. Accurate evaluation of therapy is complicated by frequent remissions that are characteristic of the disease.

The basic pathogenetic mechanism remains unknown. The disorder may occur sporadically or may be inherited as a dominant autosomal trait.[84] It has been observed in homozygotic twins and in multiple family members over several generations.[73,79,82,87]

Differential diagnosis includes the battered child syndrome,[61] ectopic bone formation with multiple congenital anomalies,[92] pseudohypoparathyroidism,[70] and dermatomyositis with multiple calcifications.[98] Dermatomyositis may also be associated with shortenings of the metacarpal and metatarsal bones, exostoses, and multiple subcutaneous ossifications.[73] Finally, as mentioned earlier, the initial noncalcified fibrous proliferation of fibrodysplasia ossificans progressiva may be mistaken for a juvenile form of fibromatosis.

EXTRASKELETAL OSTEOSARCOMA

Compared with osteosarcoma of bone, extraskeletal osteosarcoma is rare. It may be defined as a malignant mesenchymal neoplasm that produces osteoid, bone, or chondroid material and is located in the soft tissues without attachment to the skeleton, as determined by roentgenographic examination or inspection during the operative procedure. There are nearly 150 examples of this neoplasm on file at the AFIP, and there is a similar number of cases recorded in the literature. Included in our material and among the reported cases are also a number of osteosarcomas of soft tissues that developed several years after radiotherapy for carcinoma or some other malignant epithelial or mesenchymal neoplasm.

Excluded from this chapter are osteosarcomas arising in the breast,[101,121] urinary bladder,[157] prostate,[141] and other visceral organs because in many of these tumors there is a participating epithelial component suggesting carcinosarcoma. Excluded also are malignant mesenchymomas, tumors that exhibit by definition two or more well-defined malignant mesenchymal components besides the fibrous element (see Chapter 38).

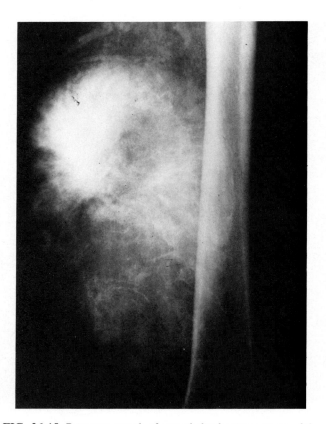

FIG. 36-15. Roentgenograph of extraskeletal osteosarcoma of the midthigh demonstrating a soft tissue mass with extensive ossification. (From *Cancer* 60:1132, 1987.)

There are few reliable data in the literature as to the incidence of extraskeletal osteosarcoma. Allan and Soule[99] encountered 26 cases among 2100 soft tissue sarcomas, an incidence of 1.24%. Lorentzon et al.,[134] in a study of the Swedish Cancer Registry, found four extraskeletal osteosarcomas (1.65%) among 242 osteosarcomas of bone. They calculated an annual incidence of two to three cases per million population.

Clinical findings

Although osteosarcomas of bone occur chiefly during the first 2 decades of life, extraskeletal osteosarcomas are rarely encountered in patients under 40 years of age. Thus in our series[113] the mean age was 54.6 years, with a range from 16 to 87 years. In Allan and Soule's report[99] the mean age was 47.5 years, with a range from 20 to 71 years. A similar age incidence was given by Fine and Stout[119] and others.[111,142] The data as to the sex incidence vary, and both male and female predominance has been reported.

There are no specific signs or symptoms. Generally the tumor presents as a progressively enlarging soft tissue mass, which is painful in about one third of patients. Large and late examples of the tumor may ulcerate through the skin, but usually only after biopsy or some other surgical procedure. The duration of symptoms varies from a few weeks to several months, with a mean of 6.5 months.[99]

Among the various anatomical sites, the muscles of the thigh and the retroperitoneum are most commonly affected; the large muscles of the pelvic and shoulder girdles are another leading location. Most of the tumors are deep seated and are fixed to the underlying tissues, but occasional lesions are freely movable and are confined to the subcutis or even the dermis.[105,113] There are also reports of extraskeletal osteosarcomas arising in the larynx,[114] pleura,[140] and in an ectopic hamartomatous thymus that was located in the pleural cavity.[148] The laboratory findings show no specific abnormalities. Alkaline phosphatase is usually normal with localized disease, but it is elevated in the presence of metastases. With conventional radiographs, CT scan, and MRI, extraskeletal osteosarcoma manifests as a soft tissue mass with spotty to massive calcifications and no evidence of bone involvement (Figs. 36-15 to 36-17, *A*).

Pathogenesis

Mechanical injury has been considered as a causative agent,[134] but, as with other neoplasms, the etiological significance of trauma is difficult to assess. Preceding trauma was reported in 12.5% of patients in our series[113] and in 13% of patients in the report of Das Gupta et al.[115] There are also reports of osteosarcoma arising at the sites of a previous injection[131] and a fracture.[108] Extraskeletal osteosarcomas arising in myositis ossificans are very rare and most of them are poorly documented.[24,26,48,55,126] Eckardt et al.[118] observed an osteosarcoma of the thigh in a 32-year-old-man that developed in a heterotopic ossification of dermatomyositis 28 years after onset of the disease. Unlike os-

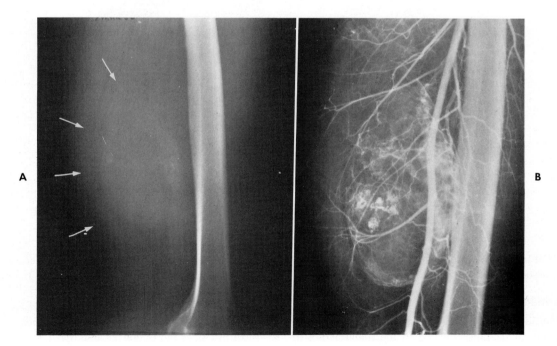

FIG. 36-16. A, Roentgenograph of extraskeletal osteosarcoma showing a soft tissue mass with areas of ossification *(arrows).* **B,** A moderate degree of vascularization in the angiogram with focal neovascularity and stretching and displacement of arteries.

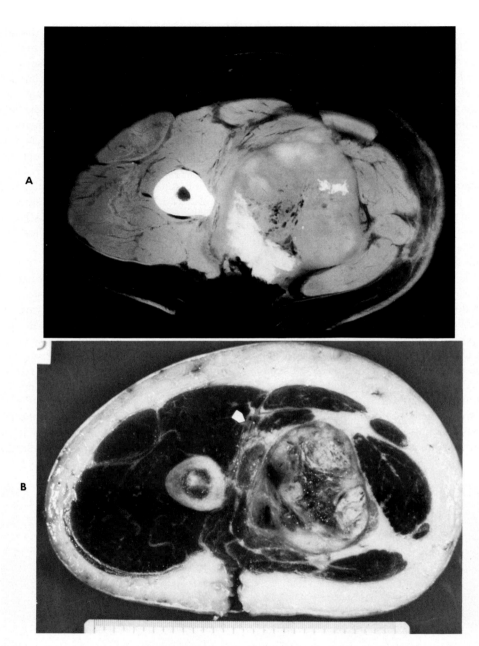

FIG. 36-17. A, CT scan and **B,** cross-section of extraskeletal osteosarcoma of the thigh. Note circumscription of the tumor, areas of hemorrhage, and absence of bone involvement.

teosarcoma of bone, the tumor has not been reported in siblings or in association with hereditary retinoblastoma.

Radiation-induced extraskeletal osteosarcoma

Since Martland[135] described the development of osteogenic sarcoma in patients engaged in the manufacture of luminous watch dials, numerous cases of osseous and extraosseous postradiation osteosarcomas have been reported in the literature.[104,111,130] Most of the extraosseous osteo-

sarcomas occurred in patients who received radiation therapy for a malignant neoplasm such as a mammary carcinoma,[100,123] uterine and ovarian carcinoma,[103,110,139] seminoma,[111] Wilms' tumor,[106] Hodgkin's disease,[112] neuroblastoma,[150] astrocytoma,[150] or retinoblastoma.[129,150] In most instances the tumor became apparent 4 or more years after radiotherapy. Assessment of these cases is facilitated by the presence of chronic radiodermatitis in the skin overlying the tumor or radiation change in the surrounding mus-

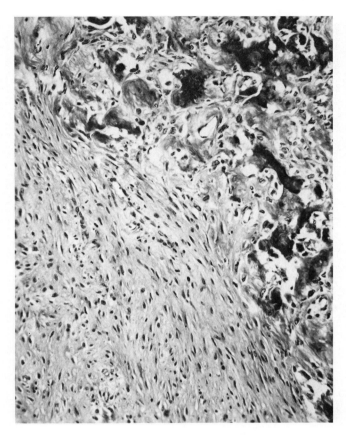

FIG. 36-18. Extraskeletal osteosarcoma with well-differentiated fibrosarcoma-like areas and formation of neoplastic osteoid and bone. (×160.)

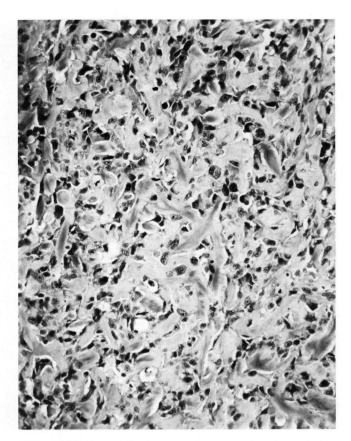

FIG. 36-19. Extraskeletal osteosarcoma showing deposition of hyalinized collagen and osteoid. (×160.)

cle tissue.[111,130] As with extraskeletal chondrosarcomas, there are also sporadic cases that developed following diagnostic procedures with radioactive thorium dioxide (thorotrast). One of these, an extraskeletal osteosarcoma of the mandibular region in a 51-year-old man, appeared 30 years after a thorotrast angiogram of the carotid artery.[122]

Pathological findings

Macroscopically, there is little that would permit a reliable diagnosis. The tumor varies in its gross appearance from a well-circumscribed mass with a distinct pseudocapsule to an infiltrating tumor without discernible borders. Frequently, it is firm to stony on palpation. Less often it presents as a soft or multicystic mass. On section it usually displays a granular white surface with yellow flecks and multiple foci of necrosis and hemorrhage. Most of the tumors measure 5 to 10 cm when excised (Fig. 36-17, B).

Microscopically, extraskeletal osteosarcomas have in common the presence of neoplastic osteoid and bone, not infrequently together with neoplastic cartilage. There is a striking variation in the relative prominence of this material and the associated osteoblastic and fibroblastic ele-

ments. Extraskeletal osteosarcomas, like osteosarcomas of bone, range from tumors that resemble fibrosarcoma or malignant fibrous histiocytoma (fibroblastic osteosarcoma) (Figs. 36-18 and 36-19) to extremely cellular tumors having an irregular round or spindle cell pattern with considerable pleomorphism and mitotic activity (osteoblastic osteosarcoma) (Fig. 36-20). Usually the osteoid is deposited in a fine, ramifying, lacelike or coarsely trabecular pattern, occasionally showing transitions toward sheaths of osteoid or mature-appearing bone (Fig. 36-21). Unlike in myositis ossificans, where the most mature portion is located at the periphery, there is often a "reverse zoning phenomenon" (i.e., central deposition of osteoid material and atypical spindle cell proliferation at the periphery).[142] Atypical cartilage of variable cellularity, with or without myxoid areas or focal bone formation, is present in many cases, but it rarely becomes a dominating feature (chondroblastic osteosarcoma) (Figs. 36-22 to 36-24, A). There is also a varying number of benign and malignant multinucleated giant cells of the osteoclastic type that are often associated with hemorrhage (osteoclastic or giant cell osteosarcoma) (Figs. 36-24, B, and 36-25). The vascular pattern varies

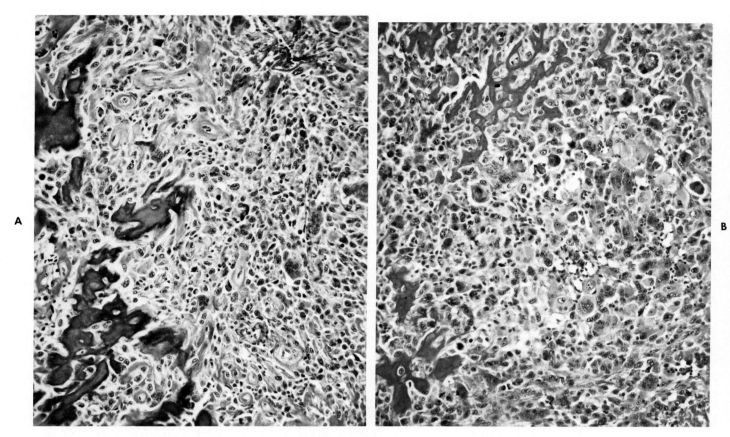

FIG. 36-20. Extraskeletal osteosarcoma consisting of small rounded osteoblasts with one or more nuclei, occasional multinucleated giant cells, and deposits of osteoid and bone. (**A** and **B**, ×160.)

substantially. Occasional examples with markedly dilated vascular spaces may resemble a vascular tumor *(telangiectatic osteosarcoma)*. Well-differentiated forms resembling parosteal osteosarcoma and tumors displaying a small cell pattern *(small cell osteosarcoma)* have also been described.[105,156] Metastatic lesions vary little in their structures from primary neoplasms. There are no specific immunohistochemical features, but osteosarcomas, like many other mesenchymal tumors, stain positively for vimentin.

Ultrastructural findings

There are only a few studies of the ultrastructural features of extraskeletal osteosarcoma, but all indicate that they are indistinguishable from those found in primary osteosarcoma of bone.[120,128] Characteristically, the tumor cells vary considerably in appearance. They possess irregularly shaped, large nuclei with crenated or indented nuclear membranes. There is a prominent endoplasmic reticulum that ranges from narrow tubular to markedly dilated structures, often enveloping mitochondria and having a finely granular content. There are also scattered free ribosomes, a well-developed Golgi complex, varying amounts

of filamentous material, and occasional lysosomes and lipid inclusions. Pinocytotic vesicles and desmosomes or tight junctions are absent or rare. Rao et al.[142] described in addition a cell with "interdigitating short processes, abundant filaments, and scarce endoplasmic reticulum." Occasionally there are multinucleated osteoclast-like giant cells with numerous mitochondria and multiple cellular processes.[132,151,152]

The extracellular spaces contain a feltwork of interlacing collagen fibers, sometimes with scattered delicate electron-dense particles and deposits of needle-shaped, crystalline hydroxyapatite.

Differential diagnosis

It is not always easy to distinguish extraskeletal osteosarcomas from other benign and malignant bone- and cartilage-forming soft tissue lesions. The differentiation from myositis ossificans and other reactive reparative processes has already been discussed. Among malignant tumors metaplastic bone is infrequently found in synovial sarcoma, epithelioid sarcoma, malignant fibrous histiocytoma, liposarcoma, malignant melanoma, and other mesenchymal

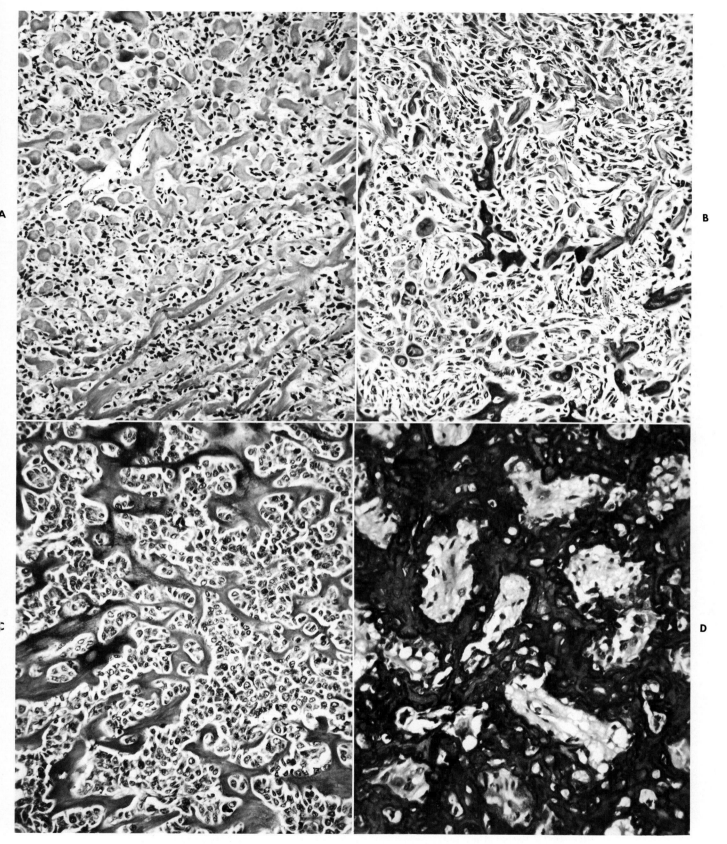

FIG. 36-21. Extraskeletal osteosarcoma. **A,** Small trabeculae of osteoid in longitudinal and cross-sections in an osteosarcoma of the retroperitoneum. (×160.) **B,** Osteoblasts and interspersed osteoid in a tumor of the neck following use of Thorotrast. (×130.) **C,** Osteoblasts separated by ribbons and trabeculae of osteoid material and bone. (×350.) **D,** Lacelike ossification. (×250.)

or epithelial neoplasms. In most of these neoplasms osteoid or bone is confined to a small portion of the tumor and is relatively well differentiated without the disorderly pattern and cellular pleomorphism of osteosarcoma. In some of them, however, it is exceedingly difficult to reach a definitive diagnosis and to exclude osteosarcoma. In fact, at times, the only distinguishing features between extraskeletal osteosarcoma and malignant fibrous histiocytoma with malignant osseous metaplasia are the relatively small amounts of neoplastic osteoid and bone in the latter tumor. According to Dorfman and Bhagavan,[109] the presence of the osseous and chondroid elements in the fibrous septa and pseudocapsule favor malignant fibrous histiocytoma. Bane et al.[105] believe that the production of any neoplastic osteoid or bone in a malignant fibrohistiocytic tumor, no matter how focal, warrants a diagnosis of osteosarcoma.

Parosteal osteosarcoma may also make its appearance as a bulky lobulated densely ossified extraosseous mass focally indistinguishable from an extraskeletal osteosarcoma. In most cases this relatively low-grade tumor can be positively identified by its greater overall differentiation, its broad attachment to a thickened cortical bone, and its tendency to encircle the shaft of the bone and cause cortical ero-

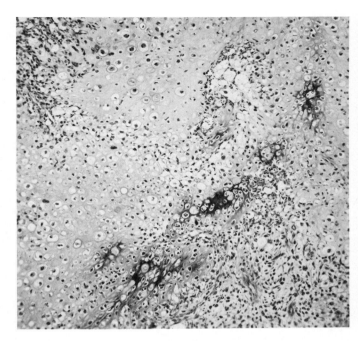

FIG. 36-22. Malignant cartilage formation in extraskeletal osteosarcoma. (×160.)

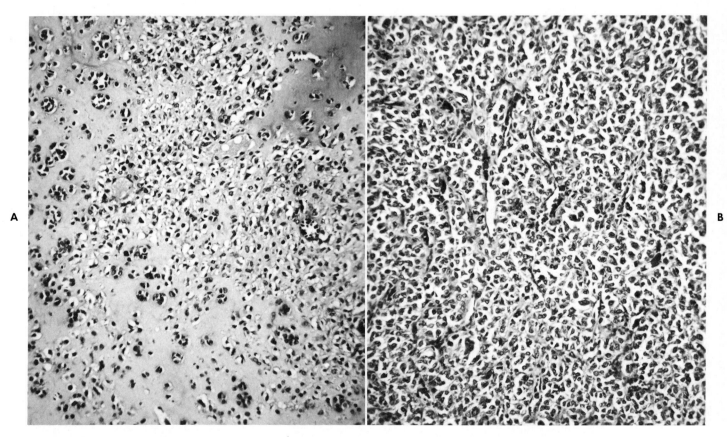

FIG. 36-23. Extraskeletal osteosarcoma with poorly differentiated chondroblastic (A) and osteoblastic (B) areas. (A and B, ×160.)

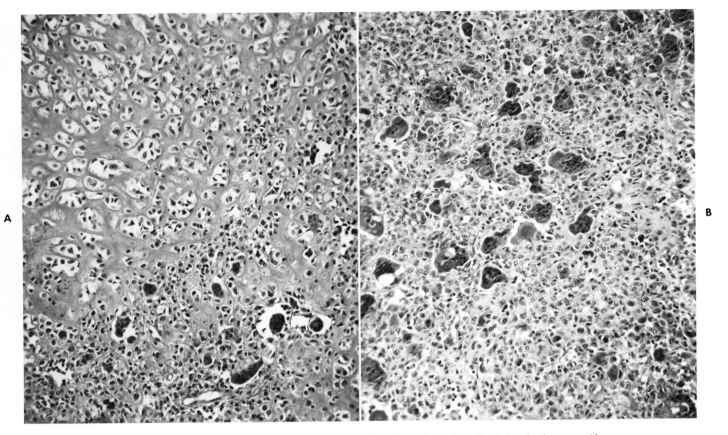

FIG. 36-24. Extraskeletal osteosarcoma. **A,** Focal cartilage formation. **B,** Osteoclastic areas. (**A** and **B,** ×160.)

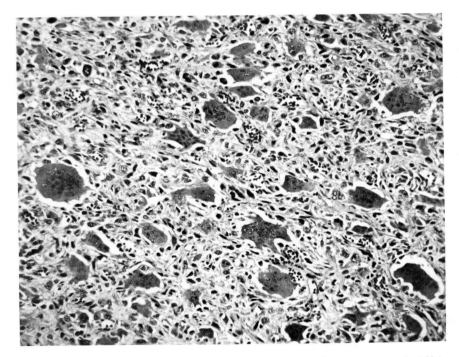

FIG. 36-25. Osteoclast-like giant cells within an extraskeletal osteosarcoma. (×160.)

sion.[117,143,146,149,153] Differential diagnostic considerations must also include periosteal osteogenic sarcoma,[147] a more aggressive and less well-differentiated osteoblastic tumor that is often marked by a prominent chondroblastic component, and the very rare "high-grade surface osteosarcoma."[154]

Prognosis

The outlook is grave and the majority of patients with this tumor succumb to metastatic growth within a period of 2 or 3 years after the initial diagnosis. Thus, in the series reported by Bane et al.,[105] 13 (50%) of 26 tumors recurred locally and 16 (61.5%) metastasized; five patients had distant metastases at presentation. Similarly, in our series of 65 patients with follow-up information, 25 (38.5%) were alive and 40 (61.5%) had died of the tumor, 36 of recurrent or metastatic disease. The most common sites of metastases were the lungs, regional lymph nodes, bone, and soft tissue. Allan and Soule[99] and Rao et al.[142] reported similar discouraging results. Nonetheless, combination therapy, radical surgery (possibly limb-sparing segmental resection as an alternative to amputation), radiotherapy, and sequential preoperative or postoperative chemotherapy should be carried out in the hope of improving survival rates.[125] Computerized assessment of tumor size and variance of nuclei has been used as a yardstick for predicting the response to chemotherapy.[102]

REFERENCES
Myositis ossificans and related lesions

1. Ackerman LV: Extra-osseous localized non-neoplastic bone and cartilage formation (so-called myositis ossificans): clinical and pathological confusion with malignant neoplasms. *J Bone Joint Surg* 40A:279, 1958.
2. Ahrengart L: Periarticular heterotopic ossification after total hip arthroplasty: risk factors and consequences. *Clin Orthop* 263:49, 1991.
3. Alling CC, Martinez MG, Ballard JB, et al: Osteoma cutis. *J Oral Surg* 32:195, 1974.
4. Asa DK, Bertorini TE, Pinals RS: Myositis ossificans circumscripta: a complication of tetanus. *Am J Med Sci* 292:40, 1986.
5. Boyd BM Jr, Roberts WM, Miller GR: Heterotopic bone formation developing in abdominal scars. *Surgery* 47:918, 1960.
6. Carney RG, Radcliffe CE: Multiple miliary osteomas of the skin. *Arch Dermatol Syph* 64:483, 1951.
7. Caulet T, Adnet JJ, Pluot M, et al: Myosite ossificante circonscrite: Edute histochemique et ultrastructurale d'un observation. *Virchows Arch (Pathol Anat)* 348:16, 1969.
8. Chalmers J, Gray DH, Rush J: Observations on the induction of bone in soft tissues. *J Bone Joint Surg* 57B:36, 1975.
9. Chaplin DM, Harrison MHM: Pseudomalignant osseous tumor of soft tissue: report of two cases. *J Bone Joint Surg* 54B:334, 1972.
10. Constance TJ: Localized myositis ossificans. *J Pathol Bacteriol* 68:381, 1954.
11. Costello FV, Brown A: Myositis ossificans complicating anterior poliomyelitis. *J Bone Joint Surg* 33B:594, 1951.
12. Dahl I, Angervall L: Pseudosarcomatous lesions of the soft tissue reported as sarcoma during a 6-year period, 1958-1963. *Acta Pathol Microbiol Scand* 85A:917, 1977.
13. Dahl I, Angervall L: Pseudosarcomatous proliferative lesions of soft tissue with or without bone formation. *Acta Pathol Microbiol Scand* 85A:577, 1977.
14. Davies CWT: Bizarre parosteal osteochondromatous proliferation in the hand: a case report. *J Bone Joint Surg* 67A:648, 1985.
15. De Smet AA, Norris MA, Fisher DR: Magnetic resonance imaging of myositis ossificans: analysis of seven cases. *Skeletal Radiol* 21:503, 1992.
16. De Smet L, Vercauteren M: Fast-growing pseudomalignant osseous tumor (myositis ossificans) of the finger: a case report. *J Hand Surg* 9:93, 1984.
17. Everett FG, Fixott HC Jr: Multiple miliary subdermal osteoma: report of a case. *Oral Surg Oral Med Oral Pathol* 24:670, 1967.
18. Fawcett HA: Hereditary osteoma cutis. *J R Soc Med* 76:697, 1983.
19. Freiberg JA: Para-articular calcification and ossification following acute anterior poliomyelitis in an adult. *J Bone Joint Surg* 34A:339, 1952.
20. Goodsell JO: Traumatic myositis ossificans of the masseter muscle: review of the literature and report of a case. *Br J Oral Surg* 2:137, 1964.
21. Hardy AG, Dickson JW: Pathological ossification in traumatic paraplegia. *J Bone Joint Surg* 45B:76, 1963.
22. Hess WE: Myositis ossificans occurring in poliomyelitis. *Arch Neurol Psychiat* 66:606, 1951.
23. Hutcheson J, Klatte EC, Kremp R: The angiographic appearance of myositis ossificans circumscripta: a case report. *Radiology* 102:57, 1972.
24. Huvos AG: The spontaneous transformation of benign into malignant soft tissue tumors (with emphasis on extraskeletal osseous, lipomatous, and schwannian lesions). *Am J Surg Pathol (suppl)* 9:7, 1985.
25. Ivey M: Myositis ossificans of the thigh following manipulation of the knee: a case report. *Clin Orthop* 198:102, 1985.
26. Järvi OH, Kvist HTA, Vainio PV: Extraskeletal retroperitoneal osteosarcoma probably arising from myositis ossificans. *Acta Pathol Microbiol Scand* 74:11, 1968.
27. Jeffreys TE, Stiles PJ: Pseudomalignant osseous tumor of soft tissue. *J Bone Joint Surg* 48B:488, 1966.
28. Johnson JTH: Atypical myositis ossificans. *J Bone Joint Surg* 39A:189, 1957.
29. Johnson LC: Histogenesis of myositis ossificans. *Am J Pathol* 24:681, 1948.
30. Johnson MK, Lawrence JF: Metaplastic bone formation (myositis ossificans) in the soft tissues of the hand. *J Bone Joint Surg* 57A:999, 1975.
31. Kransdorf MJ, Meis JM: Extraskeletal osseous and cartilaginous tumors of the extremities. *RadioGraphics* 13:853, 1993.
32. Kransdorf MJ, Meis JM, Jelinek JS: Myositis ossificans: MR appearance with radiologic-pathologic correlation. *Am J Roentgenol* 157:1243, 1991.
33. Krolls SI, Jacoway JR, Alexander WN: Osseous choristomas (osteomas) of intraoral soft tissues. *Oral Surg Oral Med Oral Pathol* 32:588, 1971.
34. Kütner H: Die Myositis Ossificans Circumscripta. *Erg Chir Orthop* 1:49, 1910.
35. Kwitken J, Branche M: Fasciitis ossificans. *Am J Clin Pathol* 51:251, 1969.
36. Lagier R, Cox JN: Pseudomalignant myositis ossificans. *Hum Pathol* 6:653, 1975.

37. Landois F: Über Knorpel und Knochengeschwülste der Muskulatur. *Virchows Arch (Pathol Anat)* 229:101, 1921.

38. Lehrman A, Pratt JH, Parkhill EM: Heterotopic bone in laparotomy scars. *Am J Surg* 104:591, 1962.

39. Lewis D: Myositis ossificans. *JAMA* 80:1281, 1923.

40. Mallory TB: A group of metaplastic and neoplastic bone and cartilage containing tumors of soft parts. *Am J Pathol* 9:765, 1935.

41. Marteinsson B, Musgrove J: Heterotopic bone formation in abdominal incisions. *Am J Surg* 130:23, 1975.

42. Miller LF, O'Neill C: Myositis ossificans in paraplegics. *J Bone Joint Surg* 31A:283, 1949.

43. Mitra M, Sen AK, Deb HK: Myositis ossificans traumatica: a complication of tetanus: report of a case and review of the literature. *J Bone Joint Surg* 58A:885, 1976.

44. Nora FE, Dahlin DC, Beabout JW: Bizarre parosteal osteochondromatous proliferation of the hands and feet. *Am J Surg Pathol* 7:245, 1983.

45. Norman A, Dorfman HD: Juxtacortical circumscribed myositis ossificans: evolution and radiographic features. *Radiology* 96:301, 1970.

46. Nuovo MA, Norman A, Chumas J, et al: Myositis ossificans with atypical clinical, radiographic, or pathologic findings: a review of 23 cases. *Skeletal Radiol* 21:87, 1992.

47. Ogilvie-Harris DJ, Fornasier VL: Pseudomalignant myositis ossificans: heterotopic new-bone formation without a history of trauma. *J Bone Joint Surg* 62A:1274, 1980.

48. Pack GT, Braund RR: Development of sarcoma in myositis ossificans. *JAMA* 119:776, 1942.

49. Paterson DC: Myositis ossificans circumscripta: report of four cases without history of injury. *J Bone Joint Surg* 52B:296, 1970.

50. Povysil C, Matejovsky Z: Ultrastructural evidence of myofibroblasts in pseudomalignant myositis ossificans. *Virchows Arch (Pathol Anat)* 381:189, 1979.

51. Reiman HM, Dahlin DC: Cartilage- and bone-forming tumors of the soft tissues. *Semin Diagn Pathol* 3:288, 1986.

52. Roth SI, Stowell RE, Helwig EB: Cutaneous ossification: report of 120 cases and review of the literature. *Arch Pathol* 76:44, 1963.

53. Rothberg AS: Tendinitis ossificans traumatica. *Am J Surg* 58:285, 1942.

54. Samuelson KM, Coleman SS: Nontraumatic myositis ossificans in healthy individuals. *JAMA* 235:1133, 1976.

55. Shanoff LB, Spira M, Hardy S: Myositis ossificans: evolution to osteogenic sarcoma. *Am J Surg* 113:537, 1967.

56. Skajaa T: Myositis ossificans traumatica. *Acta Chir Scand* 116:68, 1958.

57. Sumiyoshi K, Tsuneyoshi M, Enjoji M: Myositis ossificans: a clinicopathologic study of 21 cases. *Acta Pathol Jpn* 35:1109, 1985.

58. Wilhelmsen HR, Bereston ES: Treatment of osteoma cutis. *Cutis* 33:481, 1984.

59. Wittenberg RH, Peschke U, Botel U: Heterotopic ossification after spinal cord injury: epidemiology and risk factors. *J Bone Joint Surg* 74B:215, 1992.

60. Yagmai I: Myositis ossificans: diagnostic value of arteriography. *Am J Roentgenol* 128:811, 1977.

61. Youssef L, Schmidt TL: Battered child syndrome simulating myositis. *J Pediatr Orthop* 3:392, 1983.

Fibroosseous pseudotumor of the digits

62. Angervall L, Stener B, Stener I, et al: Pseudomalignant osseous tumor of soft tissue. *J Bone Joint Surg* 51B:654, 1969.

63. Carpenter EB, Lubin B: An unusual osteogenic lesion of a finger. *J Bone Joint Surg* 49A:527, 1967.

64. Chan KW, Khoo US, Ho CM: Fibroosseous pseudotumor of the digits: report of a case with immunohistochemical and ultrastructural studies. *Pathology* 25:193, 1993.

65. Dupree WB, Enzinger FM: Fibroosseous pseudotumor of the digits. *Cancer* 58:2103, 1986.

66. Kovach JC, Truong L, Kearns RJ, et al: Florid reactive periostitis. *J Hand Surg* 11:902, 1986.

67. McCarthy EF, Ireland DCR, Sprague BL, et al: Parosteal (nodular) fasciitis of the hand. *J Bone Joint Surg* 58A:714, 1976.

68. Nance KV, Renner JB, Brashear HR, et al: Massive florid reactive periostitis. *Pediatr Radiol* 20:186, 1990.

69. Spjut HJ, Dorfman HD: Florid reactive periostitis of the tubular bones of the hands and feet: a benign lesion which may simulate osteosarcoma. *Am J Surg Pathol* 5:423, 1981.

Fibrodysplasia (myositis) ossificans progressiva

70. Bronsky D, Kushner DS, Dubin A, et al: Idiopathic hypoparathyroidism and pseudohypoparathyroidism: case report and review of the literature. *Medicine* 27:317, 1958.

71. Caron KH, DiPietro MA, Aisen AM, et al: MR imaging of early fibrodysplasia ossificans progressiva. *J Comput Assist Tomogr* 14:318, 1990.

72. Cohen RB, Hahn GV, Tabas JA, et al: The natural history of heterotopic ossification in patients who have fibrodysplasia ossificans progressiva: a study of forty-four patients. *J Bone Joint Surg* 75A:215, 1993.

73. Connor JM, Evans DAP: Fibrodysplasia ossificans progressiva: the clinical features and natural history of 34 patients. *J Bone Joint Surg* 64A:76, 1982.

74. Connor JM, Evans DAP: Genetic aspects of fibrodysplasia ossificans progressiva. *J Med Genet* 19:35, 1982.

75. Connor JM, Skirton H, Lunt PW: A three-generation family with fibrodysplasia ossificans progressiva. *J Med Genet* 30:687, 1993.

76. Cramer SF, Ruehl A, Mandel MA: Fibrodysplasia ossificans progressiva: a distinctive bone-forming lesion of the soft tissue. *Cancer* 48:1016, 1981.

77. Dixon TF, Mulligan L, Nassim R, et al: Myositis ossificans progressiva: report of a case in which ACTH and cortisone failed to prevent reossification after excision of ectopic bone. *J Bone Joint Surg* 36B:445, 1954.

78. Dobrzaniecki W: The problem of myositis ossificans progressiva. *Ann Surg* 104:987, 1936.

79. Eaton WL, Conkling WS, Daeschner CW: Early myositis ossificans progressiva occurring in homozygotic twins: a clinical and pathological study. *J Pediatr* 50:591, 1957.

80. Illingworth RS: Myositis ossificans progressiva (Münchmeyer's disease). *Arch Dis Child* 46:264, 1971.

81. Kaplan FS, McCluskey W, Hahn G, et al: Genetic transmission of fibrodysplasia ossificans progressiva: report of a family. *J Bone Joint Surg* 75A:1214, 1993.

82. Kaplan FS, Tabas JA, Gannon FH, et al: The histopathology of fibrodysplasia ossificans progressiva: an enchondral process. *J Bone Joint Surg* 75A:220, 1993.

83. Kuebler E: Neue Gesichtspunkte bei der Beurteilung der Verlaufsformen der Myositis ossificans progressiva. *Fortschr Roentgenstrahlen* 8:354, 1954.

84. Lutwak L: Myositis ossificans progressiva: mineral, metabolic and radioactive calcium studies of the effect of hormones. *Am J Med* 37:269, 1964.

85. Maxwell WA, Spicer SS, Miller RL, et al: Histochemical and ultrastructural studies in fibrodysplasia ossificans progressiva (myositis ossificans progressiva). *Am J Pathol* 87:483, 1977.

86. McFarland GS, Robinowitz B, Say B: Fibrodysplasia ossificans progressiva presenting as fibrous scalp nodules. *Cleve Clin Q* 51:549, 1984.

87. McKusick VA: Fibrodysplasia ossificans progressiva. In *Heritable disorders of connective tissue*, ed 4, St. Louis, 1972, C.V. Mosby Co.

88. Münchmeyer E: Ueber die Myositis ossificans progressiva. *Z Rationelle Medizin* 34:9, 1869.

89. Reinig JW, Hill SC, Fang M, et al: Fibrodysplasia ossificans progressiva: CT appearance. *Radiology* 159:153, 1986.

90. Rogers JG, Dorst JP: Use and complications of high-dose disodium etidronate therapy in fibrodysplasia ossificans progressiva. *J Pediatr* 91:1011, 1977.

91. Rogers JG, Geho WB: Fibrodysplasia ossificans progressiva: a survey of 42 cases. *J Bone Joint Surg* 61A:909, 1979.

92. Rosborough D: Ectopic bone formation associated with multiple anomalies. *J Bone Joint Surg* 48B:499, 1966.

93. Ryan KJ: Myositis ossificans progressiva: a review of the literature with a report of a case. *J Pediatr* 27:348, 1945.

94. Schroeder HW, Zasloff M: The hand and foot malformations in fibrodysplasia ossificans progressiva. *Johns Hopkins Med J* 147:73, 1980.

95. Smith DM, Zeman W, Johnston CC Jr, et al: Myositis ossificans progressiva: case report with metabolic and histochemical studies. *Metabolism* 15:521, 1966.

96. Smith R, Russell GG, Woods CG: Myositis ossificans progressiva: clinical features of eight patients and their response to treatment. *J Bone Joint Surg* 58B:48, 1976.

97. Thickman D, Bonakdar-pour A, Clancy M, et al: Fibrodysplasia ossificans progressiva. *Am J Roentgenol* 139:935, 1982.

98. Young JW: Case report 314: diagnosis: juvenile dermatomyositis with changes of the hallux typical of fibrodysplasia (myositis) ossificans progressiva. *Skeletal Radiol* 13:318, 1985.

Extraskeletal osteosarcoma

99. Allan CJ, Soule EH: Osteogenic sarcoma of the somatic soft tissues: clinicopathologic study of 26 cases and review of the literature. *Cancer* 27:1121, 1971.

100. Alpert LI, Abaci IF, Werthamer S: Radiation-induced extraskeletal osteosarcoma. *Cancer* 31:1359, 1973.

101. Anani PA, Baumann RP: Osteosarcoma of the breast. *Virchows Arch (Pathol Anat)* 357:213, 1972.

102. Apel R, Delling H, Krumme H, et al: Nuclear polymorphism in osteosarcomas as a prognostic factor for the effect of chemotherapy. *Virchows Arch (Pathol Anat)* 405:215, 1985.

103. Ascenzi A, Casagrande A, Ribotta G: On radiation-induced extraskeletal osteosarcoma: report of a case. *Tumori* 66:261, 1980.

104. Auerbach O, Friedman M, Weiss L, et al: Extraskeletal osteogenic sarcoma arising in irradiated tissue. *Cancer* 4:1095, 1951.

105. Bane BL, Evans HL, Ro JY, et al: Extraskeletal osteosarcoma: a clinicopathologic review of 26 cases. *Cancer* 65:2726, 1990.

106. Belasco JB, Meadoves AC: Extraskeletal osteogenic sarcoma after treatment of Wilms' tumors. *Cancer* 50:1894, 1982.

107. Berenson RJ, Flynn S, Freiha FS: Primary osteogenic sarcoma of the bladder. *Cancer* 57:350, 1986.

108. Berry MP, Jenkin RD, Fornasier VL, et al: Osteosarcoma at the site of previous fracture: a case report. *J Bone Joint Surg* 62A:1216, 1980.

109. Bhagavan BS, Dorfman HD: The significance of bone and cartilage formation in malignant fibrous histiocytoma of soft tissue. *Cancer* 49:480, 1982.

110. Binkley JS, Stewart FW: Morphogenesis of extraskeletal osteogenic sarcoma and pseudosarcoma. *Arch Pathol* 29:42, 1940.

111. Boyer CW, Navin JJ: Extraskeletal osteogenic sarcoma: a late complication of radiation therapy. *Cancer* 18:628, 1965.

112. Catanese J, Dutcher JP, Dorfman HD, et al: Mediastinal osteosarcoma with extension to lungs in a patient treated for Hodgkin's disease. *Cancer* 62:2252, 1988.

113. Chung EB, Enzinger FM: Extraskeletal osteosarcoma. *Cancer* 60:1132, 1987.

114. Dahm LJ, Schaefer SD, Carder HM, et al: Osteosarcoma of the soft tissue of the larynx: report of a case with light and electron microscopic studies. *Cancer* 42:2343, 1978.

115. Das Gupta TK, Hajdu SI, Foote FW Jr: Extraosseous osteogenic sarcoma. *Ann Surg* 168:1011, 1968.

116. Dorfman HD, Bhagavan BS: Malignant fibrous histiocytoma of soft tissue with metaplastic bone and cartilage formation. *Skeletal Radiol* 8:45, 1982.

117. Dwinnell LA, Dahlin DC, Ghormley RK: Parosteal (juxtacortical) osteogenic sarcoma. *J Bone Joint Surg* 36A:732, 1954.

118. Eckardt JJ, Ivins JC, Perry HO, et al: Osteosarcoma arising in heterotopic ossification of dermatomyositis: case report and review of the literature. *Cancer* 48:1256, 1981.

119. Fine G, Stout AP: Osteogenic sarcoma of the extraskeletal soft tissues. *Cancer* 9:1027, 1956.

120. Ghadially FN, Mehta PN: Ultrastructure of osteogenic sarcoma. *Cancer* 25:1457, 1970.

121. Gonzalez-Licea A, Yardley JH, Hartmann WH: Malignant tumor of the breast with bone formation: studies by light and electron-microscopy. *Cancer* 20:1234, 1967.

122. Hasson J, Hartman KS, Milikow E, et al: Thorotrast-induced extraskeletal osteosarcoma of the cervical region: report of a case. *Cancer* 36:1827, 1975.

123. Hatfield PM, Schulz MD: Postirradiation sarcoma, including five cases after x-ray therapy of breast carcinoma. *Radiology* 96:593, 1970.

124. Huvos AG: Osteogenic sarcoma of bones and soft tissues in older persons: a clinicopathologic analysis of 117 patients older than 60 years. *Cancer* 57:1442, 1986.

125. Jaffe N, Robertson R, Takaue T, et al: Control of primary osteosarcoma with chemotherapy. *Cancer* 56:461, 1985.

126. Järvi OH, Kvist HTA, Vainio PV: Extraskeletal retroperitoneal osteosarcoma probably arising from myositis ossificans. *Acta Pathol Microbiol Scand* 74:11, 1968.

127. Kahn L, Wood F, Ackerman L: Fracture callus associated with benign and malignant bone lesions and mimicking osteosarcoma. *Am J Clin Pathol* 52:14, 1969.

128. Katenkamp D, Stiller D, Waldmann G: Ultrastructural cytology of human osteosarcoma cells. *Virchows Arch (Pathol Anat)* 381:49, 1978.

129. Kauffman SL, Stout AP: Extraskeletal osteogenic sarcomas and chondrosarcomas in children. *Cancer* 16:432, 1963.

130. Laskin WB, Silverman TA, Enzinger FM: Postradiation soft tissue sarcomas: an analysis of 52 cases. *Cancer* 62:2330, 1988.

131. Lee JH, Griffiths WJ, Bottomley RH: Extraosseous osteogenic sarcoma following an intramuscular injection. *Cancer* 40:3097, 1977.

132. Lee WR, Laurie J, Townsend AL: Fine structure of a radiation-induced osteogenic sarcoma. *Cancer* 36:1414, 1975.

133. Lewis RJ, Lotz MJ, Beazley RM: Extraosseous osteosarcoma. *Am Surg* 40:597, 1974.

134. Lorentzon R, Larsson SE, Boquist L: Extra-osseous osteosarcoma: a clinical and histopathological study of four cases. *J Bone Joint Surg* 61B:205, 1979.

135. Martland HS: Occupational poisoning in manufacture of luminal watch dials. *JAMA* 92:466, 1929.

136. Mayer L, Friedman M: Extraskeletal bone-forming tumor of the fascia, resembling osteogenic sarcoma. *Bull Hosp Joint Dis* 2:187, 1941.

137. Meister P, Konrad EA, Stotz S: Extraskeletal osteosarcoma: case report and differential diagnosis. *Arch Orthop Trauma Surg* 98:311, 1981.

138. Niebrugge D, Monzon C, Perry MC, et al: Osteogenic sarcoma following Hodgkin's disease. *Cancer* 48:416, 1981.

139. Paik HH, Wilkinson EJ: Peritoneal osteosarcoma following irradiation therapy of ovarian cancer. *Obstet Gynecol* 47:488, 1976.

140. Pearson KD, Rubin D, Szemes GC, et al: Extraosseous osteogenic sarcoma of the chest. *Br J Dis Chest* 63:231, 1969.

141. Rachman R, Di Massa EV: Pelvis extraskeletal osteosarcoma associated with prostatic adenocarcinoma. *Am J Clin Pathol* 44:556, 1965.

142. Rao U, Cheng A, Didolkar MS: Extraosseous osteogenic sarcoma: clinicopathologic study of eight cases and review of literature. *Cancer* 41:1488, 1978.

143. Reddick RL, Popovsky MA, Fantone JC, et al: Parosteal osteogenic sarcoma: ultrastructural observations in three cases. *Hum Pathol* 11:373, 1980.

144. Sordillo PP, Hajdu SI, Magill GB, et al: Extraosseous osteogenic sarcoma: a review of 48 patients. *Cancer* 51:727, 1983.

145. Tortora MJ, Aseltine DT Jr, Demaio JT, et al: Primary retroperitoneal extraosseous osteogenic sarcoma: a case report and review of the literature. *Am Surg* 43:755, 1977.

146. Unni KK, Dahlin DC, Beabout JW, et al: Parosteal osteogenic sarcoma. *Cancer* 37:2644, 1976.

147. Unni KK, Dahlin DC, Beabout JW, et al: Periosteal osteogenic sarcoma. *Cancer* 37:2476, 1976.

148. Valderrama E, Kahn LB, Wind E: Extraskeletal osteosarcoma arising in an ectopic hamartomatous thymus: report of a case and review of the literature. *Cancer* 51:132, 1983.

149. Van Der Heut RO, Von Ronnen JR: Juxtacortical osteosarcoma: diagnosis, differential diagnosis, treatment, and an analysis of 80 cases. *J Bone Joint Surg* 49A:415, 1967.

150. Varela-Duran J, Dehner LP: Postirradiation osteosarcoma in childhood: a clinicopathologic study of three cases and review of the literature. *Am J Pediatr Hematol Oncol* 2:263, 1980.

151. Waxman M, Vuletin JC, Saxe BI, et al: Extraskeletal osteosarcoma: light and electron microscopic study. *Mt Sinai J Med* 48:322, 1981.

152. Williams AH, Schwinn CP, Parker JW: The ultrastructure of osteosarcoma: a review of 20 cases. *Cancer* 37:1293, 1976.

153. Wold LE, Unni KK, Beabout JW, et al: Dedifferentiated parosteal osteosarcoma. *J Bone Joint Surg* 66A:53, 1984.

154. Wold LE, Unni KK, Beabout JW, et al: High-grade surface osteosarcomas. *Am J Surg Pathol* 8:181, 1984.

155. Wurlitzer F, Ayala A, Romsdahl M: Extraosseous osteogenic sarcoma. *Arch Surg* 105:691, 1972.

156. Yi ES, Shmookler BM, Malaver MM, et al: Well-differentiated extraskeletal osteosarcoma: a soft-tissue homologue of parosteal osteosarcoma. *Arch Pathol Lab Med* 115:906, 1991.

157. Young RH, Rosenberg AE: Osteosarcoma of the urinary bladder: report of a case and review of the literature. *Cancer* 59:174, 1987.

CHAPTER 37

BENIGN SOFT TISSUE TUMORS
OF UNCERTAIN TYPE

TUMORAL CALCINOSIS

Tumoral calcinosis is a distinct clinical and histological entity that is characterized by tumorlike periarticular deposits of calcium that are found foremost in the regions of the hip, shoulder, and elbow. The disorder occurs predominantly in otherwise healthy children, adolescents, and young adults, is more often multiple than solitary, and not infrequently affects two or more siblings of the same family. Unlike similar calcifications associated with renal insufficiency, hypervitaminosis D, and milk-alkali syndrome, there are no demonstrable abnormalities in calcium metabolism. Hyperphosphatemia, however, is present in many of the cases.

The term *tumoral calcinosis* was coined by Inclan[16] in 1943, but this condition was recognized as an entity much earlier. In 1899 Duret[12] observed this process in siblings: a 17-year-old girl and her younger brother who had multiple calcifications in the neighborhood of the hip and elbow joint. Later, in 1935, Teutschlaender[44] gave a detailed account of another typical case, an 11-year-old girl with multiple lesions in the shoulder and elbow regions, which had their onset at age 2 years. He thought that this process was secondary to fat necrosis and used the term "lipid calcinosis."[46] Since these descriptions, almost 100 acceptable examples of this growth have been reported under various names, mostly as tumoral calcinosis, but also as calcifying bursitis,[9-11,13] calcifying collagenolysis,[50] and Kikuyu bursa.[28] In New Guinea the natives aptly refer to it as "hip stones."[5,30,35] Among the reported cases, the majority of patients are African or American blacks.

Clinical findings

The principal manifestation of the disease is the presence of a large, firm, subcutaneous calcified mass that is asymptomatic and slowly growing, often gradually enlarging over many years; it is usually located in the vicinity of a large joint, especially the trochanteric and gluteal regions of the hip, the lateral portion of the shoulder, and the posterior elbow. It is less frequent in the hands, feet, and knees. The lesion is firmly attached to the underlying fascia, muscle, or tendon and may infiltrate these structures but is unrelated to bone. Approximately two thirds of patients have multiple lesions, some of which are bilateral and symmetrical. The mass is usually asymptomatic and only rarely causes discomfort, tenderness, or pain. The underlying joints are unaffected, and with few exceptions the patients with tumoral calcinosis are in good health. In fact, smaller and more deep-seated lesions are frequently overlooked and are often incidental findings during examination for some other cause. Large lesions, measuring 20 cm or more in diameter, are not particularly rare.[57] Association with calcifying skin lesions, dental abnormalities, and angioid retinal streaks has been reported.[3,26,41,54]

Tumoral calcinosis has its onset during the first and second decades of life, and is rare in patients older than 50 years. Males outnumber females by a narrow margin; yet elderly patients and females were mainly affected in a report of tumoral calcinosis from Somalia and Ethiopia.[18] Approximately two thirds of cases involve blacks. About half affect siblings, and in some instances several generations of the same family are involved.[41] Complications of the disease are rare. In some instances there is ulceration of the overlying skin with secondary infection, fistula formation, and discharge of a yellow-white chalky fluid.[36,57] There is no association with scleroderma or other collagen diseases such as calcinosis circumscripta and calcinosis universalis.

Laboratory examinations show no evidence of increased calcium levels, but in many patients there is slight to moderate hyperphosphatemia.[15,41,55] Calcitriol (1,25-dihydroxyvitamin D_3) may also be elevated, but serum alkaline phosphatase and uric acid levels are normal.

Roentgenological findings

Examination with radiographs or CT scan reveals a subcutaneous conglomerate of multiple, rounded opacities separated by radiolucent lines (fibrous septa)[2,6,20] (Figs. 37-1

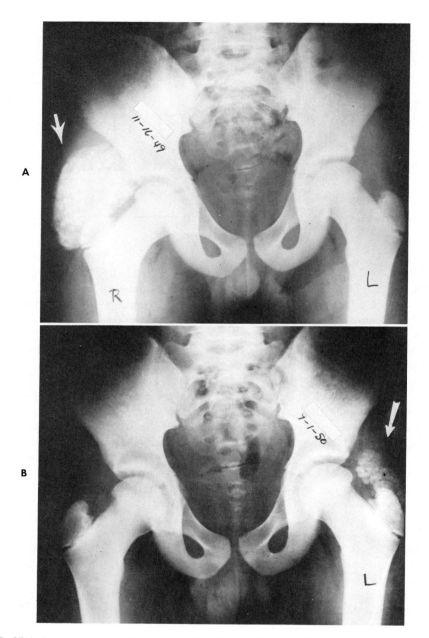

FIG. 37-1. Roentgenograph of tumoral calcinosis involving the soft tissues of both hips *(arrows)*. Nine months after the calcified mass in the right hip **(A)** was removed, a second mass developed in the left hip **(B)**.

and 37-2, *A*), with distinct fluid levels in some of the nodules.[22] There are no associated bony abnormalities, and despite the large amounts of calcium in the lesion, there is no evidence of osteoporosis in the skeleton, as in patients with renal insufficiency and secondary hyperparathyroidism. Scintigraphic examination is useful, especially in the identification of multiple lesions and assessment of therapy.[6] For instance, all of the seven patients reported by Balachan-

dran et al.[1] displayed abnormal scintigrams with increased tracer concentration.

Pathological findings

Study of the gross specimen discloses a firm rubbery mass that is unencapsulated, extends into the adjacent muscles and tendons, and usually ranges from 5 cm to 15 cm in greatest diameter. On sectioning, the mass consists of a

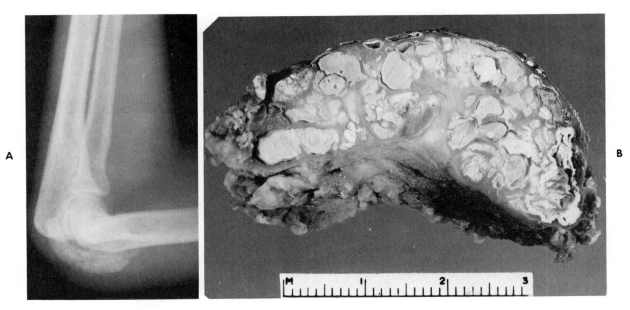

FIG. 37-2. Tumoral calcinosis occurring in the right elbow region of an 18-year-old man. **A,** Radiograph showing calcified mass in the elbow region. **B,** Cross-section of tumor revealing a conglomerate of calcified masses surrounded by dense collagenous tissue.

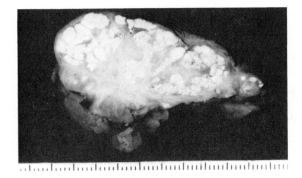

FIG. 37-3. Cross-section of tumor calcinosis of the right thigh showing multilocular calcification of densely collagenous tissue.

framework of dense fibrous tissue containing spaces filled with yellow-gray, pasty, calcareous material or chalky, milky liquid that is easily washed out, resulting in irregular cystic cavities (Figs. 37-2, *B*, and 37-3). Chemical analysis of the intra- and extracellular calcified material reveals hydroxyapatite.[6,41]

Microscopically, active and inactive phases of the disease can be distinguished, often together in the same lesion. In the active phase a central mass of amorphous or granular calcified material is bordered by a florid proliferation of mono- or multinuclear macrophages, osteoclast-like giant cells, fibroblasts, and chronic inflammatory elements (Figs. 37-4 to 37-6). In the inactive phase there is

merely calcified material surrounded by dense fibrous material extending into the adjacent tissues or a cystic space surrounded by calcium deposits (Fig. 37-7). Sometimes the calcified material forms small psammoma body–like masses with concentric layering of calcium (calcospherites) that bear a superficial resemblance to ova of parasites (Fig. 37-8). Examination with the electron microscope reveals histiocytes with and without lipid inclusions and osteoclast-like elements with multiple vacuoles containing needle-shaped hydroxyapatite crystals, crystalline aggregates with a dense central core, and laminated calcospherites.[20,24,41]

Differential diagnosis

Morphologically, identical periarticular lesions may be encountered in patients with chronic renal disease and secondary hyperparathyroidism,[17,37] but most of the patients with these lesions are older than those with tumoral calcinosis, have additional calcifications in visceral organs such as the kidney, lung, heart, and stomach, and have abnormally low calcium levels. There are also tumoral calcinosis–like lesions and vascular calcifications associated with hyperphosphatemia in patients with end-stage renal disease undergoing hemodialysis.[21,23,31,43] Similar calcifying soft tissue lesions, but associated with hypercalcemia, occur in patients with hypervitaminosis D,[4,56] hyperparathyroidism, and milk-alkali syndrome (Burnett's syndrome),[40] a rare condition associated with prolonged antacid therapy for peptic ulcer, and in patients with excessive osteolysis and mobilization of calcium in destructive neoplastic and infec-

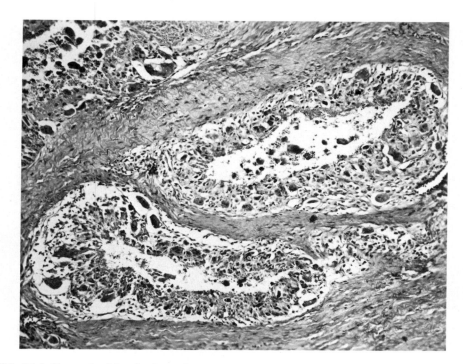

FIG. 37-4. Tumoral calcinosis. Amorphous calcified material bordered by a florid proliferation of macrophages and multinucleated, osteoclast-like giant cells. (×100.)

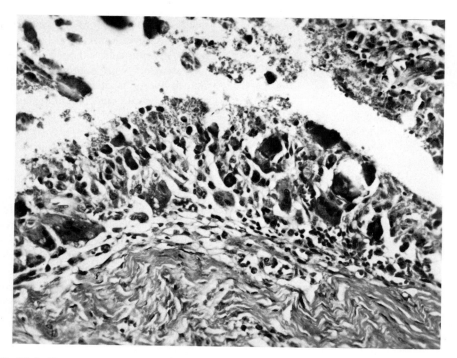

FIG. 37-5. Tumoral calcinosis showing characteristic mixture of calcified material, histiocytes, and multinucleated giant cells. (×250.)

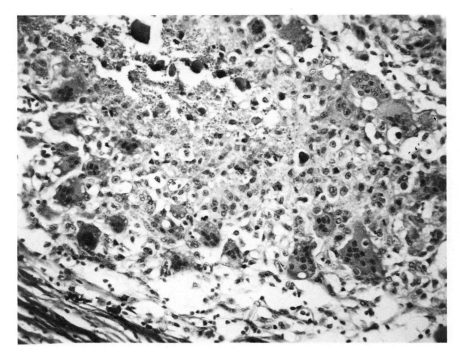

FIG. 37-6. Active phase of tumoral calcinosis composed of calcified material surrounded by histiocytes and osteoclast-like giant cells. (×160.)

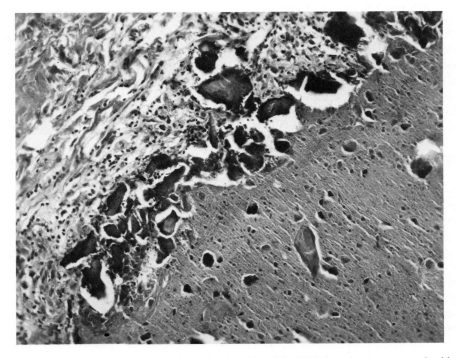

FIG. 37-7. Inactive phase of tumoral calcinosis with minimal histiocytic response and without multinucleated giant cells. (×160.)

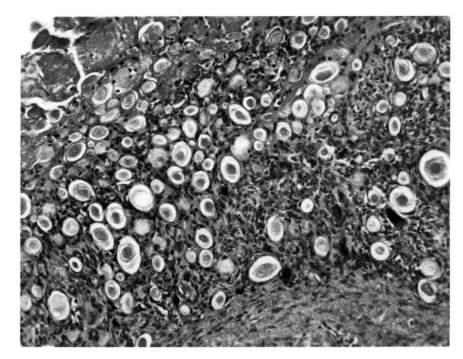

FIG. 37-8. Variant of tumoral calcinosis with numerous calcospherites simulating a parasitic infection. (×160.)

tious lesions of bone.[17] In all of these lesions a detailed clinical history will aid in reaching a reliable diagnosis.

Calcinosis universalis and calcinosis circumscripta likewise are located in the skin and subcutis and show normal serum calcium and phosphorus levels. Calcinosis universalis forms multiple nodules or plaques that occur mainly in children and are associated in about half of the cases with the manifestations of scleroderma or dermatomyositis. It may ultimately lead to limited mobility, contractures, and ankylosis. Calcinosis circumscripta, on the other hand, chiefly affects middle-aged women and most commonly involves the hand and wrist, including tendon sheaths. It is associated in a high percentage of cases with Raynaud's disease or scleroderma, sclerodactyly, or polymyositis.[19,34,53] In one such case secondary infection led to a severe and fatal amyloidosis.[53] The CREST syndrome is a related condition involving *c*alcinosis cutis, *R*aynaud's phenomenon, *e*sophageal hypomotility, *s*clerodactyly, and *t*elangiectasis.

There are also dystrophic calcifications, as in calcareous tendinitis, that show an identical microscopic picture, but are smaller, and develop in damaged tissue secondary to minor injury, ischemic necrosis, or a necrotizing infectious process.[38] Calcifications of tendons and ligaments have also been reported in patients receiving long-term etretinate therapy, a synthetic vitamin A derivative prescribed for acne, psoriasis, and various disorders of keratinization.[11] Other

forms of calcifications, such as those of the scrotal skin, are not uncommon, but the exact cause is still not clear.[29,48]

Discussion

Tumoral calcinosis is an inborn error in calcium metabolism that is inherited according to a dominant or recessive pattern.[26] Laboratory studies reveal normal calcium levels, but in many cases there is elevation of serum phosphorus levels, probably as the result of increased tubular reabsorption or reduced renal excretion of phosphorus. Calcitriol (1,25-dihydroxyvitamin D_3) levels are also increased in some of the patients.[27,32,42] Slavin et al.[41] and others[1,2,10,39] described a family in which 7 of 13 siblings developed tumoral calcinosis; all 7 had hyperphosphatemia and normocalcemia; 1 had increased phosphorus levels prior to the onset of the calcification; phosphorus levels, however, were normal in the remaining 6 siblings without calcifications. Carey et al.[8] reported massive calcification during phosphate treatment of hypercalcemia.

Trauma is rarely reported by patients with tumoral calcinosis, but minor repeated trauma and tissue injury seem to play a role in the calcifying process; it probably serves as a trigger mechanism that leads to a chain of events, beginning with hemorrhage, fat necrosis, fibrosis, and collagenization and ending with collagenolysis and ultimately massive calcification. Thomson[50] and others,[28,30] who observed tumoral calcinosis in African blacks, thought that in their patients the pressure of sleeping on the hard ground may explain the principal sites of calcification. Although collagenolyis may result in bursalike lesions there is no convincing histological evidence that this process ever originates in a true bursa.

Prognosis

The treatment of choice is surgical removal of the lesion as early as possible, when the lesion is still small and amenable to total resection. Incomplete excision may lead to recurrence, secondary infection, or abscess formation. Treatment with radiation or cortisone is largely ineffective.[24,34] Calcium deprivation and PO_4—binding antacids have been effectively employed as an alternative mode of therapy.[1,32,33] Others, however, report no response to a low-phosphorus diet and oral aluminum hydroxide gel.[42] Scintigrams are helpful in assessing the extent of the disease and the results of therapy.[1]

INTRAMUSCULAR MYXOMA

Although there are only a few reports of this entity in the earlier literature,[81,82] numerous examples of this growth have been reported during the last 30 years, including our 1964 report of 34 cases of this entity.[62,68,69] All reviewers agree that awareness of this entity is of particular importance because this lesion, which has no tendency toward recurrence and is cured by local excision, is easily mistaken for a sarcoma, especially myxoid liposarcoma and botryoid-type rhabdomyosarcoma.

Clinical findings

Intramuscular myxoma is a tumor of adult life that occurs primarily in patients between 40 and 70 years of age. In our experience it is extremely rare in young adults and virtually nonexistent in children and adolescents. Examples of myxomas in children, however, have been reported by Dutz and Stout.[60] About two thirds of the patients are women.[66,78] There is no evidence of increased familial incidence.

The clinical manifestations are nonspecific, and it is difficult to diagnose the tumor before biopsy and microscopic examination. In the majority of patients the sole presenting sign is a painless palpable mass that is firm, slightly movable, and often fluctuant. Pain or tenderness is present in fewer than one fourth of cases.[62] As one would expect, pain, as well as occasional numbness, paresthesia, and muscle weakness distal to the lesion, is mostly associated with tumors of large size. In one of our cases there was also swelling of the lower leg and foot for several months before a myxoma of the thigh was detected. Because of the relative lack of symptoms, most of the tumors are present for several months before they are excised. The rate of growth, however, varies, and there is no close relationship between size and clinical duration. In fact, in two of our cases the tumors were present for 13 and 15 years, respectively, with minimal growth after the first year. The cause is uncertain. A history of trauma is given in less than one fourth of the cases. There is also nothing in the clinical history that would indicate that the tumor is etiologically related to thyroid dysfunction, as in myxedema.

By far the most frequent sites of the tumor are the large muscles of the thigh, shoulder, buttocks, and upper arm. In a review of 147 cases from the AFIP files,[72] the thigh was involved in 66 cases, the shoulder in 17, the buttocks in 12, and the arm in 8. An additional 14 cases occurred in the head and neck region, the lower leg, and the chest wall. A similar anatomic distribution is given in the literature.[66,68] The exact location in the musculature varies: some tumors are completely surrounded by muscle tissue; others are firmly attached on one side to muscle fascia. There are also myxomas of identical appearance that seem to arise from the periosteum, the subchondral epiphysis, and the joint capsule.[110,117] Angiographical examination reveals a poorly vascularized soft tissue mass surrounded by well-vascularized muscle tissue.[63,69] Kransdorf et al.[70] and others[58,61,83] describe the CT scan and magnetic resonance imaging findings in this process.

MULTIPLE INTRAMUSCULAR MYXOMAS AND FIBROUS DYSPLASIA

Although the great majority of intramuscular myxomas are solitary, there are occasional ones in which two or more myxomas are present, usually in the same region of the body. Microscopically, these tumors are in no way different from the solitary intramuscular myxomas. Nearly all, however, are associated with monostotic or rarely polyostotic fibrous dysplasia of bone, generally in the same anatomical region where the myxomas are located.[59,64,71,73,77] Often there is a long interval between the appearances of the two processes: the fibrous dysplasia is noted during the growth period, whereas the multiple myxomas, like their solitary forms, become apparent many years later during adult life.[80,85] Some patients with these lesions also display melanotic pigmentation of the skin and endocrine abnormalities, including precocious puberty (Albright's syndrome),[74,75] but there is no evidence that this process is ever associated with neurofibromatosis. Lever and Pettingale[74] report the case of a 52-year-old woman with a single large myxoma of the right thigh, fibrous dysplasia with "shepherd's crook" deformities of both hips, macular pigmentation of the skin, and a history of hypophosphatemic osteomalacia with multiple fractures during her growth period. Miettinen et al.[78] noted minor bone abnormalities in 14 of their 16 cases of intramuscular myxoma. In the case of

Mazabraud et al.,[77] an osteosarcoma developed in a patient with fibrous dysplasia and multiple myxomas.

Pathological findings

The gross appearance is characteristic and changes little from case to case. Most tumors are ovoid or globular and have on section a glistening gray-white or white appearance, depending on the relative amounts of collagen. They consist of a mass of stringy gelatinous material with occasional small fluid-filled, cystlike spaces and are covered by bundles of skeletal muscle or fascial tissue (Figs. 37-9 and 37-10). Although on casual examination most of the tumors appear to be well circumscribed, many infiltrate the adja-

cent musculature or are surrounded by edematous muscle tissue, which may serve as a cleavage plane for the surgeon. The size varies greatly. Most measure 5 cm to 10 cm in greatest diameter, but we have also seen examples measuring as large as 21 cm.

On histological examination the tumor varies little in its appearance and is composed of relatively small numbers of inconspicuous cells, abundant mucoid material, and a loose meshwork of reticulin fibers (Figs. 37-11 and 37-12). Characteristically, mature collagen fibers and vascular structures are sparse, a feature that has also been demonstrated with microangiograms.[69] Fluid-filled cystic spaces are seen occasionally, but they are rarely a prominent feature.[79] The constituent cells have small, hyperchromatic, pyknotic-appearing nuclei and scanty cytoplasm that sometimes extends along the reticulin fibers with multiple processes, giving the cell a stellate appearance. There is little cellular pleomorphism, and there are no multinucleated giant cells (Figs. 37-13 and 37-14). In some of the cases there are also scattered macrophages with small intracellular droplets of lipid material. The small size of these droplets and the absence of nuclear deformation or scalloping afford their distinction from lipoblasts (Fig. 37-15). The cells stain positively for vimentin, but, unlike lipoblasts, they do not stain for S-100 protein.[66,78,84] Glazunov et al.[65] noted intracellular inclusion bodies in several of their cases. We have seen inclusion bodies in one case only, an intramuscular myxoma in a patient with herpes zoster.

Cells and reticulin fibers are suspended in large amounts of mucoid material, which stains positively with the alcian blue, mucicarmine, and colloidal iron stains. The mucoid material is depolymerized by prior treatment of the sections with hyaluronidase. According to Kindblom et al.,[69] the

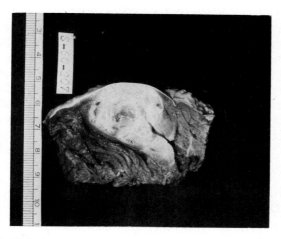

FIG. 37-9. Intramuscular myxoma firmly attached to muscle fascia. (Reproduced with permission from the *Am J Clin Pathol* 43:104, 1965.)

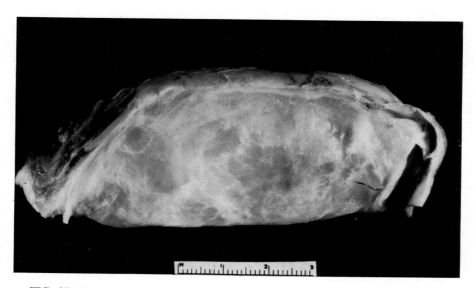

FIG. 37-10. Intramuscular myxoma showing a richly mucoid, gelatinous cut surface.

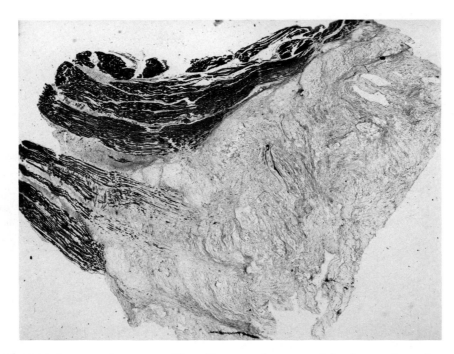

FIG. 37-11. Intramuscular myxoma. The uniform growth pattern and the absence of vascular structures are typical of this tumor. (×5.)

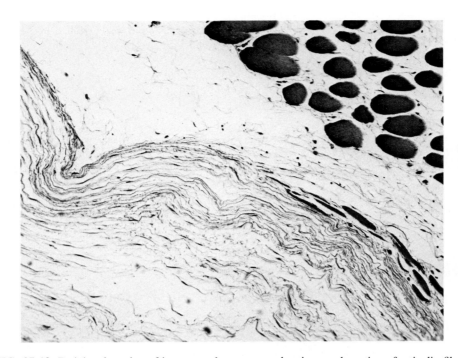

FIG. 37-12. Peripheral portion of intramuscular myxoma showing condensation of reticulin fibers and edema and atrophy of the surrounding musculature. (×110.)

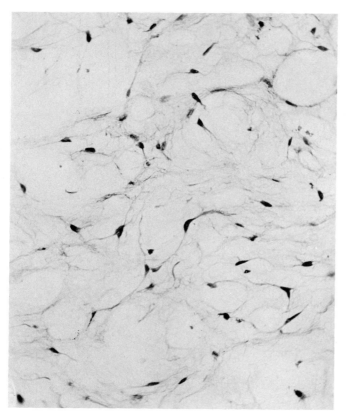

FIG. 37-13. Intramuscular myxoma. The tumor is composed of small cells with hyperchromatic nuclei and scanty cytoplasm, which often extend along the reticulin fibers with multiple processes giving the cells a stellate appearance. (×210.)

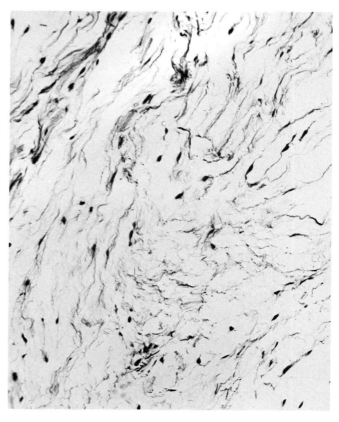

FIG. 37-14. Intramuscular myxoma characterized by a paucity of cells, abundance of mucoid material, and almost complete absence of vascular structures. (×150.)

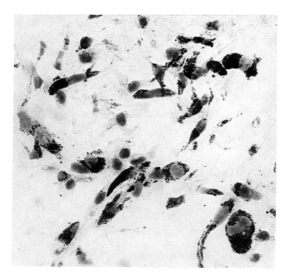

FIG. 37-15. Intramuscular myxoma with granular ORO-positive intracellular lipid material mimicking a liposarcoma. (×400.)

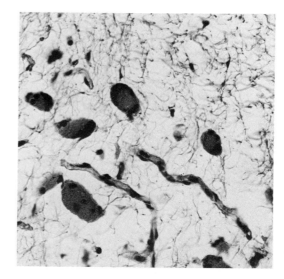

FIG. 37-16. Residual muscle cells and vessels within an intramuscular myxoma simulating a rhabdomyosarcoma. (×300.)

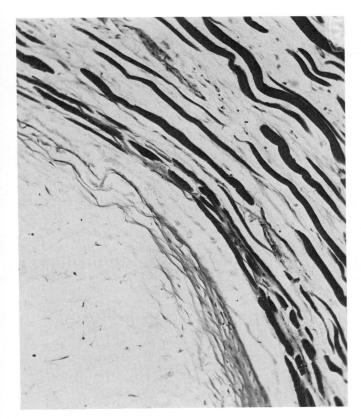

FIG. 37-17. Intramuscular myxoma surrounded by edematous, atrophic muscle tissue. (×115.)

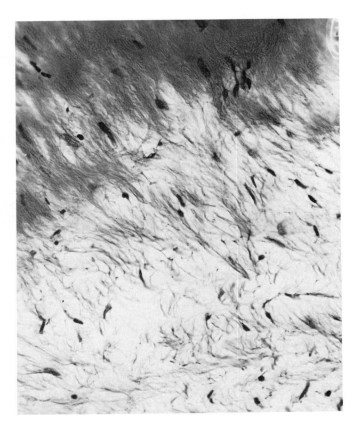

FIG. 37-18. Intramuscular myxoma showing transitions between collagenous and myxomatous areas. (×300.)

critical electrolyte concentration of the mucoid material is 0.10 M of magnesium chloride.

At the periphery, where the tumor merges with the surrounding muscle, fat cells and atrophic muscle fibers are occasionally scattered within the mucoid substance. In fact, in one of our cases residual muscle fibers were initially misinterpreted as evidence of rhabdomyoblastic differentiation, and the tumor was misdiagnosed as rhabdomyosarcoma (Fig. 37-16).

Although a distinct fibrous capsule is uncommon, even in tumors that have been present for many years, fibrous membranes are frequently found at the interface between tumor and surrounding edematous and atrophic muscle (Fig. 37-17). The borders of these fibrous structures are often frayed or fibrillated and blend with the myxoid portion of the tumor, suggesting a common cellular origin (Fig. 37-18).

Ultrastructural examination discloses predominantly fibroblast- and myofibroblast-like cells with prominent rough endoplasmic reticulum, microfilamentous material, a prominent Golgi complex, and pinocytotic and secretory vesicles, together with a mixture of amorphous and granular material and collagen fibers in the extracellular spaces

(Fig. 37-19, A). There are also macrophage-like cells with small lipid droplets or secretory vacuoles and multiple cytoplasmic processes (Fig. 37-19, B).[63,66,73]

Differential diagnosis

Numerous benign and malignant lesions are apt to be confused with intramuscular myxoma. At times the tumor may be difficult to distinguish from myxolipoma, myxoid neurofibroma, neurothekeoma, myxochondroma, and nodular fasciitis, conditions that have been discussed in previous chapters. More importantly, intramuscular myxoma may be confused with richly myxoid malignant tumors such as the myxoid variant of dermatofibrosarcoma protuberans, myxoid liposarcoma, botryoid-type rhabdomyosarcoma, myxoid malignant fibrous histiocytoma, and myxoid chondrosarcoma. All of these tumors differ from intramuscular myxoma by a much greater degree of cellularity, a more pronounced vascular pattern, and the presence of specific cellular elements such as lipoblasts, rhabdomyoblasts, or chondroblasts. Chondroblastic sarcomas also differ by the resistance of the mucoid material to depolymerization with hyaluronidase and positive staining for S-100 protein. Botryoid-type rhabdomyosarcomas occur in much younger

Table 37-1. Differential diagnosis of intramuscular myxoma

Tumor type	Pleomorphism	Vascularity	Alcian blue	Alcian blue with hyaluronidase
Intramuscular myxoma	−	−	+ +	−
Myxoid liposarcoma	−	+ + +	+ + +	−
Myxoid chondrosarcoma	−	−	+ + +	+ +
Myxoid malignant fibrous histiocytoma	+ + +	+ + +	+ +	−

A

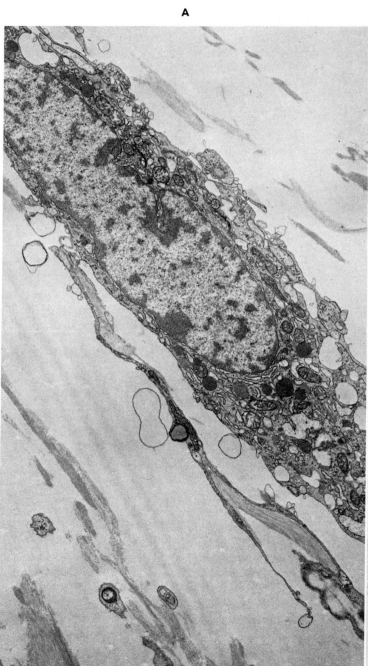

B

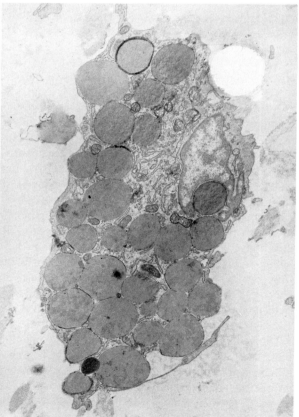

FIG. 37-19. **A,** Electron microscopic picture of intramuscular myxoma showing fibroblast-like cells with prominent rough endoplasmic reticulum and collagen fibers in the extracellular spaces. (×1800.) **B,** Electron microscopic picture of intramuscular myxoma. Macrophage-like cells with multiple membrane-bound lipid droplets. (×1800.) (**A** and **B,** courtesy Veterans Administration Hospital, Ann Arbor, Michigan.)

patients, are virtually never encountered in the musculature of the extremities, and contain cells staining positively with antibodies to actin (HHF-35) and desmin. Some of the differential diagnostic features of these tumors are further summarized in Table 37-1.

Discussion

Despite their frequent large size and prominent myxoid appearance, intramuscular myxomas are benign and very rarely recur locally.[66,69,72] In our material only one intramuscular myxoma recurred after 15 years. Microscopically, it was poorly cellular and virtually indistinguishable from the primary tumor. In the series reported by Ireland et al.,[68] two of 39 intramuscular myxomas recurred. They were described as "cellular" and "moderately cellular" and were successfully treated by reexcision.

The lack of progressive growth, the paucity of vascular structures, and the apparent immutability of the tumor cells make it highly unlikely that myxoma, as Stout[82] had suggested, is a tumor of primitive mesenchyme. Instead it seems much more likely that this tumor, as well as similar benign myxomatous lesions occurring in the corium and subcutis, arises from modified fibroblasts that produce excessive amounts of glycosaminoglycans, which in turn, as has been shown experimentally, inhibit the polymerization of normal collagen. The frequent large size of the growth, exceeding 15 cm in some instances, favors a true neoplastic process over mere mucoid degeneration of collagen. There is no convincing evidence that trauma is an important factor in the genesis of intramuscular myxoma. The oc-

casional association with fibrous dysplasia, however, suggests an underlying localized error in tissue metabolism.

MISCELLANEOUS MYXOMA-LIKE LESIONS

There are several other often ill-defined myxoid lesions, in addition to intramuscular myxoma, that are characterized by an abundant myxoid matrix, a small number of inconspicuous stellate-shaped or spindle-shaped cells, and a poorly developed vascular pattern. Most seem to be composed of modified fibroblasts that produce excessive amounts of glycosaminoglycans rich in hyaluronic acid and little collagen. Fluid-filled cystic spaces are common, but their prominence seems to depend largely on their anatomical location and their exposure to friction or repeated minor trauma.

CUTANEOUS MYXOID CYST

This lesion, which has received relatively little attention in the literature, is characterized by a soft, dome-shaped nodule located in the corium of the distal and dorsal portion of the fingers and infrequently the toes close to the nail. With the exception of small children, it occurs at virtually any age and is about twice as common in women as in men.[86] In general, the nodule is small, slow growing, and rarely exceeds 2 cm in greatest diameter.[87-89] Typically it consists of a small number of spindle-shaped and stellate-shaped fibroblasts producing small amounts of glycosaminoglycans (mucopolysaccharides) at the expense of collagen (Fig. 37-20). Many contain small fluid-filled cavities, but few of these cavities are bordered by collagenous walls

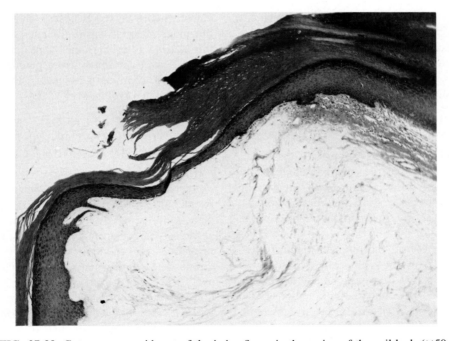

FIG. 37-20. Cutaneous myxoid cyst of the index finger in the region of the nail bed. (×50.)

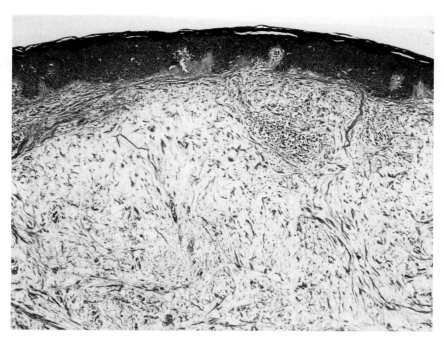

FIG. 37-21. Cutaneous focal mucinosis. (×45.)

as in ganglia. Not infrequently the nodules are covered by wartlike verrucous skin and are associated with grooving or other dystrophic changes of the nail and Heberden's nodes. Radiographic examination frequently reveals osteoarthritis in the adjacent terminal joint. Treatment may be difficult. Recurrence after incision and drainage and even excision is a common event, and some reviewers recommend wide excision with full-thickness skin grafting.[87] Others report good results with multiple injections of topical steroids (triamcinolone acetonide).[89] A morphologically similar giant fibromyxoid growth was described in association with a meningomyelocele scar and compound nevi.[90]

CUTANEOUS MUCINOSIS (CUTANEOUS MXYOMA) AND MYXEDEMA

Cutaneous focal mucinosis is an asymptomatic localized accumulation of mucinous material and scattered small spindle-shaped cells in the corium that is usually small and solitary and is found in the face, trunk, and oral region of adult patients[91,94] (Fig. 37-21). It is curable by local excision.

Localized myxedema is histologically indistinguishable from cutaneous mucinosis, but it is clinically marked by a large, discrete, often bilateral, nonpitting nodule or plaque in the pretibial region and less commonly in the dorsal aspects of the ankle and foot, often with hyperpigmentation of the overlying skin (Fig. 37-22). Characteristically, it affects patients who have hyperthyroidism or have been cured

of hyperthyroidism but continue to show exophthalmus (Grave's ophthalmopathy), probably because of blocking TSH receptor autoantibodies.[92] This process may be associated with osteoarthropathy. The term *dermal mucinosis* has been applied to myxoid change occurring in rare cases of lupus erythematosus and dermatomyositis.[96] Papular mucinosis (lichen myxedematosus), a nodular accumulation of mucinous material and proliferated fibroblasts in the dermis causing a "cobblestone" appearance of the skin, is associated with abnormal serum gamma globulins and may be a feature of mycosis fungoides, Hodgkin's disease, and non-Hodgkin's lymphoma.[93,95]

CUTANEOUS AND CARDIAC MYXOMAS, SPOTTY PIGMENTATION, AND ENDOCRINE OVERACTIVITY (CARNEY'S COMPLEX)

This triad, which has also been described as *NAME syndrome* (nevi, atrial myxoma, mucinosis, and endocrine overactivity) or *LAMB syndrome* (lentigenes, atrial myxoma, and blue nevi),[98,107] affects principally young adults and consists of cutaneous and cardiac myxomas, spotty pigmentations, and endocrine overactivity with Cushing's syndrome. The cutaneous myxomas have a predilection for the eyelids and range from small sessile papules to large pedunculated fingerlike masses; they are multiple in the majority of cases. Some of the afflicted patients have also multicentric myxoid fibroadenomas of the breast, adrenocortical hyperplasia, calcifying Sertoli cell tumors of the testis,

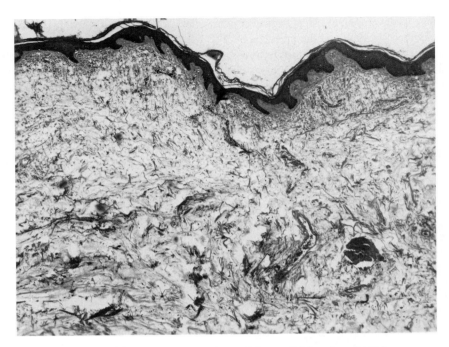

FIG. 37-22. Localized myxedema of the pretibial region. (×40.)

or psammomatous melanotic schwannomas.[102] There is no sex prevalence. The disease is inherited as a autosomal dominant trait and has been traced over several generations in some cases[99,101,105,106] (Fig. 37-23). In contrast, cardiac myxomas without associated disorders do not have an increased familial incidence and affect chiefly women.[99] All cardiac myxomas, however, may be associated with peripheral tumor emboli.[103,104] Allen et al.[97] described 30 dermal and subcutaneous myxoid tumors with and without epidermal components as *angiomyxomas*.

GANGLION

This is by far the most common and best known of the more superficially located myxoid lesions. It occurs as a unilocular or multilocular cystic or myxoid mass on the dorsal surface of the wrist in young persons, especially women, generally between 25 and 45 years of age. Less often it is found on the volar surface of the wrist or fingers and the dorsum of the foot and toes.[109,112-114,118] In about half of the cases the condition is associated with tenderness or mild pain and causes interference of function. In Carp and Stout's series,[111] a history of trauma was given by about half of the patients. Ganglia usually measure 1.5 cm to 2.5 cm in diameter. They are frequently attached to the joint capsule and tendon sheaths, and probably are due to excessive mucin production by fibroblasts rather than disintegration of preformed fibrous structures. There is no communication between the ganglion and the joint space. Some of these lesions are easily confused with myxomas, especially

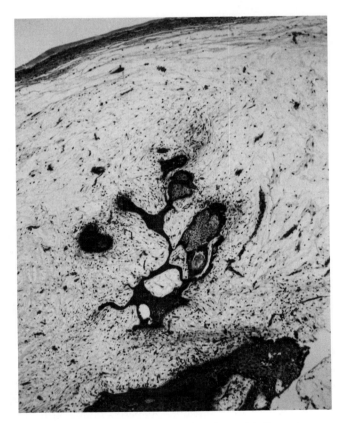

FIG. 37-23. Cutaneous myxoma in a patient with Carney's complex (cutaneous and cardiac myxomas, spotty pigmentation, and endocrine overactivity). Note residual adnexal structures within the tumor. (×60.)

in the initial myxoid stage of development. Most, however, are readily recognized by their location and the presence of multiple thick-walled cystic spaces of variable size in association with myxoid areas (Fig. 37-24). These myxoid changes, found frequently in the soft tissues outside the cystic spaces, have been misinterpreted as sarcomas. Sarpyener et al.[116] described multiple ganglia of the hands, wrists, feet, and ankles in a 4-year-old mentally retarded boy with bilateral ptosis of the eyelids. Ganglion-like lesions may also arise in the subperiosteal region or bone.[110] Intraneural ganglion-like lesions (nerve sheath ganglion) and neurothekeoma are discussed and illustrated in Chapter 31.

JUXTAARTICULAR MXYOMA

This process is marked by the accumulation of mucinous material in the vicinity of the knee and other large joints such as the shoulder and elbow joints. It occurs in adults, with a distinct prevalence for men. The growth presents as a swelling or mass that is often associated with pain or tenderness.[123,124] When occurring in the region of the knee it is frequently found together with meniscal and parameniscal cysts, small myxoma-like masses embedded within the lateral or medial semilunar cartilage (Fig. 37-25).[120-123,125,126] Like other myxomas, juxtaarticular myxoma is composed of scattered small, spindle-shaped or stellate-shaped fibroblast-like cells and a richly myxoid matrix that often contains variously sized thin- or thick-walled cystic spaces. Occasionally, there are hypercellular areas with slight cellular pleomorphism, features that may arouse the suspicion of cancer. The process involves not only the periarticular and the overlying subcutaneous fat but also the joint capsule, tendons, and, rarely, skeletal muscle.

Juxtaarticular myxoma is often associated with trauma to

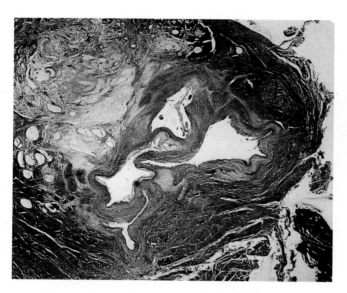

FIG. 37-24. Ganglion showing an irregular thick-walled cystic space with myxoid changes in the surrounding matrix. (×30.)

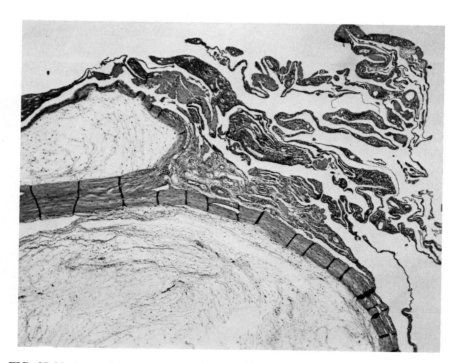

FIG. 37-25. Juxtaarticular myxoma with dense fibrous capsule and attached synovial villi.

the knee or severe osteoarthritis, and sometimes is merely an incidental finding during total knee or hip arthroplasty.[120,121,125] The cause of this condition is not clear, but most likely it is an exuberant reactive fibroblastic proliferation with overproduction of mucin. The lesion is benign but is apt to recur after incomplete excision.

MYXOMA OF THE JAWS

Although this is primarily a bone tumor, it occasionally manifests in the soft tissues as a myxomatous swelling or mass overlying a radiographically demonstrable osteolytic defect of the mandible or maxilla.[128,129,132,136] It may also displace and destroy teeth, extend into the adjacent maxillary sinus,[130] and involve the soft tissues of the face. It chiefly affects young adults, with a predilection for females, and is slightly more frequent in the mandible than in the maxilla.[135] Microscopically it is a poorly circumscribed myxoma-like mass that differs from other myxomatous lesions merely by a slightly greater degree of cellularity and cellular pleomorphism and a higher rate of mitosis. The cells are immunoreactive with antibodies against vimentin and S-100 protein but not desmin or cytokeratin.[133] Electron microscopic examination reveals the presence of fibroblasts and myofibroblasts.[131] Surgical removal of the growth is often difficult. The lesion is apt to recur, especially when it is treated by curettage rather than excision. More cellular forms may be difficult to distinguish from fibrous dysplasia and ossifying fibroma.[127]

AGGRESSIVE ANGIOMYXOMA

The term *aggressive angiomyxoma* was coined by Steeper and Rosai[144] for a morphologically distinctive and slow-growing myxoid neoplasm that occurs chiefly in the genital, perineal, and pelvic regions of adults between 25 and 60 years of age. Women are chiefly involved, but in our material and among the reported cases there are also some examples in men.[138,139,145] Tumors occurring in the vulvar region, the most common site of this process, may be initially misinterpreted as Bartholin's cysts or hernias; but unlike these lesions they grow aggressively with infiltration of perivaginal and perirectal tissues. When occurring in men they are chiefly found in the inguinal region, along the spermatic cord, or within the scrotum or pelvic cavity. Grossly, angiomyxomas are soft, partly circumscribed, or polypoid, and on cross-section have a gelatinous appearance; they range in size from a few cm to 20 cm or more. Steeper and Rosai reported an angiomyxoma of the pelvis and retroperitoneum in a 34-year-old woman that measured 60 cm by 20 cm in greatest diameter. Another huge "pelvic myxoma," measuring 75 cm in greatest diameter, was described by Alexander et al.[137] Destian and Ritchie,[140] who reported on the CT scan appearance of the tumor, emphasized the tendency of angiomyxoma to displace rather than invade neighboring structures.

Microscopically the tumor is composed of widely scattered spindle-shaped and stellate-shaped cells with ill-defined cytoplasm and variably sized, thin- or thick-walled hyalin vascular channels within a myxoid matrix that is rich in collagen fibers and, like other richly myxoid tumors, often contains foci of hemorrhage (Fig. 37-26). Occasionally, desmoplasia is prominent and leads to an angiofibroma-like picture. The cells of aggressive angiomyxoma show little nuclear atypia and virtually no mitotic activity. They are immunoreactive with antibodies against vimentin but do not stain for desmin, S-100 protein, or keratin. Electron microscopic examination shows fibroblast-like[138] or

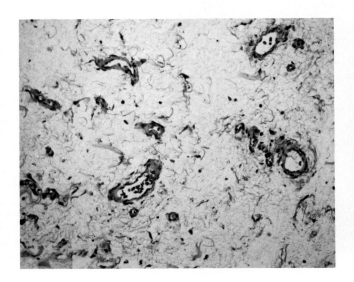

FIG. 37-26. Aggressive angiomyxoma of the paravaginal region in a 43-year-old woman. (×160.)

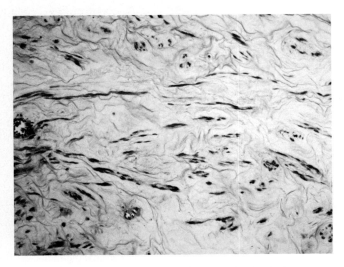

FIG. 37-27. Myxoid leiomyoma of the pelvis simulating an angiomyxoma. (×160.)

myofibroblast-like cells,[144] often with delicate cytoplasmic processes extending into the surrounding myxoid matrix consisting of a mixture of finely granular material and scattered collagen fibers.

As in other myxoid tumors differential diagnosis ranges from benign tumors such as myxolipoma, spindle cell lipoma, myxoid neurofibroma, and especially myxoid leiomyoma to myxoid liposarcoma and botryoid rhabdomyosarcoma. Myxoid leiomyoma, a tumor that may reach a very large size and is frequently found in the pelvic region, differs from angiomyxoma by its less prominent vascular pattern and the presence of widely scattered, actin- and desmin-positive smooth muscle fibers within a myxoid ma-

trix (Fig. 37-27). Angiomyofibroblastoma, a growth recently described by Fletcher et al.,[141] also occurs in the vulva and bears a close resemblance to angiomyxoma. According to the authors these tumors are better circumscribed, more cellular, and more vascular than angiomyxomas, and consist of plump cellular elements that are immunoreactive for vimentin and desmin.

Aggressive angiomyxoma tends to recur in a high percentage of cases, but there is no evidence that it is capable of metastasis. Steeper and Rosai[144] reported 5 cases with more than 12 months' follow-up, 4 of which recurred locally, 1 as late as 14 years after local excision. Begin et al.[138] described 6 cases with follow-up data, all of which

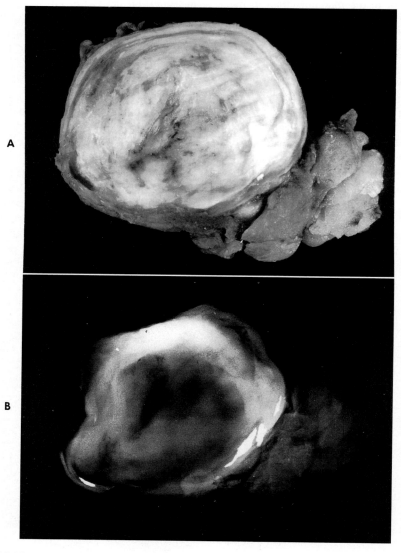

FIG. 37-28. Ossifying fibromyxoid tumor showing a well-circumscribed mass that is covered by a pseudocapsule (**A**) and displays on radiographic examination multiple areas of calcification, particularly in the capsular region of the tumor (**B**).

recurred within 9 to 84 months after excision. Since many of these tumors have infiltrative borders, complete excision may be difficult but must be attempted to prevent complications by recurrent growth.

OSSIFYING FIBROMYXOID TUMOR OF SOFT TISSUE

This tumor, which was first described in 1989,[147] usually presents as a small, painless, well-defined, often lobulated subcutaneous mass having a predilection for the upper and lower extremities (Fig. 37-28). Among the 59 reviewed cases in our material the tumor had a male predominance and almost exclusively affected adults (range of 14 to 79 years). It is composed of rather uniform round or polygonal cells arranged in a cordlike or nestlike pattern bearing some resemblance to myxoid chondrosarcoma. The surrounding matrix ranges from myxoid to hyalin and richly collagenous. Metaplastic bone is present in most cases, usually as a narrow shell at the periphery or as irregular branching spicules or trabeculae between the tumor lobules[147-151] (Figs. 37-29 to 37-31). There are also nonossifying forms and highly cellular, potentially malignant variants of the growth. Yoshida et al.[152] observed a tumor of this type in a 54-year-old man that had its onset in the right thigh and over a period of 10 years involved the upper arm and neck with invasion of the mediastinum and vertebrae.

Immunohistochemically, the cells are positive for vimen-

tin and express S-100 protein in about two thirds of cases, but the immunoreactivity for S-100 protein tends to be less intense than in benign schwannoma.[147,151] The cells do not express desmin, actin (HHF-35), or cytokeratin. Ultrastructurally, there are parallel arrays of intermediate filaments, complex cell processes, and partial, sometimes reduplicated, basal lamina (Fig. 37-32).[146,147,151]

Differential diagnosis includes benign and malignant epithelioid nerve sheath tumors (epithelioid neurofibroma, malignant epithelioid schwannoma), chondrosyringoma (mixed tumor of adnexal origin), and myxoid chondrosarcoma. The absence of epithelial markers, especially cytokeratin, helps to rule out chondrosyringoma. The lack of markers for type II collagen seems to rule out a cartilaginous neoplasm.[146] The tumors are positive for S-100 protein, but there is no evidence of nerve involvement or neurofibromatosis in the reported material.

The clinical behavior of ossifying fibromyxoid tumor varies: most of the reported tumors followed a benign clinical course, but almost one third recurred locally. One patient with three recurrences developed a second tumor in the opposite thigh, presumably a metastasis. We have also encountered a richly cellular and mitotically active example of the tumor that metastasized to the lungs after many years, indicating the existence of rare malignant forms of this tumor.

Although the exact nature of this lesion is still uncertain,

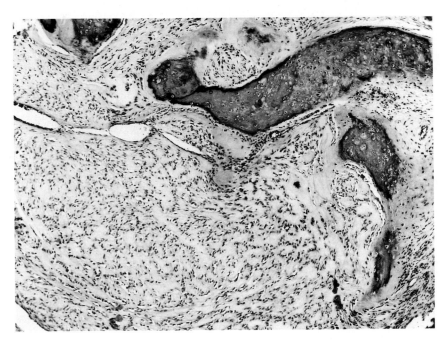

FIG. 37-29. Ossifying fibromyxoid tumor with cords of tumor cells surrounded and separated by abundant hyalinized fibrous matrix and associated with irregular trabeculae of mature bone. (×60.)

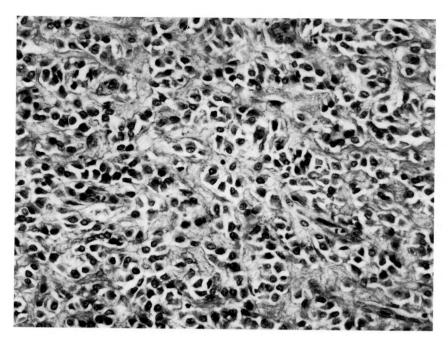

FIG. 37-30. Ossifying fibromyxoid tumor showing ill-defined nests of tumor cells with eosinophilic cytoplasm and eccentrically placed small, round vesicular nuclei. (×250.) (From *Am J Surg Pathol* 13:817, 1989.)

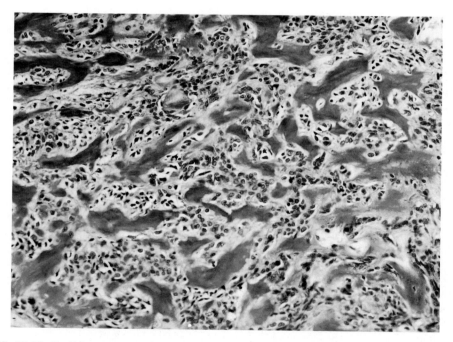

FIG. 37-31. Ossifying fibromyxoid tumor displaying cords and nests of small tumor cells within a prominent hyalinized fibrous matrix. (×260.)

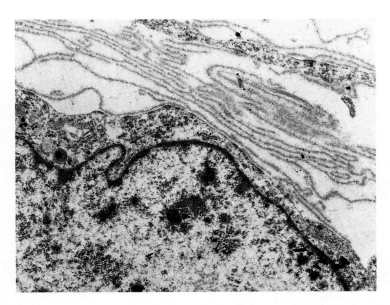

FIG. 37-32. Electron micrograph of ossifying fibromyxoid tumor showing reduplication and scroll formation of external laminae, a feature suggesting a tumor of neural origin. (×16,000.) (From *Am J Surg Pathol* 13:817, 1989.)

many of the immunohistochemical and ultrastructural features point toward an unusual neural tumor possibly of Schwann cell origin.

PARACHORDOMA

Parachordoma is a very rare tumor of characteristic histological appearance and uncertain histogenesis. It was first described by Laskowski and later, in 1977, by Dabska[153] in the English literature. It should not be confused with chordoid sarcoma, a chondroblastic tumor synonymous with extraskeletal myxoid chondrosarcoma (Chapter 35). According to Dabska's report of 10 cases, the tumor affects both adolescents and adults and predominates in the extremities, where it is usually deep seated and involves the soft tissues adjacent to tendons, synovium, and osseous structures.[153] In one of our cases the tumor arose in the lumbar region of a 53-year-old man. It had been present for 20 years and was thought to represent an epidermoid cyst. Stout and Gorman's case[155] of a deep-seated mixed tumor in the soft tissue of the left leg, which was located beneath the deep fascia and caused indention of the shaft of the tibia, may be another example of this entity.

Grossly, parachordoma forms a lobulated or multinodular mass, averaging 3.5 cm in diameter. Microscopically, it consists of small nests of pale-staining cells resembling the cells of the fetal chorda dorsalis, or notochord. The cells have vesicular or pyknotic nuclei and a vacuolated cytoplasm, and they occasionally form indistinct acinar or alveolar structures. They are embedded in a myxoid or sometimes eosinophilic hyalin matrix (Fig. 37-33). In some of the reported cases there are, in addition, undifferentiated spindle cells that blend with the myxoid areas. According to our limited experience with this tumor, the cells contain glycogen, but the interstitial mucoid material differs in its staining characteristics from cartilaginous neoplasms and chordomas. It contains large amounts of glycosaminoglycans, but the mucinous material is depolymerized by hyaluronidase. This makes it very unlikely that parachordoma is a tumor of chondroblastic or chordoid origin.

Immunohistochemical examination, carried out by Ishida et al.[154] on a parachordoma of the left calf in a 19-year-old woman, revealed positive staining for vimentin and S-100 protein; the cells did not stain for desmin, cytokeratin, epithelial membrane antigen, and carcinoembryonic antigen. Ultrastructurally, there were well-developed rough endoplasmic reticulum, abundant intermediate filaments, microvillous cytoplasmic processes, pinocytotic vesicles, and desmosome-like junctions.

The clinical course is that of a benign neoplasm. Of Dabska's 10 cases, 8 had follow-up information; 3 of the 8 recurred locally, one after 19 years, but all were cured by reexcision of the tumor.

AMYLOID TUMOR

Tumorlike localized deposits of amyloid are not only encountered in association with a variety of immunocytic dyscrasias, including multiple myeloma and lymphoplasmacytoid lymphoma, but are also associated with long-term

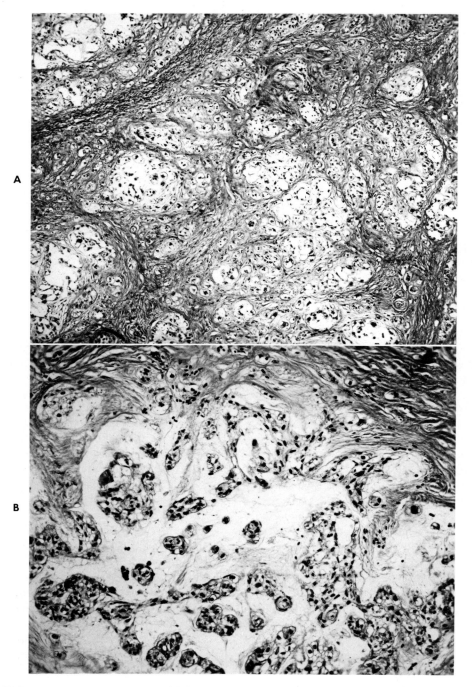

FIG. 37-33. Parachordoma consisting of nests of pale-staining cells surrounded by fibrous stroma (**A**) and aggregates of cells with vacuolated cytoplasm and pyknotic nuclei within a myxoid matrix (**B**). (**A,** ×50; **B,** ×60.)

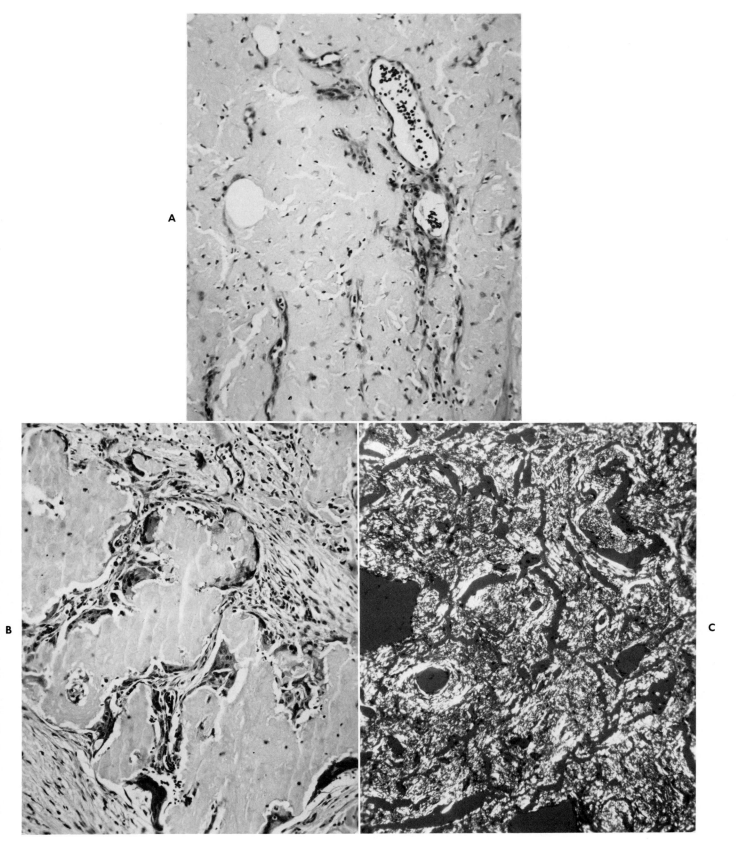

FIG. 37-34. Amyloid tumor showing amorphous deposits of amyloid surrounding dilated vascular channels **(A)**, association of deposits with foreign body–type giant cells **(B)**, and birefringence (apple-green birefringence) under polarized light **(C)**. (**A** and **B**, ×160; **C**, Congo red stain, ×160.)

hemodialysis and a variety of chronic infections or inflammatory diseases (tuberculosis, osteomyelitis, and rheumatoid arthritis).[174] There are also localized deposits of amyloid that occur without any clinical evidence of immunocytic dyscrasia or any other coexisting or preexisting disease; these lesions are rare and are found mainly in the soft tissues or as solitary or multiple nodules in the intestinal, urinary, and respiratory tracts.[120] There are only few examples of soft tissue amyloidomas in our files: one such case occurred in the soft tissues of the neck of a 46-year-old man; it was a large lobulated mass that was situated deep to the sternomastoid muscle and internal jugular vein and had been present for 6 years. Another was located in the left femoral triangle of an 84-year-old woman; it measured 6.5 cm in greatest diameter and had a mottled gray-pink cut surface. Serum proteins were normal in both cases. A small number of similar cases have been recorded in the literature: Lipper and Kahn[168] described 4 cases, 3 in the soft tissue and 1 in bone; the soft tissue tumors were located in the left groin, the abdominal wall, and the right breast of adult patients who were 40, 47, and 57 years of age, respectively. The largest measured 12 cm in greatest diameter. Follow-up information available in two of the three cases failed to reveal any associated disease. Krishnan et al.[166] reported 14 soft tissue amyloidomas, mostly from the mediastinum and retroperitoneum; 4 of the 14 displayed only reactive features; the remaining 10 cases were associated with lymphoplasmacytoid lymphoma (9 cases) or myeloma (1 case). There are also reports of localized amyloid tumors in the eyelid, conjunctiva, and orbit,[161,173] palate,[178] breast,[158,172] mediastinum,[169] and lower extremity.[170] Amyloid tumors of the skin are usually of much smaller size and occur as multiple macules or papules in the upper dermis.[160,163,170] Typical examples of visceral amyloid tumors have been observed in the parotid gland,[176] stomach,[156] and lower urinary tract,[162,177] as well as in the larynx,[165,171,175] and especially the lungs.[159,180]

Grossly, the tumor consists of a slow-growing lobulated nodule or mass with a white-yellow or pink-yellow waxy surface. Microscopic examination discloses amorphous faintly eosinophilic material that is positive for PAS and metachromatic with the crystal violet stain. The deposits are surrounded by histiocytes and multinucleated giant cells and a more or less prominent chronic inflammatory infiltrate containing polyclonal lymphocytes and plasma cells showing no evidence of immaturity or cellular atypia. In most cases the interspersed vessel walls are diffusely thickened by deposited amyloid. Elastica stains help to distinguish the tumor from elastofibroma, and the absence of a fibroblastic proliferation separates it from tumoral calcinosis. Calcification and metaplastic cartilage and bone formation, however, do occur in some amyloid tumors. The deposited amyloid stains positively with the Congo red preparation, showing an "apple-green" birefringence under polarized light (Fig. 37-34). The Congo red affinity is abolished by prior treatment of the sections with potassium permanganate (amyloid A protein [AA]) in most reactive or inflammatory forms of the disease.[172,179,181] Under the electron microscope, amyloid consists of fine straight nonbranching fibrils that measure between 70 nm and 100 nm in diameter. There is little information as to the type of amyloid in the reported cases. Three of the four reactive amyloidomas described by Krishnan et al.[166] had a long history of chronic inflammatory disorders, and the fourth had persistent antinuclear antibody positivity. In all four the Congo red staining of the amyloid was sensitive to treatment with potassium permanganate and all showed the immunohistochemical characteristics of amyloid A protein (AA), the prognostically most favorable form of the disease. Others, however, demonstrated the AL type of amyloid in bilateral amyloidomas of the breast.[172] So far there are no reports of other types of amyloid protein in amyloidoma.

REFERENCES
Tumoral calcinosis

1. Balachandran S, Abbud Y, Prince MJ, et al: Tumoral calcinosis: scintigraphic studies of an affected family. *Br J Radiol* 53:960, 1980.
2. Baldursson H, Evans EB, Dodge WF, et al: Tumoral calcinosis with hyperphosphatemia: a report of a family with incidence in four siblings. *J Bone Joint Surg* 51A:913, 1969.
3. Barton DL, Reeves RJ: Tumoral calcinosis: report of three cases and review of the literature. *Am J Roentgenol* 86:351, 1961.
4. Bauer JM, Freyberg RH: Vitamin D intoxication with metastatic calcification. *JAMA* 130:1208, 1946.
5. Berg D: Tumoral calcinosis. *Br J Surg* 59:570, 1972.
6. Boskey AL, Vigorita VJ, Spencer O, et al: Chemical, microscopic, and ultrastructural characterization of the mineral deposits in tumoral calcinosis. *Clin Orthop* 178:258, 1983.
7. Brown ML, Thrall JH, Cooper RA, et al: Radiography and scintigraphy in tumoral calcinosis. *Radiology* 124:757, 1977.
8. Carey RW, Schmitt GW, Kopald HH, et al: Massive extraskeletal calcification during phosphate treatment of hypercalcemia. *Arch Intern Med* 122:150, 1968.
9. Carnett J: The calcareous deposits of so-called calcifying subacromial bursitis. *Surg Gynecol Obstet* 41:404, 1925.
10. Clarke E, Swischuk LE, Hayden CK Jr: Tumoral calcinosis, diaphysitis, and hyperphosphatemia. *Radiology* 151:643, 1984.
11. DiGiovanna JJ, Helfgott RK, Gerber LH, et al: Extraspinal tendon and ligament calcification associated with long-term therapy with etretinate. *N Engl J Med* 315:1177, 1986.
12. Duret MH: Tumeurs multiples et singulieres des bourses sereuses (endotheliomes peut etre d'origine parasitaire). *Bull Mem Soc Anat (Paris)* 74:725, 1899.
13. Ghormley RK, Manning GF, Power MH, et al: Multiple calcified bursae and calcified cysts in soft tissues. *Trans West Surg Assoc* 51:292, 1942.
14. Hacihanefioglu U: Tumoral calcinosis. a clinical and pathological

study of eleven unreported cases in Turkey. *J Bone Joint Surg* 60A:1131, 1978.

15. Harkess JW, Peters HJ: Tumoral calcinosis. *J Bone Joint Surg* 49A:721, 1967.

16. Inclan A: Tumoral calcinosis. *JAMA* 121:490, 1943.

17. Irnell L, Werner I, Grimelius L: Soft tissue calcification in hyperparathyroidism. *Acta Med Scand* 187:145, 1970.

18. Jain SP: Tumoral calcinosis in Somalia and Ethiopia: a report of twenty-one cases and brief review of literature. *East Afr Med J* 66:476, 1989.

19. Katayama I, Higashi K, Mukai H, et al: Tumoral calcinosis in scleroderma. *J Dermatol* 16:82, 1989.

20. Kindblom LG, Gunterberg B: Tumoral calcinosis: an ultrastructural analysis and consideration of pathogenesis. *APMIS* 96:368, 1988.

21. Knowles SAS, Declerck G, Anthony PP: Tumoral calcinosis. *Br J Surg* 70:105, 1983.

22. Kolawole TM, Bohrer SP: Tumoral calcinosis with "fluid levels" in the tumoral masses. *Am J Roentgenol* 120:461, 1974.

23. Kuzela DC, Huffer WE, Conger JD, et al: Soft tissue calcification in chronic dialysis patients. *Am J Pathol* 86:403, 1977.

24. Lafferty FW, Reynolds ES, Pearson OH: Tumoral calcinosis: a metabolic disease of obscure etiology. *Am J Med* 38:105, 1965.

25. Lufkin EG, Wilson DM, Smith LH, et al: Phosphorus excretion in tumoral calcinosis: response to parathyroid hormone and acetazolamide. *J Clin Endocrinol Metabol* 50:648, 1980.

26. Lyles KW, Burkes EJ, Ellis GJ, et al: Genetic transmission of tumoral calcinosis: autosomal dominant with variable clinical expressivity. *J Clin Endocrinol Metabol* 60:1093, 1985.

27. Lyles KW, Halsey DL, Friedman NE, et al: Correlation of serum concentrations of 1,25-dihydroxyvitamin D, phosphorus, and parathyroid hormone in tumoral calcinosis. *J Clin Endocrinol Metabol* 67:88, 1988.

28. Maathuis JB, Koten JW: Kikuyu-bursa and tumoral calcinosis. *Trop Geogr Med* 21:389, 1969.

29. Malhotra R, Franks S, Bhawan J: Idiopathic calcinosis of the scrotum. *Citos* 27:396, 1981.

30. McClatschie S, Bremner AD: Tumoral calcinosis: an unrecognized disease. *Br Med J* 1:153, 1969.

31. Meltzer CC, Fishman EK, Scott WW Jr: Tumoral calcinosis causing bone erosion in a renal dialysis patient. *Clin Imaging* 16:49, 1992.

32. Mitnick PD, Goldfarb S, Slatopolsky E, et al: Calcium and phosphate metabolism in tumoral calcinosis. *Ann Intern Med* 92:482, 1980.

33. Mozzaffarian G, Lafferty FW, Pearson OH: Treatment of tumoral calcinosis with phosphorus deprivation. *Ann Intern Med* 77:741, 1972.

34. Muller SA, Brunsting LA, Winkelman RK: Calcinosis cutis: its relationship to scleroderma. *Arch Dermatol* 80:15, 1959.

35. Murthy DP: Tumoral calcinosis: a study of cases from Papua, New Guinea. *J Trop Med Hyg* 93:403, 1990.

36. Palmer PES: Tumoural calcinosis. *Br J Radiol* 39:518, 1966.

37. Parfitt AM: Soft tissue calcifications in uremia. *Arch Intern Med* 124:544, 1969.

38. Pedersen HE, Key JA: Pathology of calcareous tendinitis and subdeltoid bursitis. *Arch Surg* 62:50, 1951.

39. Prince MJ, Schaeffer PC, Goldsmith RS, et al: Hyperphosphatemic tumoral calcinosis: association with elevation of serum 1,25-dihydroxycholecalciferol concentrations. *Ann Intern Med* 96:586, 1982.

40. Randall RE Jr, Strauss MB, McNeely WF: The milk-alkali syndrome. *Arch Intern Med* 107:163, 1961.

41. Slavin RE, Wen J, Kumar D, et al: Familial tumoral calcinosis: a clinical, histopathologic, and ultrastructural study with an analysis

of its calcifying process and pathogenesis. *Am J Surg Pathol* 17:788, 1993.

42. Steinherz R, Chesney RW, Eisenstein B, et al: Elevated serum calcitriol concentrations do not fall in response to hyperphosphatemia in familial tumoral calcinosis. *Am J Dis Child* 139:816, 1985.

43. Suzuki K, Takahashi S, Perrouchoud A, et al: Tumoral calcinosis in a patient undergoing hemodialysis. *Acta Orthop Scand* 50:27, 1979.

44. Teutschlaender O: Zur Kenntnis der progressiven Lipocalcinogranulomatose der Muskulatur. *Virchows Arch (Pathol Anat)* 295:424, 1935.

45. Teutschlaender O: Lipid Calcinosis (Lipoid Kalkgicht). *Zieglers Beitr* 110:402, 1947.

46. Teutschlaender O: Die symmetrisch fortschreitende Lipocalcinogranulomatose (Hygromatosis lipocalcinogranulomatosa progrediens) und andere Schleimbeutelveränderungen (sog. "Bursitis calcarea" und Lipoma arborescens). *Zieglers Beitr* 103:499, 1939.

47. Tezelman S, Siperstein AE, Duh QY, et al: Tumoral calcinosis: controversies in the etiology and alternatives in the treatment. *Arch Surg* 128:737, 1993.

48. Theuvenet WJ, Nolthenius-Puylaert T, Giedrpcy JZL, et al: Massive deformation of the scrotal wall by idiopathic calcinosis of the scrotum. *Plast Reconstr Surg* 74:539, 1984.

49. Thomson JEM, Tanner FJ: Tumoral calcinosis. *J Bone Joint Surg* 31A:132, 1949.

50. Thomson JG: Calcifying collagenolysis (tumoural calcinosis). *Br J Radiol* 39:526, 1966.

51. Vasudev KS, Tapp L, Harris M, et al: Tumoural calcinosis in Britain. *Br Med J* 1:676, 1973.

52. Veress B, Malik OA, El Hassan AM: Tumoural lipocalcinosis: a clinicopathological study of 20 cases. *J Pathol* 119:113, 1976.

53. Wheeler CE, Curtis AC, Cawley EP, et al: Soft tissue calcification with special reference to its occurrence in the "collagen diseases." *Ann Intern Med* 36:1050, 1952.

54. Whiting DA, Simson IW, Kallmeyer JC, et al: Unusual cutaneous lesions in tumoral calcinosis. *Arch Dermatol* 102:465, 1970.

55. Wilber JF, Slatopolsky E: Hyperphosphatemia and tumoral calcinosis. *Ann Intern Med* 68:1044, 1968.

56. Wilson CW, Wingfield WL, Toone EC Jr: Vitamin D poisoning with metastatic calcification. *Am J Med* 14:116, 1953.

57. Yaghmai I, Mirbod P: Tumoral calcinosis. *Am J Roentgenol* 111:573, 1971.

Intramuscular myxoma

58. Abdelwahab AF, Kenan S, Hermann G, et al: Intramuscular myxoma: magnetic resonance features. *Br J Radiol* 65:485, 1992.

59. Blasier RD, Ryan JR, Schaldenbrand MF: Multiple myxomata of soft tissue associated with polyostotic fibrous dysplasia: a case report. *Clin Orthop* 206:211, 1986.

60. Dutz W, Stout AP: The myxoma in childhood. *Cancer* 14:629, 1961.

61. Ekelund L, Herrlin K, Rydholm A: Computed tomography of intramuscular myxoma. *Skel Radiol* 7:15, 1981.

62. Enzinger FM: Intramuscular myxoma. *Am J Clin Pathol* 43:104, 1965.

63. Feldman P: A comparative study including ultrastructure of intramuscular myxoma and myxoid liposarcoma. *Cancer* 43:512, 1979.

64. Gianoutsos MP, Thompson JF, Marsden FW: Mazabraud's syndrome: intramuscular myxoma associated with fibrous dysplasia of bone. *Aust N Z J Surg* 60:825, 1990.

65. Glazunov MF, Puckov JG: Ueber die sogenannten Muskelmyxome und Myxosarkome des Menschen mit Zelleinschlüssen. *Z Krebsforsch* 65:439, 1963.

66. Hashimoto H, Tsuneyoshi M, Daimaru Y, et al: Intramuscular myxoma: a clinicopathologic, immunohistochemical, and electron microscopic study. *Cancer* 58:740, 1986.

67. Henschen F: Fall von Ostitis fibrosa mit multiplen Tumoren in der umgebenden Muskulatur. *Verh Dtsch Ges Path* 21:93, 1926.

68. Ireland DC, Soule EH, Ivins JC: Myxoma of somatic soft tissues: a report of 58 patients, 3 with multiple tumors and fibrous dysplasia of bone. *Mayo Clin Proc* 48:401, 1973.

69. Kindblom LG, Stener B, Angervall L: Intramuscular myxoma. *Cancer* 34:1737, 1974.

70. Kransdorf MJ, Moser RP Jr, Jelinek JS, et al: Intramuscular myxoma: MR features. *J Comput Assist Tomogr* 13:836, 1989.

71. Krogius A: Ein Fall von Osteitis fibrosa mit multiplen fibromyxomatoesen Muskeltumoren. *Acta Chir Scand* 64:465, 1928.

72. Lattes R, Enzinger FM: *Soft tissue tumors.* Proceedings of the Thirty-ninth Anatomic Pathology Slide Seminar. American Society of Clinical Pathology, 1973.

73. Leung TK, Vauzelle JL, Patricot LM, et al: Etude ultrastructurale et cytochimique d'un myxome musculaire associé á une dysplasie fibreuse. *Ann Anat Pathol (Paris)* 16:417, 1971.

74. Lever EG, Pettingale KW: Albright's syndrome associated with a soft-tissue myxoma and hypophosphataemic osteomalacia: report of a case and review of the literature. *J Bone Joint Surg* 65B:621, 1983.

75. Logel RJ: Recurrent intramuscular myxoma associated with Albright's syndrome: case report and review of the literature. *J Bone Joint Surg* 58A:565, 1976.

76. MacKenzie DH: The myxoid tumors of somatic soft tissues. *Am J Surg Pathol* 5:443, 1981.

77. Mazabraud A, Semat P, Roze R: A propos de l'association de fibromyxomes des tissus mous a la dysplasie fibreuse des os. *Presse Med* 75:2223, 1967.

78. Miettinen M, Hockerstedt K, Reitamo J, et al: Intramuscular myxoma: a clinicopathologic study of 23 cases. *Am J Clin Pathol* 84:265, 1985.

79. Pettersson H, Hudson TM, Springfield DS, et al: Cystic intramuscular myxoma: report of a case. *Acta Radiol Diagn (Stockh)* 26:425, 1985.

80. Sedmak DD, Hart WR, Belhobek GH, et al: Massive intramuscular myxoma associated with fibrous dysplasia of bone. *Cleve Clin Q* 50:469, 1983.

81. Sponsel KH, McDonald JR, Ghormley RK: Myxoma and myxosarcoma of the soft tissues of the extremities. *J Bone Joint Surg* 34A:820, 1952.

82. Stout AP: Myxoma, the tumor of primitive mesenchyme. *Ann Surg* 127:706, 1948.

83. Sundaram M, McDonald DJ, Merenda G: Intramuscular myxoma. *AJR Am J Roentgenol* 153:107,1989.

84. Weiss W, Langloss JM, Enzinger FM: Value of S-100 protein in the diagnosis of soft tissue tumors with particular reference to benign and malignant Schwann cell tumors. *Lab Invest* 49:299, 1983.

85. Wirth WA, Leavitt D, Enzinger FM: Multiple intramuscular myxomas: another extraskeletal manifestation of fibrous dysplasia. *Cancer* 27:1167, 1971.

Cutaneous myxoid cyst

86. Arner O, Lindholm A, Romanus R: Mucous cysts of fingers. *Acta Chir Scand* 111:314, 1956.

87. Constant E, Royer JR, Pollard RJ, et al: Mucous cysts of the fingers. *Plast Reconstr Surg* 43:241, 1969.

88. Gross RE: Recurring myxomatous, cutaneous cysts of the fingers and toes. *Surg Gynecol Obstet* 65:289, 1937.

89. Johnson WC, Graham JH, Helwig EB: Cutaneous myxoid cyst. *JAMA* 191:15, 1965.

90. McCalmont CS, White WL, Jorizzo JL: Giant fibromyxoid tumor of the adventitial dermis: forme fruste of trichodiscoma. *Am J Dermatopathol* 13:403, 1991.

Cutaneous mucinosis

91. Buchner A, Merrell PW, Leider AS, et al: Oral focal mucinosis. *Int J Oral Maxillofac Surg* 19:337, 1990.

92. Gimlette TMD: Pretibial myxoedema. *Br Med J* 5195:348, 1960.

93. Howsden SM, Herndon JH Jr, Freeman RG: Lichen myxedematosus. *Arch Dermatol* 111:1325, 1975.

94. Johnson WC, Helwig EB: Cutaneous focal mucinosis. *Arch Dermatol* 93:13, 1966.

95. Shapiro CM, Fretzin D, Norris S: Papular mucinosis. *JAMA* 214:2052, 1970.

96. Weigand DA, Burgdorf WH, Gregg LJ: Dermal mucinosis in discoid lupus erythematosus: report of two cases. *Arch Dermatol* 117:735, 1981.

Carney's complex

97. Allen PW, Dymock RB, MacCormac LB: Superficial angiomyxomas with and without epithelial components: report of 30 tumors in 28 patients. *Am J Surg Pathol* 12:519, 1988.

98. Atherton DJ, Pitcher DW, Wells RS, et al: A syndrome of various cutaneous pigmented lesions, myxoid neurofibromata and atrial myxoma: the NAME syndrome. *Br J Dermatol* 103:421, 1980.

99. Carney JA: Differences between nonfamilial and familial cardiac myxoma. *Am J Surg Pathol* 9:53, 1985.

100. Carney JA, Gordon H, Carpenter PC, et al: The complex of myxomas, spotty pigmentation, and endocrine overactivity. *Medicine* 64:270, 1985.

101. Carney JA, Hruska LS, Beauchamp GD, et al: Dominant inheritance of the complex of myxomas, spotty pigmentation, and endocrine overactivity. *Mayo Clin Proc* 61:165, 1986.

102. Carney JA, Toorkey BC: Myxoid fibroadenoma and allied conditions (myxomatosis) of the breast: a heritable disorder with special associations including cardiac and cutaneous myxomas. *Am J Surg Pathol* 15:713, 1991.

103. Feldman AR, Keeling JH: Cutaneous manifestations of atrial myxoma. *J Am Acad Dermatol* 21:1080, 1989.

104. Gardner SS, Solomon AR: Cutaneous and cardiac myxomas: an important association. *Semin Dermatol* 10:148, 1991.

105. Koopman RJ, Happle R: Autosomal dominant transmission of the NAME syndrome (nevi, atrial myxoma, mucinosis of the skin, and endocrine overactivity). *Hum Genet* 86:300, 1991.

106. McCarthy PM, Piehter JM, Schaff HV, et al: The significance of multiple, recurrent, and "complex" cardiac myxomas. *J Thorac Cardiovasc Surg* 91:389, 1986.

107. Rhodes AR, Silverman RA, Harrist TJ, et al: Mucocutaneous lentigines, cardiomucocutaneous myxomas, and multiple blue nevi: the "LAMB" syndrome. *J Acad Dermatol* 10:72, 1984.

Ganglion

108. Angelides AC, Wallace PF: The dorsal ganglion of the wrist: its pathogenesis, gross and microscopic anatomy, and surgical treatment. *J Hand Surg* 1:228, 1976.

109. Barnes WE, Larsen RD, Posch JL: Review of the ganglia of the hand or wrist with analysis of surgical treatment. *Plast Reconstr Surg* 34:570, 1964.

110. Bauer TW, Dorfman HD: Intraosseous ganglion: a clinicopathologic study of 11 cases. *Am J Surg Pathol* 6:207, 1982.

111. Carp L, Stout AP: A study of ganglion: with especial reference to treatment. *Surg Gynecol Obstet* 47:460, 1928.

112. Englert HM: Die ganglioplastischen Tumoren oder Gangliome der Hand. *Chirurg* 44:35, 1973.

113. McEvedy V: Simple ganglia. *Br J Surg* 49:585, 1961.

114. Oertel YC, Beckner ME, Engler WF: Cytologic diagnosis and ultrastructure of fine-needle aspirates of ganglion cysts. *Arch Pathol Lab Med* 110:938, 1986.

115. Salyer WR, Salyer DC: Myxoma-like features of organizing thrombi in arteries and veins. *Arch Pathol* 99:307, 1975.

116. Sarpyener MA, Ozcurumez O, Seyhan F: Multiple ganglions of tendon sheaths. *J Bone Joint Surg* 50A:985, 1968.

117. Sime FH, Dahlin DC: Ganglion cysts of bone. *Mayo Clin Proc* 46:484, 1971.

118. Soren A: Pathogenesis, clinic and treatment of ganglion. *Arch Orthop Trauma Surg* 99:247, 1982.

119. Zachariae L, Vibe-Hansen H: Ganglia recurrence rate elucidated by a follow-up of 347 operated cases. *Acta Chir Scand* 139:625, 1973.

Juxtaarticular myxoma

120. Becton JL, Young HH: Cysts of semilunar cartilage of the knee. *Arch Surg* 90:708, 1965.

121. Bennett GE, Shaw MB: Cysts of the semilunar cartilages. *Arch Surg* 33:92, 1936.

122. Gallo GA, Sryan RS: Cysts of the semilunar cartilages of the knee. *Am J Surg* 116:65, 1968.

123. Ghormley RK, Dockerty MB: Cystic myxomatous tumors about the knee: their relation to cysts of the menisci. *J Bone Joint Surg* 25:306, 1943.

124. Meis JM, Enzinger FM: Juxtaarticular myxoma: a clinical and pathological study of 65 cases. *Hum Pathol* 23:639, 1992.

125. Noble J, Hamblen DL: The pathology of the degenerate meniscus lesion. *J Bone Joint Surg* 57B:180, 1975.

126. Zäch-Christen P: Ueber Meniscuscysten des Kniegelenkes. *Virchows Arch (Pathol Anat)* 279:273, 1930.

Myxoma of the jaws

127. Balough G, Inovay J: Recurrent mandibular myxoma: report of a case. *J Oral Surg* 30:121, 1972.

128. Byrd DL, Kindrick RD, Dunsworth AR: Myxoma of the maxilla: report of a case. *J Oral Surg* 31:123, 1973.

129. Ghosh BC, Huvos AG, Gerold FP, et al: Myxoma of the jaw bones. *Cancer* 31:237, 1973.

130. Greenfield SD, Friedman O: Myxoma of maxillary sinus. *N Y State J Med* 51:1319, 1951.

131. Hasleton PS, Simpson W, Craig RDP: Myxoma of the mandible: a fibroblastic tumor. *Oral Surg Oral Med Oral Pathol* 46:396, 1978.

132. Kangur T, Dahlin D, Tulington E: Myxomatous tumors of the jaws. *J Oral Surg* 33:523, 1975.

133. Lombardi T, Kuffer R, Bernard JP, et al: Immunohistochemical staining for vimentin filaments and S-100 protein in myxoma of the jaws. *J Oral Pathol* 17:175, 1988.

134. Simes RJ, Barros RE: Ultrastructure of an odontogenic myxoma. *Oral Surg Oral Med Oral Pathol* 39:640, 1975.

135. Slootweg PJ, Wittkampf AR: Myxoma of the jaws: an analysis of 15 cases. *J Maxillofac Surg* 14:46, 1986.

136. Zimmerman DC, Dahlin DC: Myxomatous tumors of the jaws. *Oral Surg Oral Med Oral Pathol* 11:1069, 1958.

Aggressive angiomyxoma

137. Alexander JW, Bossert LJ, Altemeier WA: Myxomas of the pelvis. *Surg Gynecol Obstet* 125:73, 1967.

138. Begin LR, Clement PB, Kirk ME, et al: Aggressive angiomyxoma of pelvic soft parts: a clinicopathologic study of nine cases. *Hum Pathol* 16:621, 1985.

139. Clatch RJ, Drake WK, Gonzalez JG: Aggressive angiomyxoma in men: a report of two cases associated with inguinal hernias. *Arch Pathol Lab Med* 117:911, 1993.

140. Destian S, Ritchie WG: Aggressive angiomyxoma: CT appearance. *Am J Gastroenterol* 81:711, 1986.

141. Fletcher CD, Tsang WY, Fisher C, et al: Angiomyofibroblastoma of the vulva: a benign neoplasm distinct from aggressive angiomyxoma. *Am J Surg Pathol* 16:373, 1992.

142. Habeck JO: Aggressive angiomyxoma of the vulva and perineum. *Zentralbl Pathol* 138:303, 1992.

143. Smith HO, Worrell RV, Smith AY, et al: Aggressive angiomyxoma of the female pelvis and perineum. *Gynecol Oncol* 42:79, 1991.

144. Steeper TA, Rosai J: Aggressive angiomyxoma of the female pelvis and perineum: report of nine cases of a distinctive type of gynecologic soft-tissue neoplasm. *Am J Surg Pathol* 7:463, 1983.

145. Tsang WY, Chan JK, Fisher C, et al: Aggressive angiomyxoma: a report of four cases occurring in men. *Am J Surg Pathol* 16:1059, 1992.

Ossifying fibromyxoid tumor of soft tissue

146. Donner LR: Ossifying fibromyxoid tumor of soft parts: evidence supporting Schwann cell origin. *Hum Pathol* 23:200, 1992.

147. Enzinger FM: Critical commentary. *Pathol Res Pract* 189:605, 1993.

148. Enzinger FM, Weiss SW, Liang CY: Ossifying fibromyxoid tumor of soft parts: a clinicopathological analysis of 59 cases. *Am J Surg Pathol* 13:817, 1989.

149. Guarner J: Ossifying fibromyxoid tumor of soft parts (letter to the editor). *Am J Surg Pathol* 14:1167, 1991.

150. Kyriakos M: Ossifying fibromyxoid tumor: something new to mull over. *Am J Clin Pathol* 95:107, 1991.

151. Miettinen M: Ossifying fibromyxoid tumor of soft parts: additional observations on a distinctive soft tissue tumor. *Am J Clin Pathol* 95:142, 1991.

152. Yoshida H, Minamizaki T, Yumoto T, et al: Ossifying fibromyxoid tumor of soft parts. *Acta Pathol Jpn* 41:480, 1991.

Parachordoma

153. Dabska M: Parachordoma: a new clinicopathologic entity. *Cancer* 40:1586, 1977.

154. Ishida T, Oda H, Oka T, et al: Parachordoma: an ultrastructural and immunohistochemical study. *Virchows Arch (Pathol Anat)* 422:239, 1993.

155. Stout AP, Gorman JA: Mixed tumor of the skin of the salivary gland type. *Cancer* 12:537, 1959.

Amyloid tumor

156. Balazs M: Amyloidosis of the stomach. *Virchows Arch (Pathol Anat)* 391:227, 1981.

157. Chaudhuri MR, Parker DJ: A solitary amyloid nodule in the lung. *Thorax* 25:382, 1970.

158. Fernandez BB, Hernandez FJ: Amyloid tumor of the breast. *Arch Pathol* 95:102, 1973.

159. Hayes WT, Bernhardt H: Solitary amyloid mass of the lung. *Cancer* 24:820, 1969.

160. Holtzman IN, Skeer J: Amyloid "tumor formation" of skin. *Arch Dermatol* 67:187, 1953.

161. Kaiser-Kupprer MI, McAdam KPWJ, Kuwebara T: Localized amyloidosis of the orbit and upper respiratory tract. *Am J Ophthalmol* 84:721, 1977.

162. Khan SM, Birch PJ, Bass PS, et al: Localized amyloidosis of the lower genitourinary tract: a clinicopathologic and immunohistochemical study of nine cases. *Histopathology* 21:143, 1992.

163. Kibbi AG, Rubeiz NG, Zaynon ST, et al: Primary localized cutaneous amyloidosis. *Intern J Dermatol* 31:95, 1992.

164. Kisilevsky R: Amyloid and amyloidosis: differences, common themes, and practical considerations. *Mod Pathol* 4:514, 1991.

165. Kramer R, Som ML: Local tumorlike deposits of amyloid in larynx. *Arch Otolaryngol* 21:324, 1935.

166. Krishnan J, Chu WS, Elrod JP, et al: Tumoral presentation of amyloidosis (amyloidomas) in soft tissue: a report of 14 cases. *Am J Clin Pathol* 100:135, 1993.

167. Lew W, Seymour A: Primary amyloid tumor of the breast: case reports and literature review. *Acta Cytol* 29:7, 1985.

168. Lipper S, Kahn LB: Amyloid tumor. *Am J Surg Pathol* 2:141, 1978.

169. Ossnoss KZ, Harrell DD: Isolated mediastinal mass in primary amyloidosis. *Chest* 78:786, 1980.

170. Potter BS, Johnson WC: Primary localized amyloidosis cutis. *Arch Dermatol* 103:448, 1971.

171. Schindel S, BenBasset H: Amyloid tumor of the larynx: case report with electronmicroscopic study. *Ann Otolaryngol* 81:438, 1972.

172. Silverman JF, Dabbbs DJ, Norris HT, et al: Localized primary (AL) amyloid tumor of the breast: cytologic, histologic, immunohistochemical, and ultrastructural observations. *Am J Surg Pathol* 10:539, 1986.

173. Smith ME, Zimmerman LE: Amyloidosis of the eyelid and conjunctiva. *Arch Ophthalmol* 75:42, 1966.

174. Sorensen KH, Christensen HE: Local amyloid formation in the hip joint capsule in osteoarthritis. *Acta Orthop Scand* 44:460, 1973.

175. Stark DB, McDonald JR: Amyloid "tumors" of the larynx, trachea, and bronchi: a histological study of 15 cases. *Am J Clin Pathol* 18:778, 1948.

176. Stimson PG, Tortoledo ME, Luna MA, et al: Localized primary amyloid tumor of the parotid gland. *Oral Surg Oral Med Oral Pathol* 66:466, 1988.

177. Takaha M, Naguta H, Sonoda T: Localized amyloid tumor of the ureter: report of a case. *J Urol* 105:502, 1971.

178. Timosca G, et al: Primary localized amyloidosis of palate. *Oral Surg Oral Med Oral Pathol* 44:76, 1977.

179. Van Rijswijk MH, Van Heusdan CW: The potassium permanganate method: a reliable method for differentiating amyloid AA from other forms of amyloid in routine laboratory practice. *Am J Pathol* 97:43, 1979.

180. Weiss L: Isolated multiple nodular pulmonary amyloidosis. *Am J Clin Pathol* 33:318, 1960.

181. Weiss SW: Tumoral amyloidosis of soft tissue (amyloidoma): new approaches to an old problem. *Am J Clin Pathol* 100:91, 1993.

CHAPTER 38

MALIGNANT SOFT TISSUE TUMORS OF UNCERTAIN TYPE

ALVEOLAR SOFT PART SARCOMA

Alveolar soft part sarcoma is a clinically and morphologically distinct soft tissue sarcoma that was first defined and named by Christopherson et al.[8] in 1952. Before their report, typical cases had been described under various designations including malignant myoblastoma,[18,22,27] paraganglioma,[23,34,47] angioendothelioma,[28] and even liposarcoma.[15] Since 1952 numerous examples of this tumor have been reported and have been studied immunohistochemically and with the electron microscope, but there is still considerable uncertainty as to the exact nature of this tumor. Smetana and Scott's contention[54] that it is an unusual variant of paraganglioma is not supported by the clinical, tinctorial, and immunohistochemical findings, but many of the more recent studies point toward striated muscle origin. Alveolar soft part sarcomas are uniformly malignant, and there is no benign counterpart of this tumor.

Alveolar soft part sarcoma is an uncommon neoplasm; its frequency among our cases is estimated as between 0.5% and 1% of all soft tissue sarcomas. It is even less common in other series. Ekfors et al.,[12] for example, found only 1 case of alveolar soft part sarcoma among 246 malignant soft tissue tumors in Finland, an incidence of 0.4%.

Clinical findings

According to a review of 143 examples of the tumor from the AFIP files and the available data in the literature,[8,30,32] the tumor occurs principally in adolescents and young adults and is most frequently encountered in patients between 15 and 35 years of age. Female patients outnumber males, especially among patients under 25 years of age. Less frequently infants and children are affected; in one of our cases the tumor was allegedly present at birth.

There are two main locations of the tumor. When occurring in adults, it predominates in the lower extremities, especially the anterior portion of the thigh. Thus of 143 patients from our files, 63 (44.1%) had tumors in the lower extremities, including 42 in the thigh.[30] Rare locations are

the cervix and uterus.[20,51] When the tumor affects infants and children, it is often located in the region of the head and neck, especially the orbit and tongue; tumors in the head and neck tend to be of smaller size, probably because of earlier detection[18,29,36,53] (Table 38-1).

Alveolar soft part sarcoma usually presents as a slow-growing, painless mass, nearly always without functional impairment. Because of the relative lack of symptoms, it is easily overlooked, and in a good number of cases metastasis to the lung or brain is the first manifestation of the disease.[9] Headache, nausea, and visual changes are often associated with cerebral metastasis. As a rule, the tumor is richly vascular, causing pulsation or a distinctly audible bruit in some instances. Massive hemorrhage is often encountered during surgical removal.[5] In rare instances there is erosion or destruction of the underlying bone.[12,33] Hypervascularity with prominent draining veins and prolonged capillary staining are usually demonstrable with angiography and CT scan.[33]

Pathological findings

The gross specimen tends to be poorly circumscribed, soft, and friable, and on section it consists of yellow-white to gray-red tissue, often with large areas of necrosis and hemorrhage. Frequently the tumor is surrounded by numerous tortuous vessels of large caliber.

The microscopic picture varies little from tumor to tu-

Table 38-1. Anatomical distribution of 143 cases of alveolar soft part sarcoma (AFIP)

Location	No. patients	Percent
Head and neck (orbit, 16; tongue, 10)	39	27.3
Trunk	16	11.2
Upper extremity	25	17.4
Lower extremity (thigh, 42)	63	44.1
TOTAL	143	100.0

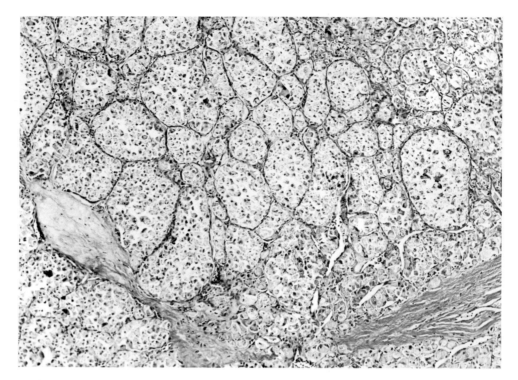

FIG. 38-1. Alveolar soft part sarcoma. Typical organoid or nestlike arrangement of tumor cells. (×50.)

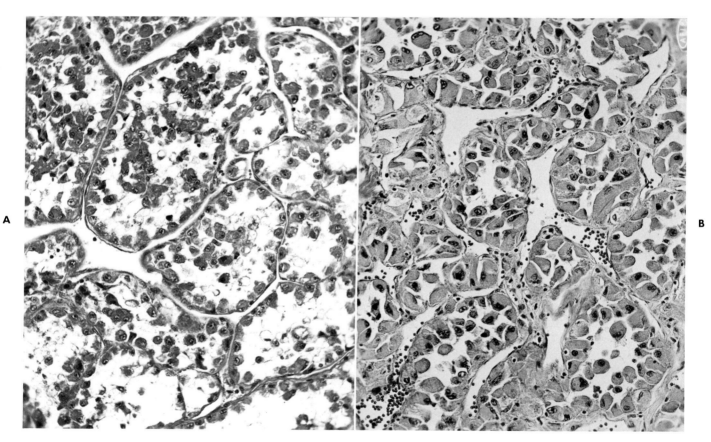

FIG. 38-2. Examples of alveolar soft part sarcoma exhibiting nests of large tumor cells with central loss of cellular cohesion resulting in a pseudoalveolar pattern. The cell nests are separated by thin-walled, sinusoidal vascular spaces. (**A,** ×210; **B,** ×180.)

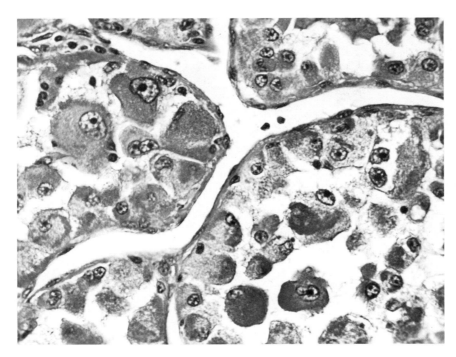

FIG. 38-3. Alveolar soft part sarcoma consisting of rounded or polygonal tumor cells with cytoplasm of varying density, vesicular nuclei, and prominent nucleoli. A basal lamina separates the tumor from the flattened endothelial cells of the intervening vascular channel. (×395.)

mor, and the uniformity of the microscopic picture is a constant and typical feature of the lesion. Characteristically, dense fibrous trabeculae of varying thickness divide the tumor into compact groups or compartments of irregular size that in turn are subdivided into sharply defined nests or aggregates of tumor cells. These cellular aggregates are separated from one another by thin-walled, sinusoidal vascular channels lined by a single layer of flattened endothelial cells. In most instances the cellular aggregates show central degeneration, necrosis, and loss of cohesion resulting in a pseudoalveolar pattern. Reticulin preparation brings out the distinctive nestlike or organoid arrangement and clearly outlines the sinusoidal vascular channels that separate the groups of tumor cells. This pseudoalveolar pattern should not be confused with the more irregular alveolar pattern of alveolar rhabdomyosarcoma (Figs. 38-1 to 38-3 and 38-7). Less frequently, the nestlike pattern is inconspicuous or absent entirely and the tumor is merely composed of uniform sheets of large granular cells with few or no discernible vascular channels. This more solid or compact type of alveolar soft part sarcoma occurs mainly in infants and children and is often associated with a more favorable prognosis (Figs. 38-4 and 38-5).

The individual cells are large, rounded, or more often polygonal and display little variation in size and shape. They have distinct cell borders and possess one or more vesicular nuclei with small nucleoli and abundant granular, eosinophilic, and sometimes vacuolated cytoplasm. Mitotic

figures are scarce. Rare pleomorphic examples of the tumor have been reported in the literature.[14]

At the margin of the tumor there are usually numerous dilated veins, a feature that is probably the result of multiple arteriovenous shunts within the neoplasm similar to hemangiopericytoma and paraganglioma. Vascular invasion is a constant and striking finding that explains the tendency of the tumor to develop metastasis at an early stage of the disease (Fig. 38-6).

PAS preparation, the most important stain for the diagnosis of alveolar soft part sarcoma, reveals varying amounts of intracellular glycogen and characteristically PAS-positive, diastase-resistant rhomboid or rod-shaped crystals, often having a sheaflike arrangement (Fig. 38-8). Masson,[35] in 1959, was the first to describe and depict these crystals as a diagnostic feature of alveolar soft part sarcoma, and Shipkey et al.,[52] in 1964, were the first to examine them with the electron microscope. According to our material, the typical crystalline material is present in at least 80% of the tumors; in the remainder there are merely PAS-positive granules, probably precursors of the crystals. The crystals are a feature of both primary and metastatic alveolar soft part sarcomas.

Immunohistochemical findings

The cells of alveolar soft part sarcoma do not stain with antibodies against cytokeratin, epithelial membrane antigen, neurofilaments, glial fibrillary acidic protein, seroto-

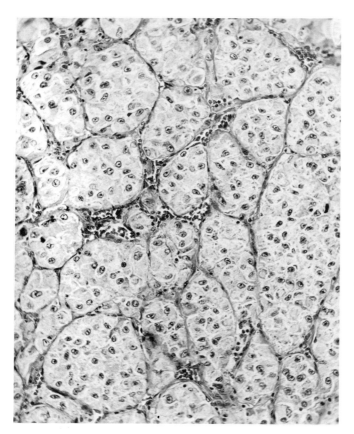

FIG. 38-4. Alveolar soft part sarcoma consisting of compact cell nests similar to those of paraganglioma. Same case as in Fig. 38-1. (×160.)

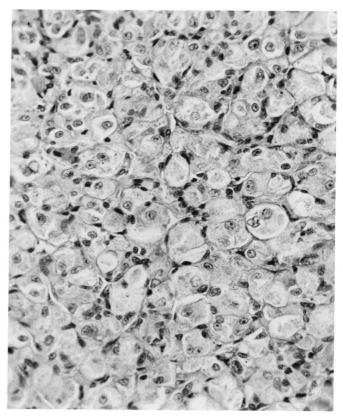

FIG. 38-5. Alveolar soft part sarcoma. Reticulin preparation outlines nests of tumor cells and intervening vascular channels. (Reticulin preparation; ×70.)

nin, synaptophysin, met-enkephalin and leu-enkephalin, but occasionally express S-100 protein and neuron-specific enolase.[1,45] The reports in regard to staining for muscle markers differ somewhat, but most investigators were able to demonstrate immunoreactivity for vimentin, muscle-specific actin, and desmin in the tumor cells*; some, however, were unable to confirm these findings.[1,31] Rosai et al.[48] reported MyoD1 protein expression in the tumor, but myoglobin expression has not been reported.[44]

Electron microscopic findings

Under the electron microscope the cells contain numerous mitochondria, a prominent smooth endoplasmic reticulum, glycogen, and a well-developed Golgi apparatus. Characteristically, there are also rhomboid, rod-shaped, or spicular crystals having a regular lattice pattern and sparse electron-dense secretory granules. Both crystals and dense granules are membrane bound and consist of crystallized and uncrystallized filaments 6 nm in diameter, suggesting transitions between the two structures. The filaments are ar-

ranged in a parallel fashion with a periodicity of 10 nm.[32,40,41] The large polygonal cells are separated from the intervening vascular channels by a basal lamina, occasional circumferentially arranged spindle-shaped cells, and collagen fibers. Rare desmosomes or hemidesmosomes are present between the individual cells and between cells and surrounding basal laminae.[12,24,39,52] There is no evidence of smooth muscle or striated muscle differentiation,[38] but Mukai et al.[41] using digital image analysis of the crystalline material, demonstrated structural similarities to actin filaments.

Differential diagnosis

The differential diagnosis chiefly includes metastatic *renal cell carcinoma, paraganglioma,* and *granular cell tumor.* Alveolar rhabdomyosarcoma is sometimes confused with alveolar soft part sarcoma but more because of the similarity in name than in the microscopic picture.

Renal cell carcinoma, primary or metastatic, often bears a striking resemblance to alveolar soft part sarcoma, but in most of the cases can be distinguished by the absence of the characteristic PAS-positive crystalline material (Fig. 38-

---

*References 10, 21, 36, 38, 39, 42, 43, 46.

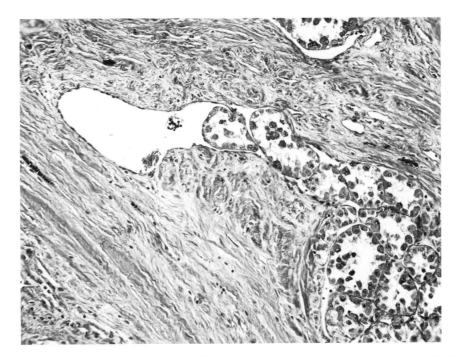

FIG. 38-6. Alveolar soft part sarcoma. Dilated peripheral vein with tumor invasion. (×140.)

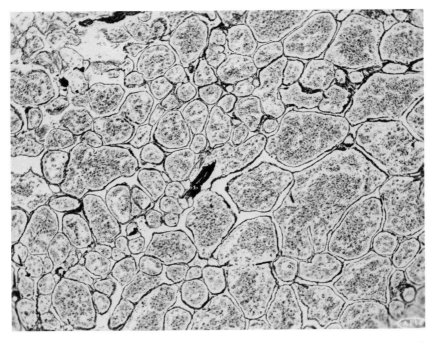

FIG. 38-7. Alveolar soft part sarcoma without the clustering or nestlike arrangement of tumor cells. This variant occurs mainly in children and often carries a more favorable prognosis. (×300.)

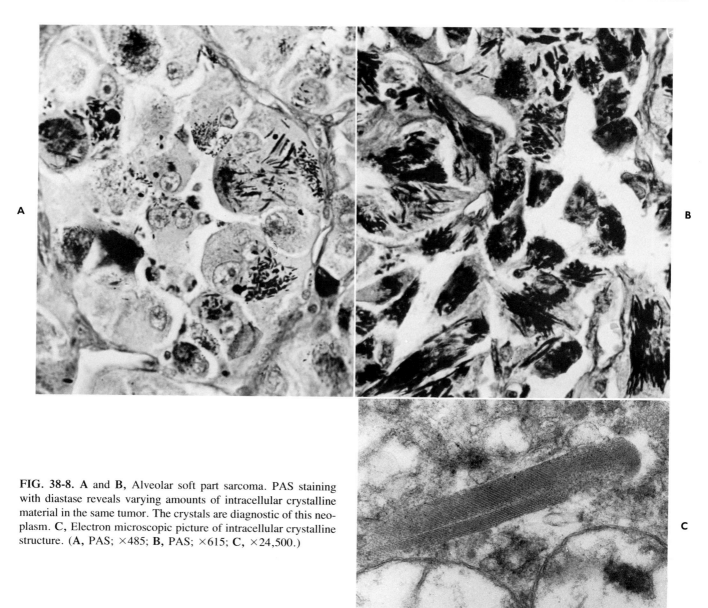

FIG. 38-8. A and **B,** Alveolar soft part sarcoma. PAS staining with diastase reveals varying amounts of intracellular crystalline material in the same tumor. The crystals are diagnostic of this neoplasm. **C,** Electron microscopic picture of intracellular crystalline structure. (**A,** PAS; ×485; **B,** PAS; ×615; **C,** ×24,500.)

9). The pale-staining cytoplasm of its cells and fat content of renal cell carcinoma are less reliable features because both may be encountered in degenerated forms of alveolar soft part sarcoma. Glycogen is present in both tumors, but it is absent in *granular cell tumor* and *paraganglioma.* It is also noteworthy that the cells of granular cell tumor are less well defined, have a distinctly granular cytoplasm, and show strongly positive immunostaining for S-100 protein; moreover, they do not display the richly vascular endocrine pattern of alveolar soft part sarcoma.

The clinical features are also of value in differential diagnosis: primary renal cell carcinomas are usually demonstrable radiographically in the retroperitoneum, and renal cell carcinoma, paraganglioma, and malignant granular cell tumor chiefly affect patients older than 40 years and are definitely rare in patients younger than 25 years. Moreover, as mentioned elsewhere, there is no record that a "bona fide" paraganglioma ever occurs in the extremities.

Discussion

Despite numerous immunohistochemical and electron microscopic studies, the exact nature and tissue type of alveolar soft part sarcoma remain uncertain. Over the years, several concepts concerning the nature of this tumor have

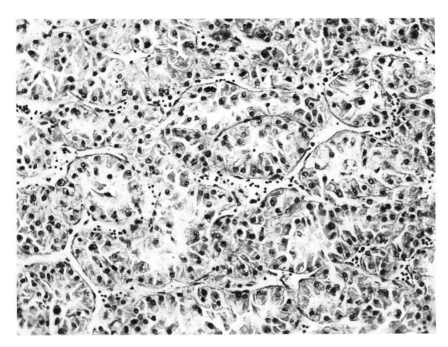

FIG. 38-9. Metastatic renal cell carcinoma simulating alveolar soft part sarcoma. (×180.)

been entertained, especially malignant granular cell tumor, paraganglioma, and tumor of skeletal muscle origin. A variant of paraganglioma was first proposed by Smetana and Scott,[54] who emphasized the morphological resemblance of this tumor and alveolar soft part sarcoma. Others also favored the concept of paraganglionic or chemoreceptor origin[23,34] and stressed the close ultrastructural resemblance between alveolar soft part sarcoma and carotid body tumor, including the presence of chief cells, peripheral spindle-shaped cells, and electron-dense secretory-like granules.[55,56] Strong evidence against this concept, however, is not only the abundance of glycogen and PAS-positive, diastase-resistant crystalline material in the tumor cells, but also the facts that the cells of alveolar soft part sarcomas are not argyrophilic with the Grimelius stain, do not stain with antibodies to neurofilaments, chromogranin, synaptophysin, serotonin, and met-enkephalin, and contain no intracellular catecholamines as indicated by the complete absence of formaldehyde vapor-induced fluorescence in the tumor cells.[12,38,39] Furthermore, alveolar soft part sarcoma differs in several clinical aspects from paraganglioma: it prevails in patients younger than 30 years, involves chiefly the extremities, and behaves in a malignant manner with frequent metastasis to lung, brain, and bone. There is also some question as to the existence of paraganglionic structures in the muscles of the extremities. We have never encountered paraganglia or related structures in the soft tissues of the limbs; nor were they detected by Karnauchow

and Magner,[25] who carried out a systematic search for such structures in the thigh.

Although there is no morphological evidence of muscle differentiation in the tumor cells such as myofilaments and cross-striations, a muscle origin or muscle differentiation is another and more likely possibility that has found growing support in the recent literature. This was first suggested by Fisher and Reidbord in 1971[17] on the basis of the resemblance of the membrane-bound crystals to those in nemaline myopathy and rhabdomyoma. More recently, this concept was considerably strengthened by immunohistochemical studies that demonstrated the potential of the tumor cells to express desmin, muscle-specific actin (HHF35), and vimentin.[19,21,38,42,45] Others, however, were unable to confirm these results or—finding only a few desmin-positive cells—questioned their significance.[1,31,37] Yet, the expression of MyoD1 protein in the tumor cells, reported by Rosai et al.,[48] seems to lend further support to the concept of skeletal muscle differentiation.

Still another concept of the histogenesis was offered by DeSchryver-Kecskemeti et al.,[11] who contended that the cytoplasmic granules of alveolar soft part sarcoma are similar to the renin granules of juxtaglomerular tumor and proposed the name "angioreninoma." There is, however, no sign of hyperreninism, such as hypertension, hypokalemia, or aldosteronism, in patients with alveolar soft part sarcoma, and, according to Mukai et al.,[39] immunostaining for renin is negative and plasma renin levels are normal. Moreover, similar PAS-positive crystals have been observed in a human muscle spindle[6] and in a variety of tumors, including rhabdomyoma, islet cell tumor, paraganglioma, schwannoma, and Warthin's tumor.

Clinical behavior and therapy

The ultimate prognosis is poor despite the relatively slow growth of the tumor. Lieberman et al.,[31] in a study of 91 cases with follow-up information, reported a 77% survival rate at 2 years, 60% at 5 years, and 38% at 10 years in patients who presented without metastasis. Only 15% of the patients were alive after 20 years. Auerbach and Brooks[1] reported an overall 5-year survival rate of 67%. Metastases tend to occur early in the course of the disease. In fact, among 36 metastatic alveolar soft part sarcomas in our files, 13 developed metastatic lesions before detection of the primary tumor. On the other hand, metastasis may also be delayed for many years; one of our patients developed pulmonary metastases 35 years after removal of the primary tumor in the parotid gland. With some exceptions, prognosis seems to be more favorable in children than in adults, but this may be related to the location of the tumor and its smaller size and better resectability.[14] Thus, 8 of the 13 patients with alveolar soft part sarcomas of the orbit reported by Font et al.[18] were alive and well; most of the tumors affected younger patients and were of small size. Yet 1 of the 13 patients died 21 years after the initial orbital surgery, indicating the need for prolonged follow-up in all cases. DNA analysis, carried out in only a small number of cases, revealed a diploid DNA distribution in typical cases but an additional tetraploid peak in a pleomorphic example of the tumor.[46]

The principal metastatic sites are the lungs, followed by the brain and skeleton. Cerebral metastases, in fact, may be the first manifestation of the disease and are more common with alveolar soft part sarcoma than with any other type of soft tissue sarcoma. Metastases to lymph nodes are infrequent.

Treatment is not particularly promising, and the relatively slow growth of the tumor must be considered when one is assessing the effect of therapy. Most reviewers recommend radical surgical excision of primary and metastatic lesions combined with radiotherapy or chemotherapy, or both. There is no consensus as to the effect of chemotherapy, and, according to Lieberman et al.,[31] there is little difference in survival rates between patients treated by postoperative radiation or chemotherapy.

EPITHELIOID SARCOMA

The term *epithelioid sarcoma* has been applied to a morphologically distinctive neoplasm that is likely to be confused with a variety of benign and malignant conditions, especially a granulomatous process, a synovial sarcoma, and an ulcerating squamous cell carcinoma. The tumor

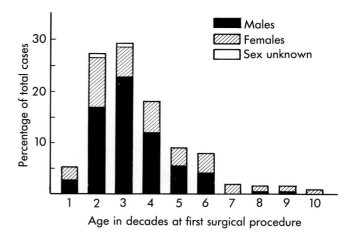

FIG. 38-10. Age and sex distribution of 241 cases of epithelioid sarcoma.

mainly afflicts young adults, and its principal sites are the fingers, hands, and forearms. More than half of the 62 tumors that we described in 1970[70] occurred at this general site. In fact, epithelioid sarcoma is the most common soft tissue sarcoma in the hand and wrist, followed by alveolar rhabdomyosarcoma and synovial sarcoma.[57] It is not surprising, therefore, that examples of this tumor were described earlier as synovial sarcoma,[58,68] sarcoma aponeuroticum,[66,84] and large cell sarcoma of tendon sheath.[60] Numerous additional articles on this subject have been published since 1970.*

Clinical findings

Information obtained from 241 cases of epithelioid sarcoma from the files of the AFIP essentially confirms the clinical data reported on our initial group of 62 cases.[64,70] The tumor is most prevalent in adolescents and young adults between 10 and 35 years of age (median age, 26 years). It is rare in children and older persons, but no age-group is exempt (Fig. 38-10). Male patients outnumber females by about 2:1. The racial distribution is similar to that in the overall population. As mentioned, the tumor has a propensity to occur in the finger, hand, and forearm, followed in frequency by the knee and lower leg, especially the pretibial region, the buttocks and thigh, the shoulder and arm, and the ankle, foot, and toe. It is extremely rare in the trunk and head and neck region with the exception of the scalp. Other unusual sites are the penis and vulva[76,81,94,101,116] (Table 38-2).

The tumor occurs in both the subcutis and deeper tissues. When located in the subcutis, it usually presents as a firm nodule that may be solitary or multiple, has a calluslike con-

---

*References 62, 79, 89, 98, 113, 115.

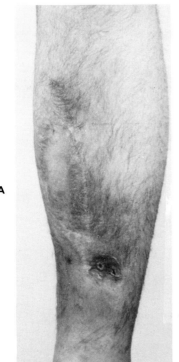

A

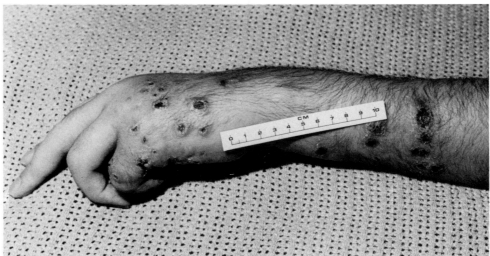

B

FIG. 38-11. A, Recurrent ulcerating epithelioid sarcoma of the anterior tibial region in a 21-year-old man. **B,** Recurrent epithelioid sarcoma of the hand and forearm with multiple, ulcerated (punched-out) satellite lesions of the skin. (**B** from Heenan P et al: *Am J Dermatopathol* 8:95, 1986.)

Table 38-2. Anatomical distribution of 215 cases of epithelioid sarcoma

Location	No. patients	Percent
Head, neck	9	4
Trunk	12	6
Shoulder, arm	20	9
Forearm, wrist	37	17
Hand, fingers	65	30
Buttock, thigh	22	10
Knee, lower leg	31	15
Ankle, foot, toes	19	9
TOTAL	215	100

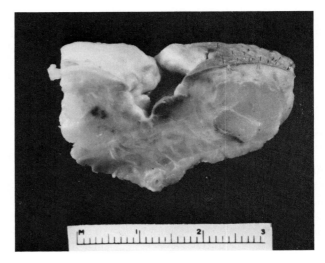

FIG. 38-12. Ulcerating epithelioid sarcoma of the hand with indurated margins.

sistency, and is often described as a "woody hard knot" or "firm lump" that is slow growing and painless. Nodules situated in the dermis are often elevated above the skin surface and frequently become ulcerated weeks or months after they are first noted. Such lesions are often erroneously diagnosed as an "indurated ulcer," "draining abscess," or "infected wart" that fails to heal despite intensive therapy (Figs. 38-11 and 38-12).

Deep-seated lesions are usually firmly attached to tendons, tendon sheaths, or fascial structures; they tend to be larger and less well defined and often manifest as areas of induration or as multinodular lumpy masses, sometimes

moving slightly with motion of the extremity (Fig. 38-13). Pain or tenderness is never a prominent symptom, with the exception of occasional tumors that encroach on large nerves. The size of the tumor varies substantially and ranges from a few millimeters to 15 cm or more. The majority of the tumors, however, measure 3 to 6 cm in diameter. Be-

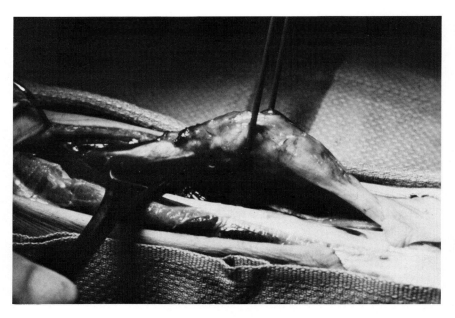

FIG. 38-13. Epithelioid sarcoma of the wrist infiltrating the tendon of the flexor carpi ulnaris in a 28-year-old man. (From Enzinger FM: *Cancer* 26:1029, 1970.)

cause many lesions are multinodular, determination of their exact size is often impossible.

Roentgenographic examination reveals mostly a soft tissue mass with an occasional speckled pattern of calcification, and with infrequent cortical thinning and erosion of underlying bone. Invasion and destruction of adjacent bone are seen occasionally.[100] Ossification is rare, but in one of our cases it was so striking that the tumor was initially mistaken for an extraskeletal osteosarcoma.

Pathological findings

Gross inspection usually shows the presence of one or more nodules measuring 0.5 to 5 cm in greatest diameter. Deep-seated tumors, attached to tendons or fascia, tend to be larger and present as firm multinodular masses with irregular outlines. The cut surface has a glistening gray-white or gray-tan mottled surface with focal yellow or brown areas caused by focal necrosis or hemorrhage.

The principal microscopic characteristics are the distinct nodular arrangement of the tumor cells, their tendency to undergo central degeneration and necrosis, and their epithelioid appearance and eosinophilia. The nodular pattern, probably the most conspicuous single feature of epithelioid sarcoma, varies somewhat: in some tumors the nodules are well circumscribed; in others they are less well defined and are often compacted into irregular multinodular masses (Figs. 38-14 to 38-16). Multiple nodules are less common in tissue obtained at the initial operation than in recurrent tumors. In rare cases the presence of multiple small superficial satellite nodules near the operative site may mimic a skin disease (Fig. 38-11, *B*).[63,79] Necrosis of the tumor nodules is a common finding; it is most prominent in the center of the nodules and at times is associated with hemorrhage and cystic change. Fusion of several necrotizing nodules results in "geographic" lesions with scalloped margins. When the tumor spreads within a fascia or aponeurosis, it forms festoonlike or garlandlike bands punctuated by areas of necrosis (Fig. 38-17). Not infrequently the tumor grows along the neurovascular bundle and invests large vessels or nerves. Vascular invasion takes place, but in our experience it is rarely a prominent feature of the tumor.

Lesions located in the dermis or extending into the dermal region often ulcerate through the skin and may simulate an ulcerating squamous cell carcinoma, especially because of the pronounced epithelioid appearance and eosinophilia of the tumor cells. This process occurs mainly in areas with small amounts of subcutaneous fat such as the fingers and the prepatellar and pretibial regions. But unlike squamous cell carcinoma, the skin surrounding the ulcerated tumor does not display any dyskeratotic change and only a moderate degree of acanthosis.

The constituent cellular elements range from large ovoid or polygonal cells with deeply eosinophilic cytoplasm, suggesting a rhabdomyosarcoma or malignant rhabdoid tumor, to plump spindle-shaped cells reminiscent of a fibrosarcoma or malignant fibrous histiocytoma. In some of the latter tumors the spindle cell pattern may predominate and may obscure the characteristic epithelioid features and nodularity.

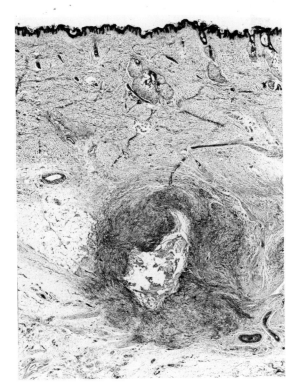

FIG. 38-14. Epithelioid sarcoma. Solitary nodules with central necrosis mimicking a necrotizing granulomatous process. (×7.) (From Enzinger FM: *Cancer* 26:1029, 1970.)

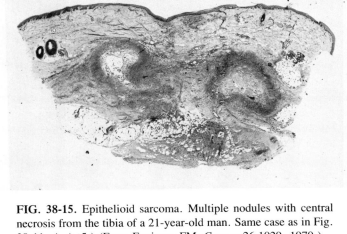

FIG. 38-15. Epithelioid sarcoma. Multiple nodules with central necrosis from the tibia of a 21-year-old man. Same case as in Fig. 38-11, *A*. (×5.) (From Enzinger FM: *Cancer* 26:1029, 1970.)

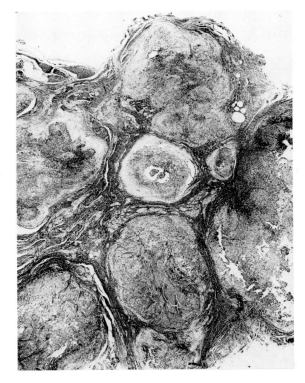

FIG. 38-16. Epithelioid sarcoma. Conglomerate of tumor nodules with central necrosis. (×10.) (From Enzinger FM: *Cancer* 26:1029, 1970.)

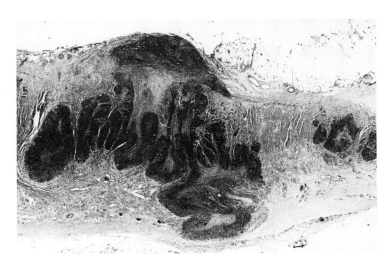

FIG. 38-17. Epithelioid sarcoma within the fascia lata forming garlandlike bands. (×11.) (From Enzinger FM: *Cancer* 26:1029, 1970.)

The "fibroma-like variants of epithelioid sarcoma" reported by Mirra et al.[93] are presumably of this type. In general, cellular pleomorphism is minimal, but pleomorphic tumors with little collagen formation were reported as possible epithelioid sarcomas.[90] In our experience multinucleated giant cells are absent or scarce.

Usually, epithelioid and spindle-shaped cells merge imperceptibly, and there is never the distinct biphasic or pseudoglandular pattern as in synovial sarcoma. In some tumors the loss of cellular cohesion and secondary hemorrhage may closely simulate an angiosarcoma; in others the presence of intracellular lipid droplets may suggest the incipient lumen formation of endothelial cells in epithelioid hemangioendothelioma. Intercellular deposition of dense hyalinized collagen is common and, together with the eosinophilic cytoplasm, contributes to the deeply eosinophilic appearance of the tumor. Calcification and bone formation do occur in 10% to 20% of cases; cartilaginous metaplasia is rare, however. Aggregates of chronic inflammatory cells along the margin of the tumor nodules are present in the majority of cases and may mimic a chronic inflammatory process (Figs. 38-18 to 38-22).

Special staining techniques contribute little to the diagnosis. The cytoplasm stains a deep red brown with the Masson trichrome stain. There is no stainable intracellular mucin, but alcian blue–positive and hyaluronidase-sensitive mesenchymal mucin is often found in the surrounding matrix. There may also be some intracellular glycogen. Almost always a dense meshwork of reticulin fibers separates the tumor cells (Fig. 38-23). Cytogenetic analysis of an epithelioid sarcoma cell line revealed a karyotype of 64 to 66 chromosomes with extensive numerical and structural rearrangements and up to 24 marker chromosomes.[104]

Immunohistochemical findings

The cells show coexpression for low-molecular-weight (45 kd and 54 kd) and high-molecular-weight (57 kd) cytokeratin, vimentin, and epithelial membrane antigen.* The degree of immunoreactivity, however, varies considerably from tumor to tumor and in different portions of the same neoplasm. Usually the presence of cytokeratin is more pronounced in epithelioid than in spindle-shaped cell areas and is enhanced by predigestion with trypsin. Staining with antibodies against desmin, FVIII, or CD-34 are uniformly negative. Antibodies directed against S-100 protein, neurofilament protein, and carcinoembryonic antigen have been reported as positive in some cases.[65,77,108]

Ultrastructural findings

Most investigators report polygonal and spindle-shaped cells with ovoid, indented nuclei having small amounts of marginally placed chromatin. The cytoplasm contains arrays of rough endoplasmic reticulum, a prominent Golgi apparatus, and free ribosomes as well as occasional mitochondria, lysosomes, and droplets of osmiophilic material. Intermediate filaments are a common and often striking fea-

---

*References 64, 67, 71, 91, 95, 98, 119.

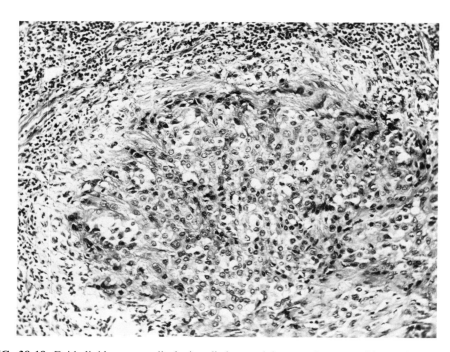

FIG. 38-18. Epithelioid sarcoma displaying distinct nodular growth pattern. Note epithelioid appearance of the tumor cells. (×165.)

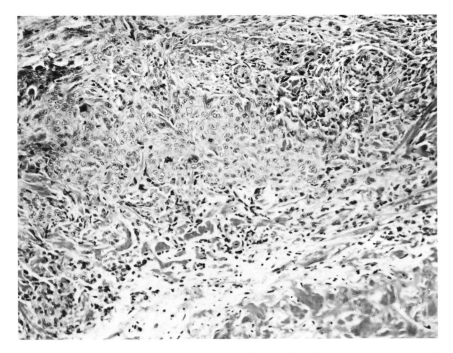

FIG. 38-19. Epithelioid sarcoma showing central necrosis of the tumor nodule. (×160.)

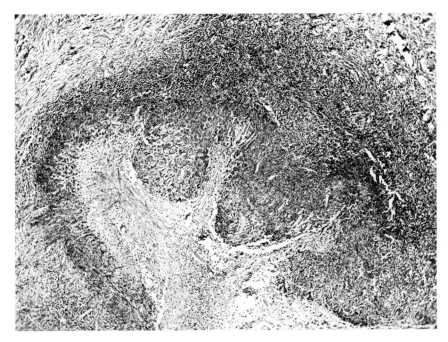

FIG. 38-20. Epithelioid sarcoma with central necrosis and a conspicuous chronic inflammatory infiltrate in the surrounding tissues.

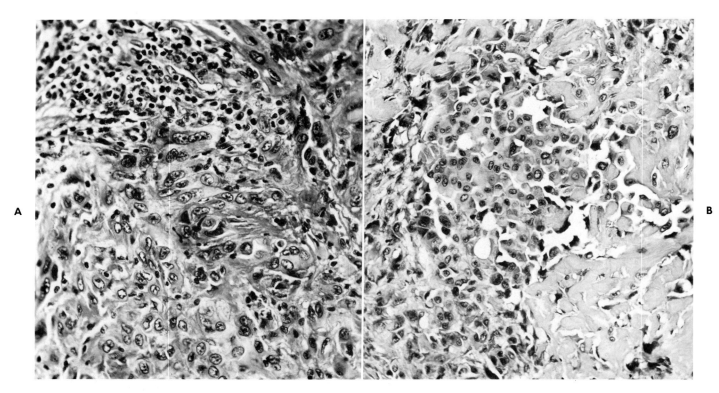

FIG. 38-21. Epithelioid sarcoma. Note the epithelioid appearance of the polygonal tumor cells **(A)** and the association of tumor cells and abundant hyalinized collagen **(B)**. (**A**, ×300; **B**, ×165.)

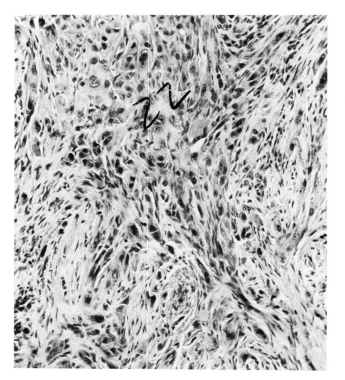

FIG. 38-22. Epithelioid sarcoma. Transition between epithelioid and spindle cells in a tumor of the right forearm of a 26-year-old man. (×165.) (From Enzinger FM: *Cancer* 26:1029, 1970.)

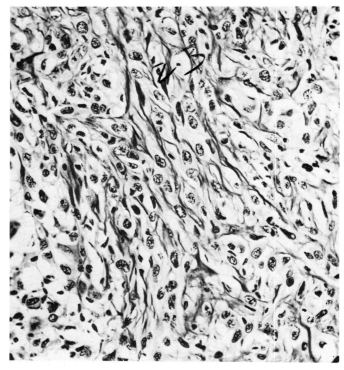

FIG. 38-23. Epithelioid sarcoma. Reticulin preparation showing a reticulin meshwork between tumor cells. (Reticulin preparation; ×145.)

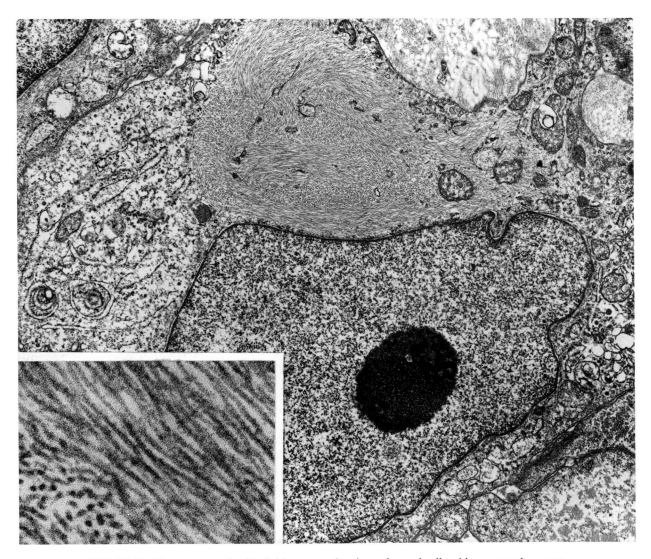

FIG. 38-24. Ultrastructure of epithelioid sarcoma showing polygonal cells with a paranuclear mass of intermediate filaments. (×15,000.) *(Inset)* High-power view of intracytoplasmic bundles of intermediate filaments ranging in diameter from 7 to 12 nm. (×150,000.) (From Mukai M, Torikata C, Iri H, et al: *Am J Pathol* 119:44, 1985.)

ture. They may be arranged longitudinally as in myofibroblasts or more often form paranuclear masses or whorls, a feature that probably accounts for the voluminous cytoplasm and the striking epithelioid appearance and eosinophilia of the tumor cells.[59,70,92,97] There are occasionally interdigitating cellular processes with maculae adherentes or intercellular desmosome-like junctions and small intercellular cystic or cleftlike spaces surrounded by filopodia. As in synovial sarcoma there may be light and dark tumor cells, but, unlike this tumor's glandular structures, intracellular cystic spaces and basal laminae are absent in epithelioid sarcoma (Fig. 38-24).[61,73,95,115]

Differential diagnosis

The frequency with which the tumor is mistaken for a benign process is chiefly a result of its deceptively harmless appearance during the initial stage of the disease. Superficially located tumors of small size with a nodular or multinodular pattern are likely to be mistaken for an inflammatory process, particularly a necrotizing infectious granuloma, necrobiosis lipoidica, granuloma annulare, or rheumatoid nodule. Yet the individual cells in epithelioid sarcoma tend to be more sharply defined than those of a granuloma. They are larger, more eosinophilic, less mature in appearance, and stain positively for cytokeratin and epithelial membrane antigen. They do not stain with anti-LCA like the large histiocytic cells in necrobiotic granuloma.[119] The epithelioid features, nodularity, and immunostaining for cytokeratin also aid in differentiating epithelioid sarcoma from nodular fasciitis, fibrous histiocytoma, and fibromatosis.

Larger neoplasms, frequently arising from tendons or fascial structures, are more readily recognizable as sarcomas, but they may be confused with synovial sarcoma, fibrosarcoma, angiosarcoma, epithelioid hemangioendothelioma, malignant extrarenal rhabdoid tumor, malignant melanoma, and other types of malignant neoplasms with a prominent epithelioid pattern. Distinction from synovial sarcoma may be difficult. It can be successfully accomplished in most cases, however, if attention is paid to the persistent absence of a biphasic pattern, pseudoglandular structures, and intracellular mucin, as well as the larger size and the prominent eosinophilia of the tumor cells. Moreover, dermal involvement and ulceration are much more common with epithelioid sarcoma than with synovial sarcoma. In some cases the location of the tumor may suggest the correct diagnosis: epithelioid sarcomas are most common in the fingers and the hand, and synovial sarcomas prevail in the vicinity of the knee and other large joints. The complete absence of keratin pearls and dyskeratosis in the adjacent epithelium nearly always allows separation from an ulcerating squamous cell carcinoma. Negative immunostaining for S-100 protein and melanoma-associated antigen permits exclusion of malignant melanoma.

Clinical course and therapy

The potential of the tumor to recur and metastasize is clearly evident from our follow-up study of 202 patients with epithelioid sarcoma from the AFIP files (Fig. 38-25).[64] Of these patients 68% were alive and 32% had died. No less than 77% developed one or more recurrences during the course of the disease. Metastases developed in 45% of the patients, most commonly to the regional lymph nodes (34%) and the lung (51%), and less frequently to the skin, central nervous system, and soft tissue. The scalp was the site of metastasis in 22% of the cases. The interval between initial surgical procedure and first recurrence averaged 1 year and 6 months in the fatal cases and 2 years and 1 month in the nonfatal cases; the time to metastasis averaged 4 years and 1 month in the fatal cases versus 3 years and 4 months in the nonfatal cases.[64]

Multiple recurrences, often as the result of marginal resection, are a characteristic feature of the tumor. One of our patients, for example, was treated for recurrent tumor growth in the left pretibial region on 11 occasions during a 16-year period. Another, a 27-year-old man, had 20 separate surgical procedures for recurrent growth within a period of 10 years. The recurrent tumor generally presents as confluent nodules in the dermis or along tendons and fas-

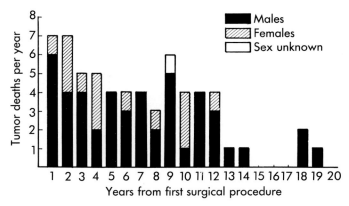

FIG. 38-25. Epithelioid sarcoma: years from first surgical procedure to death from disease. (From *Am J Surg Pathol* 9(4):241, 1985.)

cial structures at or near the original tumor site. As previously mentioned, there are also cases where the skin adjacent and proximal to the tumor is studded with small, craterlike ulcerated nodules or plaques, a striking picture unlike that of any other recurrent soft tissue sarcoma.[79] Recurrence generally develops within the first year after diagnosis, but recurrence may be late, and in one of our cases it became apparent 25 years after the primary tumor was removed by local excision.

Intravascular growth and lymph node involvement are ominous features: in one series, for instance, six of eight patients with intravenous extension of the tumor or lymph node involvement developed pulmonary metastases. Conversely, 9 of 10 patients without these features were alive from 2 to more than 13 years after diagnosis.[106] Metastasis may be early and may even manifest before detection of the primary tumor,[114] or it may be late. In one of our cases, for example, it became apparent 19 years after the initial diagnosis. Prognosis, therefore, should be rendered with considerable caution, even if the patient appears to be well and free of tumor 5 years after the initial diagnosis.

Prognosis depends on various factors, chiefly the sex of the patient, the size and depth of the tumor, the number of mitotic figures, and the presence or absence of hemorrhage, necrosis, and vascular invasion (Fig. 38-26). Moreover, tumors in the distal extremities have a more favorable prognosis than those in the trunk and proximal portions of the limbs.[64] In our series the female survival rate was 78% compared with a male survival rate of 64%. The better outcome in females was even more pronounced in the series of Bos et al.,[62] who reported a 5-year survival rate in females of 80% and in males of only 40%.

Flow cytometric DNA analysis revealed diploid (or hyperploid) and aneuploid DNA content.[82,96] In one study of 20 primary epithelioid sarcomas 40% of the tumors were

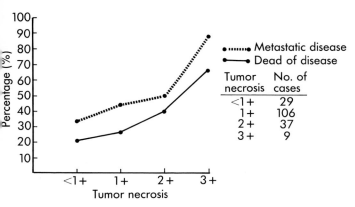

FIG. 38-26. Epithelioid sarcoma. Degree of tumor necrosis in initial biopsy or resection and clinical course. (From *Am J Surg Pathol* 9(4):241, 1985.)

hyperdiploid or tetraploid; four patients with diploid epithelioid sarcomas died of the disease.[69]

Accurate assessment and comparison of the efficacy of treatment is exceedingly difficult, especially if the cases are derived from multiple sources, as in the AFIP material. It is clearly evident, however, that the initial therapy (marginal resection) was inadequate in many cases and that a more aggressive surgical approach is required in order to prevent recurrent growth.[113] Adequate treatment requires early radical local excision or amputation if the primary tumor is situated in the fingers or toes. Amputation should also be considered as treatment for recurrent growth, but does not seem to offer any benefit to patients with distant metastasis.[117] Regional lymph node dissection should be included among the therapeutic modalities because lymph node metastasis is a fairly common occurrence in epithelioid sarcoma. In all cases surgical treatment should be combined with radiotherapy and multiagent chemotherapy over a prolonged period, similar to the chemotherapy given for other adult-type sarcomas. Shimm and Suit[111] reported local control and a low rate of recurrence with preoperative or postoperative radiation therapy and resection.

Discussion

There is still no consensus as to the exact nature and cell type of epithelioid sarcoma. Undoubtedly the tumor bears a close resemblance to synovial sarcoma, but there are several clinical and morphological differences that cast doubt on the close kinship between these two tumors. Not surprisingly, a synovial origin is often suggested in view of the intimate association of the tumor with tendons and aponeuroses, the mixture of epithelioid and spindle-shaped cell elements, and the presence of mucinous material in the surrounding ground substance. It is further supported by the immunostaining for cytokeratin,[65,75,91,95] the ultrastructural demonstration of light and dark cells and microvilli in some

of the cases, and the reported occurrence of a morphologically distinct epithelioid and synovial sarcoma that presented at two different locations in the same knee.[107] But there are also a number of distinguishing features: the predominant location of epithelioid sarcoma in the hand, the persistent absence of pseudoglandular structures and intracellular mucin droplets, and the lack of basal laminae ultrastructurally. Over the past years it has also been suggested that epithelioid sarcoma is a tumor of primitive mesenchymal cells with fibroblastic and histiocytic differentiation,[70,73,112] a primitive mesenchymal tumor with differentiation along histiocytic and synovial lines,[61] a fibrosarcoma,[72] a tumor of myofibroblasts altered by massive production of intermediate filaments,[59,99] a malignant giant cell tumor of tendon sheath,[60,71] and a tumor related to nodular tenosynovitis and arising from synovioblastic mesenchyme.[97] The last two of these suggestions appear to be most compatible with the electron microscopic features, although there is no evidence in our cases that epithelioid sarcoma ever arises in a preexisting giant cell tumor. The possible relationship to malignant extrarenal rhabdoid tumor is discussed below.

Trauma to the site of the tumor may be a contributing factor and has been reported in a large number of cases. In our series, for example, unsolicited reports of antecedent trauma were given in 20% of cases, including several foreign body–related injuries.[64,69] Prat et al.[100] report a history of trauma in 6 of 22 patients, including 1 case in which an epithelioid sarcoma of the hand developed following exposure to plutonium. Another case, reported by Bloustein et al.,[61] originated in the scar tissue of a cesarean section. Puissegur-Lupo et al.[102] observed an epithelioid sarcoma that arose in scar tissue 17 months after traumatic amputation of 3 fingers of the right hand.

MALIGNANT EXTRARENAL RHABDOID TUMOR

Malignant rhabdoid tumor, initially described in the kidney among possible variants of Wilms' tumor, superficially resembles rhabdomyosarcoma but is readily separated from this neoplasm by immunohistochemical studies.* Although extrarenal forms of this tumor are relatively rare, several deep-seated examples have been described in the soft tissues, including the neck, shoulder, trunk, and extremities.[120,126,130,137] Sporadic examples have also been reported in the prostate,[123] liver,[126,131] and central nervous system.[133] The tumor seems to be most common in infants but may also affect adolescents and adults. In the study of Kodet et al.,[128] the median age was 9 months; 11 of the 26 patients were infants less than 1 year of age. Lynch et al.[129] reported the occurrence of morphologically similar malignant rhabdoid tumors in the paravertebral regions of two female siblings during the first year of life.

---

*References 121, 127, 134, 135, 138, 139.

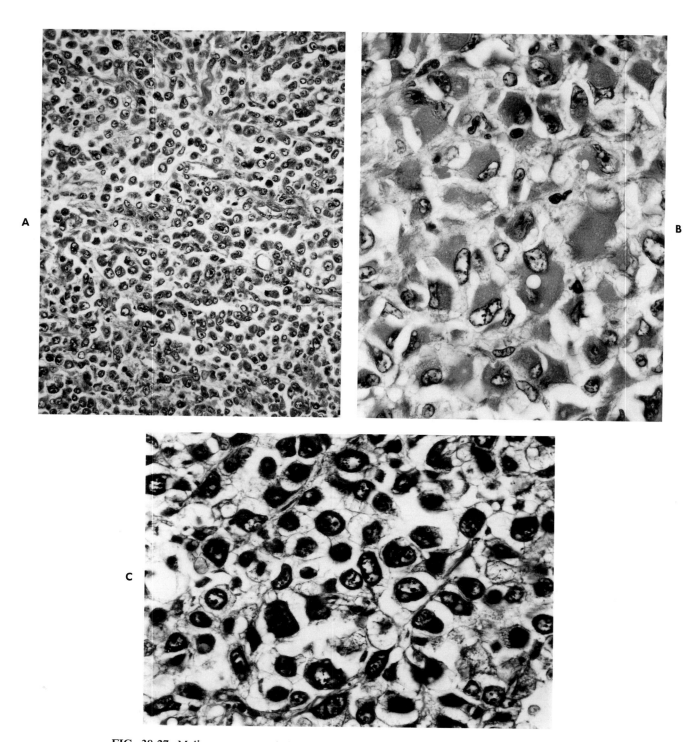

FIG. 38-27. Malignant extrarenal rhabdoid tumor composed of **A,** loosely arranged rounded or oval cells (×75), **B,** showing abundant deeply eosinophilic cytoplasm and large vesicular nuclei (×550). **C,** Unlike rhabdomyosarcoma, the cells stain positively for cytokeratin. (×350.)

Prognosis of malignant rhabdoid tumor is generally poor, with rapidly fatal course in most cases. Kodet et al.[128] report that 19 of 26 patients with this tumor died within 1 to 82 months (median time, 6 months) from the start of therapy.

Pathological findings

Microscopically, rhabdoid sarcoma is defined by three parameters: (1) round or polygonal cells with vesicular nuclei, prominent nucleoli, and abundant cytoplasm containing acidophilic and PAS-positive hyaline inclusions or globules, (2) positive staining of the intracellular acidophilic material with antibodies against keratin, epithelial membrane antigen, and vimentin; and (3) absence of demonstrable immunoreactive desmin and myoglobin, as well as lack of positive staining for S-100 protein, glial fibrillary acidic protein, and neurofilament proteins[134,137] (Fig. 38-27). Ultrastructurally, the paranuclear, intracellular masses consist of compact bundles or whorls of intermediate filaments 10 nm in length that correspond to the hyaline inclusions seen on light microscopy. Additionally, the cytoplasm contains a moderate amount of rough endoplasmic reticulum, few mitochondria, lysosomes, lipid droplets, and free ribosomes.[123,137] DNA analysis, carried out in only a few cases, revealed a diploid DNA profile.[130]

Discussion

Although extrarenal malignant rhabdoid tumor appears to be a distinct entity, considerable caution must be exercised in rendering this diagnosis, especially when it occurs as a soft tissue sarcoma. Several poorly differentiated neoplasms, especially rhabdomyosarcoma, synovial sarcoma, mesothelioma, epithelioid sarcoma, and carcinoma may show similar cellular features and in some cases differential diagnosis may be difficult, often requiring careful light microscopic, ultrastructural, and immunohistochemical assessment of the tumor.

Rhabdomyosarcoma may be very similar in appearance, but this diagnosis is readily ruled out by the demonstration of cytokeratin in the tumor cells, the absence of cross-striations and myofilaments with the light and electron microscopes, and the absence of staining for actin (HHF-35) and desmin.[128,136] Epithelioid sarcoma bears a close resemblance to rhabdoid sarcoma cytologically and immunohistochemically, but it differs from malignant rhabdoid tumor by its multinodular growth pattern with central necrosis of the tumor nodules, its predilection for the hand, wrist, and forearm of adolescents and young adults, and its less aggressive behavior with frequent recurrence but late metastasis.[122,128,130] Distinction is not always possible on these grounds, and both epithelioid sarcomas with rhabdoid features[90] and rhabdoid tumors with the features of epithelioid sarcoma[130,132] have been described. Examples of synovial sarcoma, mesothelioma, extraskeletal myxoid chondrosar-

coma, and epithelioid malignant schwannoma may also contain rhabdoid cells with globular perinuclear eosinophilic inclusions consisting of intermediate filaments. The first two of these tumors show immunostaining similar to that of rhabdoid sarcoma, but myxoid chondrosarcoma is negative for keratin and epithelial membrane antigen and stains positively with antibodies against S-100 protein.[136]

Additionally, malignant rhabdoid tumors must be distinguished from poorly differentiated carcinomas that are positive for keratin and vimentin and from malignant melanomas. The latter, however, are unlikely to be mistaken for a malignant rhabdoid tumor immunohistochemically since they stain positively for S-100 protein and melanoma-associated antigen but lack cytokeratin.

The exact nature of malignant rhabdoid tumor remains uncertain. Both mesenchymal and epithelial origin has been claimed, but it is also conceivable that the "typical" rhabdoid cells are not the hallmark of a specific single entity but are a nonspecific phenotype shared by a heterogenous group of poorly differentiated neoplasms marked by an overproduction of intermediate filaments.

DESMOPLASTIC SMALL CELL TUMOR OF CHILDHOOD

This is a recently recognized entity that was briefly described by Sesterhenn et al.[151] in 1987 as "undifferentiated malignant epithelial tumor involving serosal surfaces of scrotum and abdomen in young males" and by Gerald and Rosai[143] in 1989 as "desmoplastic small cell tumor with divergent differentiation." It is a clinically and morphologically well-defined neoplasm that chiefly affects adolescents and young adults, especially males, between 15 and 35 years of age, and occurs predominantly in the abdomen, pelvis, and omentum,[141,142,151,153] as well as the scrotum[149,151] and ovary[154]; not infrequently it is associated with multiple widespread peritoneal implants. In general, the tumor presents as a palpable, often painful mass that may cause a variety of signs and symptoms, including abdominal distention, constipation, and intestinal or ureteral obstruction or ascites, or both.[144]

Pathological findings

Grossly, the tumor forms a solid, large multilobulated mass that is white or gray-white on cross-section, sometimes distorted by cystic changes and areas of necrosis. Microscopically, it is composed of sharply demarcated nests or masses of small rounded or oval cells varying little in size and shape; in some tumors the cells have a cordlike or trabecular arrangement; in others there are irregular cystic spaces with palisading of the lining tumor cells or central foci of necrosis. Typically, the cellular aggregates are surrounded and separated by abundant fibrous connective tissue, with only a scattering of spindle-shaped fibroblasts (Figs. 38-28 and 38-29). Glandular and tubular features as

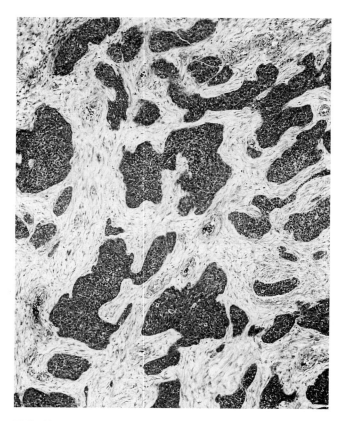

FIG. 38-28. Desmoplastic small cell tumor of childhood consisting of irregular nests of undifferentiated tumor cells surrounded by abundant fibrous stroma. The tumor cell stains positively for cytokeratin and desmin. (×75.)

well as vascular tufts with striking perivascular fibrosis are other less common features of the tumor. The tumor cells are of small to medium size and possess hyperchromatic nuclei and only small amounts of cytoplasm. Occasional cells are vacuolated or contain eosinophilic, PAS-positive inclusions reminiscent of rhabdoid cells. Cellular pleomorphism is rare.[142,154]

Immunohistochemical findings

The tumor cells react with antibodies against keratin, epithelial membrane antigen, desmin, and vimentin. Desmin frequently forms small globoid or punctate paranuclear masses within the tumor cells. Vimentin stains both tumor cells and the cells of the surrounding stroma. There is variable reactivity to neuron specific enolase, S-100 protein, Leu-7, Leu-M1, and synaptophysin. Staining for neurofilament proteins, glial fibrillary acidic protein, melanoma-associated antigen, chromogranin, and carcinoembryonic antigen is usually negative.[148,149,153,154]

DNA analysis, carried out by Ordóñez et al.,[147] revealed that among 11 cases 9 were diploid, and 1 each tetraploid and aneuploid. One of the diploid tumors metastasized to the lung.

Ultrastructural findings

The most striking ultrastructural feature of the tumor is the intracellular whorls and packets of microfilaments that are usually located near the nucleus, often compressing the nucleus or pushing it toward the periphery. There are a moderate number of mitochondria, free ribosomes, and

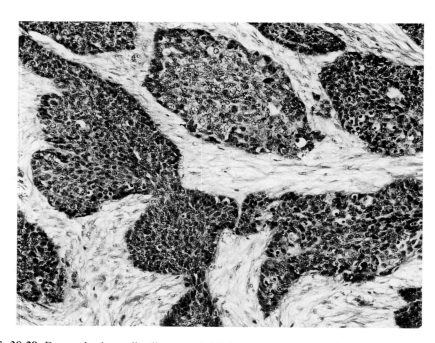

FIG. 38-29. Desmoplastic small cell tumor of childhood showing sharply demarcated nest of small rounded tumor cells separated by a prominent fibrous matrix. (×150.)

small lakes of glycogen. Dense core granules are infrequently found within the cytoplasm. The cells are closely apposed with occasional filopodia, tight cell junctions, or small desmosomes with tonofilaments. Sometimes the cell clusters are partly enveloped by a basal lamina.[142,147,154]

Cytogenetic analysis revealed a reciprocal translocation t(11;22)(q13;q12) that is very similar to the translocation t(11;22)(q24;q12) found in Ewing's sarcoma and neuroepithelial tumor (Chapter 33).[140,150]

Clinical behavior

Desmoplastic small cell tumor is a highly aggressive neoplasm with a poor prognosis. In the series reported by Ordóñez et al.,[147] 16 of the 22 patients died of the disease within 8 to 50 months after the initial therapy. Widespread metastasis is common, and most of the patients die of their disease within a few years after initial diagnosis, often despite extensive multidisciplinary and multiagent therapy. Complete excision is often impossible because of the irregular outline of the tumor and the presence of multiple implants within the peritoneum.

Discussion

The tumor must be differentiated from other small cell tumors, such as malignant neuroepithelial tumor, rhabdomyosarcoma, neuroblastoma, and extraskeletal Ewing's sarcoma. The characteristic nestlike growth pattern, desmoplasia, and absence of glycogen will aid in differentiating the tumor from Ewing's sarcoma, and the positive epithelial markers help to exclude rhabdomyosarcoma, neuroepithelioma, and neuroblastoma. Carcinoid tumor, islet cell tumor, seminoma, and trabecular (Merkel cell) carcinoma lack the intracellular globoid or dotlike staining for desmin. The exact nature of this tumor is still uncertain; both a mesenchymal and neuroectodermal neoplasm expressing mesenchymal-type microfilaments have been suggested.

MALIGNANT MESENCHYMOMA

Traditionally the term malignant mesenchymoma is applied to an intriguing but small group of malignant soft tissue tumors that do not fit into any other tumor category and are characterized by the presence of two or more different nonepithelial tissue components in the same neoplasm. Stout,[179] who coined this term in 1948, defined malignant mesenchymoma as "a malignant tumor showing two or more unrelated, differentiated tissue types in addition to the fibrosarcomatous element."[180] He applied this term to a wide variety of neoplasms, and following his initial report of 8 cases in 1948, he collected 335 cases of malignant mesenchymoma by 1959.[171] However, this tumor is rare in our material, and there is little information in the literature on this subject.[155,166,168] In 1961 Nash and Stout[171] reported their experience with 42 malignant mesenchymomas in children, including some cases that had an undifferentiated sarcoma as their second component.

Others used the term *malignant mesenchymoma* in an entirely different connotation. Symmers and Nangle[182] and Ewing and Harrison[160] employed it for a group of myxoid liposarcomas because of their lipoblastic, myxoid, and vascular components; Thomas and Kothare[185] applied it to a poorly differentiated sarcoma showing "tissue similar to embryonal mesenchyme."

Evidently, in order to avoid a meaningless "wastebasket" category, a judicious approach is mandatory in making this diagnosis, and only those tumors should be designated as malignant mesenchymoma that meet Stout's original definition of this entity. In particular, this term should not become a euphemism for poorly differentiated sarcoma, and this diagnosis should be made only if each of the two or more tissue elements is sufficiently differentiated to permit clear recognition of its histogenetic type with the light microscope, immunohistochemically or ultrastructurally. Poorly differentiated areas that are merely suggestive but not diagnostic of a certain tissue type and that display no specific immunohistochemical or electron microscopic features do not meet Stout's criteria for this diagnosis.

Review of the tumors classified at the AFIP as malignant mesenchymomas reveals a rather small and heterogeneous group of neoplasms that can be divided into two closely related categories: (1) tumors that are clearly diagnostic of malignant mesenchymoma and are characterized by the presence of coexisting myosarcomatous (rhabdomyosarcomatous or leiomyosarcomatous) and liposarcomatous elements in the same neoplasm, often in addition to a fibrosarcoma-like spindle cell component, and (2) tumors that show, in addition to a specific and clearly recognizable type of sarcoma, foci of malignant cartilaginous or osseous tissue (Figs. 38-30 and 38-31). The predominant, most readily diagnosable pattern of the latter tumors is that of rhabdomyosarcoma or liposarcoma and, less commonly, that of malignant schwannoma. In some of these tumors it is difficult to decide if the cartilaginous or osseous element is benign or malignant. Sometimes elements that appear benign and malignant are present in the same tumor. It is extremely rare, however, that the malignant cartilaginous or osseous complement constitutes the major tissue component. Although the diagnosis of malignant mesenchyoma should be applied to all of these tumors, we prefer to add the predominant tissue elements in parentheses, for example "malignant mesenchymoma (rhabdomyosarcoma with focal malignant cartilaginous differentiation)" together with the grade of the tumor.

There also remain several neoplasms that qualify as malignant mesenchymomas but that are frquently treated (rather arbitrarily) as distinct and separate entities. This group is composed of malignant schwannoma with a rhabdomyoblastic component (malignant Triton tumor), rhabdomyosarcoma-like tumors with scattered ganglionic elements (ectomesenchymoma), and liposarcoma with malignant smooth muscle, cartilaginous, or osseous differen-

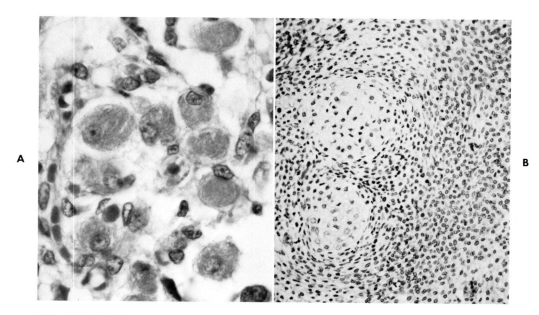

FIG. 38-30. Malignant mesenchymoma of the left calf in a 74-year-old man. Rhabdomyoblasts **(A)** and immature cartilaginous tissue **(B)** are found in the same neoplasm. **(A, ×450; B, ×160.)**

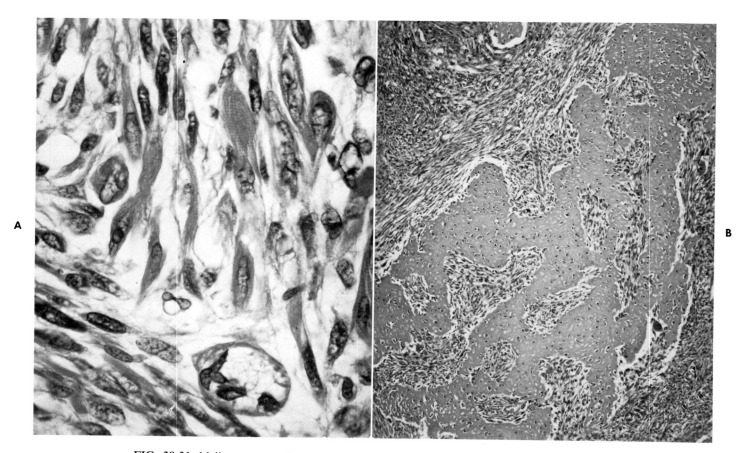

FIG. 38-31. Malignant mesenchymoma of the retroperitoneum with rhabdomyoblastic areas **(A)** and newly formed osteoid surrounded by undifferentiated fibrosarcoma-like spindle cells **(B). (A, ×630; B, ×60.)**

tiation. A richly vascular or pericytoma stromal pattern should not be counted as a separate tissue component, because the latter is a frequent feature of a variety of soft tissue sarcomas, and it is often impossible to tell whether this component is an intrinsic part of the tumor or a separate element.

As one would expect from such a heterogeneous group of tumors, the clinical setting and the manner of presentation vary widely. Most occur in patients older than 60 years of age, and only a few affect children and young adults.[165] The two major sites are the retroperitoneum and the lower extremities,[158,164,173,185] but sporadic examples of malignant mesenchymoma have also been reported at various other sites, including the larynx,[167] heart,[183] esophagus,[163] liver,[156] mesentery,[166] and urinary bladder.[184] Immunohistochemical and ultrastructural studies are often essential for diagnosis, especially for the positive identification of myoblastic (actin (HHF-35), desmin, myoglobin, and myofilaments) and chondroblastic (S-100 protein) components.

Differential diagnosis includes a variety of soft tissue sarcomas with entrapped normal muscle tissue and fat, dedifferentiated liposarcomas and leiomyosarcomas, carcinosar-

comas, malignant mixed mesodermal tumors, and other tumors with sarcomatous features such as pulmonary blastomas and immature teratomas with focal rhabdomyosarcomatous differentiation. Carcinosarcomas affect chiefly patients older than 50 years and originate in visceral organs, especially the breast,[176,187] upper aerodigestive tract,[170,189] esophagus,[162,186] lung,[175] uterus and ovary,[157,177,178] urinary bladder,[174,188] and prostate[169,172]; they are immunoreactive for cytokeratin, epithelial membrane antigen, and vimentin. In addition the sarcomatous portion of these hybrid tumors may contain cells that are immunoreactive for actin (HHF-35), desmin, myoglobin, or S-100 protein.

The clinical outcome varies, and prognosis seems to be related to type and differentiation of the prevalent mesenchymal element. The predominant and least differentiated histological component is decisive in selecting the mode of therapy. Yet there is also one report[173] indicating that some of these tumors behave much less aggressively than expected from the poor differentiation of the constituent elements. In these cases, however, additional follow-up is needed, since this assessment is based merely on five cases, with no or relatively short follow-up in four of them (0, 0.5, 2, and 3.5 years).

REFERENCES
Alveolar soft part sarcoma

1. Auerbach HE, Brooks JJ: Alveolar soft part sarcoma: a clinicopathologic and immunohistochemical study. *Cancer* 60:66, 1987.
2. Batsakis JG: Alveolar soft part sarcoma. *Ann Otol Rhinol Laryngol* 97:328, 1988.
3. Baum ES, Fickenscher L, Nachman JB, et al: Pulmonary resection and chemotherapy for metastatic alveolar soft-part sarcoma. *Cancer* 47:1946, 1981.
4. Berenzweig MS, Muggia FM, Kaplan BH: Chemotherapy of alveolar soft part sarcoma: a case report. *Cancer Treat Rep* 61:77, 1977.
5. Brunck JH: Ueber das sogenannte nichtchromaffine, maligne Paragangliom der Bauchwand und Oberschenkelmuskulatur. (Synonym: Alveoläres Weichteilsarkom, malignes granuläres Myoblastom). *Frankf Ztschft Path* 68:643, 1957.
6. Carstens HB: Membrane-bound cytoplasmic crystals, similar to those in alveolar soft part sarcoma, in a human muscle spindle. *Ultrastruct Pathol* 14:423, 1990.
7. Chaudry AP, Lin CC, Lai S, et al: Alveolar soft part sarcoma of the tongue in a female neonate. *J Oral Med* 39:2, 1984.
8. Christopherson WM, Foote FW Jr, Stewart FW: Alveolar soft-part sarcoma: structurally characteristic tumors of uncertain histogenesis. *Cancer* 5:100, 1952.
9. Cordier JF, Bailly C, Tabone E, et al: Alveolar soft part sarcoma presenting as asymptomatic pulmonary nodules: report of a case with ultrastructural diagnosis. *Thorax* 40:203, 1985.
10. Denk H, Krepler R, Artlieb U, et al: Proteins of intermediate filaments: an immunohistochemical approach to the classification of soft tissue tumors. *Am J Pathol* 110:193, 1983.
11. DeSchryver-Kecskemeti K, Kraus FT, Engleman BA: Alveolar soft-part sarcoma: a malignant angioreninoma: histochemical, immunocytochemical, and electron-microscopic study of four cases. *Am J Surg Pathol* 6:5, 1982.

12. Ekfors TO, Kalimo H, Rantakokko V, et al: Alveolar soft part sarcoma: a report of two cases with some histochemical and ultrastructural observations. *Cancer* 43:1672, 1979.
13. Enzinger FM: Recent trends in soft tissue pathology. In *Tumors of bone and soft tissue.* Chicago, 1965, Year Book Medical Publishers, Inc.
14. Evans HL: Alveolar soft-part sarcoma: a study of 13 typical examples and one with a histologically atypical component. *Cancer* 55:912, 1985.
15. Fender FA: Liposarcoma: report of a case with intracranial metastasis. *Am J Pathol* 9:909, 1933.
16. Fisher ER: Histochemical observations on alveolar soft part sarcoma with reference to histogenesis. *Am J Pathol* 32:721, 1956.
17. Fisher ER, Reidbord H: Electron microscopic evidence suggesting myogenous derivation of the so-called alveolar soft part sarcoma. *Cancer* 27:150, 1971.
18. Font RL, Jurco S III, Zimmerman L: Alveolar soft part sarcoma of the orbit. *Hum Pathol* 13:569, 1982.
19. Foschini, MP, Ceccarelli C, Eusebi V, et al: Alveolar soft part sarcoma: immunological evidence of rhabdomyoblastic differentiation. *Histopathology* 13:101, 1988.
20. Gray GF, Glick AD, Kurtin PJ, et al: Alveolar soft part sarcoma of the uterus. *Hum Pathol* 17:297, 1986.
21. Hirose T, Kudo E, Hasegawa T, et al: Cytoskeletal properties of alveolar soft part sarcoma. *Hum Pathol* 21:204, 1990.
22. Horn RC, Stout AP: Granular cell myoblastoma. *Surg Gynecol Obstet* 76:315, 1943.
23. Johnson RWP, Somerville PG: A malignant soft-tissue paraganglioma of the leg. *Br J Surg* 44:605, 1956.
24. Kamei T, Ishihara Y, Takahashi M, et al: An ultrastructural and histochemical study of alveolar soft part sarcoma with special reference to the nature of the crystals. *Acta Pathol Jpn* 34:435, 1984.

25. Karnauchow N, Magner D: The histogenesis of alveolar soft part sarcoma. *J Pathol Bacteriol* 89:169, 1963.

26. King VV, Fee WE Jr: Alveolar soft part sarcoma of the tongue. *Am J Otolaryngol* 4:363, 1983.

27. Klemperer P: Myoblastoma of the striated muscle. *Am J Cancer* 20:324, 1934.

28. Kolodny A: Angioendothelioma of bone. *Arch Surg* 12:854, 1926.

29. Komori A, Takeda Y, Kakiichi T: Alveolar soft part sarcoma of the tongue: report of a case with electron microscopic study. *Oral Surg Oral Med Oral Pathol* 57:532, 1984.

30. Lattes R, Enzinger FM: Alveolar soft part sarcoma. In Proceedings of the Thirty-ninth Annual Anatomic Pathology Slide Seminar of the American Society of Clinical Pathology, Chicago, 1973.

31. Lieberman PH, Brennan MF, Kimmel M, et al: Alveolar soft-part sarcoma: a clinicopathologic study of half a century. *Cancer* 63:1, 1989.

32. Lieberman PH, Foote FW, Stewart FW, et al: Alveolar soft part sarcoma. *JAMA* 198:1047, 1966.

33. Lorigan JG, O'Keeffe FN, Evans HL, et al: The radiologic manifestations of alveolar soft-part sarcoma. *AJR Am J Roentgenol* 153:335, 1989.

34. MacFarlane A, Macgregor AB: Malignant nonchromaffin paraganglioma of the thigh. *Arch Dis Child* 33:55, 1958.

35. Masson P: Tumeurs humaines: histologie, diagnostics et techniques, deuxiéme édition. *Paris*, 1959, Librairie Maloine.

36. Matsuno Y, Mukai K, Itabashi M, et al: Alveolar soft part sarcoma: a clinicopathologic and immunohistochemical study of 12 cases. *Acta Pathol Jpn* 40:199, 1990.

37. Menesce LP, Eyden BP, Edmondson D, et al: Immunophenotype and ultrastructure of alveolar soft part sarcoma. *J Submicrosc Cytol Pathol* 25:377, 1993.

38. Miettinen M, Ekfors T: Alveolar soft part sarcoma: immunohistochemical evidence of muscle cell differentiation. *Am J Clin Pathol* 93:32, 1990.

39. Mukai M, Iri H, Nakajima T, et al: Alveolar soft-part sarcoma: a review of the histogenesis and further studies based on electron microscopy, immunohistochemistry, and biochemistry. *Am J Surg Pathol* 7:679, 1983.

40. Mukai M, Torikata C, Iri H: Alveolar soft part sarcoma: an electron microscopic study especially of uncrystallized granules using a tannic acid containing fixative. *Ultrastruct Pathol* 14:41, 1990.

41. Mukai M, Torikata C, Iri H, et al: Alveolar soft part sarcoma: an elaboration of a three dimensional configuration of the crystalloids by digital image processing. *Am J Pathol* 116:398, 1984.

42. Mukai M, Torikata C, Iri H, et al: Histogenesis of alveolar soft part sarcoma: an immunohistochemical and biochemical study. *Am J Surg Pathol* 10:212, 1986.

43. Mukai M, Torikata C, Shimoda T, et al: Alveolar soft part sarcoma: assessment of immunohistochemical demonstration of desmin using paraffin sections and frozen sections. *Virchows Arch (Pathol Anat)* 414:503, 1989.

44. Ogawa K, Nakashima Y, Yamabe H, et al: Alveolar soft part sarcoma, granular cell tumor, and paraganglioma: an immunohistochemical comparative study. *Acta Pathol Jpn* 36:895, 1986.

45. Ordóñez NG, Ro JY, Mackay B: Alveolar soft part sarcoma: an ultrastructural and immunocytochemical investigation of its histogenesis. *Cancer* 63:1721, 1989.

46. Persson S, Willems JS, Kindblom LG, et al: Alveolar soft part sarcoma: an immunohistochemical, cytologic, and electron-microscopic study and a quantitative DNA analysis. *Virchows Arch (Pathol Anat)* 412:499, 1988.

47. Randall KJ, Walter JB: Metastasizing nonchromaffin paraganglioma of thigh. *J Pathol Bacteriol* 67:69, 1954.

48. Rosai J, Dias P, Parham DM, et al: MyoD1 protein expression in alveolar soft part sarcoma as confirmatory evidence of its skeletal muscle nature. *Am J Surg Pathol* 15:974, 1991.

49. Rosenbaum AE, Gabrielsen TO: Cerebral manifestations of alveolar soft part sarcoma. *Radiology* 99:109, 1971.

50. Rubenfeld S: Radiation therapy in alveolar soft part sarcoma. *Cancer* 28:577, 1971.

51. Sahin AA, Silva EG, Ordóñez NG: Alveolar soft part sarcoma of the uterine cervix. *Mod Pathol* 2:676, 1989.

52. Shipkey FH, Lieberman PH, Foote FW, et al: Ultrastructure of alveolar soft part sarcoma. *Cancer* 17:821, 1964.

53. Simmons WB, Haggerty HS, Ngan B, et al: Alveolar soft part sarcoma of the head and neck: a disease of children and young adults. *Int J Pediatr Otorhinolaryngol* 17:139, 1989.

54. Smetana HF, Scott WF: Soft tissue tumors of peculiar character and uncertain origin. (Malignant tumors of nonchromaffin paraganglia.) *Milit Surg* 109:330, 1951.

55. Unni K, Soule E: Alveolar soft part sarcoma. *Mayo Clin Proc* 50:591, 1975.

56. Welsh RA, Bray DM III, Shipkey FH, et al: Histogenesis of alveolar soft part sarcoma. *Cancer* 29:191, 1972.

Epithelioid sarcoma

57. Ahmed MN, Feldman M, Seemayer TA: Cytology of epithelioid sarcoma. *Acta Cytol* 18:459, 1974.

58. Berger L: Synovial sarcomas in serous bursae and tendon sheaths. *Am J Cancer* 34:501, 1938.

59. Blewitt RW, Aparicio SGR, Bird CC: Epithelioid sarcoma, a tumour of myofibroblasts. *Histopathology* 7:573, 1983.

60. Bliss BO, Reed RJ: Large cell sarcomas of tendon sheath. *Am J Clin Pathol* 49:776, 1968.

61. Bloustein PA, Silverberg SG, Waddell WR: Epithelioid sarcoma: case report with ultrastructural review, histogenetic discussion, and chemotherapeutic data. *Cancer* 38:2390, 1976.

62. Bos GD, Pritchard DJ, Reiman HM, et al: Epithelioid sarcoma: an analysis of fifty-one cases. *J Bone Joint Surg* 70A:862, 1988.

63. Bryan RS, Soule EH, Dobyns JH, et al: Primary epithelioid sarcoma of the hand and forearm. *J Bone Joint Surg* 56A:458, 1974.

64. Chase DR, Enzinger FM: Epithelioid sarcoma: diagnosis, prognostic indicators, and treatment. *Am J Surg Pathol* 9:241, 1985.

65. Chase DR, Enzinger FM, Weiss SW, et al: Keratin in epithelioid sarcoma: an immunohistochemical study. *Am J Surg Pathol* 8:435, 1984.

66. Dabska M, Koszarowski T: Clinical and pathologic study of aponeurotic (epithelioid) sarcoma. *Pathol Annual* 17:129, 1982.

67. Daimaru Y, Hashimoto H, Tsuneyoshi M, et al: Epithelial profile of epithelioid sarcoma: an immunohistochemical analysis of eight cases. *Cancer* 59:134, 1987.

68. De Santo DA, Tennant R, Rosahn PD: Synovial sarcoma in joints, bursae, and tendon sheaths. *Surg Gynecol Obstet* 72:951, 1941.

69. el-Naggar AK, Garcia GM: Epithelioid sarcoma: flow cytometric study of DNA content and regional DNA heterogeneity. *Cancer* 69:1721, 1992.

70. Enzinger FM: Epithelioid sarcoma: a sarcoma simulating a granuloma or a carcinoma. *Cancer* 26:1029, 1970.

71. Fisher C: Epithelioid sarcoma: the spectrum of ultrastructural differentiation in seven immunohistochemically defined cases. *Hum Pathol* 19:265, 1988.

72. Fisher ER, Horvat B: The fibrocytic derivation of the so-called epithelioid sarcoma. *Cancer* 30:1074, 1972.

73. Frable WJ, Kay S, Lawrence W, et al: Epithelioid sarcoma: an electron microscopic study. *Arch Pathol* 95:8, 1973.

74. Freilinger G, Konrad K: Epithelioid sarcoma. *Plast Reconstr Surg* 73:462, 1984.

75. Gabbiani G, Fu YS, Kaye GI, et al: Epithelioid sarcoma: a light

and electron microscopic study suggesting a synovial origin. *Cancer* 30:486, 1972.

76. Gallup DG, Abel MR, Morley GW: Epithelioid sarcoma of the vulva. *Obstet Gynecol* 48(suppl 1):14S, 1976.

77. Gerharz CD, Moll R, Meister P, et al: Cytoskeletal heterogeneity of an epithelioid sarcoma with expression of vimentin, cytokeratins, and neurofilaments. *Am J Surg Pathol* 14:274, 1990.

78. Graham RM, James MP: Epithelioid sarcoma of Enzinger. *J Roy Soc Med* 77(suppl 4):24, 1984.

79. Heenan PJ, Quirk CJ, Papadimitriou JM: Epithelioid sarcoma: a diagnostic problem. *Am J Dermatopathol* 8:95, 1986.

80. Heppenstall RB, Yvars MF, Chung SMK: Epithelioid sarcoma: two case reports. *J Bone Joint Surg* 54A:802, 1972.

81. Huang DJ, Stanisic TH, Hansen KK: Epithelioid sarcoma of the penis. *J Urol* 147:1370, 1992.

82. Ishida T, Oka T, Matsushita H, et al: Epithelioid sarcoma: an electron-microscopic, immunohistochemical, and DNA flow cytometric analysis. *Virchows Arch (Pathol Anat)* 421:401, 1992.

83. Kächemann K: Epithelioid sarcoma. *Beitr Path* 155:84, 1975.

84. Laskowski J: Sarcoma aponeuroticum. *Nowotwory* 11:61, 1961.

85. Linell F, Myhre-Jensen O, Ostberg G, et al: Epithelioid sarcoma: report and review of two cases. *Acta Pathol Microbiol Scand* 236:21, 1973.

86. Lo HH, Kalisher L, Faix JD: Epithelioid sarcoma: radiologic and pathologic manifestations. *Am J Roentgenol* 128:1017, 1977.

87. Lombardi L, Rilke F: Ultrastructural similarities and differences of synovial sarcoma, epithelioid sarcoma, and clear cell sarcoma of the tendons and aponeuroses. *Ultrastruct Pathol* 6:209, 1984.

88. Males JL, Lain KC: Epithelioid sarcoma in XO/XX Turner's syndrome. *Arch Pathol* 94:214, 1972.

89. Manivel JC, Wick MR, Dehner LP, et al: Epithelioid sarcoma: an immunohistochemical study. *Am J Clin Pathol* 87:319, 1987.

90. Meis JM, Mackay B, Ordonez NG: Epithelioid sarcoma: an immunohistochemical and ultrastructural study. *Surg Pathol* 1:13, 1988.

91. Miettinen M, Lehto VP, Vartio T, et al: Epithelioid sarcoma: ultrastructural and immunohistologic features suggesting a synovial origin. *Arch Pathol Lab Med* 106:620, 1982.

92. Mills SE, Fechner RE, Bruns DE, et al: Intermediate filaments in eosinophilic cells of epithelioid sarcoma: a light microscopic, ultrastructural, and electrophoretic study. *Am J Surg Pathol* 5:195, 1981.

93. Mirra JM, Kessler S, Bhuta S, et al: The fibroma-like variant of epithelioid sarcoma: a fibrohistiocytic/myoid cell lesion often confused with benign and malignant spindle cell tumors. *Cancer* 69:1382, 1992.

94. Moore SW, Wheeler JE, Hefter LG: Epithelioid sarcoma masquerading as Peyronie's disease. *Cancer* 35:1706, 1975.

95. Mukai M, Torikata C, Iri H, et al: Cellular differentiation of epithelioid sarcoma: an electron-microscopic, enzyme-histochemical, and immunohistochemical study. *Am J Pathol* 119:44, 1985.

96. Pastel-Levy C, Bell DA, Rosenberg AE, et al: DNA flow cytometry of epithelioid sarcoma. *Cancer* 70:2823, 1992.

97. Patchefsky AS, Soriano R, Kostianovsky M: Epithelioid sarcoma: ultrastructural similarity to nodular synovitis. *Cancer* 39:143, 1977.

98. Persson S, Kindblom LG, Angerval L: Epithelioid sarcoma: an electron-microscopic and immunohistochemical study. *Appl Pathol* 6:1,1988.

99. Pisa R, Novelli P, Bonetti F: Epithelioid sarcoma: a tumor of myofibroblasts, or not. *Histopathology* 8:353, 1984.

100. Prat J, Woodruff JM, Marcove RC: Epithelioid sarcoma: an analysis of 22 cases indicating the prognostic significance of vascular invasion and regional lymph node metastasis. *Cancer* 41:1472, 1978.

101. Puiblitz S, Mora-Tiscareno A, Meneses-Garcia AA, et al: Epithelioid sarcoma of penis. *Urology* 28:246, 1986.

102. Puissegur-Lupo ML, Perret WJ, Millikan LE: Epithelioid sarcoma: report of a case. *Arch Dermatol* 121:394, 1985.

103. Ramon Y, Cajal S Jr, Ispizua I, et al: Morfologia naturaleza y evolucion del sarcoma epitelioide de Enzinger. *Rev Esp Oncol* 24:311, 1977.

104. Reeves BR, Fisher C, Smith S, et al: Ultrastructural, immunocytochemical, and cytogenetic characterization of a human epithelial sarcoma cell line (RM-HS1). *JNCI* 78:7, 1987.

105. Roitzsch E, Irmscher J: Das epithelioide Sarkom. Bericht ueber drei Fälle mit Literaturübersicht. *Zentralbl Allg Pathol* 120:417, 1976.

106. Santiago H, Feinerman LK, Lattes R: Epithelioid sarcoma: a clinical and pathological study of nine cases. *Hum Pathol* 3:133, 1972.

107. Schiffman R: Epithelioid sarcoma and synovial sarcoma in the same knee. *Cancer* 45:158, 1980.

108. Schmidt D, Harms D: Epithelioid sarcoma in children and adolescents: an immunohistochemical study. *Virchows Arch (Pathol Anat)* 410:423, 1987.

109. Schwartz HS, Pritchard DJ, Sim FH, et al: Epithelioid sarcoma. *Orthopedics* 10:1299, 1987.

110. Seemayer TA, Dionne PG, Tabah EJ: Epithelioid sarcoma. *Can J Surg* 17:37, 1974.

111. Shimm DS, Suit HD: Radiation therapy of epithelioid sarcoma. *Cancer* 52:1022, 1983.

112. Soule EH, Enriquez P: Atypical fibrous histiocytoma, malignant histiocytoma, and epithelioid sarcoma: a comparative study of 65 tumors. *Cancer* 30:128, 1972.

113. Steinberg BD, Gelberman RH, Mankin HJ, et al: Epithelioid sarcoma in the upper extremity. *J Bone Joint Surg* 74A:28, 1992.

114. Sugarbaker PH, Auda S, Webber BL: Early distant metastases from epithelioid sarcoma of the hand. *Cancer* 48:852, 1981.

115. Tsuneyoshi M, Enjoji M, Shinohara N: Epithelioid sarcoma: a clinicopathologic and electron microscopic study. *Acta Pathol Jap* 30:411, 1980.

116. Weissman D, Amenta PS, Kantor GR: Vulvar epithelioid sarcoma metastatic to the scalp: a case report and review of the literature. *Am J Dermatopathol* 12:462, 1990.

117. Whitworth PW, Pollock RE, Mansfield PF, et al: Extremity epithelioid sarcoma: amputation vs local resection. *Arch Surg* 126:1485, 1991.

118. Wick MR, Manivel JC: Epithelioid sarcoma and epithelial hemangioendothelioma: an immunocytochemical and lectin-histochemical comparison. *Virchows Arch (Pathol Anat)* 410:309, 1987.

119. Wick MR, Manivel JC: Epithelioid sarcoma and isolated necrobiotic granuloma: a comparative immunochemical study. *J Cut Pathol* 13:253, 1986.

Malignant extrarenal rhabdoid tumor

120. Balaton AJ, Vaury P: Paravertebral malignant rhabdoid tumor in an adult: a case report with immunocytochemical study. *Pathol Res Pract* 182:713, 1987.

121. Beckwith JB, Palmer NF: Histopathology and prognosis of Wilms' tumor: results from the first National Wilms' Tumor Study. *Cancer* 41:1937, 1978.

122. Chase DR: Rhabdoid versus epithelioid sarcoma (letter to the editor). *Am J Surg Pathol* 14:792, 1990.

123. Ekfors TO, Aho HJ, Kekomaeki M: Malignant rhabdoid tumor of the prostatic region: immunohistological and ultrastructural evidence for epithelial origin. *Virchows Arch (Pathol Anat)* 406:381, 1985.

124. Enzinger FM: Letter to the case. *Pathol Res Pract* 182:713, 1987.

125. Frierson HF, Mills SE, Innes DJ Jr: Malignant rhabdoid tumor of the pelvis. *Cancer* 55:1963, 1985.

126. Gonzalez-Crussi F, Goldschmidt RA, Hsueh W, et al: Infantile sarcoma with intracytoplasmic filamentous inclusions: distinctive tumor of possible histiocytic origin. *Cancer* 49:2635, 1982.

127. Haas JE, Palmer NE, Weinberg AG, et al: Ultrastructure of malignant rhabdoid tumor of the kidney. *Hum Pathol* 12:646, 1981.

128. Kodet R, Newton WA Jr, Sachs N, et al: Rhabdoid tumors of soft tissues: a clinicopathological study of 26 cases enrolled in the Intergroup Rhabdomyosarcoma Study. *Hum Pathol* 22:674, 1991.

129. Lynch HT, Shurin SB, Dahms BB, et al: Paravertebral malignant rhabdoid tumor in infancy: in vitro studies of a familial tumor. *Cancer* 52:290, 1983.

130. Molenaar WM, DeJong B, Dam-Meiring A, et al: Epithelioid sarcoma or malignant rhabdoid tumor of soft tissue? Epithelioid immunophenotype and rhabdoid karyotype. *Hum Pathol* 20:347, 1989.

131. Parham DM, Peiper SC, Robicheaux G, et al: Malignant rhabdoid tumor of the liver: evidence for epithelial differentiation. *Arch Pathol Lab Med* 112:61, 1988.

132. Perrone T, Swanson PE, Twiggs L, et al: Malignant rhabdoid tumor of the vulva: is distinction from epithelioid sarcoma possible? A pathologic and immunohistochemical study. *Am J Surg Pathol* 13:848, 1989.

133. Satoh H, Goishi J, Sogabe T, et al: Primary malignant rhabdoid tumor of the central nervous system: a case report and review of the literature. *Surg Neurol* 40:429, 1993.

134. Schmidt D, Harms D, Zieger G: Malignant rhabdoid tumor of the kidney: histopathology, ultrastructure, and comments on differential diagnosis. *Virchows Arch (Pathol Anat)* 398:101, 1982.

135. Sotelo-Avila C, Gonzalez-Crussi F, de Mello D, et al: Renal and extrarenal rhabdoid tumors in children: a clinicopathologic study of 14 patients. *Semin Diagn Pathol* 3:151, 1986.

136. Tsuneyoshi M, Daimaru Y, Hashimoto H, et al: The existence of rhabdoid cells in specified soft tissue sarcomas: histopathological, ultrastructural, and immunohistochemical evidence. *Virchows Arch (Pathol Anat)* 411:509, 1987.

137. Tsuneyoshi M, Daimaru Y, Hashimoto H, et al: Malignant soft tissue neoplasm with the histologic features of renal rhabdoid tumors: an ultrastructural and immunohistochemical study. *Hum Pathol* 16:1235, 1985.

138. Ugarte N, Gonzalez-Crussi F, Weinberg AG, et al: Wilms' tumor: its morphology in patients under one year of age. *Cancer* 346, 1981.

139. Vogel AM, Gown AM, Caughlan J, et al: Rhabdoid tumors of the kidney contain mesenchymal specific and epithelial specific intermediate filament protein. *Lab Invest* 50:232, 1984.

Demosplastic small cell tumor of childhood

140. Biegel JA, Conard K, Brooks JJ: Translocation (11;22)(p13;q12): primary change in intraabdominal small round cell tumor. *Genes Chromosom Cancer* 7:119, 1993.

141. Cheung NYA, Khoo US, Chan KW: Intraabdominal desmoplastic small round-cell tumour. *Histopathology* 20:531, 1989.

142. Gerald WL, Miller HK, Battifora H, et al: Intraabdominal desmoplastic small round-cell tumor: report of 19 cases of a distinctive type of high-grade polyphenotypic malignancy affecting young individuals. *Am J Surg Pathol* 15:499, 1991.

143. Gerald WL, Rosai J: Desmoplastic small cell tumor with divergent differentiation. *Pediatr Pathol* 9:177, 1989.

144. Gonzalez-Crussi F, Crawford SE, Sun CCJ: Intraabdominal desmoplastic small-cell tumors with divergent differentiation: observations on three cases of childhood. *Am J Surg Pathol* 14:633, 1990.

145. Layfield LJ, Lenarsky C: Desmoplastic small cell tumors of the peritoneum coexpressing mesenchymal and epithelial markers. *Am J Clin Pathol* 96:536, 1991.

146. Norton J, Monaghan P, Carter RL: Intraabdominal desmoplastic small cell tumour with divergent differentiation. *Histopathology* 19:560, 1991.

147. Ordóñez NG, el-Naggar AK, Ro JY, et al: Intraabdominal desmoplastic small cell tumor: a light microscopic, immunocytochemical, ultrastructural, and flow cytometric study. *Hum Pathol* 24:850, 1993.

148. Ordóñez NG, Zirkin R, Bloom RE: Malignant small-cell epithelial tumor of the peritoneum coexpressing mesenchymal type intermediate filaments. *Am J Surg Pathol* 13:413, 1989.

149. Prat J, Matias-Guiu X, Algaba F: Desmoplastic small round-cell tumor (letter). *Am J Surg Pathol* 16:306, 1992.

150. Sawyer JR, Tryka AF, Lewis JM: A novel reciprocal chromosome translocation t(11;22)(p13;q12) in an intraabdominal desmoplastic small round-cell tumor. *Am J Surg Pathol* 16:411, 1992.

151. Sesterhenn I, Davis CJ, Mostofi K: Undifferentiated malignant epithelial tumors involving serosal surfaces of scrotum and abdomen in young males (abstract). *J Urol* 137:214, 1987.

152. Variend S, Gerrard M, Norris PD, et al: Intraabdominal neuroectodermal tumour of childhood with divergent differentiation. *Histopathology* 18:45, 1991.

153. Yeoh G, Russell P, Wills EJ, et al: Intraabdominal desmoplastic small round cell tumor. *Pathology* 25:197, 1993.

154. Young RH, Eichhorn JH, Dickersin GR, et al: Ovarian involvement by the intraabdominal desmoplastic small round cell tumor with divergent differentiation: a report of three cases. *Hum Pathol* 23:454, 1992.

Malignant mesenchymoma

155. Bleisch VR, Kraus FT: Polypoid sarcoma of the pulmonary trunk: analysis of the literature and report of a case with leptomeric organelles and ultrastructural features of a rhabdomyosarcoma. *Cancer* 46:314, 1980.

156. Cozzutto C, De Bernardi B, Comelli A, et al: Malignant mesenchymoma of the liver in children: a clinicopathologic and ultrastructural study. *Hum Pathol* 12:481, 1981.

157. de Brito PA, Silverberg SG, Orenstein JM: Carcinosarcoma (mixed mullerian [mesodermal] tumor) of the female genital tract: immunohistochemical and ultrastructural analysis of 28 cases. *Hum Pathol* 24:132, 1993.

158. DePaolo CJ, Foster WS, Dabezies EJ, et al: A case report of malignant mesenchymoma with discussion of musculoskeletal tumor staging: the Enneking system. *Orthopedics* 11:1263, 1988.

159. Ellis GL, Langloss JM, Enzinger FM: Coexpression of keratin and desmin in a carcinosarcoma involving the maxillary alveolar ridge. *Oral Surg Oral Med Oral Pathol* 60:410, 1985.

160. Ewing MR, Harrison CV: Mesenchymoma. *Br J Surg* 44:408, 1956/57.

161. Gaynor WB, DeLashmutt RE: Malignant mesenchymoma arising in the scar of a thermal burn: report of a case. *Am J Clin Pathol* 28:74, 1957.

162. Guarino M, Reale D, Micoli G, et al: Carcinosarcoma of the oesophagus with rhabdomyoblastic differentiation. *Histopathology* 22:493, 1993.

163. Haratake J, Jimi A, Horie A, et al: Malignant mesenchymoma of the esophagus. *Acta Pathol Jpn* 34:925, 1984.

164. Hauser H, Beham A, Schmid C, et al: Malignant mesenchymoma: a very rare tumor of the peritoneum: case report with a review of the literature. *Langenbecks Arch Chir* 376:38, 1991.

165. Holdsworth Mayer CM, Favara BE, Holton CP, et al: Malignant mesenchymoma in infants. *Am J Dis Child* 128:847, 1974.

166. Hyde WR, White JE, Stout AP: Mesenchymoma of the mesentery. *Cancer* 3:653, 1950.

167. Kawashima O, Kamei T, Shimizu Y, et al: Malignant mesenchymoma of the larynx. *J Laryngol Otol* 104:440, 1990.

168. Klima M, Smith M, Spjut H, et al: Malignant mesenchymoma: case report with EM study. *Cancer* 36:1086, 1975.

169. Lauwers GY, Schevchuk M, Armenakas N, et al: Carcinosarcoma of the prostate. *Am J Surg Pathol* 17:342, 1993.

170. Nakleh RE, Zarbo RJ, Ewing S, et al: Myogenic differentiation in spindle cell (sarcomatoid) carcinomas of the upper aerodigestive tract. *Appl Immunohistochem* 1:58, 1993.

171. Nash A, Stout AP: Malignant mesenchymomas in children. *Cancer* 14:524, 1961.

172. Nazeer T, Barada JH, Fisher HA, et al: Prostatic carcinosarcoma: case report and review of the literature. *J Urol* 146:1370, 1991.

173. Newman PL, Fletcher CD: Malignant mesenchymoma: clinicopathologic analysis of a series with evidence of low-grade behavior. *Am J Surg Pathol* 15:607, 1991.

174. Ro JY, Ayala AG, Wishnow KI, et al: Sarcomatoid bladder carcinoma: clinicopathologic and immunohistochemical study of 44 cases. *Surg Pathol* 1:359, 1988.

175. Ro JY, Chen JL, Lee JS, et al: Sarcomatoid carcinoma of the lung: immunohistochemical and ultrastructural studies of 14 cases. *Cancer* 69:376, 1992.

176. Spagnolo DV, Shilkin KB: Breast neoplasms containing bone and cartilage. *Virchows Arch (Pathol Anat)* 400:287, 1983.

177. Spanos WJ, Taylor Wharton J, Gomez L, et al: Malignant mixed muellerian tumors of the uterus. *Cancer* 53:311, 1984.

178. Sternberg WH, Clark WH, Craft-Smith R: Malignant mixed müllerian tumor (mixed mesodermal tumor of the uterus): a study of twenty-one cases. *Cancer* 7:704, 1954.

179. Stout AP: Mesenchymoma: the mixed tumor of mesenchymal derivatives. *Ann Surg* 127:278, 1948.

180. Stout AP: Tumors of the soft tissues. In *Atlas of tumor pathology*, Armed Forces Institute of Pathology, 1953, section 2, fascicle 5, p 118.

181. Stout AP, Lattes R: Malignant mesenchymoma. Tumors of the soft tissues. In *Atlas of tumor pathology*, Armed Forces Institute of Pathology, 1967, second series, fascicle one, p 172.

182. Symmers WSC, Nangle EJ: An unusual recurring tumor formed of connective tissues of embryonic type (so-called mesenchymoma). *J Pathol Bacteriol* 63:417, 1951.

183. Tanaka T, Bunai Y, Nishikawa A, et al: Malignant mesenchymoma of the heart. *Acta Pathol Jpn* 32:851, 1982.

184. Terada Y, Saito I, Morohoshi T, et al: Malignant mesenchymoma of the bladder. *Cancer* 60:858, 1987.

185. Thomas A, Kothare SN: Malignant mesenchymomata of soft tissues. *Indian J Cancer* 11:227, 1974.

186. Wang ZY, Itabashi M, Hirota T, et al: Immunohistochemical study of the histogenesis of esophageal carcinosarcoma. *Jpn J Clin Oncol* 22:377, 1992.

187. Wargotz ES, Norris HJ: Metaplastic carcinomas of the breast. III. Carcinosarcoma. *Cancer* 64:1490, 1989.

188. Young RH: Carcinosarcoma of the urinary bladder. *Cancer* 59:1333, 1987.

189. Zarbo RJ, Crissman JD, Venkat H, et al: Spindle-cell-carcinoma of the upper aerodigestive tract mucosa: an immunohistologic and ultrastructural study of 18 biphasic tumors and comparison with seven monophasic spindle cell tumors. *Am J Surg Pathol* 10:741, 1986.

INDEX